Essentials of Midwifery and Obstetrical Nursing

Essentials of Midwifery and Obstetrical Nursing

BT Basavanthappa
MSc (N) PhD

Professor and Principal (Retired)
Government College of Nursing, Bengaluru, Karnataka, India
PhD Guide for Research Work

Member
Faculty of Nursing, RGUHS, Karnataka
Academic Council, RGUHS, Karnataka

Examiner
UG and PG Courses on Nursing, Various Universities

Ex-Programme In-charge
IGNOU, BSc Nursing Course, Karnataka and Goa, India

Life Member
Nursing Research Society of India, New Delhi
Trained Nurses Association of India, New Delhi

President
RGUHS, Nursing Teachers Association, Karnataka, India

Winner
Bharat Excellence Award and Gold Medal
Vikas Ratan Gold Award
UWA Life Time Achievement Award
Shree Veeranjaneya "Shrujanashri" Award

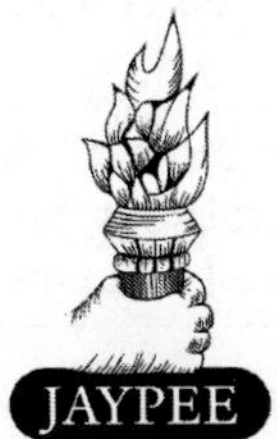

JAYPEE BROTHERS MEDICAL PUBLISHERS
The Health Sciences Publisher
New Delhi | London

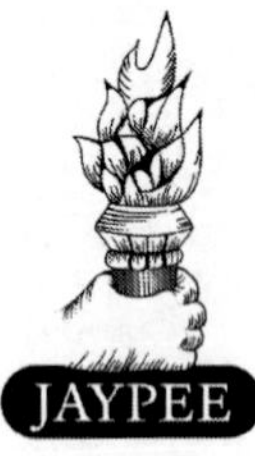

Jaypee Brothers Medical Publishers (P) Ltd

Headquarters
EMCA House
23/23-B, Ansari Road, Daryaganj
New Delhi - 110 002, India
Landline: +91-11-23272143, +91-11-23272703
+91-11-23282021, +91-11-23245672
E-mail: jaypee@jaypeebrothers.com

Corporate Office
4838/24, Ansari Road, Daryaganj
New Delhi - 110 002, India
Phone: +91-11-43574357
Fax: +91-11-43574314
E-mail: jaypee@jaypeebrothers.com

Overseas Office
J.P. Medical Ltd
83 Victoria Street, London
SW1H 0HW (UK)
Phone: +44 20 3170 8910
E-mail: info@jpmedpub.com

EU GPSR Authorised Representative
Logos Europe, 9 rue Nicolas Poussin
17000, La Rochelle, France
Phone: +33 (0) 6 67 93 73 78
E-mail: contact@logoseurope.eu

Website: www.jaypeebrothers.com
Website: www.jaypeedigital.com

Essentials of Midwifery and Obstetrical Nursing

© 2011, Jaypee Brothers Medical Publishers

All rights reserved. No part of this publication should be reproduced, stored in a retrieval system, or transmitted in any form or by any means: electronic, mechanical, photocopying, recording, or otherwise, without the prior written permission of the author and the publisher.

This book has been published in good faith that the material provided by author is original. Every effort is made to ensure accuracy of material, but the publisher, printer and author will not be held responsible for any inadvertent error(s). In case of any dispute, all legal matters to be settled under Delhi jurisdiction only.

First Edition: 2011, Reprint: **2026**

ISBN 978-93-5025-163-8

Typeset at JPBMP typesetting unit

Printed at: Samrat Offset Pvt. Ltd.

To
my parents
and
my nursing profession
and
my dear students

Preface

It gives me immense pleasure and satisfaction to introduce *Essentials of Midwifery and Obstetrical Nursing* to nursing community. In offering this text, I remain grateful to reader who supported all my 12 titles on nursing and who have provided constructive feedback as well as encouraging comments.

It has been observed that there is increase in maternal and infant mortality in home and abroad. It was stressed that nurses and midwives had a significant role to play in addressing the prioritized health problems in order to promote wellbeing of human beings, i.e. the problems will include reducing the burden of sickness and suffering resulting from communicable diseases, quality health care to children, adolescents and women, and reduction of maternal mortality and morbidity and so on; the key issues leading to changes in nursing and midwifery education and practices; the changing roles of health care professionals, competencies required for nurses and midwives. The goal of nursing education is to prepare today's student to meet the challenges of tomorrow. Keeping these views in mind, this book is designed to provide students with the knowledge and skills to practice in the area of midwifery and obstetrical nursing. It has been written in accordance with the needs of existing curriculum prescribed for the nursing courses at degree level. The information provided is based on established knowledge and practices. Every attempt has been made to maintain simplicity and lucidity of language and style.

I am aware of manifold reasons, errors might have crept in. I shall feel obliged, if such errors are brought to my notice. I sincerely, welcome constructive criticism from readers that would help me to enrich myself and good suggestions will be incorporated in the next edition.

I hope, this book will add growing understanding of midwifery and obstetrical nursing.

BT Basavanthappa

Acknowledgements

I owe a great deal of thanks to many who encouraged and supported me with their time and encouragement throughout.

- Shri G Basavannappa, Former Minister of Karnataka State for having initiated and supported me to take up this "Noble Nursing Profession" as my career.
- Dr (Mrs) Manjula K Vasundhra, Former Professor and HOD of Community Medicine, Bangalore Medical College, who continuously encouraged me to write texts in the field of nursing since nursing is a major force in medical and health services.
- My father Shri Thukkappa, who continuous to grace for the progress of my career and all-round development of my personality for the welfare of the community.
- My mother Smt Hanumanthamma who continues to be a bright spot in the lives of all who knew her and whose grace gave me strength to progress of my life.
- My wife Smt Lalitha, who gives meaning to my life in so many ways. She is the one whose encouragement keep me motivated, whose support gives me strength and whose gentleness gives me comfort.
- My lovely children BB Mahesh and BB Gaanashree, for all the joy they provided me and all the hope that they instill me and who bear with patient throughout my works of the nursing texts. They keep me young at heart.
- Finally my warmest appreciation goes to M/s Jaypee Brothers Medical Publishers (P) Ltd, New Delhi, for sharing my vision for this book and giving me the chance to turn vision into reality.

Contents

Introduction to Midwifery and Obstetrical Nursing

INTRODUCTION

According to dictionary, "to nurse" means to foster or cherish ("to nurse one's meager talents"), to treat or handle with adroit care ("to nurse one's nest egg"), to bring up, train or nurture; to clasp or handle carefully or fondly ("to nurse a memento"); to preserve ("to nurse a drink"). 'Nurse' suggests attendance and service; its antonym is 'neglect'. In the noun form, a nurse is "a person, especially a woman", who takes care of sick or infirm; a woman, who has the general care of a child or children, a woman employed to suckle an infant, or any fostering agency or influence. Thus nurse is a person formally educated in the care of the sick or infirm, especially registered nurse.

Nurses with highly specialised training would be involved in the high technology tertiary care. At the same time nurses with broad education will play essential role in directing role and public services particularly conduct safe delivery, as well as development of women health care programmes that could include family planning, nutrition and healthy child birth. Many countries in the west as well as the south-east region have such nurses who are expert in handling midwifery cases. In India rural scenario where the majority of deliveries are handled by dais where obstetricians are not available these nursing personnel posted at primary health centre/community health centre. It may turnout with the lifesaving strategy for woman in labour.

Since midwifery specialists have to be accountable for their actions and decisions taken by them independently, regulatory bodies like Indian nursing council have to enact such regulation enable the specialist midwives to redirect their practice to meet the changing health care needs. For example, these midwives should be licensed to undertake essential life saving emergency measures when necessary. The new category nurses may be named as "Nurse Midwife Practitioners" who will pave the way for change by establish autonomy are independent practice nursing.

An individual who provides health care also will be called as "Nurse" This statement is not very clarifying. The nurse's extent of participation in health care varies from simple patient care tasks to the most expert professional techniques necessary in acute life-threatening situations. The ability of a nurse to function in making self-directed judgements and to act independently will depend on his or her professional background, motivation and opportunity for professional development. The roles of nurses constantly change in patterns of demand for health services, and the evolution of professional relationships among nurses, physicians and other health professionals.

Nursing is not different from other licensed professions, including medicine, licensor is usually sought by the profession to protect its own interest. For example, the one definition of medical practice states that "practice of medicine", means the diagnosis, treatment, prevention, cure, or relieving of human disease, ailment, defect, complaint, or other physical or mental condition, by attendance, advice, device, diagnostic test or other means, or offering, understating attempting to do, or holding oneself out as able to do, any of these acts". Whereas, the practice of the profession of nursing is defined as diagnosing and treating human responses to actual or potential health problems through such services—as casefinding, health teaching, health counselling and provision of care supportive to the restorative of life and well-being; An inclusion of the diagnostic function would authorise the nursing practitioner to make nursing diagnoses, not medical diagnoses. Whereas, the diagnostic function as an intellectual process is central to the practice of any number of professions including medicine and nursing, the focus in medicine is the nature and degree of pathology or deviation from normalcy; Within nursing the focus is the "individual response to an actual or potential health problems and the nursing needs arising from such responses that emphasise on original responses."

Hence, the practice of nursing means the performance for compensation of professional service requiring substantial specialised knowledge of the biological, physical, behavioural, psychological, and sociological sciences and of nursing theory as the basis for assessment diagnosis, planning, intervention and evaluation in the promotion and maintenance of health; the case finding and management of illness, injury or infirmity; the restoration of optimum functions or the achievement of a dignified death. Nursing practice includes, but it is not limited to administration, teaching, counselling, supervision, delegation and evaluation of practice and execution of the medical regiment including the administration of medications and treatments prescribed by any person authorised by state law to prescribe. Each registered nurse is directly accountable and responsible to the consumer for quality of nursing care rendered.

According to Florence Nightingale 'a nurse means any person in charge of the personal health of another. Nursing ought to assist the reparative process; for nightingale believed that all diseases at some period or other of its course, is more or less a reparative process", and that the symptoms or the sufferings generally considered to be inevitable and incidental to the disease are very often not symptoms of the disease at all but of something quite different- of the want of fresh air, light, warmth, quiet, cleanliness, punctuality and care in the administration of diet, of each of or all of these. She further states that the word "Nursing" has been limited to signify little more than the administration of medicines and the application of policies. It ought to signify the proper use of fresh air, light, warmth, cleanliness, quiet, and the proper selection and administration of diet— all at the least expense of vital power to the patient. Accordingly what nursing has to do is to put the patient in the best condition for nature to act upon him/her.

Virginia Henderson viewed "the unique function of the nurse is to assist the individual, sick or well, in the performance of those activities contributing to health or its recovery (or to peaceful death) that he would perform unaided and to do this in such with way as to help him gain independence as rapidly as possible." Accordingly this unique function of the nurse is the care of nursing from which all other things spring and which must be protected. Henderson translates this unique function as "the nurse is temporarily the consciousness of the unconscious, the love of life for the suicidal, the leg of the amputee, the eyes of the newly blind, a means of locomotion for the infant, knowledge and confidence for the young mother, the voice for those too weak or withdrawn to speak."

Today the role of nurses as givers of "primary health care" as those who diagnose and treat when a doctor is unavailable, even as the nurse midwife function in the absence of an obstetrician/nurse may be general care providers of primary care. Obstetrical nurses or midwives have been universally recognised worldwide as the providers of primary care for mothers and newborns. They diagnose and treat as well as "care". Nursing roles have expanded because the talent is there and because there is a need, whether the need is for people to manage the care of the chronically mentally ill, manage the care of rape victims, including testifying in court or devise and manage care for patients awaiting heart transplants. When nurses do it, it is nursing.

TRENDS IN MIDWIFERY AND OBSTETRICAL NURSING

Owing to the fact that childbirth was commonly regarded in India as a time of impurity, it followed that only those whose caste was low could attend a woman of such time. From time immemorial, the presiding genius at the birth of children was the hereditary dai (Midwife). Such women were quite untrained and that only knowledge consisted in what was passed on by their predecessors or learned by experience. They had no idea of the mechanism of Labour or of the danger of sepsis, and in any difficulty, their remedy was force, often with disastrous consequences.

When medically qualified women started their practice in India, they realised the importance of establishing some system of training of these traditional midwives (dais). This was by no means an easy task, because the dais themselves for the most part, opposed any scheme for training, and refused to attend classes when arranged. They were suspicious, and there was some trap in the scheme to out them from their means of livelihood. Another factor which militated against their coming forward for training was that their patients also did not realise the need for a higher standard of skill in their attendants at childbirth and were content to continue in the way of their forbears. One of the first attempts to train these women was made by Miss Hewlett, a missionary in America, in 1886. She persuaded them to attend her classes by paying them a fee for each attendance, the funds being supplied by the Municipality of Amritsar. After a certain length of training, the dais were given an examination, and those who were successful in the examination received a certificate. A hold over them was maintained by requiring them to report every case as soon as the confinement was over, upon which Miss Hewlett or her assistant then visited the case. If all was well, the dai (Traditional midwife) was given a rupee, and although the dais had no enthusiasm for reporting the case, they were glad to win the rupee, and the system worked well. Similar attempts were made in a few other places by medical missionaries and were usually attended with some success.

In Madras (now Chennai) Tamil Nadu State, the object consistently aimed at, has been to oust the indigenous dais by means of training a superior class midwife.

'Midwife' means "with woman" or in France, "wise woman." Throughout the ages, women have depended upon a skilled person, usually another woman, to be with them during childbirth. Now-a-days, in response to women seeking alternatives to physician-hospital services, there has been rebirth of the 'lay midwife (traditional midwife), the empirically trained midwife. She is usually a mother who learned by apprenticing to another who lay midwife and is responding primarily to women who seek to give birth at home. Unlike "granny midwife" of old, today's lay midwife is usually middle class, well educated, articulate, and wellpaid for her services. As she gained experience and confidence, she questions the need for prerequisite of nursing by these new midwives. They allege that nursing education promulgates the medical model of pregnancy as an illness and birth as a medical event. They further allege that nursing education teaches subservience to medical doctrine even when the doctrine is not supported by scientific research.

The views of individual nurse midwives are divided and the profession has avoided taking a stand on whether it is essential to be a nurse before becoming a midwife. However, most agree that if not a prerequisite, the inclusion of aspects of nursing education are desirable. The expanded opportunities for practice are creating an increased demand to educate nurse-midwives. It is clear that professionals trained exclusively in medical institutions experience discomfort practising in the maternity homes (birth centres) setting. Therefore, if nurse-midwives are to be the primary care providers for childbearing families and birth centres a place for practice of midwifery, a new approach to the education and training of nurse-midwife is called for. Maybe, realizing these views, in India, Midwifery course replaced by two years Auxiliary-Nurse Midwifery course (Now Female Health Worker Training course) and sick nurse training replaced by three and half years General Nursing and Midwifery course. In addition, four years BSc Nursing course curricula included the major components of Midwifery, Obstetrics and Gynaecological nursing. And there is such speciality in Master degree in Nursing and Doctoral degree in Nursing.

Now nurse-midwives are recognised as the experts and lead caregivers in normal childbirth. Hence, the nurse-midwife is a person who, having been regularly admitted to a nursing/midwifery education, duly recognised in the state, or country, in which it is located, has successfully completed the prescribed course of studies in nursing and midwifery and has acquired the requisite qualifications to be registered and/or legally licensed to practise nursing and midwifery.

The nurse-midwife must be able to give the necessary supervision, care and advice to women during pregnancy, labour and the post-partum period, to conduct deliveries, on her own responsibility and to take care for the newborn and the infant. This care included preventable measures, the detection of abnormal conditions in mother and child, the procurement of medical assistance and the execution of emergency measured in the absence of medical help. The nurse-midwife has an important task in health counselling and education, not only for the woman, but also within the family and the community. The work should involve antenatal education and preparation for parenthood, and extends to certain areas of gynaecology, family planning and childcare. She may practise in hospitals, clinics, health units, domiciliary conditions or in any other service.

The activities of nurse-midwives includes:

- To provide sound family planning information and advice.
- To diagnose pregnancies and monitor normal pregnancies to carry out examination necessary for the monitoring of the development of normal pregnancies.
- To prescribe or advise on the examinations necessary for the earliest possible diagnosis of pregnancies at risk.
- To provide programme of parenthood preparation and complete preparations for childbirth including advise on hygiene and nutrition.
- To care for and assist the mother during labour and to monitor the condition of the foetus *in utero* by the appropriate clinical and technical means.
- To conduct spontaneous deliveries including where required an episiotomy and in urgent cases of breech delivery.
- To recognise the warning signs of abnormality in the mother or infant which necessitate referral to a qualified medical doctor and to assist the latter where appropriate; to take the necessary emergency measures the medical doctor's absence, in particular the manual removal of placenta, possibly followed by manual examination of the uterus.
- To examine and care for the newborn infant, to take all initiatives, which are necessary in case of need and to carry out where necessary immediate resuscitation.
- To care for and monitor progress of the mother in the postnatal period and to give all necessary advice to the mother on infant care to enable her to ensure the optimum progress of the newborn infant.
- To carry out the treatment prescribed by a medically qualified doctor.
- To maintain necessary records.

Today nurses serve in hospital, railway service, military service, community health centres and clinics and patient homes, maternity and nursing homes and some even hang out their own shingle in private practice, for which nurses have studied and have and update their knowledge and skill in specialized areas which includes and child health. Maternal and child health also includes subspecialities like obstetrics and gynaecological nursing, neonatal nursing, paediatric nursing, etc.

New nurses are attracted to and stay in positions that enable them to practise in their desired nursing speciality. About half of them cited the ability to practise their speciality as the primary source of their satisfaction, and almost one-third cited it as the reason for selecting their current position. Most nurses work in hospital settings. Hospitals vary widely in size, services offered, and geographic location. In general, nurses in hospital, work with patients who have medical or surgical conditions, with children, with women and their newborn, with cancer patient, with people who have had severe traumas (injuries) or burns in operating rooms or emergency rooms, and in many other capacities. In addition to direct patient care roles, nurses in hospitals serve as educators, managers, and administrators, who teach or supervise others and establish the directions of nursing hospitalwise.

Obstetrical nursing is one of the specialised area in nursing which focuses on women and their infants and families during the child bearing cycle. It deals with women's health nursing, and reproductive health nursing. Brief description of these terminology are as follows:

Obstetrical nursing focuses on the case of child-bearing and their families through all stages of pregnancy and childbirth and during first-six weeks after birth. Throughout the prenatal period, nurses and nurse-midwives provide care for women in clinics, and health centres and teach classes to help families to prepare for childbirth. They also care for childbearing families during labour and birth in hospitals, birth centres (maternity homes) and less frequently the home. Nurses with special training may provide intensive care for high-risk neonates in special care units and high-risk mothers in antepartum units, in critical care obstetric units, or at home. Maternity nurses teach about pregnancy, the process of labour, birth and recovery, and parenting skills. Investment in health promotion during child bearing can make a significant differences in the health of women and their infants.

Women's health nursing focuses on the physical, psychologic and social needs of women throughout their lives. The term "women's health" emphasises the overall experience of women diseases, child bearing functions, and general, physical and psychologic well-being. Women's health nurses specialise in and investigate conditions unique to women (such as reproductive malignancies and menopause) and socio-cultural and occupational factors that may be related to women's health problems (such as poverty, lower wages, rape, incest, sexual harassment and family violence).

Nurses caring for women have helped make the health care system more responsive to women's needs. The changing health care delivery system offers opportunities for nurses to alter nursing practice and improve the way of care, is delivered through managed care, integrated delivery systems and redefined roles. Nurses have been critically important in developing strategies to improve the well-being of women and their infants. Still, there are serious problems related to the health and health care of mothers and infant exist. Access to pre-pregnancy and pregnancy-related care for all women and the lack of reproductive health services for adolescents are major concerns. Nurses can influence national health policy by actively participating in the education of the public and states and union governments.

Reproductive Health and Maternity form an important aspect of women's health and are considered and element of primary health care, especially as they relate to maternal-child health. Also, women usually enter the health care system for reporductive care. In a number of countries maternal mortality rates remain at alarmingly high levels, as does the low nutritional status of women throughout their reproductive cycles. It has been estimated that there are at least half a million maternal deaths in the world per year that are preventable. This maternal mortality is not evenly distributed in different parts of the world, for example, women in Bangladesh face a risk of dying 400 times greater than that of women in Scandinavia and 50 times greater than that of women in Portugal. In India, 1.1% of all deaths in the country in 1991 were due to maternal causes (SRS). At a crude death rate of 9.8 per 1000 an estimated 8,29,3770 deaths occurred of which 91,231 were related to pregnancy and childbirth. Based on these numbers the estimated maternal mortality rate would be around 62.9 per 100,000 women in the reproductive age group of 15 to 44 years or a maternal mortality ratio of 3.4 per 1000 deliveries.

In India, more than 2 crore 70 lakhs pregnancies take place every year. Of these more than half are attended by untrained birth attendants or relatives. To improve the quality of ante-natal, natal and post-natal care in domiciliary deliveries, it is important that every health worker including nurses builds up a rapport with the Traditional Birth Attendants (TBAs) leading to a community based midwifery service in close conjunctions with the TBAs, Anganawadi workers and the community. It is estimated that of all pregnancies 15% will develop some complications requiring treatment at a hospital, out of which 5% may need an operation to deliver the child and to save mother. In such a situation, it is essential that all the maternal service at the community level are organised in a way that every pregnant woman received adequate care and identification of complications is done during ante-natal, natal and post-natal period. Appropriate referral of complicated cases is most crucial to save the mother and newborn from disease or death related to pregnancy.

Maternal and child health care which is now also being described as "Reproductive and Child Health" is a very important component of the family welfare programme in India. Reproductive and Child Health (RCH) can be defined as a state in which "people have the ability to reproduce and regulate their fertility; women are able to go through the pregnancy and child birth safely, the outcome of pregnancy is successful in terms of maternal and infant survival and well-being, and couples are able to have sexual relations free of the fear of pregnancy and contracting disease. This means that every couple should be able to have child when they want and that the pregnancy, the mother and the child are safe and well, and contraceptives by choice are available to prevent pregnancy and of contracting disease." The need for and underlying principles of reproductive health as an approach to solve the population issues were duly highlighted and agreed upon by participating countries during the International conference on "Population and Development" held in Cairo in 1994. In agreement to this decision, the

Govt of India has formally launched the Reproductive and Child Health (RCH) programme on October 15, 1997.

RCH Programme has envisaged a major shift in certain components, approach and emphasis of the already existing Family Welfare Programme in India. Major focus in this programme is delivery of need based client centred, good quality, comprehensive reproductive and child health services to all the beneficiaries in an integrated manner. In India, the RCH services are to be delivered through the existing primary health care infrastructure with necessary referral and supervisory support from the secondary and teritary level institutions. Capacity building among the personnel involved in the delivery of RCH services through in-service training, is considered as an essential prerequisite for the successful implementation of the programme. Strengthening of task performance skills for delivery of RCH service is particularly felt as required. Accordingly integrated skill development training of primary health care personnel being organised, in which they are trained in these components in an integrated manner throughout the country. The staff nurses placed at primary health centres and community health centres are also covered under this integrated skill training.

As already stated, reproductive health and maternity form an important aspect of women's health and is considered an element of Primary Health Care, especially as they relate to Maternal Child Health. Women often enter the health care system because of reproductive issues or problems.

HISTORICAL PERSPECTIVES AND CURRENT TRENDS IN INDIA

All health activities in the community are concerned with the wellbeing of all people irrespective of age, sex, race, or other characteristics. However, two groups, i.e., women in the reproductive age group and children especially underfives merit special attention. In India, women of the childbearing age (15-44 years) constitute 19 per cent, and children under 15 years of age about 40 per cent of the total population. Together, they constitute nearly 59 percent of the total population. By virtue of their number, mothers and children are the major consumers of health services. These groups are subjected to marked physical and physiological stress, which, if not cared for, may cause serious deviation from normal health. Mother and children are not only constitute a large group, but they are also a "vulnerable" or "special risk group." The risk is connected within the case of infants and children, since they are exposed to unusual risks of widespread infection, poor nutrition, and hazardous delivery, which may cause death or impairment of health.

According to the available sources, 50 per cent of all deaths in the developing world are occurring among people over 70 years, the same proportion of death occurring among children during the first-five years of life in the developing world. Global observation shows that in developed regions maternal mortality ratio is in averages at 30 per 100,000 live births; in developing regions the figure is 480 for the same number of live births.

The problems affecting the health of the mother and child are multifactorial. Despite current efforts, the health of the mother and child still constitute one of the most serious health problems affecting the community, particularly in the developing countries including India.

The protection of the health of the expectant mother and her children is of prime importance for building of a sound and healthy nation.

The maternal and child welfare movement in India started with attempts to train indegenous "dai" (Traditional birth attendant, TBA) by Miss Hewlett of the Church of England Zenana Mission in India 1866. Wives of officials returning from foreign countries started some services through voluntary societies in big towns, such as holding of mothers, classes and training of indigenous dais. Lady Chelmsford was much interested in this work and she established the "All India League of Maternity and Child Welfare" in 1919 and opened Health Schools for training of health visitors in many big towns. Later on the League became incorporated with the Redcross Society. Training of Midwives, Assistant Midwives and Dais was also conducted at some places. Till 1953, the MCH services in the districts were patchy and were rendered through Maternity homes and trained Midwives. The latter were under the control of the Civil Surgeons and their services mostly curative and institutional. From 1955 onwards, MCH services are rendered through MCH centres or maternity homes run by local bodies.

Today's health care environment is distinctively different from that of the past. The increasing emphasis on health care reform, cost effective treatment, shorter or eliminated hospital stays, and improved quality of care has changed where is health care delivered, how is it delivered, and by whom does it change in health care delivery in the last decade have resulted in significant alterations in the traditional approaches to career pathways for nurses. The expanded opportunities for practice are creating an increased demand to educate nurse-midwives. Keeping in view of the above changes in India, long back, we have introduced Midwifery, Obstetrics, and Gynaecological components in the curricula of ANM, LHV, GNM, BSc and MSc. Nursing courses longback to meet the future changing health needs of the community accordingly. So, the nursing practice must change in response to health care system changes, and consumer demands.

In any nation, mother and children constitute a priority group which consists about 70 per cent population, in India, women of the child bearing age (15-44 years) constitute 19 per cent and children under 15 years of age about 40 per cent of the total population. Together they constitute nearly 59 per cent of the total population. By virtue of their numbers, mothers and children are the major consumers of health services. And they are also a vulnerable or special risk group. The risk is connected with child bearing in the case of women, and growth and development, and survival in the case of infants and children. Whereas, 50 per cent of all death in the developed world are occurring among people over 70 and the same proportion of death occurring among children during the first-five years of life in the developing world. Much of the sickness and death among mothers and children is largely preventable.

In practice, mother and child must be considered as one unit. It is because:

- During ante-natal period, the foetus on the part of the mother, the period is about 280 days. During this period, the foetus obtains all the building material and oxygen from the mother's blood.
- Child health is closely related to maternal health. A healthy mother brings forth a healthy baby; there is a less chance for a premature birth, still birth, or abortion.
- Certain diseases and conditions of the mother during pregnancy (e.g., Syphilis, German measles, drug intake) are likely to have their effects upon the foetus.
- After birth, the child is dependent upon the mother. At least upto the age of 6 to 9 months, the child is completely dependent on the mother for feeding. The mental and social development of the child is also dependent upon the mother. If mother dies, the child's growth and development are affected (Maternal deprivation syndrome).
- In the care cycle of women, there are few occasions when service to the child is not simultaneously called for.
- The mother is also the first teacher of the child.

It is for these reasons, the mother and child are treated as one unit. Maternal and child health services were first organised in India in 1921, by a committee of "The Lady Chelmsford League" which collected funds for child welfare and established demonstration services on an All India basis. In 1931, Indian Red Cross Society started maternity centres in different parts of the country through its "Maternal and Child Welfare Bureau". In 1946, the Health Survey and Development Committee headed by Sir Joseph Bhore, emphasised the need for maternal and child welfare services and recommended that priority should be given for MCH services in the National Health Service.

The constitution of India envisages the establishment of new social order based on equality, justice, and dignity of the individual. Among others, it directs the state to record improvement in the public health in one of the primary duties and aims at securing the health and strength of the workers, men and women, and the tender age of children are not abused and that citizens are not forced by economic necessities to enter avocations unsuited to their age or strength and that children are given opportunities and facilities to develop in a healthy manner in conditions of freedom and their childhood and youth are protected against exploitation and against moral and material abandonment (Article 39). And the state shall regard the raising of the level of nutrition and standard of living of its people and improvement of public health as among its primary duties (Article 47).

National Policy for Children (1977): It shall be the policy of the State to provide adequate services to children, both before and after birth and through the period of growth to ensure their full physical, mental and social development. The state shall progressively increase the scope of such services so that within a reasonable time all children in the country enjoy optimum conditions for their balanced growth. It has been also indicated priority in programme formulations. In formulating programmes in different sectors, priority shall be given to programmes relating to:

a. Preventive and promotive aspects of child health.
b. Nutrition for infants and children in the preschool age.
c. Maintenance education and training of orphans and destitute children.
d. Creches and other facilities for the care of children of working and ailing mothers.
e. Care, education, training and rehabilitation of handicapped children.

The policy on Family Welfare Programme (1977) also stated that "it is of utmost importance that adequate, ante-natal and post-natal care is made available to pregnant mothers. To this end a comprehensive scheme of training of indigenous midwives (Dais) will be implemented. Under it, maternity services will be made available to all mothers who may need them. The programme of immunising children against common diseases, such as whooping cough, diphtheria, and tetanus will be expanded further. We expect that the State Government will give necessary cooperation and assistance in this direction since health is a state subject.

And there is direct correlation between the illiteracy and fertility, and between infant and maternal mortality, and the age at marriage is well established by demographic studies. While on the other hand, government will pursue its policy to the improvements of women's education level, both through formal and nonformal channels according high priority. It will also bring legislation for raising the minimum age of marriage for girls to 18 and for boys to 21 years." This has been done through Child Marriage Restraint Act 1978.

The joint conference of Central Councils of Health and Central Family Welfare Council at its meeting held in April 1979, among other things have resolved that" as a part of the package of family welfare, we have to mount gigantic efforts to radically reduce infant and child mortality to at least 50 per cent of the present levels in the shortest possible time. This calls for not only much more expanded immunisation and prophylaxis against nutritional deficiency diseases but also efforts to combat major causes of such mortality namely diarrhoeal and respiratory diseases and malnutrition.

Alma-Ata Declaration on Primary Health Care (1978) stated "that primary health care includes at least education concerning prevailing health problems and the methods of prevailing and controlling them; promotion of food supply and proper nutrition; adequate supply of safe water and basic sanitation; maternal and child health care, including family planning; immunisation against major infectious diseases; prevention and control of total endemic diseases; appropriate treatment of common diseases and injury and provision of essential drugs."

In the month of 1980, the Government of India signed the Charter for Health Development proposed by the World Health Organization. The preamble of the Charter reads.

"A nation's greatest asset is people, the more so, when they are endowed with the highest obtainable standard of health, which promotes creativeness, dynamism, determination, productivity, and self confidence to move ahead." Health is a basic requirement not only for fulfillment of human aspirations but also for the enjoyment of all mankind of a better quality of life. It is also indispensable for a balanced development of the individual within the family and as part of the community and the nation. There is an urgent need to mobilise and make effective use of all the human resources available in our countries if we are to make rapid economic and social progress. Therefore to meet this need, we the Government, represented by the undersigned, have come together to draw up an effective plan for improving the status of health of our people. Article 6 spells out the specific objectives...(6) The reduction of mortality and morbidity among infants, and children, the improvement of the health of women, especially mothers, and the regulation of fertility, so as to achieve better health and implement national population policy.

According to *World Health Organization*, the MCH Services should ensure that:

"Every child, wherever possible, lives and grows up in a family unit, with love and security, in healthy surroundings, receives adequate nourishment, health supervision and efficient medical attention, and is taught the elements of healthy living."

"Every expectant and nursing mother maintaining good health, learns the art of child care, has a normal delivery, and bears healthy children." Maternity care in the narrower sense, consist in the care of the pregnant women, safe delivery, post-natal care, care of her newly born infant, and the maintenance of lactation. In the wider sense, it begins much earlier in the measures aimed to promote the health and well being of the young who are potential parents, and to help them to develop the right approach to family life and to the place of family in the community. It should also include guidance in parent-craft and in problems associated with infertility and family planning.

Under the constitution of India, the subject of health facilities, including their planning, establishment and administration, falls under the purview of respective governments of States of the Union. However, Government of India has from time to time introduced National Health Programme, which are either centrally sponsored, i.e., part of expense is met by the Central Government, or wholly funded by the centre. Ministry of Health, Government of India, with the help of Central Councils of Health and Family Welfare has taken several initiatives in launching programmes, aimed at controlling or eradicating diseases which cause considerable morbidity and mortality in India. New programmes are being added and existing ones modified, in response to changing epidemiology of disease, host or parasites.

NATIONAL PROGRAMME RELATED TO MOTHER AND CHILD HEALTH

The important National Health Programmes are as follows:

1. Maternal and Child Health Programme (MCH)
2. Integrated Child Development Service Scheme (ICDS)
3. Child Survival and Safe Motherhood Programme (CSSM)
4. Reproductive and Child Health Programme (RCH).

National Programmes Related to Communicable Diseases

Disease Eradication Programmes

1. National Malaria Eradication Programme
2. National Leprosy Eradication Programme
3. National Yaws Eradication Programme
4. National Polio Eradication Programme
5. National Small Pox Eradication Programme (succeeded)
6. National Guinea Worm Eradication Programme (succeeded).

Disease Control Programmes

7. National Filaria Control Programme
8. National Tuberculosis Control Programme
9. National AIDS Control Programme
10. National STD Control Programme
11. National Diarrhoeal Disease Control Programme
12. National ARI Control Programme
13. National Cholera Control Programme
14. National Trachoma Control Programme
15. National Anti Malaria Programme.

National Programmes related to Control of Nutritional Deficiencies and Disorders

1. Vitamin A Prophylaxis Programme
2. Nutritional Anaemia Control Programme
3. National Iodine Deficiency Disorders Control Programme
4. Special Nutrition Programme
5. Balawadi Nutrition Programme
6. Integrated Child Development Scheme (ICDS)
7. School Mid-day Meal Programme.

National Programmes related to Control of Noncommunicable Diseases

1. National School Health Programme
2. National Cancer Control Programme
3. National Mental Health Programme
4. National Diabetes Control Programme
5. National Drug-de-addiction Programme
6. National Programme for Control of Blindness.

MATERNAL AND CHILD HEALTH PROGRAMMES

Women of the reproductive age groups (15-44 years) and children (male and female below 15 years of age) constitute almost 60 per cent of the population. Mothers and children are considered as a special group for the following reasons:

a. By virtue of their numbers, mothers and children are major consumers of health service. They comprise of approximately two-thirds of the population in the developing countries. In India, women in the child-bearing age (15 to less than 45 years) constitute 22.8 per cent and children under 15 years of age 37.1 per cent of the total population. Thus together they constitute nearly 60 per cent of the total population.

b. These groups are subjected to marked physical and physiological stress, which if not cared for, may cause serious deviation from normal health.
c. They are exposed to unusual risks of widespread infection, poor nutrition, and hazardous delivery, which may cause death or impairment of health. The high occurrence of morbidity among women and children is reflected in a seven village study (Trackrov PL, L.Kapoor J.D 1990 NIHFW).

The protection of the health of the expectant mother and her children is of prime importance for building of a sound and healthy nation.

Maternal and Child Health (MCH) refers to preventive and curative health care activities for mothers and children. The objectives of MCH are:

- To reduce maternal, infant and childhood mortality and morbidity.
- To promote reproductive health.
- To promote physical and psychological development of children and adolescent.

The mother and child should be considered and treated as one unit for providing health services because of the following reasons:

- During antenatal period the foetus is part of the mother, The period of development of the foetus is about 40 weeks. During this period it obtains all necessary supplies to nutrients and oxygen from the mother's blood.
- The health of the child is intricately linked to the mother's health.
- Certain diseases inflicting the mother during pregnancy can have that deleterious effect on the health of the foetus.
- Even after birth, the child is dependent for its feeding upon the mother, at least in the first year of life.
- During the first few years of life, the child usually accompanies the mother during her visits to the health facilities and there are few occasions when services to the mothers and children are not simultaneously called for.
- The mental and social development of the child is also dependent on the mother. The mother is the earliest teacher of the child. The death of the mother causes a maternal deprivation syndrome in the child.

The policy guidelines for implementation of MCH programme are:

1. Effective use should be made of existing resources and infrastructures available in the community.
2. The services should be delivered as close to the homes of beneficieries as possible.
3. Services for mothers and children should be delivered, in an integrated manner.
4. Child survival programmes should serve as a sugar-coating for delivery of the family planning programmes which in general are not popular.
5. Voluntary agencies working in the area should be involved in providing MCH services.

World Health Organization (WHO) in 1989 gave call for child survival and safe motherhood (CSSM) programme which was implemented by the Govt. of India. This programme was initiated in 1992. It is yet another exercise of renaming old programmes which have existed for several years and repacking them with a new name. The different components of the CSSM Programme are: advice on breastfeeding, care of the newborn infant, resuscitation of the neonate, care of low birth weight infant and also services to pregnant women. The CSSM Programme with an integrated package of intervention for improving the health status of women and children and reducing the maternal infant and child mortality rates. The services under this programme provided to pregnant women, infants and children under 5 years of age include:

Pregnant women

- Essential care for all:
  - Register by 12 to 16 weeks.
  - Antenatal check up at least 3 times.
  - Immunisation with TT.
  - Give IFA-large tablet to all (1 tablet a day for 100 days).
  - Treat those with clinical anaemia (2 tablets a day for 100 days).
  - Deworm with mebendazole (during 2nd/3rd trimesters in a case where prevalence rates of hookworm infestation are high.
  - Care and clean delivery services.
  - Prepare the woman for exclusive breast feeding and timely weaning.
  - Postnatal care, including advice and services for limiting and spacing births.
- Early detection of complications:
  - Clinical examination to detect anaemia.

- — Bleeding indicating APH or PPH.
- — Weight gain of more than 3 kg in a month or systolic BP of 140 mmHg or more diastolic BP of 90 mmHg or more.
- — Fever 39°C and above after delivery or after abortion.
- — Prolonged or obstructed labour (labour pain for more than 12 hours).
- Emergency care for those who need it:
  - — Early identfication of obstretric emergencies.
  - — Provide initial management and refer to identified referral unity.
  - — Use fastest availiable mode of transport.
- Women in the reproductive age group.
  - — Counselling on:
    - Optimal timing and spacing of birth.
    - Small family norms.
    - Use and choice of contraceptives.
  - — Information on availability of:
    - MTP services.
    - IUD and sterilization services.

The package of services under CSSM Programme are:

For the mothers
- Immunisation.
- Prevention and treatment of anaemia.
- Antenatal care and early identification of maternal complications.
- Deliveries by trained personnel.
- Promotion of Institutional deliveries.
- Management of obstetric emergencies.
- Birth spacing.

For children
- Essential newborn care.
- Immunisation.
- Appropriate management of diarrhoea.
- Appropriate management of ARI
- Vitamin A prophylaxis.
- Treatment of anaemia.

Infants
- Newborn care
  - — Birth weight for all new borns.
  - — Resuscitation of asphyxiated babies.
  - — Care of low birth weight babies.
  - — Prevention of hypothermia.
  - — Exclusive breastfeeding within 1 hour of delivery.
  - — Referral of newborns who show signs of illness.
  - — Advice to mother on essential newborn care, prevention of hypothermia, and infections, nutrition (breastfeeding and weaning), immunisation, Vitamin 'A' prophylaxis and early signs when to seek help.
- Immunisation
  - — BCG 1 dose at birth.
  - — DPT 3 doses beginning 6 weeks at monthly intervals
  - — Polio '0' dose at birth for all institutional deliveries 3 doses beginning 6 weeks at monthly interval.
  - — Measles 1 dose at completion of 9 months of age.
  - — Vitamin A First dose (100,000 IU) with measles vaccination.

Children (1-3 years)
- Immunisation.
  - — DPT/OPV booster dose at 16 to 18 months.
  - — Vitamin A Second dose (200,000 IU) at 16 to 18 months along with DPT/OPV booster.
  - — Third dose to 5th dose (200,000 IU each) at 6 months interval

Children (1-6 years)
- Prevention of anaemia.
  - IFA-small tablets of child has clinical signs of anaemia.
  - Stool examination for hookworm infestations (where facilities are available).
  - Deworm with mebendazole (during 2nd/3rd trimester) in areas where prevalence rates of hook-worm infestation are high.
- Prevention of deaths due to diarrhoeal diseases.
- Correct care management for all cases of diarrhoea.
- Advice mothers.
  - — To give increased volume of fluids (ORS or HAF (Home Available fluids) as soon as diarrhoea starts).
  - — How to prepare ORS solution.
  - — Continue feeding the normal diet.
  - — To recognise signs when to seek help.
- Prevention of deaths due to pneumonia.
- Correct case management for all cases of acute respiratory infections.
- Early initiation of cotrimoxazole to children with signs of pneumonia.
- Referral of children with severe pneumonia or very severe illness.

The rapidly growing population had been a major concern for health planners and administrators in India since independence. The result was the launching of the National Family Planning Programme by the Government of India in 1952, which later became Family Welfare Programme. India is the first country to have taken up the family planning programme at the national level. Poor health status of women and children in terms of high mortality and morbidity was also a other priority in India. Health facilities like hospitals and health centres were established for providing MCH care through ante-natal, intra-natal and post-natal services.

In addition, a number of special programmes and schemes like immunisation against vaccine preventable diseases, nutritional intervention like IFA distribution and Vitamin A supplementation, diarrhoeal disease control programme through Oral Rehydration Therapy (ORT). Acute Respiratory Infections (ARI) Control Programme, etc. were implemented over the past. In order to ensure maximum benefits from these programmes and to provide services in an integrated manner to this vulnerable group the CSSM Programme was implemented.

Despite all these efforts, the desired impact on the population growth and health, and development of women and children in the country could not be achieved, and the need for a new approach to the problem was felt. International conference on population and development (ICPD) held at Cairo in 1994, the nations of the world agreed to give special attention to reproductive health issue. ICPD recommended that new approach needs to be adopted to tackle the problem. Under this approach, it was decided that family planning services should be provided as a component of the comprehansive reproductive health care. ICPD defined reproductive health as *a state of complete physical, mental and social wellbeing and not merely the absence of disease or infirmity, in all matters relating to the reproductive system*. Reproductive health approach implies that men and women be well informed about and have access to safe and effective contraceptive methods as well as women can go through pregnancy and childbirth safely and that couples are provided with best chance of having a healthy infant.

Following the recommendations of ICPD, being one of the 180 countries which participate in the conference, the Government of India took the decision to launch a "Reproductive and Child Health (RCH) Programme in the 9th Five Year plan. Accordingly to adopt the reproduction health approach to the population issues, India officially launched the Reproductive and Child Health Programme in October 1997. In India, the RCH approach has been defined as "people have the ability to reproduce and regulate their fertility, women are able to go through pregnancy and child birth safely, the outcome of pregnancies is successful in terms of maternal and infant survival and wellbeing and couples are able to have sexual relations free of pregnancy and of contracting diseases."

The basic elements of Reproduction and Child Health Programme are:

- Family planning
- Maternal and child health.
- Safe abortion services.
- Effective control of STD and RTS
- Prevention and management of infertility and
- Prevention, detection cum treatment of reproductive tract malignancies.

The major factors affecting RCH are as follows:

- Socioeconomic condition.
- Status of women.
- Educational opportunities.
- Family environment.
- Nutrition
- Gender relationship and
- Traditional and legal structure of society.

An extrinsic factor affecting RCH care service is the following:

- Adolescent health.
- Maternal mortality.
- Unsafe abortion.
- RTIs
- STDs
- AIDS
- Infertility
- Cancer
- Empowerment of women.

THE PACKAGE OF SERVICES PROVIDED UNDER THE RCH PROGRAMME

RCH approach means that every couple should be able to have children when they want, that the pregnancy is uneventful, that safe delivery services are available, that at the end of pregnancy, the mother and the child are safe and contraception by choice are available to prevent pregnancy and contracting diseases.

Child Survival and Safe Motherhood

1. *For the mothers*
   - Essential care for all
   - Early detection of complications
   - Emergency care for those who need it.
2. *For the children*
   - Essential new born care
   - Exclusive breastfeeding and weaning
   - Immunisation
   - Appropriate management of diarrhoea
   - Appropriate management of ARI
   - Vitamin 'A' Prophylaxis
   - Treatment of anaemia
3. *For eligible couples*
   Prevention of pregnancy through contraception services. safe abortion.
4. Prevention and management of Reproductive Tract Infection (RTI) and Sexually Transmitted Infections (STI's)
5. Adolescent health services including counselling of family life and reproductive health

SERVICES

Essential Care for All

- Register by 12-16 weeks.
- Antenatal check-up at least 3 times during pregnancy (20,32,36 weeks) The purpose of antenatal check-up is to monitor progress of the pregnancy and to identify and refer high-risk cases for appropriate treatment at a hospital.
- Tetanus toxoid immunisation should be given to all pregnant women as early as possible during pregnancy with two doses at one month interval. If already immunised during the previous pregnancy, she should receive one dose of TT.
- Give 1 tablet of IFA (Large) daily for 100 days to all pregnant women.
- Treat those with clinical signs of anaemia with 2 tablets of IFA (large tablets for 100 days).
- Deworm with mebendazole (during 2nd/3rd trimester) in areas where hookworm infestation is common.
- Safe and clean delivery services.
- Prepare the woman for exclusive breastfeeding and timely weaning.
- Postnatal care, including advice and services for limiting and spacing births.

Early Detection of Complications

- Clinical examination to detect anaemia. Anaemia is not only a major cause for maternal mortality and morbidity but is also major contributory factor for birth of a low birth-weight baby.
- If there is bleeding before (APH) and excessive bleeding after delivery (PPH), she should be referred to the nearest hospital by the quickest mode of transport.
- Weight gain of more than 3 kg in a month or systolic blood pressure of 140 mmHg more should arouse suspicion of pre-eclampsia. Such cases may also get fits (Eclampsia). All these cases are medical emergencies and should be referred to the nearest hospital.
- Fever 39°C and above after delivery or after abortion are normally due to infections and some times can be fatal. They would also require treatment at a hospital.
- Prolonged or obstructed about (labour pain for more than 12 hours) can lead to rupture of uterus. It is, therefore, essential to take them to the nearest hospital where facilities for caesarian section are available.

Emergency Care for those Who Need it

- Early identification of obstetric emergencies.
- Provide initial management and refer to identify referral hospitals minimum time should be wasted, as delay can be fatal.
- Use fast available mode of transport. The health workers must know the hospital where such cases can be treated and properly guide the attendants so that they can shift the patient by locally available quickest mode of transport by taking shortest route.
- While transporting such cases the patient should lie on her left side. In case the patient has fits, a roll of cloth should be placed between teeth to avoid tongue bite.

Women in the Reproductive Age Group

- Counselling on:
  — Importance of care of girl child.
  — Optimal timing and spacing of birth.
  — Small family norms
  — Use and choice of contraceptives
  — Prevention of RTIs/STDs.

- Information on availability of
  - MTP services.
  - IUD and sterilisation services.
- Provide family planning services.
  - Condom distribution
  - Oral contraceptives.
  - IUD
- Recognition and referral of RTIs/STDs

Provision of Clean and Safe Delivery Practices at the Community Level

- Create awareness in the community on need for 5 cleans and safe deliveries.
- Deliveries by trained personnels
- Provision of Disposable Delivery Kits (DDKs) to all pregnant women.
- Promotion of institutional deliveries.
- Identification and referral of high-risk cases at the community level trained Dais.

Infants

New Born Care

- Take birthweight of all new borns; Normal birth weight is above 2,500 gm. Babies whose weight is between 2,000 to 2,500 gm would require special care. Such babies are to be covered well with clothes and put close to the mothers, breastfeed well and not to be handles by too many people in order to prevent infections. If the birth weight is less than 2,000 gm the new born must be referred to a medical officer for further examination and management.
- Resuscitation of asphyxiated babies; The mucus trapped in the mouth should be gently sucked with the help of a mucus sucker and give mouth-to-mouth respiration if necessary.
- Prevention of hypothermia: Newborns are susceptible to catch cold.
  After birth the newborn should be wiped dry and covered well with soft clean cotton cloth, which has been washed with soap and dried in sun.
- Exclusive breastfeeding within 1 hour of delivery; it is essential that the newborn is given the first milk as it contains many essential nutrients and helps in developing immunity against diseases. The infant should be breastfed exclusively and no other fluid need to be given till the age of 4 to 6 months when semisolid food should also be given.
- Referral of newborns, who signs of illness.
- Advise the mother on essential newborn care, prevention of hypothermia and infections, nutrition (breastfeeding and weaning), immunisation, vitamin A and early signs when to seek help.

Immunisation

- BCG — 1 dose at birth
- DPT — 3 doses beginning at 6 weeks at monthly interval.
- Polio — '0' dose at birth for all institution deliveries, 3 doses beginning at 6 weeks at monthly interval.
- Measles — 1 dose at completion of 9 months of age.
- Vitamin A — First dose (100,000 IU) with measles vaccination.

Children

Immunisation

- DPT/OPV booster dose at 16 to 18 months.
- Vit. A
  - 2nd dose (2,000,000 IU) at 16 to 18 months along with DPT/OPV booster.
  - 3rd to 5th doses (2,000,000 IU) each at 6 monthly intervals.
- IFA
  - Small tablets if child has clinical signs of anaemia.
- If suspected treatment for hookworm infestation.

Prevention of Deaths due to Diarrhoeal Diseases

- Correct case management for all cases of diarrhoea
- Advise mother:
  - To give increased volume of fluids (ORS or HAF) as soon as diarrhoea starts.
  - How to prepare ORS solution.
  - Continue feeding the normal diet.
  - To recognise signs, when to seek help.

Prevention of Deaths due to Pneumonia

- Correct case management for all cases of acute respiratory infections.
- Early initiation of cotrimoxazole to children with signs of pneumonia.
- Referral of children with severe pneumonia or very severe illness.

Reproductive Tract Infection (RTI)/Sexually Transmitted Infection (STI)

RTIs include a variety of bacterial, viral and protozoal infections of the lower and upper reproductive tract of both sexes. RTIs pose a threat to women's lives and wellbeing throughout the world. A high incidence of infertility, tubal pregnancy, and poor reproductives outcome is an indirect reflection of high prevalence of RTIs/STIs in India.

Vaginal discharge is amongst the first 25 per cent to consult a doctor. Forty per cent gynaecological OPD attendance is because of RTIs and 16% of gynaecological admissions are due to pelvic inflammatory disease (PID)

Causes of Reproductive Tract Infection

- Infections caused by overgrowth of organism normally found in the vaginal tract is known as endogenous infections. These infections are associated with inadequate personal, sexual and menstrual hygiene practices.
- Sexually Transmitted Diseases (STDs) are a specific group of communicable diseases that are transmitted through sexual contact.
- Infections which are due to inadequate medical procedures such as unsafe abortion, unsafe delivery or unhygienic IUD insertion are known as iatrogenic infections.

Signs and Symptoms associated with RTIs

In women

- Increased discharge from the vagina that looks and smells different from (change in amount, colour and smell).
- Pain or burning while urinating.
- Painful or painless sores, blisters or warts on or near the genitals.
- Pain on one or both sides of lower abdomen.
- Irregular menstrual periods.
- Pain or bleeding during intercourse.
- Rash on the entire body or just on the palms and soles.
- Swelling on one or both sides of the groins.

In men

Symptoms usually appear within 2 to 3 days or a couple of weeks or even months after having sex with an infected partner are:

- Pus or discharge from the penis.
- Burning or pain while urinating.
- Painful or painless sores, blisters or warts on or near the penis.
- Pain in one or both the testicles.

Prevention of RTIs and STI

- Identify the women with RTI/STI.
- Refer the women to medical officer of PHC promptly for examination and treatment.
- Identify sexual partners and ensure their treatment.
- Advice correct use of condom during every sexual act.
- Provide counselling/health education to individuals, family and community.
- Observe infection prevention measures amongst the health personnel.

A comprehensive RTI/STI control programme requires three levels of action:

- Primary prevention.
- Secondary prevention.
- Tertiary prevention.

Primary prevention

Avoiding acquisition of infection through infected sexual partners. Strategy of primary prevention includes education and counselling about safe sex practices, sexual hygiene and promotion of condom use. Use of condom prevents transmission of RTIs/STIs.

Secondary prevention

Secondary prevention aims at early detection of signs and symptoms and early referral of RTIs/STIs, so that spread of infection to others is decreased. In the peripheral health care setting currently treatment is based on syndromic management. Counselling and education to motivate health seeking behaviour in community by reducing the number of sexual partners, ideally sticking to single faithful sexual partner. Use of most appropriate antibiotics, practising proper asepsis during reproductive interventions and education of sex partners.

Tertiary prevention

Tertiary prevention includes controlling complications of RTI. Strategies for tertiary prevention includes active screening for presence of infection in high-risk group and appropriate management.

— Clinical management of septic abortion.
— Transport for ectopic pregnancy.
— Management for infertility.
— Cervical cancer screening.

Under the RCH Programme RTI/STI clinics are being set up in the FRU's and PHCs phase wise. The ANMs/LHVs will be trained to provide RTI/STI services to the community.They will identify the RTI/STI cases and refer them to the PHCs and to the nearest RTI/STI clinics. At the district level STD clinics will now treat RTI patient and are being assisted by NACO. To make them client- friendly and easily accessible to women, district hospitals are asked to provide RTI services in the gynaecology ward/post-partum centre.

CHILD WELFARE SERVICES IN INDIA

Child Welfare covers the entire spectrum of needs of children who by reason of handicapped—social, economic, physical, or mental—are unable to avail of services, provided by the community. Child Welfare Programmes that seek to provide supportive services to the families of those children because one of the important responsibilities of the society and state, is to assist the family in its natural obligations for the welfare of the children. In India, we have a number of child welfare agencies, the important ones are:

- Indian Council for Child Welfare.
- Central Social Welfare Board.
- Kasturba Gandhi Memorial Trust.
- Indian Redcross society.

These agencies have got branches all over the country and they get financial aid from the government to organise child welfare services in the country by arranging day care services, holiday homes, and recreation facilities for children.

In addition to national agencies, some international agencies also are interested in child welfare services, which include:

- UNICEF
- World Health Organization.
- International Union of Child Welfare.
- CARE
- FAO
- UNO

INTEGRATED CHILD DEVELOPMENT SERVICES (ICDS)

The most important scheme in the field of child welfare is the Integrated Child Development Services (ICDS) scheme, which was initiated in India in the Ministry of Social and Women's Welfare in 1975, in pursuance of the National Policy for Children.

The ICDS seeks to lay a solid foundation for the development of the nation's human resources by providing an integrated package of early childhood services. These consist of:

- Supplementary nutrition.
- Immunisation.
- Health check-up.
- Medical referral services.
- Nutrition and health education for women.
- Non-formal education of children upto the age of 6 years and pregnant and nursing mothers in rural, urban and tribal areas.

ICDS scheme is designed both as a preventive and development effort. The objectives of the ICDS scheme are:

- To improve the nutritional and health status of children in the age group 0 to 6 years.
- To lay the foundations for proper psychological, physical and social development of the child.
- To reduce mortality and morbidity, malnutrition and school dropout.
- To achieve an effective coordination of policy and implementation among the various departments working for the promotion of child development.
- To enhance the capability of the mother and nutritional needs of the child through proper nutrition and health education.
- To achieve the above objectives the ICDS aims as providing the following package of services:

Beneficiary	**Services**
Pregnant women	– Health check-up – Immunisation against tetanus – Supplementary nutrition. – Nutrition and health education
Nursing mothers	– Health check-up – Supplementary nutrition – Nutrition and health education
Other women 15-45 years	– Nutrition and health education
Children less than 3 years	– Supplementary nutrition. – Immunisation. – Health check-up – Referral Services.

Children in age group 3 to 6 years	– Supplementary nutrition.
	– Immunisation
	– Health check-up
	– Referral services.
	– Nonformal education.

The strategy adopted in ICDS is one of the simultaneous delivery of early childhood services. While the health component forms a major component, ICDS is much more than a mere health programme for delivery of social service input for development. The administrative unit of an ICDS project is the community development block in rural areas, the tribal development block in tribal areas and a group of slums in urban areas. The focal point for the delivery of integrated early childhood services under the ICDS scheme, is the trained local women known as "Anganawadi Worker" (AWW). Other functionaries in ICDS scheme are CDPO, who is in-charge officer for supervisors (Mukhya Sevikas) of 100 AWW.

NUTRITION PROGRAMMES

The Government of India have initiated several large scale supplementary feeding programmes, and programmes aimed at overcoming specific deficiency of diseases through various ministries to combat malnutrition including the Ministry of Health and Family Welfare, the Ministry of Social Welfare and the Minsitry of Education.

The major factors leading to malnutrition in India include inadequate intake of calories and proteins, deficiency of certain micronutrients (like iron, vitamin A, calcium or iodine), maldistribution of essential food commodities, low purchasing power, lack of knowledge about balanced nutrition and limited access to health care facilities. The vicious cycle of poverty malnutrition and ill-health has to be combated through the integrated efforts of socio-economic development, better nutrition is widely prevalent, especially amongst those who live below poverty line. The worst hit are pregnant and lactating mothers and children below six years of age, because of additional requirements and their vulnearable condition, they are more prone to infection and malnutrition.

Dietary survey in the low socio-economic groups have shown a dietary deficit of 500 to 600 calories in women, and 1000 to 1100 calories in pregnant and lactating mothers. This maternal malnutrition leads to "Low birth weight" babies. The average birth weight of newborn in the lower socio-economic groups 2.7 kg as compared with 3.1 kg in higher socio-economic groups. Low birth weight babies have a worse mortality experience, being more vulnearable to infection. Malnutritions directly or indirectly responsible for over 50 per cent die of severe protein calorie malnutrition every year. And 50 per cent pregnant women in the third trimester have a haemoglobin level of less than 10 grams per cent, anaemia in pregnancy is directly responsible for 20 per cent of all maternal deaths, and indirectly for 20 per cent of all maternal deaths, and indirectly for a much larges proportion. Over 60 per cent of children under 6 years of age suffer from some form of nutritional anaemia and PEM. Vitamin A deficiency is responsible for at least 25,000 children becoming blind every year. About 40 millions people are estimated to be affected by goitre in India.

In view of the high prevalence of malnutrition in India, the Government has launched several nutritious programmes at the national level. The following are the major nutrition programmes that are being implemented in India:

- ICDS Scheme
- National Nutritional Anaemic Prophylaxis Programme
- National Goitre Control Programme
- National Programme for Prevention of Nutritional Blindness due to Vitamin A deficiency.
- Mid-day Meal Programme.
- Special Nutrition Programme
- Allied Nutrition Programme
- Chief Minister's Noon Meal Programme (Tamil Nadu).

ICDS Scheme

ICDS scheme already explained in earlier. It is morc than a mere nutrition programme and aims at total development of the child. ICDS consists of growth monitoring, and supplementary nutrition is given for 300 days a year, by on-the-spot feeding as far as possible. All beneficieries receive daily ration of 300 kilocalories and 8 to 10 grams protein.

Severely malnourished children and pregnant and lactating mothers receive daily supplementary nutritions providing 60 kcal. and 18 to 20 grams of protein. In this programme, Vitamin 'A' prophylaxis and IFA distribution also are included.

Special Nutrition Programme (SNP)

Special nutrition programme was launched in 1970, as a crash programme to provide supplementary nutrition to children below 6 years of age, and pregnant and lactating mothers. The socially and economically handicapped are to be reached through this programme, as well as those in slums, drought prone and flood affected areas. It is now envisaged that the special Nutrition programme should include some of the components of the ICDS, in order to render it more effective. Properly selected target groups of mothers and children are to be supported with basic health inputs, including nutrition and health education.

The objectives of the programme is to improve the nutritional status of pregnant and lactating mothers and children below 6 years of age in the weakest sections and most vulnerable areas. The objectives are now to include a reduction in mortality and morbidity in children below 6 years, enhance the capacity of mothers to look after the daily health and nutritional needs of children and to strengthen the supportive services. The main activities of the programme are:

- To provide supplementary nutrition
- To provide health services including supply of vitamin A solution and iron and folic acid tablets (Since 1976).

This programme is for the nutritional benefits of children below 6 years of age, pregnant and nursing mothers and is in operation in urban slums, tribal areas, and backward rural areas. The supplementary food supplies about 30 kcal and 10 to 12 grams of protein child per day. The beneficiary mothers receive daily 500 kcal and 25 grams of proteins. This supplement is provided to them for 300 days in a year. This programme is gradually merged into ICDS.

National Nutritional Anaemia Prophylaxis Programme (NNAPP)

Nutritional anaemia is one of the important health problems, affecting women and children in India. ICMR study (1965) shows that about 50 per cent of children under 5 years and 50 per cent pregnant and lactating mothers have haemoglobin level less than 10.5 grams per cent. To start with, the NNAPP had no set goals. Under this programme, anaemia mothers and children are given IFA tablets. The tablets for mother contain 60 mg iron and 500 micrograms folic acid and those for children contain 20 mg iron and 100 micrograms folic acid. Tablets are distributed to mothers and children if their haemoglobin is below 10 gm% and 8 gm% respectively. For young children who cannot swallow, liquid preparations containing the same amount of IFA (2 ml at a time) is given. The good progress have been achieved through this programme. The specific objectives as identified from general description of the programme are as follows:

- To assess the baseline prevalence of nutritional anaemia in mothers and young children through estimation of Hb levels.
- To put the mothers and children with low Hb levels (less than 10 gm% and less than 8 gm%) on anti-anaemic treatment.
- To put the mothers with Hb levels more than 10 g/dl and children with more than 8 gm/dl on the prophylaxis programme.
- To monitor continuously the quality of the tablets, distribution and consumption, and to assess periodically the Hb levels of the beneficieries.
- To motivate mothers, through relevant education, to consume the IFA tablets and to give the same to their children.

National Goitre Control Programme (NGCP)

The government of India realising the magnitude of endemic goitre launched the NGCP in 1962. It aimed at replacement of ordinary salt by iodised salt, particularly in goitre endemic regions. Surveys indicated that the problem of the goitre and iodine deficiency disorders was more widespread than it was thought earlier, with nearly 145 million people estimated to be living in known endemic areas of the country. As a result, the programme was mounted in 1986 with objective to replace the entire edible salt by iodine salt in a phased manner by 1992. The objectives of NGCP are:

- Initial survey to assess the magnitude of the iodine deficiency disorders.
- Supply of iodised salt in place of common salt to the entire country by 1992.
- Repeat surveys to assess the impact of iodised salt after 5 years.

Accordingly the programme has been implemented, and shown some progress. But reveals strengthening of NGCP in the areas related to:

i. Irregular distribution of iodised salt for varying periods.
ii. Lack of supportive supervision for the quality of iodised salt distributed.
iii. Failure of lifting of the allotted quotas of iodised salt by wholesale agents for further distribution to retailers.
iv. Poor interpersonal relationship between salt dealers and food inspectors, the implementation of PFA act.
v. Co-ordination between department of food and civil supply, health and wholesale dealers.

National Programme for Prophylaxis against Blindness due to Vitamin 'A' Deficiency

The National Programme for Prophylaxis against Blindness due to Vitamin 'A' deficiency was launched in 1970 under the Ministry of Health as a part of MCH Programme. Studies have been shown that in the southern and eastern parts of the country, about 30 to 50 per cent pre-school children have eyes problems as a result of Vitamin 'A' deficiency. It is estimated that 2 per cent of the total blindness in India is caused by Vitamin 'A' deficiencies.

The specific objective of the programme in reduction of disease and prevention of blindness due to vitamin 'A' deficiency; An evaluation of the programme has shown than in areas where it has been implemented well there was significant reduction in the prevalence of signs of vitamin 'A' deficiency. The reasons for poor coverage have been inadequate supplies of vitamin 'A' and adoption of clinic approach instead of house-to-house visit for the distribution. As a part of RCH Programme (earlier CSSM) attention now focussed upon children upto 3 years of age.

Balawadi Nutrition Programme

The Balawadi Nutrition Programme was started in 1970-71, with the pre-school child as its target. It is operated through Balawadis and day care centres, and is under the charge of the Social Welfare Department.

The objective of the programme is to supply one-fourth of the calorie requirements and half of the protein requirements of the pre-school child as a measure to improve the nutritional status. It is to be a supplement to what the child receives at home. As far as possible, locally available food stuff is to be utilised. Children belonging to the lower socio-economic group would be selected. Community involvement would be encouraged.

The nutrition supplement providing 300 calories and 10 grams of protein per child per day for 270 days a year, in provided in Balawadis or day care centres where some non-formal education of the pre-school child is given. It is envisaged that a package including basic health components are to be included as in the ICDS.

This programme is directed by the Ministry of Social Welfare through several voluntary organization. Balawadi is managed by Balsevikas assisted by helper, coordination committees at the centre, state, district, block along with the community, are to ensure regular supply of resources and effective management.

Mid-day Meal Programme (MDMP)

The Mid-day Meal Programme started in India in 1925 in Chennai as part of the People's movement. It picked up momentum and the Government on a nationwide basis, stepped it up in 1962-63. Care started assisting the programme in 1961. The Mid-day Meal Programme gives supplementary food to children aged 6 to 11 years in primary schools. Food is given for 200 days a year and ration of 38 lb per year per child.

The objectives of the programme is to providing food to meet the gap in nutritional requirements particularly in poor children. This would help the children, not only improving the nutritional status, but also improve their performance at school. It would indirectly act as an incentive for sending children to school.

In this programme, each primary school child is given food for 200 days. This is to be an addition to what the home provides. This programme is co-ordinated and implemented by the Ministry of Education.

As stated earlier, the major objectives of the programme is to attract more children for admission to schools and retain them so that literacy improvement of children could be brought about. In formulating mid-day meals for school children, the following broad principles should be kept in mind:

- The meal should be a supplement and not a substitute to the home diet.

- The meal should supply at least one-third of the total energy requirement and half of the protein need.
- The cost of the meal should be reasonably low.
- The meal should be such that it can be prepared easily in schools; no complicated cooking process should be involved.
- As far as possible, locally available foods should be used, this will reduce the cost of the meal.
- The menu should be frequently changed to avoid monotony.

A model menu for a mid-day school meal will be:

Food stuff	*gram/day/child*
Cereals and millets	75
Pulses	30
Oils and fats	8
Leafy vegetables	30
Non-leafy vegetables	30

This Mid-day Meal Programme become the part of the Minimum Needs Programme in the fifth FYP.

Applied Nutrition Programme (ANP)

Improvement in nutritional status depends largely upon awareness and knowledge as well as availability of food. The erstwhile expanded programme of nutrition started in India in 1960. It was started first in Orissa and Andhra Pradesh, and extended in 1960 to Tamil Nadu and in 1962 to Uttar Pradesh. In 1963, the ANP was extended to the whole country through the Government of India, along with aid from UNICEF with the active participation of the states.

The programme was launched in 1963 to combat malnutrition in vulnearable groups, particularly mothers and children in rural areas. The programme was basically an education oriented programme, operational at the village and family level.

The main objectives of the programme are:

- To make people conscious of their nutritional needs.
- To increase production of nutritious foods and their consumption.
- To provide supplementary nutrition to vulnerable groups through locally produced foods.

The main components of the ANP are:

- Production of protective foods.
- Training of functionaries involved in the production of these foods.
- Nutrition education and demonstration (demonstration of improved technique of cooking and feeding were also used).

The programme is coordinated by the Ministry of Rural Reconstruction.

At the state level the Panchayatraj and community development is generally in-charge of the programme and in the field, block development officer's incharge of the programme.

The activities of the Applied Nutrition Programme will include:

- Kitchen gardens, school gardens and community gardens are set up to promote the concept of a balanced diet, as well as to increase production
- Fishery units and poultry units are set up. This gives employment, added income and more production of food (poultry farming, beehive keeping), etc.
- Providing better seeds as well as well-breed cattle were provided.
- Supplementary feeding, through local food production was given to vulnerable pregnant in lactating mothers and children.
- Panchayats, Yuvak and Mahila Mandals were to be involved to promote community participation.
- Training for horticulture and pisciculture were given.
- Non-formal pre-school education.

Evaluation studies showed that ANP has not generated the desired awareness for production and consumption of protective foods. The community kitchen gardens and school gardens could not function properly due to lack of suitable land, irrigational facilities and low financial investments. The scheme of setting up of poultry units and pisciculture also did not make much headway. The adequate infrastructure for co-ordination implementation and monitoring was not developed at the field and district level. Therefore, the programmes lacked effective supervision and has almost become defunct.

CHAPTER 2

Anatomy and Physiology of Reproductive System

INTRODUCTION

Nurses providing health care to women require a greater knowledge of female and male anatomy and physiology than is usually taught in general courses. Knowledge of the anatomy and physiology of female and male structures involved in reproduction is basic to planning, implementing and evaluating nursing care of the maternity and women's health clients and their families.

Although the male and female reproductive systems differ in appearance, their structures are homologous (have the same embryonic origin). Each structure performs a vital role in continuing the human species. Expressing sexuality, and generating and maintaining secondary sexual characteristics. Through hormonal influences the genitals, pelvis, and breasts acquire the unique adaptations necessary for childbearing. Female and male reproductive system consist of the following four principal components:

1. External genitals.
2. A pair of primary sex glands (gonads).
3. Ducts leading from the gonads to the body's exterior.
4. Secondary (accessory) sex glands.

FEMALE REPRODUCTIVE SYSTEM

The female reproductive system consists of internal organs, located in the pelvic cavity and supported by the pelvic floor, and external genitals, located in the perineum. The female's internal and external reproductive structures develop and mature in response to oestrogens progesterones starting in foetal life and continuing through puberty and childbearing years. The reproductive structures atrophy (decrease in size) with age or a drop in ovarian hormone production. An extensive and complex innervation and a generous blood supply, support the functions of these structures. The appearance of the external genitals varies greatly among women. Heredity, age, race, and the number of children a women has born determine the size shape and colour of her external organs.

The normal female pelvis has a bowl-shaped cavity, encouraging the foetus to assume a well-flexed occiput anterior position and enhancing the normal progress of labour. These views show the relationship between the vertebral column and bony pelvis. Enlargements clarify how the bones work together to provide support for the foetus yet allow for birth.

External Structures

The external structures, also called the vulva, are presented in the following order: mons pubis (mons veneris), labia majora and minora, clitoris, prepuce of clitoris, vestibule, fourchette, and perineum. These external genitals are shown in Figures 2.1A and B.

Mons Pubis

The mons pubis, or mons veneris, is the rounded soft fullness of subcutaneous fatty tissue and loose connective tissue over the symphysis pubis. The mons contains many sebaceous (oil) glands and develops coarse, dark, curly hair at pubarche (about 1 to 2 years before the onset of the menses), menarche (the onset of menses) occurs about the age of 13 years. Characteristics of pubic hair vary from sparse and fine among Asian women to thick coarse, and curly among African-American women. The mons plays a role in sensuality and protects the symphsis pubis during coitus (sexual intercourse). As a woman

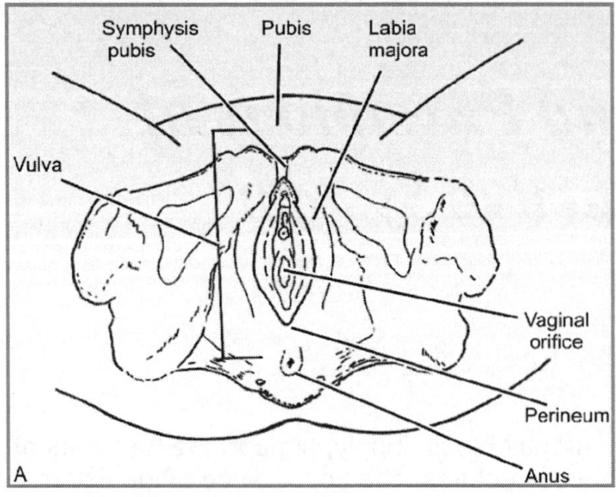

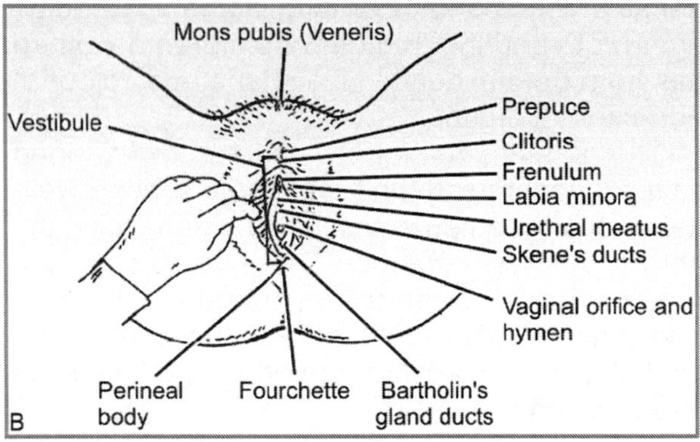

Figs 2.1A and B: The external female genitalia important structures can be visualized only after the labia are gently spread by the examiner's fingers

age increases, the amount of fatty tissue found in her body decreases and pubic hair becoming thins.

Labia Majora

The labia majora are two rounded, lengthwise folds of skin covered fat and connective tissue that merge with the mons. They extend from the mons downward around the labia minora. The labia majora protect the labia minora, urinary meatus, and vaginal introitus. In the woman who has never experienced vaginal child birth the labia majora lie close together in the mildline, covering the underlying structures. Some labial separation and even gaping of the vaginal introitus occur after childbirth and perineal or vaginal injury. Later in a woman's life, declining hormone production causes the labia majora to atrophy.

On the lateral surfaces, labial skin is thick, usually pigmented darker than surrounding tissues, and covered with coarse hair (similar to that of the mons) that thins out towards the perineum. The medial surfaces of the labia majora are smooth, thick, and hairless. These surfaces contain an abundant supply of sebaceous and sweat glands, are highly vascular, and have an extensive nerve network. The labia majora protect the inner surfaces of the vulva and enhance sexual arousal.

Labia Minora

The labia minora, located between the labia majora, are narrow, lengthwise folds of hairless skin. The lateral and anterior aspects of the labia are usually pigmented. The medial surfaces are similar to vaginal mucosa, and are pink and moist. The rich vascularity of these surfaces gives them a reddish colour and permits noticeable turgenscence (swelling) of the labia minoris with emotional or physical stimulation. The glands in the labia minora lubricate the vulva. A rich nerve supply makes the labia minora sensitive, thereby enhancing the erotic function. The space between the labia minora is called the *vestibule*.

Clitoris

The clitoris is a short, cylindrical, erectile organ located just beneath the arch of the pubis; the visible portion is about 6 × 6 mm or less in the unaroused state. The tip of the clitorial body is called the glands and is more sensitive than its shaft. Whenever a woman is sexually aroused, the glans and shaft increase in size.

Sebacious glands of the clitoris secrete smegma, a cheese like fatty substance with a distinctive odour that serves as a pheromone (an organic compound that provides olfactory communication with other members of the same species to elicit a certain response, which in this case is erotic stimulation of the human male). The term *clitoris* comes from a Greek word meaning "key" because the clitoris was seen as the key to female sexuality. Its rich vascularity and innervation make the clitoris highly sensitive to temperature, touch and pressure sensation. The main function of the clitoris is to stimulate and elevate the levels of sexual tension. Some cultural groups practice ritual removal of the clitoris during childhood (see cultural consideration).

Cultural Consideration

Female circumcision Female circumcision occur in women of many different ethnic, cultural, and religious back-grounds. Although circumcision is usually performed during childhood, some communities circumcise infants or older females.

The procedure involves the removal of a portion of the clitoris but may extend to the removal of the entire clitoris and labia minora.

Additionally, the labia majora, which are often stitched together over the urethral and vaginal openings may be affected.

The extent of the circumcision site affects the seriousness of complications. Common complications include bleeding, pain, local scarring, keloid or cyst formation, and infection. Impaired drainage of urine and menstrual blood may lead to chronic pelvic infections, pelvic, and back pain, and chronic urinary tract infections. Some women may require surgery before vaginal examination, intercourse, or childbirth if the vaginal opening is obstructed.

Nurses are providing care to a growing number of women who have emigrated from the Middle East, Asia, and Africa, where female circumcision is more common. Nurses need to be sensitive to the unique needs of these clients, especially if these women have concerns about maintaining or restoring the intactness of the circumcision after childbirth.

Prepuce of Clitoris

Near the anterior junction, the right and left labia minora separate into medial and lateral portions. The lateral portions unite above the clitoris to form its prepuce, which is a hoodlike covering the medial portions unite below the clitoris to form its frenulum. Sometimes the prepuce covers the clitoris. As a result, this area looks like an opening that can be mistaken for the urethral meatus is the nurse does not identify vulvar structures carefully. Attempts to insert a catheter into this sensitive area can cause considerable discomfort.

Vestibule

The vestibule is an oval-shaped area formed among the labia minora, clitoris and fourchette. The vestibule contains opening in the urethra, para urethral (lesser vestibular or skene's glands, vagina and paravaginal (greater vestibular, vulvovaginal, or Bartholin's glands). The thin almost mucosal surface of the vestibule is easily irritated by chemicals (for example, feminine deodorant sprays, bubble bath salts), heat, discharges, and friction (for example, from wearing tight jeans).

Although not a true part of the reproductive system, the urinary (urethral) meatus is considered here because of its closeness and relationship to the vulva. The meatus is a pink or reddened opening that varies in shape and often has slightly puckered margins. The meatus marks the terminal (distal) part of the urethra. It is usually located about 2.5 cm (1 inch) below the clitoris.

The lesser vestibular (paraurethral or skene's) glands are short tubular structures situated posterolaterally just inside the urethral meatus at about the 5 o'clock and 7 o'clock positions around the meatus.

These glands are not usually visible but produce a small amount of mucus, which functions as lubrication.

The hymen (see Fig. 2.1B) is a partial, rarely complete, elastic but tough mucosa-covered fold around the vaginal introitus (opening to the vagina). In virginal females the hymen may be an impediment to vaginal examination, insertion of menstrual tampons, or coitus. The hymen may be elastic and allow distention, or it may be torn easily. Occasionally the hymen covers the orifice completely, resulting in an imperforate hymen that prevents passage of menstrual flow, use of instrumentation (for example, a speculum), or coitus. A hymenotomy may be necessary in some cases. After instrumentation, use of tampons, coitus or vaginal delivery residual tags of the torn hymen (hymenal caruncies or carunculae myrtiformes) may be seen.

One common myth is that the condition of the hymen can disclose whether a female is a virgin. Sexually active and even parous females may have intact hymens. For other women, the hymen may be torn during strenuous physical work or exercise, masturbation, or use of tampons. Therefore, the "test for virginity" (evidence of bleeding after sexual intercourse) is an unreliable criterion.

The greatest vestibular (vulvovaginal or Bartholin's) glands are two compound glands located at the base of the labia majora, one on either side of the vaginal orifice. Several ducts about 1.5 cm long drain each gland. Each duct opens into the groove between the hymen and labia minora. Usually the gland openings are not visible or palpable. The galnds secrete a small amount of clear, viscid (sticky) mucus, especially during coitus. The alkaline pH of the mucus is supportive of sperm.

Fourchette

The fourchette is a thin, flat, transverse fold of tissue formed where the tapering labia majora and minora merge in the midline below the vaginal orifice.

Perineum

The perineum is the skin-covered muscular area between the vaginal introitus and anus. The perineum forms the base of the perineal body (Fig. 2.2).

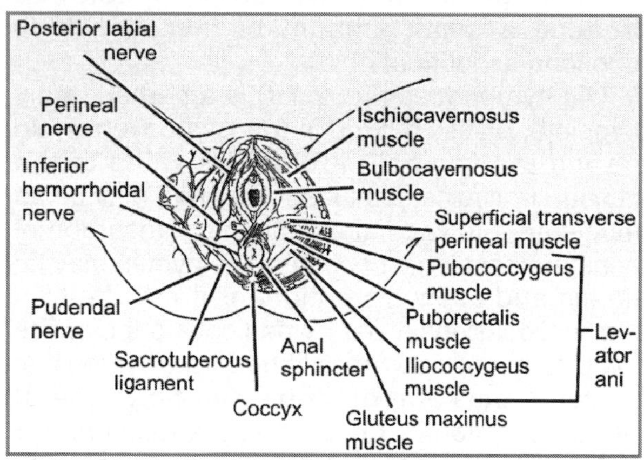

Fig. 2.2: The pudendal nerve and vessels. They provide the major innervation and blood supply to the area

Internal Structures

The internal reproductive organs are discussed in the order that reflects the path of the ovum. Supportive tissues are discussed with the internal reproductive organs that they support. Internal organs include the ovaries, uterine (fallopian) tubes, uterus, and vagina. The following provides a brief description of the pelvic floor and bony pelvis:

Ovaries

One ovary is located on each side of the uterus below and behind the uterine tubes. The ovaries are held in place by two ligments, the mesovarian portion of the uterine broad ligament, which suspend the ovaries from the lateral pelvic side walls at about the level of the anterosuperior iliac crest, and the ovarian ligaments (Fig. 2.3) which anchor the ovaries to the uterus. The ovaries are movable with palpation.

The ovaries are similar in origin (homologous) to the testes in the male. Each ovary resembles a large almond in size and shape (Fig. 2.3).

Uterus

Between birth and puberty the uterus gradually descends into the true pelvis from the lower abdomen. After puberty the uterus is usually located in the midline in the true pelvis posterior to the symphysis pubis and urinary bladder and anterior to the rectum.

For most women, with the urinary bladder empty, the uterus is anteverted (tipped forward) and slightly anteflexed (bent forward), with the corpus (body), lying over the top of the posterior wall of the bladder. The cervix is directed downwards and backwards towards the tip of the sacrum so that it is usually at approximately a right angle to the plane of the vagina. For other women, the uterus may be in the midposition or tipped backward (retroverted), A uterus that is bent more than usual so that the fundus (top) is closer to the cervix is called *'Anteflexed or Retroflexed'*.

A full bladder pushes the uterus back towards the rectum. A full rectum moves the uterus forward against the bladder. Uterine postion also change depending on the woman's position (for example, laying supine, prone, on her side, or standing), her age, and a pregnancy state. The free mobility permits the uterus to rise slightly during the sexual response cycle so that the cervix is placed in a position to increase the likelihood of fertilization.

Ligaments and muscles of the pelvic floor, including the perineal body, support the uterus. a total of 10 ligaments stabilize the uterus within the pelvic cavity (see Figs 2.6A and B). These 10 ligments include the followings four paired ligaments—broad, round, uterosacral and cardinal (transverse or Mackenrodt) and two single ligaments—anterior (pubocervical) and posterior (recto-vaginal). The posterior ligament forms the deep recto-uterine pouch known as the Cul-de-sac of Douglas.

The uterus is a flattened, hollow, muscular, thick walled organ that looks somewhat like an upside-down pear. In the adult woman who has never been pregnant the uterus weighs 60 g (2 oz).

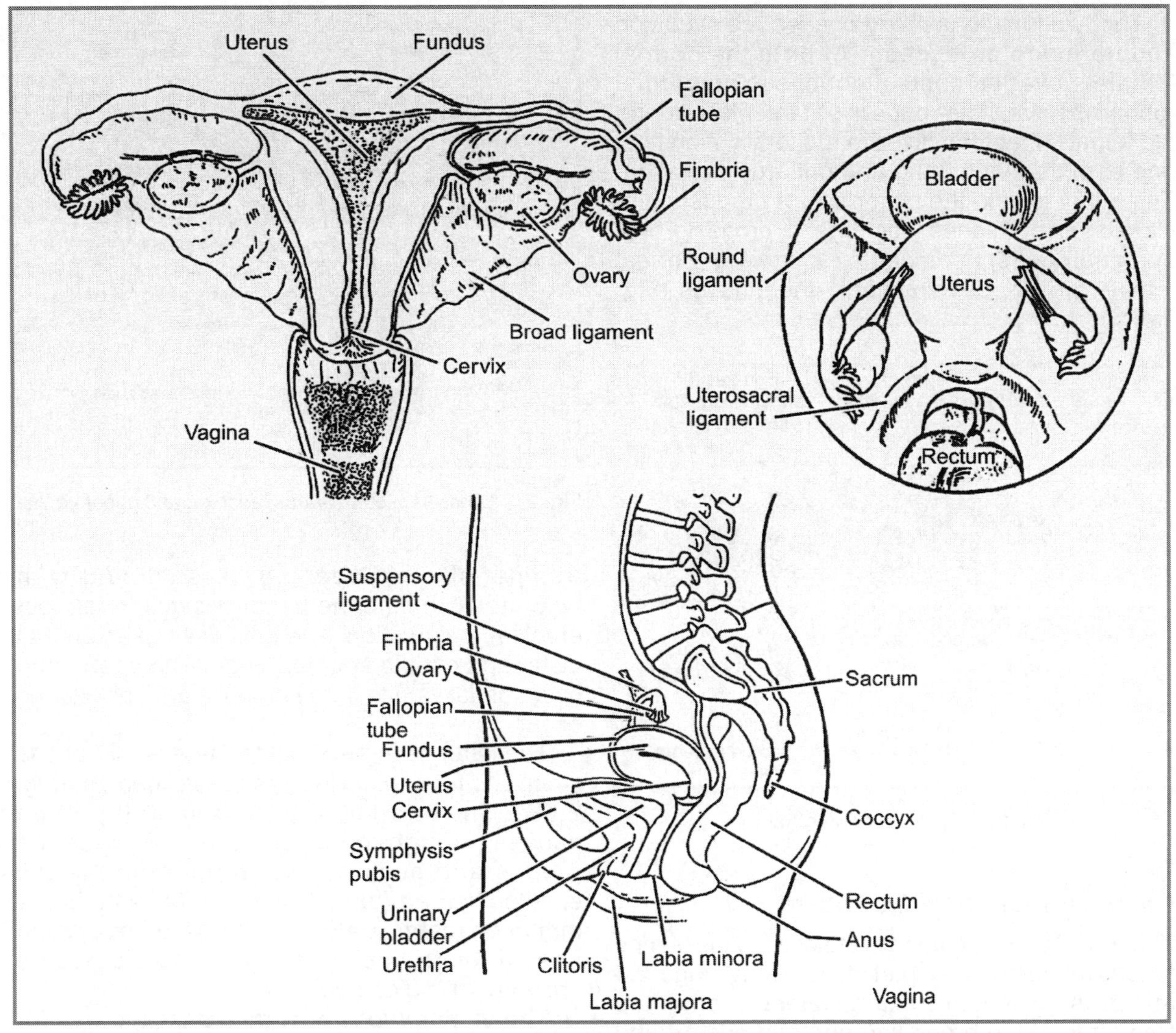

Fig. 2.3: Internal structure of female reproductive organs provide for great flexibility that accommodates both the nonpregnant state and a growing foetus

The uterus normally is symmatric and non-tender, smooth, and firm to the touch. The degree of firmness varies with several factors; for example, the uterus is spongier during the secretory phase of the meanstrual cycle, softer during pregnancy, and firmer after menopause.

The uterus has three parts (see Fig. 2.6A)—the fundus, which is the upper, rounded prominence above the insertion of the uterine tubes, the corpus, or main portion, encircling the intrauterine cavity; and the isthmus which is the slightly constricted portion joining the corpus to the cervix and called the lower uterine segment during pregnancy.

The three functions of the uterus are cyclic, menstruation with rejuvenation of the endometrium, pregnancy and labour. These functions are essential to reproduction but not necessary for a woman a physiologic survival.

Each ovary is whitish and rounded but flattened, weights about 3 g, and measures approximately 3 cm x 2 cm x 1 cm. At the time of ovulation, ovarian size may double temporarily. The oval-shaped ovaries are firm in consistency and slightly tender. The surface of the ovary is smooth before menarche. After sexual maturity, scarring from repeated follicle rupture during ovulation roughens the surface.

The two functions of the ovaries are ovulation and hormone production. At birth the normal female's ovaries contain countless primordial (primitive) ova. After puberty, at intervals during the female's reproductive life (generally monthly), one or more ova mature and undergo ovulation. The ovary is also the major site of production of steroid sex hormones (oestrogens, progesterone, and androgens) in amounts required for normal female growth, development, and function (Fig. 2.4).

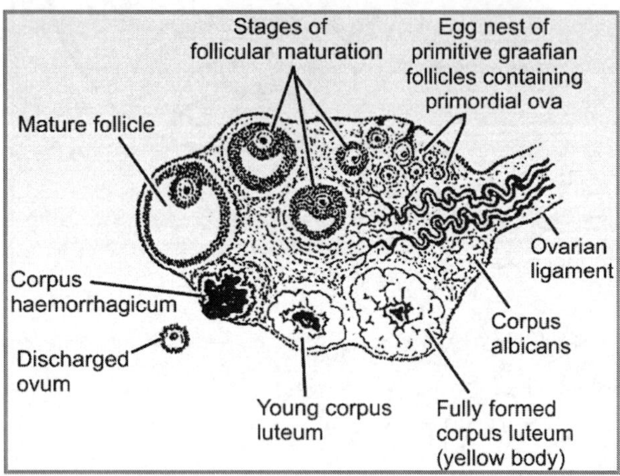

Fig. 2.4: Cross section of ovary

Fallopian Tubes (Uterine Tubes)

The paired uterine tubes are attached to the uterine fundus (upper rounded part of the uterus) (Figs. 2.5 and 2.6A). The tubes extend laterally, enter the free ends of the broad ligment, and curl around each ovary.

The tubes are approximately 10 cm (4 inches) long and 0.6 cm (1/4 inch) in diameter. Each tube has an outer coat of peritoneum a middle, thin, muscular coat; and an inner mucosa. The mucosal lining consists of columnal cells, some of which are ciliated and others of which are secretory. The mucosa is at its thinnest during the time of menstruation. Each tube and its mucosa are continuous with the mucosa of the uterus and vagina.

The structures of the uterine tube changes along its length. The following four distinctive segments can be identified (see Figs. 2.5 and 2.6A); the infundibulum, ampulla, isthmus, and interstitial. The infundibulum is the most distal portion of the tube. The uterine tubes funnel, or

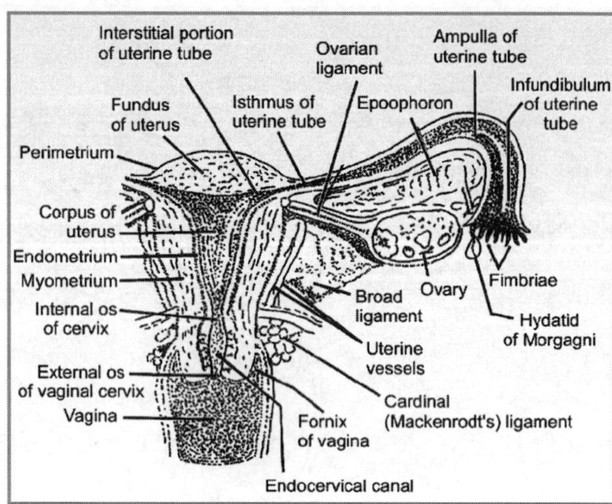

Fig. 2.5: Cross section of uterus, adnexa, and upper vagina

trampet-shaped opening, is encircled with fimbriae. The fimbriae become swollen (almost erectile) at ovulation. The ampulla makes up that distal and middle segment tube. The sperm and ovum usually unite in the ampulla and fertilization occur.

The isthmus is proximal to the ampulla and is small and firm, much like the round ligament (Fig. 2.6B). The interstitial (or intramural) portion passes through the myometrium between the fundus and body of the uterus and has the smallest lumen (tunnel), measuring less than 1 mm in diameter. Before the fertilized ovum can pass through this lumen, it has to discard its crown of granulosa cells.

The uterine tubes provide a passage way for the ovum. The finger-like projections (fimbriae) of the infundibulum pull the ovum into the tube with waveline motions. The ovum is propelled along the tube, partially by the cilia but primarily by the peristaltic movements of the muscular coat, towards the uterine cavity. Peristaltic motion is influenced by oestrogen and prostaglandins. Peristaltic activity of the uterine tubes and the secretory function of the mucosal lining of the uterine tubes are greatest at the time of ovulation. The columnar cells secrete a nutrient to sustain the ovum while it is in the tube.

Uterine Wall

Three layers comprise the uterine wall—the endometrium, the myometrium, and a partial outer layer of parietal peritoneum (see Fig. 2.7).

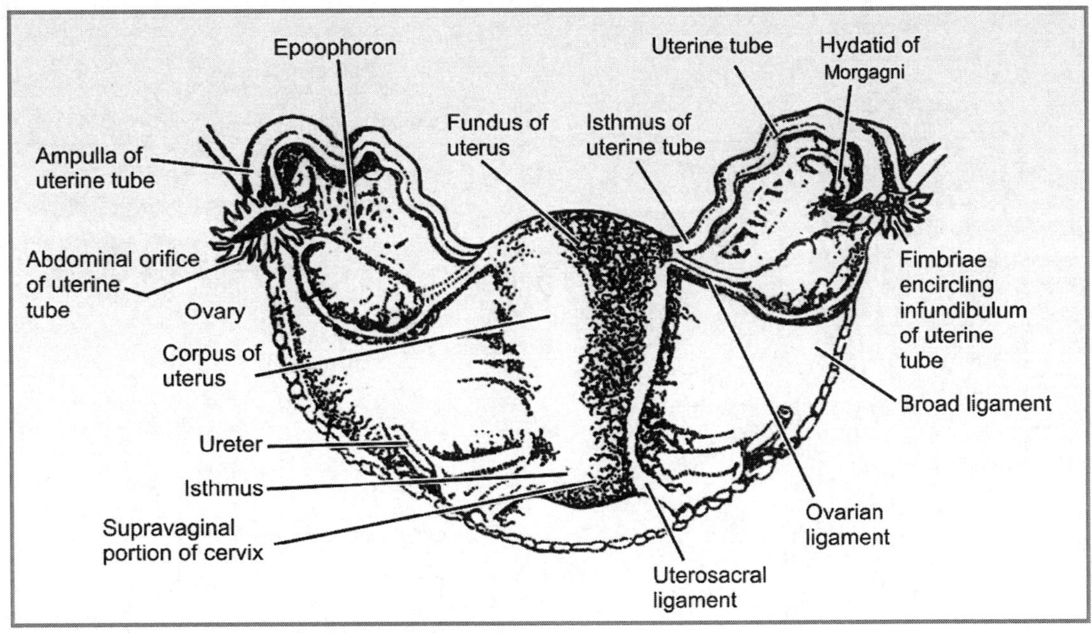

Fig. 2.6A: Posterior view of uterus and adnexa

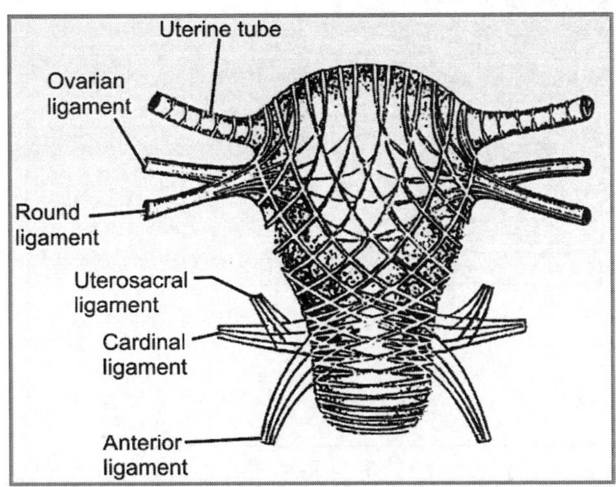

Fig. 2.6B: Arrangement of directions of muscle fibers. Uterine muscle fibers are continuous with supportive ligaments of uterus

The highly vascular endometrium is a lining of mucous membrane composed of three layers—a compact surface layer, a spongy middle layer of loose connective tissue, and a dense inner layer that attaches the endometrium to the myometrium. (The upper two layers are also referred to as the functional layer, and the inner layer is also called the basal layer). During menstruation and after birth, the compact surface and middle spongy layers slough off. Just after menstrual flow ends, the endometrium is 0.5 mm thick, near the end of the endometrial cycle and just before menstruation begins again, the endometrium is about 4 mm (less than 1/4 inch) thick.

Layers of smooth muscle fibres that extend in three directions (longitudinal, transverse and oblique) make up thick myometrium (Fig. 2.7). The smooth muscle fibres interlace with elastic and connective tissues and blood vessels throughout the uterine wall and blend with the dense inner layer of the endometrium. The myometrium is particularly thick in the fundus, thins out as it nears the isthmus, and is thinnest in the cervix.

Longitudinal fibres comprise the outer myometrial layer, found mostly in the fundus, which makes this layer well-suited for expelling the foetus during the birth process. In the thick middle myometrial layer the interlaced music fibres form a figure-eight pattern encircling large blood vessels. Contraction of the middle layer produces a haemostatic action (Fig. 2.7). Only a few circular fibres of the inner myometrial layer in the interlaced muscle fibres form a figure-eight pattern encircling large blood vessels. Contraction of the middle layer produces haemostatic action (Fig. 2.7). Only a few circular fibres of the inner myometrial layer are found in the fundus. Most of the circular fibres are concentrated in the cornua (the place where the uterine tubes join the uterine body) and around the internal os. The blood out the uterine tubes

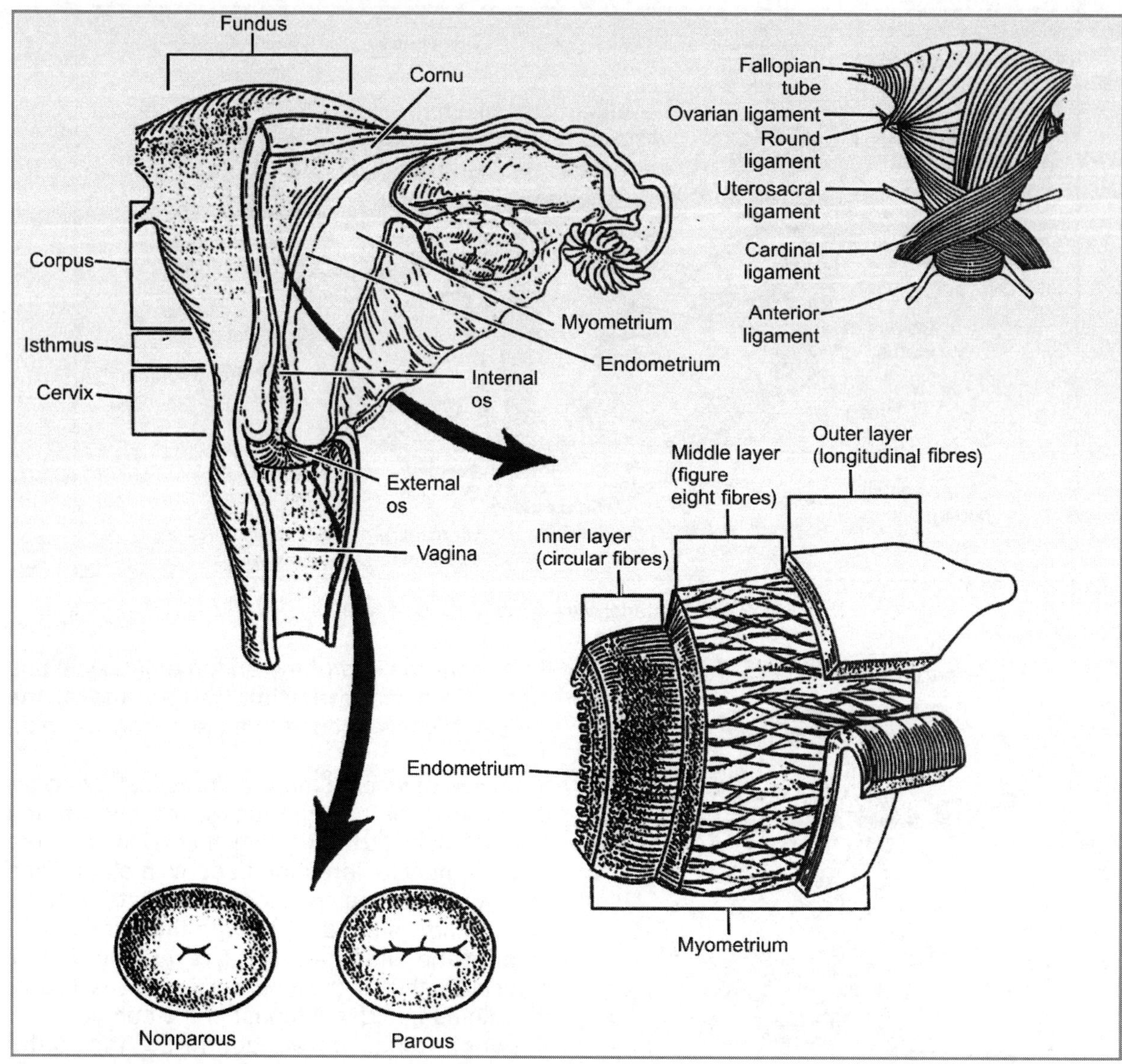

Fig. 2.7: The uterus is a unique muscular organ supported by a complex pattern of ligaments: Its size can increase by 16 times (70 g to 1100 g) during pregnancy, after vaginal delivery the appearance of the external cervical os shows marked change

during menstruation. This sphincter action around the internal cervical os helps retain the uterine contents during pregnancy. Injury to this sphincter can weaken the internal os and result in an internal cervical os that opens prematurely.

Although each muscle layer and its function were described individually, the myometrium works as a whole. The structure of the myometrium, which gives strength and elasticity, presents as example of adaptation to function:

1. The fundus must contract with the most force to thin out, pull up, and open the cervix and push the foetus out of the uterus.
2. Contraction of interlacing smooth muscle fibres that surround the blood vessels controls blood loss after abortion and childbirth. Because of their ability to close off (ligate) blood vessels between them, the smooth muscle fibres of the uterus are called the living ligature (see Fig. 2.7).

The parietal peritoneum, a serous membrane, coats all the uterine corpus except for the lower one-fourth of the anterior surface, where the bladder and the cervix is attached. Diagnostic tests and surgery involving the uterus can be performed without entering the abdominal cavity because parietal peritoneum does not completely cover the uterine corpus.

Cervix

The lowermost portion of the uterus is the cervix, or neck. The attachment site of the uterine cervix to the vaginal vault divides the cervix into the longer supravaginal (above the vagina) portion (see Figs 2.5 and 2.6A) and the shorter vaginal portion (see Fig. 2.5). The length of the cervix is about 2.5 to 3 cm, of which about 1 cm protrudes into the vagina in nonpregnant women.

The cervix is primarily composed of fibrous connective tissue with some muscle fibres and elastic tissue. The cervix of a nulliparous woman is a rounded, almost conical, rather firm, spindle-shaped body. The narrowed opening between the uterine cavity and endocervical cannal (the canal inside the cervix that connects the uterine cavity with the vagina) is the internal os. The narrowed opening between the endocervix and vagina is the external os, a small circular opening in women who have not delivered children. Childbirth changes the circular os to a smal transverse opening that divides the cervix into an anterior and a posterior lip (Figs 2.5 and 2.6A).

When a woman is not ovulating or pregnant, the tip of the cervix feels firm, much like the end of the nose, with a dimple in the center. The dimple marks the site of the external os.

The most significant characteristic of the cervix is its ability to stretch during vaginal childbirth. Several factors contribute to cervical elasticity—high connective tissue and elastic fiber content, numerous infoldings in the endocervical lining, and a 10 per cent muscle-fibre content.

Canals

The two cavities within the uterus are known as the uterine and cervical canals (see Fig. 2.5). The uterine canal in the nonpregnant state is compressed by thick muscular walls so that it is only a potential space, flat and triangular. The fundus forms the base of the triangle. The uterine tubes open into both ends of the base. The apex of the triangle points downwards and forms the internal os of the cervical canal.

The endocervical canal with its many infoldings has a surface layer of tall, columnar, mucus producing cells. Columnar epithelium is beefy red, deeper, and rougher looking than the epithelial outer covering or the cervix. After menarche, squamous epithelium covers the outside of the cervix (ectocervix). This external covering of flat cells gives a glistening pink colour to the cervix. A deeper bluish-red colour is seen if a women is ovulating or pregnant. A reddened (hyperemic) cervix may indicate inflammation.

The two types of epithelium meet at the squamo-columnar junction. This junction line usually lies just inside the external cervical os but may be found on the ectocervix in some women. The squamo-columnar junction is the most common site of neoplastic cellular changes. Therefore cells used for cytologic study (for example, the Papanicolaou test) are scraped from this juction.

The columnar-epithelial cells produce odourless and nonirritating mucus in response to the stimulation of oestrogen and progesterone.

Blood Vessels

The abdominal aorta divides at about the level of the umbilicus and forms the two iliac arteries. Each iliac artery divides to form two arteries, the major one of which is the hypogastric artery. The uterine arteries branch off from the hypogastric arteries. The closeness of the uterus to the aorta ensures an ample blood supply to meet the needs of the growing uterus and conceptus.

In addition, the ovarian artery is a direct subdivision of the aorta. It first supplies the ovary with blood and then joins the uterine artery, thereby further adding to the blood supply (Fig. 2.8).

In the nonpregnant state, uterine blood vessels are coiled and tortuous (twisted). With advancing pregnancy and an enlarging uterus, these blood vessels straighten. The uterine veins follow along the arteries and empty into the internal iliac veins.

UTERINE BLOOD SUPPLY

- Hormonal triggers cause uterine blood supply to expand or contract.
- During the Proliferative phase of the female reproductive cycle, there is a two-to-three fold

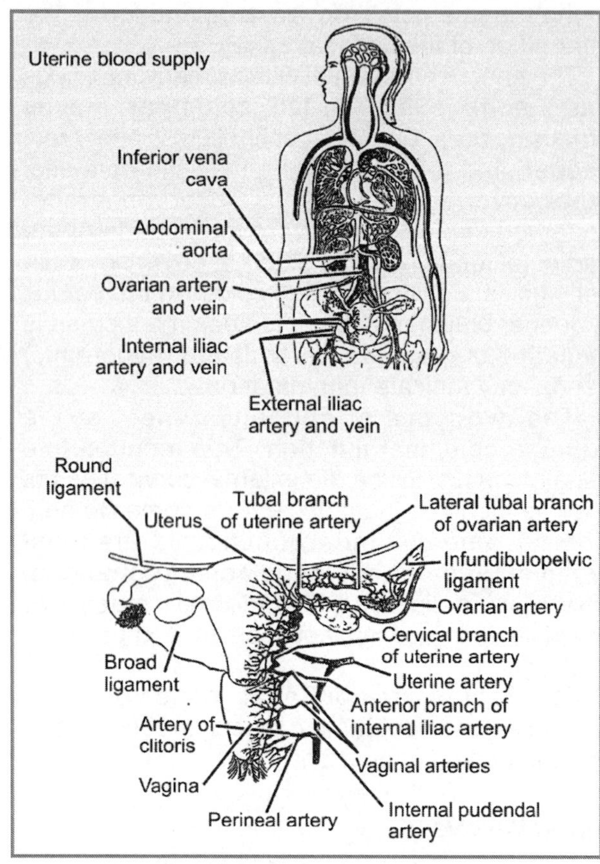

Fig. 2.8: Pelvic and uterine blood supply in relation to the circulatory system

increase in endometrium thickness as spiral arteries elongate.

- In the secretory phase, spiral arteries grow into coiled spongy and compact layers.
- A blastocyte can implant in this prepared endometrium.
- When fertilization does not occur, the blood supply is reduced as spinal arteries become restricted during the ischaemic phase.

Innervation

The internal genitals have a rich supply of afferent and efferent autonomic nerves. These autonomic nerves are motor and sensory.

Parasympathetic fibres from the sacral nerves are probably responsible for producing vasodilation and inhibiting muscular contraction. Efferent sympathetic motor nerves arise from the ganglia of T-5 (thoracic-5) to T-10, come together over the sacrum, and reach the uterus through ganglia lying near the base of the uterosacral ligaments. These efferent sympathetic motor nerves are believed to cause vasoconstriction and muscular contraction. The autonomic nerves described (para-sympathetic and efferent sympathtic motor) regulate the action of the uterus, but the uterus has an intrinsic motility (that is, the uterus can contract and relax even if nerves leading to it are cut). Even if a woman suffers an accidents that injures the spinal cord at or above T-5, she may still be able to have uterine contractions sufficient to give birth to an infant vaginally.

Sensory fibres carrying pain sensation from the uterus come together in the paracervical areas and proceed upward to pass just below the division (bifurcation) of the aorta and then travel to the spinal cord at the level of T-11 and T-12. Because of this arrangement, pain originating in the ovary or ureters may mimic pain that originates in the uterus, any of which may be felt in the flank and down to the inguinal and vulvar areas.

Vagina

The vagina, a tubular structure located in front of the rectum and behind the bladder and urethra (see Fig. 2.2) extends from the introitus, which is the external opening in the vestibule between the labia minora of teh vulva, and the cervix. If a woman is standing, the vagina slants backwards and upwards. The vagina is mainly supported by its attachments to the pelvic floor musculature and fascia.

The vagina is a thin-walled, collapsible tube capable of great distention. Because of the way the cervix protrudes into the uppermost portion of the vagina, the length of the vagina's interior wall is only about 7.5 cm whereas the length of the posterior wall is about 9 cm. The recesses formed around the protruding cervix are called fornics—right, left, anterior and posterior. The posterior fornix is deeper than the other three (see Fig. 2.5).

Glandular mucous membranes line the smooth muscle walls. During the reproductive years this mucosa is arranged in transverse folds called rugae.

The vaginal mucosa promptly responds to oestrogen and progesterone stimulation. The mucosa loses cells, especially during the menstrual cycle and pregnancy. Cells scraped from the vaginal mucosa can be used to estimate steroid sex hormone levels.

Vaginal fluid is derived from the lower or upper genital tract. The fluid is ordinarily slightly acidic.

Interaction between vaginal lactobacilli and glycogen, maintains acidity. If the pH rises above 5, the incidence of vaginal infection increases. The continuous flow of fluid from the vagina maintains relative cleanliness of the vagina. Therefore vaginal douching under normal circumstances is neither necessary nor recommended.

The copious blood supply to the vagina is derived from the descending branches of the uterine artery, vaginal artery, and internal pundendal arteries (see Fig. 2.8).

The vagina is relatively insensitive. Some innervation exists from the pudendal and haemorrhoidal nerves to the lowest one-third of the vagina. Because of this minimal innervation and lack of special nerve endings, the vagina is the source of little sensation during sexual excitement and coitus, and it causes less pain during the second stage of labour than if this tissue were well supplied with nerve endings.

The G-spot is an area on the anterior vaginal wall beneath the urethra and is defined by Graefenberg as analogous to the male prostate gland. During sexual arousal the G-spot may be stimulated to the point of organ with ejaculation into the urethra of fluid similar in nature to prostatic fluid.

The vagina functions as the organ for coitus, passage way for menstrual flow, and birth canal.

Pelvic Floor and Perineum

The pelvic diaphragm, urogenital diaphragm or triangle, and muscles of the external genitals and anus compose the pelvic floor and perineum. The perineum is sometimes defined as including all the muscles, fascia, and ligaments of the upper (pelvic) and lower (urogenital) diaphragms. The perineal body adds strength to these structures.

The upper pelvic diaphragm composed of muscles and their fascia and ligaments, extends across the lowest part of the pelvic cavity like a hammock (Fig. 2.9). The largest and most significant portion of the diaphragm is formed by the pair of broad, thin levator animuscles that extend in sheets between the ischial spines and coccyx and the sacrum. The levator ani group of muscles is made of three muscle pairs; puborectalis, iliococcygeus, and pubo-coccygeus muscles. The pubococcygeus muscle is particularly significant for women. It plays a role

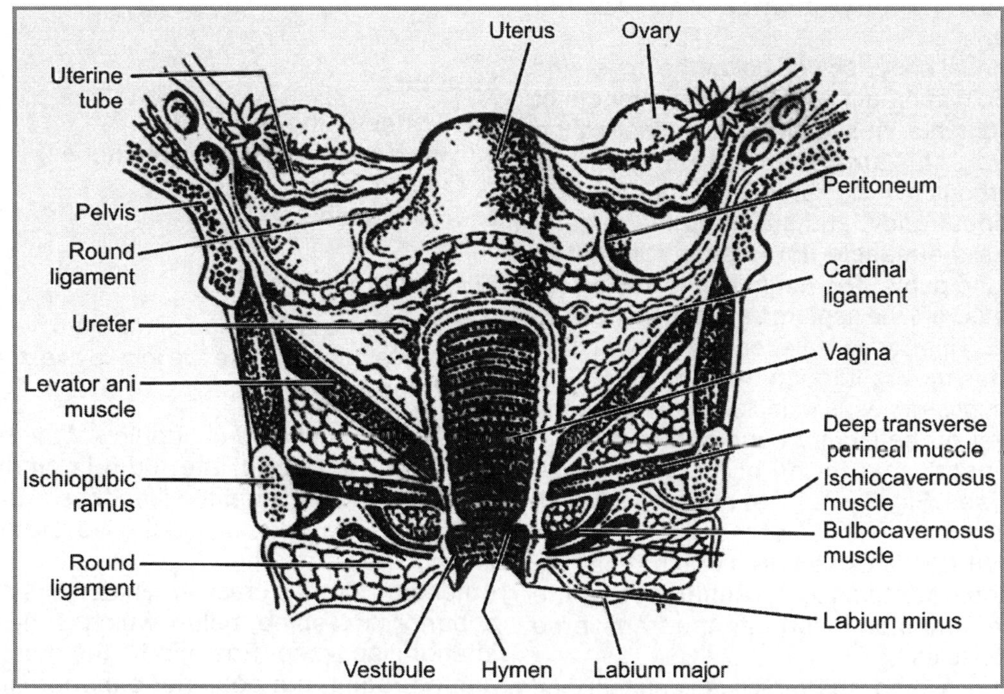

Fig. 2.9: Anterior view of levator ani muscles in the upper pelvic diaphragm and urogenital (lower pelvic) diaphragm

in sexual sensory function, bladder control, control of the perineal relaxation during labour and expulsion of the foetus during birth.

The second paired muscles of the upper pelvic diaphragm are the closely joined coccygeus muscles. These muscles extend from the ischial spines to the coccyx and lower sacrum. The several parts of the pelvic diaphragm provide a sling like support to abdominal and pelvic viscera.

The strength and resilience of this sling are derived from the way in which the layered parts of this sling are interwoven and interlaced. The layers are not fixed; that is, they slide over each other. This unique arrangement strengthens the supportive capacity of the pelvic diaphragm, allows for dilatation of the vagina during the birth process and its closure after birth, and assists with constriction of the urethra, vagina and anal canal, which pass through the diaphragm.

The lower pelvic diaphragm is located in the hollow of the pubic arch and consists of the transverse perineal muscles, which originate at the ischial tuberosities and insert into the perineal body. The strong muscle vagina during birth. The deep transverse perineal muscles join to form a central seam, or raphe. Some of their fibres encircle the urinary meatus and vaginal sphincters.

The perineal body, located below the upper and lower pelvic diaphragm reinforces the strength of the pelvic diaphragm and aids in constricting the urinary vaginal and anal openings. The bulbocavernous muscle fibres (Fig. 2.9) originate in the perineal body, and surround the vaginal opening as the muscle fibres pass forward to insert into the pubis. The perineal body (Fig. 2.9) is continuous with the septum between the rectum and vagina. This tissue is flattened and stretched as the foetus moves through the birth canal.

The ischiocavernosus muscles originate in the tuberosities of the ischium and continue at an angle to insert next to the bulbocavernosus muscles (see Fig. 2.9). These muscle fibres contract to cause exection of the clitoris.

Anal sphincter muscle fibres originate at the coccyx, separate to pass on either side of the anus, fuse, and then insert into the transverse perineal muscles.

The bulbocavernousus transverse perineal, and anal sphincter muscle fibres can be strengthened through Kegel exercises.

THE BONY PELVIS

The bony pelvis is a basin-like structure which connects the spine to the lower limbs (Fig. 2.10). In life, it contains and protects the female reproductive organs and other structures listed below:

1. The reproductive organs, namely the vagina, the uterus, the Fallopian tubes and the ovaries.
2. The bladder and the urethra.
3. The pelvic colon, the rectum and the anal canal.

The bony pelvis is the canal through which the foetus passes during labour.

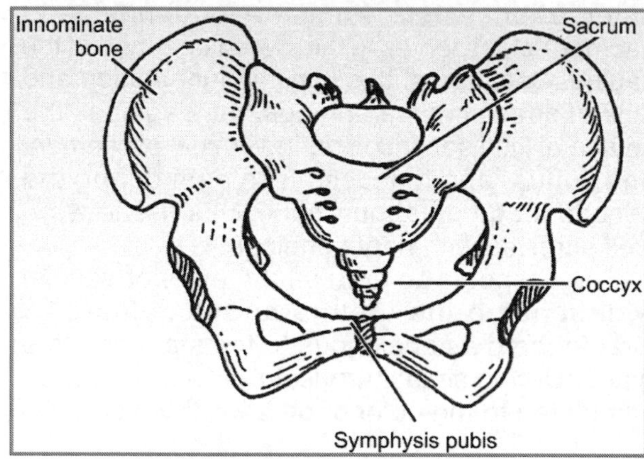

Fig. 2.10: Female pelvis

Structure

The bones of the pelvis are:

1. Two hip bones (innominate bones).
2. One sacrum.
3. One coccyx.

The Hip Bone (Fig. 2.11)

Each hip bone is made up of the ilium, the ischium and the os pubis. These are joined at a depression called the acetabulum.

The ilium is the flared-out portion of the hip bone. The inner aspect of the ilium is smooth and concave and is called the iliac fossa. Below the iliac fossa is a ridge called the ilio-pectineal line and above it is another ridge called the iliac crest. Anteriorly, the iliac crest terminates at the anterior superior iliac spine, below which is the anterior inferior iliac spine. Posteriorly, the crest ends at another point, the posterior superior iliac spine above and posterior inferior iliac spine below Beyond the posterior inferior iliac spine is a curve

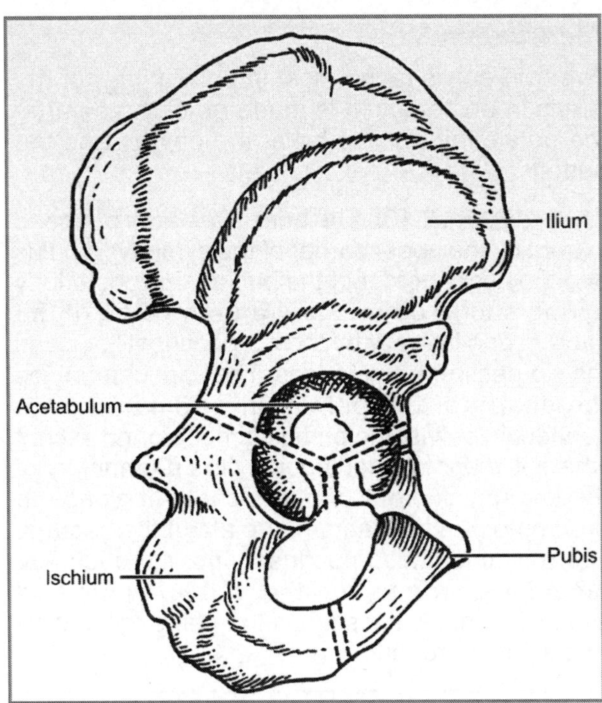

Fig. 2.11: Posterior aspect of the right innominate bone

called the greater sciatic notch. The ilium articulates with the sacrum at the sacro-iliac joint.

Pubic bone: Each of the pubic bones has a body and two rami. The two pubic bones form the anterior aspect of the pelvis. The horizontal or the upper ramus joins the ischium at a thick point called the ilio-pectineal eminence. The descending ramus forms part of the pubic arch, and also forms part of the obturator foramen. The bodies of the pubic bones articulate at the symphysis pubis.

The ischium: This is the thickest and the lowest of the hip bones. It forms two-fifths of the acetabulum. The thick portion of the ischium below the acetabulum is the ischial tuberosity on which the body rests in the sitting position. Above and behind the ischial tuberosity is a sharp protrusion called the ischial spine. This spine separates the greater and the lesser sciatic notches. A small shaft of the ischium goes into the formation of the pubic arch.

The Sacrum

The sacrum is a wedge-shaped bone which forms the back of the pelvis. It is made up of five sacral vertebrae which have fused together. The anterior surface of the sacrum is concave and the posterior surface is convex. The concavity is called the hollow of the sacrum (Fig. 2.12). The midline protuberance of the first sacral vertebra which overhangs the hollow of the sacrum is called the promontory of the sacrum. The first sacral vertebra articulates with the fifth lumbar vertebra at the lumbosacral joint. The lateral masses of bone on either side of the first sacral vertebra are the alae or wings of the sacrum and they articulate with the ilium at the sacro-iliac joints.

The four foramina on each side of the sacrum are for the passage of nerves and blood vessels. The small canal on the posterior aspect of the sacrum is called the sacral canal. It contains the cauda equina, the sacral and the coccygeal nerves.

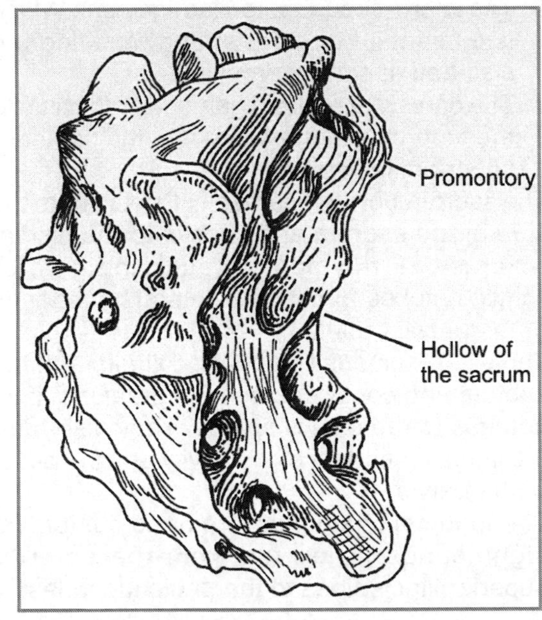

Fig. 2.12: Lateral view of the sacrum

The Coccyx

The coccyx consists of four rudimentary coccygeal vertebrae. The first of these vertebrae articulates with the fifth sacral vertebra at the sacro-coccygeal joint. The coccyx bends backward at this joint during parturition to increase the antero-posterior diameter of the pelvic outlet.

The Pelvic Joints

The important ones which have been underlined are:

- The sacro-iliac joints
- The symphysis pubis
- The sacro-coccygeal joint.

Normally, there is little or no movement in these joints. But during pregnancy, especially towards term, there is relaxation of ligaments of the joints resulting in a certain degree of movement in them. This movement may cause some difficulty in walking and some backache, especially in multiparous patients. There is also a little widening of the joints during labour and delivery and this is referred to as the 'give' of the pelvis.

The Pelvic Ligaments

These are:

1. The sacro-iliac ligaments which comprise:
   a. The interosseous sacro-iliac ligament: Which is a ligament of great strength uniting the iliac and sacral tuberosities.
   b. The dorsal sacro-iliac ligaments: Which unite the tubercles of the sacrum to the posterior superior iliac spine.
2. The sacro-tuberous ligaments: Stretch from the side of the sacrum and coccyx to the ischial tuberosity. They pass through the greater sciatic notches forming the lateral boundaries of the pelvic outlet.
3. The sacro-spinous ligaments: Extend from the sacrum and coccyx across the greater sciatic notches to the ischial spines. They also form the lateral boundary of the cavity and the outlet of the pelvis.
4. The inguinal ligaments: Are of no obstetrical significance. They run from the anterior superior iliac spines to the pubic tubercles.

The Pelvis as a Whole

The pelvis is divided into:

a. The false pelvis.
b. The true pelvis.

The False Pelvis

This consists of the iliac fossae laterally, the fifth lumbar vertebra posteriorly, the abdominal wall and the inguinal ligaments anteriorly. The false pelvis is of no obsterical importance except that it provides certain landmarks for external pelvimetry.

The True Pelvis

The true pelvis is the most important part of the pelvis in obstetrics. It is made up of three parts- the pelvic inlet or the brim, the cavity, and the outlet.

The brim (Fig. 2.13): The brim is the area bounded in front by the upper border of the symphysis pubis and the upper border of the pubic rami, posteriorly by the sacral promontory and the alae of the sacrum and laterally by the ilio-pectineal lines and the ilio-pectineal eminences. The brim determines the shape of the pelvis. In a female or the gynaecoid pelvis, the brim is almost round except where it is encroached upon by the promontory of the sacrum. A piece of paper cut to fit along the promontory of the sacrum, the ala of the sacrum, sacro-iliac joint, ilio-pectineal line, ilio-pectineal eminence, ramus of the pubic bone and symphysis pubis constitutes the plane of the brim and it will be round.

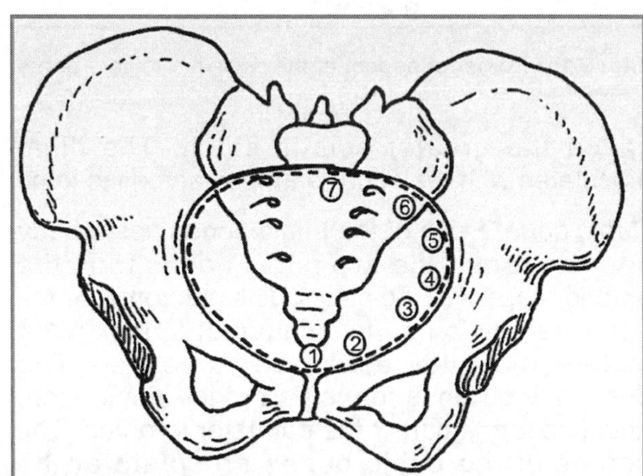

Fig. 2.13: The brim or inlet of the female pelvis. (i) Symphysis pubis, (2) Pubic crest, (3) Ilio-pectineal eminence, (4) Ilio-pectineal line , (5) Sacro-iliac joint, (6) Ala of the sacrum, (7) Promontory of the sacrum

The cavity: The cavity lies between the inlet and the outlet. Its boundaries are: anteriorly—the pubic bones 3.8 cm deep: posteriorly—the sacral hollow 11.4 cm deep; laterally—the bodies of the ischium and part of the ilium, the greater sciatic notches and the obturator foramina.

A flat surface cut to fit along the second and third sacral vertebrae, the sacrospinous ligaments, the body of the ischium on both sides, and the mid-parts of the obturator foramina and the symphysis pubis constitutes the plane of the cavity and this is round.

The outlet: Two pelvic outlets could be described.

1. The anatomical outlet which is bounded by the landmarks: the tip of the coccyx and the sacrotuberous ligament posteriorly, the ischial tuberosity laterally, the pubic arch and the lower border of symphysis pubis anteriorly.
2. The obstetrical outlet is the area the foetal head negotiates as it is being born (Fig. 2.14). It is a segment of the pelvis between the anatomical outlet and a line drawn along the sacro-coccygeal joint, and sacro-spinous ligament, the ischial spine across to the obturator foramen, and the lower border of the symphysis pubis. The flat surface marked by this line is the plane of the outlet.

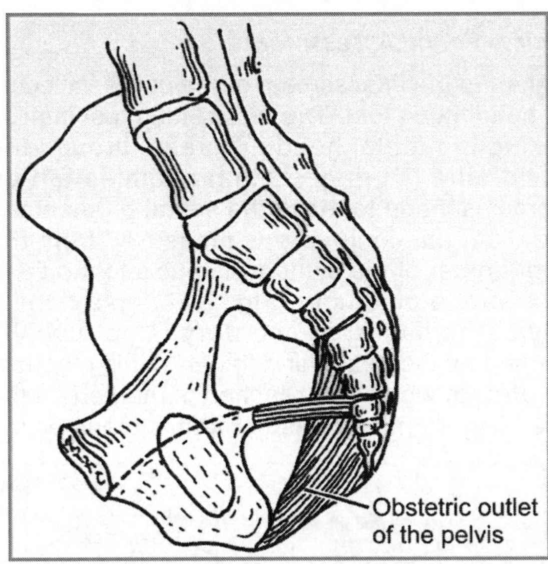

Fig. 2.14: Obstetric outlet of the pelvis

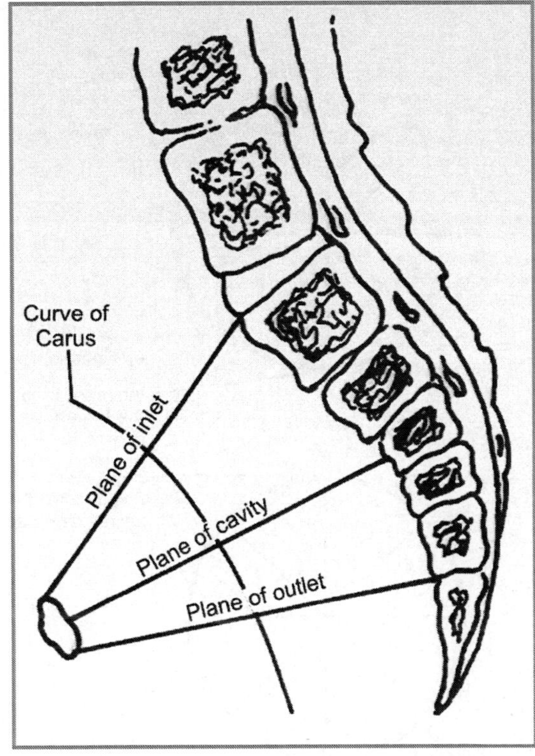

Fig. 2.15: The planes of the pelvis

Dimensions of the Pelvis

These are often referred to as diameters which are measurements taken on the planes of the brim, cavity and the outlet of the pelvis (Fig. 2.15).

Diameter of the brim (Fig. 2.16): The antero-posterior diameter of the brim is measured from the centre of the sacral promontory to the top of the symphysis pubis. It measures 11.4 cm. This is the true conjugate and it differs from the obstetrical conjugate which is measured from the sacral promonotory to a point 1.25 cm down the posterior surface of the symphysis pubis. It measures 10.2 cm. In life, this obstetrical conjugate is assessed by estimating the diagonal conjugate on vaginal examination. The diagnoal conjugate is the distance between the lower border of the symphysis pubis and the sacral promontory. It measures 12 cm; 1.25 cm is deducted for the width of the pubic bone.

The oblique diameters of the brim are estimated from the sacro-iliac joint on one side to the ilio-pectineal eminence on the opposite side-each measures 12 cm. They take their names from the sacro-iliac joints, hence the right oblique diameter is from the right sacro-iliac joint to the left ilio-pectineal eminence and vice versa.

The transverse diameter of the brim is between the furthest points on the ilio-pectineal lines and it measures 13.5 cm.

The sacrocotyloid diameter of the brim which extends from the sacral promontory to the ilio-pectineal eminence; it measures 8.8 cm.

Diameter of the cavity (Fig 2.16): The antero-posterior diameter of the cavity is measured from the midpoint of the symphysis pubis to the junction of the second and third sacral vertebrae. It measures 12 cm. Since the plane of the cavity is a circle, all the other diameters measure 12 cm.

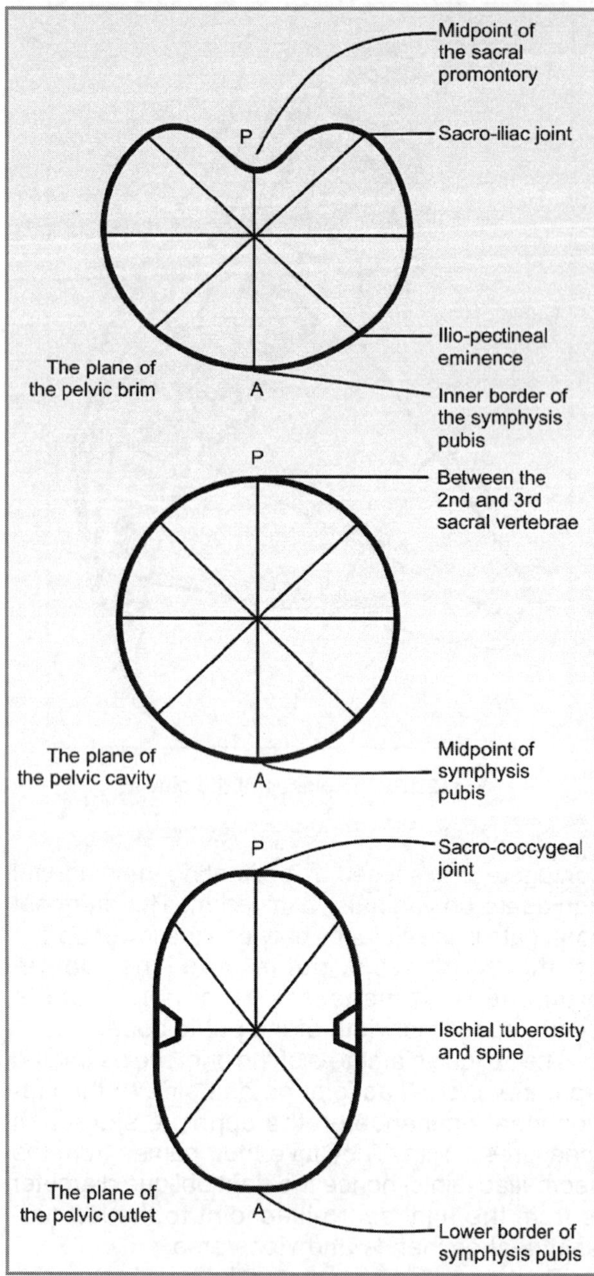

Fig. 2.16: Diagram showing shape and diameters of the pelvic brim cavity and outlet

Diameters of the outlet: The antero-posterior diameter is measured from the lower border of the symphysis pubis to the sacro-coccygeal joint. It measures 12 cm. During delivery it may be slightly increased by the backward displacement of the coccyx over the sacro-coccygeal joint.

The transverse diameters are taken or estimated between the ischial spines or tuberosities. Each measures 10.2 cm. If the ischial spines are prominent, the inter-spinous diameter is reduced and it is, therefore, of greater obstetrical importance than the intertuberous diameter. The intertuberous diameter is easily assessed by the nurse midwife, by placing four knuckles of her hand between the tuberosities. The oblique diameters are parallel to the other oblique diameters and measure 12 cm.

Pelvic Assessment

External Pelvic Measurements

These are not accurate and are, therefore, no longer used. To a nurse midwife, the foetal head is the best pelvimeter and to get the head to pass through the pelvic brim (that is, to engage) is more significant than pelvimetry.

Clinical Pelvic Assessment

It refers to the assessment of the pelvis including the head fitting test. The head fitting test implies making the foetal head progress through the pelvic brim. During vaginal examination an attempt is made to reach the sacral promontory. The diagonal conjugate is measured from the lower border of the symphysis pubis to the tip of the sacral promontory (Fig. 2.17). In a normal pelvis, the sacral promontory is not usually reached by the examining finger. If it is reached, the point at which it is reached is marked on the index finger and a measurement is made with a

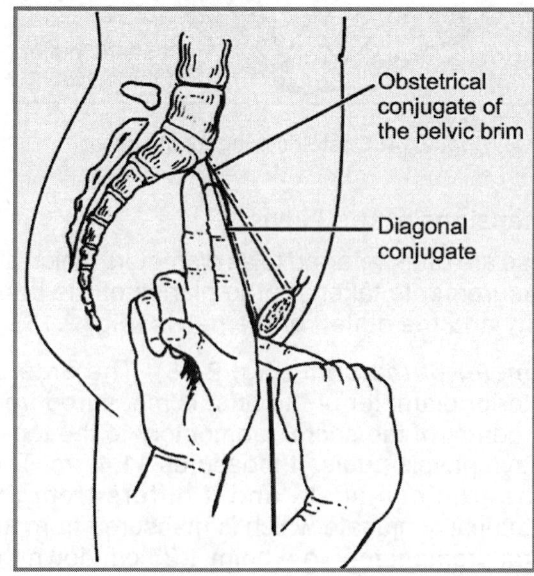

Fig. 2.17: Estimation of the diagonal conjugate

ruler tape when the finger is withdrawn. The measurement obtained gives the diagonal conjugate of that pelvis. Before the examining fingers are withdrawn, an attempt is made to assess the span of the pelvis by running the fingers down on either side of the pelvic wall. The concavity of the sacrum is also assessed. If the sacrum is flat instead of being concave, a note is made of this. The ischial spines are felt and the degree of their prominence is observed. The subpubic arch is assessed by inserting two or three fingers beneath the lower border of the symphysis pubis between the pubic rami. The pubic arch in a normal gynaecoid pelvis admits three finger breadths. The distance between the two ischial tuberosities is measured by putting three or four knuckles between the two tuberosities. The normal pelvis takes 3 1/2 to 4 knuckles. If a pelvis is normal in shape and size, a baby weighing 3.2 kg should pass through it without great difficulty provided the head is well flexed. However, pelvis differ even within the normal limits, and varieties of pelvis are described.

Different Types of Pelvis

The main types of pelvis are described below:

The Gynaecoid Pelvis

The normal female pelvis is gynaecoid in shape. The brim of the true pelvis is round or almost oval in shape.When the patient is standing, the pelvic inlet or the brim is inclined at an angle of 50°-60° to the horizontal. The true conjugate should measure at least 11.5 cm. The greatest transverse diameter of the brim bisects the antero-posterior diameter of the brim at its midpoint. This greatest transverse diameter (also referred to as available transverse diameter) measures 13.5 cm.

The sacrum is well curved and is concave inwards from above downwards, and from side to side. The sacro-sciatic notches are wide and shallow. All the diameters (antero-posterior, transverse and oblique diameters) of the midcavity are about the same in size and each of them measures approximately 12 cm.

The antero-posterior diameter of the pelvic outlet is at least 11.5 cm. It is usually measured from the lower border of the symphysis pubis to the tip of the sacrum. The transverse diameter of the outlet may be measured between the tips of the ischial spines or between the inner aspects of the ischial tuberosities. It measures at least 10.2 cm. The coccyx is freely mobile. This further helps to increase the antero-posterior diameter of the pelvic outlet.

The subpubic arch is wide and can allow a foetal head whose biparietal diameter is 9.5 cm to pass through. The waste space, that is, the distance between the circumference of the foetal head and the highest point of the pubic arch, is usually not more than 1 cm.

Effect on labour: The foetal head often engages in the transverse diameter of the brim in an anterior position. The course and mechanisms of labour are normal. Therefore, the gynaecoid pelvis is the best for child bearing.

The Android Pelvis

This is the male type of pelvis (Fig. 2.18). The brim is triangular or heart shaped and is more roomy posteriorly. The pelvic cavity is deep and funnel-shaped because the sacrum is straight and the side walls converge inwards. The great sciatic notch is narrow. The subpubic angle is narrow. The ischial spines are prominent and the transverse diameter is usually reduced.

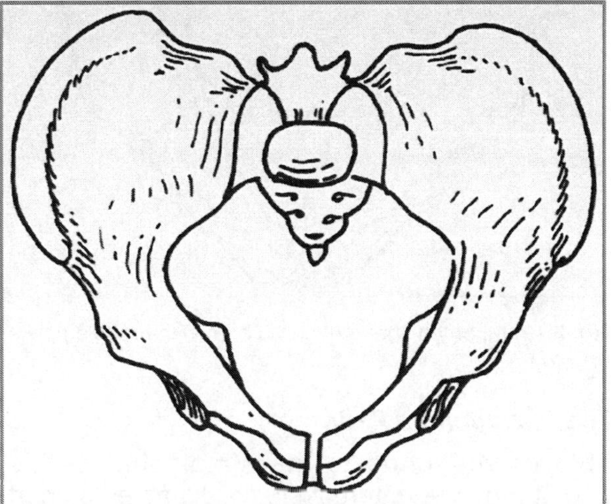

Fig. 2.18: Inherited shape of pelvic brim—android pelvis

Effect on labour: The foetal head often engages in the transverse diameter of the pelvic brim or in a posterior position because the biparietal diameter is more easily accommodated in the posterior segment of the heart-shaped brim. Deep transverse arrest of the head often occurs because of the prominent ischial spines. The acute pubic arch forces the head backwards into the posterior segment of the outlet causing much bruising or laceration of the pelvic floor and the perineum.

The Anthropoid Pelvis

This type of pelvis resembles the pelvis of the ape (Fig. 2.19). The brim is oval in shape with an increase in the antero-posterior diameter and a corresponding decrease in the transverse diameter. The sacrum is long and narrow and may contain six vertebra.

Effect on labour: The head often engages in the antero-posterior diameter, sometimes with the occipit-posterior. The head may descend through the pelvis in the occipito-posterior and be born face to pubes. Generally, the pelvis is so large that labour is easy.

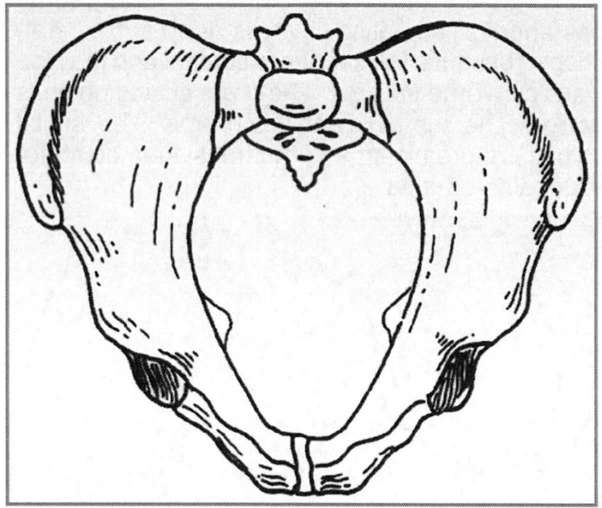

Fig. 2.19: Inherited shape of pelvic brim—anthropoid pelvis

The Platypelloid Pelvis

This corresponds to the simple flat pelvis (Fig. 2.20). The anteroposterior diameter is short but transverse diameter is wide. The sacro-sciatic notch is narrow. The sacrum is flat and displaced forward, therefore the antero-posterior narrowing of the pelvis continues in the cavity and outlet. The subpubic angle is wide.

Effect on labour: The head will engage in the transverse diameter of the brim. Rotation of the head may be restricted and deep transverse arrest of the head may occur.

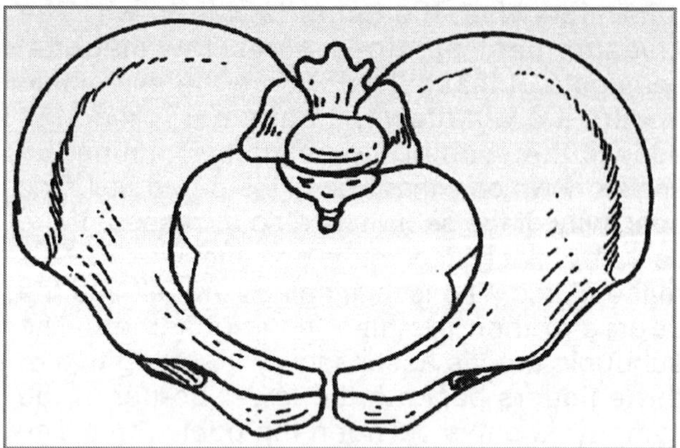

Fig. 2.20: Inherited shape of pelvic brim—platypelloid pelvis

The Contracted Pelvis

A contracted pelvis is one in which one or more diameters are much reduced, interfering with the normal mechanisms of labour (Fig. 2.21). The usual varieties of contracted pelvis are as follows:

The justo minor pelvis: This is gynaecoid type of pelvis in which all the pelvic measurements are diminished but are in correct proportion. Women with this type of pelvis are short in stature and are usually not more than 150 cm tall. These women tend to develop pre-eclampsia during pregnancy and their pregnancy may go beyond term. Occasionally, this type of pelvis may be found in a woman of normal stature.

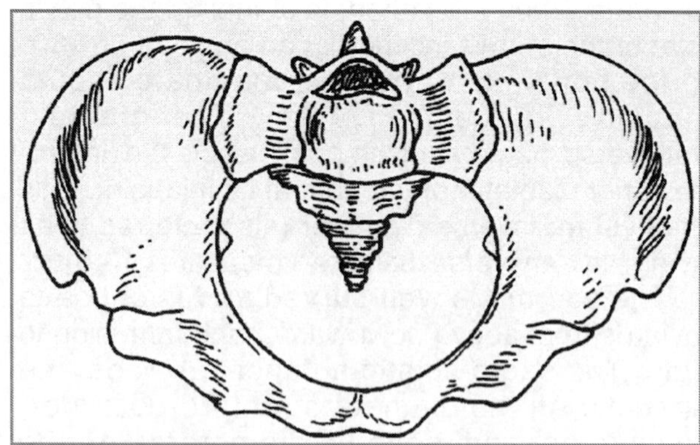

Fig. 2.21: Generally contracted pelvis

Effect on labour: The difficulty encountered will depend on the degree of cephalo-pelvic disproportion and will persist throughout the first and second stages of labour. The mechanism of labour proceeds in the usual way, but there will be exaggerated flexion of the head. If vaginal delivery is thought possible, a trial of labour is carried out. Caesarean section may be necessary, but fortunately these women often have small babies.

The funnel-shaped pelvis is a form of contracted pelvis. It usually leads to obstructed labour if there is cephalo-pelvic disproportion.

The anthropoid and the platypelloid pelves are also types of contracted pelvis.

The Rachitic Pelvis

This pelvic deformity is due to rickets which affects the patient in early childhood. Clinical signs of rickets may be evident in the patient such as bow legs and deformities of the spine. The only pelvic diameters diminished are the obstetrical conjugate and the sacro-cotyloid diameter. All the other diameters are increased. The brim is kidney-shaped, because the sacral promontory projects far forwards. The sacrum lacks the normal curve and, in some cases, is straight and the coccyx bends acutely forwards. The ischial tuberosities are further apart, so the pubic arch may be greater than a right angle, the outlet is, therefore capacious.

Effects on labour: The head enters the brim with the sagittal suture in the transverse diameter and is incompletely flexed. Caesarean section will be neccessary, if the degree of contraction is severe. In minor or moderate degrees, a trial of labour may be carried out. Many hours will elapse before the head passes through the pelvic brim, but when this is accomplished the remainder of the labour is rapid.

Face presentation, prolapse of the cord and foetal distress are complications to be anticipated during labour.

Asymmetrical Pelvis

This may be due to congenital dislocation of one hip or may follow poliomyelitis. In this type of pelvis one side is distorted.

Effect on labour: The effect on labour is the same as for Robert's pelvis discussed below.

Robert's Pelvis (Fig. 2.22)

This is a very rare type of pelvic deformity in which the alae of the sacrum are either absent or poorly developed.

Effect on labour: The pelvis is grossly contracted and there is usually a major degree of cephalo-pelvic disproportion necessitating delivery of the baby by caesarean section.

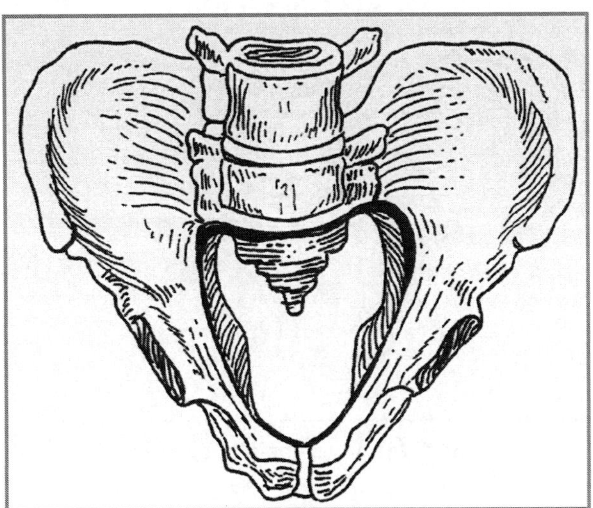

Fig. 2.22: Robert's pelvis

Nägele's Pelvis (Fig. 2.23)

In this type of pelvis, the sacrum has only one wing, probably due to maldevelopment or disease of the sacro-iliac joint with ankylosis occurring during infancy. The brim is obliquely contracted.

Effect on labour: The effect on labour is the same as for Robert's pelvis.

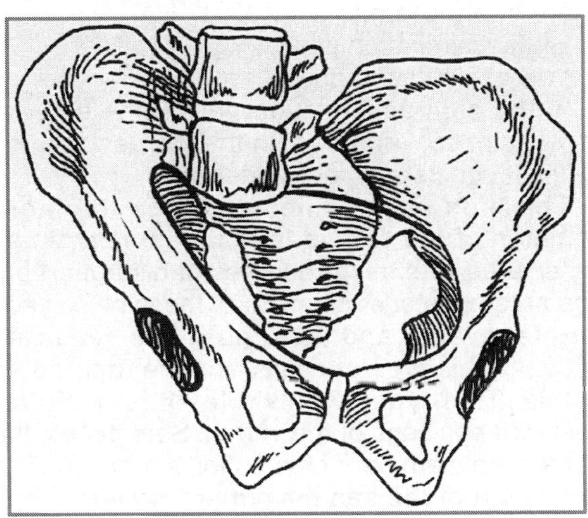

Fig. 2.23: Nägele's pelvis

Osteomalacic or Maacosteon Pelvis (Fig 2.24)

This extreme deformity is due to osteomalacia. It occurs in multiparae and is due to a deficient diet

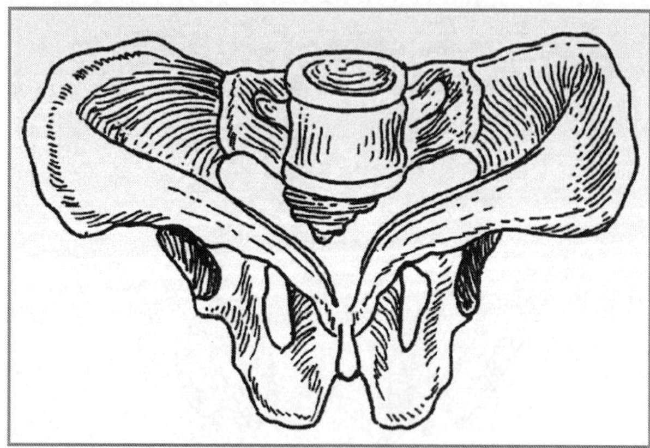

Fig. 2.24: An osteomalacic pelvis

and lack of vitamin D and sunlight. All the skeletal bones soften and the sides of the pelvic canal are squashed together until the brim becomes a mere Y-shaped slit. Osteomalacic pelvis was commonly seen in China and India but is now disappearing.

Effect on labour: A major degree of cephalo-pelvic disproportion is usually present and the foetal head will not descend. Labour will obstruct, if the patient attempts to deliver at home. Caesarean section is the only way out.

Assimilation Pelvis

There are two forms:

a. High assimilation pelvis;
b. Low assimilation pelvis.

In the high assimilation pelvis, the sacrum consists of six vertebrae. In the low assimilation pelvis it consists of four vertebrae.

The high assimilation pelvis is the more common of the two varieties. It is sometimes associated with minor degrees of disproportion. The anteroposterior diameter of the inlet exceeds the transverse and thus there is a similarity between this type of pelvis and the anthropoid pelvis. This type of pelvis favours occipito-posterior positions of the vertex. Sometimes, the transverse diameter of the outlet is reduced. The lower part of the sacrum curves forwards thus further reducing the size of the outlet and causing a degree of funnelling of the pelvis.

Other Types of Pelvic Contraction

Sometimes, pelvic deformities are secondary to disease of the spinal column such as rickets or tuberculosis. Pelvic deformities leading to gross reduction in diameters may result from accident, e.g. fractured pelvis, or fractured femur causing shortening of the affected limb. A few other examples of pelvic deformities secondary to disease follow:

Kyphosis

Kyphosis is a condition in which the antero-posterior curve of the spinal column is affected in such a way that there is a localized bulging backwards or prominence in the spinal column. The thoracic or the lumbar vertebrae may be involved. In thoracic kyphosis, nature usually compensates and the pelvic diameters may not be reduced. In cases involving the lower thoracic and lumbar vertebrae, no compensation takes place. The result is that the upper part of the sacrum is pushed backwards and the lower part is pushed forwards. Because of this, the antero-posterior diameter of the pelvic brim is increased whilst the same diameter in the outlet is reduced. All the transverse diameters are reduced. This type of deformity leads to funnelling of the pelvis.

Scoliosis

This is due to lateral curvature of the spinal column. It may be due to rickets. If it involves only the upper dorsal vertebrae, the pelvic shape may not be affected.

Spondylolisthesis

In this condition the fifth lumbar vertebra projects beyond the promontory of the sacrum (Fig. 2.25). The fifth lumbar vertebra is displaced downwards and forwards. It leads to a false promontory and may produce extreme contraction of the true conjugate.

Diagnosis of Contracted Pelvis and Cephalo-Pelvic Disproportion

Patients whose height is 150 cm or less should be suspected of having contracted pelvis. It is true that not all short women have contracted pelvis but the height of the patient is the best yardstick for sorting out cases.

The diagnosis of contracted pelvis can be confirmed by:

1. External pelvic assessment or external pelvimetry.

2. Clinical internal pelvic assessment or internal pelvimetry.
3. Radiological pelvic assessment or X-ray pelvimetry.

Nurse midwives should not depend on external pelvic measurements, since the method is grossly inaccurate and is not used in modern obstetrics.

Internal pelvimetry is carried out by vaginal examination. The best time to assess the pelvis internally is a time as near to term as possible. For primigravidae internal pelvic assessment should be carried out at about 38 weeks gestation. Multigravidae who have spontaneously delivered babies weighing 3 to 4 kg are not likely to have a contracted pelvis. Those who have delivered smaller babies should have a through pelvic assessment at about the 38th week.

Procedure for Internal Pelvic Assessment

Two fingers (the index and middle fingers) are passed high into the vagina and an attempt is made to reach the sacral promontory. Later the fingers are swept to the left and to the right in an attempt to reach the lateral margins of the pelvic brim. If they are not reached or are only reached with difficulty, the examiner can safely presume that there is no gross pelvic deformity or contraction. If, on the other hand, the examining fingers reach the sacral promontory and lateral margins of the pelvic brim very easily, then a gross degree of pelvic contraction should be presumed.

The pelvic cavity is assessed by feeling the two ischial spines and estimating the distance between them. The curve of the sacrum is examined. The fingers are swept round on either side to palpate the pelvic side walls for evidence of convergence of these walls. If the sacrum is straight instead of being concave, if the ischial spines are prominent and the distance between them is short, and finally if the pelvic side walls are convergent, then it can be presumed that the midcavity is small. If there is no prominence of the ischial spines, if the distance between them is reasonable, if the sacrum is well curved and concave and if the pelvic side walls do not converge, then the nurse midwife can reasonably assume that the midcavity is adequate.

The pelvic outlet is measured by noting the shape of the subpubic arch. Usually, the subpubic angle is about 90 or more and two or three fingers of the examining hand can be accommodated in the subpubic angle. A narrow subpubic arch diminishes the antero-posterior and transverse diameters of the pelvic outlet. The distance between the two ischial tuberosities in a pelvis with a normal outlet should take three to four knuckles of the clenched fist. If this bi-ischial tuberous diameter is reduced, the transverse diameter of the outlet is also reduced. The distance between the sacrum and the subpubic angle is also roughly estimated and if this is small the antero-posterior diameter of the outlet is small. An attempt is made to determine whether the coccyx is mobile over the sacro-coccygeal joint. A fixed coccyx decreased the antero-posterior diameter of the outlet.

Head Fitting Test and Cephalometry

The nurse midwife should rely on the head fitting test to diagnose disproportion. It should be done between the 37th and the 38th week. After the 38th week of pregnancy there is relatively little increase in the foetal head circumference and an accurate assessment of the relationship of the foetal head to the maternal pelvis can be obtained.

Method: The patient should be propped up in a semi-recumbent position with her weight being supported by her elbows. If an assistant is present, she is asked to help support the patient. The nurse midwife then tries, either by Pawlik's or the pelvic grip, to determine whether or not the head will go into the pelvis. If the head goes through the brim, it can safely be presumed that there is no disproportion. If the head fails to enter the pelvis, the degree of overlap should be assessed. A major degree of overlap signifies gross cephalo-pelvic disproportion. On the other hand, if the overlap is minor, it is reasonable to presume that with good uterine contractions and moulding, tho foetal head may enter the pelvis. It must, however, be emphasized that all cases of disproportion minor or major should be referred to the doctor. It is only in cases where the head goes into the pelvis that the midwife should attempt to deliver the patient.

Sometimes, the head fitting test may be done with the patient in the squatting position. This position is, however, not a very comfortable one for the patient.

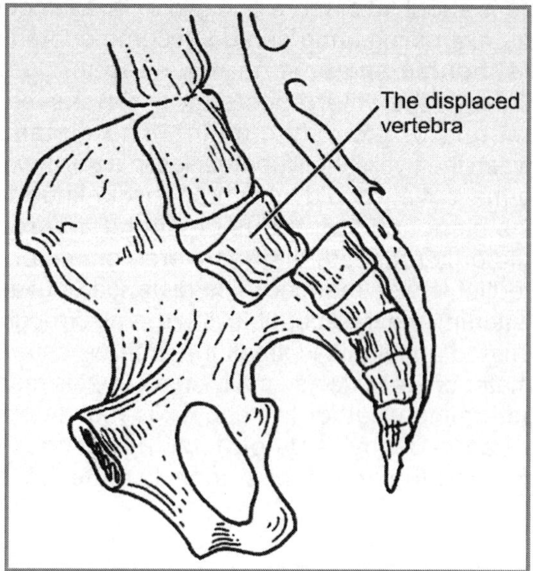

Fig. 2.25: The pelvis in spondylolisthesis

Cephalo-pelvic Disproportion

Cephalo-pelvic disproportion is a disparity between the foetal head and the maternal pelvis. It means that the particular head is too big for the particular pelvis through which it must pass. It may be due to a contracted pelvis with a normal sized head, or a normal pelvis with a large baby, or a combination of a large baby and a contracted pelvis. Cephalo-pelvic disproportion cannot be diagnosed before the 36th week of pregnancy because before then the foetal head is too small for comparison with the pelvis.

Degrees of disproportion: There are three degrees of disproportion:

1. *Minor degree*—In minor degree of disproportion, the head does not engage or pass through the pelvic brim, but it may be possible to push it through the brim. The head is at the same level as the anterior border of the symphysis pubis.
2. *Moderate degree*—In moderate degree of disproportion the head cannot be made to engage at the pelvic brim. The head slightly overlaps the anterior edge of the symphysis pubis.
3. *Major degree*—In major degree of disproportion the head greatly overlaps the anterior edge of the symphysis pubis.

Diagnosis of disproportion: Disproportion should be suspected in short primigravid women. It is uncommon in multigravid women with a previous history of spontaneous vaginal delivery of babies weighing more than 3.4 kg. Its presence must, however, be looked for in all women because of the tendency for subsequent babies to be larger than the previous ones. A pendulous abdomen should lead to the suspicion of disproportion. If the head cannot be made to engage by the 38th week of pregnancy, the patient should be referred to a doctor for an opinion chiefly to exclude the possibility of disproportion. Non-engagement of the head in a primigravida at 36 weeks in Caucasians is regarded as an ominous sign of cephalo-pelvic disproportion. In the African the foetal head does not usually engage until the 40th week or even towards the end of the first stage of labour. The head can, however, be made to engage by the head fitting test already described. The doctor will decide whether disproportion is present and determine its degree by estimating the following:

1. The degree of overlap of the head over the pelvic brim at the symphysis pubis.
2. By internal pelvic assessment at previously described.
3. By X-ray pelvimetry as described above.

Methods of determining the degree of disproportion: There are many methods of determining the degree of disproportion but only two of these will be described.

1. *The left-hand grip method* The patient is made to lie on her back with arms to her side. The nurse midwife stands facing the patient's feet. She grasps the foetal head with the left hand, the thumb being on the patient's right side. The first two fingers of the right hand mark the brim and are placed across the anterior border of the symphysis pubis. The head is pushed in a downward and backward direction. The two fingers of the right hand assess any overlap at the symphysis pubis.
2. *Muller-Munro-Kerr method* The Muller-Munro-Kerr method is employed by the doctor to determine the degree of disproportion. The patient is placed in the lithotomy position. Two fingers of the gloved right hand are inserted into the vagina. The left hand grasps the head abdominally and applies a downward pressure on it. The amount of descent is detected by the fingers in the vagina. The thumb of the hand in the vagina feels the degree of overlap at the summit of the symphysis pubis.

Patients with major and moderate degrees of disproportion are delivered by caesarean section. Patients with minor degrees of cephalo-pelvic disproportion are allowed trial of labour with the aim of achieving vaginal delivery.

FEMALE GENITAL TRACT

The Vulva External Genitalia

The structures forming the vulva are described below (Fig. 2.26):

The mons veneris: The mons veneris (mons pubis) is a mount of fat situated in front of the symphysis pubis. It is covered by skin and hair which has a typical distribution.

Labium majus: The labium majus (one on either side) is a fold of fat and skin lying below the mons veneris. It extends downwards and backwards and disappears into the perineal body. It contains sweat and sebaceous glands. There is hair on the outer surface of the labium majus. The inner surface is smooth.

Labium minus: The labium minus (one on either side) is a smaller fold of skin under the labium majus. It also contains sweat and sebaceous glands. Anteriorly, it unites with the other labium minus to form the prepuce above and the frenulum below. These form the hood which surrounds the clitoris.Both the labia minora enclose the vestibule and the vaginal orifice and they are united posteriorly by a thin fold of skin called the fourchette.

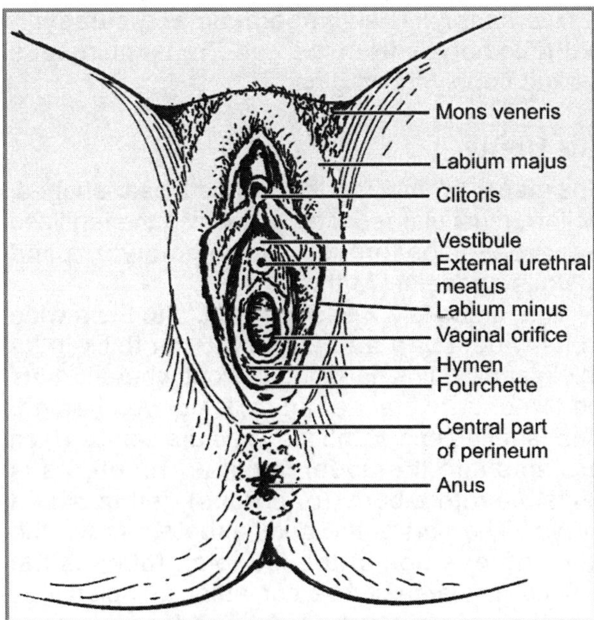

Fig. 2.26: External genital organs

The clitoris: The clitoris is the counterpart of the male penis in the female. It is a small, sensitive, highly vascular organ made of erectile tissue.

The vestibule: This is the area between the labia minora. Two orifices open below.

The external urethral meatus: This lies an inch below the clitoris. If looks like a 'slit' with two dimples on either side. These dimples are the openings of Skene's tubules or ducts.

The vaginal orifice or introitus vaginae: This occupies the lowest third of the vestibule and is covered in the virgin by an incomplete membrane- the hymen. After marriage and childbirth, the hymen is torn leaving small tags called the carunculae myrtiformes.

The Bartholin's glands: These are the size and shape of a small bean on either side of the vaginal orifice. Their ducts open onto the surface external to the hymen and medial to the labia minora. They secrete mucus which lubricates the vulva.

Blood supply: The vulva is supplied by branches of the internal pudendal arteries which are branches of the internal iliac arteries. Corresponding veins drain into the iliac veins.

Lymphatic drainage: The lymphatics of the vulva drain into the inguinal and femoral lymph nodes and from there to the iliac nodes.

Nerve supply: Nerve supply is by the pudendal nerve which divides in the pudendal canal into three terminal branches to supply the perineum, vulva, vagina, etc. The vulva is also supplied by the ilio-inguinal nerve from L1.

The Vagina

General Description

The vagina is a muscular tube extending from the vulva to the cervix. It passes into the pelvis in an upward and backward direction. The walls of the vagina are in close contact. The cervix of the uterus enters the vagina making a right angle with the anterior vaginal wall which is 7.5 cm in length. The posterior wall is 10 cm long. The recesses of the vagina extending above the cervix are called fornices. There are four fornices, namely the anterior, the posterior (which is the largest) and the two lateral fornices.

Structure

This consists of (from inside out):

a. A layer of squamous epithelium which is modified skin thrown into small transverse folds called rugae. The rugae allow for enlargement of the vagina during delivery.
b. Elastic connective tissue with numerous blood vessels which give the vagina its pinkish colour.
c. Smooth muscle layer. There are two muscle layers-the inner circular layer and the outer longitudinal layer.
d. The outer encircling layer of connective tissue which contains blood vessels, nerves and lymphatics.

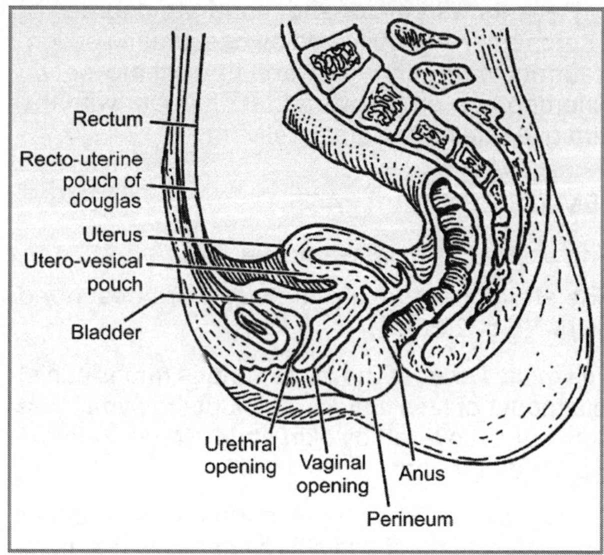

Fig. 2.27: Illustration showing the relationship of the pelvic organs

Lubrication

The vagina is always warm and moist. The small amount of fluid in the vagina is from the secretions of the cervical glands and the exudates from the wall of the vagina. The reaction of the vagina is acidic—this is due to the presence of the Doderlein's bacilli which act on the glycogen from the vaginal walls forming lactic acid. This acidity prevents the growth of pathogenic bacteria in the vagina. In the pre-pubertal girl and in elderly women, the reaction of the vagina is less acid. This tends to cause vulvovaginitis. During pregnancy, the acidity is increased. The upper third of the vagina is sterile, the middle third and lower third are unsterile.

Relations of Vagina (Fig. 2.27)

The anterior wall of the vaginal is related to the urethra and the base of the bladder. Each occupies 1.2 cm of its length.

The lower one-third of the posterior vaginal wall is related to the perineum, the middle one-third to the rectum and the upper one-third to the pouch of Douglas. Above the vagina are the cervix and the uterus. Below, the hymen (or its remnant) is related to the vagina. The lateral relations are the pelvic fascia, ureters and the levatores ani muscles which are inserted to the lower third of the vagina.

Blood supply: The blood supply is by the descending branch of the uterine artery. The vaginal artery and branches of the pudendal artery also supply the vagina.

The venous drainage: The venous drainage is by the corresponding veins.

The lymphatic drainage: The lymphatics from the upper two-thirds of the vagina drain into the sacral and internal iliac glands. The lymphatics from the lower third drain into the inguinal glands.

Nerve supply: The sympathetic and parasympathetic nerves from the Lee-Frankenhauser's plexus supply the vagina.

The Uterus

The uterus (womb) is a thick-walled, pear-shaped, hollow, muscular receptacle in which the fertilized ovum develops throughout the embryonic and foetal stages until birth.

The uterus is 7.5 to 9 cm long, 5 to 6 cm wide in its widest part and 2.5 to 3.5 cm thick in its thickest part. It is flattened in front where it rests on the urinary bladder and it is convex behind. The tapering end of the uterus is the cervix which projects into the upper vagina. The uterus is divisible into a body (or corpus), isthmus and cervix. The part of the body situated above the level of insertion of the fallopian tubes is the fundus. The area of insertion of the fallopian tube into the uterus is the cornu. The tapering area before the cervix is the isthmus. The body (with the fundus) measures 5 to 6 cm and the cervix measures 2.5 cm.

The cavity of the uterus is triangular in shape when seen from the front (Fig. 2.28). It communicates with the vagina through the cervical canal and with the Fallopian tubes at the cornua. The opening of the cervix into the vagina is known as the external os. The constriction marking the junction of the cervical canal and uterine cavity proper is the anatomical internal os of the cervix. The external os of the cervix is usually round until the birth of the first child. After the first child, it becomes a transverse slit with an anterior and a posterior lip.

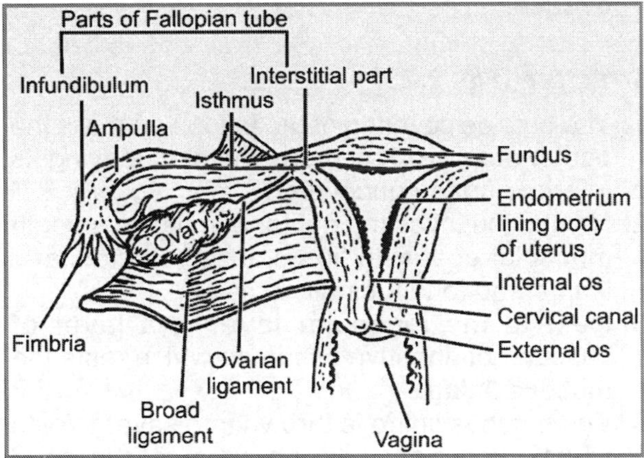

Fig. 2.28: Section of reproductive organs showing the component parts

Structure

The uterus has three coats-serous, muscular and mucous. The muscle coat of the uterus is known as myometrium. It is about 1.5 cm thick and consists of interlacing bundles of smooth muscles running in a criss-cross fashion. It is this arrangement that facilitates the arrest of haemorrhage after delivery of a baby. The serous (peritoneal) coat of the body of the uterus is closely adherent to the uterus except at the sides where it passes into the broad ligaments. The mucous lining of the uterus is known as the endometrium. It is thick and is lined with columnar cells, many of which are ciliated. The endometrium also possesses numerous tortuous glands which extend to the muscle coat.

The muscle fibres of the cervix are circularly arranged. These are not as thick as the muscles of the body of the uterus. The mucous membrane of the cervix is thrown into branching folds and it is lined with columnar mucous secreting cells.

The isthmus: The isthmus is a small annular zone about 0.6 cm from top to bottom which lies between the body of the uterus and the cervix. It is important because it is believed that it becomes the lower uterine segment during pregnancy and labour.

The position of the uterus: When viewed from the side, the uterus is bent forwards on itself in a state of anteflexion and this bend is situated at the level of the internal os. The cervix is inclined forwards at an angle of 90 to the vagina, giving rise to a state of anteversion of the uterus. In about 10 percent of women, the uterus is retroverted.

Relation of the Uterus

a. In front—These are the utero-vesical and bladder.
b. Behind—The pouch of Douglas (recto-uterine pouch of peritoneum) and coils of intestine. The posterior fornix of the vagina lies behind the cervix.
c. At the sides—The broad ligaments with their important contents-the uterine arteries and the lower portions of the ureters.
d. Above—The intestines.
e. Below—The vagina.

Blood supply: The uterus is supplied by the uterine arteries (branches of the internal iliac artery) and partly from the ovarian artery (a branch of the abdominal aorta).

Venous drainage: Venous drainage is through the veins in the broad ligaments, namely the uterine veins, the ovarian veins, the vaginal veins and the vertebral plexuses.

Lymphatics: These drain into the paracervical, external and internal iliac, obturator and sacral lymph nodes.

Nerve supply: The uterus is supplied from the pelvic autonomic nerves of the Lee-Frankenhauser plexus.

The Supports of the Uterus

The uterus is supported by the vagina, the cardinal (transverse cervical or Mackenrodt's) ligaments, the utero-sacral ligaments, the round ligaments, the broad ligaments and to some extent the levator ani muscles which are inserted into the vagina.

The cardinal (transverse cervical or Mackenrodt's) ligaments are condensations of pelvic cellular tissue. They run from the supra-vaginal cervix (the portion of the cervix above the vagina) and vaginal vault to the side walls of the pelvis.

The utero-sacral ligaments: These are the inner edges of the cardinal ligament. They sweep backwards on either side of the rectum to the sacrum. They, together with the round ligaments, keep the uterus in an anteverted position.

The round ligament: This is a fibro-muscular cord which extends from the cornu of the uterus to the internal abdominal ring through which it enters the inguinal canal to be inserted into the subcutaneous tissue of the foreparts of the labium majus. The two round ligaments (one on either side) together with the utero-sacral ligaments keep the uterus in an anteverted position.

The broad ligament: Each broad ligament, if a double fold of peritoneum and subperitoneal fibro-muscular tissue stretching across from the uterus to the side wall of the true pelvis. The fallopian tube is enclosed in the upper free edge of the broad ligament. The mesentery of the ovary (the mesovarium) is attached to the posterior leaf of the broad ligament. The infundibulo-pelvic ligament is the portion of the broad ligament which lies between the infundibulum (outer end of the fallopian tube) and the pelvic wall. The part of the broad ligament between the fallopian tube and the level of attachment in the ovary is known as the mesosalpinx.

The contents of the broad ligament: The lower part of the broad ligament contains loose cellular tissue, the cardinal ligament, the terminal part of the ureter, the uterine artery, nerves and lymphatics. The upper part contains the fallopian tube below which are the ovarian vessels and nerves.

Fallopian Tubes

General Description

These are two tubes which extend from the cornua of the uterus to the ovaries. Each fallopian tube is 10 to 11 cm long and has a small lumen which communicates with the uterine cavity medially and opens into the peritoneal cavity laterally.

Division

Each tube is divided into:

a. The interstitial portion—which is the narrowest portion of the tube lying within the thickness of the uterine wall. It is 1 to 2 cm long.
b. The isthmus—If another narrow portion, 2 to 3 cm from the cornu of the uterus.
c. The ampulla—Is the dilated portion which extends for about 5 cm from the isthmus to the infundibulum.
d. The infundibulum—Is the last 2.5 cm of the fallopian tube. It is made up of finger-like processes called fimbrae. One of the fimbrae extends to the ovary and is called the fimbria ovarica.

Structure (Fig. 2.29)

1. The outside covering of the fallopian tube is the peritoneum which is draped over it, leaving its inferior surface uncovered.
2. Next to the investing peritoneum is the smooth muscular coat with fibers arranged circularly inside and longitudinally outside.
3. Next to the muscular layer is a layer of vascular connective tissue on which rests the mucous lining.
4. The mucous lining is thrown into several folds which almost occlude the lumen of the tube. These folds are called plicae and are more abundant in the ampulla where they help slow down the passage of the ovum.

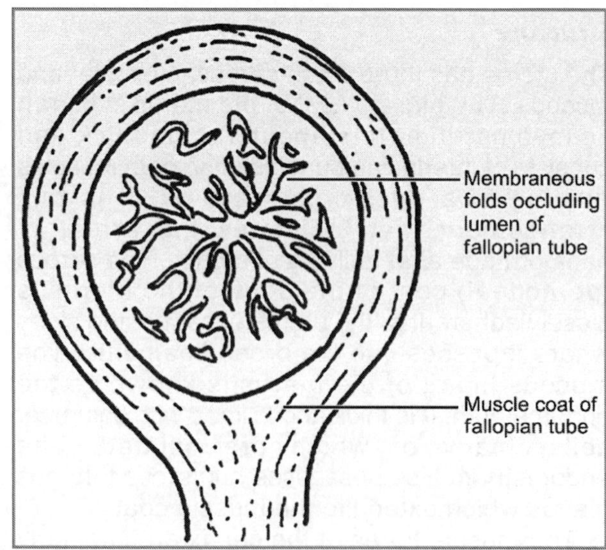

Fig. 2.29: Cross-section of fallopian tube

Many of the cells of this lining are ciliated, others secrete mucus into the lumen of the tube.

Relations of Fallopian Tubes

Both fallopian tubes open into the peritoneal cavity at their distal ends and into the uterus proximally. The broad ligament and the ovaries are below the tubes. Lateral to the tubes are the infundibulo-pelvic ligaments, and other contents of the pelvic side wall.

Blood supply: Branches of the uterine and ovarian arteries supply the fallopian tubes and they are drained by the corresponding veins. The lymphatics drain into the lumbar glands.

Nerve supply: This is from the ovarian plexus.

The Ovaries

General Description

The ovaries are the female sex glands. There are two ovaries, one on either side of the pelvic wall. Each ovary is a solid body measuring about 3.5 cm in length and 1.5 to 2.5 cm in thickness. It weighs about 4 to 8 g. The right ovary is slightly larger than the left.

The ovary is attached to the back of the broad ligament by the mesovarium. The point of attachment of the mesovarium to the ovary is known as the hilum. All nerves and blood vessels entering and leaving the ovary pass through the hilum.

The ovary is suspended from the cornu of the uterus by the ovarian ligament. Apart from the points of attachment to the mesovarium and ovarian ligament, the ovary projects freely into the peritoneal cavity. It is the only abdominal organ not covered by the peritoneum. It is covered by thick connective tissue known as tunica albuginea. The surface of the ovary of an adult looks scarred and pitted. The surface of the ovary of the newborn baby Is smooth. Later in life, scarring and pitting appear. The ovary of the post-menopausal woman is smooth, shrivelled and consi-derably smaller than that of a young woman.

Blood supply: The ovaries are supplied by the ovarian arteries (branches of the abdominal aorta) and the uterine arteries (branches of the internal iliac arteries.)

Venous drainage: The venous drainage is through the ovarian and uterine veins and the pampiniform plexus.

Lymphatic drainage: The lymphatic vessels follow the course of the ovarian vessels and drain into the aortic lymph nodes and also into the external iliac nodes.

Nerve supply: The ovary is supplied by branches from the 10th thoracic nerve.

Relations of the Ovary

The ovary is very closely related to the fallopian tube. Together with their mesenteries the ovary and fallopian tube are collectively referred to as the adnexum or the appendage. The ovary lies behind the fallopian tube and the broad ligament.

Structure of the Ovary (Fig. 2.30)

The ovary has an outer zone and an inner zone. The outer zone is called the cortex and the inner zone the medulla.

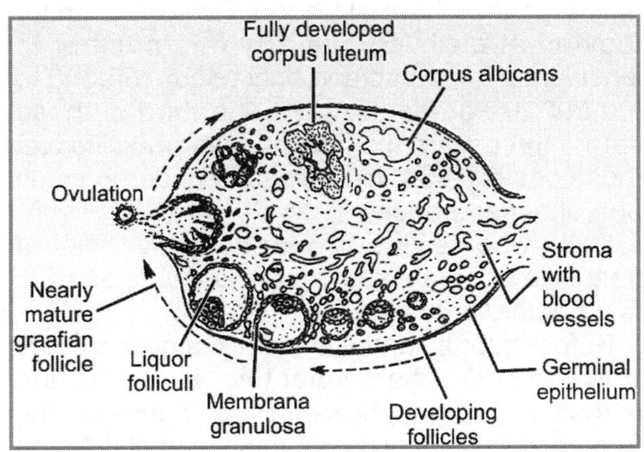

Fig. 2.30: Cross-section of the ovary showing its contents

The cortex: The cortex has a stroma of connective tissue in which Graafian follicles, blood vessels and nerves are found. The Graafian folicles are in varying stages of development. Primordial follicles are seen in large numbers in the cortex. The cortex in early life is covered with germinal epithelium lined with cubical cells. Later the cortex is covered by thick connective tissue- tunica albuginea.

The medulla: The medulla has connective tissue stroma in which numerous blood vessels, nerves and Graafian follicles are found. The cortex contains nearly all the primordial follicles and these are not usually found in the medulla.

The Graafian follicle: The Graafian follicle is lined on the outside by theca externa and on the inside by theca interna. Internal to the theca interna many layers of granulosa cells form the membrana granulosa. The membrana granulosa points inward to form the discus proligerus or cumuluscophorus. In the centre of the discus proligerus is the ovum surrounded by a clear zone—the zona pellucida. The granulosa cells immediately around the ovum form the corona radiata.

Functions of the Ovary

The ovary has two main functions:

1. The production of ova for the purpose of procreation
2. The production of hormones.

Production of ova: The ovary of a newborn female baby contains all the primary oocytes, also known as oogonia, which it will ever possess. It is estimated that there are about 500,000 primary oocytes at birth. By puberty this number is considerably reduced and only about 150,000 to 200,000 are present. About one-third of these mature throughout the patient's reproductive life. Those oocytes that do not mature undergo some form of degeneration.

Each oocyte is surrounded by a layer of granulosa or pregranulosa cells and is referred to as a primordial follicle.

Before puberty and during childhood the ovary grows in size. The connective tissue stroma increases. There is, however, no ripening of the primordial follicles and no ovulation until the time of menarche. Ovulation may, however, be delayed until the age of 15, 16, or 17 years.

Ovulation: Ovulation is the process by which an ovum is discharged from a mature Graafian follicle to form a gamete (secondary oocyte). Each month the two ovaries take it in turn to shed an ovum. Ovulation usually continues until the age of 45 to 50 years.

The adult ovary undergoes a cycle of activity which usually lasts 28 days. The cycle starts on the first day of menstruation and can be divided into two phases. The first phase which lasts approximately 14 days is the follicular phase. This is a phase during which ripening of the ovum takes place. The second phase is the luteal phase. It lasts approximately 14 days. During this phase the corpus luteum (yellow body) is formed. It functions but later degenerates in the absence of pregnancy. The follicular phase and luteal phase are separated by ovulation. The ovarian cycle is under the control of the anterior pituitary gonadotrophic hormones.

The secretion of follicle stimulating hormone (FSH) by the anterior pituitary causes the Graafian follicle to ripen and the level of oestrogen in the blood to rise. Oestrogen depresses the secretion of FSH and encourages the secretion of the luteinizing hormone (LH) by the anterior pituitary. When the correct ratio of LH to FSH is attained, LH brings about the formation and function of the corpus luteum. The corpus luteum secretes oestrogen in small quantities and progesterone in large quantities. If pregnancy does not occur the level of LH falls and the corpus luteum begins to degenerate. This causes a fall in the level of oestrogen and progesterone and releases FSH, which in turn brings about the ripening of a Graafian follicle and so the cycle continues.

The Ovarian Hormones

Under the influence of the anterior pituitary gland the ovaries secrete principally two hormones-oestrogen and progestogen. A third hormone—androgen or male sex hormone—is also secreted by the ovaries but in very small quantities.

During the follicular phase under the influence of the FSH of the anterior pituitary, oestrogen is secreted in large quantities by the ripened Graafian follicle. When a sufficient amount of oestrogen has been secreted the secretion of FSH by the anterior pituitary is inhibited. Luteinizing hormone is then secreted and this stimulates the formation and function of the corpus luteum (yellow body). The corpus luteum secretes both oestrogen and progestogen. When the optimal level of progestogen has been attained the anterior pituitary is inhibited from producing LH. The corpus luteum begins to degenerate and there is fall in the blood level of oestrogen and progestogen. This fall in hormonal level causes the endometrium to break down and leads to menstruation. With the fall in the level of oestrogen and progestogen, the anterior pituitary is released from its inhibition. Follicle stimulating hormone is secreted and this brings about the ripening of a Graafian follicle and the production of oestrogen and thus the cycle previously described is repeated.

The actions of ovarian hormones:

Action of Oestrogen

Oestrogen induces oestrus or sexual heat in the lower animals. This is how it received its name. In woman it plays very little part in sexual desire.

Oestrogen stimulates the secondary sex organs such as the vulva, vagina, uterus, fallopian tubes and breasts. It plays a major role in the development of the breasts at puberty. It is responsible for the development of feminine characteristics such as shyness, feminine curves, profuse growth of scalp hair.

Action of oestrogen on the vulva and vagina: It maintains the healthy state of the vulva and vagina by promoting the laying down of glycogen in the vaginal epithelium. Doderlein's bacilli act on the glycogen to produce lactic acid which maintains the acidity of the vagina and prevents infection of the vagina and vulva. Oestrogen increases the vascularity of the vulva and vagina.

Uterus: Oestrogen increases the vascularity of the uterus. It causes hypertrophy of the myometrium and proliferation of the endometrial glands. Oestrogen does not cause a secretory endometrium. However, it plays a part in the growth and secretory activity of the cervical glands. It modifies the consistency of the cervical mucus.

Fallopian tubes: The actions of oestrogen on the fallopian tubes are similar to its actions on the uterus.

Breast: The effect of oestrogen is to increase the vascularity of the breast and to bring about the pigmentation of the areola. It causes growth of the nipples.

Actions of Progestogen

Progestogen maintains pregnancy in animals. This is how it derived its name. During pregnancy, large quantities of progestogen are produced, initially by the corpus luteum and after the third month by the placenta.

The action of progestogen on the secondary sex organs is dependent on the priming of these organs by oestrogen. Under the influence of oestrogen, progestogen causes a secretory endometrium. It helps oestrogen to bring about an increase in the size and number of the muscle fibres of the myometrium. In the breasts, progestogen acts in conjunction with oestrogen to bring about the changes seen at puberty. It also causes growth of the acini of the breasts. It relaxes the smooth muscles of the ureter, blood vessels and the alimentary tract. This may well explain why hydroureter, Varicose veins, haemorrhoids and constipation are common in some women in pregnancy.

The Pelvic Floor

The soft tissues which fill the pelvic outlet constitute the pelvic floor (Fig. 2.31)

These are mainly muscles and their fascial coverings. A coronal section of the pelvis shows these tissues in the order mentioned below:

a. Peritoneum—which is the broad ligament.
b. The pelvic fascia—some of which forms the cervical ligaments.
c. The levator ani muscles.
d. The superficial perineal muscles.
e. Some fat.
f. Outside covering of skin.

It is important for the nurse midwife to know the muscular structure of the pelvic floor so that she can appreciate the damage which may occur to it during labour. The muscular structure consists of two layers:

1. Deep layer which comprises the levator ani muscles.
2. Superficial layer which comprises the superficial perineal muscles.

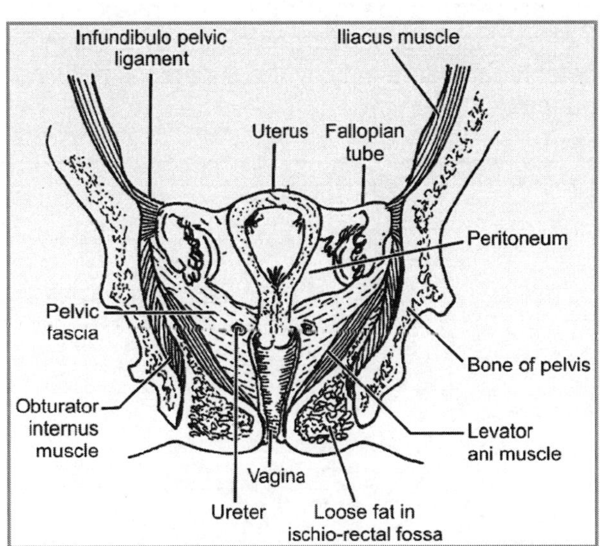

Fig. 2.31: Transverse section of pelvis showing formation of the pelvic floor

Levator Ani Muscles

The levators ani are a pair of muscle sheets arising from around the brim of the pelvis (Fig. 2.32). They converge in a downward and inward direction forming a gutter-shaped slope. Where these muscle sheets meet in the middle are three orifices, the urethra, vagina and anal canal.

The muscle fibres of the levator ani are arranged in three pairs, namely:

a. *The pubo-coccygeus fibres* Arise from the bodies of the pubic bones, pass beneath the bladder, the lowest one-third of the vagina and are inserted into the perineal body and the coccyx.
b. *The ilio-coccygeus fibres* Arise from the white line which is a condensation of the fascia of the obturator internus and iliacus muscles. The white line lies slightly below the ilio-pectineal line. The ilio-coccygeus muscle fibres are fanned out along the white line and then pass inwards to be inserted in the sacrum and coccyx.
c. *The ischio-coccygeus fibres* These are situated in front of the sacrospinous ligament. They arise from the ischial spines and pass downwards and inwards to be attached to the coccyx and the lowest part of the sacrum.

The internal or upper surface of the levator ani muscle is gutter-shaped, that is, concave, and the posterior or undersurface is convex. This undersurface is occupied posteriorly by the ischio-rectal fat and anteriorly by the superficial perineal muscles.

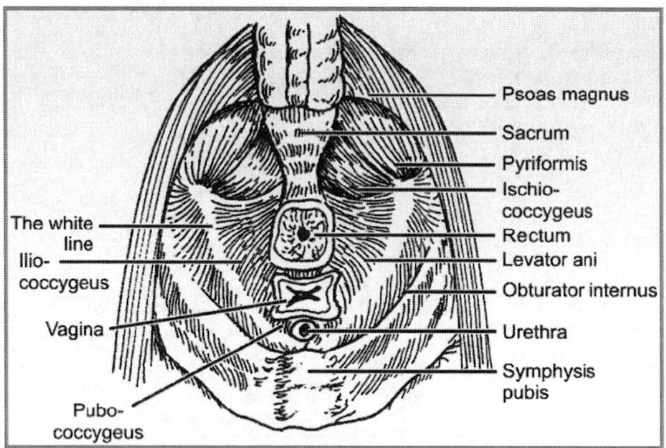

Fig. 2.32: The levator ani muscles of the pelvic floor seen from above

The superficial perineal muscles consist of these groups of muscles (Fig. 2.33):

a. *The transverse perineal muscles* They originate from the ischial tuberosities and meet horizontally at the perineum.
b. *The bulbo-cavernosus* Arises from the perineum and passes forwards around the vagina to be inserted into the corpora cavernosa (spongy-like bodies on either side of the clitoris).
c. *The ischio-cavernosus* Arises from the ischial tuberosities and passes upwards and inwards along the pubic arch to end at the corpora cavernosa. The following groups of muscle fibres are considered part of the pelvic floor. They are:
   1. The external sphincter muscle of the anus. This muscle encircles the anal canal and goes into the formation of the perineal body.
   2. Membranous sphincter of the urethra. Though this is not a true sphincter, it can occlude the urethral orifice when it contracts. It arises from one pubic bone, passes below and above the urethra to the other pubic bone.

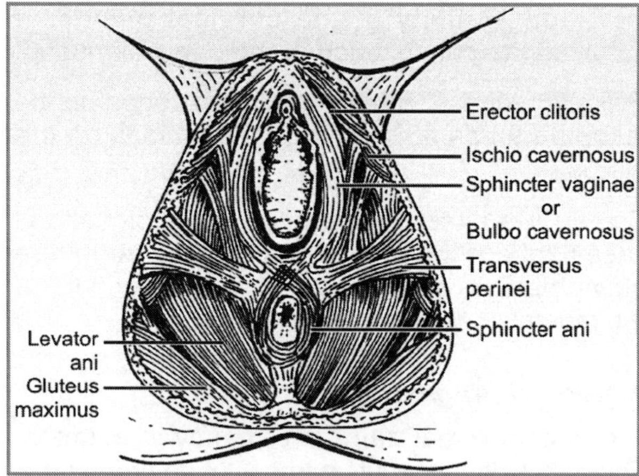

Fig. 2.33: The superficial muscles of the pelvic floor

The Perineal Body

The perineal body is a wedge-shaped tissue between the anal canal behind and vagina in front. Laterally, it lies between the ischial tuberosities. Its deeper half consists of fibres from the levatores ani and the superficial half is made up of the bulbo cavernosus and the transverse perineal muscles. There is then the outer skin covering the perineum. The perineal body is of great importance to the nurse midwife as it is likely to be injured during the delivery of a baby. The injury is often in some form of laceration described in degrees—first, second and third (see perineal laceration).

Blood supply—Pudendal arteries and veins supply and drain the perineum.

The lymphatics—The lymphatics drain to the inguinal glands.

Nerve supply—Nerve supply is by the pudendal nerve.

Functions—The levatores ani form a hammock across the pelvis and thus give support to the abdominal organs. Some of the pelvic floor fascia condenses round the cervix and forms the ligamentory support of the uterus. This explains why extra strain on the pelvic floor during labour and parturition weakens these supports and results in prolapse of the uterus. During labour, the pelvic floor contracts when the foetal head reaches it; this action directs the head forward (described as internal rotation of the head).

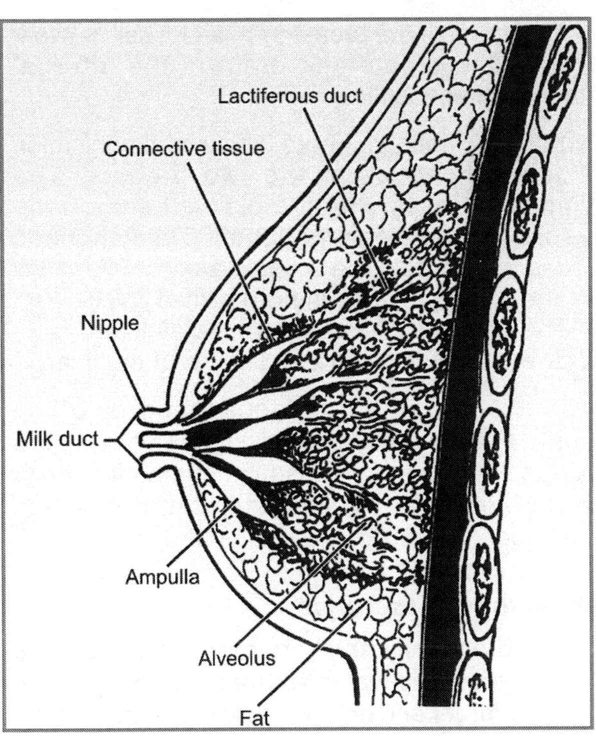

Fig. 2.34: Section through the breast showing its attachment to the chest wall

The Breasts

The breasts are accessory glands of the female reproductive system. They are situated on the superficial fascia of the pectoralis major and serratus anterior muscles in the anterior chest wall. The size and shape of the breasts vary in individuals. They are usually hemispherical in the young nulliparous girl but they are often flat and pendulous in the multiparous woman.

The breast extends vertically from the second to the sixth rib (Fig. 2.34). Horizontally, it extends from the axilla to the lateral margin of the sternum. The part of the breast which extends up into the axilla reaching as high as the third rib is called the axillary tail of spence.

Structure

The breast consists of a central protuberance called the nipple. The nipple is made up of erectile tissue. It is covered and surrounded by a pigmented area called the areola. The areola extends for a distance of about 2.5 cm around the nipple. There are sebaceous glands at the edges of the areola. These sebaceous glands secrete sebum to keep the nipple supple. The other gross structures of the breast are glands, some fat and smooth muscle, and an outer skin covering.

Microscopic structure: The breast is divided into 18 to 20 lobes which radiate outwards from the areola. Each lobe is a complete unit and is separated from the next lobe by fibrous connective tissue.

A lobe consists of glandular tissues and ducts. Each gland is called an alveolus and is a milk-secreting unit lined by milk-making cells called acini. A little duct empties each alveolus. The small ducts run into one another uniting to form bigger ducts. The bigger ducts also unite to form a big lactiferous duct with runs along the lobe. The lactiferous duct dilates underneath the areola to form a reservoir for milk. This reservoir is called an ampulla. The ampullae narrow as they enter the nipple and terminate as minute openings on its surface.

The blood supply: The breast is supplied with blood by the following:

1. The internal mammary artery which is a branch of the subclavian artery.
2. The external mammary artery—a branch of the axillary artery.
3. The intercostal arteries which originate from the aorta.

The veins of the breast form a circular network around the nipple and drain to the internal mammary and axillary veins.

Lymphatic drainage: There is free communication of the lymphatics of the two breasts. The lymphatic vessels form a plexus beneath the areola and between the lobes. The lymphatic nodes which drain the breasts are:
1. The axillary glands in both axillae.
2. The glands in the anterior mediastinum.
3. The glands in the portal fissure of the liver.

Nerve supply: The cutaneous branches of the fourth, fifth and sixth thoracic nerves supply the skin of the breast for sensation but the functions of the breasts are controlled by hormones, viz, oestrogen, progesterone and prolactin.

Physiology of Lactation

During pregnancy, the hormones oestrogen and progesterone activate the breasts. The breasts become larger and produce fluid called colostrum. During the puerperium they are expected to secrete milk which is different from the colostrum. The secretion or production of milk is known as lactation.

The hormone which initiates lactation is called prolactin. It is a secretion of the anterior pituitary gland. Prolactin is antagonized by the hormone oestrogen. For this reason, prolactin does not function until the level of oestrogen in the blood is low. The reduction in the level of oestrogen occurs within the first two days of the puerperium. This explains why milk is secreted from about the third day of the puerperium. The effect of prolactin wears off after eight days. Further production of milk and maintenance of lactation are as discussed below:

Maintenance of Lactation

The breasts should be able to produce enough milk for full or partial feeding of the baby for nine months postpartum. In order to achieve this the following factors are necessary:
1. Maternal good health—A mother should be physically and mentally well and she should be free from anxiety.
2. Stimulation of the breasts by the sucking reflex of the baby. The baby should suckle at the breasts at regular intervals.
3. Adequate emptying of the breasts by the baby sucking on them or by manual expression of the breasts.

The sucking action of the baby on the breast stimulates the posterior pituitary gland to release an oxytocic or pressor factor. The oxytocic or pressor factor causes the plain muscles of the breast to contract thereby propelling the milk from the alveolae along the lactiferous ducts into the ampullae. The rhythmic compression of the baby's sucking action of the ampullae will empty the breasts. As the breasts are emptied the acini cells are stimulated to produce more milk.

The draught or 'let down' reflex is a term used to describe the effect of the oxytocic factor on the breast. It is demonstrated by the dripping of milk from one breast as the baby sucks on the other breast. Again if one removes the baby's mouth from the breast during feeding, a shower of milk will escape via the nipples. It should be noted that the oxytocic released during breast feeding also causes uterine contractions, hence 'after pain' is felt more during feeding times. It is also for the above reason that breast feeding is said to aid involution of the uterus.

CONCEPTION AND FOETAL GROWTH

The event of conception, the union of the male sex cell (sperm) and the female sex cell (ovum), sets into motion a period of growth unequalled at any other time in the life of the individual. Just after fertilization or conception, the ovum is not quite as large as the period used to complete a sentence, but with 266 days or approximately 9 calender months, that particle of the life will increase in size approximately 200 billion times and becomes the highly complex structure and personality known as a baby.

Between conception and birth, health care begins for the prospective mother and the growint foetus. Many factors are involved in the growth and development of the infant as a separate and unique individual, including the configuration of genes from both parents, intrauterine environment, and external environmental influences.

It is important to distinguish between growth and development. Growth is an increase in size and number of cells that causes an organism to gain weight.

Development refers to the changes that occur in primitive cells as they differentiate into tissues that will perform specific functions.

When prospective parents inquire about the formation, growth, and development of their infant, nurse will be in an ideal position to encourage their interest and help them to understand factors that can affect the health of the foetus.

Cellular Reproduction

In all body tissue, cells multiply by a process called mitosis. To divide, the parent cell duplicates each chromosome so each new cell is an exact replica (copy) of it. First, there is separation to the opposite sides of the cell before division; an indentation develops in the center so two identical cells result.

In contrast, a special type of cell division, meiosis must take place in the ovum and sperm to assure that there will be exactly 23 pairs or 46 chromosomes in the new embryo's cells. Meiosis causes each oocyte and spermatocyte to contain one member of each pair of chromosomes. This reduction in chromosomes is made possible by a two-step process. The first meiotic division begins much earlier than fertilization. During this step, the primary oocyte and primary spermatocyte duplicate their deoxyribonucleic acid (DNA) and double their chromosomes, producing double strands or chromatids.

At the same time, the two members of a chromosome pair often exchange segments of genetic material. During this "crossing over" between homologous chromosomes, paternal and maternal genetic material is randomly recombined so that the genes passed to the infant may be quite different from those in either parent. This is one of the reasons a child may not look or act like either parent. After the exchange, the chromosomes divide into two new cells. Thus two non-identical daughter cells result from this division.

Double strands of genetic material are still in these cells however In the second meitoic division, the double-structured chromosomes divide, and the reduction is completed. The resulting cells are ready for fertilization. Each of the four cells that resulting from the two oocyte maturational divisions contain 22 autosomes (body cell chromosomes) and one X (sex) chromosome. Only one of these cells develops into a mature oocyte. The other three become polar bodies, which receive chromosomes that eventually degenerate and dissolve. In contrast, a spermatocyte divide into four types of cells, two containing 22 autosomes and one X chromosome and two containing 22 autosomes and one Y chromosome. All these cells become active sperm.

Oogenesis

During embryonic life, the primary oocytes undergo only a part of the first meiotic division. Then these same primary oocytes enter a resting phase may vary from 12 to 50 years, providing ample opportunity for damage to the oocytes genetic material. When puberty begins, these primary oocytes complete the first meiotic division to ovulation can occur in monthly patterns. Each month, usually a single primary oocyte begins to increase in size and thickness and develops a protective membrane, the *zona pellucida*. The graafian follicle enlarges, and follicle cells form a thick, fluid-filled layer around the oocyte. As soon as the graafian follicle matures, the oocyte resumes a meiotic division to produce two cells of unequal size; the secondary oocyte and the first polar body. The secondary oocyte receives all the cytoplasm and enters into the second meiotic division. This second division is completed only if the ovum is fertilized. Otherwise, the ovum degenerates and is passed out of the body.

Spermatogenesis

Spermatogenesis starts as puberty begins and can continue well into the eighth decade of life. Once it begins, it is a continuous process, no cyclical. It takes about 72 hours for a primary spermatocyte to develop into a mature sperm. Primary spermatocytes begin the first meiotic division, which results in two secondary spermatocytes. Immediately, the secondary spermatocytes undergo the second meiotic division to result in four spermatids. These spermtids contain half the number of chromosomes of the primary spermatocyte. Several stages of the process may occur simultaneously in different parts of the seminiferous tubules.

Mature sperm have virtually no source of nutrition when separated from the semen. Therefore, after ejaculation only some will survive as long as 72 hours.

Fertilization

Many factors are necessary for effective fertilization of the ovum. Coitus causes an average of 200 to 300 million sperm to be deposited in the vaginal canal close to the cervical os. After ejaculation, the life span of sperm is relatively short, and they must quickly move towards the outer distal portion of the fallopian tube where fertilization normally occurs. Many factors may impede the journey, a distance of about 21 cm. These factors include incompatible vaginal or cervical fluids, an extremely acidic environment, or possible narrowing of the cervix, uterus, or tubes. Yet, the oestrogenic influences that help to change cervical mucus properties to allow for easier sperm penetration are at a peak at ovulation.

At the same time, the peristaltic actions of the uterine and tubal muscles foster the movement of sperm towards the tube and move the ovum towards the sperm. Prostaglandins found in semen might aid in the rapid transport of sperm towards the tube by affecting the smooth muscle contractions of the uterus. Approximately 2000 sperms reach the fallopian tubes.

Normally, only one of the many sperm reaching the ovum will enter it. The others secrete hyaluronidase, an enzyme found in the acrosome or outer covering of the head of each sperm that helps to penetrate the zona pellucida. As fertilization occurs, a process called syngamy acts to protect the fertilized ovum. During syngamy, the ovum completes its second maturational division and extrudes a polar body. A reaction that causes the membrane to form a barrier preventing other sperm from entering the cell occurs in the oocyte cytoplasm just below the cell membrane. The tail of the sperm disappears, and the nucleus becomes larger, revealing its chromosomal content. At this point, the structure becomes known as the *male pronucleus*, the sperm nucleus before it fuses with the nucleus of the ovum. The *female pronucleus*, the nucleus of the ovum before it fuses with the nucleus of the sperm, swells. The pronuclei gravitate towards one another and fuse, thus completing fertilization by restoring the full diploid number of chromosomes to the fertilized ovum, which is now the zygote. At this point, the genetic foundation is laid for the growth and development of the infant.

Determination of Sex

The twenty-third pair of chromosomes are the sex chromosomes (either XX or XY). Females have two X chromosomes; males have X-and a Y-chromosome (Fig. 2.35).

The sex of an individual is determined by the presence or absence of the Y chromosome. The scientists did not discover that embryos carrying the Y chromosome developed as males; embryos lacking a Y chromosome developed as females until 1959.

A *testes determining factor* is thought to be a single gene on the Y chromosome. Before 6 weeks, the male and female genitalia are undifferentiated or in the *indifferent stage*. Then it is thought that the gene triggers signals that lead to development of the Lydig's cells that produce

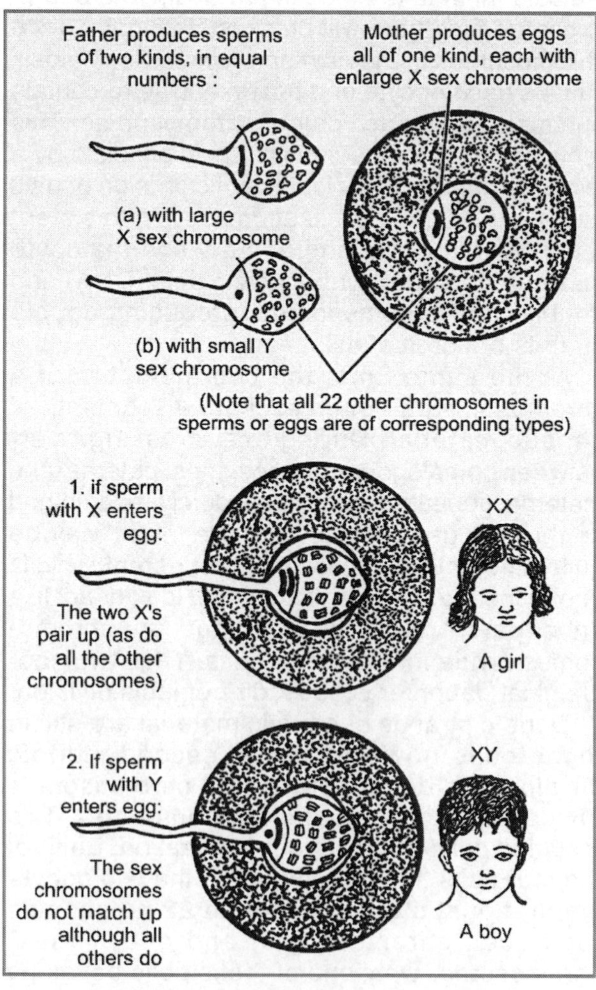

Fig. 2.35: How sex is determined

testosterone to induce masculinization of the external genitalia. In the absence of the gene (regardless of whether there is a Y chromosome) the embryo becomes a female. Similarly, there may be a single gene on the X chromosome to control a chain of events that triggers feminization of external genitalia.

Gestational vs Fertilization Age

When clinicians calculate the embryo's age from the first day of its mother's last menstrual period (LMP), they are calculating its gestational age, or menstrual age. Calculating its gestational age, is easy because most women are able to remember when their LMP began. However, calculating the time of ovulation, the fertilization age, is difficult because the duration of the follicular phase of the menstrual cycle varies from month-to-month and woman-to-woman.

Prior to proceed details about foetal growth nurse should understand anatomy and physiology of the foetal, i.e. foetal skull and foetal physiology.

ANATOMY OF THE FOETUS

The Foetal Head

The foetal head is the most important part of the foetus because it contains the brain, which is a vital organ. About 95 percent of babies present by the head. The nurse midwife must know which area of the foetal head causes least problem during labour and delivery. If the nurse midwife is familiar with the landmarks on the foetal head, she will be able to diagnose abnormal presentations and positions as well as conduct delivery with minimal injury to the mother. The foetal head consists of the scalp, the skull and its contents.

The Scalp

The scalp is the outer soft part of the head. It consists of the following:
- Skin on which some hair grows.
- Connective tissue on which the skin rests.
- Aponeurosis with some muscle fibres which are situated mainly to the sides of the head.
- Loose connective tissue.
- Periosteum which covers the bones of the skull.

The Skull

The skull is the skeleton of the foetal head and consists of the dome-shaped portion called the vault, underneath which is the base of the skull and the face (Fig. 2.36).

The constituent bones of the foetal skull are the same as those of the adult. The bones of the face and the base of the skull are ossified and fixed before birth. These are the sphenoid, the ethmoid and the temporal bones which form the base of the skull while the orbital bones; the maxillae and the mandibles constitute the bones of the face.

The bones of the vault are not well ossified before birth. The vault starts as a sheet of membrane in which five centres of ossification appear. These centres develop to form the occipital bones ,the two parietal bones and the two frontal bones. A portion of the temporal bone forms part of the vault. The membranous ends of these bones are known as sutures and where two or more sutures meet, a fontanelle is formed. The five original centres of ossification are the eminences on the skull, namely:
- One occipital protuberance;
- Two parietal eminences;
- Two frontal eminences.

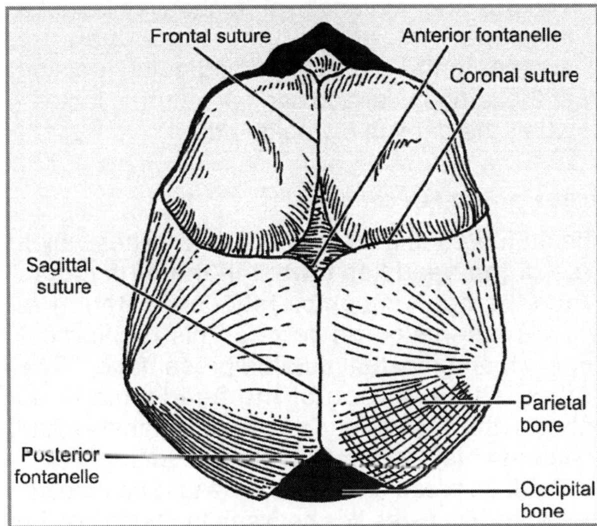

Fig. 2.36: Superior view of the foetal skull

The Sutures

The sutures are of great obstetrical importance in that they allow for the overlapping of the bones of the vault during labour and birth of the baby. The overlapping of the bones is known as moulding.

The suture close gradually after birth. The important sutures are listed below:

1. Frontal suture lies between the two frontal bones and extends from the root of the nose to the anterior fontanelle.
2. Sagittal suture extends from the anterior to the posterior fontanelle. It lies between the two parietal bones.
3. Coronal suture runs transversely between the frontal and the parietal bones and extends from one temporal bone to the other.
4. Lambdoidal suture separates the parietal and the occipital bones.

Fontanelles

Fontanelles are membranous spaces at the point of junction of the sutures. The following two are of obstetrical significance:

1. The anterior fontanelle or the bregma formed at the junction of the frontal, coronal, and sagittal sutures. It is diamond-shaped, measuring 2.5 cm in length and 1.25 cm in breadth. The pulsations of the cerebral vessels can be felt on the bregma. It is usually not closed till the baby is 18 months old, after which becomes completely ossified.
2. The posterior fontanelle or lambda is triangular in shape with less definite space than the anterior fontanelle. It is formed at the junction of the lambdoidal and sagittal sutures. It close when the baby is 6 weeks old.

Areas of the Foetal Head

The attitude of the foetal head determines which area of the head lies lowest in the birth canal. When the head is completely flexed, the area which presents is the vertex. This is the most common and most favourable presentation. The vertex is that portion of the head which lies between the anterior and posterior fontanelles and is bounded laterally by the parietal eminences.

The face presents when the head is completely extended. This area lies between the bridge of the nose and the chin.

The brow or sinciput, comprising the two frontal bones, presents when the head is partially extended. The sinciput extends from the bridge of the nose to the anterior fontanelle.

The occipital area comprises the occipital bone only and it extends from the posterior fontanelle to the foramen magnum.

Diameters of the Foetal Head

Diameters are straight distances between any two points on the foetal head (Fig. 2.37) The largest diameter laying across the pelvis in a presentation is called the engaging diameter. The length of an engaging diameter depends on the presentation and the attitude of the head (Fig. 2.38). Table 2.1 shows the relationship of the attitude of the head with the presentation and the engaging diameter.

Other diameters of the foetal head are (Figs 2.39 and 2.40):

1. Biparietal diameter 9.5 cm, the distance between the parietal eminences;
2. Bitemporal diameter is 8.3 cm long. It passes through the lower ends of the coronal suture;
3. Sub-mento vertical diameter is 11.4 cm and is taken from where the chin joins the neck to the highest point on the vertex.

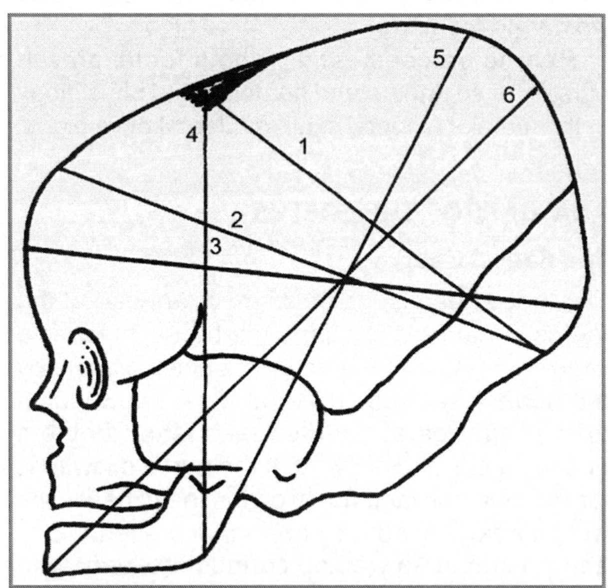

Fig. 2.37: Side view of the foetal skull showing diameters. (1) Sub-occipito bregmatic, (2) Sub-occipito frontal, (3) Occipito frontal, (4) Sub-mento bregmatic, (5) Sub-mento vertical, (6) Mento vertical

Internal Structures of the Head

The brain with its covering, the meninges, occupies the skull. A double layer of menings called the flax cerebri divides the cerebrum into two hemispheres. The flax cerebri extends from the root of the nose, along the frontal and sagittal sutures to the occipital protuberance. It is sickle-shaped and contains large blood sinuses.

Table 2.1: Various attitudes of foetal head

Attitude of the head	*Presentation*	*Engaging diameter and length*	*Extent of the engaging diameter*
1. Complete flextion	Vertex	Sub-occipito bregmatic (Fig. 2.39A) 9.5 cm	Estimated from below the occipital protuberance to the midpoint of the bregma
2. Poorly flexed head or deflexed head	Vertex (occipito-posterior position)	Sub-occipito frontal (Fig. 2.39A) 10 cm	From below the occipital protuberance to the midpoint of the frontal suture
3. Head in a military attitude associated	Crown (persistent occipito-posterior)	Occipito frontal (Fig. 2.39B) 11.4 cm	From occipital protuberance to the midpoint of the frontal suture
4. Head partially extended	Brow	Mento vertical (Fig. 2.40A) 13.3 cm	From the chin to the highest point on the vertex
5. Head fully extended	Face	Sub-mento bregmatic (Fig. 2.40B) 9.5 cm	From where the chin joins the neck to the bregma

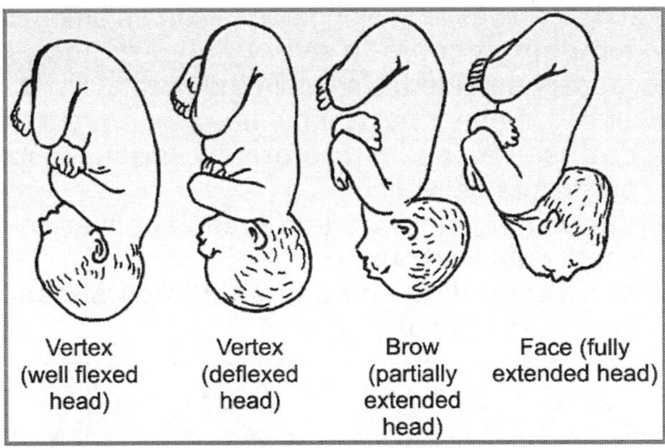

Fig. 2.38: Various attitudes of foetal head with corresponding presentations

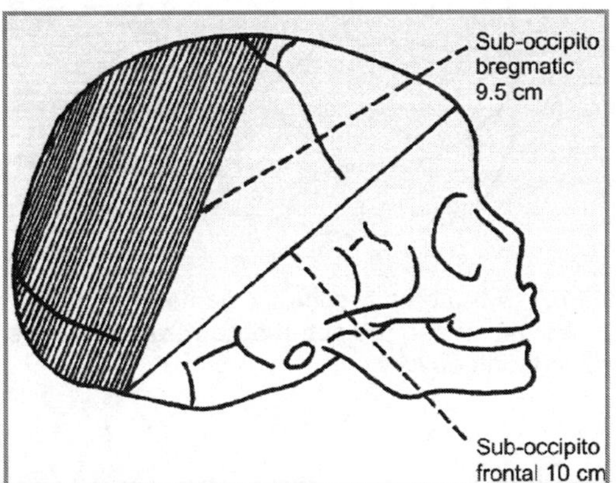

Fig. 2.39A: Sub-occipito bregmatic is the engaging diameter in a vertex presentation while sub-occipito frontal distends the perineum during delivery

Another double layer of meninges called the tentorium cerebelli separates the cerebri from the cerebellum.It lies horizontally across the occiput extending from one temporal bone to the other. It is attached in its midpoint to the posterior part of the falx cerebri. There are blood sinuses also in the tentorium (Fig. 2.40).

The blood sinuses in the meninges are as listed below:

1. The superior sagittal sinus which lies along the upper edge of the falx cerebri.
2. The inferior sagittal sinus which lies along the lower border of the falx cerebri.
3. The straight sinus is found at the base of the falx cerebri.

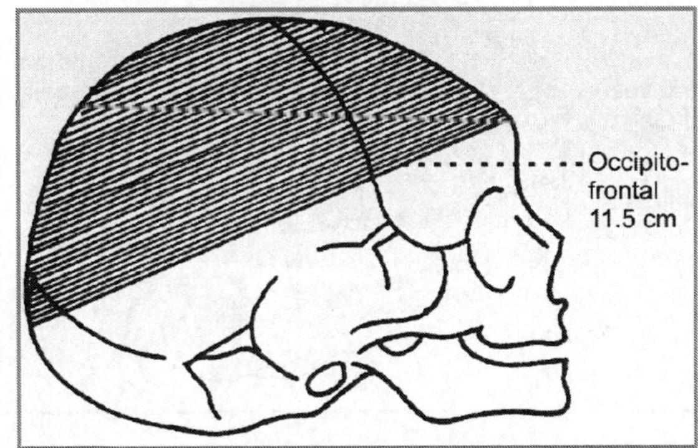

Fig. 2.39B: Occipito frontal diameter engages when the head is deflexed as occurs in occipito posterior position

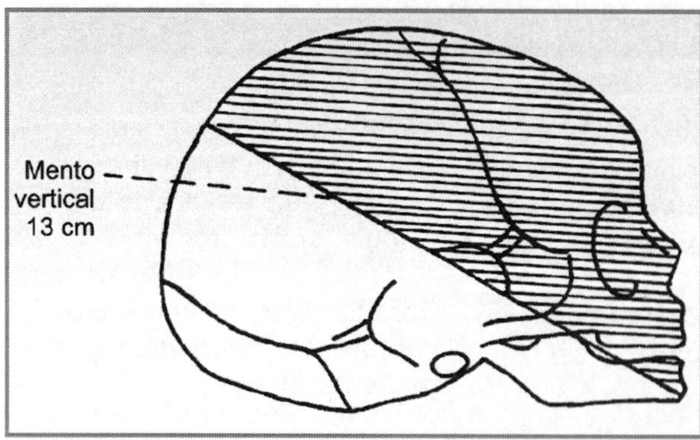

Fig. 2.40A: Mento vertical diameter engages in brow presentation and may result in obstructed labour

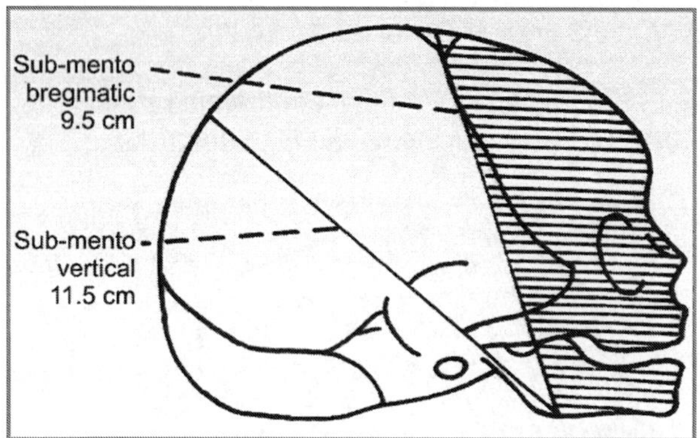

Fig. 2.40B: Sub-mento bregmatic diameter engages in a face presentation and the sub-mento vertical sweeps the perineum during delivery

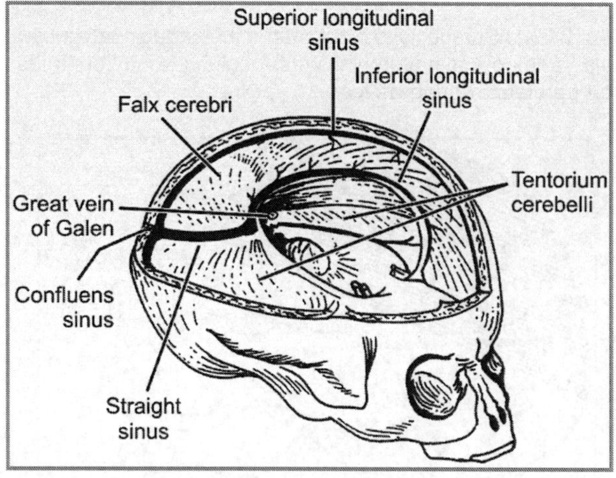

Fig. 2.41: Interior view of the skull showing the falx cerebri, tentorium cerebelli and venous sinuses

4. The confluens sinus is at the junction of the superior sagittal sinus and the straight sinus.
5. The great vein of Galen joins the inferior sagittal and the straight sinuses at a point where the union of the tentorium and the falx is weak. This sinus drains the brain substance and is the most susceptible to injury because of its situation.

Changes which Occur on the Foetal Head as a Result of Labour

Moulding: Moulding is the alteration in the shape of the foetal head to facilitate its easy passage through the birth canal (Fig. 2.42) it is achieved by the slight overriding of the vault bones aided by the sutures and the fontanelles. The end result is the shortening of the engaging diameter and the elongation of the one at right angles to it. For example, in a vertex presentation, the engaging diameter of sub-occipito bregmatic of 9.5 cm diminishes in length and the mento vertical, which is at right angles to it, elongates. A certain amount of moulding occurs in every delivery and is necessary provided it is within the normal limits. Moulding is abnormal when it is:

a. *Excessive*, as in prolonged labour and premature delivery;
b. *Sudden*, as may occur in breech delivery or caesarean section;
c. In a wrong direction as found in persistent occipito-posterior position.

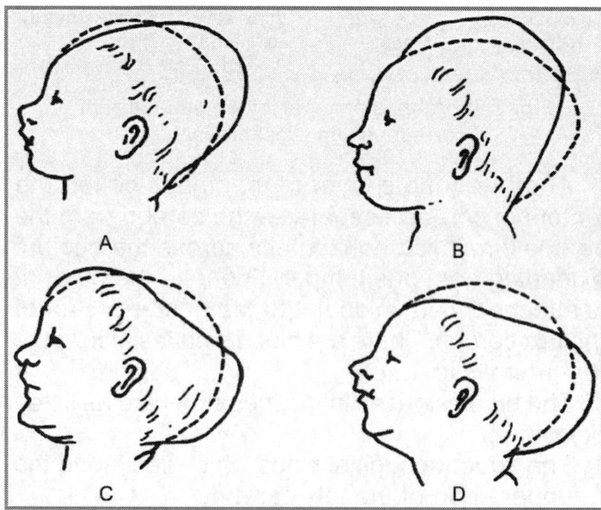

Fig. 2.42: Moulding of the head. Dotted lines indicate the normal shape of the head. **A.** Normal vertex, **B.** Occipito posterior, **C.** Brow, **D.** Face

Caput succedaneum: This is a collection of tissue fluid (or oedema) under the scalp (Fig. 2.43A). It occurs as a result of pressure on the part of the foetus which lies over the cervical os. It is thus present at birth and could be present on any presenting part head or breech and tends to shrink in size after birth. It pits on pressure; it is usually unilateral. Caput succedaneum usually disappears within 24 hours of birth without treatment.

Cephalhaematoma: A collection of blood under the periosteum, it occurs as a result of damage to the fine capillaries under the periosteum (Fig. 2.43B). This may be the effect of a difficult labour. The haematoma is confined to the affected bone and does not cross the sutures. It tends to grow bigger after birth and it does not pit on pressure. It may be on one or both sides of the head. Cephalhae matoma usually appears 24 hours after birth and usually requires no treatment. It persists for about six weeks. It may be absorbed or it may calcify.

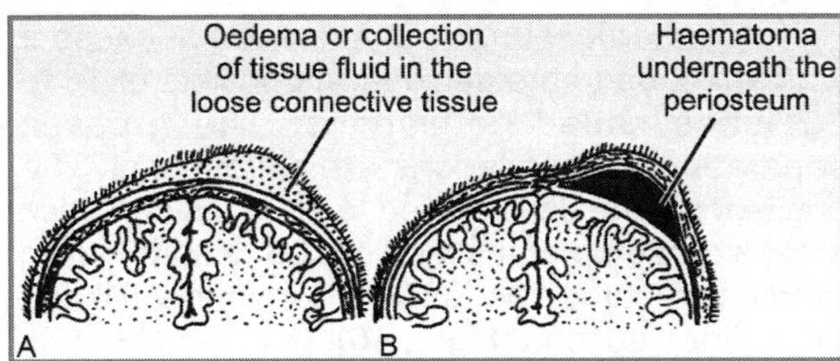

Figs 2.43A and B: Caput succedaneum and Cephalhaematoma

Injury to the inner structures: Injury to the inner structures of the foetal skull is often referred to as cerebral injury and it may be in the form of:

a. Anoxia of the brain cells;
b. Tearing the falx or tentorium and subsequent bleeding into the brain tissue.

These injuries often occur as a result of:

1. Abnormal moulding.
2. Prolonged and excessive pressure on the head.
3. Congestion of the blood vessels as a result of anoxia.

PHYSIOLOGY OF THE FOETUS FUNCTIONS OF THE PLACENTA

During intrauterine life, the foetus does not breathe or eat, so its requirements for survival are provided by the mother via the placenta. The placenta is able to provide these requirements because it is the only link between the mother and the foetus and because of its structure. The placenta is mainly a collection of chorionic villi and each villus is surrounded by maternal blood and carries a foetal capillary in its cavity (Fig. 2.44). The wall of the villus has a semipermeable membrane called the Langhan's layer and the foetal capillary inside the villus also has a semipermeable wall. The maternal and foetal blood are, therefore, separated by these semipermeable membranes. In this way, diffusion and osmosis are possible and substances like oxygen, nutrients, etc., pass from the maternal blood into the foetal blood for circulation. Oxygen is carried in the maternal blood in the form of oxyhae-moglobin-an unstable compound. When the maternal blood gets to the intervillous space, the oxyhaemoglobin breaks up into haemoglobin and oxygen. The oxygen diffuses through the Langhan's layer and the capillary wall, and is picked up by the foetal red blood cells. The oxygen is conveyed in the foetal circulation to supply the foetal tissues. Carbon dioxide is in a soluble form in the foetal blood. It diffuses through the capillary wall and the Langhan's layer into the maternal circulation for subsequent excretion.

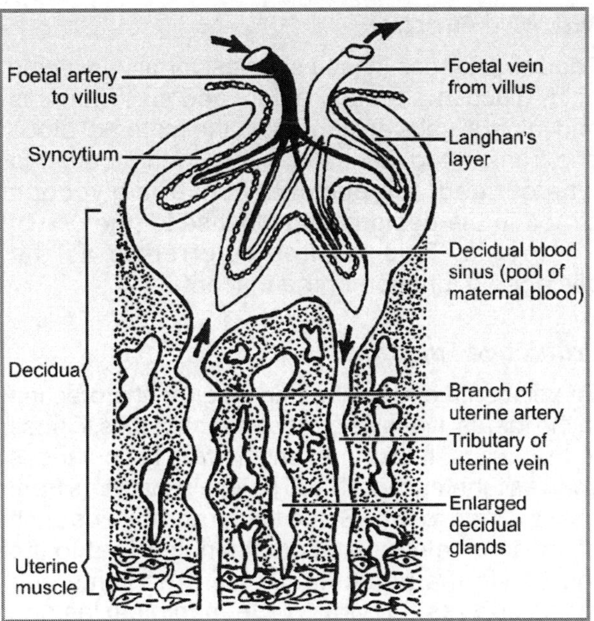

Fig. 2.44: One chorionic villus in a pool of maternal blood sinus

Nutritive Function

Food substances in their simplest forms, as amino acid, glucose and fatty acids, and also vitamins and mineral salts are carried in the maternal blood and transmitted via the placenta to the foetus. In time of need, the placenta converts glycogen stored in the decidua into glucose for the use of the foetus. This is often referred to as the glycogenic function of the placenta.

Protective Function

The placenta offers a certain amount of protection to the foetus. It allows protective antibodies to pass to the foetus. It also prevents harmful substances such as tubercle bacilli and poliomyelitis virus from getting to the foetus. Some toxins and toxoids such as those of tetanus and diphtheria can get to the foetus via the placenta. Some organisms and toxins such as the virus of German measles and *Treponema pallidum* can cross the placental barrier and affect the foetus in utero. Drugs such as morphine, pethidine, and inhalation anaesthetics do cross the placental barrier.

Hormonal Function

The placenta produces chorionic gonadotrophic hormones (anterior pituitary-like hormones). These stimulate the placenta itself to produce oestrogen and progesterone. Another hormone, similar in action to progesterone, called relaxin is also produced by the placenta. Some of these endocrine secretions are readily transmitted to the foetus via the placenta.

Excretory Function

Waste products of metabolism are excreted in the company of carbon dioxide from the foetus via the maternal circulation.

Appearance of the Placenta at Birth

The placenta is a flat, circular organ with a diameter of 20 to 25 cm. It weighs approximately 45 grams or one-sixth of the baby's weight. The umbilical cord and the membranes are attached to the placenta. The placenta has two surfaces:

1. The dark red irregular surface is called the maternal surface.
2. The greyish surface with blood vessels running in different directions is called the foetal surface (Fig. 2.45).

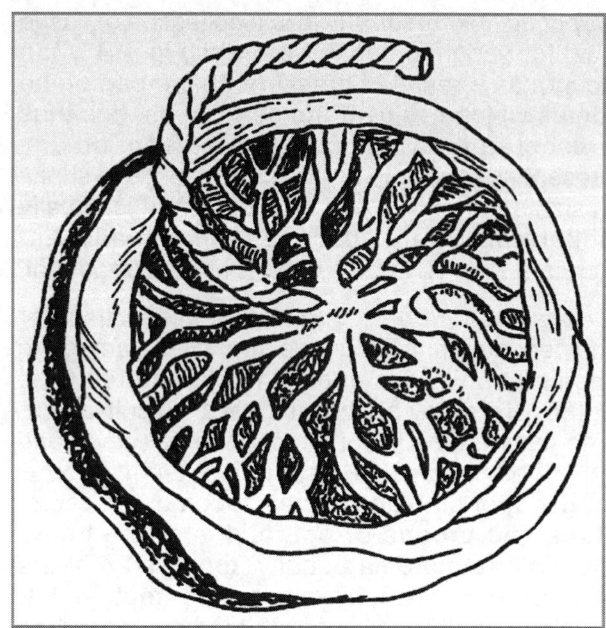

Fig. 2.45: The placenta; foetal surface

The maternal surface is so called because it was attached to the decidua. It consists of 15 to 20 lobes called cotyledons. The grooves separating the cotyledons are called sulci. The cotyledons are also referred to as lobes and each lobe is made up of masses of chorionic villi. The reddish colour is due to the blood in the villi and intervillous spaces (Fig. 2.46).

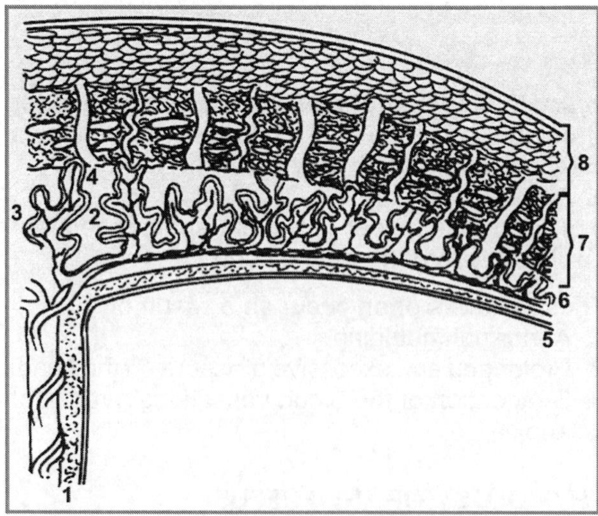

Fig. 2.46: Cross-section of the placenta showing its component parts. (1) Umbilical cord, (2) Intervillous space containing maternal blood, (3) Villi with foetal blood vessels, (4) Maternal blood sinus, (5) Amnion, (6) Chorion with blood vessels, (7) Decidua, (8) Uterine muscular wall

The foetal surface of the placenta is part of the amniotic cavity. It is covered by the amnion and the umbilical cord is inserted into it . The blood vessels, which are mainly foetal, radiate from the point of the cord insertion to the edge of the placenta where they disappear into the placental tissue.

The membranes attached to the placenta consist of amnion—a tough transparent membrane—and the chorion. The amnion forms the bag enclosing the foetus, and lines the foetal surface of the placenta and the umbilical cord. The amnion is often referred to as the foetal membrane.

The Chorion

The chorion is attached to the edge of the placenta and it is adherent to the amnion. It is the membrane which was in direct contact with the decidua. The chorion is soft and friable. It is thicker than the amnion. It can be stripped from the amnion to the edge of the placenta but it is not continuous with the cord.

The Umbilical Cord (Funis)

The umbilical cord at term is about 50 cm long and varies in thickness from 1.2 to 2 cm.

It consists of:

a. One large umbilical vein through which flows oxygenated blood from the placenta to the foetus.
b. Two umbilical arteries which carry deoxygenated blood from the foetus to the placenta.

These vessels are wrapped in a jelly-like material known as Wharton's jelly. The umbilical cord is covered on the outside with a layer of stratified cubical cells, continuous with the foetal epidermis at one end of the cord and the amniotic epithelium at the other.

The cord is not always of uniform thickness. Local accumulation of Wharton's jelly known as false knots are sometimes present. True knots rarely occur and are invariably due to foetal movements in the liquor.

Liquor Amnii

Liquor amnii is the fluid that fills the amniotic sac in which the foetus swims. Its origin is not known but it is believed to be a secretion of the amniotic cells. The foetal micturition and transudates from the foetal and maternal vessels, the cord, placenta and decidua are supposed to augment the quantity of the liquor amnii.

The liquor amnii is a clear fluid in which solids are both dissolved and suspended. Glucose, sodium chloride and protein are dissolved in it while vernix caseosa, lanugo hair and desquamated cells from the foetus float in the liquor amnii.

The quantity of the liquor amnii increases steadily as pregnancy advances but relative to the foetus, it is most abundant in mid-pregnancy. About 1 to 1.5 litres of liquor is regarded as normal, especially towards the end of pregnancy. The liquor is not stagnant, it is continually changed during pregnancy. In fact, the whole volume is said to be changed every two to three hours. It is removed by the swallowing action of the foetus and it is absorbed into the foetal circulation and carried to the placenta.

Functions of the liquor amnii:

a. It permits foetal movements and uniform development of the foetus.
b. It maintains equal pressure and provides constant temperature for the foetus.
c. It protects the foetus from trauma.
d. During labour, it prevents compression of the foetus by the contracting uterus; it acts as a sterile douche when the membranes rupture.

Abnormalities of the Placenta

Abnormalities of the placenta may be structural or as a result of disease, as stated below.

Battledore Placenta

In battledore placenta, the cord is inserted at the margin of the placenta.

Placenta Succenturiata (Figs 2.47A and B)

In this condition, one or more small accessory lobules are developed in the membranes at some distance from the periphery of the main placenta. Thus there is a bridge of membranes between the main placenta and the accessory lobe with vessels running across the membraneous bridge. Occasionally, there are no vessels on the membranes and the condition is known as placenta spuria.

Placenta succenturiata is of great clinical importance because the accessory lobe may be

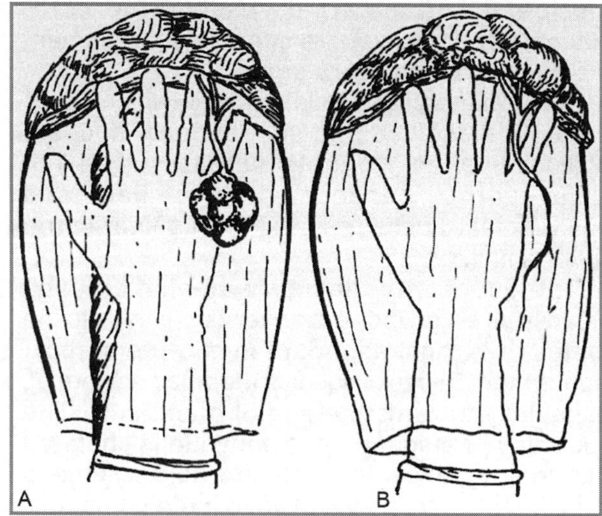

Figs 2.47A and B: A. Placenta succenturiata, **B.** Torn membrane. The missing succenturiate lobe is in the uterus

left in the uterus after the expulsion of the main placenta and thereby lead to very severe post-partum haemorrhage (Fig. 2.47B). This condition must always be borne in mind when examining the placenta especially in deliveries complicated by unexplained postpartum haemorrhage.

Placenta Circumvallata

Placenta circumvallata has a depression in the centre of the foetal surface surrounded by a thickened whitish ring. The ring is composed of a double layer of amnion and chorion which has undergone infarction. When the ring coincides with the placental margin, it is described as plancenta marginata. The placental vessels which show no abnormality do not extend beyond the margin of the ring. The cord is usually inserted centrally.

Placenta Membranacea

Placenta membranacea results from the failure of the chorion leave in contact with the decidua capsularis to degenerate. The bulk of the chorion laeve takes part in the formation of the placenta. The placenta is not therefore limited to the decidua basalis, but becomes a thin membraneous structure occupying the entire periphery of the chorion. There is no interference with the nutrition of the ovum. Difficulties usually occur during the third stage of labour because the placenta does not separate easily and manual removal may be necessary. Post-partum haemorrhage may result.

Placenta Velamentosa

In placenta velamentosa, the placenta has developed at some distance from the original attachment of the umbilical cord. The blood vessels divide on the surface of the membranes and may lie on the os to reach the placenta. This condition may lead to ante-partum haemorrhage during artificial or spontaneous rupture of the membranes.

Placenta Bipartita (Dimidiata)

In this condition, the division of the placenta into two distinct lobes is incomplete. The umbilical vessels extend from one lobe to the other before they unite to form the umbilical cord.

In placenta duplex, the two lobes may be separated and the vessels are perfectly distinct and do not unite until just before they enter the umbilical cord. The above mentioned abnormalities are thought to result from abnormalities in the blood supply of the decidua.

Placenta Fenestrata

In this condition, the placenta is oblong with an aperture of varying sizes near its centre. This is a rare condition. What frequently happens is the division of the placenta into two lobes.

Diseases of the Placenta

Hydatidiform Mole

This is proliferative cystic degeneration of the chorionic villi (see bleeding in early pregnancy).

Calcareous Degeneration

This is associated with normal degenerative processes of the placenta. The maternal surface is rough to touch and white gritty substances like broken egg shells form plaques on it.

Infarcts

These are necrosed or dead choronic villi. They are whitish in colour and appear as white patches, on the maternal surface. Infarcts result from placental insufficiency.

Oedematous Placenta

This is associated with hydrops foetalis. The placenta is large and pale.

Syphilitic Placenta

This is greasy-looking and may weigh as much as one quarter of the weight of the foetus.

THE FOETAL CIRCULATION (FIG. 2.48)

To understand the foetal circulation, it must be appreciated that the foetus develops its own blood and that at no time does the foetal and maternal blood mix unless some pathological process is present. The foetus produces its own red and white blood corpuscles. During intra-uterine life the foetal gastrointestinal and respiratory systems are not functioning, so the maternal blood furnishes the necessary nutrients and oxygen through the placenta, which in this case acts as the organ of respiration.

There are four temporary structures in the foetal circulation, and if the student nurse midwife learns their functions she will be able to understand how the foetal circulation differs from that of the adult and the changes which take place at birth.

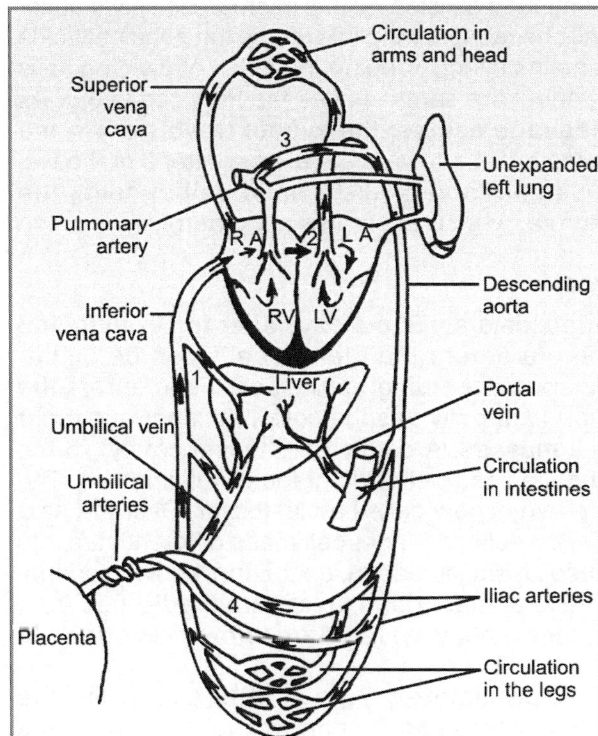

Fig. 2.48: Foetal circulation:
→ Direction of blood flow
== Temporary structures namely:
(1) Ductus venosus,
(2) Foramen ovale,
(3) Ductus arteriosus,
(4) Hypogastric arteries

The four temporary structures are as follows:

1. *The ductus venosus (from a vein to a vein)*: This vessels from the umbilical vein to the inferior vena cava carries replenished oxygenated blood to the foetal heart for circulation throughout the foetus.
2. *The foramen ovale*: A temporary opening between the two atria in the foetal heart, allows the replenished blood to enter the left atrium and be pumped out through the aorta.
3. *The ductus arteriosus (from an artery to an artery)*: This vessel from the pulmonary artery to the descending arch of the aorta carries deoxygenated blood returned from the head and upper limbs, thereby bypassing the pulmonary circulation.
4. *The hypogastric arteries*: These two vessels branch off from the internal iliac arteries and are known as the umbilical arteries when they enter the umbilical cord. They return deoxygenated blood to the placenta for oxygenation and replenishment.

Blood which has been circulated throughout the foetus requires to be oxygenated and replenished, so it is carried by the two umbilical arteries in the umbilical cord to the placenta, where an interchange takes place between the foetal and maternal blood by a process of osmosis and diffusion, as well as by the selective action of the vital (Langhan's) layer of the chorionic villi. Four layers separate the foetal blood from the maternal blood. These are syncytium, Langhan's layer, mesoderm and the capillary wall. Carbon dioxide and other excretory products are given off into the maternal blood; nutritional substances and oxygen are picked up. It is important to realize that the blood which circulates within the foetal, umbilical and placental vessels is foetal in origin.

The replenished blood returns to the foetus by the umbilical vein in the umbilical cord which goes directly to the liver, but before reaching that organ a large branch, the ductus venosus, splits off and this empties the purified blood to the heart via the vena cava, which is returning the impure blood to the heart from all the vellels below the diaphragm, including the portal vein. Oxygenated blood is, therefore, mingled with deoxygenated blood.

The foetal heart has a temporary opening, known as the foramen ovale, situated between the two atria so that the oxygenated blood returning from the placenta via the inferior vena cava is shunted from the right into the left atrium and not into the right ventricle which is the route after birth. It is thought that the force exerted by the Eustachian valve in the inferior vena cava directs the oxygenated blood through the foramen ovale into the left atrium. The blood then passes from the left atrium to the left ventricle where it is pumped out through the aorta. This blood has the highest oxygen content in the foetal circulation, and the major portion of it goes via branches of the aorta to the great vessels of the neck that supply the brain, and to the upper limbs. A smaller quantity passes down the descending arch of the aorta.

The deoxygenated blood from the head and upper limbs returns to the heart via the superior vena cava and passes from the right atrium to the right ventricle (as it does after birth), and leaves the right ventrcle by the pulmonary artery.

The pulmonary circulation functions very slightly before birth, most of the blood leaving the right ventricle of the foetus is, therefore, diverted from the lungs via a temporary vessel-the ductus arteriosus. A small quantity of blood is carried by the pulmonary artery to the lungs to nourish them and is returned by the pulmonary veins. The ductus arteriosus conveys the blood from the pulmonary veins. The ductus arteriosus conveys the blood from the pulmonary artery to the descending arch of the aorta where it is distributed to the abdominal and pelvic viscera and to the lower limbs, but the greater proportion of it is returned to the placenta via the hypogastric arteries which are branches of the internal iliac arteries.

The hypogastric arteries enter the umbilical cord and are then known as the umbilical arteries.

Changes in Circulation at Birth

The changes which occur are not due to the trying off of the umbilical cord, but rather to the establishment of respiration. When the infant cries, the lungs expand and their vascular field is increased so the blood which has been passing through the ductus arteriosus to the aorta now flows through the pulmonary arteries to the lungs for oxygenation. Within five minutes, the ductus arteriosus is half closed. It eventually becomes a cardiac ligament. In a very small number of cases the ductus arteriosus remains patent.

The increased flow of blood to the lungs reduces the pressure in the right side of the heart and increases the tension in the left side, causing the valve-like foramen ovale to close . If this does not occur, the venous blood in the right atrium will mix with arterial blood in the left atrium of the heart.

The part of the umbilical vein lying under the abdominal wall becomes thrombosed and occluded soon after the cord is tied and forms a fibrous cord, the ligamentum teres of the liver. The ductus venosus becomes the ligamentum venosum which supports the attachment of the portal vein to the vena cava. The hypogastric arteries atrophy and form a ligament between the bladder and umbilicus.

EMBRYONIC PERIOD

Cleavage

About 24 to 48 hours after fertilization, the zygote divides; the daughter cells resulting from this mitosis are half the size of the fertilized ovum. Continued division results in progressively smaller cells because during this phase the zona pellucida remains intact, keeping the mass of dividing cells at about the same size as the fertilized ovum. As cleavage occurs, the zygote travels down the fallopian tube toward the uterus. After 3 or 4 days, it begins to look like a solid ball of cells, the morula, which resembles a mulberry.

Implantation

Approximately 3 to 4 days after fertilization, the morula enters the uterus, cells can be distinguished according to function. Fluid enters the morula and divides the cells into inner and outer cell masses. A cavity (blastocyst cavity) forms and the zona pellucida gradually disappears. The embryo is now called a blastocyst. Over the next 2 1/2 weeks the inner cell mass differentiates into three layers: ectoderm, endoderm, and mesoderm. These primary germ layers are the tissues from which all body systems are formed are shown in Table 2.2.

Approximately 7 days after ovulation, the trophoblast begins to burrow into the lining of the uterus; this burrowing is called implantation or nidation. Trophoblastic cells secrete enzymes that digest or liquefy endometrial tissue. The blastocyst sinks deep into the endometrum, which becomes the decidua basalis. Finger-like projections, villi, of trophoblast "dig into" and break down tissue and firmly anchor the blast cyst in the decidua basalis, an area with a rich source of

Table 2.2: Organs and tissues derived from germ layers

Ectoderm	*Mesoderm*	*Endoderm*
• Central nervous system • Peripheral nervous system • Sensory epithelium of sense organs • Epidermis of hair, nails subcutaneous glands • Hair follicles • Lens of eye • Enamel of teeth • Hypophysis • Mammary glands	• Heart • All connective tissue layers • Bone • Muscles • Cartilage • Blood • Kidneys • Urinary tract • Lymphatic system • Gonadal system • Spleen	• Gastrointestinal tract • Epithelium of respiratory tract, pharynx, tongue, thyroid, parathyroids • Liver • Pancreas • Epithelial lining of bladder and urethra

nourishment a oxygen. This may be confused with a menstrual period. Some women may experience slight vaginal bleeding at this time. However, by the ninth or tenth day, the epithelium, now called the DECIDUA CAPSULARIS, has beg to heal over the area in which the blastocyte became embedded.

By day 13, the trophoblast has become the chorion, and the villi have become the chorionic villi. By the end of the third month when the growth of the embryo causes the decidua capsularis and decidua parieta (uterine lining farthest from the implantation site) to compress one another, the chorionic villi (also called the chorion frondosum) remain only in the decidua basalis. These chorionic Villi make up the foetal portion of the placenta.

Chorion

The chorion from the trophoblast and is the outermost membrane and closest to the uterine lining. The trophoblast infiltrates maternal tissues with chorionic villi, which are embedded the decidua basalis. These willi form the foetal side of the placenta. Thus the villi become bathed with maternal blood rich in oxygen and nutrients.

Exchange of foetal and maternal material takes place through osmosis, diffusion, active transport, and pinocytosis (ameboid-like action). There are also other complex transfer mechanisms. There is no direct mingling of foetal and maternal blood. However, there may be very isolated exchanges of foetal and maternal blood cells when small leaks occur in the trophoblast or during threatened abortion or diagnostic tests such as chorionic villus sampling (CVS) and amniocentesis.

The chorionic villi enlarge by the end of the fourth and fifth months to form 15 to 20 visible placental partitions (cotyledons or little trees).

In addition, part of the chorion produces hCG, which helps to sustain pregnancy by preventing the involution of the corpus luteum.

Amnion

The amnion appears very early in embryonic life, even before the embryo has taken form. At first, the amnion is small, but as it fills with fluid and the embryo grows, it becomes much larger and eventually surrounds the embryo and umbilical cord. Later in pregnancy, the amnion expands to fill the entire space and adheres to the other membrane, the chorion. Together, the amnion and chorion are known as the foetal membranes.

At term, the amniotic sac contains almost a litre of amniotic fluid, which forms from amniotic cells, urine, and secretions from the lungs and skin of the foetus. This fluid contains albumin, urea, creatinine, lecithin, sphingomyelin, bilirubin, fat, fructose, lanugo hairs, uric acid and inorganic salts and is slightly alkaline. It cushions the foetus against injury, prevents adhesions of the sticky skin and umbilical cord compression, equalizes pressure, and provides thermal regulation, a medium for foetal movement, and fluid for the foetus to swallow. The fluid is replaced approximately every 3 hours. This secretion and reabsorption is regulated by the amnion cells and foetal swallowing and urinating.

At term, this fluid provides a "wedge" to help to soften and dilate the cervix during labour. Amniotic fluid can also provide the physician with valuable diagnostic information when its components are analyzed in high risk pregnancies. Volumes of amniotic fluid greater (hydramnios) or less (oligohydramnios) than average are significant because these variations may be associated with foetal abnormalities.

Placenta

The development and circulation of the placenta occurs during the third week. It is formed at the site of attachment of the chorion to the uterine wall. The placenta and membranes are completely functional by the twelfth week. The placenta expands until it covers about half of the internal surface area of the uterus by the twentieth week.

The placenta secretes hormones essential for maintaining pregnancy. By the third month, it takes over production of progesterone from the corpus luteum. It also secretes oestriol, an oestrogen.

Human placental lactogen (hPL), a hormone similar to prolactin, is also produced by the placenta. hPL stimulates changes in the mother's metabolic process to ensure that the mother's body is prepared for lactation.

The placenta grows until late in the eighth month. Towards the end of pregnancy, it begins to age, secreting hormones in decreasing amounts and becoming gradually less able to effectively exchange nutrients, oxygen, and wastes. Placental aging may be assessed during ultrasound examination.

The placental barrier is composed of layers of foetal tissue (trophoblast, connective tissue, basement membrane, and foetal capillary endothelium). It provides some protection to the foetus, but as pregnancy progresses the membrane becomes thinner.

The pregnant woman must understand that placental exchange is by simple diffusion for oxygen, carbon dioxide, fat-soluble vitamins, lipids (including narcotics, anesthetics, and barbiturates that are fat soluble). Facilitated diffusion and active transport govern glucose, amino acids. calcium, iron, and water soluble vitamins, pinocytosis controls larger molecules such as globulins, viruses and antibodies. Other substances pass by additional means. Some larger molecules such as IgM, heparin, insulin, or complex cells such as blood cells do not cross the placenta unless there is damage to the placental membrane.

Umbilical Cord

While the placenta develope, the umbilical cord is also forming. Blood vessels establish a connection between the developing embryo and the placenta via the body stalk. Together the body stalk and remnants of the yolk sac form the primitive umbilical cord.

Originally there are four cord vessels. Early in gestation, one vein atrophies, leaving one larger vein to carry blood from the placenta to the foetus and two small arteries to return deoxygenated blood to the placenta. Approximately 400 ml/ min flows through the cord, this flow helps to stabilize the soft cord. The cord vessels also are supported by a substance. Wharton's jelly, made up of connective tissue, mucopolysaccharides, and covered by amnion that extends up from the foetal side of the placenta and ends at the skin of the abdomen of the foetus. The amount of Wharton's jelly varies widely; it is especially influenced by foetal nutrition, activity and gestational age. Cord vessels may be constricted in response to stimuli or drugs. The surface of the cord contains no pain receptors; thus cutting the cord is painless.

Development of the Embryo

The time between fertilization and the first 14 days of development is the preembryonic period. It is a time of rapid cell division, with differentiation of tissues and the development of the primary germ layers, the ectoderm, endoderm, and mesoderm. These three germ layers are the tissues from which all body structures are formed (Table 7.2).

At the third week, the mass of growing cells becomes an embryo. The embryonic period is marked by rapid growth and further tissue differentiation, including organogenesis, the differentiation and formation of organs. Many organs are developed before the mother realizes she is pregnant. This period is also characterized by extreme susceptibility to adverse environmental influences such as radiation, infection, drugs, or smoking. The shape of the embryo changes dramatically.

By the end of the third week, germ layers have begun to form distinct tissue. The ectodermal layer develops into the organs and structures such as the central nervous system and brain that maintain interaction with the outside world. The mesodermal layer develops into the supporting tissues of the body (muscle and bone) and the vascular and urinary tract systems so the body can maintain movement and internal function. Finally, the endodermal layer provides for the epithelial linings of most of the system of the body.

EMBRYOLOGY

Early Beginnings

Conception normally takes place in the fallopian or uterine tube. The single cell soon divides into two, then four, then eight cells, and continues to multiply until a cell count would be impossible, The fertilized egg, or zygote, assumes the bumpy apearance of a mulberry and for the reason is called a morula as its journeys down the tube in search of a warn, safe place to grow. The journey from ovary to uterine cavity, where nesting or implantation occurs, involves about 7 days. At the end of the time the zygote, now a hollow, fluid-filled blastocyst, burrows into the soft uterine lining. Its outer surface becomes covered with finger-like tissue projections called chorionic villi, which aid in the process of implantation into the endometrium (known as the decidua during pregnancy). Implantation may cause limited bleeding, which may be reported as "spotting." The villi also manufacture the human chorionic gonadotropin (hCG) that initially signals the corpus luteum in the ovary to continue to manufacture progesterone and oestrogen to prevent menstruation and additional ovulation. The aggregation of cells begins to form a definite pattern. The microscopic embryonic disc develops, and primitive beginnings of the child and his basic support system appear.

Of course, the possibility of intentional alteration in the initiation and early development of selected pregnancies exists. In 1978 an ovum obtained from a woman's ovary, fertilized by her husband' s sperm in a laboratory and placed in her uterus as a blastocyst, resulted in the birth of an apparently normal, healthy infant girl. At this writing, *in vitro* fertilization has made possible the birth of many infants including twins, to women who were denied biologic parenthood because of blocked fallopian tubes.

Placental Development and Role

After implantation of a zygote, a supply and disposal system across the uterine wall is initiated through a special intermediary organ called the placenta, or after birth. The placenta a miraculous structure, develops from part of the chorionic villi that extended from the outside of the egg. Attached to the uterine wall, it manufactures estrogen, progesterone, chorionic gonadotropin, and various other hormones and enzymes that apparently influence the growth and maintenance of the pregnancy and maternal preparation for birth and lactation. Using various complex molecular processes, the placenta also transports the food and oxygen necessary for foetal growth and hormones and protective substances called antibodies from the mother's blood to the foetus by way of the umbilical cord. Also, the placenta handles waste products brought to its tissues from the foetus; it allows carbon dioxide and other metabolic wastes to pass from the foetal circulation to the maternal bloodstream. The mother and foetus do not share a common bloodstream. The mother and foetus do not share a common bloodstream. The mother and foetus do not share a common bloodstream; the foetus manufactures its own blood. Normally the whole blood of the mother and that of the foetus stay within their separate, closely related channels. Blood flows from the placenta to the foetus through a large umbilical vein in the umbilical cord. The two arteries in the umbilical cord are wound around the umbilical vein and carry the waste to the placenta.

Bag of Waters

As the embryo develops, the chorionic villi that face the interior of the uterus and are not involved in the formation of the placenta detach from the spherical covering and leave a transparant sac made up of two membranous layers called the chorion and the amnion. The inner layer, the amnion, contains a salty liquid known as amniotic fluid, in which the foetus may float. The amniotic fluid helps control the environmental temperature of the foetus and shield it from trauma and infection. Perhaps weightlessness is not such an extraordinary condition for mankind after all. This amniotic sac is commonly known as the "bag of waters," or the membranes. Normally, it remains intact until the time of labour and birth.

The Foetus

From the eighth week of growth, the embryo is recognizable as a small, unfinished human and is called a foetus, meaning 'young one'. The foetus is less than 2 inches (about 3 cm) long and weights a fraction of anounce. Rudimentary body systems are formed and working, and the skeleton is becoming established.

At 12 weeks: By the end of the third lunar month, the sex of the foetus is clearly fiscernible. Needless to say, parents are curious regarding the sex of the developing foetus. However no completely safe procedure exists to determine the sex of the foetus before birth. A technique called amniocentesis makes sex identification possible before birth is this information is genetically important. Amniotic fluid is aspirated from the bag of waters and examined for cellular content and chromosome determination later in the pregnancy.

The foetus is most susceptible to malformation from the effects of maternal drug ingestion, radiation, or infection in the first trimester (the first 13 weeks of pregnancy), when basic organs and systems are being formed. It is possible for certain drugs to distort foetal development within 11 days of conception, before the woman realizes that she may be pregnant. Such an "assault at an early gestational period usually causes foetal death. Drugs or conditions that produce foetal structural defects are termed teratogenic. They are currently the object of much concern and study.

At 16 weeks: At 16 weeks of intrauterine development, the foetus has increased in size considerably. It is approximately 7½ inches (19 cm) long and weighs about 3 ounces (100 g). The uterus is correspondingly larger, and the expectant mother may make her debut in maternity clothes. At 16 to 18 weeks GA, pregnant women usually report feelings of life, or quickening. Elbows, feet, and hands punch and twitch as the foetus attempts more vigorous exercise in the confining uterus.

At 20 Weeks: At 20 weeks of growth, the foetus is about 8 1/4 inches (22 cm) long and weighs approximately 10 ounces (300 g) at this time. At 20 weeks GA, the uterus is at or slightly above the mother's umbilicus, and the foetal hearbeat is heard using a standard foetoscope.

Some state laws declare that the legal threshold of viability is 24 weeks of GA; others use 20 weeks GA as the lower limit. However, the true length of a pregnancy may be difficult to determine and can lead to moral-ethical dilemmas involving the rights and responsibilities of the parents and the community, as well as consideration for the life and well-being of the developing foetus. Infants diagnosed as less than 24 weeks of GA have made postnatal respiratory efforts. Special neonatal care units employing exceptional techniques suporting or moni-toring body warmth, ventilation, cardiac function, and nutrition have been able to save foetuses of increasingly shorter gestations. Nevertheless, when all births are evaluated, such survivals must be considered a rare occurrence.

The characteristics of the premature infant and his grip on life depend on his genetic endowment, the length and quality of his prenatal environment, and his immediate postnatal care. Assuming his prenatal environment and personal condition are satisfactory, each additional day the foetus is able to remain in the uterus until maturity, which is approximately 38 weeks in length, is beneficial. Each day increases his ability to withstand the demands of extrauterine life and to adjust to the tremendous circulatory, respiratory, and digestive alterations that must take place at birth.

Foetal Circulation (Fig. 2.38)

A diagram of foetal circulation is shown in Figure 2.38 to give a better understanding of the circulorespiratory changes. The umbilical vein within the umbilical cord carries blood from the placenta to the foetus and enters the body at the umbilicus. It travels upward, dividing to form a bypass of the liver called the ductus venosus, which eventually joins the inferior vena cava. The rich oxygenated blood from the umbilical vein mixes with the oxygenpoor blood flowing form the lower extremities and abdominal cavity toward the heart. The blood enters the heart by way of the right atrium, as in postnatal circulation. Because the pulmonary circulation is unnecessary to oxygenation, much of the blood entering the heart from the inferior vena cava crosses directly to the left atrium through the foetal shunt, or interatrial opening, called foramen ovale. This blood is then guided into the usual circulation pattern, left atrium, left ventricle, aorta.

Blood from the head and upper extremities enters the right atrium via the superior vena cava, flows primarily into the right ventricle, and is eventually pushed into the pulmonary artery.

However, the trip to the lungs is superfluous at this time, and another shunt, the ductus arteriosus, is employed. This short duct leads from the pulmonary artery to the aorta. Relatively little blood flows to the lung fields and back to the left heart by way of the pulmonary veins.

The blood that flows downward through the aorta is eventually channelled into the iliac arteries to the hypogastric arteries that join with the umbilical arteries leading to the umbilical cord and placenta.

The pulmonary circulation becomes established within a relatively short time after birth. The umbilical cord is clamped and cut, and the blood vessels it contains become occluded. Because of the changes in thoracic pressures initiated by postnatal expansion of the lungs, the foramen ovale begins to close, and the ductus arteriosus collapses and becomes a ligament without within a period of days or weeks.

Because the maturity of an infant is important to survival outside the uterus, improved techniques to determine intrauterine growth as well as general health *in utero* have become very helpful. Before labour, types of tests that help assess foetal age, size, maturity and well-being have included; amniocentesis—an examination of amniotic fluid aspirated transabdominally from the amniotic sac under sterile conditions; ultrasonography—unlike X-ray examination, appears to be a safe technique for the foetus and mother at any stage of pregnancy maternal blood and urine analysis; chorionic villi sampling—a new test providing early diagnosis of some genetic diseases; and foetal heart monitorinig. During labour the immediate status of the baby may be evaluated though simultaneous monitoring of the foetal heart rate and contraction patterns, observation of the colour of the amniotic fluid and in certain cases, by foetal blood sampling.

Respiratory System: Development and Function

In utero the placenta is a substitute for the nonfunctioning foetal lungs. Oxygenated blood comes to the foetus from the placenta via the umbilical vein. Although lungs are not being used for ventilation and oxygenation, the normal foetus makes respiratory movements in utero. These movements have been demonstrated by real time ultrasound and are one of the parameters of the biophysical profile. These "practice" respiratory movements normally do not draw amniotic fluid into the foetal lungs; they are merely small movements of the chest wall. The respiratory system develops from the endoderm (the same tissue that will give rise to the gastrointestinal system) during day 24 of embryonic life. Bronchi are formed by the sixteenth week of foetal development, and there are primitive lungs by 23 weeks. However, these can function only with great difficulty, since there are not enough alveoli for the necessary exchange of gases. Blood flow to the lungs is also inadequate at this time.

Two distinct types of cells are found in the lungs; type 1 cells, which allow for exchange of gases, and type 2 cells, which produce surfactant at 20 to 24 weeks of gestational age. Surfactant is composed of surface-active compounds that stabilize the alveoli and prevent their collapse with each exhalation. There are two pathways of surfactant production. The first pathway functions from 20 to 24 weeks and continues until birth. However, it is an unstable pathway easily inhibited after birth by hypoxia, hypothermia and acidosis. The second pathway is much more resistant to these stressors but does not fully mature until 35 to 37 weeks of foetal life. Interestingly, stresses on the health of the mother, such as hypertension, pre-eclampsia, or heroin use, can stimulate the production of surfactant. It is thought that increased amounts of steroids are produced by a mother who is stressed. Pulmonary maturity can be accelerated by giving steroids to a mother before term if enough time is available before delivery of the infant.

Respiration is regulated by the respiratory center in the brainstem. Maturation of the central nervous system progresses as pregnancy continues, with coordination of feeding, and respiration occurring at about 34 weeks of gestation. All of these developmental milestones are vital to the discussion of foetal viability. The foetus is considered to have reached the age of viability at 20 weeks gestation, although extrauterine survival at this stage of development is currently almost impossible. When an infant of 20 weeks seems to be surviving, it is often because there is a discrepancy between the expected date of birth and the real gestational age. The lungs become capable of borderline support of extrauterine respiration some time after 23 weeks of gestation. Adequate respiratory function also depends on maturation of surfactant production and neurologic control of respiration. There is great variation between humans; therefore there is no "magic week of gestation" during which pulmonary maturity is certain.

Cardiovascular System: Development and Function

With blood circulating by the end of the third week of gestation, the cardiovascular system is the first system to function in the embryo. This is necessary because the rapidly growing embryo requires a large quantity of nutrients and produces an equally large amount of waste products Humans, unlike other animals, have a small yolk sac for nutritional support during early gestation.

The first indication of cardiac development is seen on day 18 to 19 in the cardiogenic area where cells cluster to form the cardiogenic cords. These are two tubes, which fuse and then develop strictures and outpouchings that form the primitive heart chambers and vessels. By the end of the fifth week, cells around the heart tubes differentiate into myocardial and pericardial cells. The primitive heart begins beating by day 22, even before the four chambers are well defined. Cardiac muscle develops from mesenchyme, which is around the embryonic cardiac tubes.

Some of these cells will later form Purkinje's cells, which are the conducting system.

The three purposes for foetal circulation are accomplished through the following specialized foetal structures and their functions:

1. To decrease blood flow to the foetal lungs.
2. To increase blood flow to the head and the heart.
3. To direct blood to the placenta.

Foetal circulation differs from adult circulation in several ways. Blood pressure in the adult is lower in the lungs (pulmonary blood pressure) than it is in the rest of the body (systemic blood pressure). In foetal life, this condition is reversed. Foetal pulmonary blood pressure is higher because foetal pulmonary blood vessels are constricted divert blood away from the nonfunctioning foetal lungs. Foetal systemic blood pressure, however, is lower because flow leads to the placenta through blood vessels that are not constricted. The following is the description of foetal circulation:

1. Highly oxygenated blood comes to the foetus from the placenta VIA;
2. The umbilical vein;
3. This is shunted past the liver via the ductus venosus and;
4. Continues through the inferior vena cava to the right atrium;
5. Poorly oxygenated blood from the lower body flows from the inferior vena cava through the liver and also continues through the inferior vena cava to the right atrium;
6. Most of the highly oxygenated blood from the inferior vena cava is diverted to the left atrium through the foramen ovals, a flap that allows blood to flow only from the right to left sides of the heart ("right to left shunt");
7. Poorly oxygenated blood from the upper body flows through the tricuspid valve into the right ventricle and through;
8. The pulmonary artery to the foetal lungs, but;
9. Increased pressure caused by foetal pulmonary constriction directs most of this blood away from the pulmonary vessels and to the aorta throgh the ductus arteriosus; this is another "right-to-left shunt;"
10. Simultaneously, highly oxygenated blood in the left atrium, mixed with a small amount of blood from the nonfunctioning foetal lungs, flows through the mitral valve into the aorta. This allows highly oxygenated blood to be directed to the myocardium and the brain, a major benefit;
11. Blood from the ductus arteriosus and the aorta mixes and supplies the rest of the body;
12. The two umbilical arteries (branches of the internal iliac arteris) carry mixed blood back to the placenta for reoxygenation.

Metabolic Control

Thermal Control

The foetus produces heat *in utero*, which is dissipated through the placenta to the mother if the mother's temperature is less than that of the foetus (the maternal-foetal-thermal gradient). The temperature of the foetus is about 0.5°C (0.9°F) above maternal core temperature, which ranges from 37.6°C to 37.8°C (99.8°F to 100.0°F). If the mother becomes febrile, this mechanism can fail, allowing foetal core temperature to rise. Maternal hyperthermia may not be related to illness. Strenuous exercise or increased environmental temperatures such as those found in hot tubs, saunas, and steam baths can lead to foetal hyperthermia. It has been suggested that early foetal/maternal hyperthermia may cause central nervous system defects such as anencephaly.

Newborns produce most of their body heat by metabolizing a specialized tissue called brown fat, which develops progressively during the last trimester of pregnancy. Sites for brown fat storage in the term infant; the nape of the neck, between the scapulae, in the mediastinum, and surrounding the kidneys.

The control center for heat regulation is located in the hypothalamus and is fully functional in the healthy newborn. It is therefore the lack of brown fat and not the lack of temperature control that places healthy but premature and growth retarded infants at risk for hypothermia. An insulating layer of fat (white fat) is also deposited during the third trimester. With maturation of the hypothalamus, central control of temperature is further developed. However, the neonate does not adapt well to extremes of temperature; mechanisms for maintaining temperature are still immature at birth.

Glucose and Calcium

Foetal energy requirements are supplied by maternal metabolism in the form of glucose, lactate, free fatty acids, and amino acids; foetal gluconeogenesis also contributes to energy supplies. This energy is used for both foetal growth and storage of energy for future needs. The rate of energy storage increases toward term as glycogen is stored in the foetal liver and cardiac muscle.

Calcium is supplied to the foetus via active transport mechanisms in the placenta that facilitate transfer from the maternal circulation. Foetal calcium levels are maintained 1 mg/100 ml of blood higher than maternal levels. Maternal calcium levels drop slightly towards term because of foetal needs. Because the growing foetus needs calcium for development of the bony skeleton, during the last trimester of pregnancy, foetal calcium content increases four fold as bone density progresses. Thus the infant who is delivered prematurely will have decreased calcium stores. If nutritional intake of calcium is inadequate, foetal calcium needs will be taken from maternal stores.

Integumentary System: Development and Function

Although the skin is considered a single organ, it arises from two separate embryologic germ layers. The epidemis, or outermost layer, develops from the surface ectoderm. The dermis is derived from mesenchyme. The skin and its products (mainly vernix caseosa) function mainly in foetal life as protection for underlying structures. Tactile sense is present *in utero*—a foetus accidentally touched by the needle during amniocentesis will move away from it.

During gestation, cells from the epidermis proliferate, are shed and replaced. These cells part of the vernix caseosa, a white cheesy substance that products the skin *in utero*. The amount of vernix decreases as gestation proceeds, until at term only a small amount is seen in the thigh and axillary creases. Therefore, nurse will observe the extent and location of any vernix when nurse assess the infant's gestational age.

During the eleventh week of gestation, cells proliferate downward and form epidermal ridges in a pattern or grooves and ridges on the soles, fingers and plams. A unique, genetically determined, permanent design forms by 17 weeks of gestation dermatoglyphics, or the study of epidermal ridges and lines, is part of the examination of infants with possible genetic disease, because distinct patterns are sometimes associated with specific syndromes.

Skin colour begins to develop prentally as some cells differentiate into melanoblasts and then melanocytes. The amount of melanin produced *in utero* varies with race. Infants of black parents may vary in skin colour from very light to very dark, with darker skin found nearest the nail beds and on the scrotum.

The hair that becomes visible during the twentieth week of foetal life, has fine downy quality and is called LANUGO. Lanugo is found over the entire foetal body and then recedes with increasing gestational age. By 36 weeks it can be found only on the foetal shoulders and forehead. By term most is gone.

Sebacious glands develop along with the hair follicles. Sweat glands develop as growths from the epidermis downward into the dermis.

Nails begin to appear at the tips of digits during the tenth week of gestation, with fingernails appearing before toe nails (Arm development proceedes leg development as well.) Nail growth is used to assess gestational age; at 32 weeks the finger nails are at the finger-tips; by 36 weeks the toenails have reached the ends of the toes.

The teeth arise from two embryologic layers. The enamel is derived from ectoderm; all other tissues have the mesenchyme as their source. Teeth begin to appear in the parimitive jaws during the sixth week of gestation. Early proliferations of cells, or tooth buds, will later become the primary or deciduous teeth, which are shed during childhood. Each jaw contains 10 tooth buds that start developing from the anterior region of the jaw with progression posteriorly. Some precursors to the permanent teeth appear later in gestation, at 10 weeks, while others appear even later in the pregnancy. Tooth buds for second and third permanent molars, however, do not appear until after birth, during the fourth month and fifth year.

Mammary glands develop along the mammary ridges, commonly called the milk lines, during the sixth week of gestation. Normally, only those breast buds located in the pectoral region persist. The mammary buds that remain divide and develop the main lactiferous ducts. Furthers development of lactiferous ducts in the female is postponed until the onset of puberty and continues during pregnancy under the influence of oestrogen and progesterone.

Gastrointestinal System: Development and Function

The gastrointestinal tract or gut, appears during the fourth week of gestation as the embryo folds on itself and incorporates part of its yolk sac. Epithelium, glands, muscles, and fibrous tissues are derived from separate foetal germ layers. Because of the separate arterial supply of each, the gastrointestinal tract is divided into three anatomic areas; foregut, midgut, and hindgut.

The mouth first appears as a slight depression on the embryo's surface. The lips and palate arise from separate tissue masses of the head and face that grow inward and merge in the midline of the foetus. Cleft in lips or palate occur when either of these masses fails to merge competely. The oesophagus grows from the foregut and a partition, the tracheoesophageal groove, divides it from the beginning trachea. The stomach begins as a dilated area in the foregut as it nears its caudal end. The duodenum forms just past this joint, at the junction between the foregut and midgut. The liver, pancreas, and spleen develop from specialized layers of foregut and midgut. All structures from the common bile duct to the proximal part of the transferse colon are midgut derivatives. The hindgut gives rise to the distal colon, rectum, part of the anal canal, and the urogenital system.

The anus and rectum develop from the cloaca (end of the hindgut) as it is divided by the urorectal membrane into the rectum posteriorly and urogenital sinus. The cloaca is covered externally by the cloacal membrane, which must rupturs to establish a route for excretion.

Development of digestive enzymes continues throughout gestation. Intestinal disaccharidase function develops earliest, with mature levels of maltase and sucrase observed at 6 to 8 months of gestation and mature levels of lactase only at term. However, if an infant is born premature, lactase levels will reach normal levels soon after delivery. Production of some enzymes responsible for protein metabolism does not reach mature levels until term, making an external source of some amino acids vital.

The foetus will "rehearse" later feeding behaviour by swallowing amniotic fluid. This does not provide any nutrition to the foetus but the cellular components of amniotic fluid contribute to the production of meconium. Coordination of suck and swallow reflexes does not occur until about 34 weeks of gestation, but this does not stop the foetus from swallowing amniotic fluid. A foetus will also turn toward his or her finger if they brush the face (the rooting reflex) and begin to suck on them. Another reflex important for successful feeding without aspiration is the gag reflex. This does not fully mature until the 8th month of gestation.

Meconium, a tarry black substance, begins to form in the foetal intestine during weeks 13 to 16 of gestation. It consists of secretions from the gastrointestinal tract, including bile pigments, foetal cells and hair contained in swallowed amniotic fluid, and cells sloughed from the intestinal walls.

Although meconium is formed early in foetal life, there should be no passage of it *in utero*. During a breech position delivery, meconium may be passed as the infant's abdomen is compressed by the maternal tissues and perhaps other foetal parts. During times of stress, especially hypoxic stress, the foetal and sphincter may relax and meconium may be passed, causing the amniotic fluid to become "meconium stained."

Genitourinary System

Renal Development and Function

Developmental problems of the renal and reproductive systems are relatively common because they develop in close proximity to each other and derive from several common sources of tissues; therefore, malformations of either system may occur together.

Kidneys

The kidneys develop low in the pelvis and seem to move up as they develop, but their location only seems to move because of the growth of the lower part of the body. At about 12 weeks of gestation the foetal kidneys start to produce hypotonic urine, which contributes to amniotic fluid volume. Absent or malformed kidneys lead to a decrease in amniotic fluid volume, or oligohydramnios. This is an important observation during the antepartal period. Although urine production has begun *in utero*, the placental and maternal kidney functions eliminate foetal waste products.

At birth, the term newborn has all the nephrons that will be produced during his or her lifetime. Further growth of the kidney is by hypertrophy not hyperplasia.

Bladder and Urethra

The cloaca is a dilation at the caudal and of the hindgut, divided into the rectal/anal canal and the urogenital sinus by the urorectal septum. The bladder and urethra develop from the urogenital sinus, with additional contributions from surrounding tissues. In the male production of androgens is vital to the closure of tissues around the urethral tube. If this tube closes abnormally, the urethral meatus will be located on the dorsal (hypospadias) or ventral (epispadias) surface of the penis, rather than at the tip. In very rare instances, the abdominal wall fails to close around the bladder, causing extrophy of the bladder.

Adrenal Development and Function

The adrenal glands, although in direct contact with the kidneys, have different embryologic origins. Even the cortex and medulla are derived from separate germ layers. The adrenal glands, although in direct contact witht the kidneys, have different embryologic origins. Even the cortes and medulla are derived from separate germ layers. The adrenal cortex, which secretes corticosteroids and some androgenic hormones, arise from the mesoderm, while the adrenal medulla which secretes neuro hormones (epinephrine and norepinephrine) has the neuroectoderm as its source. The adrenal glands also secrete androgens. Adrenal hyperplasia during gestation can cause masculinization of the female foetus because of the increased amounts of androgens secreted.

During the first half of pregnancy the foetal adrenal glands are large but they decrease in size as term approaches. Foetal adrenal function may be vital to maintenance of the pregnancy through the active production of steroids. Foetal lung maturity is accelerated by increased foetal steroid production, which occurs during pregnancies complicated by hypertension or pre-eclampsia and also during labour. Development of the foetal adrenals depends on a functoning hypothalamic pituitary axis. A foetus with major defects in cerebral development, such as an encephaly, also has adrenal hypoplasia.

Reproductive Development and Function

The reproductive system develops along with the urinary system. Testes develop in the foetal abdomen can be recognized after 7 weeks of gestation. By week 30 of gestation, testes begin to descend through the inguinal canal into the scrotum. Ovaries develop in the abdomen and remain in the pelvic cavity.

Sexual development continuous throughout gestation as the external genitalia change in appearance.

Bony Pelvis

The pelvis serves three primary purposes: (1) Its bony cavity produces a protective cradle for pelvic structures, (2) its architecture is of special importance in accommodating a growing foetus throughout pregnancy and during the birth process, and (3) its strength provides stable anchorage for the attachment of supportive muscle, fascia, and ligaments.

The following structures and landmarks of the bony pelvis are especially important

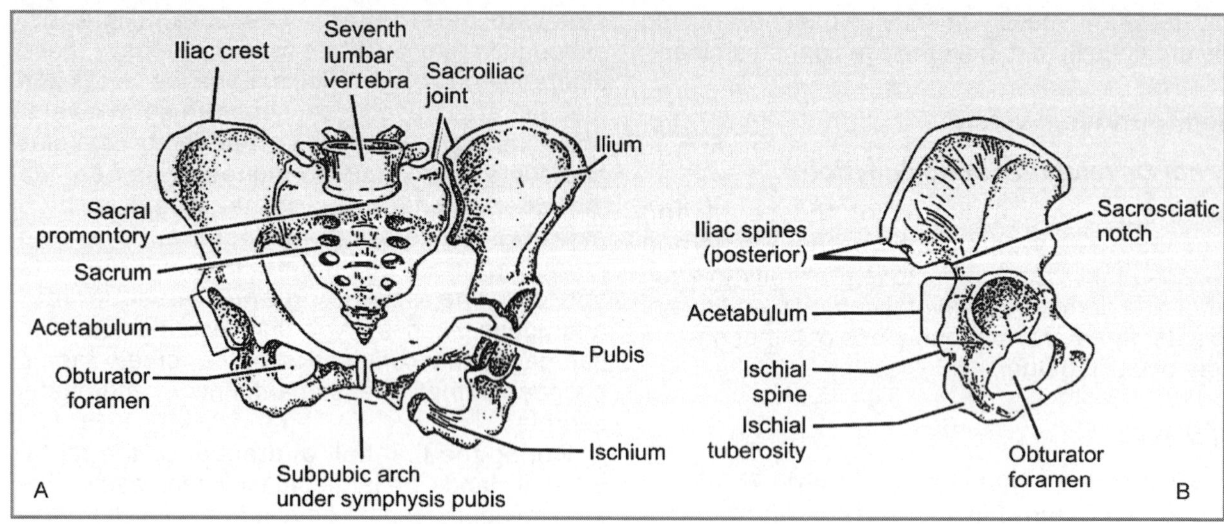

Figs 2.49A and B: Adult female pelvis. **A.** Anterior view. The three embryonic parts of the left innominate bone are lightly shaded, **B.** External view of right innominate bone (fused)

(Fig. 2.39A and B); iliac crest and superior anterior iliac spine, sacral promontory, sacrum, coccyx, symphysis pubis, subpubic arch, ischial spines and ischial tuberosities.

The pelvis (Fig. 2.50) is made of four bones; the right and left innominate bones, each of which comprises the right or left pubic bone, ilium, and ischium, which fuse after puberty, the sacrum, and the coccyx. The two innominate bones (hip bones) form the sides and front of the bony passage, and the sacrum and coccyx form the back.

Below the ilium is the ischium, a heavy bone terminating posteriorly in the rounded protuberances known as the ischial tuberosities (Fig. 2.49B). The tuberosities bear the body's weight in the sitting position. The ischial spines, the sharp projections form the posterior border of the ischium into the pelvic cavity, may be blunt or prominent.

Forming the front portion of the pelvic cavity, the pubis is located beneath the mons. In the midline the two pubic bones are joined by strong ligments and a thick cartilage to form the joint called the symphysis pubis. In the female the angle formed by the subpubic arch optimally measures slighly more than 90 degrees.

The sacrum is formed by five fused vertebrae. The upper anterior portion of the body of the first sacaral vertebra, the promontory forms the posterior margin of the pelvic brim.

The coccyx (tail bone), composed of three to five fused vertebrae, articulate with the sacrum. The coccyx projects downwards and forwards from the lower border of the sacrum.

The pelvis is divided into two sections, the shallow upper basin, or false pelvis, and the deeper lower, or true, pelvis (Fig. 2.50). The false pelvis lies above the linea terminals (brim or inlet) and varies considerably in size in different women. The true pelvis consists of the brim, or inlet and the area below.

The pelvic planes include the planes of the inlet, midpelvis, and outlet. The cavity of the (true) midpelvic resembles an irregularly curved canal (Fig. 2.50) with unequal anterior and posterior surfaces. The anterior surface is formed by the length of the symphysis. The posterior surface is formed by the length of the sacrum.

Age, gender, and race are responsible for the greatest variations in pelvic shape and size. The pelvis changes considerably during growth and development. Pelvic ossification is complete at about 20 years of age or slightly later. Smaller people have smaller, lighter bones than larger people.

Breasts

The breasts are paired mammary glands between the second and sixth ribs (Fig. 2.51A and B). About two-thirds of the breast overlies the pectoralis major muscle between the sternum and midaxillary line, with an extension to the axilla referred to as the *tail of spence*. The lower one-

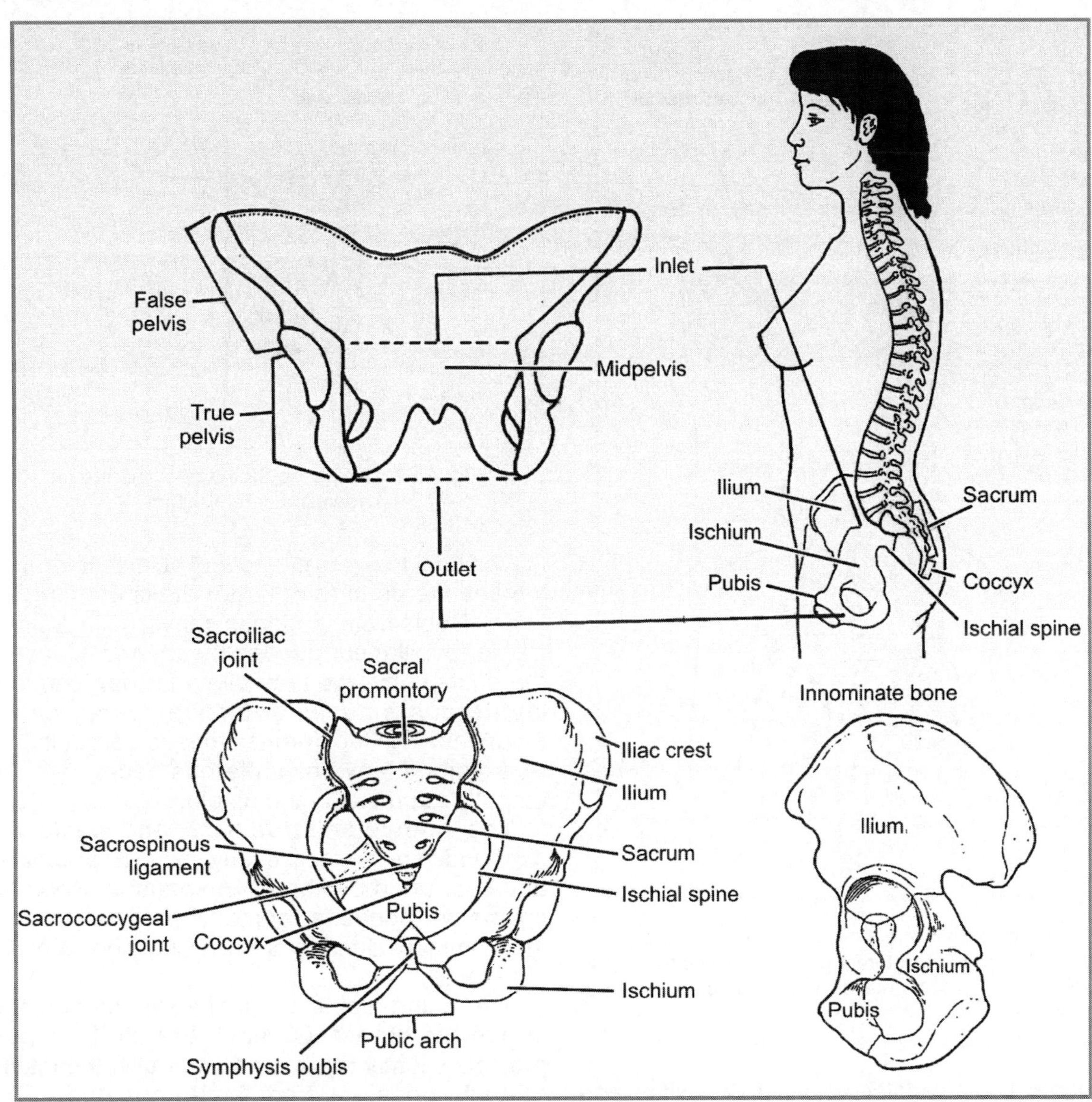

Fig. 2.50: Bony pelvis

third of the breast overlies the serratus anterior muscle. The breasts are attached to the muscles by connective tissue or fascia.

The breasts of healthy mature women are approximately equal in size and shape but are often not absolutely symmetric. The size and shape depending on the woman's age, heredity, and nutrition. However, the contour should be smooth with no retractions, dimpling or masses.

True glandular tissue is called parenchyma, supporting tissues, the fat, and fibrous connective tissue are called stroma. The relative amount of stroma determines the size and consistency of the breast.

Oestrogen stimulates growth of the breast by inducing fat deposition in the breasts, development of stromal tissue (that is, increase in its amount and elasticity), and growth of the extensive ductile system, oestrogen also increases the vascularity of breast tissue.

Once ovulation begins in puberty, progesterone levels increase. The increase in progesterone levels causes maturation of mammary gland tissue, specifically the lobules and acinar

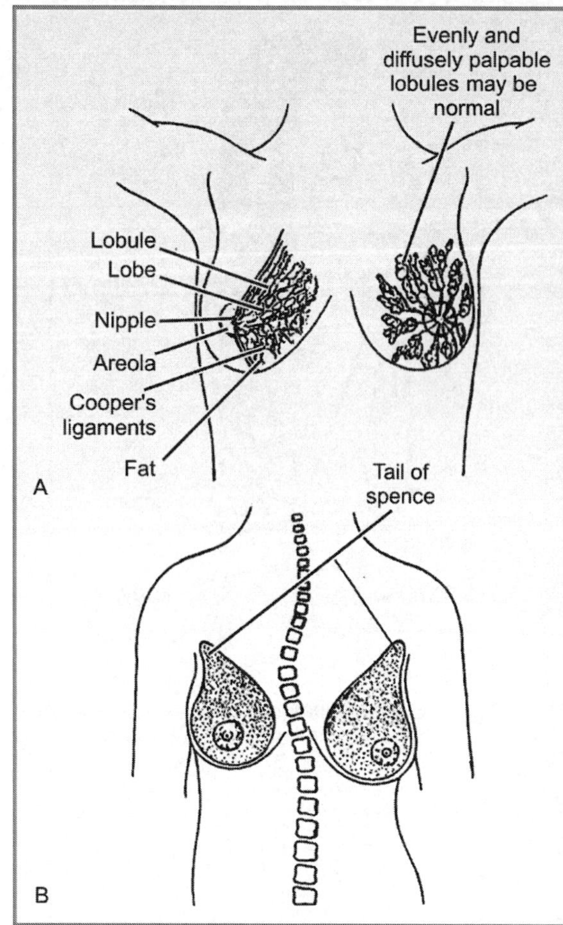

Figs 2.51A and B: Female breast anatomy. **A.** Internal tissues and support structures, **B.** Tail of spence extends to support axilla. Note normal asymmetry of breasts due to scoliosis

structures. During adolescence, fat deposition and growth of fibrous tissue contribute to the increase in the size of the gland. Full development of the breast is not achieved until after the end of the first pregnancy or in the early period of lactation.

Each mammary gland is made of 15 to 20 lobes divided into lobules. Lobules are clusters of acini. An acinus is a sacline terminal part of a component gland emptying through a narrow lumen or duct. In discussions of mammary glands the correct anatomic term (*Acinus*), is often used interchangeably with alveolus. The acini are lined with epithelial cells that secrete colostrum and milk. Just below the epithelium is the myoepithelium (myo, or muscle). Which contracts to expel milk from the acini (Figs 2.52 and 2.53).

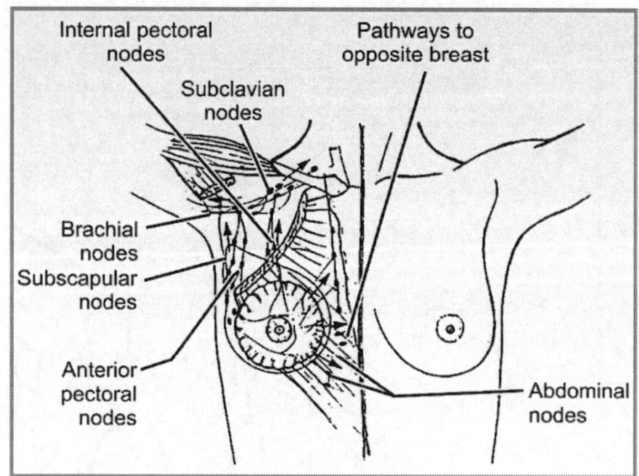

Fig. 2.52: Lymphatic drainage of the breast. Arrows indicate direction

The duct from the clusters of acini that form the lobules merge to form larger ducts draining the lobes. Ducts from the lobes converge in a single nipple (papilla) surrounded by an areola. Just as the ducts converge they dilate to form common lactiferous sinuses, which are also called ampullae. The lactiferous sinuses serve as milk reservoirs. Many tiny latiferous ducts drain the ampullae and exit in the nipple.

The glandular structures and ducts are surrounded by protective fatty tissue and separted and supported by fibrous suspensory Cooper's ligaments. Cooper's ligaments provide suport to the mammary glands while allowing mobility on the chest wall.

The round nipple is usually slightly elevated above the breast. On each breast the nipple projects slightly upward and laterally. It contains 15 to 20 openings from lactiferous ducts. The nipple (mammary papilla) is surrounded by fibromuscular tissue and covered by wrinkled skin. Except during pregnancy and lactation, there is usually no discharge from the nipple.

The nipple and surrounding areola are usually more deeply pigmented than the skin of the breast. The rough appearance of the areola is caused by sebaceous glands. Montgomery tubercles (Fig. 2.53) located directly beneath the skin. These glands secrete a fatty substance thought to lubricate the nipple. Smooth muscle fibres in the areola contract to stiffen the nipple, making grasping easier for the infant during breastfeeding. Sexual stimulation can also cause the nipple to become erect.

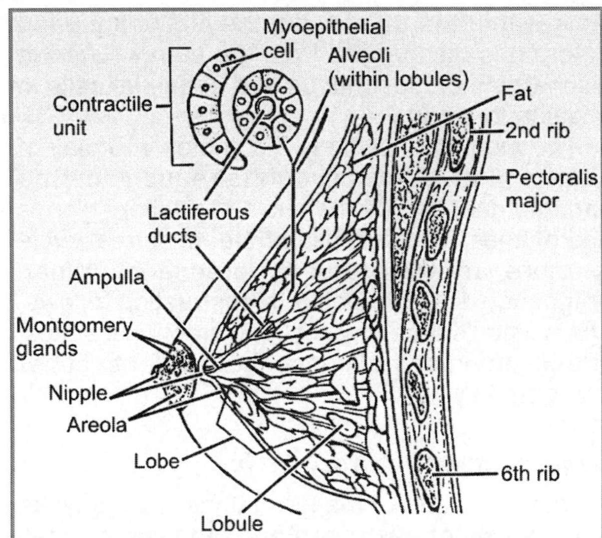

Fig. 2.53: The breast, or mammary gland, has 15 to 25 lobes: Lobes radiate from the areola like a wheel, cushioned by varying amounts of fat, under hormonal influence the alveoli secrete milk

The vascular supply to the mammary gland is abundant. In the nonpregnant state, the skin may not have an obvious vascular pattern and is smooth without tightness or shineness. During pregnancy, the skin of the breasts displays increased vascularity. As breast tissue increases, the skin becomes stretched and tight as the breasts become fuller.

The skin covering the breasts contain an extensive superficial lymphatic network that serves the entire chest wall and is continuous with the superficial lymphatics of the neck and abdomen. In the deeper portions of the breasts the lymphatics also form a rich network. The primary deep lymphatic pathway drains laterally towards the axillae.

Besides their function fo lactation, breasts function as organs for sexual arousal in the mature adult.

Breasts change in size and nodularity In response to cyclic ovarian changes throughout reproductive life. Increasing levels of oestrogen and progesterone 3 to 4 days before menstruation increase vascularity of the breasts, induce growth of the ducts and acini, and promote water ratention. The epithelial cells lining the ducts proliferate, the ducts dilate, and the lobules distend. The acini become enlarged and secretory, and lipid (fat) is deposited in their epithelial cell lining. As a result, breast swelling tenderness, and discomfort are common just before the onset of menstruation. After menstruation, cellular proliferation regresses, the size of acini decrease, and retained water is lost.

After breasts have undergone changes numerous times in response to the ovarian cycle, the proliferation and involution (regression) are not uniform throughout the breast. In time, after repeated hormonal stimulation, small persistent areas of nodulation may develop. This normal physiologic change must be considered when breast tissue is examined. Nodules may develop just before and during menstruation times when the breast is most active. The physiologic alterations in breast size and activity reach their minimal level about 5 to 7 days after menstruation stops. Therefore breast self examination is best carried but during this phase of the menstrual cycle.

Physiology of Menstrual Cycle

Knowledge of the menstrual cycle is important for nurses providing care to women across the life span. Menstrual myths, menarche, the endometrial cycle, the hypothalamic-pituitary cycle, the ovarian cycle, other cyclic changes, and the climacterium are discussed in the following section.

Menstrual Myths

Many myths have their origin in the mystery that surrounded the woman, her hidden reproductive organs, and her uniqueness in adding new members to society. Consequently, a vast store of folklore, fancies, and superstitions has evolved. Because of their recurrence and similar sequence, menstrual cycles were thought to be under the control of the moon. Before the discovery of ovulation in humans, an egg was thought to be produced during menstruation only when fruitful intercourse had occurred. Knowledge about the existence of the human egg, ovulation, and ovarian functioning was not attained until the nineteenth century.

As late as the second-half of this century the many behavioural changes falsely attributed to women during their menstrual cycles have been used to question women's capabilities. Historical literature contains many references to dangers attributed to menstruating women. If a menstruating woman walked through a farmer's fields, the crops would not grow and the flowers would wilt; if she tried to bake bread, the dough would not rise. The danger also existed for her husband, physical contact, especially sexual intercourse, was and in some places still is prohibited. In many cultures the menstruating woman is kept in a separate menstrual hut or in separate quarters. After a ritualized "cleansing" the woman returns to her place in her family.

Menarche

Although young secretes well, rather constant amounts of oestrogen, a marked increase occurs between 8 and 11 years of age. Moreover increasing amounts and variations in gonadotropin and oestrogen secretion develop into a cycle pattern at least a year before menarche or the first menstrual period. This occurs in most girls in India about 13 years of age (with the range of onset being 10 to 16 years of age).

Initially periods are irregular, unpredictable, painless, and an ovulatory in the majority of young girls. After one or more years a hypothalamic-pituitary rhythm develops and adequate cyclic oestrogen is produced by the ovary to produce mature ova. Ovulatory periods tend to be regular. In some women, ovulatory periods are associated with dysmenorrhoea (painful uterine cramping), which may be an effect of production of progesterone, prostaglandins, or both. This discomfort is rarely serious and is readily relieved by heat, exercise, or simple analgesics. This slight cramping may be heat, exercise, or simple analgesics. This slight cramping may be reassuring to the girl and her parents as an indication of normal ovulatory function.

Although pregnancy may occur in exceptional cases of true (constitutional) precocious puberty, most pregnancies in young girls occur well after the normally timed menarche. All girls can benefit from knowing that pregnancy can occur at any time after the onset of menses.

Menstruation is periodic uterine bleeding that begins approximately 14 days after ovulation. The first day of the cycle is the first day of bleeding or menses. The average duration of menstrual flow is 5 days (range of 3 to 6 days), and the average blood loss is approximately 50 ml (range of 20 to 80 ml), but great variation exists.

For about 50 per cent of women, menstrual blood does not appear to clot. The menstrual blood clots within the uterus, but the clot is liquefied before it is discharged from the uterus. Uterine discharge includes mucus and epithelial cells in addition to blood.

The menstrual cycle is a complex interplay of events that occur simulataneously in the endometrium, hypothalamus and pituitary glands and ovaries. The purpose of the menstrual cycle is to prepare the uterus for pregnancy. When pregnancy does not occur, menstruation follows. The woman's age, physical and emotional status, and environment influence the regularity of her menstrual cycles.

Hypothalamic Pituitary Cycle

Towards the end of the normal menstrual cycle, blood levels of oestrogen and progesterone fall (Fig. 2.54). Low blood levels of these ovarian hormones stimulate the hypothalamus to secrete gonadotropin releasing hormone (Gn-RH). Gn-RH in turn stimulates anterior pituitary secretion of follicle stimulating hormone (FSH). FSH stimulates development of ovarian graafian follicles and their production of oestrogen. Oestrogen levels begin to fall, and hypothalamic Gn-RH triggers the anterior pituitary release of luteinizing hormone (LH). A marked surge of LH and a smaller peak of oestrogen on day 12 (Fig. 2.55) precede the expulsion of the ovum from the ovarian follicle by about 24 to 36 hours. LH peaks about the thirteenth or fourteenth day of a 28 day cycle. If fertilization and implantation of the ovum have not occurred by this time, regression of the corpus luteum follows. Therefore, the levels of progesterone and oestrogen decline, menstruation occurs, and the hypothalamus is once again stimulated to secrete Gn-RH. This is called the hypothalamic-pituitary cycle (Fig. 2.55).

Ovarian Cycle

The primitive graafian follicles contain immature oocytes or primordial ova. Before ovulation, 1 to 30 follicles begin to mature in each ovary under the influence of FSH and oestrogen. The preovulatory surge of LH affects a selected follicle. Within the chosen follicle, the oocyte matures, ovulation occurs, and the ovum is released. After ovulation, the empty follicle begins its transformation into the corpus luteum. This follicular phase or preovulatory phase (Fig. 2.55) of the ovarian menstrual cycle varies in length

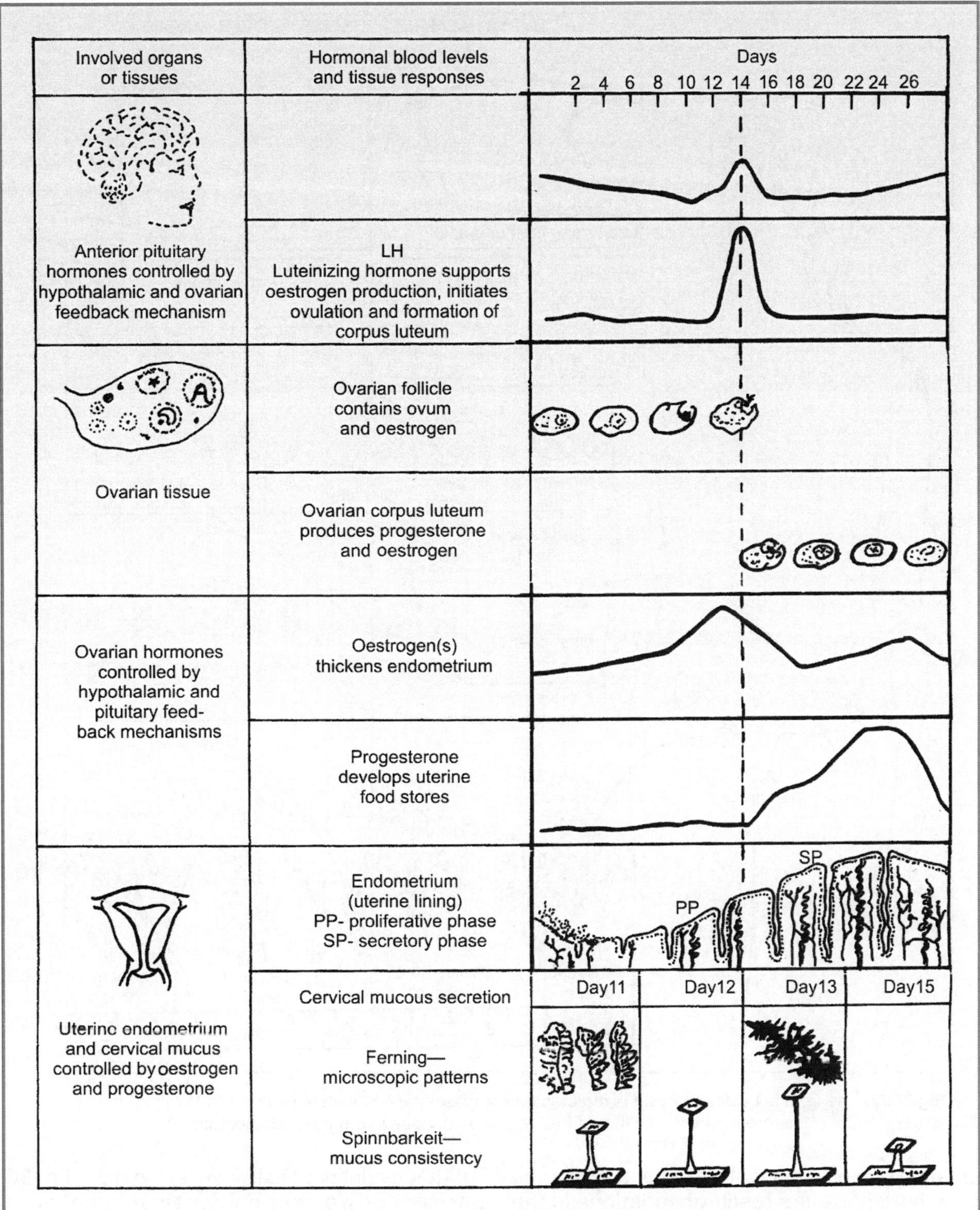

Fig. 2.54: Normal menstrual cycle schematically depicted to highlight hormone production, ovulation, endometrial response, and changes in cervical mucus

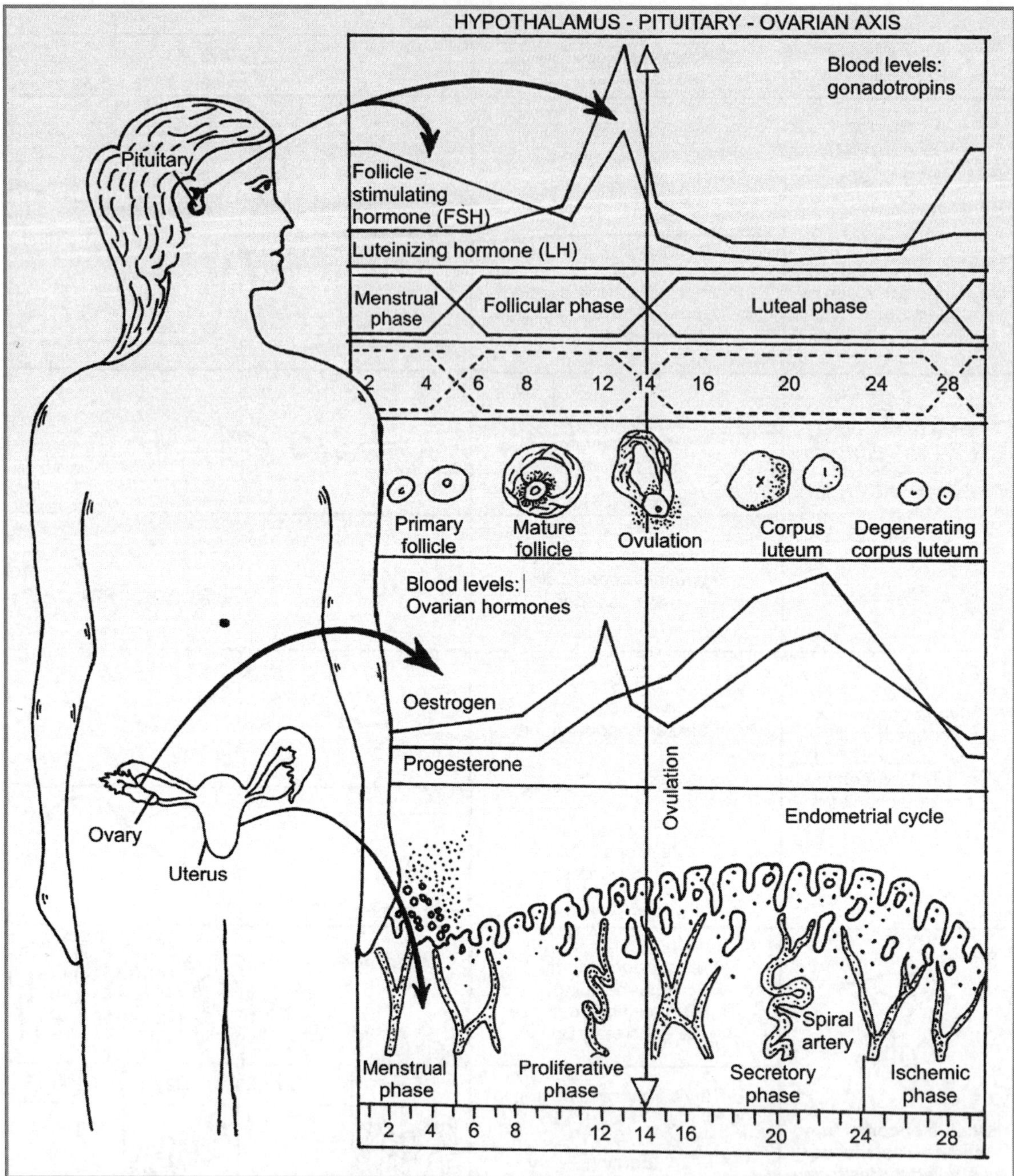

Fig. 2.55: The female ovulatory cycle is directed by complex inter-relationships between levels of hormone, secretion, development of follicles, and changes in uterine endometrium

among women. Almost all variations in ovarian cycle length are the result of variations in the length of the follicular phase. On rare occasions (approximately 1 in 100 menstrual cycles), more than one follicle is selected and more than one oocyte matures and undergoes ovulation.

After ovulation, oestrogen levels drop. For 90 per cent of women, only a small amount of withdrawal bleeding occurs, so this event usually is unnoticed. In 10 per cent of women, bleeding is visible, resulting in what is known as midcycle bleeding.

The luteal phase begins immediately after ovulation and ends with the start of menstruation. This post-ovulatory phase of the ovarian cycle usually requires 14 days (range of 13 to 15 days). The corpus luteum reaches its peak of functional activity 8 days after ovulation, secreting both of the steroids oestrogen and progesterone. Coincident with this time of peak luteal functioning, the fertilized egg is implanted in the endometrium. If no implantation occurs, the corpus luteum regressed and steroid levels drop. If fertilization and implantation do not occur, the functional layer of the uterine endometrium is shed through menstruation 2 weeks after ovulation.

Endometrial Cycle

The four phases of the endometrial cycles are (1) menstrual, (2) proliferative, (3) secretory, (4) ischaemic (Fig. 2.55). During the menstrual phase, shedding of the functional two-thirds of the endometrium (the compact and spongy layers) is initiated by periodic vasoconstriction of spiral arterioles in the upper layers of the endometrium. The basal layer is always retained, and regeneration begins near the end of cycle from cells derived from the remaining glandular remanants or stromal cells in the basal layer.

The proliferative phase is a period of rapid growth that extends from about the fifth day to the time of ovulation (for example, day 10 of a 24-day cycle, day 14 of a 28-day cycle, or day 18 of a 32-day cycle). The endometrial surface is completely restored in approximately 4 days or slightly before bleeding cases. From this point an eightfold to tenfold thickening occurs, with a levelling off growth at ovulation. The proliferative phase depends on oestrogen stimulation derived from ovarian follicles.

The secretory phase lasts form the day of ovulation to about 3 days before the next menstrual period. After ovulation, larger amounts of progesterone are produced. An edematous, vascular, functional endometrium is now apparent.

At the end of the secretory phase the fully matured secretory endometrium reaches the thickness of heavy, soft velvet. It becomes luxuriant with blood and glandular secretions, a suitable protective and nutritive bed for a fertilized ovum.

Implantation (nidation) of the fertilized ovum generally occurs about 7 to 10 days after ovulation. If fertilization and implantation do not occur, the corpus luteum (yellow body), which secretes oestrogen and progesterone, regresses. With the rapid fall in progesterone and oestrogen levels, the spiral arteries go into a spasm. During the ischemic phase the blood supply to the functional endometrium is blocked and necrosis develops. The functional layer separates from the basal layer, and menstrual bleeding begins, marking day 1 of the next cycle.

Other Cyclic Changes

When the hypothalmic-pituitary-ovarian axis functions properly, other tissues undergo predictable responses. Before ovulation the woman's basal body temperature (BBT) is lower, often below 98.6° F (37°C) after ovulation, with rising progesterone levels, her BBT rises. Changes in the cervix and cervical muscus follows a generally predictable pattern (Table 2.3). Preovulatory and postovulatory mucus is viscous (sticky), and sperm penetration is discouraged. At the time of ovulation, cervical mucus is thin and clear. It looks, feels, and stretches like egg white. This stretchable quality is termed spinnbarkeit. Some women experience localized lower abdominal pain called mittelschmerz that coincides with ovulation.

These and other cyclic changes enhance fertility awareness and form the basis for the symptothermal method used for conception and contraception. The subjective and objective signs are biologic markers of the phases of the menstrual cycle (Table 2.3).

Examination of women with impaired fertility includes a through documentation of the presence or absence of these biologic markers.

Prostaglandins

Prostaglandins (PGs) are oxygenated fatty acids now classified as hormones. The different kinds of PGs are distinguished by letters (PGE, PGF), numbers (PGE_2) and letters of the Greek alphabet ($PGF_{2\alpha}$).

PGs are produced in most organs of the body but most notably by the prostate and endometrium. Therefore semen and menstrual blood are potent PG sources. PGs are metabolized quickly by most tissues. They are biologically acitive in minute amounts in the cardiovascular, gastrointestinal, respiratory, urogenital, and nervous

Table 2.3: Signs and symptoms of the phases of the menstrual cycles

Sign	*Preovulation*	*Ovulation*	*At least 2 days after ovulation upto menses*
Subjective signs			
Physical Discomfort			
Breasts	Unreported	Unreported	Heaviness, fullness enlarged and tender
Abdomen	Dysmenorrhoea, Uterine cramping; nausea,vomiting and diarrhoea, dizziness	Instrumental pain (mittle-schmerz) occurring 1-7 days after peak of cervical mucus and 2-5 days before increase in BBT	Premenstrual syndrome backaches, feeling of increasing pelvic fullness
General	Increased weight, feeling of heaviness	Unreported	Headache, acne
Affective changes			
Moods	Some depression possibly persisting from premenses	Sense of well-being	Premenstrual syndrome (PMS); increased irritability, passivity, depression
Libido	Unreported	Increased sexual desire	Unreported
Energy levels	Unreported	Unreported	Spurt of energy followed by fatigue
Objective signs			
BBT	Individualized, often below 98.6° F (37°C)	Slight drop in BBT	Rise of about 0.4° to 0.8° F (0.2° to 0.4° C)
Respiration	Unreported	Unreported	Hyperventilation with decrease in alveolar pCO_2
Heart rate	Unreported	Unreported	Increased slightly
Breasts	Time of least hormonal effect and smallest breast size	Increased nipple erectility, increased areolar pigmentation	Increased nodularity
Cervix	"Dry" (no mucus) progressing to viscous, opaque; no ferning	A bundant, thin, clear (egg-white) mucus with spinnbarkeit (4 cm, often upto 10 cm) that dries in a fern pattern (arborization), facilitation of sperm transport	Cloudy, sticky, impenetrable to sperm; drying in granular pattern (no ferning)
Mucus pH	About 7.0	7.5	Unreported
Os	Gradual, progressive widening	Open, with mucus seen spilling out	Gradual closing of Os
Colour of ecto-cervix	Pink	Hyperemic (red)	Gradual return to pink
Body	Firm to touch (like tip of nose)	Soft (like earlobe)	Gradual return to firm

systems. They also exert a marked effect on metabolism, particularly on glycolysis. PGs play an important role in many physiologic, pathologic, and pharmacologic reactions. PGF2, RPGE1 and PGE2 are most commonly used in reproductive medicine.

PGs affect smooth muscle contractility and modulation of hormonal activity. Indirect evidence supports their effects on ovulation, fertility changes in the cervix and cervical mucus that affect receptivity to sperm, tubal and uterine motility, sloughing off endometrium (menstruation), onset of abortion (spontaneous and induced), and onset of labour (term and pre-term) After exerting their biologic actions, new synthesized PGs are rapidly metabolized by tissues in organs such as the lungs kidneys and liver.

PGs may play a key role in ovulation. If PG levels do not rise along with the surge of LH, the ovum remains trapped within the graafian follicle. After ovulation, PGs may influence production of oestrogen and progesterone by the corpus luteum.

The introduction of PGs into the vagina or uterine cavity (from ejaculated semen) increased the motility of uterine musculature, which may assist the transport, of sperm through the uterus and into the oviduct. A high concentration of PGs in the semen may be necessary for normal fertility in males.

PGs produced by the woman cause regression of the corpus luteum, regression of the endometrium, and sloughing off the endometrium, which results in menstruation. PGs increase myometrial response to oxytocic stimulation, enhance uterine contractions, and cause cervical dilatation PGE2, PGF2?, or both may be factors in initiating or maintaining labour. In addition, PGE may be involved in the following pathologic states; male infertility, dysmenorrhoea, premenstrual syndrome, hypertensive states pre-eclampsia-eclampsia, and anaphylactic shock.

Climacterium

The climacterium (perimenopause) is a transitional phase during which ovarian function and hormone production decline. This phase spans the years from the onset of premenopausal ovarian decline to the postmenopausal time when symptoms stop. Menopause (from the Latin MENTS, "month, "and the Greek PAUSIS, "to cease") refers only to the last menstrual period. However, unlike menarche, menopause can be dated with certainty only at one year after menstruation ceases. The average age at natural menopause is 51.4 years with an age range of 35 to 60 years.

URINARY SYSTEM

Urinary system has some links with the reproductive system, it is better to have brief knowledge of the same.

The Kidney

The kidneys are situated in the posterior part of the abdomen on each side of the vertebral column, behind the peritoneum. They extend from approximately the 12th thoracic vertebra above to the third lumbar vertebra below. The right kidney is usually slightly lower than the left, probably due to the considerable amount of space occupied by the liver.

The kidneys are described as bean-shaped organs and are approximately 10.5 cm in length, 5 to 7.5 cm in width, and 2.5 to 3.5 cm thick. They are embedded and held in position by a mass of adipose tissue termed the renal fat.

Relations of organs in association with the kidneys (Fig. 2.56).

The Right Kidney

Superiorly: The right suprarenal gland which rests on the upper border of the kidney.

Anteriorly: The right lobe of the liver lies in front of the lateral border of the kidney. The duodenum is in contact with the medial border of the kidney. The right colic flexure is in contact with the part of the anterior surface of the kidney.

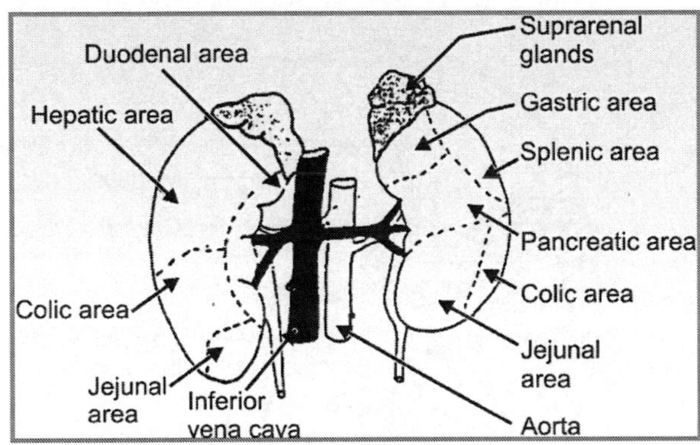

Fig. 2.56: Impressions on the kidneys of related organs

Posteriorly: The right kidney lies upon the diaphragm and the muscles of the posterior abdominal wall.

The Left Kidney

Superiorly: The left suprarenal gland lies on its upper border.

Anteriorly: The upper two-thirds of the lateral aspect is related to the spleen and medial to this is the stomach. the middle of the anterior surface is occupied by the pancreas and its blood vessels; below this area the jejunum and the left colic flexure of the large intestine are in contact with the kidney.

Posteriorly: The organs in association with the left kidney are the same as for the right kidney, that is, the diaphragm and the muscles of the posterior abdominal wall.

Gross Structure of the Kidney (Fig. 2.57)

The kidneys are enclosed in a capsule of fibrous tissue which can be easily stripped off. Underlying the capsule is the cortex of the kidney, reddish-brown in colour. Internal to the cortex is the medulla. The medullary substance is made up of pale conical striations known as the renal pyramids. Medial to the medulla is a concave fissure which is known as the hilum of the kidney. At the hilum, the renal artery and nerves enter the kidney and the renal vein leaves the kidney. It is here also that the expanded part of the ureter known as the pelvis leaves the kidney.

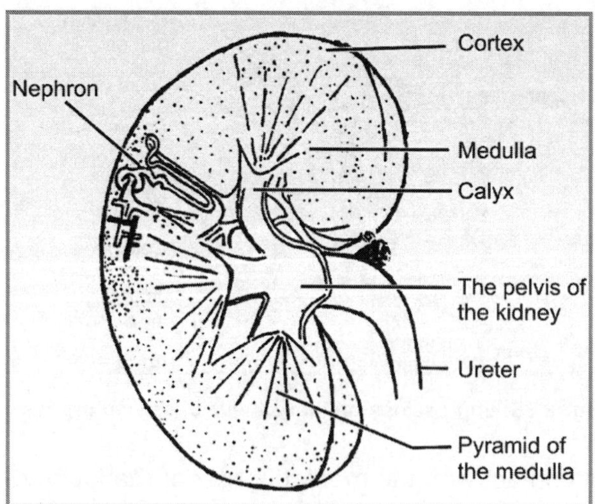

Fig. 2.57: Cross section of kidney showing component parts and one nephron

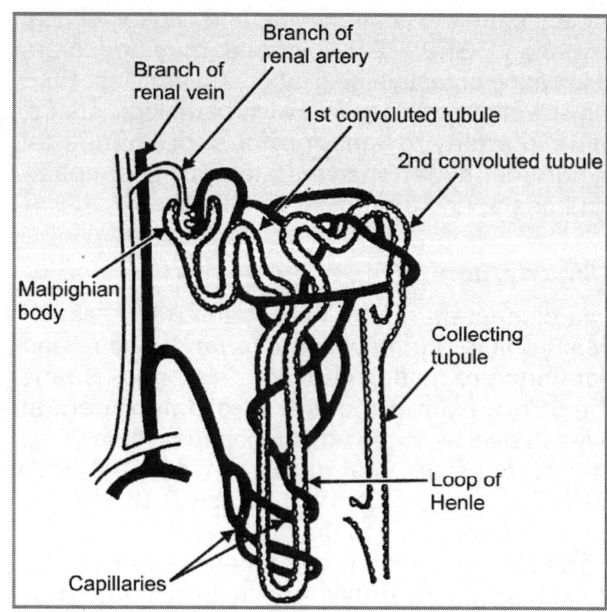

Fig. 2.58A: A nephron

Beyond the hilum is central cavity known as the renal sinus. The blood vessels and the pelvis of the ureter are within the renal sinus. The pelvis of the ureter divides into two or three branches called large calyces. The large calyces divide into smaller branches—small calyces. The apices of the renal pyramids converge towards the small calyces where they form prominent papillae which project into the small calyces.

Blood Supply

The kidneys receive their arterial supply from the renal arteries which are branches of the abdominal aorta.

The venous drainage is through the renal veins. The right renal vein drains into the inferior vena cava. The left drains into the vena azygos.

Microscopic Structure of the Kidneys

The kidney substance is composed of a large number of minute microscopic structures known as nephrons and collecting tubules. The nephrons are the functioning unit of the kidney (Fig. 2.58A). Just before the renal artery enters the kidney it breaks up into smaller arteries which pass into the hilum of the kidney. These arteries traverse the kidney substance breaking up into smaller and smaller branches finally becoming arterioles in the cortex. Each arteriole is now described as an afferent vessel. This afferent vessel entwines itself within a cup-shaped structure known as the glomerular or Bowman's capsule. The entwined vessel within the capsule forms a tuft of blood vessel which is termed the glomerulus. The blood vessel leading away from the glomerulus is known as the efferent vessel. Continuing from each glomerular capsule is the renal tubule which is divided into three parts:

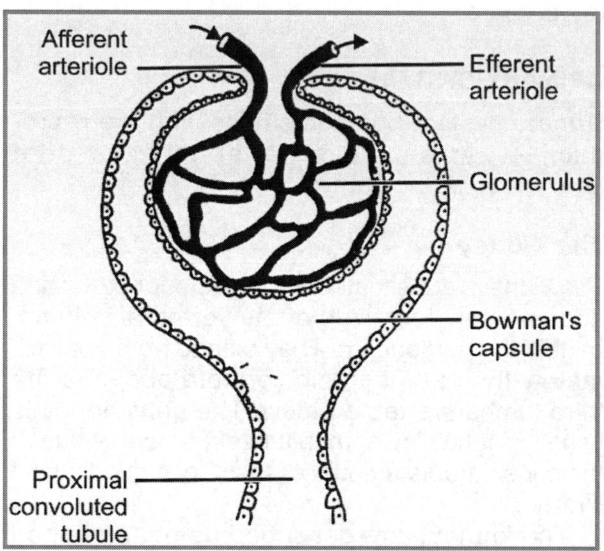

Fig. 2.58B: Malpighian body magnified

a. The proximal convoluted tubule
b. The loop of Henle
c. The distal convoluted tubule.

The Bowman's capsule, proximal convoluted tubule, loop of Henle and the distal tubule, all form the functional unit or nephron of the kidney. The distal convoluted tubule opens into a collecting tubule which with others forms the medullary substance of the kidney, giving it a striated appearance.

Structure of a Nephron and Malpighian Body (Figs 2.58A and B)

The glomerulus is made up a single layer of flattened epithelial cells. The glomerular or Bowman's capsule is also made up of a single layer of flattened epithelial cells.

The proximal and distal convoluted tubules are formed by cells somewhat columnar in shape. Some of the cells forming the loop of Henle are flattened and some are columnar in shape. The nephrons are supported by connective tissue known as the interstitial tissue. The efferent vessel which is smaller in calibre than the afferent vessel entwines itself round the tubules in a network of capillaries and, having given its oxygen into these structures, eventually forms venous capillaries which join capillaries from other nephrons to form the renal vein which empties into the inferior vena cava.

Functions of the Kidney

The kidneys are important to the health of the human body. Their function is to form urine and pass the urine to the ureters and urinary bladder for excretion. In doing this, other vital body functions are carried out.

Maintenance of water balance: The kidneys excrete water, thus maintaining the water balance of the body. If a large quantity of water is taken and the individual is not sweating noticeably then more urine is excreted. On the other hand if hardly any fluid is taken, the urinary output is less and the urine is usually darker in colour. Again in hot weather when one tends to lose fluid by perspiration, less urine is excreted. The reverse happens in cold weather that is more urine is excreted because one hardly perspires in cold weather.

Regulation of the acidity and alkalinity of the blood and other body fluids: The kidneys are responsible for maintaining the acid-base balance of body fluids because they are the route by which inorganic cat–ions such as sodium and potassium, and anions such as chloride and sulphate are excreted. In this regard the most importantions concerned in the regulation of the acidity or alkalinity of the blood and body fluids are the H+ (hydrogen ion) and OH-(hydroxy ion).

Excretion of toxins and drugs: The waste products of many of the drugs we take are excreted by the kidneys. The kidney, through some chemical processes, sometimes helps to maintain normal arterial blood pressure. As referred to above, an important function of the kidneys is the formation of urine.

Formation of urine: Urine is formed by the nephrons of the kidney. The process of urine formation occurs: 1.by simple filtration; 2.by selective re-absorption.

Simple filtration: Simple filtration takes place between the glomerulus and Bowman's capsule. The pressure in the glomerulus is higher than that of the capsule; thus substances pass from the area of higher pressure to the area of lower pressure through semi-permeable membranes. Most substances and components of the blood except the red blood cells, white blood cells and plasma proteins are filtered through.

Selection and reabsorption: Selection and re-absorption of substances in order to maintain alkalinity of the blood takes place in the convoluted tubules. The selection and re-absorption consists of the return to the capillaries of substances which the body cannot afford to lose. Examples of these are glucose, fatty acids, amino acids and hormones. Water, urea, uric acid and some salts remain in the tubule.

Water Balance

Regulation of the water balance is due to the ability of the tubule and the loop of Henle to return water to the capillary network. If the kidneys excreted all the water filtered into the tubules, dehydration would result. Anti diuretic hormone, secreted by the posterior pituitary gland, controls the amount of water re-absorbed.

The Ureters

These are two tubes which convey the urine from the kidneys to the urinary bladder. Each ureter measures 25-30 cm. It commences from the pelvis of the kidney, passes downwards through the abdominal cavity behind the peritoneum and in front of the psoas muscle into the pelvic cavity. Here it opens into the posterior aspects of the urinary bladder. The ureter passes obliquely through the bladder wall. In this way, when the bladder is distended with urine, the walls of the ureters are pressed together thus preventing regurgitation of urine.

The ureters are composed of :

i. An outer coat of fibrous tissue continuous with the fibrous capsule of the kidney;
ii. A middle muscular coat, consisting of involuntary muscle fibres disposed of in two layers of outer longitudinal muscle fibres and inner circular muscle fibres;
iii. An inner lining of mucous membrane covered with transitional epithelium.

The function of the ureters is to propel the urine from the kidney into the bladder. The driving force consists of waves of rhythmic contractions (peristalsis) which force the urine downwards.

The Female Bladder

The bladder is a muscular distensible organ which acts as a reservoir for urine. It is a pelvic organ with a capacity of 500 ml, but it could contain more urine under pathological conditions. When the bladder is over distended, it becomes an abdominal organ. When empty, the bladder is almost pyramidal in shape.

Structure (Fig. 2.59)

The bladder consists of:

a. An upper surface over which is the utero vesical pouch;
b. The side walls which rest on the levator ani muscles;
c. The base or trigone which is the sensitive portion of the bladder and is adjacent to the upper half of the vagina. It is triangular in shape with the base directed upwards. The two lateral angles at the base consists of the ureteric orifices while the apex is occupied by the urethral orifice.

The walls of the bladder consist of the following, starting from inside outwards:

i. A lining of transitional epithelium thrown into called rugae. The rugae allow for the distension of the bladder and are absent at the trigone.

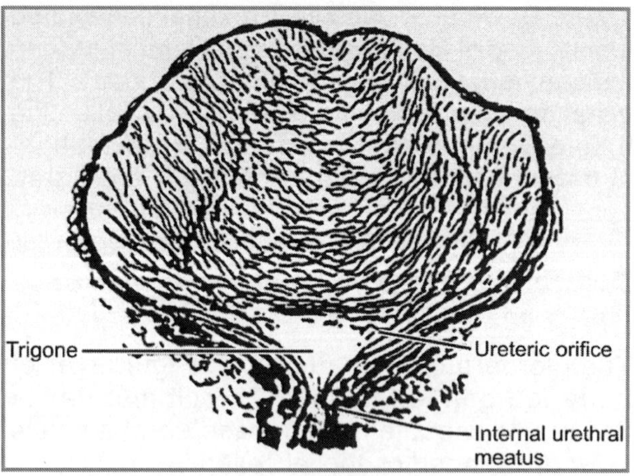

Fig. 2.59: Dissection of the bladder showing trigone, the ureteric orifices and the internal urethral meatus

ii. A layer of areolar tissue on which rests the epithelial lining.
iii. The muscle coat, known as the detrusor muscle. It helps inthe expulsion of urine. It is a smooth muscle with the fibres arranged in three layers, namely: the inner longitudinal, the middle circular and the outer longitudinal layers. Some of the circular fibres become thickened around the internal urethral meatus to form the internal sphincter of the bladder.

The muscular arrangement at the trigone is different. The muscle fibres between the ureteric orifices fold into a band called the Mercier's bar and the fibres between the ureteric orifices and the internal urethral meatus also form folds called Bell's muscles. Bell's muscles pull open the internal meatus during micturition. The outer surface of the bladder is covered by the pelvic facia except at the upper surface which is covered by peritoneum.

The Urethra

The urethra is a narrow tube about 3.5 cm long, which lies along the lower half of the anterior vaginal wall. It opens onto the vestibule 2.5 cm below the clitoris from the internal meatus of the bladder.

Structure of the urethra from within outwards: The upper half of the urethra is lined by transitional epithelium and the lower half by the squamous epithelium. These rest on vascular connective tissues. The muscle coat is thickened where it leaves the bladder to form the internal urethral sphincter. The fibres are arranged longitudinally and circularly. The urethra is covered on the outside by the pelvic connective tissue.

Relations of the bladder and urethra: Anteriorly, the pubic bone is separated from the bladder by a space of areolar tissue known as the retropubic space or the cave of Retzius. The retropubic space allows the bladder to fill and empty without hindrance. A dense plexus of veins (vesical plexus) lies in the areolar tissue in front of the bladder and separates it from the retropubic space.

Posteriorly the bladder is related to the cervix. The ureters pass laterally on either side of the bladder to enter the trigone. There is also the anterior wall of the vagina to which the base of the bladder and the urethra are related.

The lateral relations of the bladder are the retropubic space and the pelvic side walls. Superiorly is the body of the uterus. Inferiorly is the urethra which opens into the vestibule.

Blood Supply

Arteries: The superior and inferior vesical arteries supply the bladder and urethra. In addition the pudendal artery supplies a part of the urethra.

Veins: The veins drain into the vesical plexus and from there into the internal iliac veins.

Lymphatic drainage: The lymphatic drainage of the bladder is into the external iliac gland and the obturator glands. The lymphatic drainage of the urethra is into the internal iliac glands.

Nerve supply: The nerve supply is from the sympathetic and parasympathetic of the Lee-Frankenhauser's plexus. The external urethral sphincter is under voluntary control via the pudendal nerve.

HUMAN SEXUALITY

Sexuality encompasses far more than just the gender of person or sexual activity. It involves physical emotional and cultural factors and in an intrinsic part of each human being. Sexuality begins at conception, with sex determination, grows in infancy and childhood as the infant learns to relate to the people and the world around him or her, and continues until death.

The term 'sexuality' is often linked only with romance and genital activity; however, sexuality is intrinsic and influences every aspect of a person's life. The product of many factors, it impinges on a person's choice of career as well as sexual partner, friends as well as interests, and both selfperception and how that person is viewed by others. Sexuality enervates, motivates, defines, and also grows and changes with the individual person. Gender identity, sexual roles, and choice of sex partners are all parts of that on going process.

The term "Sexuality" refers to a persons perceptions, thoughts, feelings and behaviours related to sexual identity and sexual interaction with others. Expression of sexuality are not limited to sexual intercourse or coitus but include the manner in which people project themselves as sexual beings, and the way they respond to others as sexual beings.

Adult sexuality has been broadly classified as procreative and non-procreative. Procreative expressions of sexuality are associated with reproduction or child-bearing. In women, these expressions cease with menopause. Non-procreative sexuality refers to behaviours involving sexual satisfaction that are noted in persons of all ages, whether or not they involve sexual relationship with others.

Sexuality is influenced by a person's lifelong attitudes and reflects individual perceptions and behaviours related to sexual identity. Although reproductive development and function are determined genetically, reproductive patterns are influenced by perceptions of maleness and femaleness and by social and cultural norms.

HUMAN SEXUAL RESPONSE

The hypothalamas and anterior pituitary gland in females and males regulate the production of FSH and LH. The target tissue for these hormones is the gonads: an ovary or testis. In females the ovary produces ova and secretes oestrogen and progesterone and small amounts of testosterone; in males the testis produces sperm and secretes testosterone. A feedback mechanism controlling hormone secretion from the gonads, hypothalamus, and anterior pituitary aids in the control of the production of sex cells and steroid sex hormone secretion (Fig. 2.60).

Physiologic Response to Sexual Stimulation

Although the first outward appearance of maturing sexual development occurs at an earlier age in females, both females and males achieve physical

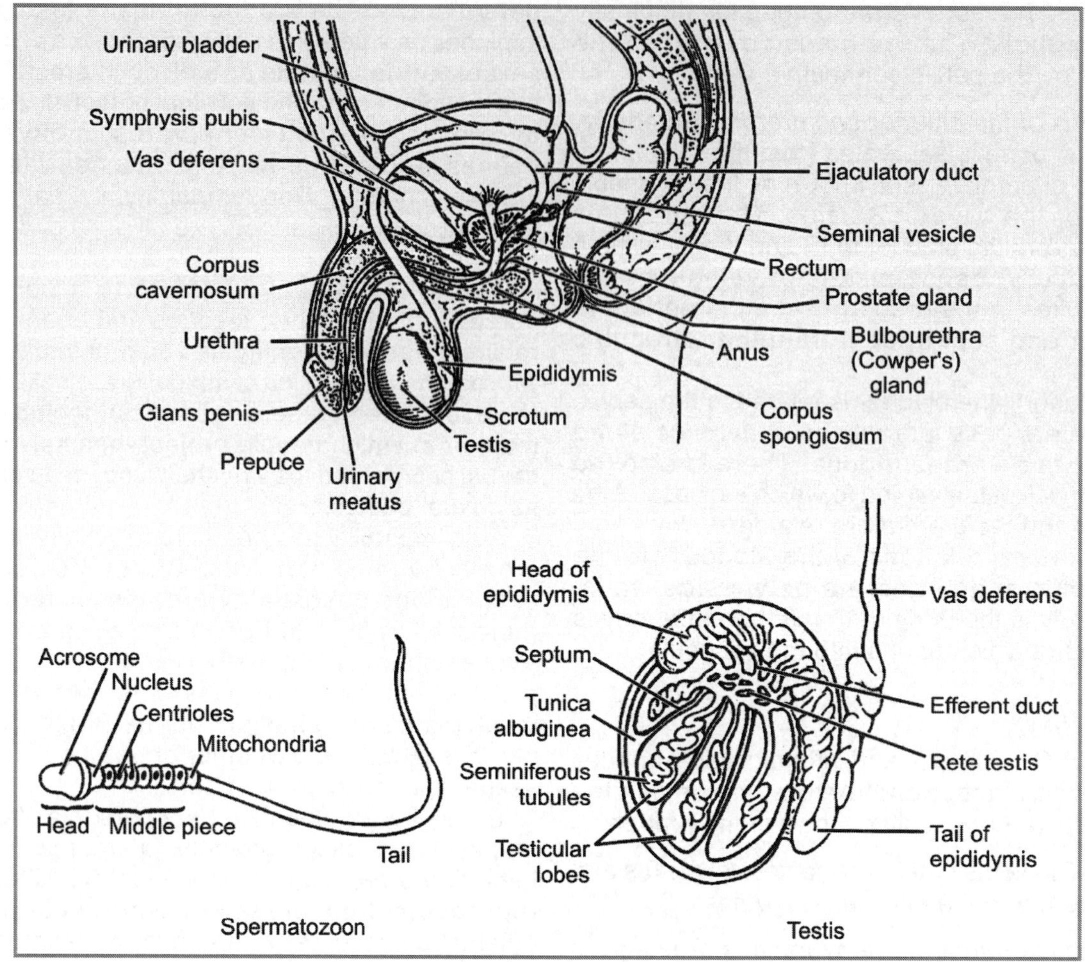

Fig. 2.60: Male reproductive organs with enlargements of a spermatozoon and testis

maturity at approximately age 17 years. Individual rates of development vary greatly. Anatomic and reproductive differences not withstanding, women and men are more alike than different in their physiologic response to sexual excitement and orgasm. For example, the glans clitoris and glans penis are embryonic homologues (Figs 2.1 and 2.60). Female and male sexual responses differ little, and the physical response is essentially the same whether the source of stimulation is coitus, fantasy or mechanical/manual.

According to Masters and Johnson (1966), sexual response can be physiologically analyzed in terms of two processes, vasocongestion and myotonia.

Sexual stimulation results in a vasocongestive reflex dilation of penile blood vessels (erection in the male) and circumvaginal blood vessels (lubrication in the female), causing engorgement and distention of the genitals. Venous congestion is localized primarily in the genitals, but it also occurs to a lesser degree in the breasts and other parts of the body.

Arousal is characterized by myotonia (increased muscular tension), which results in voluntary and involuntary rhythmic contraction. Examples of sexually stimulated myotonia are pelvic thrusting, facia grimacing and spasms of the hands and feet (carpopedal spasms).

This *sexual response cycle* is arbitrarily divided into four phases—excitement, plateau, orgasmic and resolution. The four phases occur progressively with no sharp dividing line between any two phases. Specific body changes take place in sequence. The time, intensity, and duration for cyclic completion also vary for individuals and situations. Body changes during each phase of the sexual response cycle explained in the chapter on Sexual Health and Nursing.

Psychosocial Aspects of Sexuality

Sexuality is a complex phenomenon influenced by a variety of biophysical psychologic, sociocultural, and ethical factors. Biologic gender is determined at conception through the combination of egg and sperm. However, the development of sexuality begins in utero and extends throughout the life span.

In a culture characterized by a rapid increase in knowledge and technology, many people are still misinformed about sexuality. The following are common myths about expressions of sexuality and reproduction.

1. A couple must have simultaneous climaxes (orgasms) for conception to take place.
2. A woman can become pregnant only through penile penetratioin or artificial insemination.
3. Urination by the woman after coitus or having sexual intercourse in a standing position will prevent pregnancy.
4. The woman determines the sex of the child.
5. Excessive masturbation is harmful.
6. Sex during menstruations unclean and harmful.
7. Advancing age means the end of sex.
8. Oral and anal intercourse are perverted or dangerous practices.

Men and women tend to view sexuality differently. For example, men may think of sexuality in term of specific numbers of activities, whereas women may focus on the meaning of a particular activity. However, no two people (man or woman) experience or express their sexuality in the same way. Sexuality is unique and individual and changes based on a person's sexual and life experiences.

Sexuality consists of at least four components—sexual response, sexual desire, view of self, and presentation of self *sexual response* refers primarily to the biophysical component of sexuality and includes the physical ability to engage in and respond to sexual activity sexual desire (Libido) refers to the urge (or lack there of) for sexual activity. The intensity of sexual desire varies throughout the life span and is affected by hormonal changes (for example, child bearing and menopause), fatigue, change of relationship with a partner, illness, and disability and medication.

View of self (gender identity) and presentation of self (sex role) are two other important aspects of sexuality. Gender identity and sex role behaviours develop early in life (from 2 to 4 years of age) as children identify with same-gender parents and mimic the behaviours of that parent. The feelings that children develop about themselves as sexual beings (heterosexual, homosexual, or bisexual) are related to these early experiences.

Expressions of gender identity and sex role behaviours with age and reflect the child's cognitive development (Piaget, 1950) and personality development

For example, a toddler may dress up and "play mommy" whereas an adolescent may actively seek a maternal role. Selected expressions of gender identity and sex role behaviours may also give some information about gender preferance—same gender, other gender, or both. However, sexuality is dynamic, the way sexuality is expressed during childhood may be different later in life.

Nursing Implications

The nurse is in a unique position to provide counselling and guidance to sexually maturing and sexually active individuals, as well as expectant and new parents. The role of educator is an important one for nurses working with families during the child-bearing and child-bearing hears. Parents often need help with teaching their children about sex because adults are commonly misinformed and fell uncomfortable about many aspects of sexuality, reproduction, and body function. Accurate sex information helps parents to provide a supportive environment for sexual development and teach their children to be healthy, responsible sexual beings.

Parents with adolescents require additional help and information as the adolescent confronts body image concerns, attempts to establish independence and mature relationships, explores sexuality and develops socially responsible behaviours. Nursing interactions with adolescents should provide accurate information privately, confidentially, and nonjudgmentally and should reflect an awareness of peer and family influences and ethnocultural background.

Besides helping with childhood and adult sexuality, the nurse can help prepare clients of the sexual concerns and changes occuring with age. Many nurses have not been aware of the importance of sex education for older people because of the myth that older adults are no longer interested in sex.

Sexual dysfunction problems often begin after children are born. The mother especially may become so involved with child rearing that her relationship with her partner suffers. At the same time the partner may be actively involved in career establishment, thereby leaving little energy for home life. The nurse needs to be awared of the way parenting demands can adversely affect relationships. Simple counselling provided during these early years, may prevent serious problems later.

The older woman in particular who has been able to move gracefully into old age and who continues to recognize herself as a sexual being is probably better able to accept the sexuality of the young. The pregnancy of a daughter may then be accepted as a continuation of her own sexuality rather than as a threat or reminder of her lost youth.

Knowledge about and comfort with sexuality are important for the establishment of therapeutic relationships. A nonjudgmental nurse who recognizes personal sexual biases can contribute a great deal to the sexual health of families. A sensitivity to alternative lifestyles can help the nurse to provide comprehensive care to a lesbian/gay family for example. Many lesbian/gay families are choosing to parent, whether through insemination, intentional heterosexual encounter, adoption, or a previous heterosexual relationship (Deevey 1995). The nurse can recognize potential problems and intervene or refer family members to other professionals or agencies.

SEXUAL DEVELOPMENT

An individual's sexual development evolves from conception through adolescence. Following the teenage years, sexuality represents for many the expression of knowledge acquired throughout childhood.

Stages of Sexual Development

From one perspective, human sexual development can be viewed within the context of three stages. These stages are gender assignment at birth (actually initiated at conception); reproductive maturation, together with the individual's gender identity and gender role, and the development of the sensual aspects of sexuality.

Gender Assignment

Sexual development begins at birth with the assignment of a gender. At birth, human sexuality expresses itself with a sameness and lack of individuality that will never again be witnessed during a person's lifetime. From this point, each individual's sexual behaviour and form of sexual expression will differ.

At fertilization, chromosomes provide genetic coding for core gender development. This genetic coding, however, remains undifferentiated until 6 to 12 weeks of embryonic growth. Until then, the foetus is female. With out androgenization, occurring at 6 to 7 weeks of gestation, the undifferentiated foetus will remain female regardless of its genetic coding.

Homologous organs have been found to respond similarly during the sexual response cycle and generally respond to similar stimulation. For example, the testes and ovaries originate from the same embryonic tissue and will respond similarly when examinations exceed pressure tolerance levels. This information is relevant to questions asked by adolescents and adults about what feels good sexually to their heterosexual partners. Even in our gender differences, there is much sameness.

Gender Identity and Role

Gender identity and role, together with a reproductive or biologic maturation, mark the second stage of sexualization. Gender identity pertains to how the individual feels about being male or female and gender role addresses how these feelings about being male or female are translated into the child's interaction in the world. Gender identity and role are influenced by messages of parents and society attach to sexual roles. Sexual orientation is one of the expressions of gender identity and role. The process of individual internalization of one's sexual identity is, therefore, largely shaped by the culturally defined sense of femininity and masculinity, as well as by other environmental influences, such as family, parents, media, school, religion, and socio-economic status.

Sexual development of early childhood takes place at age 3 years, and certainly by adolescence, individuals have already shaped most of their sexual identity and orientation. Few adjustments are made in sexual identity after this point.

Views of Adolescent Sexual Behaviour

The most widely held view is that adolescents, particularly of high-school age, may be biologically ready for sexual intercourse, but are psychologically and socially too immature to cope with the complexity, it introduces into a relationship.

Biologically, the adolescent is experiencing changes in hormonal secretions, rate of skeletal growth, and temporary imbalances in body structure and function. Basic instinctual forces are given impetus by these physiologic changes, leading to an increase in energy that may override the thought processes and control mechanisms. This increase in energy may discharge itself through impulsive behaviour often related to the alleviation of sexual tensions.

Erikson describes identity formation as the period of adolescence during which the integration of the biologic and psychosocial aspects of past experience leads greater stability, the individual gains sufficient ego strength and sex-role identity to experience, leads to greater stability in the individual's sense of self. Through this stability, the individual gains sufficient ego, strength and sex-role identity to experience intimacy without risk of identity diffusion. Sexual intimacy prior to identity formation may result in a crisis of premature commitment and may introduce complexities with which the young person is not prepared to deal.

Hamburg describes the onset of puberty as the young adolescent's first encounter with life in which he or she confronts challenges of both a biologic and psychosocial nature and is unable to draw upon analogous past experience as a guide. Piaget describes the intellectual development and are still relying upon past or present converte experiences, they will have difficulty considering alternatives, concerning sexual behaviour because they have little or no past experience upon which to rely and because they are also unable to comprehend casual relationships.

An opposing and less common held view of adolescent sexuality suggests that former sexual mores are outdated. Teenagers are not only believed to be biologically ready for sexual intercourse while psychosocial development continues, but are also believed to need the experience to establish their sexual identity and to learn to develop healthy relationships with the opposite sex.

Maddock argues that adolescent sexual expression may provide the possibility to experience intimacy prior to the achievement of identity, and might be used by adolescents who are engaged in a mutual search for identity. He believes that some forms of sexual expression could precede identity formation without danger of identity diffusion.

Contrary to Erickson, who believes that intimacy, especially sexual intimacy, is possible only after identity is achieved, sexual expression might very well be seen as a normative form of interaction between adolescents who are engaged in a mutual search for identity.

Influence of Peer Group

As young adolescents struggle to emancipate themselves from parental control, the peer group provides a sense of belonging and a source of empathy. This close, more intense relationship with peers compensates for the "loss" felt by young people during the transition from dependence to independence. It also provides a safe environment in which adolescents rehearse different roles, attitudes, and behaviours during their evolution of self-identity and personal value system. Most adolescents will go to great lengths to conform to the group's modes and peer group pressures may strongly influence an individual's decisions about sexual behaviour.

Influence of Parental Values

Childhood internalisation of parental values and attitudes and the struggle against these mores mark the adolescent's efforts to formula personal life goals and a separate identity. This is an important factor in attempts to make decisions about sexual 'behaviour'. Sexual acting out as a form of rebellion against parents may be used in efforts to separate.

Critical to the development of sexuality througout childhood are the messages received regarding the child's body, reactions to childhood sex play, sexual role modeling of adults, and the type of communication encountered regarding sexual attitudes and behaviour.

An example is the expected roles placed on the male child beginning at birth. Accompanying the announcement, "It's a boy" are numerous expectations and the beginning of conditioning. Boys are expected to be strong, virile, assertive, and in control of all things, including their emotions. The expectation for males to perform, succeed and protect, and other messages about sexual interactions will increase with age and peak during adolescence.

Of course, all men do not ascribe to all of these descriptive terms. The male role, defined in childhood primarily by the family, will generally represent the culture within which the family resides and is modeled by the father and/or significant male figure within the extended family. Sons generally reflect the parental role exhibited to them, although knowledge acquired through experience is also important. Also, as women continue to redefine their sexual role in society, men's roles are affected, often causing confusion for males.

Role Rehearsal

Childhood and adolescence serve as a rehearsal time for learning and acting out roles, including sexual roles, which are then assumed in adulthood. Childhood is dominated by the learning process, which is stimulated in such childhood games as playing house, playing mommy and daddy, and show and tell games. The games may be played alone or with groups of friends, of the same sex or the oposite sex. They are nature, the child does not necessarily perceive them in this manner, since sexuality has not been separated out as a completely distinct children internalize the adult context of sexuality and will become more clandestine in their interactions and games.

SEXUALLY RELATED DEVELOPMENT IN ADOLESCENTS

At each stage of development, adolescents differ in the types of questions asked. To design health-education and promotion topics that appropriately address their needs, a closer look at each of the three stages of adolescence is helpful.

Early Adolescence

Characteristic of early adolescence are individual questions, about questions, about changing bodies and the development of a new body image. Alternating embarrassment and pride about the adolescent's new body still continue until most physical maturation is completed in middle adolescence. The rate of growth and maturation of visible sexual characteristics varies widely. This can cause much concern and confusion, especially during physical education classes, where individuals reaching adult status early may feel embarrassed, as may those whose development has just begun. Discussing their maturational process will help to alleviate anxiety.

Girls will begin experiencing vaginal lubrication. This normal physiologic response occurs at two different stages before menarche in conjunction with changing hormonal levels and again with the establishment of ovulatory cycles. This brings as much concern to girls as did budding breasts and menstruation. The permenarchal stage of vaginal lubrication and discharge probably results, in part, from the same feedback system causing spontaneous erections in boys.

In boys, spontaneous erections, nocturnal emissions, and masturbation are common to this age-group. Males need to understand the normalcy of these actions and have myths surrounding those functions dispelled.

Masturbation

Approximately one half of boys and one-third of girls have masturbated by age 15 years. This rate continues to increase with age, until by 20 years, approximately 85 per cent of males and 60 per cent of females have masturbated.

There is general agreement among professionals that the fear and guilt formerly associated with masturbation is now declining. However, considerable embarrassment by adolescents when they are relating information about their masturbatory activities.

To talk about sex is often considered by teenagers to represent being "in the know" or "more mature." Seldon, however, do they voluntarily discuss their concerns about masturbating. It is often possible to elicit serious concerns if, during a group presentation of the harmless effects of masturbation to make an appointment to discuss these concerns in private. This approach is very effective in work with young adolescents, especially at the high-school level.

Most adolescents, if misinformed or worried, will be relieved to hear that masturbation is a common and normal practice among both males and females. It can be an outlet for accumulated sexual tension and may provide a means of experimenting with developing biologic capacities and enhance the future development of healthy heterosexual relationships.

Petting Experience

Petting, flirtations, and "puppy love" are typical behaviours in early and middle adolescence, as teenagers begin experimenting with intimacy and coupling. These behaviours should be taken seriously by parents, friends and professionals and not joked about with the teenager.

Heavy petting, often leading to orgasm (more often for males than females), is believed by some to provide youth with an outlet for sexual needs and an opportunity to experiment with sex in a heterosexual relationship without fear of pregnancy. However, one might speculate that these young persons will be experimenting with sexual intercourse within a short period of time, and might be a target group for the teaching of contraceptive methods along with a discussion of the responsibility involved.

Those adolescents who report having had no petting experience are found primarily in the under-15 age-group. These young people, in the early stage of adolescence may be physiologically less mature and may not yet experience the need for more independence from their parents and closer communication with their opposite sex peers. Religious attitudes also are a factor in the decision not to engage in petting and to delay sexual activity.

Sexual Intercourse

Sexual intercourse is probably too stressful an event to contemplate during early adolescence, while adolescents are adapting to their bodily changes. Several elements contribute to this. First, those in early adolescence are egotistically focused. Second, changes in skeletal and muscle growth are often disproportionate to the rest of the bodily changes. Third, the differences in onset and duration of biologic growth between the sexes are sources of awkwardness for teenagers. This coupled, with the wide variance between individuals of the same sex at any given age in early and middle adolescence, contributes to selfconscious feelings and a strong identification and conformity with one's own sex. This is especially true in early adolescence, when physical and verbal experimentation with the safe sex begins.

In certain cultures and with in certain socioeconomic groups, sexual intercourse in early adolescence may be considered normal. It may also represent acting out behaviour, especially when coupled with low self-esteem and other behaviour such as decline in school performance, running away from home, delinquent problems, or attempted suicides. Careful evaluation of the motives for sexual behaviours can help to distinguish pathologic problems from behaviour examplifying a curious explorative nature.

Middle Adolescence

As teenagers move from the family to their peer group as the source of moral attitude and guidelines, it is often difficult for them to obtain information about actual sexual behaviour. Societal messages, increased communications, discussions about sexuality and boasting often create distortions in perceptions of sexual behaviour among adolescents. Middle adolescence is a difficult time to encourage individuality, as teenagers strive for sameness among themselves. Yet it is important for health providers and educators to encourage and support the adolescent's individual decision making, especially with respect to their sexual development.

Middle adolescence also marks the height of psychological growth, with concrete thinking maturing to abstract deducation. Until this developmental process is intact, it is difficult for the sexual adolescent to make responsible decisions. Under stress or during illness, the ability for abstract deduction reverts to concrete thinking. Thus, when discussing sensitive issues surrounding sexuality, providing information in concrete (literal-minded) format is essential. Their narcissistic omnipotent viewpoint and psychological development do not enable teenagers in middle adolescence to project current behaviours (such as sexual intercourse) into future consequences. This has a major effect upon approach to contraception.

Heterosexual Attitudes and Behaviours

During middle adolescence, approximately 30 to 40 per cent of teenage boys and 20 to 30 per cent of teenage girls have sexual intercourse. The peer culture has historically served as a support group for teenagers to rhearse new personal values, identities, and behaviour. In the 1960s, birth-control methods advanced technically and became legally available, bringing a new dimension to sexual choice. Teenagers now may use the option for sexual intimacy as a means for mutually seeking their identities, supported by their peer culture. However, many adolescents do not condone early sexual behaviour. They emphasize, rather, that the acceptability of sexual expression depends on the closeness and meaningfulness of the relationship and the emotion involved. Contrary to much popular opinion the attitudes of younger adolescents are more conservative than attitudes of those on the verge of adulthood. Pathologic motivations underlie sexual behaviour engaged in for nonsexual reasons; such motivations are representative of personality disorders or are exploitative and manipulative in nature. The incidence of pathologic motivations in those who are sexually active decreased with age, especially as teenagers approach late adolescence.

Dating Behaviours

Dating among teenagers, once considered to be an important aspect of the couting process, now appears to be an end in itself and a socially approved outlet for heterosexual experience. It would appear that, for the sexually active young woman, going steady is a much more serious and intimate affair, whereas the sexually inactive young woman seems to be experimenting with a variety of relationships on a less intense level.

Many teenagers choose to be sexual without including intercourse, and they require support for their decision. This behavioural standard is generally prevalent among their chosen peer group. Other deterrents to the choice of sexual intercourse include sexual knowledge, with the ability to discuss feelings with parents; self-esteem; strong family orientation and unity; and career aspirations However, deterrent and sexual decision making among adolescents are poorly understood.

Options for sexual interactions without intercourse, especially prior to age 15 years, are often not presented or supported in discussions with teenagers. If professionals and adults are to guide today's youth, options such as communications and forms of sexual expression other than intercourse must also be discussed. These behaviours provide safe alternatives that do not interfere with the normal sexual development or denote negative sexual messages.

In early or middle adolescence, as questions about sexual functioning arise, it is time to begin discussing social-sexual communications and sexual attitudes and to help provide some beginning social skills and options with respect to sexual interactions. One area of discussion is the social-sexual response cycle. Each of the stages—vague unrest, options, negotiations, agreement, and anticipation—can provide the basis for discussing myths sexual feelings, sexual options excluding intercourse and emotions. Role playing with teenagers to explore negotiations and communications of desires and needs is helpful. Enabling the teenager to verbalize thoughts and feelings about each of these stages can provide insight to both the teenager and the adult from this point, further discussion can evolve.

It has been suggested a communication exercise appropriate for teenagers as they begin dating. "Tell me something that you like about me. Tell me something that you think we agree on. Tell me something that you think I should know about you." Each person takes 5 minutes with each question, and the receiver only listens and acknowledges what is being said by a nod of the head or a simple thank you, but does not discuss the consent. Discover of feelings and thoughts about the communication will open doors to further discussion. This type of communication begin in adolescence and continue through adulthood, will increase the individual's ability to express concerns, feelings and needs.

Another exercise addresses traditional stereotypical roles by discussing the role of money including the question: Does the person paying for the date make the rules? "The exercise alternates between partners, with each taking the responsibility for "a date." It allows each individual to experience "walking in the other person's shoes." From this experience, each individual can identify what he or she enjoyed or disliked, and can creat guidelines for future dating behaviour.

The rates for premarital intercourse have risen sharply in the past years, and it is occurring at younger ages. Positive attitudes towards education, and greater educational aspirations among high school students tend to lower the rate of intercourse, or at least the total number of sexual partners, during adolescence. Feelings of guilt and anxiety over sexual behaviour may be an indication of the lasting effect of internalized parental values. A close relationship with both parents may be associated with low-levels of sexual intercourse, and an unsatisfactory relationship, with increased sexual activity.

Late Adolescence

Late adolescence presents a less complicated picture, biologic and psychological maturation is near completion for both sexes, and social maturation is the central focus at this stage. Such tasks as career aspirations, economic autonomy, and intimacy issues addressed. Pairing is common, enabling teenagers to test out new values, communication skills, and intimacy levels while they continue to rely on their peer culture for support and recognition. Partner involvements as well as psychological maturation result in more responsible decision making affecting sexual interactions. One example is consistent use of an effective contraceptive.

Also, once career aspirations are embarked upon, sexual issues may decrease in priority.

Sex Education

As their bodies begin to reflect the maturational changes of puberty, the interest and curiosity of adolescents is directed towards gaining information in order to adjust. They may recognize parental discomfort in discussing sexual matters and thus turn to their peers for information, although their preference during preadolescence and adolescence for source of sex information remains family based. Unfortunately this often leads to misconceptions and misinformation and prevents adolescents from fully understanding the way in which their bodies will function when they become physically mature. Within their peer group, curiosity may be intense, with examination of their own bodies and those of their friends, secret conversations, and exchange of information gleaned from magazines, novels, or television.

When children have learned throughout childhood that their parents answer questions without evasion or obvious discomfort, they will be more likely to approach them when they feel a need for knowledge at this time. As children learn more biologic and social facts, they will become motivated to bring more questions and ideas to their parents for discussion. When parents have accepted this curiosity before adolescence, children will seek further help from them when sexual feelings become reawakened. Then, much of their concern will be centered on learning to deal with their impulses in the company of the opposite sex.

NURSING MEASURES TO PROMOTE SEX EDUCATION

Nurses should incorporate sex education as a preventive and continuing approach to the nursing care of adolescents. It is essential for nurses to examine carefully their own attitudes and values regarding teenage sexual activity. A judgmental negative attitude may be conveyed to teenagers unwittingly, if the nurse is not aware of her prejudices. This will certainly affect the degree of openness and compliances the adolescent shows in discussing this issue. If a nurse feels that her attitude interferes with fostering an objective, open attitude in the adolescent, then this area should be discussed with the teenager by someone else who is more comfortable with the topic.

Girls can understand descriptions of the menstrual cycle or explanations of the female generative tract that will reassure them that their bodies are responding normally, if their menstruation begins at a different time from that of their friends.

As the girl approaches adolescence, she will need to have her own supplies and to know the approximate length of a period. She should also know that menstrual irregularity is characteristic during early adolescence. If she accepts menstruation as a natural feminine function, which should not interfere with daily activities, transition into adolescence will be smoother.

At menarche, girls should be encouraged to keep records of their menstrual cycles. There are several benefits in keeping such records. First, the major female reproductive organs are hidden deep within the pelvis and are not visible. It is therefore difficult for the girl to become acquainted with them and understand how they relate to her. Systemic illnesses, major weight changes, life crises, travel (especially if includes air travel), and changes in environment will affect the length of a menstrual cycle and ovulation. Awareness of how these factors individually affect her body, increased her body awareness, making possible an increased ability to formulate a new body image. Record keeping will also provide knowledge of ovulatory or anovulatory cycles and hence, fertility. Although natural family planning is not well used by teenagers, record keeping provides the vehicle for increased options at any point when other birth control methods are contraindicated. Increased information about menstrual cycles should serve to increase positive attitudes about a bodily function that is steeped in negative messages and will emphasize the fact that is, is a normal body function.

Involuntary discharge of semen that occur during sleep (wet dreams) are as natural for boys as menstruation is for girls. Unless boys understand this natural phenomenon, they may be frightened and thin, that it is caused by masturbation or disease or is a sign of weakness. Seminal emissions require acceptance, as do the boy's spontaneous erections in early adolescence, changing voice, growth of a beard and spurt in physical growth. Boys may worry needlessly about their rate of maturation unless they are reminded that normally there are wide variations in the time when adolescence begins.

Gynaecomastia, or development of breast tissue, occurs in approximately two-third of boys. This may be of great concern, particularly when accompanied by adiposity of the lower torso. Boys are often embarrassed to ask anyone about this development. Although generally transient, disappearing within a year but sometimes lasting 3-years, such physical characterstics may cause real distress and stimulate bisexual fantasies leading the boy to question his masculinity.

SEXUAL RESPONSE PATTERN

Each person experiences sexual desire in a way unique to him or herself and many different stimuli can trigger the feeling. For some people simply sitting next to someone they find attractive will be enough to initiate sexual interest. It has been well documented that reading about sex or looking at photos or erotic films can stimulate sexual feelings, but even the sound of someone's voices or smell of their clothes may be enough to initiate feelings of sexual desire.

Both males and females respond to any sexual stimulation by experiencing a cycle of events. Masters and Johnson (1966) were sexologists, were the first to explain in detail how human beings respond to sexuality. Their four stages, sexual cycle describes the physical changes that body experiences at different level of arousal. In their theory, after an initial period of desire, men and women go through four phases; excitement, plateau, orgasm and resolution. These phases are the result of vasocongestion and myotonia, which are the basic physiological responses of sexual arousal. Vasocongestion in the pooling of blood in the genitals and female breasts during sexual arousal.

In women this reaction leads to vaginal lubrication, tumescence (swelling) of the clitoris and the labia minora and majora, and engorgement of the outer third of the vagina. In men, vasocongestion leads to erection of the penis. Myotonia, or neuromuscular tension, gradually increases throughout the body during excitement and plateau phases. It peaks during orgasm, result in involuntary contractions of the arm, leg, facial and gluteal muscles. Corpopedal spasms of spastic contractions of the muscles of the hands and feet, may occur. After orgasm, the body returns to prearousal levels.

The Stages of Sexual Response (Table 2.4)

Once the mind has recognized a conscious or subconscious sexual attraction, the sexual responses of the body follow; One explanation of sexual response, concentrates on how the mind perceives and responds to arousal. The psychological charges that takes place during arousal are more or less the same for men and women. The seduction stage consists of personal experience of a conscious or subconscious sexual attraction to someone (whether a new or existing partner) and his or her attempt to interest or attract them. *Sensation* is the stage, when the five senses —sight, hearing, taste, touch and smell— send signals of sexual pleasure and arousal to their brain.These sansations are their processed and can be acted upon consciously. The *surrender* stage describes the mental "letting go" that is necessary, for orgasm to take place. Finally the reflection stage involves thinking about the physical events that have taken place. If the feelings are positive, there will be a subconscious or conscious desire to repeat the cycle.

Masters (1960) studied male and female subjects and was able to describe sexual

Table 2.4: Four phases of sexual response

Reactions common	*Female reactions*	*Male reactions*
1. ***Excitement phase*** Heart rate and blood pressure increase. Nipples become erect. Myotonia begins	Clitoris increases in diameter and wells. External genitals become congested and darken. Vaginal lubrication occurs; Upper two-thirds of vagina lengthen and extend. Cervix and uterus pull upward. Breast size increases.	Erection of penis begins; penis increases in length and diameter. Scrotal skin becomes congested and thickens. Testes being to increase in size and elevate toward body.
2. ***Plateau phase*** Heart rate and blood pressure continue to increase. Respirations increase Myotonia becomes pronounced; grimacing occurs.	Clitorial head retracts under clitoral hood. Lower one-third of vagina becomes engorged. Skin colour changes occur—redflush may be observed across breasts, abdomen or other surfaces.	Head of penis enlarge slightly. Scrotum continues to grow tense and thicken. Testes continue to elevate and enlarge. Preorgasmic emission or 2 or 3 drops of fluid appear on head of penis.
3. ***Orgasmic Phase*** Heart rate, blood pressure, and respirations increase to maximum levels. Involuntary muscle spasms occur. External rectal sphincter contracts.	Strong rhythmic contractions are felt in clitoris vagina and uterus Sensations of warmth spread through pelvic area.	Testes elevate to maximal level. Point of "inevitability" occurs just before ejaculation and is an awareness of fluid in urethra. Rhythmic contraction occur in penis. Ejaculation of semen occurs.
4. ***Resolution Phase*** Heart rate, blood pressure and respirations return to normal Nipple erection subsides Myotonia subsides	Engorgement in external genitalia and vagina resolves Cervix and uterus descend to normal position. Breast size decreases. Skin flush disappears.	Approximately 50 per cent of erection is lost immediately with ejaculation, penis gradually returns to normal size. Testes and scrotum return to normal size. Refractory period (time needed for erection to occur again) varies according to age and general physical condition.

response in relation to genital tissue charges, extragenital changes and subjective or feeling stages related to sexual arousal. He determined that the sexual response cycle has four stages (as stated earlier), excitement, plateau, orgasm and resolution. Normal variations were noted between men and women as well as among the persons of the same sex. For example, some women experience multiple orgasms following sexual arousal and other don't reach orgasm at all.

3 Review of Genetics and Embryology

INTRODUCTION

Human Genetics deals with human variation: its nature, extent, origin and maintenance, its distribution in families and populations; its interaction with the environment, and its consequences for normal development. Unprecedented scientific and technologic advances are rapidly expanding service capabilities; the capacity to undertake mass screening to identify carriers, if deleterious genes, the opportunities for prenatal diagnosis, the technology to sustain the lives of seriously ill and malformed newborns and the ability to increase the life expectancy of people affected by genetic disorders. In rapid developments, genetics have also resulted in heightened public awareness and concern for enhanced health and optimal reproduction.

Human embryology is the study of development of an individual before birth. Every individual spends first nine months (266 days or 38 weeks to be exact) of its life within the womb (uterus) of its mother. During this period, it develops from a small one-celled structure to an organism having billions of cells. Numerous tissues and organs are formed and start to function in perfect harmony. The most spectacular of these changes occur in first two months. We call the developing individual an "embryo". From the third month until birth, we call it a "foetus". This embryology is the study of the formation and development of the embryo (or foetus) from the moment of its inception upto the time when it is born an infant.

GENETICS

Human development is a complicated process that depends on the systematic unraveling of instructions found in the genetic material of the egg and sperm. Development from conception to birth of a normal healthy baby occurs without incident in most cases; occasionally, however, some anomaly in the genetic code of the embryo creates a birth defect or disorder. Parents are then left to wonder what went wrong, which parent might be "responsible" or most significantly, what are the chances of the problem recurring with the next pregnancy. The science of genetics seeks to explain the underlying causes of congenital disorders (disorders present at birth) and the patterns in which inherited disorders are passed from generation to generation. A basic understanding of genetics helps the professional nurse, assist families to locate the genetics helps, the professional nurse assist families to locate the right sources (often genetic counsellors) to help them cope with the questions and fears surrounding birth defects.

Genes and Chromosomes

The hereditary material carried in the nucleus of each somatic (body) cell, determines in individual's physical characteristics. This material, called deoxyribonucleic acid (DNA), forms thread-like strands known as "chromosomes". Each chromosome is composed of many smaller segments of DNA referred to as *genes*. Genes are combinations of coded information that determines an individual's unique characteristics. The "code" is found in the specific linear order of the molecules that combine to form the strands of DNA.

All normal human somatic cells contain 46 chromosomes arranged as 23 pairs of homologous (matched) chromosomes, one chromosome of each pair is inherited from each parent. There are 22 pairs of autosomes, which control most traits in the body, and one pair of sex chromosomes, which determine gender and other traits. The large female chromosome is the X, the tiny male chromosome is the Y. When X and Y chromosomes are present, the embryo develops as a male. When two chromosomes are present, the embryo develops as a female.

Because each gene occupies a specific chromosome location and because chromosomes are inherited as homologous pairs, each person has two genes for every trait. In other words; if an autosome has a gene for hair colour, its partner will also have a gene for hair colour—in the same location on the chromosome. However, although both genes code for hair colour—in the same location on the chromosome. However, although both genes code for hair colour, they may not code for the same hair colour. Different genes coding for different variations of the same trait are called alleles. An individual having two copies of the same allele for a given trait is said to be homozygous for that trait, with two different alleles, the person is heterozygous for the trait.

Some genes are dominant, and their characteristics are expressed even if another allele is present on the other chromosome. Other genes are recessive, and their characteristics will be expressed only if they are carried by both homologous chromosomes. For example, the gene for brown eyes is dominant over the gene for blue eyes. Thus a person with one gene for brown eyes and one gene for blue eyes will have brown eyes. When an egg and a sperm unite, the combination of alleles becomes that individual's entire genetic make up, or genotype, which includes all the genes that the person carries and that can be passed to offspring. The genotype determines the persons physical appearance, or phenotype, but this is affected by the nature of the dominant or recessive allele. To continue the above example, an individual with two brown eyes alleles at the gene for eye colour will have the same phenotype as one with one brown eyes and one blue eyes allele; that is, both individuals will have brown eyes.

The pictorial analysis of the number, form, and size of an individuals chromosomes is known as a karyotype. A karyotype can be obtained from a blood sample specially treated and stained to make the replicating chromosomes visible under a microscope. The photographed chromosomes are cut out and arranged in a specific numeric order according to their length and shape. Figures 3.1A and B illustrate the chromosomes in a body cell and a karyotype. Karyotypes can be used to determine the sex of a child and the presence of any gross chromosomal abnormalities.

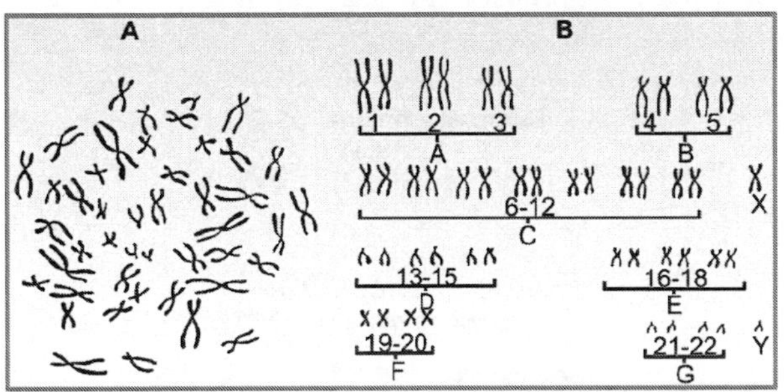

Figs 3.1A and B: Chromosomes during cell division. **A.** Example of photomicrograph, **B.** Chromosomes arranged in karyotype; female and male sex-determining chromosomes

Cell Division

Cells are reproduced by two different methods mitosis and meiosis. In mitosis, the body cells replicate to yield two cell with the same genetic make up as the parent cell. First the cell makes a copy of its DNA, then it divides, and each daughter cell receives one copy of the genetic material. The purpose of mitotic division is for growth and development or cell replacement (Fig. 3.2).

Meiosis produces gametes (eggs and sperm). Each homologous pair of chromosomes contains one chromosome received from the mother and one from the father; thus meiosis results in cells that contain one of each of the 23 pairs of chromosomes. Because these germ cells contain 23 single chromosomes, half the genetic material of a normal somatic cell they are haploid. When the female gamete (egg or ovum) and the male gamete (spermatozoan) unite to form the zygote, the diploid number of human chromosomes (46, or 23 pairs) is restored.

The process of DNA replication and cell division in meiosis allows different alleles for genes to be distributed at random by each parent and then rearranged on the paired chromosomes. The chromosomes then separate and proceed to different gametes. Because parents have genotypes derived from four different grandparents, many combinations of genes on each chromosome are possible. This random missing

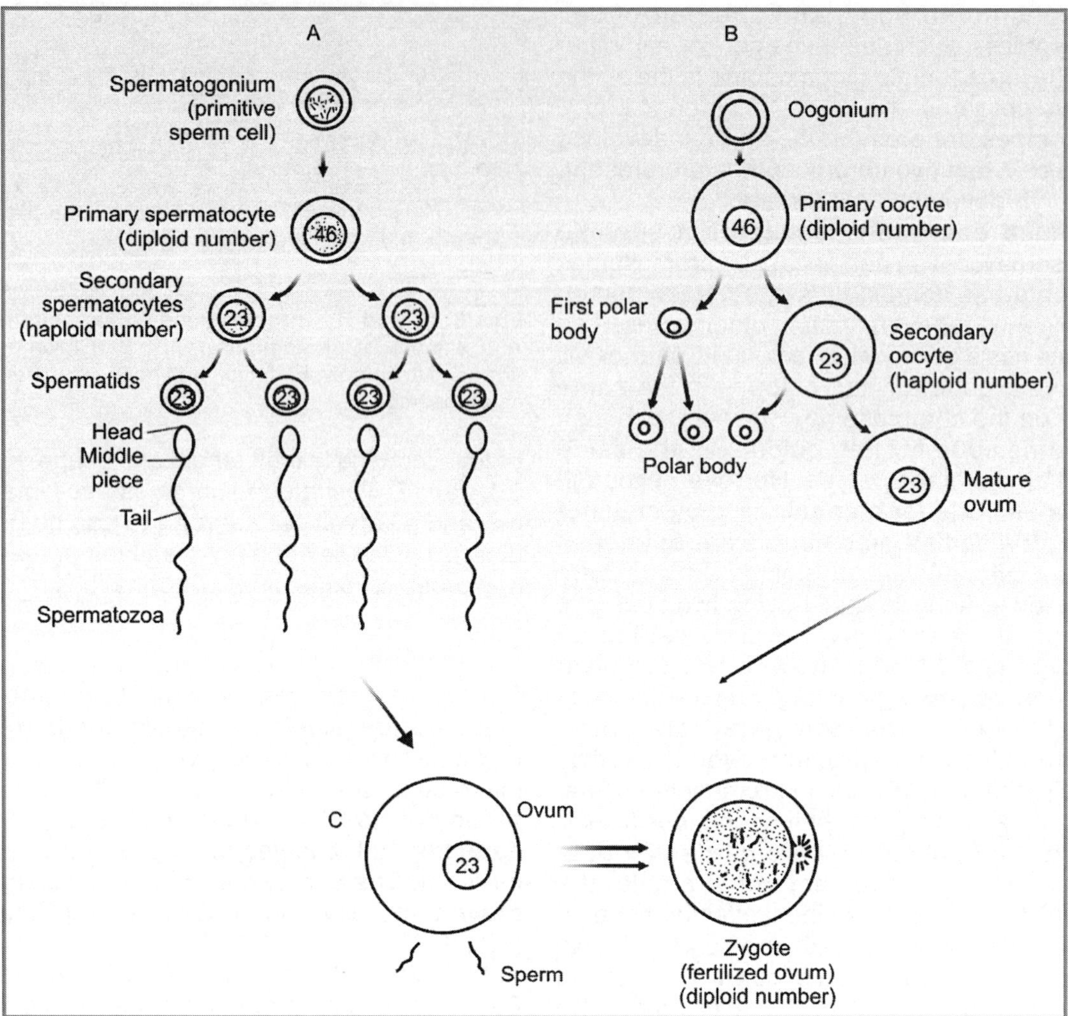

Figs 3.2A to C: A. Spermatogenesis: gametogenesis of the male produces four mature gametes, the sperm. **B.** Oogenesis: gametogenesis in the female produces one mature ovum and three polar bodies. Note the relative difference in overall size between the ovum and sperm. **C.** Fertilization results in the single-cell zygote and restoration of the diploid number of chromosomes

of alleles accounts for the variation of traits seen in the offspring of the same two parents.

Gametogenesis (Fig. 3.2A)

When a male reaches puberty, his testes begin the process of spermatogenesis. The only cells that undergo meiosis in the male are spermatocytes. The primary spermatocyte, which undergoes the first meiotic division, contains the diploid number of chromosomes. The cell has already copied its DNA before division, so four alleles for each gene are actually present. Because the copies are bound together—one allele plus its copy on each chromosome—the cell is still considered diploid.

During the first meiotic division, two haploid secondary spermatocytes are formed, each containing 22 autosomes and one sex chromosome; one contains the X-chromosome (plus its copy) and the other the Y-chromosome (plus its copy). During the second meiotic division, the male produces too gametes with an X-chromosome and two gametes with a Y-chromosome, all of which will develop into viable sperm (Fig. 3.2A).

Oogenesis (Fig. 3.2B)

Oogenesis, the process of egg (ovum) formation, begins during the foetal life of the female. All the cells that may undergo meiosis in a woman's lifetime are contained in her ovaries at birth. The majority of the estimated 2 million primary oocytes (the cells that undergo the first meiotic division) degenerate spontaneously. Only 400 to 500 ovum will mature during the approximately 35 years of a woman's reproductive life. The primary oocytes begin the first meiotic division (that is, they replicate their DNA) during foetal life but remain suspended at this stage until puberty. Then, usually monthly, one primary oocyte matures and completes the first meiotic division, yielding two unequal cells the secondary oocyte and a small poles body both contain 22 autosomes and one X sex chromosome.

At ovulation, the second meiotic division begins. However, the ovum does not complete the second meiotic division unless fertilization occurs. Fertilization produces a second polar body and the zygote (the united egg and sperm) (Fig. 3.2C). If fertilization does not occur, the ovum degenerates (Figs 3.2 and 3.3).

Chromosomal Abnormalities

Errors resulting in chromosomal abonormalities can occur in mitosis or meiosis. These occur in either the autosomes or sex chromosomes. Even without the presence of obvious structural malformations, small deviations in chromosomes can cause problems in foetal development.

Autosomal Abnormalities

Autosomal abnormalities involve differences in the number or structure of chromosomes resulting from unequal distribution of the genetic material during gamete formation.

Abnormalities of Chromosome Number

Abnormalities of chromosome number, aneuploidy are most often caused by non-disjunction. Non-disjunction occurs during meiosis when a pair of chromosomes fails to separate and one resulting cell contains both chromosomes and the other contains none. The product of the union of a normal gamete with a gamete containing an extra chromosome is a trisomy. The resulting individual has 47 chromosomes in each cell.

The most common trisomal abnormality is Down's syndrome, or trisomy 21. The affected individual has an extra chromosome 21. The

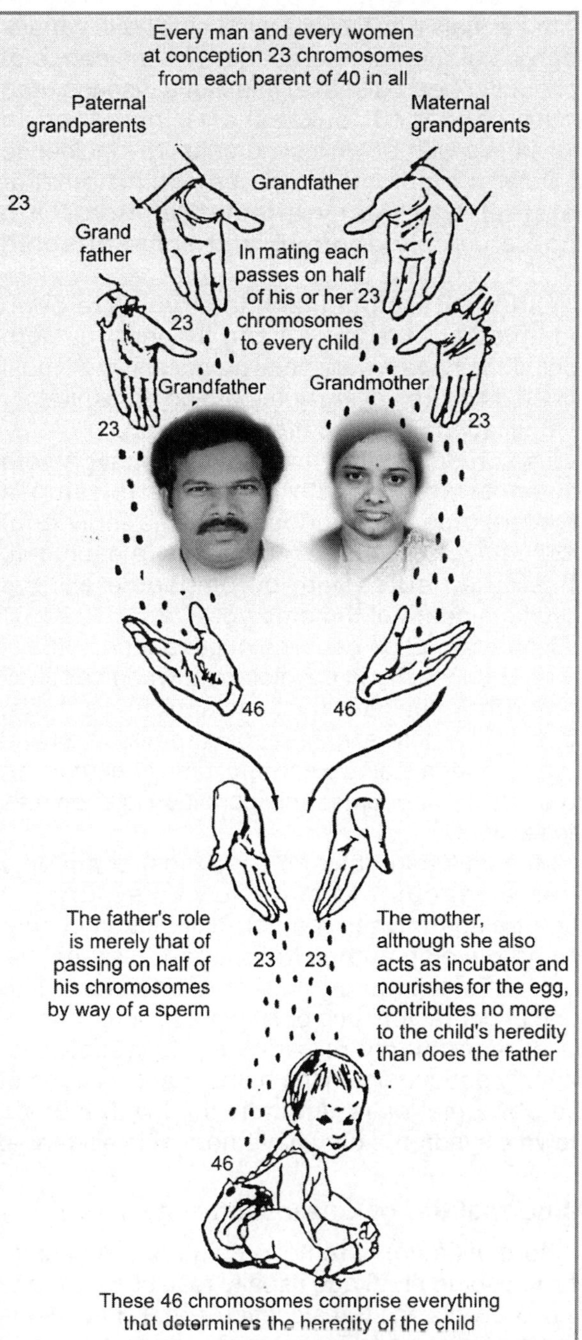

Fig. 3.3: The hereditary process

clinical characteristics of Down's syndrome include a broad, small skull; flat facial profile; epicanthal folds with slanted palpebral fissures in the eyes, flat, low-set ears protruding tongue; a short neck with fat pads at the nape, short, broad hands with a single transverse (simian) crease, and hypotonic muscles with hypermobility of joints.

Individuals with Down's syndrome have various degrees of mental retardation. The incidence of congenital heart disease, infectious disease, and acute childhood leukaemia is increased in individuals with Down's syndrome. The incidence of Down's syndrome increases with maternal or paternal age. Many affected embryos are spontaneously aborted, and some affected foetuses are stillborn.

Other autosomal trisomies that have been identified are trisomy 18 and trisomy 13. Both conditions have a very poor prognosis, with most affected children dying from cardiac or respiratory complications within 6 months of birth.

The product of the union of a normal gamete (ovum or sperm) with a gamete missing a chromosome is a monosomy. This individual would have only 45 chromosomes in each cell. Missing an autosomal chromosome always results in death of the embryo.

Non-disjunction can also occur during mitosis. If this occurs early in development when cell lines are forming, the individual has a mixture of cells, some with a normal number of chromosomes and others either missing a chromosome or containing an extra chromosome. This condition is known as mosaicism.

Mosaicism in autosomes is most commonly seen as another form of Down's syndrome. Depending on when the non-disjunction occurs during development, different body tissues will have different numbers of chromosomes. The clinical characteristics of Down's syndrome may be present mildly or with varying degrees of severity depending on the number and location of the abnormal cells. An individual with mosaic Down's syndrome may have normal intelligence.

Abnormalities of Chromosome Structure

Abnormalities of chromosome structure involve chromosome breakage usually resulting from one of two events: (1) translocation and, (2) additions and/or deletions. Translocation occurs when genetic material is transferred from one chromosome to another different chromosome. Thus instead of two normal pairs of chromosomes, the individual has one normal chromosome of each pair and a third chromosome that is a fusion of the each pair and a third chromosome that is a fusion of the other two chromosomes. As long as all genetic material is retained in the cell, the individual is unaffected but is carrier of a balanced translocation.

If a gamete receives the two normal chromosomes or the fused chromosomes of the fused chromosome, the resulting off spring are clinically normal. If the gamete receives one of the two normal chromosomes and the fused version, the resulting off spring have an extra copy of one of the chromosomes. This condition is called an unbalanced translocation and often has serious clinical effects.

Whenever a portion of a chromosome is deleted from one chromosome and added to another, the gamete produced may have either extra copies of genes or too few copies. The clinical effects produced may be mild or severe depending on the amount of genetic material involved. Two of the more common conditions that have been described are the deletion of the short arm of chromosome 5 (cri du chat syndrome) and the deletion of the long arm of chromosome 18. (cri du chat syndrome) , so named after the typical mewing cry of the affected infant, causes severe mental retardation with microcephaly and unusual facial appearance. Deletion of the long arm of chromosome 18 causes psychomotor retardation with multiple organ malformations.

Sex Chromosome Abnormalities

Several sex chromosome abnormalities have been identified, that are caused by non-disjunction during gametogenesis in either parent. The most common deviation in females is Turner's syndrome, or monosomy X. The affected female is missing an X-chromosome and exhibits juvenile external genitalia with undeveloped ovaries. She is usually short and has webbing of the neck. Intelligence may be impaired. Most affected embryos abort spontaneously.

The most common deviation in males is Klinefelter's syndrome or trisomy XXY of the sex chromosomes. The affected male has an extra X-chromosome and exhibits poorly developed secondary sexual characteristics and small testes. He is infertile, usually tall, and effeminate. Males who are mosaic for Klinefelter's syndrome may be fertile. Subnormal intelligence is usually present.

PATTERNS OF GENETIC TRANSMISSION

Heritable characteristics are those that can be passed on to offspring. The patterns by which genetic material is transmitted to the next generation are affected by the number of genes involved in the expression of the trait. Although many phenotypic characteristics result from two or more genes on different chromosomes acting together (referred to as multifactorial inheritence), others are controlled by a single gene (referred to as unifactorial inheritance).

Unlike chromosomal abnormalities, defects at the gene level cannot determined by conventional laboratory methods such as karyotyping. Instead, genetic counsellors predict the probability of the presence of an abnormal gene from the known occurrence of the trait in the individual's family and the known patterns by which the trait is inherited.

Multifactorial Inheritance

Most common congenital malformations result from multifactorial inheritance: a combination of genetic and environmental factors. Examples are cleft lip, cleft plate, congenital heart disease, neural tube defects, and pyloric stenosis. Each malformation may range from mild to severe depending on the number of genes for the defect present or the amount of environmental influence. A neural tube defect may range from spina bifida, a bony defect in the lumbar region of the vertebrae with little or no neurologic impairment, to anencephaly, absence of brain development, which is always fatal. Some malformations occur more often in one sex. For example, pyloric stenosis and cleft lip are more common in males. Multifactorial disorders also tend to occur in families.

Unifactorial Inheritance

If a single gene controls a particular trait, disorder or defect, its pattern of inheritance is referred to as unifactorial mendelian, or single gene inheritance. The number of unifactorial abnormalities far exceeds the number of chromosomal abnormalities. This is understandable considering that 50,000 to 100,000 genes in the haploid number (23) of chromosomes are passed on to an offspring from each parent.

Unifactorial or single gene disorders follow the inheritance patterns of dominance, segregation, and independent assortment described by Mendel and include autosomal dominant, autosomal recessive, and X-linked dominant and receive modes of inheritance.

Autosomal Dominant Inheritance

Autosomal dominant inheritance disorders are those in which the abnormal gene for the trait is expressed even when the other member of the pair is normal. The abnormal gene may appear as a result of a mutation, a spontaneous and permanent change in the normal gene structure, in which case the disorder occurs for the first time in the family. Usually, an affected individual comes from multiple generations having the disorder. An affected parent who is heterozygous for the trait has a 50 per cent chance of passing the abnormal gene to each offspring. Males and females are equally affected.

Autosomal dominant disorders are not always expressed with the same severity of symptoms. The parents may have a minor abnormality that had not been diagnosed until the birth of a more severely affected child. Predicting whether an affected will have a minor or severe abnormality is not possible.

Examples of common autosomal dominantly inherited disorders are Marfan's syndrome (a disorder of connective tissue resulting in skeletal, occular, and cardiovascular abnormalities), achondroplasia (dwarfism), polydactyl (extra digits), Huntington's chorea and polycystic kidney disease.

Autosomal Recessive Inheritance

Autosomal recessive inheritance disorders are those in which both genes of a pair must be abnormal for the disorder to be expressed. Heterozygous individuals have only one abnormal gene and are unaffected clinically because their normal gene overshadows the abnormal gene. They are known as carriers of the recessive trait because these recessive traits are inherited by generations of the same family, an increased incidence of the disorder occurs in consanguineous mating (closely related parents). For the trait to be expressed, two carriers must each contribute the abnormal gene to the offspring. The chance of the trait occurring in each child is 25 per cent. A clinically normal offspring may be a carrier at the gene. Males and females are equally affected.

Most recessive disorders tend to have severe clinical manifestations and affected offspring do not often reproduce. If they do, all their offspring will be carriers, for the disorder.

Most in born errors of metabolism, such as phenylketonuria (PKU), galactosemia, maple syrup urine disease. Tay-Sachs disease, sickle cell anaemia, and cystic fibrosis, are autosomal recessive inherited disorders.

X-Linked Dominant Inheritance

X-linked dominant inheritance disorders occur in males and heterozygous females. Because the females also have a normal gene, the effects are less severe than in affected males. Affected males transmit the abnormal gene only to their daughters on the X-chromosome. heterozygous females have a 50 per cent chance of transmitting the abnormal gene to each offspring. An example of these extremely rare disorders is vitamin D-resistant rickets.

Fragile-X syndrome is a relatively recent diagnosis. The 'fragile site' on the X-chromosome was identified in a central nervous system disorder affecting males and is also seen in heterozygous carrier females. Affected individuals are mentally handicapped.

X-Linked Recessive Inheritance

Abnormal genes for X-linked recessive inheritance disorders are carried on the X-chromosome. Females may be heterozygous or homozygous for traits carried on the X-chromosome because they have two X-chromosome. Males are hemizygous because they have only one X-chromosome carrying genes with no alleles on the Y-chromosome. Therefore X-linked recessive disorders are most commonly manifested in the male with the abnormal gene on his single X-chromosome. Haemophilia, colour blindness, and Duchenne muscular dystrophy are X-linked recessive disorders.

The male receives the defective gene from his carrier mother on her affected X-chromosome. Female carriers (those heterozygous for the trait) have a 50 per cent probability of transmitting the abnormal gene to each offspring. An affected male can pass the abnormal gene only to his daughters on the X-chromosome but not to his sons. The daughters will be carriers of the trait if they receive a normal gene on the X-chromosome from their mother. They will be affected only if they receive an abnormal gene on the X-chromosome from both their mother and father.

Inborn Errors of Metabolism

Disorders of protein, fat, or carbohydrate metabolism reflecting absent or defective enzymes generally follow a recessive pattern of inheritance. Enzymes, the actions of which are genetically determined, are essential for all the physical and chemical processes that sustain body systems. Defective enzyme action interrupts the normal series of chemical reactions from the affected point onward. The result may be an accumulation of a damaging product such as phenylmelanin or the absence of a necessary product such as thyroxin or melanin.

Phenylketonuria (PKU) is an uncommon disorder caused by autosomal recessive genes. A deficiency in the liver enzyme phenylalanine hydroxylase results in failure to metabolize the amino acid phenylalanine, allowing its metabolities to accumulate in the blood. The incidence of the disorder is 1 in every 10,000 to 20,000 births. Screening for PKU is routinely performed on all infants through a blood test.

Tay-Sachs disease, inherited as an autosomal recessive trait, results from a deficiency of hexosaminidase. It occurs primarily in Jewish families. Until 4 to 6 months of age, infants appear normal; in fact, their facial features are considered very beautiful. Then the clinical symptoms appear; apathy and regression in motor and social development and decreased vision. Death occurs between 3 and 4 years of age. No known treatment exists for Tay-Sachs' disease.

Cystic fibrosis (mucoviscidosis or fibrocystic disease of the pancreas) is inherited as an autosomal recessive trait characterized by generalized involvement of exocrine glands. Clinical features are related to the altered viscosity of mucus-secreting glands throughout the body. This serious chronic disease occurs primarily in white populations but can appear in people of mixed ancestry. The overall incidence is 1 in every 2000 births. The incidence of the carrier state is estimated at 1:20 to 1:25. Advances in diagnosis and treatment have improved the prognosis, so many affected individuals now live to adulthood. Some affected women have borne children, but men are generally sterile. If the mother has cystic fibrosis and the father has no family history of the disease, the offspring have a 50 per cent chance of inheriting the gene for cystic fibrosis.

Meconium ileus occurs in about 10 per cent of newborns with cystic fibrosis.Although an initial stool may be passed from the rectum with none thereafter, usually no meconium is passed during the first 24 to 48 hours. The abdomen becomes increasingly distended and eventually the newborn requires a laparotomy for diagnosis and treatment of the condition.

EMBRYO FORMATION

Conception, defined as the union of a single egg and sperm, marks the beginning of a pregnancy. Conception does not occur in isolation; a series of events surrounds it. These events include gamete (egg and sperm) formation, ovulation (release of the egg), and union of the gametes (which results in an embryo). Implantation of the embryo in the uterus is the next event in the sequence.

Ovum

As discussed previously, meiosis in the female produces an egg, or ovum. This process occurs in the ovaries, specifically in the ovarian follicles. Each month one ovum matures with a host of surrounding supportive cells.

At the time of ovulation (Fig. 3.4) the ovum is released from the ruptured ovarian follicle. High oestrogen levels increase the motility of the uterine tubes so that their cilia can capture the ovum and propel it through the tube towards the uterine cavity. The ovum cannot move by itself.

Understanding Ovulation (Fig. 3.4)

- A dynamic relationship exists between the pituitary and gonadal hormones and the cyclic nature of the normal reproductive process
- At any time, an ovary contains ova in various stages of development
- A complex series of changes must occur which cause the final maturation of the ovum and the decomposition of the collagenous layer of the follicular wall
- Around the time of ovulation the fimbria actually sweeps gently across the ovary.

Two protective layers surround the ovum (Fig. 3.5). The first layer is a thick acellular layer, the zona pellucida. The outer layer, the corona radiata, is composed of elongated cells.

Ova are considered fertile for about 24 hours after ovulation. If unfertilized by a sperm, the ovum degenerates and is reabsorbed.

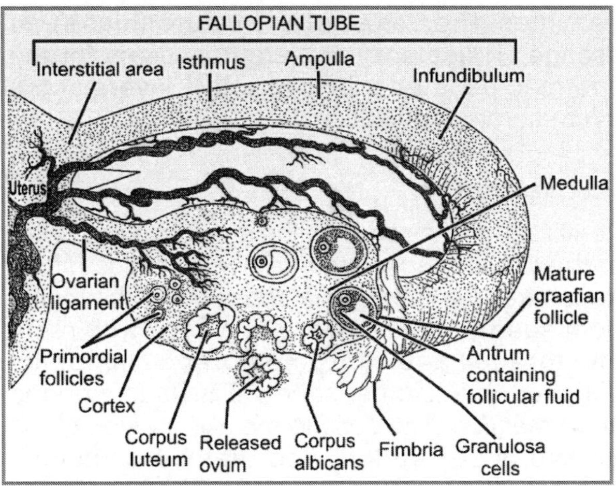

Fig. 3.4: Cross section of the human ovary shown in relation to the uterus and fallopian tubes

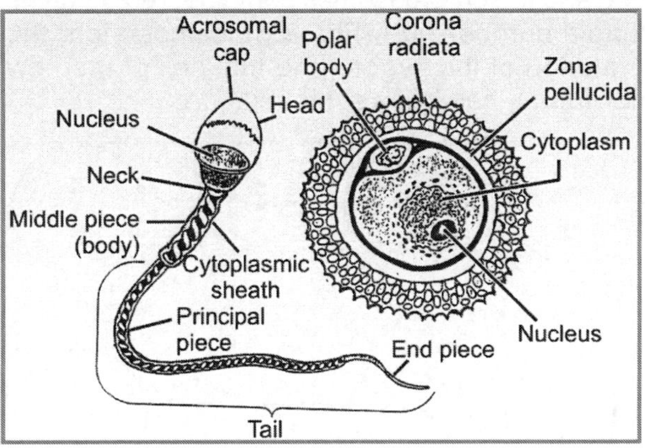

Fig. 3.5: Sperm and ovum

Sperm

Ejaculation during sexual intercourse normally propels almost a teaspoon of semen containing as many as 200 to 500 million sperm into the vagina. The sperm swim with the flagellar movement of their tails. Some sperm can reach the site of fertilization within 5 minutes, but average transit time is 4 to 6 hours. Sperm remain viable within the woman's reproductive system for an average of 2 to 3 days. Most sperm are lost in the vagina, within the cervical mucus, or in the endometrium, or they enter the tube that contains no ovum.

As the sperm travel through the uterine tubes, enzymes are produced to aid in capacitation of the sperm. Capacitation is a physiologic change that removes the protective coating from the heads of the sperm. Then small perforations form in the acrosome (a cap on the sperm) and allow enzymes (For example, hyaluronidase) to escape. These enzymes are necessary for the sperm to penetrate the protective layers of the ovum before fertilization.

Fertilization

Fertilization takes place in the ampulla (outer third) of the uterine tube. When a sperm successfully penetrates the membrane surrounding the ovum, both sperm and ovum are enclosed within the membrane and the membrane becomes impenetrable to other sperm. This is termed the *zona reaction*. The second meiotic division of the oocyte is completed, and the ovum nucleus becomes the female pronucleus. The head of the sperm enlarges to become to the male pronucleus, and the tail degenerates. The nuclei fuse and the chromosomes combine, restoring the diploid number (46) (Fig. 3.6). Conception, the formation of the zygote (the first cell of the new individual), has been achieved.

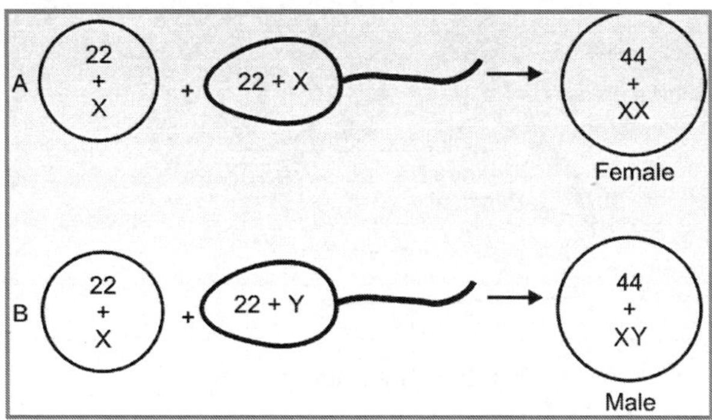

Fig. 3.6: Fertilization. **A.** Ovum fertilized by X-bearing sperm to form female zygote. **B.** Ovum fertilized by Y-bearing sperm to form male zygote

Mitotic cellular replication, called cleavage begins as the zygote travels the length of the uterine tube into the uterus. This voyage takes 3 to 4 days because the fertilized egg divides rapidly with no increase in size, successively smaller cells, blastomeres, are formed with each division. A 16-cell *morula*, a solid ball of cells, is produced within 3 days (Fig. 3.7). The morula is still surrounded by the protective zona pellucida. Further development occurs as the morula floats freely within the uterus. Fluid passes through the zona pellucida into the intercellular spaces between the blastomeres. A cavity forms within the cell mass as the spaces come together, forming a structure called the *blastocyst*. The outer layer of cells surrounding the cavity is the *trophoblast*.

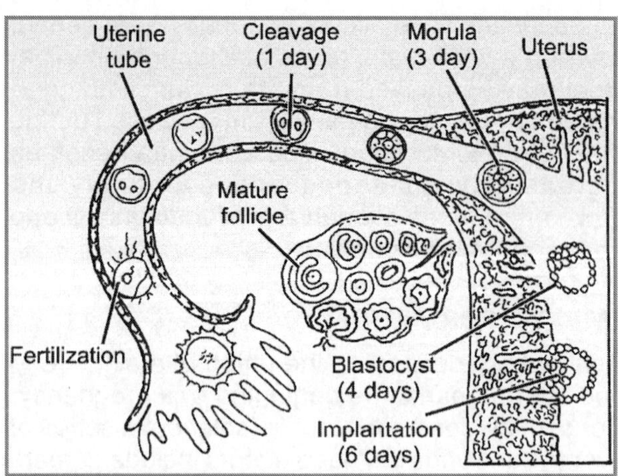

Fig. 3.7: First week of human development. **A.** Follicular development in the ovary, ovulation, fertilization, and transport of the early embryo down the uterine tube and into the uterus where implantation occurs

Implantation

The zona pellucida degenerates, and the trophoblast attaches itself to the uterine endometrium, usually in the anterior or posterior fundal region. Between 6 and 10 days after conception, the trophoblast secretes enzymes that enable it to borrow into the endometrium until the entire blastocyst is covered. This is known as *implantation*. Endometrial blood vessels erode, and some women experience slight implantation bleeding (slight spotting or bleeding during the time of the first missed menstrual period) chorionic villi, finger-like projections develop out of the trophoblast and extend into the blood filled spaces of the endometrium. These villi are vascular processes that obtain oxygen and nutrients from the maternal blood-stream and dispose of carbon dioxide and waste products into the maternal blood.

After implantation, the endometrium is called the decidua. The portion directly under the blastocyst which is where the chorionic villi tap the maternal blood vessels, is the decidus basalis. The portion covering the blastocyst is the decidua capsularis, and the portion lining the rest of the uterus is the decidua vera (Figs 3.8 and 3.9).

The Embryo and Foetus

Pregnancy lasts approximately 10 lunar months, 9 calendar months, 40 weeks or 280 days. Length

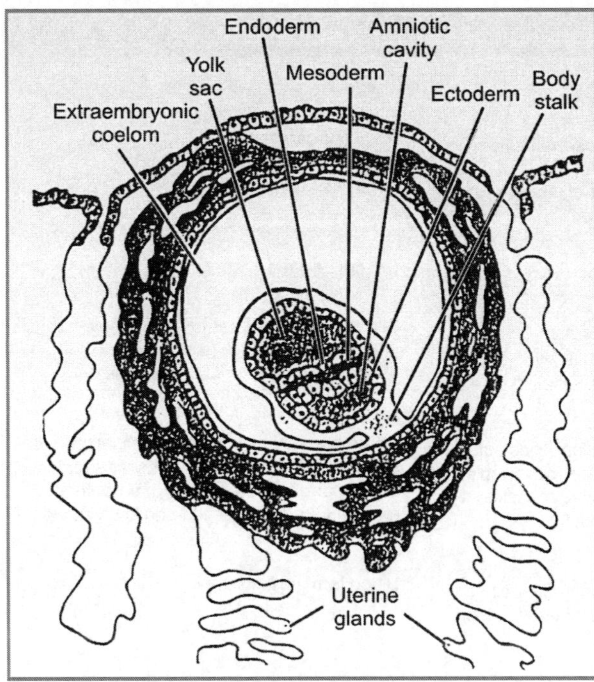

Fig. 3.8: Blastocyst embedded in endometrium. Germ layers forming

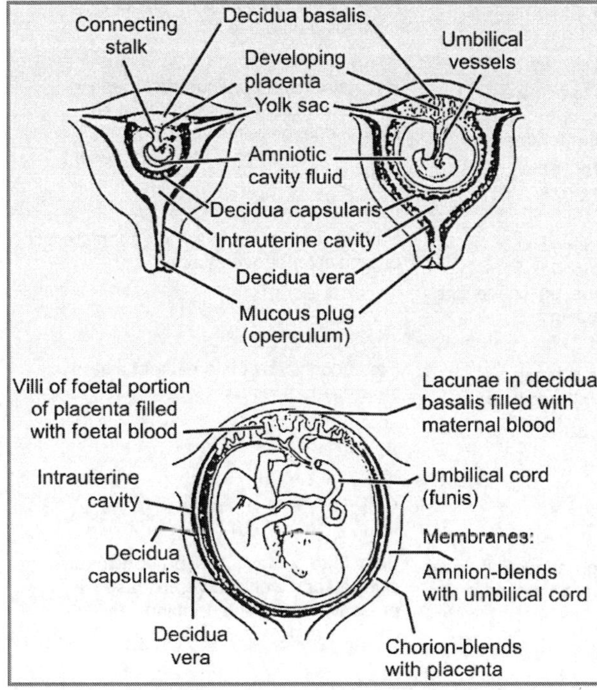

Fig. 3.9: Development of foetal membranes. Note gradual obliteration of intrauterine cavity as decidua capsularis and decidua vera meet. Also note thinning of uterine wall. Chorionic and amniotic membranes are in apposition to each other but may be peeled apart

of pregnancy is computed from the first day of the last menstrual period (LMP) until the day of delivery. However, conception occurs approximately 2 weeks after the first day of the LMP.

Thus the post-conception age of the foetus is 2 weeks less for a total of 266 days or 38 weeks. Post-conceptional age is used in the discussion of foetal development.

Intrauterine development is divided into three stages. ovum or pre-embryonic, embryo, and foetus (Table 3.1 summarizes this development).

The stage of the ovum lasts from conception until day 14. This period covers cellular replication, blastocyst formation, initial development of the embryonic membranes, and establishment of the primary germ layers.

DEVELOPMENT OF THE EMBRYO

The stage of the embryo lasts from day 15 until approximately 8 weeks after conception or until the embryo measures 3 cm (1.2 inches) from crown to rump. This stage is the most critical time in the development of the organ systems and the main external features. Developing areas with rapid cell division are the most vulnerable to malformation by environmental teratogens (a substance or exposure that causes abnormal development). At the end of the eighth week all organ systems and external structures are present and the embryo is unmistakably human.

Membranes

At the time of implantation two foetal membranes that will surround the developing embryo to form. The chorion develops from the trophoblast and contains the chorionic villi on its surface. The villi burrowing into the decidua basalis increase in size and complexity as the vascular processes develop into the placenta. The chorion becomes the covering of the foetal side of the placenta. It contains the major umbilical blood vessels as they branch out over the surface of the placenta. As the embryo grows, the decidua capsularis stretches. The chorionic villi on this side atrophy and degenerate, leaving a smooth chorionic membrane.

The inner cell membrane, the amnion, develops from the interior cells of the blastocyst. The cavity that develops between the inner cell mass and the outer layer of cells (trophoblast) is the amniotic cavity (Fig. 3.8) As it grows larger, the amnion

Table 3.1: Milestones in human development before birth since LMP

4 weeks	8 weeks	12 weeks
External appearance Body flexed, C-shaped, arm and leg buds present head at right angles to body	Body fairly well formed; nose flat eyes far apart; digits well formed, head elevating; tail almost disappeared; eyes, ears, nose and mouth recognizable	Nails appearing resembling a human, head erect but disproportionately large, skin pink, delicate
Crown-to-rump measurement, weight 0.4-0.5 cm, 0.4 gm	2.5-3 cm, 2 gm	6.9 cm, 9 gm
Gastrointestinal system Stomach at midline and fusiform, conspicuous liver, oesophagus short, intestine a short tube	Intestinal villi developing, small intestines coiling within umbilical cord; palatal folds present, liver very large	Bile secreted, palatal fusion complete, intestines withdrawn from cord and assuming characteristic positions
Musculoskeletal system All somites present	First indication of ossification—occiput mandible, and humerus, embryo capable of some movement, definitive muscles of trunk, limbs, and head well represented	Some bones well outlined ossification spreding; Upper cervical to lower sacral arches and bodies ossifying, smooth muscle layers indicated in hollow viscera
Circulatory system Heart developing; double chambers visible, beginnig to beat, aortic arch and major veins completed	Main blood vessels assuming final plan, enucleated red cells predominate in blood	Blood forming in marrow
Respiratory system Primary lung buds appearing	Pleural and pericardial cavities forming, branching bronchioles nostrils closed by epithelial plugs	Lungs acquiring definite shape, vocal chords appearing
Renal system Rudimentary ureteral buds appearing	Earliest secretory tubules differentiating bladder urethra separation from rectum	Kidney able to secrete urine, bladder expanding as a sac
Nervous system Well-marked midbrain flexure, no hindbrain or cervical flexure groove closed	Cerebral cortex beginning to acquire typical cells, differentiation of cerebral cortex meninges, ventricular foramens, cerebrospinal fluid circulation spinal cord extending entire length of spine	Brain structural configuration roughly complete, cord showing cervical and lumbar enlargements ventricle foramens developed, stucking present
Sensory organs Eye and ear appearing as optic vessel and otocyst	Primordial choroid plexus developing ventricles large relative to cortex development progressing, eyes converging rapidly, internal ear developing.	Earliest taste buds indicated characteristic organization of eye attained
Genital system Genital ridge appearing (fifth week)	Testes and ovaries distinguishable, external genitals sexless but beginning to differentiate	Sex recognizable, internal and external sex organs specific
16 weeks	*20 weeks*	*24 weeks*
External appearance Head still dominant; face looking human eyes, ears, and nose approa-ching typical appearance on gross examination; arm-leg proportionate; scalp hair appearing	Vernix caseosa and latingo appearing, legs lengthening considerably, sebaceous glands appearing	Body lean but fairly well proportioned, skin red and wrinkled,vernix caseosa present sweat gland forming

Contd...

Contd...

16 weeks	*20 weeks*	*24 weeks*
Crown-to-Rump measurement, weight		
11.5-13.5 cm, 100 gm	16-18.5 cm, 300 gm	23 cm, 600 gm
Gastrointestinal system		
Meconium in bowel some enzyme section anus open	Enamel and dentine depositing ascending colon recognizable	
Musculoskeletal system		
Most bones distincty indicated through-out body, joint cavities appearing, muscular movements detectable	Sternum ossification foetal movements strong enough for mother to feel	
Circulatory system		
Heart muscle well developed, blood formation active in spleen		Blood formation increasing in bone marrow and decreasing in liver
Respiratory system		
Elastic fibers appearing in lungs, terminal and respiratory bronchioles appearing	Nostrils reopening primitive respiratory like movements beginning	Alveolar ducts and sacs present, lecithin beginning to appear in amniotic fluid (weeks 26 to 27)
Renal system		
Kidney in position and attaining typical shape and plan		
Nervous system		
Cerebral lobes delineated, cerebellum assuming some prominence	Brain grossly formed, cord myelination beginning, cord ending at level S-1	Cerebral cortex layered typically, neuronal proliferation in cerebral cortex ending
Sensory organs		
General sense organs differentiated	Nose and ears ossifying	Ability to hear
Genital system		
Testes in position for descent into scrotum, vagina open		Testes at inguinal ring in descent to scrotum
28 weeks	30-31 weeks	36 weeks
External appearance		
Lean body, less wrinkled and red; nails appearing	Subcutaneous fat begining to collect, more rounded appearance, skin pink and smooth, assumption of birth position (Fig. 5.16)	Skin pink, body rounded, general lanugo disappearing, body usually plump
Crown-to-rump measurement weight		
27 cm, 1100 g	31 cm, 1800-2100 gm	35cm, 2200-2900gm
Gastrointestinal system		
Musculoskeletal system		
Astragalus (talus, ankle bone) ossification; weak, fleeting movements minimum tone	Middle fourth phalanges ossification, permanent teeth primordia visible able to turn head to side	Distal femoral ossification centers, present, sustained, definite movements, fair tone, able to turn and elevate head
Circulatory system		
Respiratory system		
Lecithin forming on alveolar surfaces	L/S ratio=1:2:1	L/S ratio $\geq$ 2:1
Renal system		
		Formation of new nephrons ceasing. Ending of spinal cord at level (L3), definite sleep-wake cycle

Contd...

Contd...

16 weeks	*20 weeks*	*24 weeks*
Nervous system Appearance of cerebral fissures, convolutions fast appearing: indefinite sleepwave cycle; cryweek or absent weak suck reflex		
Sensory organs Eyelids reopening: retinal layers completed, light receptive, pupils able to react to light	Sense of taste present awareness of sounds outside mother's body	
Genital system	Testes descending to scrotum	
40 Weeks		
External appearance Skin smooth and pink, scant vernix caseosa, moderate to profuse hair, lanugo on shoulders and upper body only, nasal and alar cartilage apparent.		
Crown-to-rump measurement, weight: 40 cm, 3200 gm *Gastrointestinal system* *Musculoskeletal system* Active, sustained movement; good tone		
Circulatory system		
Respiratory system Pulmonary branching only two-thirds complete		
Renal system		
Nervous system Myelination of brain beginning, patterned sleep-wake cycle, strong suck reflex		
Sensory organs		
Genital system Testes in scrotum, labia majora well developed		

forms on the side opposite the developing blastocyst (Fig 3.9) The developing embryo draws the amnion ground itself, forming a fluid filled sac. The amnion becomes the covering of the umbilical cord and covers the chorion on the foetal surface of the placenta. As the embryo grows larger, the amnion enlarges to accommodate the embryo-foetus and surrounding amniotic fluid. The amnion eventually comes in contact with the chorion surrounding the foetus.

Amniotic Fluid

Initially, the amniotic cavity derives its fluid by diffusion from the maternal blood. The amount of fluid increases weekly, so that at term, between 800 and 1200 ml of transparent liquid is normally present. The amniotic fluid volume changes constantly. The foetus swallows fluid, and fluid flows into and out of the foetal lungs. The foetus urinates into the fluid, greatly enhancing its volume.

The volume of amniotic fluid is important factor in assessing foetal well-being. The presence of less than 300 ml of amniotic fluid (ligohydramnios) is associated with foetal renal abnormalities; more than 2L (hydramnios) is associated with gastrointestinal and other malformations.

Many functions are served by amniotic fluid for the embryo-foetus. Amniotic fluid helps maintaining a constant body temperature. It serves as a source of oral fluid and repository for waste. It cushions the foetus from trauma by blunting and dispersing the forces. It allows freedom of movement for musculo-skeletal development. It keeps the embryo from tangling with the membranes which facilitates symmetric growth. If the embryo does interact with the membranes, amputations of extremities or other deformities can occur from constricting amniotic bands.

Amniotic fluid contains albumin, urea, uric acid, creatinine, lecithin, sphingomyelin, bilirubin, fructose, fat, leukocytes, proteins, epithelial cells, enzymes, and lanugo hair. Study of foetal cells in amniotic fluid through amniocentesis yields much information about the foetus. Genetic studies (karyotyping) provide knowledge about the gender and normality of chromosome number and structure. Other studies determine the health or maturity of the foetus.

Yolk Sac

At the same time the amniotic cavity and amnion are forming, another blastocyst cavity has formed on the other side of the developing embryonic disk. This cavity becomes surrounded by a membrane, forming the yolk sac. The yolk sac aids in transferring maternal nutrients and oxygen, which have diffused through the chorion to the embryo. Blood vessels form to aid transport. By the third week, blood cells and plasma are manufactured in the yolk sac. At the end of the third week, the primitive heart begins to beat to circulate the blood through the embryo, connecting stalk, chorion and yolk sac.

The folding in of the embryo during the fourth week results in part of the yolk sac being incorporated into the embryo's body as the primitive digestive system. Primordial germ cells arise in the yolk sac and move into the embryo. The shrinking remains of the yolk sac degenerate (Fig 3.9). By the fifth or sixth week, the remnant has separated from the embryo.

Primary Germ Layers

During the third week after conception, the embryonic disk differentiates into three primary germ layers; the ectoderm, mesoderm, and endoderm or entoderm (Fig. 3.9). All tissues and organs of the embryo develop from these three layers.

The ectoderm, the upper layer of the embryonic disk, gives rise to the epidermis, glands, nails and hair, central and peripheral nervous systems, lens of the eye, tooth enamel, and floor of the amniotic cavity.

The middle layer the mesoderm, develops into the bones and teeth, muscles (skeletal, smooth, and cardiac), dermis, connective tissue, cardiovascular system and spleen, urogenital system.

The lower layer, the endoderm, gives rise to the epithelium lining the respiratory tract and digestive tract, including the oropharynx, liver and pancreas, urethra, bladder, and vagina. The endoderm forms the roof of the yolk sac.

Umbilical Cord

By day 14 after conception, the embryonic disk, connecting stalk. During the third week, the blood vessels develop to supply the embryo with maternal-nutrients and oxygen. During the fifth week, after the embryo has curved inward on itself from both ends, bringing the connecting stalk to the ventral side of the embryo, the connecting stalk becomes compressed from both sides by the amnion forming the narrower umbilical cord (Fig. 3.9). Two arteries carry blood from the embryo to the chorionic villi and one vein returns blood to the embryo. Approximately 1 per cent of umbilical cords contain only two vessels; one artery and one vein. This occurrence is sometimes associated with congenital malformations.

The cord rapidly increases in length. At term, the cord ranges from 30 to 90 cm long (average 55 cm) and is 2 cm in diameter. It twists spirally on itself and loops around the embryo foetus. A true knot is rare, but false knots occur as folds or kinks in the cord. Connective tissue called Wharton's jelly prevents compression of the blood vessels to ensure continued nourishment of the embryo-foetus. Compression can occur if the cord lies between the foetal head and pelvis or is twisted around the foetal body. When the cord is wrapped around the foetal neck, it is called a nuchal cord.

As the placenta develops from the chorionic villi, the umbilical cord is usually located centrally. A peripheral location is less common and is known as a battledore placenta (Fig. 3.9). The blood vessels are arrayed out from the center to all parts of the placenta.

Placenta Development (Figs 3.10A to D)

Structure

During the third week after conception the trophoblast cells of the chorionic villi continue to

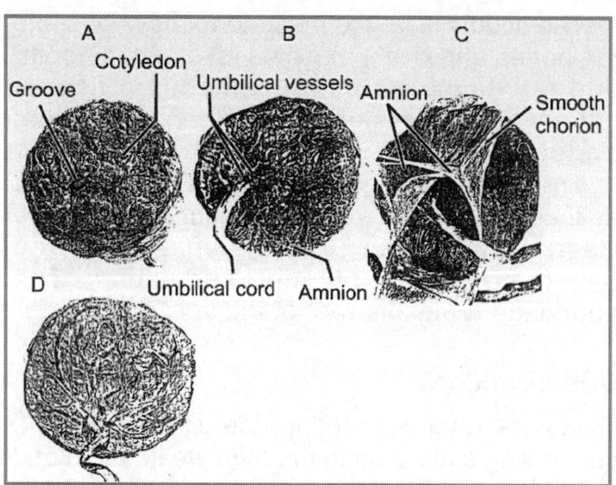

Figs 3.10A to D: Full-term placentas. **A.** Maternal (or uterine) surface, showing cotyledons and grooves. **B.** Foetal (or amniotic) surface, showing blood vessels running under amnion and converging to form umbilical vessels at attachment of umbilical cord. **C.** Amnion and smooth chorion are arranged to show that they are fused and continuous with margins of placenta. **D.** Placenta with a marginal attachment of the cord, often called a battledore placenta because of its resemblance to bat used in medieval game of battledore and shuttlecock

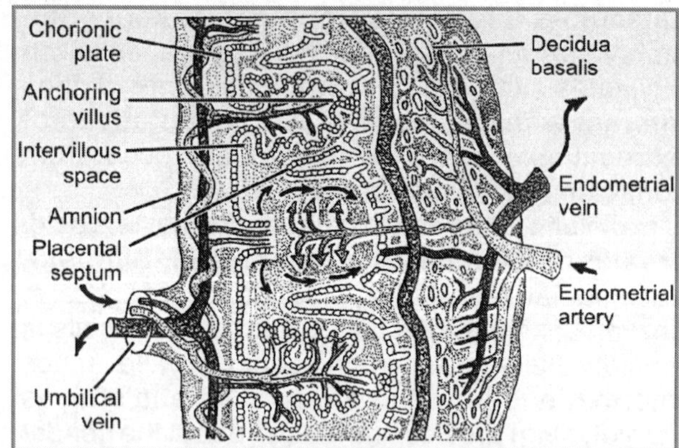

Fig. 3.11: Flow the placenta supplies oxygen and nutrition to the embryo and removes its waste products. Deoxygenated blood leaves the foetus in the umbilical arteries and enters the placenta where it is oxygenated. Oxygenated blood leaves the placenta in the umbilical vein, which enters the foetus via the umbilical cord

invade the decidua basalis. As the uterine capillaries are tapped, the endometrial spiral arteries fill with maternal blood. The chorionic villi grow into the spaces with two layers of cells; the outer syncytium and the inner cytotrophoblast. A third layer develops into anchoring septa, dividing the projecting decidua into separate areas called cotyledons. In each of the 15 to 20 cotyledons, the chorionic villi branch out and a complex system of foetal blood vessels forms. Each cotyledon is a functional unit. The whole structure is the placenta (Fig. 3.10A).

The maternal-placental-embryonic circulation is in place by day 17, when the embryonic heart starts beating. By the end of the third week, embryonic blood is circulating between the embryo and chorionic villi. In the intervillous spaces, maternal blood supplies oxygen and nutrients to the embryonic capillaries in the villi (Fig. 3.11). Waste products and carbon dioxide diffuse into the maternal blood.

Functions

The placenta functions as a means of metabolic exchange. Exchange is minimal at this time because the two cell layers of the villous membrane are too thick. Permeability increases as the cytotrophoblast thins and disappears by the fifth month, leaving only the single layer or syncytium between the maternal blood and foetal capillaries. The synctium is the functional layer of the placenta. By the eighth week, genetic testing may be done by obtaining a sample of chorionic villi by aspiration biopsy; however, limb defects have been associated with chorionic villus sampling done before 10 weeks. The structure of the placenta is complete by the twelfth week. The placenta continues to grow wider until 20 weeks when it covers about one half of the uterine surface. It then continues to grow thicker. The brancing villi continue to develop within the body of the placenta, increasing the functional surface area.

One of the early functions of the placenta is as an endocrine gland that produces four hormones necessary to maintain the pregnancy and support the embryofoetus. The hormones are produced in the syncytium.

The protein hormone human chorionic gonadotropin (hCG) can be detected in the maternal serum by 8 to 10 days after conception, shortly after implantation. This hormone is the basis for pregnancy tests. The hCG preserve the function of the ovarian corpus luteum, ensuring a continued supply of oestrogen and progesterone needed to maintain the pregnancy. Spontaneous abortion occurs if the corpus luteum stops functioning before the placenta is producing sufficient oestrogen and progesterone. The amount of hCG reaches its maximum level at 50 to 70 days and then begins to decrease.

The other protein hormone produced by the placenta is human placental lactogen (hPL). This substance is like a growth hormone and stimulates maternal metabolism to supply needed nutrients for foetal growth. This hormone increases the resistance to insulin, facilitates glucose transport across the placenta membrane, and stimulates breast development to prepare for lactation.

The placenta eventually produces more of the steroid hormone progesterone than the corpus luteum does during the first few months of pregnancy. Progesterone maintains the endometrium, decreases the contractility of the uterus, and stimulates development of breast alveoli and maternal metabolism.

By 7 weeks, the placenta is producing most of the maternal oestrogens, which are steroid hormones. The major oestrogen secreted by the placenta is oestradiol, whereas the ovaries produce mostly oestradiol. Measurement of oestradiol levels is a clinical assay for placental functioning. Oestrogen stimulates uterine growth and uteroplacental blood flow. It causes a proliferation of the breast glandular tissue and stimulates myometrial contractility. Placental oestrogen production increases markedly towards the end of pregnancy. One theory for the cause of the onset of labour is the decrease in circulating levels of progesterone and the increased levels of oestrogen.

The metabolic functions of the placenta may be summarized as respiration, nutrition, excretion, and storage. Oxygen diffuses from the maternal blood across the placental membrane into the foetal blood, and carbon dioxide diffuses in the opposite direction. In this way the placenta functions as lungs for the foetus.

Carbohydrates, proteins, calcium, and iron are stored in the placenta for ready access to meet foetal needs. Water, inorganic salts, carbohydrates, proteins, fats and vitamins pass from the maternal blood supply across the placental membrane into the foetal blood, supplying nutrition. Water and most electrolytes with a molecular weight less than 500 readily diffuse through the membrane. Hydrostatic and osmotic pressures aid the flow of the transfer of glucose, amino acids, calcium, iron and substances with higher molecular weight. Amino acids and calcium are transported against the concentration gradient between the maternal blood and foetal blood.

The foetal concentration of glucose is lower than the glucose level in the maternal blood because of its rapid metabolism by the foetus. This requires transport of larger amounts of glucose from the maternal blood than would be supplied by sample diffusion alone.

Pinocytosis is a mechanism used for transferring large molecules, such as albumin and gamma globulins, across the placental membrane. This mechanism conveys the maternal immunoglobulins that render early passive immunity to the foetus.

Metabolic waste products of the foetus cross the placental membrane from the foetal blood into the maternal blood. The maternal kidneys then infect the foetus.

Many viruses can cross the placental membrane and infect the foetus. Some bacteria and protozoa first infect the placenta and then infect the foetus.

Drugs can also cross the placental membrane and may harm the foetus. Caffeine, alcohol, nicotine, carbon monoxide and other toxic substances in cigarette smoke, and prescription and recreational drugs (such as cocaine and marijuana) readily cross the placenta. For example of the drugs that cross the placental membrane are listed later in this chapter.

Although no direct link exists between the foetal blood in the vessels of the chorionic villi and the maternal blood in the intervillous spaces, only one cell layer separates them. Breaks in the placental membrane occasionally occur. Foetal erythrocytes then leak into the maternal circulation, and the mother may develop antibodies to the foetal red blood cells. This is often the way an Rh-negative mother becomes sensitized to the erythrocytes of her Rh-positive foetus.

Even though the placenta and foetus are living tissue transplants, they are not destroyed by the host mother. The placental hormones suppress the immunologic response, or the tissue evokes no response.

Placental function depends on the maternal blood pressure supplying circulation. Maternal arterial blood, under pressure in the small uterine spiral arteries, spurts into the intervillous spaces. As long as rich arterial blood continues to be supplied, pressure is exerted on the blood already in the intervillous spaces, pushing it towards drainage by the low-pressure uterine veins. At term gestation, 10 per cent of the maternal cardiac outputs goes to the uterus.

If interference with the circulation to the placenta occurs, the placenta cannot supply the embryofoetus. Vasoconstriction, such as that caused by hypertension and cocaine use, diminishes uterine blood flow. Decreased maternal blood pressure or cardiac outputs also diminishes uterine blood flow. When a woman lies on her back with the pressure of the uterus compressing the vena cava, blood return to the right atrium is diminished. Excessive maternal exercise that diverts blood to the muscles away from the uterus compromises placental circulation. Optimal circulation is achieved when the woman is laying at rest on her left side.

Braxton-Hicks contractions appear to enhance the movement of blood through the intervillous spaces, aiding placental circulation. However, prolonged contractions or too-short intervals between contractions during labour reduce blood flow to the placenta.

Foetal Maturation

The stage of the foetus lasts from 9 weeks until the pregnancy ends. Changes during the foetal period are not as dramatic, since refinement of structure and function are taking place. The foetus is less vulnerable to teratogens except for those affecting central nervous system functioning (Fig. 3.12).

Viability refers to the capability of the foetus to survive outside the uterus. In the past, the earliest age at which foetal survival could be expected was 28 weeks after conception. With modern technology and advancements in maternal and neonatal care, viability is now possible at 20 weeks after conception (22 weeks since LMP, foetal weight of at least 500 gm). The limitations on survival outside the uterus are based on central nervous system function and oxygenation capability of the lungs.

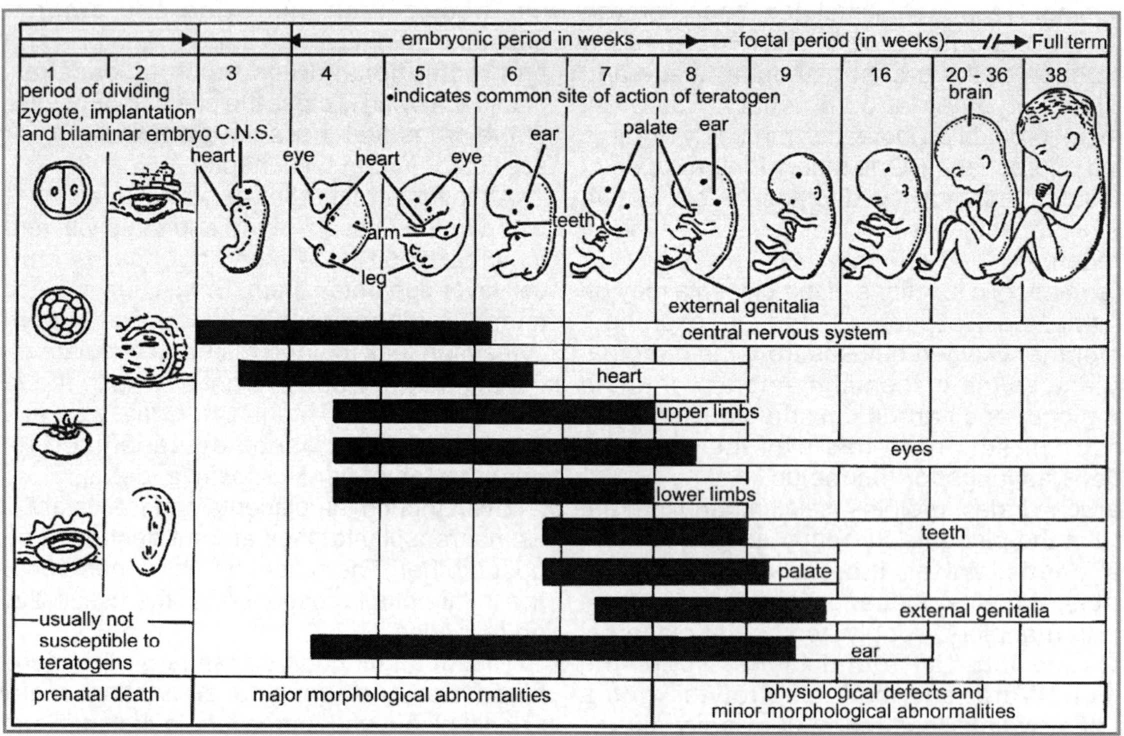

Fig. 3.12: Schematic illustration of the sensitive or critical periods in prenatal development. Dark boxes denote highly sensitive periods: light boxes indicate states that are less sensitive to teratogens

Foetal Circulatory System

The cardiovascular system is the first organ system to function in the developing human. Blood vessel and blood cell formation begins in the third week to supply the embryo with oxygen and nutrients from the mother. By the end of the third week the tubular heart begins to beat and the primitive cardiovascular system links the embryo, connecting stalk, chorion, and yolk sac. During the fourth and fifth weeks the heart develops into a four-chambered organ. By the end of the embryonic stage the heart development is complete.

The foetal lungs do not function for respiratory gas exchange, so a special circulatory pathway exists that by passes the lungs. Oxygen-rich blood from the placenta flows rapidly through the umbilical vein into the foetal abdomen (Fig. 3.13). When the umbilical vein reaches the liver, it divides into two branches. One circulates some oxygenated blood through the liver. Most of the blood passes through the *ductus venosus* into the inferior venacava. There it mixes with the deoxygenated blood from the foetal legs and abdomen on its way to the right atrium and through the *foramen ovale*, an opening into the left atrium. There it mixes, with the small amount of blood returning deoxygenated from the foetal lungs through the pulmonary veins.

The blood flows into the left ventricle and is squeezed out into the aorta. Here the arteries supplying the heart, head, neck and arms receive the major part of the oxygen-rich blood. This pattern, supplying the highest levels of oxygen and nutrients to the head, neck and arms receive the major part of the oxygen-rich blood. This pattern, supplying the highest levels of oxygen and nutrients to the head, neck, and arms, enhances the cephalocaudal (head to rump) development of the embryo-foetus.

Deoxygenated blood returning from the head and arms enters the right atrium through the superior vena cava. This blood is directed downward into the right ventricle, where it is squeezed into the pulmonary artery. A small amount of blood circulates through the resistant lung tissue, but the majority follows the path with less resistance through the ductus arteriosus into the aorta, distal to the point of exit of the arteries supplying the head and arms with oxygenated blood. The oxygen poor blood flows through the abdominal aorta into the internal iliac arteries, where the umbilical arteries direct most of its back through the umbilical cord to the placenta. There, the blood gives up its wastes and carbon dioxide in exchange for nutrients and oxygen. The blood remaining in the iliac arteries flows through the foetal abdomen and legs, ultimately returning through the inferior vena cava to the heart.

There are three special characteristics that enable the foetus to obtain sufficient oxygen from the maternal blood:

1. Foetal hemoglobin carries 20 per cent to 30 per cent more oxygen than maternal haemoglobin.
2. The haemoglobin concentration of the foetus is about 50 per cent greater than that of the mother.
3. The foetal heart rate (FHR) is 120 to 160 beats per minute, making the cardiac output per unit of body weight higher than that of an adult.

Haematopoietic System

Haematopoiesis, the formation of blood, occurs in the yolk sac (Fig. 3.14) beginning in the third week, haematopoietic stem cells seed the foetal liver during the fifth week and haematopoiesis begins there during the sixth week. This accounts for the relatively large size of the liver between the seventh and ninth weeks, stem cells seed the foetal bone marrow, spleen and thymus, and lymph nodes between weeks 8 and 11.

The antigenic factors that determine blood type are present in the erythrocytes soon after the sixth week. For this reason, the Rh-negative longer than 6 weeks after fertilization.

Respiratory System

The respiratory system begins development during embryonic life and continues through foetal life and into childhood. The development of the lungs begins between weeks 5 and 17 with the formation of trachea, bronchi and lung buds. Between 16 and 24 weeks the bronchi and terminal bronchioles enlarge and vascular structures and primitive alveoli are formed. Between 24 weeks and term birth, more alveoli form. Specialized alveolar cells secrete pulmonary surfactants to line the interior of the alveoli. After 32 weeks, sufficient surfactant is present in developed alveoli to provide infants with a good chance of survival.

LMP

Day 1 of menses

EARLY DEVELOPMENT OF OVARIAN FOLLICLE

MENSTRUAL PHASE → PROLIFERATIVE PHASE

COMPITION OF DEVELOPMENT OF TOUCLE → Oocyte — Ovulation

CONTINUATION OF PROLIFERATIVE PHASE

AGE (eks)							
1	1 Stage 1 — Fetilization	2 Stage 2 begins — Zygote divides	3 Morula	4 Stage 3 begins — Early blastocyte	5 Late blastocyte	6 Stage 4 implantation begins	7 Stage 5 begins

SCRETORY PHASE OF MENSTRUAL CYCLE

AGE (eks)							
2	8 Amniotic cavity — Bilaminar disc	9 Lacunae appear insyncyliotropho blast — Primitive yolk sac	10 Blastocyst completely implanted — Epithelium growing over surface defect	11 Primitive placental circulation established	12 Extraembryonic mesoderm — Coelom	13 Stage 6 begins Primary rill	14 Dorsal aspect of embryo — Prochordal Plate — Embry-onic disc
3	15 First missed menstrual period — Primitive streak	16 Stage 7 begins — Noto boardal process	17 Intra embroynic mesoderm — Tulaminar embryo	18 Stage 8 begins — Nural plate — Primitive streak — Length: 1.5 mm	19 Neural fold — Notochord — Embryonic coelom	20 Stage 9 begins — Brain — Neural groove — Somile — Thyroid begins to develop	21 Neural groove — Somile — Heart tubes about to fuse
4	22 Stage to begins — Heart begins to beat — Neural folds fusing	23 Rostral neuropore — Primordia of eye and ear present — Posterior neuropore	24 Stage 11 begins — Heart bulge — Rostral neuropore closes — Two pales of branchial arches	25 Otic pit — Three pairs of branchial arches	26 Stage 12 begins — Arm bud — Indicates actual size	27 Four pairs of branchial arches arm and leg buds present — CR - crown rump length	28 Stage 13 begins — CR: 4.0 mm
5	29 CR: 5.0 mm	30 Lens pits optic cups nasal pits forming	31 Developing eye — Nasal pit — Primitive mouth	32 Stage 14 Hand plates (paddle-shaped) — Lens pits and optic cups formed	33 Stage 15 begins — CR : 7.0 mm	34 Head much larger relative to trunk — Cerebral vesicles distinct — Leg buds (paddle-shaped)	35 CR : 13.0 mm
6	36 Oral and nasal cavities conliuent	37 Stage 16 begins — CR : 90 mm	38 Upper bp formed	39 CR : 10.0 mm	40 Arms bent at elbow Finger rays and auricular hillocks distinct — Palate developing	41 Stage 17 begins — Finger rays — Ventral view	42 CR :13.0 mm
7	43 CR : 16.0 mm	44 Stage 18 begins — Eyelids beginning	45 Tip of nose distinct toe rays appear Ossilication may begin — CR : 17.0 mm	46 Loss of villi Smooth chorion forms	47 General tubercle — Urogenital membrane — Anal membrane — ♀ or ♂	48 Stage 19 begins — Trunk elongating and straightening	49 CR : 13.0 mm
8	50 Upper limbs longer and bent at elbows — Fingers distinct	51 Anal membrane perforated utrogenital membrane degenerating testes and ovanes distinguishable	52 Stage 21 begins	53 Stage 21 — External genitals still in sexless state but have begun to differentiate	54 Stage 22 begins — Genital tubercle — Urethral groove — Anus — ♀ or ♂	55 Beginnings of all essential external and internal structures are present	56 Stage 23 — CR : 30 mm
9	57 Beginning of fetal period	58	59 Genitals show some 8 characterstics but still easily confused with &	60 Phallus — Urogenital fold — abioscrotal fold — Perineum — ♀	61 Genitals show fusion of urethral folds — Urethral groove extends into phallus	62 Phallus — Urogenital fold — abioscrotal fold — Perineum — ♂	63 CR : 50 mm
0	64 Face has human prollie — Note growth of chin compared to day 44	65	66 Face has human appearance	67 Clitoris — Labium minus — Urogenital groove — Labium majus ♀	68 Genitals have 9 to 4 characteristics but still not fully formed	69 Glans penis — Urethral groove — Scrotum — ♂	70 CR : 61 mm

Fig. 3.13: Time table of human prenatal development from LMP and weeks 1 to 10 after fertilization. Within large boxes are small boxes with numbers in upper left corner. These numbers refer to days since fertilization

Pulmonary Surfactants

The detection of the presence of pulmonary surfactants, surface active phospholipids, in amniotic fluid has been used to determine the degree of foetal lung maturity, or the ability of the lungs to function after birth. Lecithin is the most critical alveolar surfactant required for postnatal long expansion. It increases in amount after the twenty-fourth week. The level of another pulmonary phospholipid, sphingomyelin, remains constant. Thus the measure of lecithin (L) in relation to sphingomyelin (S), or the L/S ratio of 2:1, is used to determine foetal lung maturity. This occurs at approximately 35 weeks of gestation.

Certain maternal conditions after the development of the foetal lungs. Those conditions that accelerate lung maturity generally cause decreased maternal placental blood flow. The resulting foetal hypoxia apparently stresses the foetus, increasing blood levels of corticosteroids that accelerate alveolar and surfactant development. Conditions such as maternal hypertension, placental dysfunction, infection, and corticosteroid use accelerate foetal lung maturity. Conditions such as gestational diabetes and chronic glomerulonephritis can retard foetal lung maturity.

The use of intrabronchial synthetic surfactant in the treatment of respiratory distress syndrome in the newborn has greatly improved the chances of survival of preterm infants.

Foetal respiratory movements have been seen on ultrasound as early as the eleventh week. These foetal respiratory movements may aid in development of the chest wall muscles and regulate lung fluid volume. The foetal lungs produce fluid that expands the air space in the lungs. The fluid drains into the amniotic fluid or is swallowed by the foetus.

Before birth, secretion of lung fluid decreases. The normal birth process squeezes out approximately one-third of the fluid. Infants of caesarean births do not benefit from this squeezing process, thus they have more respiratory difficulty at birth. The fluid remaining in the lungs at birth is usually reabsorbed into the infant's blood stream within 2 hours of birth.

Renal System

The permanent kidneys form during the fifth week. Urine formation is present during the third month. Urine is excreted into the amniotic fluid and forms a major part of the amniotic fluid volume oligohydraminos, an abnormally small amount of amniotic fluid, is indicative of renal dysfunction. Because the placenta acts as the organ or excretion and maintains foetal water and electrolyte balance, the foetus does not need functioning kidneys while *in utero*. However, at birth, the kidneys are required immediately for excretory and acid-base regulatory functions.

A foetal renal malformation can be diagnosed *in utero*. Corrective or palliative foetal surgery may treat the malformation successfully, or plans can be made for treatment immediately after birth.

At term, the foetus has fully developed kidneys. However, the glomerular filtration rate (GFR) is low, and the kidneys lack the ability to concentrate urine. This makes the newborn more susceptible to overhydration and dehydration.

Most newborns void within 24 hours of birth. With the loss of the swallowed amniotic fluid and metabolism of nutrients provided by the placenta, voidings for the first days of life are scanty until fluid intake increases.

Neurologic System

The nervous system originates from the ectoderm at 18 days after fertilization. The open neural tube forms during the fourth week. It initially closes at what will be the junction of the brain and spinal cord, leaving both ends open. The embryo folds in on itself length wise at this time, forming a head fold in the neural tube closes and then the caudal end closes. During fifth week, different growth rates cause more flexures in the neural tube, delineating three brain areas the forebrain, midbrain, and hindbrain.

The forebrain develops into the eyes (cranial nerve II) and cerebral hemispheres. The development of all areas of the cerebral cortex continues throughout foetal life and into childhood. The olfactory system (cranial nerve I) and thalamus also develop from the forebrain. Cranial nerves III and IV (oculomotor and trochlear) form from the midbrain. The hindbrain forms the medulla, pons, cerebellum, and remainder of cranial nerves. Brain waves can be recorded on an electroencephalogram by eighth week.

The spinal cord develops from the long end of the neural tube. Another ectodermal structure, the neural crest, develops into the peripheral nervous system. By the eighth week, nerve fibres traverse throughout the body. By week 11 or 12 the foetus makes respiratory movements, moves all extremities and changes position *in utero*. Thumb sucking is possible, and the foetus can swim in the amniotic fluid pool, turn somersaults, and sometimes tie a knot in the umbilical cord. The major types of foetal movements are described as given below:

Major Types of Foetal Movements

General movements: These slowgross movements involve the whole body. Their duration is from several seconds to a minute.

Startle movements: These quick (less than 1 second); generalized movements always start in the limbs and may spread to the trunk and neck.

Hiccups: These are repetitive phasic contractions of the diaphragm. About may last several minutes.

Foetal breathing movements: These are paradoxical movements in which the thorax moves inward and the abdomen outward with each contraction of the diaphragm.

Isolated arm or leg movements: These movements of extremities occur without movement of the trunk.

Hand to face contact: This occurs any time the moving hand makes contact with the face or mouth.

Retroflexion of the head: This is a slow to jerky backward bending of the head.

Opening of mouth: This isolated movement may be accompanied by protrusion of the tongue.

Yawn: The mouth is slowly opened and rapidly closed after a few seconds.

Sucking: This burst of rhythmical jaw movements is sometimes followed by swallowing. With this movement the foetus may be drinking amniotic fluid

Stretch: This complex movement involves over extension of the spine, retroflexion of the head, and elevation of the arms.

Sometime between 16 and 20 weeks, when the movements are strong enough to be perceived by the mother as "the baby moving" quickening has occurred. The perception of movement occurs earlier in the multipara than in the nullipara. The mother also becomes aware of the sleeping and waking cycle of the foetus.

Sensory Awareness

Purposeful movements of the foetus have been demonstrated in response to a firm touch transmitted through the mother's abdomen. Invasive procedures to be done on a foetus require anaesthesia.

Foetus respond to sound by 24 weeks. Different types of music evoke different movements. The foetus can be soothed by the sound of the mother's voice. Acoustic stimulation can be used to evoke an FHR response. The foetus does become accustomed to noises heard repeatedly.

The foetus is able to distinguish taste. By the fifth month, when the foetus is swallowing amniotic fluid, a sweetener added to the fluid causes the foetus to swallow twice as fast. The foetus also reacts to temperature changes. A cold solution placed into the amniotic fluid can cause foetal hiccups.

The foetus can see. Eyes have both rods and cones in the retina by the seventh month. A bright light shown on the mother's abdomen in late pregnancy causes abrupt foetal movements. During sleep time, rapid eye movements (REMs) have been observed similar to those occurring in children and adults while dreaming.

At term, the foetal brain is approximately one-fourth the size of an adult brain. Neurologic development continues. Stressors on the foetus and neonate, such as chronic poor nutrition or hypotic drugs, environmental toxins, trauma, and disease, cause damage to the central nervous system long after the vulnerable embryonic time for malformations in other organ systems. Neurologic insult can result in cerebral palsy, neuromuscular impairment, mental retardation, and learning disabilities.

Gastrointestinal System

During the fourth week, the embryo changes from almost straight to a "C" shape as both ends fold in towards the ventral surface. A portion of the yolk sac is incorporated into the body from head to tail as the primitive gut (digestive system).

The foregut produces the pharynx, part of the lower respiratory tract, the oesophagus, the stomach, the first half of the duodenum, the liver, the pancreas, and the gallbladder. These structures evolve over the fifth and sixth weeks. The malformations that can occur in these areas are oesophageal atresia, hypertrophic pyloric stenosis, duodenal stenosis or atresia and biliary atresia.

The midgut becomes the distal half of the duodenum, jejunum and ileum, caecum and appendix, and proximal half of the colon. The midgut loop projects into the umbilical cord between weeks 5 and 10. A malformation (omphalocele) results if the midgut fails to return to the abdominal cavity and intestines protrude from the umbilicus. Mechel's diverticulum is the most common malformation of the midgut. It occurs when a remnant of the yolk stalk that has failed to degenerate, attaches to the ileum, leaving a blind sac.

The hindgut develops into the distal half of the colon, rectum and parts of the anal canal, urinary bladder, and urethra. Anorectal malformations are the most common abnormalities of the digestive system.

The foetus swallows amniotic fluid beginning in the fifth month. Gastric emptying and intestinal peristalsis occur. Foetal nutrition and elimination needs are taken care of by the placenta. As the foetus nears term, foetal waste products accumulate in the intestines as dark green to black, tarry meconium. Normally, this substance is passed through the rectum within 48 hours of birth. Sometimes with a breech presentation or foetal hypoxia, meconium is passed *in utero* into the amniotic fluid. The failure to pass meconium after birth can be indicative of atresia somewhere in the digestive tract, an imperforate anus, or a meconium ileus with a firm meconium plug blocking passage. Meconium ileus is seen in infants with cystic fibrosis.

The metabolic rate of the foetus is relatively low, but the infant has great growth and development needs. Beginning in week 9, the foetus synthesizes glycogen for storage in the liver. Between 26 and 30 weeks the foetus begins to lay down stores of brown fat in preparation for extrauterine cold stress. Thermoregulation in the neonate requires increased metabolism and adequate oxygenation.

The gastrointestinal system is mature by 36 weeks. Digestive enzymes except pancreatic amylase and lipase are present in sufficient quantity to facilitate digestion. The neonate cannot digest starch or fat efficiently. Little saliva is produced.

Hepatic System

The liver and biliary tract develop from the foregut during the fourth week of gestation. Haematopoiesis begins during the sixth week, requiring that the liver be large. The embryonic liver is prominent and occupies most of the abdominal cavity. Bile, a constituent of meconium, begins to form in the twelfth week.

Glycogen is stored in the foetal liver beginning at week 9 or 10. At term, glycogen stores are twice those of the adult. Glycogen is the major source of energy for the foetus and neonate who is stressed by *in utero* hypoxia, extrauterine loss of the maternal glucose supply the work of breathing or cold stress.

Iron is stored in the foetal liver. If the material intake is sufficient, the foetus can store enough iron to last for 5 months after birth.

During foetal life, the liver does not have to conjugate bilirubin for excretion because the unconjugated bilirubin is cleared by the placenta. Therefore the glucoronyl transferase enzyme needed for conjugation that is present in the foetal liver is less than is required after birth. This predisposes the neonate to hyperbilirubinemia.

Coagulation factors II, VII, IX, and X cannot be synthesized in the foetal liver because of the lack of vitamin K synthesis in the sterile foetal gut. This coagulation deficiency persists after birth for several days and is the rationale for the prophylactic administration of vitamin K to the newborn.

Endocrine System

The thyroid gland develops with structures in the head and neck during the third and fourth weeks. The secretion of thyroxine begins during the eighth week. Maternal thyroxine does not readily cross the placenta; therefore the foetus who does not produce thyroid hormones will be born with congenital hypothyroidism. If untreated hypothyroidism can result in severe mental retardation. All neonates should be screened for hypothyroidism with a blood test after birth.

The adrenal cortex is formed during the sixth week and produces hormones by the eighth or ninth week. As term approaches, the foetus produces more cortisol. This is believed to aid in initiation of labour by decreasing the maternal progesterone and stimulating production of prostaglandins.

The pancreas forms from the foregut during the fifth through eighth weeks. The islets of Langerhans develop during the twelfth week. Insulin is produced by the twentieth week. In infants of mothers with uncontrolled diabetes, maternal hyperglycaemia produces foetal hyperglycaemia, stimulating hyperinsulinaemia and islet-cell hyperplasia. This results in a macrosomic (large) foetus. The hyperinsulinaemia also blocks lung maturation, placing the neonate at risk for respiratory distress and hypoglycaemia when the maternal glucose source is lost at birth. Control of the maternal glucose source is lost at birth. Control of the maternal glucose level before and during pregnancy minimizes problems for the infant.

Reproductive System

Until the seventh week, there is no sex differentiation in the embryo. When a Y chromosome is present, testes are formed. By the end of the embryonic period, testosterone is being secreted and causes formation of the male genitalia. By week 28, the testes begin descending into the scrotum. After birth, low-levels of testosterone continue to be secreted until the pubertal surge.

The female, with two X chromosomes, forms ovaries and female external genitalia. Female and male external genitalia are indistinguishable until about the twelfth week. By the sixteenth week, oogenesis has been established. At birth, the ovaries contain the female's lifetime supply of ova. In the female, most female hormone production is delayed until puberty, however the foetal endometrium responds to maternal hormones and withdrawal bleeding or vaginal discharge (pseudomenstruation) may occur at birth when these hormones are lost. The high-level of maternal oestrogen also stimulates mammary engorgement and secretion of fluid (witch's milk in newborn of both sexes).

Immunologic System

During the third trimester, albumin and globulin are present in the foetus. The only immunoglobulin that crosses the placenta is IgG, providing passive acquired immunity to specific bacterial toxins. The foetus produces IgM by the end of the first trimester. These are produced in response to blood group antigens, gram-negative enteric organisms, and some viruses, IgA is not produced by the foetus. However colostrum, the precursor to breast milk, contains large amounts of IgA and can provide passive immunity to the neonate who is breastfed.

The normal term neonate can fight infection but not as effectively as an older child. The preterm infant is at much greater risk for infection.

Musculoskeletal System

Bones and muscles develop from the mesoderm by the fourth week of embryonic development. At that time the cardiac muscle is already beating. The mesoderm next to the neural tube forms the vertebral column grow towards each other to enclose the developing spinal cord. Ossification or bone formation begins. If a defect in the bony fusion is present, spina bifida may occur. A large defect affecting several vertebrae may allow the membranes and spinal cord to pouch out from the back, producing neurologic deficits and skeletal deformity.

The flat bones of the skull develop during the embryonic period, and ossification continues throughout childhood. At birth, connective tissue sutures exist where the bones of the skull meet. The areas where more than two bones, called fontanels, are especially prominent. The sutures and fontanels allow the bones of the skull to mould, or move, during birth, enabling the head to pass through the birth canals.

The bones of the shoulders, arms, hips, and legs appear in the sixth week as continuous skeleton with no joints. Ossification continues through childhood to allow growth. Beginning during the seventh week, muscles contract spontaneously. Arm and leg movements are visible on ultrasound, although the mother does not perceive them until the sixteenth to the twentieth week.

Integumentary System

The epidermis begins as a single layer or cells derived from the ectoderm at 4 weeks. By the seventh week, two layers of cells are present. The cells of the superficial layer are sloughed and become mixed with the sebaceous gland secretions to form the white greasy vernix caseosa, the material that protects the skin of the foetus. The vernix is thick at 24 weeks but becomes scant by term.

The basal layer of the epidermis is the germinal layer, which replaces the lost cells. Until 17 weeks, the skin is very thin and wrinkled, with underlying blood vessels visible. The skin thickens, and all layers are present at term. After 32 weeks as subcutaneous fat is deposited under the dermis, the skin becomes less wrinkled and red.

By 16 weeks the epidermal ridges are present on the palms of the hands, fingers, bottom of the feet, and toes. This makes the hand and footprints unique.

Hairs form hair bulbs in the epidermis that project into the dermis. Cells in the hair bulb keratinize to form the hair shaft. As the cells at the base of the hair shaft proliferate, the hair grows to the surface of the epithelium. The very fine hairs, called Lanugo appear first at 12 weeks on the eyebrows and upper lip. By 20 weeks, they cover the entire body. At this time, the eyelashes, eyebrows and scalp hair are beginning to grow. By 28 weeks, the scalp hair is longer than the lanugo, which is thinning and may disapper by term gestation.

Fingernails and toenails develop from thickened epidermis of the tips of the digits beginning during the tenth week. They grow slowly. Fingernails usually reach the fingertips by 32 weeks, and toenails reach toetips by 36 weeks (Figs 3.12 and 3.13).

MULTIFOETAL PREGNANCY (FIGS 3.14 TO 3.16)

Twins

When two mature ova are produced in one ovarian cycle, both can be fertilized by separate sperm. This results in two zygotes, or *dizygotic twins* (Fig. 3.14) Two amnions two chorions and two placentas that may fused together are always present. These dizygotic or fraternal twins may be the same sex or different sexes and are genetically no more alike than siblings born at different times. Dizygotic twinning occurs in families, more often among African-American women than white women, and least among Asian women. The incidence increases with maternal age upto 35 years, parity and the use of fertility drugs.

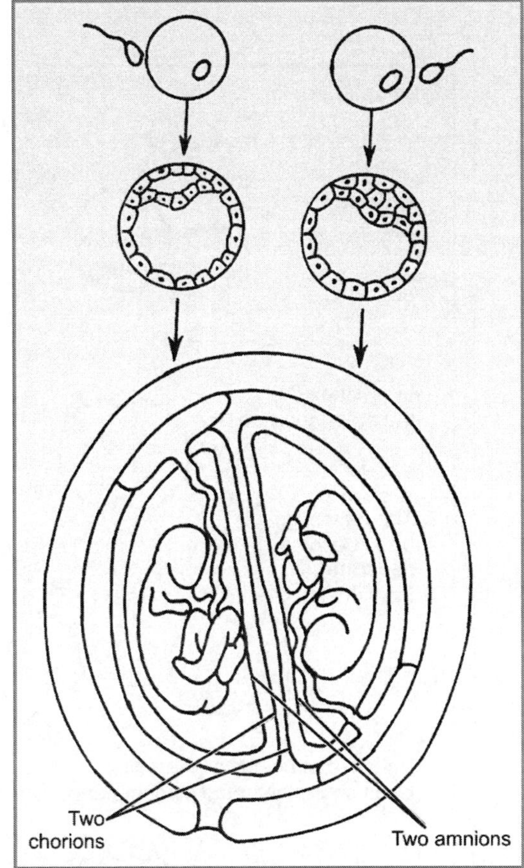

Fig. 3.14: Formation of dizygotic twins. There is fertilization of two ova, two implantations, two placentas, two chorions, and two amnions

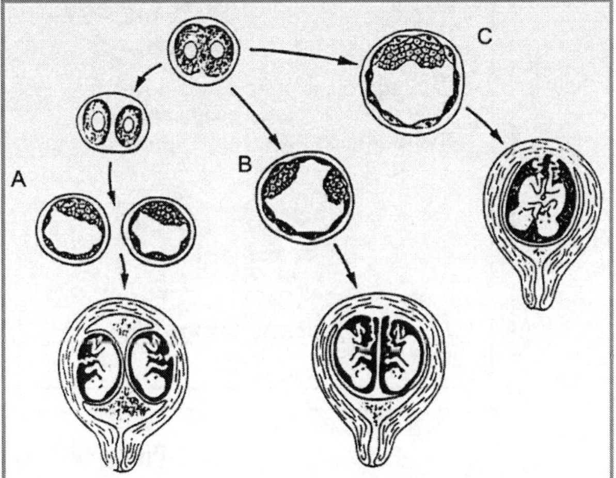

Fig. 3.15: Formation of monozygotic twins. **A.** On fertilization: blastomeres separate, resulting in two implant: two placentas, and two sets of membranes. **B.** One blastomere with two inner cell masses, one fused placenta, one chorion and separate amnions, **C.** One blastomere with incor separation of cell mass resulting in conjoined twins

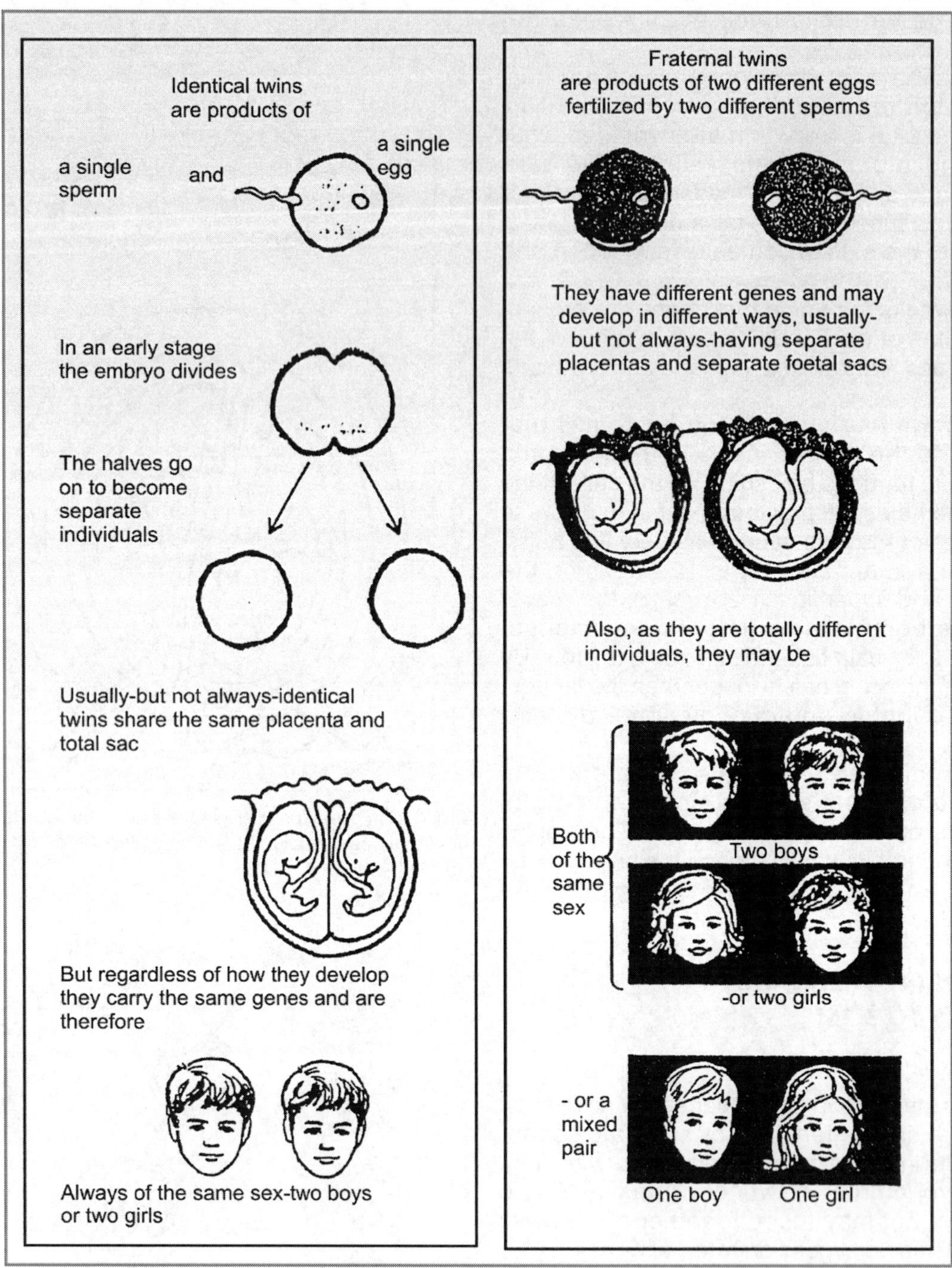

Fig. 3.16: The two types of twins

Identical twins develop from one fertilized ovum, which then divides, (hence the term *monozygotic twins*) (Fig. 3.16). They are the same sex and have the same genotype. If division occurs soon after fertilization, two embryos, two amnions, two chorions, and two placentas that may be fused develop. Most often, division occurs between 4 and 8 days after fertilization, and two embryos, two amnions, one chorion and one placenta result. Rarely does division occur after the eighth day after fertilization. In this case, two embryos are within a common amnion and a common chorion with one placenta. This frequently causes circulation problems because the umbilical cords may tangle together and one or both foetuses may die. If division occurs very late, cleavage may not be complete and conjoined, or "Siamese" twins result.

Monozygotic twinning occurs in approximately 1 of 250 births. No association with race, heredity, maternal age, or parity has been established. Fertility drugs do increase the incidence of multiple births.

Other Multifoetal Pregnancies

The occurrence of multifoetal pregnancies with three or more foetuses has increased with the use of fertility drugs and *in vitro* fertilization. Triplets occur once in about 7600 pregnancies. They can occur from the division of one zygote into two, with one of the two dividing again, producing identical triplets. Triplets can also be produced from two zygotes, one dividing into a set of identical twins and the second zygote a single fraternal sibling, or from three zygotes. Quadruplets, quintuplets, sextuplets, and so on have similar possible derivations.

GENETIC COUNSELLING

Rapid expansion in the identification, understanding, and diagnosis of genetic disease has been accompanied by effective medical and surgical therapies in a small number of cases. For the majority of genetic conditions, therapeutic or preventive measures are nonexistent or disappointly limited. Consequently, the most useful means of reducing the incidence of these disorders is by preventing their transmission. With the accumulation of knowledge about genetic disorders, the probability of recurrence can be predicted with increased accuracy. At present the best means for reducing the number of children born with genetic defects is for health professionals to provide families with genetic information and services.

The Nature and Characteristics of Genetic Counselling

Genetic counselling has been defined as a communication process which deals with the human problems associated with the occurrence, or the risk of occurrence, of a genetic disorder in a family. This process involves an attempt by one or more appropriately trained persons to help the individual or family (1) comprehend the medical facts, including the diagnosis, the probable course of the disorder and the available management; (2) appreciate in specified relatives; (3) understand the options for dealing with the risk of recurrence; (4) choose the course of action which seems appropriate to them in view of their risk and family goals and act in accordance with that decision; and (5) make the best possible adjustment to the disorder in an affected family member and/or to the risk of recurrence of that disorder.

This definition is broad and encompasses the long-term physical, psychological and sociologic adaptations that accompany the occurrence of a genetic disorder in an individual and the family.

The usefulness of genetic counselling depends partly on the timing of information provided to families. Since many emotions are involved in a genetic disorder, it is not always helpful to provide genetic counselling soon after the birth of an affected child or soon after a serious diagnosis has been made in a family member. During the initial early stages of a genetic diagnosis, information may be directed to explaining the nature of the disorder, describing the short-term prognosis, and providing support services for on going counselling. Parents for example, will often feel that their child's defect is a sign that they themselves are abnormal in some way and may benefit by having these feelings aired. Once the initial crisis is over and the parents become aware of the long-term significance of their baby's defect and wonder about its cause and whether it may happen again, specific genetic counselling may be offered.

Examples of the kinds of families that are likely to be referred for genetic assessment and counselling, are couples who have a child with a birth defect or known genetic disorder; those who are known carriers of a specific genetic disorder, those who have a known or suspected inherited condition in the family; those who have experienced reproductive problems, such as multiple miscarriages or stillbirth; those with exposure to environmental agents during pregnancy; those with ethnic backgrounds at high-risk for genetic disease; and women 35 years of age or older.

Genetic counselling is best provided in a multidisciplinary team setting that enables individuals and families to receive expert care from a variety of professionals who specialize in the management and counselling of genetic and related disorders. Because of rapid advances in human genetics and the need for clients to have access to the latest methods of genetic diagnosis and treatment, this team approach to the delivery of genetic care is especially crucial. An effective geneticist team includes expertise in genetic analysis, diagnosis, and treatment; skills in objective and subjective data collection; experience in information presentation; and family support. Accordingly, the team may be composed of a medical geneticist, cytogeneticist, biochemical geneticist, genetic counsellor, paediatrician, obstetrician, nurse, social worker, and psychologist. Other specialists, such as a neurologist or endocrinologist, may be consulted as needed. In one study of prenatal management of foetal anomalies, team counselling was found effective in offering a clear definition of the problem, avoiding unnecessary confusion and anxiety for families, and providing a supportive environment during the crisis.

Genetic Counselling Process

There are five major steps in the process of genetic counselling; obtaining a family history, establishing a diagnosis, establishing the recurrence risk, communicating information, and following up. The family history, in association with a physical examination and various confirmatory or supplementary tests, forms the basis on which a articular diagnosis is made. In taking a detailed family history, both members of a couple should be present, if possible, to obtain accurate information about both sides of the family. Information should be recorded about relatives as far back as three generation, including grand parents siblings, half-siblings, parents, offspring, aunts, uncles, and cousins. Among the kinds of information to be gathered are names, ages, and health status; early infant deaths, stillbirths, or miscarriages; parental consanguinity; ethnic origin; and presence of birth defects, retardation, and familial traits in the various family members. If a child is affected, information about the pregnancy and birth history should be noted with particular attention to maternal infections and fever; metabolic disorders; X-ray, drug and chemical exposures; labour and delivery details Apgar scores; and birth weight, head circumference, and other relevant data. Information collected from the history should be assembled in the form of a pedigree or family tree. Tests that may be necessary to help confirm or establish a diagnosis are, for examples, chromosome analysis, X-ray studies, skin or muscle biopsy, electromyography, immunologic studies, and biochemical tests appropriate to the disorder in question. Photographs may also be useful for consulting with experts about a rare or unknown disorder.

Establishing the recurrence risk involves placing the disorder in one of several categories; single-gene, chromosome aberration, multifactorial or major environmental agents. The risk can then be calculated either from mendelian ratio or by selection of the appropriate empirical estimate. Once the recurrence risk is estimated, the next step is to inform the individual or couple about the condition, its consequences, the risk figures, and therapeutic and reproductive options available for dealing with the problem. The communication of information must take into account the educational level of the couple. Since most people have little knowledge of the medical or genetic aspects of the disorder for which they are receiving counselling, the counsellor must take adequate time to explain information in simple terms and repeat content in different ways. Explaining information which the use of pictures and diagrams is useful. A follow-up letter summarising the information provided is also helpful, as it gives the couple something tangible to refer to when needed.

Follow-up visits may be needed to make sure that individuals understand and remember the information they are given. Many families are seen by a genetics team for a period of years for ongoing treatment, to keep current on new therapies and diagnostic procedures, or when new family members develop the disorder or want information to assist them in reproductive planning. As part of follow-up, parents should be informed about community agencies that can assist in the care of an affected infant, such as infant stimulation programmes, physical therapy, and support groups. Home visits by a nurse are also beneficial to assess coping and family adjustment, identify problems, clarify information, and answer further questions.

Clients Seeking Genetic Counselling

The reasons people seek genetic counselling vary, and those who are counselled may not be affected themselves. Those who seek counselling commonly fall into the following categories:

1. People who want to know whether they have or are carriers of a genetic disorder.
2. People who are concerned out being at risk for giving birth to a child with a specific genetic disorder.
3. People who are planning parenthood and who want to know the implications (prognosis and treatment) of a genetic disorder affecting one or both partners.
4. People seeking help in making a decision about prenatal diagnosis, selective abortion, artificial insemination by donor, or adoption.
5. People seeking help for a child affected with a genetic disorder.

For all pregnancies, assessing for heritable disorders to identify potential problems is standard practice. The interviewer inquires about the health status of family members, abnormal reproductive outcomes, history of maternal disorders (for example, diabetes, PKU, and cystic fibrosis), drug exposures, and illness. Advanced maternal and paternal ages are noted.

Ethnic origin should be recorded because some disorders appear more frequently in some groups.

Purposes

The purposes of genetic counselling are to (1) advise couples before conception of the probability of conceiving an infant with a genetic disorder, (2) advise couples after conception and foetal screening of whether the foetus has a genetic disorder, and (3) inform the couple options available to them including choosing not to become pregnant. The information should be presented in language the couple can understand and the risks should be placed in the proper perspective in relation to a random risk situation. The decision is never right or wrong, the counsellor should be supportive of the decision the family makes.

Counselling Services

The most efficient counselling services are associated with the larger universities and major medical centers where support services are available (for example, biochemistry and cytology laboratories) and consist of a group of specialists under the leadership of a physician trained in medical genetics. Many of these regional centers maintain satellite clinics or services in outlying areas to provide contact with consumers and health professionals. A number of specialized groups provide clinics and services for people with a specific genetic disorder such as cystic fibrosis, muscular dystrophy, haemophilia and diabetes. Health professionals should become familiar with people who provide genetic counselling and places in which counselling services are available to clients in their area of practice.

All nurses, especially those involved in the care of mothers and children, need to (1) have an understanding of genetic theory and the nature of more common genetic disorders to recognize cues that may indicate a genetically related problem. (2) help families obtain counselling services, and (3) augment the counselling process, and be aware of the legal and ethical issues involved. Nurses assist with preparation of clients for procedures and counselling and with diagnostic procedures and therapeutic programmes. Nurses also interpret and reinforce counselling, maintain follow-up care, support the family's coping capacities and assist family members in their problem solving. Nurses with advanced preparation in genetics and counselling may be genetic counsellors.

Management of Genetic Disorders

Currently, genetic disorders cannot be cured, although remedies can be implemented to prevent or reduce the harmful effects of a few disorders. Structural defects can sometimes be modified to produce normal or near normal function. Research is being conducted to devise methods to influence or change the genes directly by placing substitute DNA in the cells of those with a genetic mutation, thereby preventing or curing the disease process or relieving symptoms. Successful treatment of adenosine deaminase deficiency and cystic fibrosis has been reported.

The major emphasis in therapy is modification of the internal or external environment to minimize the effects of the disorder.

Surgical therapy is used for congenital heart defects and cosmetic defects such as cleft lip, Advances in foetal surgery are occurring foetal malformations treatable by open foetal surgery will include:

- Posterior urethral valves
- CAM (cystic adenomatoid malformation of the lung)
- CDH (congenital diaphragmatic hernia)
- Twin-twin transfusion syndrome
- Sacrococcygeal teratoma
- Complete heart block.

Other conditions are treated with product replacement (thyroid for hereditary cretinism), diet modification (low phenylalanine diet for PKU), and corrective devices for missing limbs.

People with some disorders, such as glucose-6-phosphate dehydrogenase (GPD) deficiency or the porphyrias, can prevent the disease by avoiding the specific chemical agent that precipitates the symptoms. Avoiding circumstances that reduce tissue oxygenation can reduce the sickling of red blood cells in sickle cell anaemia.

Researchers continue to develop therapies for heritable diseases. Some possible methods of future management include replacement or stabilization by oral or parenteral medications or other methods, altering of intracellular DNA, and other projected features of genetic engineering. Molecular techniques provide infinite possibilities for altering human genes through gene splicing. Thus using altered genes in ova and sperm for *in vitro* fertilization will be possible.

Process

The counselling process begins with an accurate diagnosis and a careful detailed family history. The diagnosis is frequently made on the basis of clinical manifestations but may require special biochemical or cytologic tests, especially in very rare or unusual cases. An accurate diagnosis is essential number of diseases have similar manifestations but different modes of inheritance. The mode of inheritance determines the recurrence risks and sometimes the prognosis.

Estimation of Risk

The risks are determined by the mode of inheritance. The risk of recurrence for disorders caused by a factor that segregates during cell division (genes and chromosomes) can be estimated with a high degree of accuracy by application of Mendelian principles. In a dominant disorder the risk is 50 per cent or 1 in 2, that a subsequent offspring will be affected; an autosomal-recessive disease carries a 1 in 4 risk of recurrence; and an X-linked disorder is related to the sex of the child as described in X-linked inheritance. Translocation chromosomes have a high-risk of recurrence.

Disorders in which a subsequent pregnancy carries no more risk than that for any pregnancy (estimated at 1 in 30) include those resulting from isolated incidences not likely to be present in another pregnancy, such as maternal infections (for example, rubella and toxoplasmosis), maternal ingestion of drugs, most chromosomal abnormalities, and a disorder determined to be the result of a fresh mutation.

The risk of recurrence for multifactorial conditions can be estimated empirically. An empiric risk is not based on genetic theory but on experience and observation of the disorder in other families. Recurrence risks are determined by applying the frequency of a similar disorder in other families to the case under consideration.

Interpretation of Risk

Counsellors explain the risk estimates to clients without making recommendations or decisions and avoid allowing their own biases to interfere. Counsellors provide appropriate information about the nature of the disorder, the extent of the risks in the specific case, the probable consequences, and (if appropriate) alternative options available, but the final decision must be left to the family. An important nursing role is reinforcing the information the families are given and continuing to interpret this information on their level of understanding.

Because most clients have limited knowledge of genetics and human biology, the complex concepts of cell division, segregation, and recombination are often difficult to explain. However, most people have some understanding of games of chance and have had experience with flipping coins, lotteries, and various other games based on probabilities. These are effective devices for illustrating monogenic disorders, weather forecasts and horse racing handicaps are excellent example of empiric-risk estimates.

The most important concept that must be emphasized to families is that each pregnancy is an independent event. For example, in monogenic disorders in which the risk factor is 1 in 4 that the child will be affected, the risk remains the same no matter how many affected children are already in the family. Families often erroneously assume that the presence of one affected child ensures the next three will be free of the disorder. However "chance has no memory." The risk is 1 in 4 for each pregnancy.

On the other hand, in a family in which a child is affected with a disorder with multifactorial causes, the risk increases with each subsequent child born with the disorder.

Role of the Nurse in Genetic Counselling

Nurses with advanced preparation are assuming an increasingly important role in counselling people about genetically transmitted or genetically influenced conditions. Diagnosis and treatment of genetic disorders require medical skills; the complexities of determining risk factors for many disorders and individual circumstances require the expertise of a geneticist. Nurses are usually the ones who provide follow-up care and maintain contact with clients. They are in the best position to sustain a close relationship with families; for example, community health nurses may have already established rapport with families.

Counselling and diagnosis usually involve some well-established processes. The nurse is responsible for having a beginning understanding of these processes and the impact they may have on the family. In this way, they will be better prepared to provide supportive care.

Preparation for Counselling

The initial interview or intake visit is often conducted by a nurse. At this time, a detailed family history is obtained including information about the social aspects of their lives and the meaning that disorder has for this particular erson or family. The family is told what to expect during the counselling process, procedures to be performed, and the personnel with whom they well be involved. The interview serves as an opportunity to assess the client's or family's needs and reduce anxiety. Most people who come for genetic counselling are nervous and apprehensive because they are not only concerned about a genetic condition but also know that the outcome of the counselling and the decisions made may significantly alter their lives, Therefore, a distraction-free atmosphere should be provided. This may require care for small children whose restlessness and behaviour can divert attention from what is being said. An ample amount of time is allotted to provide the family with as much information as possible.

The people involved need to know where and how the service is conducted and structured, including such aspects as the numbers and timing of visits the family members who should come, and some concepts of what the family can expect during the process. Most families have only vague or confused ideas of what a genetic counselling service can do for them. Some have unrealistic expectations. Instructions should be clear and specific and may need to be repeated. The counsellor will need information about the family, their needs and pertinent aspects of the case that may facilitate the counselling process.

Families are often sensitive about or even ashamed of their genetic problem. They may avoid keeping appointments. Part of their preparation is reassurance, which may require several telephone calls or visits before the family feels secure enough to follow through with counselling.

Diagnostic Tests and Procedures

The family and others directly involved with diagnostic procedures need to know the purpose of each test, what they can expect, and what they can do to facilitate the process. They may be concerned about whether the test will be painful, whether they will be required to undress, and whether they can be accompanied by a family member. Nurses can do a great deal to allay, fears and to supply support and reassurance.

The tests are not usually performed at the time of the initial interview but at a subsequent visit or visits. This gives the family time to assimilate information and explanations presented during the first visit. These visits provide an opportunity to obtain additional information, clarify misconceptions, and explore some of the thoughts generated by information from the previous visit. Several visits may be required before a definitive diagnosis can be made.

A pregnant woman who has chorionic villus sampling or amniocentesis for detection of genetic disease in a foetus is particularly anxious. Although the physical risk to the foetus and mother is almost neglible (approximately 1 per cent), the procedure may be fraught with emotional issues and sequelae. When the foetus is found to be free of the disorder for which the test was performed the parents need only a thorough explanation of the procedure and support during the test.

Follow-up Care

Maintaining contact with the family after genetic counselling testing or therapy is one of the most important nursing responsibilities, since the success of counselling is measured by the way the family uses the information presented to them. Most counselling services try to schedule at least one post-diagnostic or post-counselling visit to assess how well the family is beginning to incorporate this new information into their lives and value systems. Follow-up visits to the counselling service or visits to the home provide additional opportunities to re-explore all aspects of the situation and answer any questions that may have occurred to the family since the previous contacts. Clarifying information is an important nursing function.

A newly diagnosed disorder may require the implementation of a therapeutic regimen. For example, the disorder may be an in born error of metabolism, such as PKU or galactosaemia, and require consistent and rigid adherence to a diet. The family may need help in securing the necessary formula and counselling from dietetic services. The importance of maintaining the diet. Keeping an adequate supply of special preparations, and avoiding unauthorized substitutions must be impressed on the family.

Referral to appropriate agencies is another essential part of the follow-up management. Numerous parent groups with whom the family can share experiences and derive mutual support from other families with similar problems are also available. Nurses should become familiar with services available in their community that provide assistance and education to families with these special problems.

Emotional Support

Probably the most important of all nursing functions is providing emotional support of the family during all aspects of the counselling process. Feelings generated under the real or imagined threat posed by a genetic disorder vary as much as the people being counselled. Responses may include several stress reactions, including apathy, anger, hostility, fear, embarrassment, grief, and loss of self-esteem.

Guilt and selfblame universal reactions. Many look on the disorder as a stigma—especially if the disorder is visible to others. People involved with the family are often able to dispel fears and even absolve the family from guilt simply by explaining the random nature of cell division and segregation and pointing out that everyone carries defective genes that, when combined with the same genes in a partner, can produce undesirable consequences. Old wive's superstitions, and longheld misconceptions are factors that may influence a family's reaction to a genetic disorder.

The attitude of other family members and relatives can have a significant impact on some people—especially in situations in which the cause can be identified (such as a dominant or an X-linked disorder). Recessive disorders are less likely to cause blaming, since both partners carry the defective gene.

Unfortunately, most families tend to view a genetic disorder as a cause for shame, and its presence in a family may because to alter plans for marriage or child bearing even when the probability of recurrence is no more than a random risk. The way a family views the probability of recurrence varies tremendously. For example, one family will consider a 10 per cent risk as reasoning, whereas another may consider it too great a risk to contemplate marriage or childbearing.

The nature of a genetic condition also influences the way families respond to a disorder. Factors such as the severity or chronicity of a disease, the age of onset, the threat of early death, a lengthy period of deterioration, presence or absence of pain, mental retardation, and cosmetic disfiguration determine the reaction, that a condition will produce in a family. One family may risk a child with a disorder that produces a minor defect or even an early death but will not risk having a child with a lifelong physical or mental disability.

Factors such as religious beliefs, intellectual level, and prior attitudes towards the disorder affect the way families respond to counselling information. Sometimes counsellors and other health personnel create barriers through their own attitudes towards a specific disorder. Being nonjudgemental and objective is often difficult, and nurses may intentionally or unintentionally influence families in making decisions. This is especially true when the intellectual level of family members makes it difficult or impossible for them to comprehend the ramifications of a situation. Even people who can repeat information accurately often fail to grasp its significance in their case. Families may pressure the nurse to make decisions for them with questions such as "What would you do if you were me?"

Families and individuals need education, guidance, and support throughout the counselling process. They should be given the facts and possible consequences and all the assistance they need in problem solving, but the final decision regarding a course of action must be their own.

NONGENETIC FACTORS INFLUENCING DEVELOPMENT

Not all congenital disorders are inherited, congenital simply means that the condition was present at birth. Some congenital malformations may be the result of teratogens, defined as environmental substances or exposures that result in functional or structural disability. In contrast to other forms of developmental disabilities, disabilities caused by teratogens are theoretically totally preventable. Known human teratogens are drug and chemicals and for embryonic foetal effects—infections exposure, radiation, and certain maternal conditions.

A teratogen has the greatest effect on the organs and parts of an embryo during the periods of rapid differentitation. This occurs during the embryonic period, specifically from days 15 to 60. During the first-two weeks of development, teratogens have no effect on the embryo or the effects are so severe that they cause spontaneous abortion. Brain growth and development continue during the foetal period, and teratogens can severely affect mantal development throughout gestation.

In addition to the genetic make up and influence of teratogens, the adequacy of maternal nutrition influences development. The embryo and foetus must obtain the nutrients needed from the mother's diet; maternal reserves cannot be tapped. Malnutrition during pregnancy produces lowbirth-weight newborns who are susceptible to infection. Malnutrition also affects brain development during the latter half of gestation and may result in learning disabilities in the child.

CHAPTER 4

Assessment and Management of Pregnancy (Antenatal)

INTRODUCTION

Prenatal nursing is the care of the woman during pregnancy. The prenatal period is a time of physical and psychological preparation of birth and parenthood. Becoming a parent is a time of intense learning both for parents and for those close to them. The prenatal period provides a unique opportunity for nurses and other members of the health care team to influence family health. During this period, essentially healthy women seek regular care and guidance. The nurse's Health-Promotion-Intervention can affect the well being of the women, her unborn child and the rest of her family for many years.

The term "antepartal or prenatal care" as used by physicians and nurses refers to the planned examination, observation and guidance of an expectant mother. The extension of prenatal care is probably the primary factor in the improvement of maternal morbidity and mortality statistics. Society needs to appreciate its importance. The primary aims of antenatal or prenatal care is to achieve at the end of a pregnancy a healthy mother and a healthy baby. Ideally this care should begin soon after conception and continue throughout pregnancy.

The objectives of prenatal nursing are as follows:

1. To have a pregnancy with a minimum mental and physical discomfort and a maximum of gratification.
2. To promote, protect and maintain good physical and mental health, during pregnancy.
3. To monitor progress of pregnancy.
4. To detect early and treat appropriately, medical and obstetrical conditions, that would endanger the life or impair the health of pregnant woman and/or baby.
5. To ensure delivery of a mature, live and healthy infants birth under the best circumstances possible (a normal, well baby).
6. To prepare woman for delivery, breastfeeding and subsequent childcare nutrition, personal hygiene and environmental sanitation.
7. To sensitize the mother to the need for family planning including advice to cases seeking MTP.

Regular prenatal visits, ideally beginning soon after the first missed menstrual period, offer opportunities for the nurse and other health care providers to ensure the health of the expectant mother and her infant. This is achieved by supervising the course of pregnancy. Prenatal health supervision permits the diagnosis and treatment of pre-existing maternal disorders or disorders that may develop during pregnancy. This supervision is designed to monitor the growth and development of the foetus and identify abnormalities that may interfere with normal labour. The woman and her family can also seek support to reduce stress and learn parenting skills at these prenatal visits.

Before understanding the details about nursing of normal pregnancy it is better to understand the anatomy and physiology specific with bony pelvis and female genital tract, for better learning.

PHYSIOLOGICAL CHANGES DURING THE PREGNANCY PROCESS

Pregnancy triggers a complex chain of events. Energy is required to fuel the rapidly dividing cells on the journey towards implantation and development. At the same time, hormones begin sending messages throughout the body, preparing the organ systems for the changes of accommodation during pregnancy.

Table 4.1: Laboratory values during pregnancy

Determination	Value
Cardiovascular system	
Blood volume	+ 30%-50% + 1500-2000 ml
RBC mass	+ 30% (250 to 450+), 3.75^6-4.5^6/mm^3
Hematocrit (Hct)	34%-40%
Hemoglobin (Hb)	11.5-14 g/dl
White blood cells	5000-15000/mm^3
Heart rate (HR)	+ 15-20 beats/min
Cardiac output (co)	+30%-50% (to 61/min)
First-Stage labour	+ 60%
Second-stage labour	+ 80%
Blood pressure (BP) Second trimester	90/60-128/79 mmHg
Mean arterial pressure. (MAP)-second trimester	
Adult	< 100 mmHg
Adolescent	< 85 mmHg
Respiratory system	
PaO_2	104-108 mmHg
$PaCO_2$	27-32
pH 7.40-7.45	
Sodium bicarbonate ($NaHCO_3$)	18-22 mEg/L

Cardiovascular System

Blood volume expansion is one of the earliest and most basic of changes in pregnancy (Table 4.1). Values higher for multiple pregnancy.

It occurs to provide circulation to all the developing organs and body parts. To accommodate the expansion, progesterone causes relaxation of smooth vascular tissue. The intravascular space is expanded, allowing greater blood volume to meet the increased needs of the mother and foetus. The average increase of 45 per cent may occur as early as 6 weeks, although it generally rises slowly in the first trimester, reaching a peak around 30 to 34 weeks. Most of the increased volume (1200-1500 ml) is plasma, with about 300 to 450 ml composed of red blood cells (RBCs). Because of this Imbalance, the ratio of RBCs to plasma (the haematocrit) will decrease. This is called haemodilution of pregnancy. What appears to resemble anaemia is a normal event. The RBC count may fall from a prepregnancy count of 4.0 to 5.5 million/mm3 to 3.75 to 4.5 million/mm3 (written on laboratory reports as 3.756, meaning six places to the right of the decimal point, which takes place with a comma 3,750,000). The haematocrit decreases from a ratio of 37 to 45 per cent falling. Haemoglobin levels also may drop slightly because of the demand for extra iron.

During pregnancy, there is an increase in platelets, fibrin, fibrinogen, and coagulation factors, especially factors 7, 8, 9 and 10. These changes are necessary to protect the mother from bleeding at the time of delivery. However, this hypercoagulability makes her more susceptible to thrombus development during pregnancy and the puerperium, the postbirth period.

The normal white blood cell count in the nonpregnant state is between 5000 and 10000/mm^3. The count begins to rise during the second month to about 10000 mm3 and by late pregnancy and labour can reach levels of 18000 or more. This count is within normal limits for pregnancy and recovery. An increase in the granulocytes particularly neutrophils (which are polymorphonuclear (PMN) cells), causes this increase. Neutrophils which normally constitute more than half of the white blood cells profile, increase in the body in response to inflammation, pain, anxiety, stress, and labour and delivery protect against invading organisms, engulfing them through phagocytosis, and debride the decidual tissues of dead cells during the healing process.

Pulse and Blood Pressure

The heart makes several adaptations to accommodate these changes. Viewed during X-ray examination, it is more prominent because of its increased work load. The heart rate (HR) increases by 15 to 20 beats/min; the cardiac output (CO), the amount of blood pumped from the heart in 1 minute, increases by 30 to 50 per cent very early in pregnancy. Cardiac output is determined by multiplying the stroke volume with times the heart rate in 1 minute:

CO = Stroke volume × Heart rate per minute

The stroke volume does not usually increase, but the heart rate increases resulting in the increased cardiac output.

Blood pressure (BP) in the first 24 weeks usually decreases 5 to 10 mmHg systolic and 10 to 15 mmHg diastolic, producing a widening of the pulse pressure. These changes are caused by (1) relaxation of the vascular smooth muscle layer and (2) formation of new peripheral vascular beds in the breasts, uterus, and placenta, BP levels usually rise to stabilize at nonpregnancy levels by the time labour begins.

Mean Arterial Pressure

The mean arterial pressure (MAP) is computed by the following formula, which was the systolic (S) and diastolic (D) readings:

$$MAP = D + \frac{(S - D)}{3} \text{ (pulse pressure)}$$

In the second trimester, a mean arterial pressure (MAP-2) of more than 100 mmHg after 20 weeks can be interpreted as hypertension. Adolescents with lower baseline pressures may have hypertension with an MAP after 20 weeks on be interpreted as hypertension. Adolescents with lower baseline pressures may have hypertension with an MAP after 20 weeks of > 85. These figures are general guide lines; remember that BP readings must be measured against a woman's baseline. Accuracy of readings can be ensured by consistent measurement on the same arm (and during labour, between contractions). Readings also are influenced by maternal factors such as anxiety, pain, and drug use.

Vena Caval Compression

Maternal position can cause the enlarging uterus to compress the inferior vena cava, impeding venous return, thus decreasing the CO and lowering BP. This problem occurs more often in the later stages of pregnancy, particularly when the woman is lying in the supine position. This resultant supine hypotension occurs in upto 10 percent of women, who experience dizziness, light-headedness, nausea, pallor, clumsiness of skin, and even syncope, or fainting. Treatment consists of changing the maternal position from supine to left side-lying and explaining to the woman the cause of the symptoms. This problem also is referred to as the vena caval syndrome (VCS) or supine hypotension syndrome (SHS) and must be avoided during pregnancy.

Femoral Venous Pressure

An increase in femoral venous pressure is related to the weight of the uterus. Venous return from the femoral veins venous pressure rises in the legs upto 18 mmHg from a normal of below 10 mmHg. This contributes to a feeling of fullness in the legs and to dependent oedema, which is more noticeable in the evening or after standing or sitting a long time. Varicose veins may appear early in the second trimester and worsen as pregnancy progresses.

Varicose veins of the saphenous system and of the vulva and rectum (haemorrhoids) are affected primarily by the rising venous pressure in the lower extremities. Varicosities usually are more common and pronounced in the multigravida but may occur for the first time in a young primigravida with a family history of varicose veins. In addition to being unsightly, these enlarged superficial veins may be painful and throbbing, especially those in the vulva and rectal/anal area.

Walking and positional change to facilitate venous return is helpful. A woman with a tendency towards varicosities should wear support hose during pregnancy to give support and counter pressure to the walls of the distended veins.

Dependent oedema of the lower extremities also is related to venous return. Standing or sitting for long periods of time and pressure of the uterus on large veins returning from the legs tend to hinder the venous return (against gravity). Positional change to facilitate venous return helps reduce this gravity-based oedema. The side lying position during sleep and rest provides maximal kidney blood flow and function. Oedema that persists is a warning signal to report to the physician.

Orthostatic Hypotension

A decrease in the CO caused by the interference of venous return can result from the effects of orthostatic hypotension, which occurs when a woman moves from a recumbent to a standing position. Normal, uncomplicated pregnancies usually can withstand this stress without harm to the foetus. However, it might cause problems in pregnancies with pre-existing utero placental insufficiency. For such women, bed rest is recommended.

Respiratory System

Oxygen Demands

Changes in the respiratory system are caused by the increased need for oxygen intake and carbon dioxide (CO_2) discharge. Increased oxygen consumption of 20 to 30 per cent during pregnancy is the result of cardiac work, renal performance, respiratory performance, and breast, uterine, and placental demands.

Progesterone lowers the CO_2 threshold in the respiratory centre, thus increasing sensitivity to CO_2. This hormone decreases pulmonary resistance, thereby promoting an environment for increased alveolar function, allowing the thoracic cage to expand and the diaphragm to become more mobile. The result is a 30 to 40 per cent increase in tidal volume; thus the lungs have a greater capacity to exchange gases. Although these events increase the depth of respiration, the rate remains stable.

Blood Gases

To facilitate CO_2 transfer from the foetus, the pregnant woman is in a state of compensated respiratory alkalosis with a lowered carbon dioxide pressure (pCO_2) and an elevated oxygen pressure (pO_2). Maternal pO_2 increases to 100 to 108 mmHg during pregnancy. At that level, 100 per cent of material hemoglobin is oxygen saturated, thereby readily allowing maternal red cells to give up oxygen to the foetus. Foetal oxygen levels are much lower, 25 to 35 mmHg. Foetal hemoglobin (HbF) however, has an extremely high affinity for oxygen, and the maternal-foetal oxygen gradient promotes foetal uptake.

Maternal $PaCO_2$ values are decreased from 35 to 45 mm Hg to about 27 to 32 mmHg during pregnancy, which promotes elimination of foetal waste CO_2. To maintain a milk alkalosis, the concentrations of sodium bicarbonate ($NaHCO_3$) become lower in pregnancy, averaging 18 to 22 mEq/L. The maternal pH remains stable at about 7.4 to 7.42 because bicarbonate is efficiently eliminated from the kidneys.

Hyperemia

Nasopharyngeal congestion occurs as more blood enters the system. Secretions increase and sometimes cause discomfort because of oedema in the upper airway, care must be taken to prevent damage or bleeding if any manipulation of the passage is necessary, such as with intubation or suctioning at the time of delivery. A few women complain of chronic nasal stuffiness and may have a hoarse voice. The pitch of the voice may change. These women feel as if they always have a cold. A humidifier may help this discomfort. The symptoms recede without treatment in the post-birth period.

Renal System

The kidneys increase in size and weight to enable greater filtration volume and reabsorption. No real increase in output occurs in spite of the 50 per cent increase in flow. Changes occur because of increased CO, decreased renal vascular resistance, plasma volume expansion, decreased viscosity of the blood, and other endocrine changes. The pelvis, calyces and ureters are dilated because of hormonal stimuli and the physical presence of a more filtered load.

Haemodynamic Changes

Hemodynamic changes include increases in the glomerular filtration rate (GFR), renal plasma flow (RPF), excretion of amino acids, and eliminiation of water-soluble vitamins. Early in pregnancy, creatinine excretion levels also increase, and there is increased reabsorption of sodium chloride, and water. A trace of glycosuria and proteinuria may develop. Any greater amounts should be investigated because they could signal other disorders.

Positional changes affect kidney function. In the supine position the uterus presses on renal veins and arteries, reducing effective flow. Best function is produced during rest in a side-lying position.

Frequency of Urination

Some common urinary complaints during pregnancy arise from physiologic adaptations. Urinary frequency usually occurs in the first and third trimesters. In the first trimester, the enlarging uterus presses or impinges on the bladder, stimulating the sensation of needing to void even though the bladder is not full. During the second trimester the uterus rises out of the pelvic cavity and into the abdominal cavity, reducing pressure on the bladder. Later, during the third trimester, the uterus rises out of the pelvic cavity and into the abdominal cavity and into the abdominal cavlty reducing pressure on the bladder. Later, during the third trimester when lightening, or descent of the presenting part, occurs, the enlarged uterus will again compress the bladder.

Nocturia

The horizontal position for sleep promotes renal flow, with the result that more urine is produced during rest and sleep. This may be a positive benefit in reducing lower extremity oedema, or it may be a problem because sleep is interrupted several times during the night. The woman can plan to avoid fluid intake after the evening meal to help the number of times she must void during the night.

Urinary Tract Infections

Although only a small number of women are affected by urinary tract infection with symptoms, many more women may have asymptomatic bacteriuria, that is bacteria in the urine. The changes of pregnancy promote growth of bacteria because of (1) obstruction of free flow of urine by the pressure of the uterus on the ureters and (2) the relaxing effect of progesterone on smooth muscle. The bladder may contain residual urine, and the ureters loop and dilate. Stasis of urine provides a medium for bacterial growth. Nursing interventions include teaching and symptoms of urinary tract infections: dysuria, pain, blood in urine, and urgency. Because there may be a strong link with preterm labour, some physicians treat bacteriuria with antibiotics.

Gastrointestinal System

Pregnancy causes profound changes in the gastrointestinal (GI) system; many of these changes result in the common discomforts women report. Progesterone causes the GI system to relax, and the growing foetus causes crowding of the surrounding organs.

Several changes occur in the mouth. The gums become more vascular and are more likely to bleed when the woman brushes her teeth or even eats crunchy foods. Dental care is important for the treatment of gingivitis, which is common. There is no evidence to support the myth that dental caries is more common at this time. The production of saliva and its pH usually are unchanged during pregnancy. However, some women experience Ptyalism, an increased secretion of saliva. These women usually experience extreme discomfort from nausea, and the amount of saliva is increased. Women wipe their mouths frequently and complain of an enlarged reddened tongue. This discomfort is related to increased circulation to peripheral tissues and cannot be reversed.

Changes within the stomach are the result of smooth muscle relaxation, which decreases motility and cardiac sphincter control. Gastric emptying time is diminished, and acid reflex into the oesophagus may cause hearburn. The normal amount of gastric secretions is somewhat lower in the first and second trimesters but increases dramatically in the third. Throughout gestation, however, mucus production increases, which produces a soothing, protective effect on the gastric lining. The mucosa needs this effect because delayed emptying time means that irritating gastric juices remain in the stomach longer. Acid indigestion, or pyrosis (heartburn) may include burping and an acidic taste in the mouth.

Motility is reduced in the small bowel. Absorption of nutrients generally is unchanged; the absorption of iron, however is increased.

The size of the liver and blood flow to it are unchanged during pregnancy. Normal function is altered, mostly from the influence of progesterone. Serum albumin levels fall gradually; serum alkaline phosphatase and serum cholesterol levels rise by the end of pregnancy. Serum concentrations of many proteins also are elevated.

Nausea and Vomiting

Nausea and vomiting in about 50 per cent of all pregnancies generally are attributed to changes within the GI tract and higher systemic hormone levels. The problem usually surfaces early in the first trimester, around 4 to 6 weeks, and persists until the early part of the second trimester. The incidence of nausea parallels the curve of human chorionic gonadotropin (hCG) and the increase in steroidal hormones. By 100 days most nausea has subsided. A study using ultrasonography determined that the corpus luteum was on the right ovary in most women who complained of nausea. It is possible that ovarien steroid hormone concentration increased because of the more direct blood flow from the right ovary through the portal vein to the liver; in contrast, blood flow from the left ovary carries steroids through the circulatory system before they reach the liver. It has been found that women who have been pregnant more than once are more prone to morning nausea and noted that the same women may feel nausea in one pregnancy but not in another.

Constipation

Women may find constipation a major discomfort. During pregnancy some relaxation of the intestinal smooth muscle results in slowing of motility with removal of more water from the lower bowel. In later pregnancy, displacement of the bowel by the enlarging uterus may intensify the problem. If the women is taking prescribed iron supplements, constipation may be further aggravated unless medication contains a stool softener, such as ferrous fumarate plus docusate sodium (Ferro-Sequels). Increasing fluid intake to 8 glasses a day, as well as increasing the exercise level and intake of fibre, may help alleviate constipation.

Diarrhoea

Diarrhoea during pregnancy may precipitate haemorrhoids. It usually does not last long and is usually related to a food source or a viral infection. If it does not subside within 24 hours, medical attention should be sought. Over the counter (OTC) medications should not be taken without medical advice.

Diarrhoea may occur normally as labour begins and uterine activity increases. Uterine contractions stimulate bowel activity, causing frequent bowel movements. For this reason the routine enema in early labour has largely been abandoned, except for constipated women.

Haemorrhoids

Haermorrhoids are painful outpouchings of varicose veins in the lower rectal and anal area. Because of increased femoral and portal venous pressure and increased femoral and portal venous pressure and increased blood volume, haemorrhoids may worsen towards the end of pregnancy. The following interventions should be encouraged to prevent or minimize haemorrhoids and varicose veins in the pelvic area.

1. Elevate legs and the lower pelvis to facilitate venous return.
2. Use support hose, take more frequent rest intervals, decrease standing and increase walking.
3. Use sitz baths or sit in a bathtub in 2 to 3 inches of warm water as needed.
4. Insert a glycerin suppository before stooling.
5. Apply witch hazel wipes to anal area.
6. Perform frequent perineal hygiene.
7. With lubricated glove, replace external haemorrnoids after each bowel movement.

If additional medication is needed, it is prescribed for constipation, and as a local anaesthetic in ointment or suppository form may ease evacuation.

Integumentary System

Vascular Changes

As a result of higher oestrogen levels, superficial vascular changes related to increased blood flow can occur. Spider angioma, commonly seen in light-skinned women, consists of tiny vessel networks that appear mainly on the face, chest and arms. Many women notice erythema or redness of the palms and soles of the feet. Nose bleeds nasal congestion, and increased bleeding of the gums also can occur. In addition, many women who are usually intolerant of cold weather are more comfortable during pregnancy because of increased peripheral circulation.

Striae Gravidarum

Striae gravidarum commonly called stretch marks appear as pink or purpellines on the breasts, lower abdomen, or thighs. In time, they become brown or silvery but never completely disappear. There is no preventive treatment; striae occur in women who are genetically predisposed to these changes, regardless of the amount of weight gained.

Glandular Changes

Sweating and the excretion of sebum increase during pregnancy, necessitating more frequent cleansing for comfort. Oily skin and sometimes acne may recur in women with a history of this problem. In contrast, some women complain of pruritus (itching) caused by dry skin. If it persists, the women should be evaluated for liver function.

PUPPP

Pruritic urticarial papules and plaques of pregnancy (PUPPP) is epidermatologic condition that may affect a primigravida in her third trimester. The condition is thought to occur in 1 in 200 pregnancies. The rash usualy starts as eruptions in the stretch marks (striae) and spreads across the abdomen and buttocks to the arms and legs.

The rash resembles poison ivy rash, according to one affected mother. Women affected by this pruritic rash tend to have excessive weight gain.

Treatment consists of oatmeal baths, topical ointment, and antihistamines, usually diphenhydramine (Benadryl). The eruptions usually clear within a few days of delivery. It has been reported spontaneous clearing within 3 weeks after birth.

Hormonal Changes

The actions of hormones during pregnancy spur increased pigmentation, especially on the nipples and areolae, umbilicus, axillae and perineum. On the lower portion of the abdomen, the line between the symphysis and the umbilicus, the linea alba, will darken, to become the linea nigra. melasma, a blotchy, irregular hyperpigmentation of the forehead, cheeks nose, and upper lip, commonly referred to as the "mask of pregnancy" occurs more frequently in women with dark complexions. This condition, which formerly was called chloasma fades after delivery, but in some women, it never disappears completely. Pigmented nevi are stimulated and become darker and larger; new moles may even appear but usually regress after delivery.

Growth of hair and nails is accelerated during pregnancy. Hair growth quickens, and more follicles become active. After delivery, this rate slows, the follicles cease activity, and hair loss increases. Some women are frightened by this and must be reassured that their prepregnancy hair-growth pattern will return.

Musculoskeletal System

As pregnancy progresses, the skeleton makes several adjustments to accommodate the growing uterus and to prepare for delivery. Progressive lordosis (abnormal increased degree of forward curvature) of the spine develops to keep the centre of gravity over the woman's legs. Although this measure allows her to maintain her upright posture, the abnormal curvature causes backache. Posture is affected by the hormonal changes and the weight of the uterus. The hormone relaxin loosens the cartilage and connective tissues of the symphysis pubis and sacroiliac joints to facilitate vaginal delivery. The relaxation however can lead to pelvic discomfort, particularly in late pregnancy.

As a result of these adjustments, the pregnant woman acquired a characteristic carriage and gait. The compensatory changes, although helpful, do not allow her to maintain full control of balance and mobility a situation distressing to many women, who want to be active throughout pregnancy.

Calcium Metabolism

Although maternal calcium levels fall during pregnancy, the serum ionized calcium concentration remains at nonpregnancy levels, probably a result of the increased action of maternal parathyroid hormone (PTH). PTH acts on the intestines to increase absorption of calcium and in the kidneys to decrease filtration. As a result, more calcium is recovered from dietary sources, thereby ensuring a supply for maternal and foetal needs. There is no loss of bone density from pregnancy.

Leg Cramping

Muscle cramping is a common complaint. It occurs later in pregnancy and often at night. The cause may be related to a change in electrolyte, calcium and phosphorus levels. Usually medical intervention is not indicated. The woman may stretch the muscle by sitting up and pulling, hard on her toes or by standing at the bedside and, with her foot flat, flexing the foot to stretch the calf muscle. Gentle massage of the muscle also seems to help. Some women occasionally are treated with calcium lactate or vitamin B complex, but no standard intervention exists.

Backache and Neuralgia

Strain on weak abdominal muscles and lower back muscles and increased weight of the uterus may cause backache. A few women have a serious problem with backaches or with pain radiating along the nerve to the leg. Sacroiliac joint strain is common, with tenderness over the posterior aspect of the joint. Separation of the symphsis pubis is uncommon but very distressing. The woman has pain while walking, and the pubic joint is tender to touch. This problem may appear at the time of childbirth, and a client who reports severe pain during ambulation should be examined for symphysis separation.

Exercise to strengthen the lower back is basic to improved status. Some women need to wear a supportive girdle. Warmth to the affected area and physical therapy may be advised. Remember, pain during pregnancy is a sign of a problem. The woman should be referred for evaluation.

Sacroiliac Joint Strain

Sacroiliac joint strain, which is affected by relaxin, also is common in pregnancy. Very few women have sciatic nerve pressure with significant pain.

Bed rest is required in these cases. Others have carpal tunnel syndrome the radial side of the hand may be numb or painful. The median nerve is compressed in the fibrous tunnel through which it passes. Treatment to moderate the condition is not given until after childbirth, when it may disappear. The lateral cutaneous nerve of the thigh also runs in a restricted space under the inguinal ligament and may be compressed during later pregnancy, resulting in sensory changes.

Strain on weak abdominal and lower back muscles because of the weight of the uterus may lead to lordosis and backache. Women should be instructed to recognize postural changes, to use low-heel, comfortable shoes, and to strengthen lower back muscles with exercise. She should be taught proper body alignment for standing, stooping, and lifting. Squatting instead of stooping is beneficial; yet women who are unaccustomed to squatting, fall when they attempt that posture. Women find squatting, very comfortable, and a number of these women give birth in this position. Walking upstairs also is a function that demands good posture.

To balance and compensate for the weight at the front of the body, the woman should learn appropriate ways to get out of a chair or out of bed. In this technique, she moves to the edge of the chair and leans forward until the weight of her body is over the feet. To arise from a bed, she should move to the edge of the bed while lying on her side. She pushes up with her dependent elbow and opposite hand to a sittig position and waits for dizziness to pass before standing upright.

Posture

Proper posture, good body mechanics, and exercise cannot be ignored by the expectant mother. Women need to recognize the value of good body condition. Although many participate in exercise programs, others are not active and become less so during pregnancy.

Exercise

In health conscious society, there has been a surge of interest in physical fitness and exercise programmes. Aware of the difficulties produced by the changing body, frustrated in their attempts to lead an active life-style, and motivated to be physically fit for vaginal delivery, women have extended this pursuit to pregnancy. In most communities exercise classes are readily available through fitness centres and child birth educators. Swimming is a recommended activity during pregnancy.

Physiologic Responses to Exercise

Exercise physiology is a new field that explores the effects of exercise on pregnancy and the foetus. Current guidelines are based on extensive studies and anecdotal observations surround the increased oxygen consumption and cardiac workload needed for exertion before and during pregnancy; there is also concern about the effect on the foetus of the temperature increase produced during a workout.

During exercise, vasodilation to the heart, muscle, and brain occurs thus decreasing the blood supply, particularly to the viscera. Stress is placed on joints already weakened by hormonal influence. Oxygen uptake is increased to meet the demands of the heart and muscles. The respiratory rate, tidal volume, heart rate, cardiac output, body temperature, and metabolic rate rise. If exercise is prolonged and strenuous, the oxygen supply may be exceeded, leading from aerobic (with oxygen) to an anaerobic (without oxygen) state. If the latter occurs, metabolic acidosis arises, which may compromise the foetus.

Foetal Responses to Exercise

Foetal responses to maternal exercise can be transitory or long-term. Foetal heart rate and breathing movements increase with moderate exercise. The greatest concern is that regular strenuous exercise particularly in the first trimester could rise the body temperature core sufficiently to manifest the teratogenic effects of heat on the growing embryo. For this reason, moderation is advised during this period.

Another concern for the foetus is the adequacy of uteroplacental blood flow. Studies of working mothers and those who have engaged in active fitness programmes have shown that birth weights are consistently somewhat lower. Because of design limitation, these studies cannot be judged as definitive; however, most physicians advise limiting activity for women with known utero-placental deficiency problems such as hypertension and intra-uterine growth retardation. In addition, women who engage in strenuous activity should be monitored for signs of compromise before continuing regular exercise.

Basic Exercises

Basic exercises to strengthen the abdominal muscles and lower back are curl-ups or partial sit-ups and and the pelvic tilt. The nurse should inform the woman of the guidelines of exercise and inquire about her exercise posture, and fatigue at each clinic visit. In addition, conditioning exercises for childbirth preparation should be encouraged. The woman should be taught Kegel exercises in preparation for birth and recovery. To perform Kegel exercises, the woman should sit or lie supine and alternately tighten and then relax the muscles of the pelvic diaphragm and perineum for 6 seconds at a time.It has been suggested that women increase the tightening time to 12 seconds per exercise and work up to at least 12 minutes of exercise a day.

The comparison exercising with non-exercising women and found that women who exercised had significantly higher self-esteem and lower rating for physical discomforts than did the non-exercising group. This study's findings point to the importance of exercise during pregnancy.

Guidelines: The proposed guidelines for exercise during pregnancy and suggests that strenuous exercise be limited to 15 minutes. Before a pregnant woman begins a new exercise programme or considers a strenuous new activity, risks and benefits must be presented to her as well as precautions.

The Guidelines for Exercise during Pregnancy and Postpartum are:

Pregnancy and postpartum

1. Regular exercise (at least three times per week) is preferable to intermittent activity. Competitive activities should be discouraged.
2. Vigorous exercise should not be performed in hot, humid weather or during a period of febrile illness.
3. Ballistic movements (jerky, bouncy motions) should be avoided. Exercise should be done on a wooden floor or a tightly carpeted surface to reduce shock and provide sure footing.
4. Deep flexion or extension of joints should be avoided because of connective tissue laxity. Activities that require jumping, jarring motions, or rapid changes in direction should be avoided because of joint instability.
5. Vigorous exercise should be preceded by a 5-minute period of muscle warm-up. This can be accomplished by slow walking or stationary cycling with low resistance.
6. Vigorous exercise should be followed by a period of gradually declining activity that includes gentle stationary stretching. Because connective tissue laxity increases the risk of joint injury, stretches should not be taken to the point of maximum resistance.
7. Heart rate should be measured at times of peak activity. Target heart rates established in consultation with the physician should not be exceeded.
8. Care should be taken to gradually rise from the floor to avoid orthostatic hypotension. Some form of activity involving the legs should be continued for a brief period.
9. Liquids should be taken liberally before and after exercise to prevent dehydration. If necessary, activity should be interrupted to replenish fluids.
10. Women who have led sedentary life-style should begin with physical activity of very low intensity and advance activity levels very gradually.
11. Activity should be stopped and the physician consulted if any unusual symptoms appear.

Pregnancy only

1. Maternal heart rate should not exceed 140 beats/min.
2. Strenuous activities should not exceed 15 minutes in duration.
3. No exercise should be performed in the supine position after the fourth month of gestation is completed.
4. Exercises that employ the Valsalva manoeuvre should be avoided.

5. Caloric intake should be adequate to meet not only the extra needs of pregnancy but also of the exercise performed.
6. Maternal core temperature should not exceed 38°C (100.4°F).

For example, activities that require the supine position and could lead to supine hypotensive syndrome should be avoided. High impact aerobics and aggressive contact sports also should be questioned because low impact aerobics are safer for the pregnant woman and provide equal benefit. Sky diving, scuba diving, and similar activities in which atmospheric and oxygen pressure changes occur should be avoided during pregnancy.

Exercise in moderation benefits both the mother and foetus. Pregnant women should be encouraged to engage in some form of exercise or activity programme to promote physical and psychologic well being. The following exercises help woman to relieve some discomfort:

Pelvic Rock (Fig. 4.1A)

Purpose

- Improves muscle tone.
- Relieves backache.

Instructions

1. Lie on your back with your knees bent, exhale, rolling your waist upward, toward your chest. Then inhale as you relax back to the starting position.
2. On your hands and knees, exhale as you pull your stomach up. Inhale as you relax.
3. Stand against a wall, pull your stomach in, and roll your hips forward and upward, tucking your buttocks under. Practice pressing the small of your back against the wall.

Tips for performing this exercise

- Do not exaggerate the curve of your back when relaxing.
- Gradually increase from 10 to 30 repetitions daily.

Tailor Stretch (Fig. 4.1B)

Purpose

- Stretches the muscles that pull the legs together
- Loosens, the perineum
- Reduces back strain.

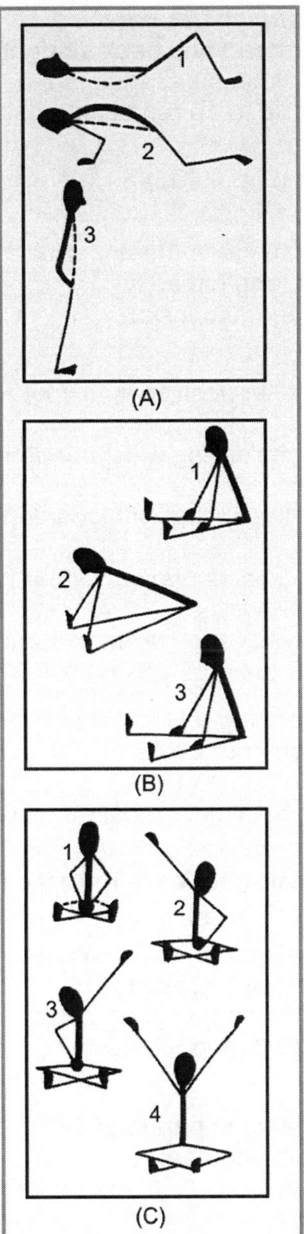

Figs 4.1A to C: These conditioning exercises prepare the woman's muscles for labour and relieve some of the discomforts of late pregnancy **A.** Pelvic Rock, **B.** Tailor Stretch, **C.** Tailor Reach

Instructions

1. Sit on the floor with your, legs spread comfortably apart.
2. Exhale as you stretch your hands down toward your ankles.
3. Inhale as you relax back to the starting position.

Tips for performing this exercise
- Keep your head and back straight
- Keep your knees flat against the floor
- Do slowly up to 10 repetitions daily.

Tailor Reach (Fig. 4.40C)

Purpose
- Relieves fatigue in the upper back
- Increases lung capacity
- Aids rib cage expansion.

Instructions
1. Sit in the tailor position with your arms in your lap.
2. Reach for the ceiling with your right hand, then relax.
3. Reach for the ceiling with your left hand, then relax.
4. Reach for the ceiling with both hands, then relax.
5. Inhale as you reach up to expand your lungs and ribs. Exhale as you relax.

Tips for performing this exercise
- Do not arch your back
- Look straight ahead
- Begin with 5 repetitions daily and work up to 10.

Phase 1: Tension Release in Large Muscles

Technique
- Tense one large muscle area at a time
- Feel the tension spread
- Release the tension gradually and smoothly
- Count to 10 during release.

Muscle areas

Do each of these separately:
1. Face, neck, shoulders
2. Upper back
3. Lower back
4. Abdomen
5. Buttocks
6. Pelvic floor
7. Legs
8. Arms.

Practice positions

Use different positions to provide for good circulation and body weight distribution:

Chaise lounge—lie flat on back with shoulders and head elevated to comfort with pillows; legs slightly apart, arms at sides, elbows bent, palms down, head to one side.

Sims lateral—lie on side with pillows under head; place one pillow under bent, upper leg; make arms comfortable.

Phase 2: Tension Release in Small Muscles

Technique

Use slow, comfortable, natural breathing rate. Allow one complete breath for each activity. For each of the exercises listed below, follow these steps:
1. Inhale
2. Exercise
3. Exhale
4. Release tension.

Exercises

Do the following exercises in sequence; concentrate on release of all tension:
1. Pull toes downward, upward
2. Turn ankles inward, outward
3. Bend knees slightly
4. Straighten knees
5. Stretch, extend left leg from lip
6. Repeat with right leg
7. Squeeze thighs together
8. Tighten buttocks
9. Tighten pelvic floor
10. Roll legs inward, outward
11. Make fists
12. Extend fingers
13. Bend wrist downward, backward
14. Bend elbows slightly
15. Straighten elbows
16. Raise shoulder toward left ear
17. Repeat with right shoulder
18. Squeeze chest (shoulders forward)
19. Squeeze shoulder blades (shoulders back)
20. Expand chest
21. Arch lower back slightly
22. Erase curve in lower back slowly
23. Bend neck forward, chin to chest
24. Bend neck backward, erase curve

On completion of exercises, take several deep breaths and get up slowly.

ENDOCRINE SYSTEM AND METABOLISM THYROID FUNCTION

In the first trimester the thyroid gland increases in size and is readily palpable. This results in a normal increase in thyroid hormons (triiodothyronine (T3) and thyroxine (T4) synthesis to support gestational growth. In spite of this increase, the hypothalamic-pituitary-thyroidal relationship remains stable.

Normal pregnancy mimics a mild hyperthyroid state; the basal metabolic rate (BMR), CO, heat intolerance, and emotional lability increase, and menses stop. The BMR rises gradually during pregnancy to a 25 per cent increase. The thyroid hormones function to increase the production of initracellular proteins and energy, which increases the rate of consumption of carbohydrates, fats, and oxygen, resulting in increased heat production. Because of increased heat production and expanded vascular supply many women complain of being warm and flushed. This change is normal and subsides after childbirth.

Adrenals

The adrenal glands produce glucocorticoids during pregnancy.

Free plasma cortisol levels rise to 2.5 times higher at full term than they were before pregnancy. Cortisol regulates carbohydrate metabolism and influences insulin production.

Pancreas

The insulin producing cells of the pancreas increase in size and number during pregnancy. Thus an accelerated starvation effect is produced by maternal fasting. During fasting, the woman's blood glucose levels will drop 15 to 20 mg/dl below nonpregnancy levels as a result of foetal drain on the maternal supply. The fasting levels of insulin also are lower, resulting in the potential for ketosis. Ketosis must be avoided because ketone bodies have been implicated in foetal brain damage.

Maternal eating, on the other hand, produces an extreme opposite response. Blood sugar levels rise sharply, as do insulin and triglycerides, and there is decreased tissue sensitivity to the action of insulin. This diabetogenic response, or insulin antagonism, is heightened by the action of human placental lactogen (hPL) and, to a lesser extent, is related to the higher levels of oestrogen, progesterone, and free cortisols. This is the reason for encouraging six small meals a day in place of three large meals.

Pregnancy impairs insulin action, and the decreased responsiveness of tissue to the effect of insulin results in elevated glucose levels. Although maternal insulin does not cross the placenta, the foetus relies on facilitated diffusion of maternal glucose for energy needs. If maternal hyperglycaemia is present, foetal levels are elevated.

Parathyroid

Activity of the parathyroid glands increases during pregnancy. With more parathyroid hormones (PTH) released, the body is able to absorb more calcium from the GI tract, ensuring sufficient calcium for maternal and foetal needs.

Pituitary

Because the menstrual cycle has been interrupted, the anterior pituitary gland ceases its release of follicle-stimulating hormone (FSH) and luteinizing hormone (LH). After birth, prolactin or leuteotropic hormone (LTH) is secreted in response to nipple stimulation and breast-feeding. The posterior pituitary secretes small amounts of oxytocin late in pregnancy, which simulates uterine contractions of labour. After delivery, nipple stimulation with breast feeding triggers release of oxytocin (1) to contract uterine muscle and thus prevent bleeding, (2) to release prolactin, and to (3) contract the ducts, which causes the let-down reflex whereby milk is ejected as the baby sucks on the nipple.

REPRODUCTIVE SYSTEM

Hormones

Oestrogen: Oestrogen is secreted by the ovary at the beginning of pregnancy and then by the placental cells. Oestrogenic effects on most of the body systems have been indicated earlier. Acting alone or in conjunction with other hormones, it stimulates the following groups of actions:

- Alteration in vaginal pH and glucose levels
- Increase in uterine size and weight
- Breast and mammary duct development and changes in nipple consistency and colour.
- Various skin changes, including darker colouration of melana-influenced cells.
- Nasopharyngeal oedema.
- Diabetogenic response, partially as the result of oestrogen levels.
- Increased blood flow to tissues, stimulated by oestrogen.

Progesterone: The hormone that maintains the pregnancy is named for its action-progestation.

Progesterone inhibits uterine motility, increasing potential for implantation, allowing the uterus to contain the foetus. Progesterone is first secreted by the corpus luteum in the ovary, but by the twelfth week it is secreted primarily by the placental tissue. It maintains the decidual lining, relaxes smooth muscle throughout the body, and contributes to the vascular changes. The following categories of effects are seen:

- Cardiovascular system: Relaxed vessels allow for blood expansion
- Respiratory system: Decreasing pulmonary resistance
- Renal system: Relaxing its structures to allow for high volume
- Breasts: Development of lobes and alveoli in preparation for breastfeeding
- Liver: Decreasing levels of serum albumin and increasing level of serum phosphatase and cholesterol
- Pancreas: Contributes to diabetogenic effects.
- Gastrointestinal system: Reducing motility.

Human chorionic gonadotropin: Human chorionic gonadotropin (hCG) is secreted by the trophoblastic layer of the blastocyst. This hormone maintains the corpus luteum until the placental tissue can produce adequate amounts of pregnancy hormones. This hormone has been implicated in the cause of morning sickness; nausea of pregnancy follows closely the curve of hCG in the first trimester hCG levels in urine or serum provide the basis for pregnancy tests. The hormone also may be referred to as urinary chorionic gonadotropin (UCG).

Relaxin: Relaxin is secreted during pregnancy, first by the corpus luteum and then by the placenta. Its actions are not precisely known, but it appears to work in conjunction with progesterone, quieting uterine muscular activity and preventing loss of the conceptus. It may contribute to the fatigue and tiredness experienced early in pregnancy. Later in pregnancy it may relax the connective tissue, especially in the sacroiliac ad symphysis pubis in preparation for labour. Softening of the cervix also is partially attributed to relaxin.

Human placental lactogen: When human placental lactogen (hPL) was first isolated from the placenta, its similarity to both human growth hormone (hGH) and prolactin was noted. Because its effect on the mammary gland is greater than its effect on growth, it is called hPL. Later, because it possessed somatropic and lactogenic properties, the name human chorionic somatomammotropin (hCS) was proposed. Both names are still used.

hPL prepares the body for lactation by stimulating the development of the breast and milk production. Other possible effects are attributed to this hormone; it may assit hCG in prolonging the life and activity of the corpus luteum. It has been suggested then other influences of hPL, including enhancement of carbohydrate metabolism, promotion of fat storage, increase of free circulating fatty acids, and stimulation of erythropoiesis (erythrocyte production) and aldosterone secretion.

Prolactin: Prolactin (PRL, PL) is secreted by the chorionic layer of the placenta and the pituitary gland. Its major influence is indicated by its name, prolactin (for lactation), although the hormone also is known as galactopoietic hormone, lactogenic hormone, luteotropic hormone (LTH), and mammotropin.

Prolactin has 82 groups of actions, including breast growth, osmoregulation, reproductive activity, itegumentary action, synergism with steroids, and lactogenesis. Medications, exercise, and anaesthesia can influence its release.

Serum levels rise from 30 mg/ml in the first trimester to a high of 200 ng/ml at term. Amniotic fluid contains 5 to 10 times more prolactin than does maternal serum. After delivery, prolactin levels diminish in 1 week if bottle feeding is chosen. If the mother chooses breast feeding, levels remain high during the first week and rise even higher after a feeding. After lactation is established, however, the base level is lower, with continued peaks of release within 30 minutes of suckling by the infant. There is indication that prolactin plays some part in inhibiting ovulation during the period of breastfeeding by inhibiting release of LH by the anterior pituitary. Continued release of prolactin occurs in response to infant suckling, but levels eventually decrease and menses resumes. Thus frequent nursing and vigorous sucking of the infant seem to be the key to preventing the return of ovulation for at least 3 to 6 months after birth.

Uterus

To accommodate the growing foetus, the smooth muscles of the uterus enlarge, stretching to at least eight times the prepregnant size. As already noted, the nonpregnant uterus weighs approximately 60 g (2 Oz). The once pear-shaped organ enlarges first to a globular shape and then to an ovoid or egg shape weighing more than 1000 g. The increase in size depends on foetal size, the shape of the placenta, and the volume, of amniotic fluid. Most of the increase is in the fundal portion and is due not to an increase in the number of cells but rather to cell size. This hypertrophy contributes to the remarkable changes just after the birth.

Uterine growth follows a pattern, and measurement of the height of the uterine fundus gives clues to deviations that may indicate a problem with pregnancy. By week 12 the uterus is palpable at the symphysis pubis, by week 20 the fundus should reach the umbilicus, and by week 36 it should be at the xiphoid process within 2 weeks of birth, as the foetus settles into position for birth, the uterus shifts position and moves away into a more forward angle, relieving pressure on the diaphragm. This final shift in position is known as lightening for the sense of relief that is experienced.

The myometrium is thick and firm and becomes progressively stretched and thinner in the second half of gestation. Toward the end of pregnancy, it is thin enough to allow the foetal head and extremities to be palpated easily.

The isthmus or juncture between the body of the uterus and the cervix is softened by hormonal influence. By bimanual examination, the isthmus can be compressed to almost paper thinness, a condition called Heggar's sign. Another early sign of pregnancy is Ladin's sign, a softening of a spot on the anterior portion just above the uterocervical juncture.

Cervix

The nonpregnant cervix has the firmness and feel of the tip of a nose, because of expanded blood circulation and hormonal activity, it becomes increasingly soft. The softening is known as goodell's sign, One of the early indications of pregnancy. The cervical os is lined with mucus-secreting glands that enlarge to secrete a thick tenacious mucus that effectively closes the os for the duration of pregnancy. This seal or mucous plug prevents ascending infection from contaminating the foetus. In the few weeks before birth the cervix becomes gradually softened or it pens. Toward the beginning of labour, it gradually shortens (effaces) and begins to open (dilates). As the uterus begins the work of labour to pen and thin the cervix, the mucous plug (called "show") is expelled from the cervical canal. The show is one of the the first indications that effective labour has begun. Because small capilaries in the cervix may be broken, blood mixes with the mucus and hence the term bloody show.

Vagina

During pregnancy, the vaginal rugae enlarge and become more elastic in preparation for the passage of the foetus and placenta. Because of hormones, especially oestrogen, there is increased sloughing of cells from the cervical and vaginal walls. Causing increased amounts of vaginal mucus and leucorrhea. Leucorrhea may be thin and milky or thick and sticky but should not cause itching or irritation to tissues unless infection such as trichomonas or *Candida albicans* is present. The vaginal pH changes from a low of 4 to 5 to a less acidic 5 to 6. This change, with increased glycogen content in cells, may foster growth of organism in the vagina. Circulation to the vaginal and cervical tissues increases, and the vaginal mucosa and cervix take on a bluish purple-blue; this change is Chadwick's sign and can be seen by the eighth week of pregnancy. Vaginal birth weakens the circum-vaginal muscles (CVM), and Kegel's exercises can help to strengthen the CVM.

Breast Changes

For many women, one of the first signs of pregnancy is a fullness or tingling of the breasts very similar to the fullness and tingling experienced during the pre-menstrual period. During pregnancy, however, the fullness can cause discomfort. The tenderness continues for some time because the hormones of pregnancy, particularly oestrogen and progesterone, prepare the body for breast-feeding: most changes are influenced by both hormones. Oestrogen influences the development of the ducts, whereas progesterone influences alveolar and lobule development. Blood vessels in the breast enlarge and become prominent, showing visible, blue, twisting patterns. The enlargement and mobility of the nipple and darkening and enlargement of the tubercle of Montgomery are attributed in part to the action of oestrogens.

Additional hormones are necessary for breast development; these include pituitary hormones (prolactin, adrenocorticotropic hormone (act high FSH, LH, thyroid stimulating hormone TSH, and hCS).

Colostrum, a fluid full of nutrients and antibodies is secreted in small amounts as early as the second trimester. Some authors suggest no breast preparation or expression of colostrum during pregnancy. Experts, however, recommends that nipple preparation and prenatal breast massage be begun in the third trimester to more quickly establish lactation.

Breast stimulation during later pregnancy has been out of favour because nipple stimulation triggers the release of oxytocin from the posterior pituitary. Oxytocin is a factor in the initiation of labour. There is doubt about stimulation or if the woman is threatened with labour, such a practice is not recommened in the last few weeks of pregnancy.

NURSING CARE PLAN (TABLE 4.2/4.3)

Diagnosis of Pregnancy

The professionals who have contact with the pregnant woman and her family will include a cross section of health workers such as nurses, physicians, midwives, nutritionists, and social workers. These people must collaborate to provide holistic care for the client. The case management model, which makes use of care maps and critical pathways, is one system that promotes comprehensive care with little or no overlap in services.

The initial visit of the woman to the health care provider is important in setting the tone for her care. The woman needs to feel welcomed and important. This initial visit may include diagnosing the pregnancy and establishing the data base, depending on the duration of gestation. If pregnancy is too early and cannot be verified, the woman's next appointment is scheduled for 2 weeks later.

The woman's desire for pregnancy is evaluated. If she is pregnant and does not wish to be, she is counselled about her options. If she is not pregnant and does not wish to be, she is counselled about fertility management. If appropriate. If the woman is pregnant, and plans to carry the pregnancy to term, prenatal health supervision should be started and continued until the birth of the infant.

Pregnancy spans nine calendar months or 10 lunar months,or approximately 40 weeks. Pregnancy is divided into three month periods or TRIMESTERS. The first trimester extends from weeks 1 through 13, the second from weeks 14 through 26, and the third from week 27 through term (38 to 40 weeks). The prenatal care rendered during each trimester includes different aspects of care. This chapter focuses on meeting the needs of the pregnant woman during the first trimester.

Many women come to the first prenatal visit after a home pregnancy test result proved positive. However, the clinical diagnosis of pregnancy before the second missed period may be uncertain in at least 25 to 30 per cent of women. Such things as physical variability, lack of relaxation, obesity, and tumours may make a difficult even for the experienced obstetrician, nurse practitioner, or midwife to diagnose pregnancy. The accuracy of the diagnosis is important because the emotional, social, medical or legal consequences of an inaccurate diagnosis, positive or negative, can be extremely serious to correct date for first day of the LMP, dates of intercourse or BBT record may be of great value in accurately diagnosing pregnancy.

All the activity initiated within the uterus with the onset of pregnancy cannot be kept a secret for long. Widespread changes take place in the body, creating various signs and symptoms that possess varying degrees of importance in the diagnosis of pregnancy. These signs and symptoms are usually arranged according to their accuracy into three groups, the presumptive, the probable, and the positive signs of pregnancy. However, no universal agreement exists regarding the contents of these categories. Events are noted using Gestational Age (GA).

Presumptive Signs and Symptoms

The presumptive signs and symptoms of pregnancy are those that could easily be an indication of other condition. They usually include the following:

Amenorrhoea: Although absence of menses may be an early sign of developing pregnancy, it is not always an indication. Amenorrhoea may occur as a result of sudden changes in environment of occupation, emotional upset, malnutrition, fatigue, hormonal disorders, extensive exercise and menopause.

Table 4.2: Nursing care plan of women adjusting to the pregnant state

Problem	*Objective*	*Nursing interventions*
Anxiety related to emotional responses to pregnancy	Anxiety is reduced. Woman discusses her feelings and uses positive coping mechanisms to deal with her emotional responses to pregnancy Specific plans for selected problems are described below:	Provide realistic reassurance that responses are normal and encourage open discussion of concerns
A. Early phase of maternal adaptation to pregnancy evidences by ambivalence about being pregnant *Clinical manifestations*: Expresses surprise at being pregnant Responses to news includes mixed emotions: "Who me? Not now!"	Woman verbalizes her concerns and exhibits positive behaviors towards pregnancy status, e.g., tells others about being pregnant, buys/wears maternity clothes	Ask how she feels about being pregnant Give permission to express positive or negative feeling about pregnancy, e.g., "many women find that they do not feel quite ready when they learn that they are pregnant" Provide appropriate place to talk Explain near universality of ambivalence in early pregnancy
B. Alteration in self-concept: change in body image *Clinical manifestations*: Feelings range from very positive to extremely negative May worry that she is seen as fat. Feels large, heavy, and awkward as pregnancy advances	Enlarging abdomen and other body changes are accepted as normal	Provide information: hormonal and uterine changes, and what outcomes can be expected, e.g., most changes revert after delivery; striae don't disappear but do fade; weight can be lost, muscle tone regained with exercise Observe for indications that the woman is not coping well with pregnancy's impact on her body, e.g. wears constrictive clothing; repeated referral to self as "fat" or "ugly" or "look what this baby is doing to me"; overly concerned with striae or pigment changes of the skin. Arrange counselling for these women to avoid inappropriate self-care and psychologic stresses. Explain possible causes of discomfort or lack of responsiveness in pregnancy, e.g., fatigue, nausea, and vomiting; breast tenderness in first trimester Fatigue and enlarging abdomen in third trimester
Altered patterns of sexual expression related to physical changes of pregnancy, sexual desire, or fear of injury to fetus *Clinical manifestations*: Woman may ask questions about effect of pregnancy. on sexuality but, more often, will not	Woman and partner understand the reason for these changes and concerns and will maintain a mutually satisfying sexual relationship	Determine impact on sexuality of pregnancy on woman and her partner, need of couple to share concerns Suggest alternative sexual activities and positions Discuss issues of safety: there is no evidence that sexual intercourse during normal pregnancy can cause harm to foetus. Intercourse can be safely continued until membranes rupture unless physician advises otherwise

Nausea and vomitings: Nausea and vomiting often occur in the morning, but are not limited to this time. Nausea and vomiting, presumably caused by changes in hormone levels in the body, in the first weeks of pregnancy, are not confined to this cause, since they are a common occurrence during gastrointestinal tract irritation and emotional stress.

Frequent urination: Frequent urination usually of small amounts, is common during the first and last weeks of pregnancy because of pelvic congestion and the particular pressure of the uterus on the bladder. Urinary frequency may also be present because of excitement, large fluid intakes, or irritation of the urinary tract. Increased urination is also associated with diabetes mellitus.

Breast changes: Tingling, swelling and tenderness involving the breasts are also found early in pregnancy. These symptoms may also be experienced during each menstrual cycle just before menses.

Changes in shape of abdomen: Increased abdominal size and shape are usually noted the eighth to tenth week of pregnancy. However, the contour of a woman's abdomen may depend on dietary will power rather than gestation. Increased abdominal size may also be influenced by the growth of tumours of hernias.

Changes in the skin and mucous membranes: Increased abdominal size may be accompanied by pink to purplish "stretch marks," known technically as striae gravidarum. It is now thought that their presence is probably more related to increased production or sensitivity to adreno-cortical hormones during pregnancy than to weight gain alone. Such skin changes are also noted in patients with Cushing's disease and, to a lesser degree, in patients with sudden weight gains not associted with pregnancy.

Another pigmentation characteristic of pregnancy is a bronze type of facial colouration called chloasma, or the mask of pregnancy, often seen on dark-haired women. Development of a dark line (linea nigra), extending from the sternum to the pubis in the midline is quite common. These changes in skin colouration are probably related to hormonal alterations.

Most references list the violet colouration of the vagina, cervix, and vulva, which is apparent at about 6 to 10 weeks gestation (Chadwick's sign), as a presumptive indication of pregnancy. It is caused by increased circulation to the area may be associated with any cause of pelvic congestion.

Quickening: Quickening, meaning the first time life or foetal movement is felt by the woman, can sometimes be imitated by peristalsis or gas and be misinterpreted. By the time quickening is felt (at approximately 16 weeks by women who have already had children and 18 weeks or more by women who are experiencing their first pregnancy), other more definite signs should be manifested.

Fatigue: Fatigue, often included on the list, is a widespread complaint.

Probable signs and symptoms: The probable signs of pregnancy are more certain than presumptive signs, but not foolproof. Listed enlargement of the uterus, certain other changes in the reproductive anatomy and physiology, and positive pregnancy tests. The increasing accuracy of selected pregnancy tests has led some physicians to consider their positive results equal to positive signs.

Certain presumptive signs found in a woman who has never experienced pregnancy usually are considered probable. They are depened pigmentation of the breasts, production of breast secretion (colostrum), and the presence of the linea nigra. However, these may have little diagnostic value for women who have had children recently or have been nursing their infants.

Changes in reproductive organs: Enlargement of the uterus, rather than an increase in abdominal circumference, is a definitive sign of pregnancy. Nevertheless, uterine tumours or inflammation may cause an increase in abdominal size. At 6 to 8 weeks' gestation a special softening of the region of the uterus between the body and the cervix, called the isthmus, occurs. It is determined by a simultaneous abdominal and vaginal examination, a bimanual maneuver illustrated. This softening is termed Hegar's sign. Another softening of the uterus affecting the cervix is detected by the examiner's finger. In the nonpregnant state, the cervix feels somewhat like the cartilage at the tip of a nose. During pregnancy, the cervix changes in consistency to resemble the pliability of the ear lobe to lips (Goodell's sign).

Basal body temperature elevation: Basal body temperature elevation is one of the earliest diagnostic observations possible and is considered to have 97 per cent accuracy. However, for the basal or waking temperature to have meaning the woman must have taken her temperature consistently, using proper technique both before and after ovulation to detect the persistent relative increase in basal reading.

Ballottement: The French term ballotement describes "tossing a ball in the air and catching it on its return. "Near midpregnancy the small foetus is enclosed in a relatively large fluid-filled sac or bag of waters. When an examiner taps the baby's head or body, it characteristically floats away and then rebounds to nudge the examiner's fingertips. Rarely this ball-lip rebound may be mimicked by the movement of a utering tumour or polyp; therefore it represents only a probable sign.

Positive Biologic and Immunochemical Pregnancy Tests

Pregnancy tests are based on the fact that the chorionic villi of an implanted ovum or of the developing placenta secrete human chorionic gonadotropic hormone (hCG) which is excreted in small amounts in urine and blood. The first pregnancy tests were biologic. A concentrated urine sample obtained from a morning specimen, voided after a period of fluid limitation, was injected into a laboratory animal. The animal was then observed for changes inits reproductive cycle. Rabbits, mice, and frogs were used. Immunochemical tests that no longer require laboratory animals are now employed.

Although the excretion of urinary hCG during pregnancy shows significant individual variations, within 48 hours of implantation hCG levels increase rapidly. Immunologic pregnancy tests have become more accurate and easier to read and have a very high level of sensitivity. Recently URINE tests involving the use of monoclonal antibodies have demonstrated very accurate results as early as 1 week after implantation. The use of these tests in increasing.

If pregnancy tests that have been designed for use in the home are employed, the need to follow directions carefully must be emphasized. Tests are usually done 3 days after the missed menstrual period and must be repeated if negative. A relatively low false-positive rate but a high (about 25%) false-negative result has been reported. The use of client-performed tests continues to be controversial.

Special blood tests known as radioimmunoassays (RIAs) may also be used to obtain pregnancy confirmation. The RIA for Beta subunit of hCG is said to be capable of diagnosing pregnancy as early as two days before the first missed period.

Most pregnancy tests are only about 95 to 99 per cent accurate, depending on when they are performed, the method used, and the presence of factors that may cause both false negatives and positives. For these reasons, "positive" results are usually considered probable and not positive signs of pregnancy. Although a firm diagnosis of pregnancy can often be made after the eighth week without any special chemical tests, there is a growing tendency to use the tests to help detect pregnancy as soon as possible. The earlier that pregnancy can be documented, the sooner that prenatal care can be initiated and an accurate estimated date of birth established. The results of pregnancy tests are especially helpful in diagnosing pregnancy outside the uterine cavity (ectopic pregnancy) or a suspected abnormal growth of the fertilized ovum (hydatidiform mole). They are strategic in planning surgery involving anaesthesia; diagnostic or therapeutic radiation; prescription of medications potentially toxic to a developing pregnancy; or abortion.

Positive Signs

Seeing With ultrasound techniques, a gestation sac may be visible as early as 3 to 4 weeks after conception. Foetal form and motion become progressively more apparent with real-time sonography as the pregnancy advances.

Conventional X-ray usually reveals the skeleton of a foetus by the latter half of pregnancy. However, this method is not purposefully used today because of possible radiation injury to the foetus or the mother.

Hearing: A foetal heart tone is usually heard after 18 to 20 weeks by conventional auscultation with a standard fetoscope. Up until the 20th weeks the foetal heart rate is heard best at the centre of the pubic hairline. Foetal heart tones are usually detected by 10 to 12 weeks after conception using ultrasonic or Doppler effect techniques.

The presence of the funic souffle, a rapid repetitive whistle like sound not synchronized with the maternal pulse can be evidence of the foetal heart rate. However, this sound, caused by pulsations of blood in the baby's cord is not always heard. Another occasional sound called the uterine souffle, a swish-like tone occuring at the same rate as the maternal pulse is not diagnostic of pregnancy. It originates from the mother's pulsating uterine arteries and may also be detected in the presence of large vascular pelvic tumours.

Feeling: Foetal movement is detected by a trained examiner after about 20 weeks' gestation.

Progressive Foetal Growth

With the growth of the embryo and foetus, the contours and silhouette of the expectant mother change progressively. The fundus, or top of the uterus, is felt about halfway between the top of the pubic bone and the umbilicus at approximately 16 weeks. The fundus is found near the umbilicus at about 20 weeks. When near full term, the fundus is almost at the level of the tip of the sternum. A woman expecting her first baby usually experiences a sudden relief from shortness of breath about 2 weeks before her delivery when the foetus 'drops' and lightening occurs, taking pressure off the diaphragm.

The increasing size of the fundus puts greater demands on the woman's respiratory, circulatory and urinary systems. Her intestines and stomach become crowded and compressed. Increasing size necessitates changes in wardrobe and creates a typical posture of pregnancy, which makes the simple process of tying shoes almost impossible. The onset of labour terminates the long period of waiting and is usually a welcome event.

Estimated Date of Birth

After pregnancy is diagnosed the woman's first question usually concerns when she will give birth. This date has traditionally been termed the *estimated date of confinement* (EDC), but to promote a more positive perception of pregnancy and birth, the term estimated date of birth (EDB) is now customarily used. Because the precise date of conception is usually inexact, many formulas or rules of thumb have been suggested for calculating the EDB. None of these rules of thumb is the method commonly used. To better estimate the EDB, it is important to obtain an accurate menstrual history plus information about the woman's contraceptive history and the results of previous pregnancy tests (both these tests performed at home and in a laboratory).

Menstrual history

- First day of last normal menstrual period (LNMP) date, duration, amount.
- First day of previous menstrual period (before LMP) PMP; date, duration amount.
- Menarche: date, interval, duration
- History of menstrual irregularity.
- Contraceptive history.
  - Type contraceptive used.
  - When stopped.
- Pregnancy test
  - Date
  - Type
  - Result
- Clinical evaluation.

Once the information is obtained, a more accurate EDB can be computed using Nagele's rule.

Naegele's rule: Naegele's rule is applied as follows: Add 7 days to the first day of the LMP, subtract 3 months, and add 1 year, if appropriate. That is, EDB- (LMP + 7 days) – 3 months) + 1 year. For example, if the first day of the LMP was july 10, the EDB is April 17. Another method is to add 7 days to the LMP and count forward 9 months. Nagele's rule assumes that the woman has a 28-day cycle and that the pregnancy occurred on the fourteenth day. An adjustment is necessary if the cycle is longer or shorter than the number of days should be subtracted from the EDB; if it is longer than 28 days the difference should be added to the EDB. Using Nagele's rule, only about 4 per cent to 10 per cent of pregnant women ultimately give birth spontaneously on the EDB. Most women give birth during the 7 days before or 7 days after the EDB.

For women who do not have regular menstrual cycles, or who cannot provide an accurate menstrual history, ultrasound studies can be used to estimate gestational age. The length of the embryo can be measured by a weeks gestation.

SIGN AND SYMPTOMS OF PREGNANCY

Several weeks and for two months may pass a woman suspects she is pregnant because early symptoms may be confusing. Although fatigue and breast changes often are the earliest symptoms, amenorrhoea or scanty, brief menstrual flow usually signals possible pregnancy. Other women report nausea or taste and olfactory disturbances as early clues.

Possible Signs and Symptoms

Signs that indicate a growing embryo might also occur with another condition. In the past the term presumptive referred to signs most likely to indicate pregnancy; this distinction no longer is necessary. If pregnancy is suspected, it may be verified by a urine test for the presence of hCG or by ultrasound examination. Table 4.4 summarizes signs and symptoms of pregnancy by trimester.

Subjective Signs

Breast tingling: Tender breasts occur because of increased blood supply. Nipples and areolae darken and become more prominent. By 14 weeks, colostrum, the precursor of breast milk, is being produced. Many women experience breast tenderness or tingling as one of the first symptoms (Table 4.5).

Nausea is experienced by approximately 50 per cent of pregnant women. It is easy to identify and often occurs on awakening. With onset about the fourth week nausea usually lasts until the thirteenth week.

Frequency of urination occurs during the first trimester because of the enlarging uterus. With no other signs of infection, frequency usually indicates pregnancy.

Abdominal enlargement does not become evident until the second trimester. By the sixteenth week a woman will find it difficult to wear her normal waistband size. The rise of the uterus into the abdominal cavity is gradual and reaches the symphysis pubis by the twelfth week. From that time the height of the fundus becomes a guide to the progress of foetal growth. Measurements are changed by obesity, multiple pregnancy, and a smaller or larger than average amount of amniotic fluid.

There are a few cases of pseudocyesis, or pseudo pregnancy, when a woman believing strongly that she is pregnant, appears to have all the early signs. The physiologic basis for such a condition was documented and showed that the corpus luteum can remain active under the influence of stress-induced hormones, although conception has not occurred. Of course ultrasound examination would confirm the absence or presence of an embryo.

Quickening occurs by the sixteenth to eighteenth week and certainly by the midpoint of pregnancy. A woman will feel the baby move- "feeling life". It is a significant point in pregnancy for many women. Even the woman who is anxiously waiting for the signs may mistake if for flatulence because foetal movement is so slight at the beginning.

Objective Signs

Breast enlargement under the influence of hormones and with increased vascular supply, begins soon after the woman becomes pregnant. By term the breast may have doubled in size. Superficial veins become more prominent.

Amenorrhoea is a sign that may be caused by other factors such as stress anaemia, illness and approaching pre-menopause. Also, some women may have spotting during the early weeks of pregnancy, particularly at the time of implantation or expected menstrual period.

Uterine and cervical changes occur as a result of hormonal activity and increased blood supply to these tissues. The isthmus or juncture between the body of the uterus and cervix is softened under hormonal influence. On bimanual examination the isthmus may be compressed to almost paper thinness, a condition called Hegar's sign. Because of expanded blood circulation and hormonal activity, the cervix becomes increasingly soft, known as Goodell's sign. Today, with the use of ultrasound, these tests are used less frequently for determining pregnancy status.

Vaginal hyperemia results from increased circulation in the pelvic area that causes the tissues to take on a bluish-purple hure. The colour change of vaginal mucosa and cervix is called Chadwick's sign.

Pregnancy tests based on isoimmunologic reactions are in common use. Kits available OTC provide a 70 to 85 per cent accuracy rate. A fresh urine sample is tested together with hCG-coated particles and antiserum. As early as 15 to 20 days after conception, if enough hCG is present in the

Table 4.3: Nursing care plan of client with normal physiologic changes during pregnancy

Problem/objective	*Nursing interventions*	*Rationale*
1. Health-seeking behaviours related to normal pregnancy		
Woman will communicate her understanding of changes that take place in her body during pregnancy. woman will verbalize telephone number to call as questions arise	1. Encourage woman to write down questions to ask her health-care provider	1. Many women are nervous during early prenatal visits, and they often forget to ask questions; if there are language barriers, they need to be addressed
	2. Answer questions during prenatal visits	2. Answers to questions reduce a woman's anxiety and promote a more relaxed and enjoyable pregnancy
	3. Clearly identify problems about which woman should immediately call	3. Not all changes during pregnancy are normal, and the woman should clearly understand danger signals that require immediate attention. (see Box 5-1)
	4. Provide printed material for woman to take home for reference and to share with "significant other"	4. Printed material needs to be in native language of client; this provides reference if woman forgets and/or for review later if questions arise
2. Knowledge deficit related to common problems of pregnancy		
Woman is able to identify causes of discomfort/problem	1. Explain physiologic causes of discomforts according to knowledge level of woman	1. Woman will not interpret normal discomforts as dangerous ; she is able to distinguish between normal and abnormal
Woman states appropriate measures to alleviate problems	2. Provide suggestions for self-help measures to reduce discomforts:	
(i) Nasal stuffiness and epistaxis	a. Teach woman to improve humidity in house by cool -air vaporizer	a. Humidity reduces drying nasal mucosa, which alleviate some causes of epistaxis
	b. Teach woman to blow nose gently	b. This prevents trauma to membranes and vessels of nose
	c. When bleeding occurs, instruct woman to apply pressure to nostrils and to place ice over nose	c. Most epistaxis occurs in anterior part of the septum; pressure and ice compresses produce vasoconstriction, which may decrease bleeding
	d. Instruct woman to call healthcare provider if bleeding continues for longer than 5 min	d. These measures generally stop bleeding; however, nasal packing may be required
(ii) Increased blood volume	a. Explain that dizziness or a clammy feeling that may occur when lying flat on the back is relieved by rolling onto left side	a. Enlarging uterus may cause pressure on vena cava, which interferes with returning blood flow and cardiac output ; this produces a marked decrease in blood pressure, termed *supine hypotensive syndrome*
(iii) Constipation	a. Instruct woman to increase daily fluid intake by 4-6 glasses	a. Delay in emptying time of intestine, due to decreased muscle tone, allows more water to be absorbed from the bowel; during pregnancy, peristaltic action of gastrointestinal tract is reduced because of increase in progesterone

Contd...

Contd...

Problem/objective	*Nursing interventions*	*Rationale*
	b. Teach woman to eat a well balanced diet with whole grains, fruits, and vegetables	b. Roughage promotes peristalsis
	c. Encourage woman to respond immediately to urge to defecate	c. This helps to promote regularity
(iv) Heartburn	a. Teach woman to eat small Meals at more frequent intervals throughout day	a. Cardiac sphincter of stomach relaxes, causing gastric contents to enter esophagus; small meals prevent further pressure
	b. Instruct sit up for 30 min following meals	b. Sitting up may prevent reflux
(v) Frequency in urination	a. Explain to woman that pressure on bladder during 1st trimester is due to expansion of uterus in pelvic area; in 3rd trimester, pressure is due to developing foetus	a. As long as other symptoms of urinary tract infection are not present, frequency is considered normal during 1st and 3rd trimester
	b. Teach woman signs and and symptoms of actual infection, i.e., burning, pain and fever	b. Early detection prevents complications
	c. Teach woman to avoid caffeine, which can be found in tea, cofee cocoa, chocolate, some over-the-counter drugs such as anacin and some prescription drugs	c. Caffeine is a stimulant that increases urination; its half-life triples during pregnancy because of impeded caffeine clearance; the foetus faces a higher risk of exposure because of this. Pregnant woman consults with health-care provider before taking any over-the-counter or previously prescribed medication
(vi) Skin changes	a. Reassure woman that darkened skin areas are temporary and will gradually disappear after birth of of baby	a. Changes in skin pigmentation are stimulated by elevated levels of melanocyte stimulating hormone, which may be caused by increased levels of estrogen and progesterone; these include chloasma, linea nigra, spider nevi, striae, darkened nipples and areolae, and increased pigmentation of palms of hands
	b. Softening oils and creams may reduce stretch marks but do not completely prevent them	b. Applying softeners together may enhance closeness of couple
(vii) Backache	a. Advise woman to wear low healed shoes	a. Joints of pelvis relax during pregnancy as a result of hormonal changes, causing lumbosacral lordosis; changes in posture also occur as a result of shifts in woman's center of gravity due to enlarging uterus. Excessive weight gain also puts strain on back
	b. Demonstrate good body mechanics	b. Good posture and good body mechanics prevent additional strain

Table 4.4: Subjective and objective signs during pregnancy

Subjective	*Objective*
FIRST TRIMESTER	
Weeks 1-4	
Fatigue, thought to be due to relaxin Nausea, peaking 60 to 100 days After conception Soreness, tingling of breasts	Amenorrhoea, but possible spotting at time of expected period. Elevated hCG levels. Elevated BBT because of progeste -rone secretion.
Weeks 5-8	
Enlarging uterus causing pressure on bladder and frequency of urination Possible decrease in desire for sexual relations.	Breast enlargement, darkening of areolas, enlarged Montgomery's tubercles *Signs (weeks 5-7);* Ladin's Goodell's Hegar's Positive pregnancy test for hCG Using isoimmunologic methods Chadwick's
Weeks 9-13	
Nausea subsiding by 13 weeks Frequency of urination subsiding By 12 weeks Gingivitis and hypertrophy of gums	Weight gain or 0-3 lb but also possible weight loss Height of fundus at the symphysis pubis, rising about 1 cm/wk Thereafter 9-12 weeks—detection of fetal pulse by ultrasonic techniques
SECOND TRIMESTER	
Weeks 14-20	
Breastfullness Headaches	Colostrum present. Mucous plug formation in cervical canal, Leucorrhoea; report if pruritus Or foul odor develops. CANDIDA ALBICANS, trichomonal infections. Abdominal appearance of pregnancy Height of fundus between symphysis And umbilicus. Increase in total blood volume contributing to lightheadedness or fainting, occurs by 10-14 weeks; Peaks at 8 ½ months (34-36 weeks)
Weeks 20-24	
Quickening Often increased sexual desire	Haemodilution of pregnancy resulting from increased plasma (40%) and Shall red blood cell increase ; Hb of 11-12 g and possible Hct of 33%-35%

Contd...

Contd...

Subjective	*Objective*
	Fundus at umbilicus (20 weeks) Pelvic joints relaxing because of hormone relaxin. Possible pigment changes in skin; Melasma, linea nigra, striae gravidarum. increased perspiration, oily secretions dilation of right ureter as a result of pressure from dextrorotated uterus.
Weeks 25-28 Leg cramps caused by decreased Calcium when phosphorus level is increased.	Constipation and haemorrhoids because of slowed peristalsis and pressure of uterus on lower colon and rectum
Fatigue THIRD TRIMESTER	
Weeks 29-33 Fatigue Anxiety about future bad, Fearful dreams Possible faintness in supine position from pressure on inferior vena cava.	Heartburn caused by pressure of uterus on stomach, causing mild hiatus hernia and regurgitation of stomach acid into oesophagus. BP returning to prepregnancy level After slight drop as a result of vasodilation.
Decrease in sexual desire because of physical discomfort	Pulse rate at 15 beats / min over normal from increase in cardiac work Braxton Hicks contractions (painless, intermittent contractions) Fundus midway between umbilicus and xiphoid.
Weeks 34-38 Backache, change in gait Impatience for end of pregnancy Mood swings because of ambivalence about future.	Increase in shortness of breath and other pressure symptoms (heartburn, feeling of fullness after eating, constipation, varicose veins, dependent oedema, haemorrhoids).
Just before labour lightening aching in lower abdomen	Fundus just below diaphragm until lightening, then appears to tip forward

urine, the particles will not agglutinate. The later the test is performed, the more accurate it will be, with positive results reflective higher levels of hCG. Monoclonal antibody tests are more accurate but more costly.

Positive Signs and Symptoms

Visualization of the foetus by ultrasonic examination will demonstrate the amniotic sac, foetal parts, and heart rate movements. It also is used at 16 to 18 weeks to confirm the expected date of childbirth.

Auscultation of first foetal heartbeat may be noted at 9 weeks with a Doppler scan or foetal monitor. Auscultation with a stethoscope must wait until 18 to 20 weeks.

Palpation of the foetal outline by the use of Leopold's manoeuvres (Fig. 4.6A to D) allows the examiner to feel for parts of the foetus, including the head, knees and back. By week 20 an observer also may see foetal movements by watching the surface of the abdomen when the foetus is active.

Foetal Maturity

Gestational age The preterm or premature infant is born after week 20 and before the end of week 37. The term of mature infant has developed for 266 to 287 days, or 38 to 41 weeks. The postterm or postmature infant gestational age is 42 weeks or longer.

The previable period extends to week 20 ; if the pregnancy ends, the foetal product is an abortion, even if it occurs spontaneously. To be considered viable or able to live, the foetus must weigh more than 499 g. After 20 to 24 weeks a foetus is considered potentially viable. Therefore any foetus who dies in utero after 20 weeks of gestation is considered a still birth that must be recorded in the statistics of foetal mortality. Very few premature infants survive intact (that is without residual problems) between weeks 20 and 28. By week 28, the foetus's chances have improved.

These facts reinforce the importance of determining the gestational age of the pregnancy. Because the first phase of the menstrual cycle may be longer or shorter than 14 days, women often do not give birth on their predicted days.

Estimating duration of pregnancy: Because the exact day of fertilization rarely is known, calculation is based on the first day of the last menstrual period (LMP). Thus approximately 14 extra days are added to the conception age; as a result the gestational age is based on 280 days from the LMP. All calculations are based on a 28-day cycle in which ovulation occurs 14-2 days after the menstrual period begins, even though 50 per cent of all women have a shorter or longer interval between menses.

The full-term date is indicated by many terms, most commonly estimated date of childbirth (EDC), estimated date of birth (EDB) and due date (DD).

Several methods are used to calculate the EDB. Using Nagele's rule, for example (first formulated in 1812), the EDB is calculated by adding 7 days to the first day of LMP and then subtracting 3 months from the month of LMP. Using the LMP date of July 5, the following calculation is made:

	Day	Month (July)
LMP	5	7
	+ 7	– 3
	—	—
	12	4

EDB = April 12

Remember to account for the number of days in a month. For instance, if a calculation resulted in the figure July 32, move forward to August 1. A newer method uses + 9 days + 9 months from LMP. This measure is the method of nines.

A simple guide to the progress of pregnancy is to measures from the symphysis pubis to the top of the fundus and to add 12 weeks to the centimeter reading on the tape. The fundus rises about 1 cm per week after the twelfth week. When it reaches the umbilicus 20 weeks should have elapsed; when it reaches the xiphoid process, 36 weeks should have elapsed. Another quick and simple means to determine DD is by using the birthing wheel.

A more precise estimation is possible by ultrasound evaluation of the biparietal diameter of the foetal head or of the length of the femur commonly performed at 16 weeks by use of a table of expected measurements, ultrasound evaluation is accurate to ± days. In any case the woman should know that the EDB is approximate so she will not worry unnecessarily.

Terminology of Pregnancy

Terms are used in obstetrics to refer to a woman's obstetric history. gravidity means that a woman has conceived a baby or has been pregnant, regardless of the length of time she is or was pregnant, it refers only to the number of conceptions, not to the number of babies born. Parity refers to the delivery of any foetus older than 20 to 24 weeks. If a woman miscarried before week 20 of gestation, it is recorded with her gravidity but not in her parity. Parity does not refer to the number of babies, just the number of times a woman has delivered. Thus multiple births still count as one parity.

In an effort to clarify and provide more detail in describing obstetric history, a second system was developed. In this system, parity is listed in four categories.

Full-term (F/T) delivery : 38 + weeks.
Preterm (P) delivery : 20 to 37 completed weeks.
Abortion (A) : Loss of pregnancy before viability (Spontaneous or elective)
Living offspring (L) : Number of children, whether or not living with the family (covers multiple gestations)

If a child has died, however the notation will seem inaccurate, and additional comments must be made to explain the (L) column. Occasionally a fifth column is added to detail the outcome of multiple pregnancies. Try transferring between systems for the examples in Table 4.6.

Maternal and Foetal Blood Incompatibility

A major concern during pregnancy is maternal-foetal blood incompatibility. An antigen-antibody reaction to the mixing of foetal blood into the maternal circulation may occur in the same way that a reaction to a poorly typed blood transfusion may occur. The mechanism of becoming sensitized or forming antibodies against antigens from the same species is isoimmunisation, or alloimmunisation. When two parents have different blood types, their infant may inherit from the father an RBC group that differs from the mother's. As a result specific antibodies may be produced in the mother's serum if the foetal erythrocytes enter her system, and these antibodies can cross the placenta to destroy foetal erythrocytes.

Table 4.5: Signs and symptoms of pregnancy

Possible signs and symptoms

Subjective
- Breast tingling
- Nausea
- Frequency of urination
- Fatigue
- Increased abdominal girth
- Quickening.

Objective
Breast enlargement
- Amenorrhoea
- Changes in uterus and cervix
- Vaginal hypermia
- Positive pregnancy tests.
- Ballottement.

Positive signs
- Ultrasonic visualisation of moving embryo or foetus and foetal heart movements.
- Auscultation of foetal heartbeat.
- Foetal parts or movement palpated by examiner.

Rh Factor Incompatibility

The Rh factor is a group made up of the C, D and E factors of the red cell (there are more than 50 blood factors). The Rh group is referred to with C, D and E typing; other countries may refer to the Rh-Hr system (Table 4.7).

The D factor (positive or dominant) is the major stimulus, although in rare instances, the infant may be affected by C or E alone.

Because the Rh-negative cell group is inherited as a recessive trait a child must inherit the same gene from both parents to show Rh negativity. This is why only approximately 15 per cent of the white population has the Rh-negative factor.

Mechanism: The placenta is usually in effective barrier to the transfer of foetal red blood cells. Minute breaks in the placental interface may occur in cases of infection of the placenta, trauma during abortion, ectopic pregnancy, or birth; or small tears occurring as the placenta separates from the wall of the uterus. Intermingling of maternal and foetal blood also may occur during or after amnioentesis. In another way an Rh-negative woman may build up anti-Rh antibodies after receiving even a brief transfusion of Rh-positive blood. The antibody build-up is detrimental to an Rh-positive infant.

Table 4.6: Comparison of gravidity and parity

Case A: A woman is pregnant; she has had one delivery at term, and this child is living.
Case B: A woman is not pregnant; she has had one delivery at term, one abortion (spontaneous or induced), and has one living child.
Case C: A woman is pregnant; she has had three delivery at term one preterm delivery, and two abortions, she has four living children.
Case D: A woman is not pregnant, she has had one preterm delivery (at 33 weeks) and has two living children.

	System 1				System 2 (Parity only)	
Case	Gravidity	Parity	Term	Preterm	Abortion	Living
A	II	I	1	0	0	1
B	II	I	1	0	1	1
C	VII	IV	3	1	2	4
D	I	I	0	1	0	2 (twins)

Prevention: The best solution is prevention of the intial reaction. Today, few cases of Rh incompatibility are seen in woman, who receive adequate medical care during their reproductive lives. Women, particularly those who have immigrated from other countries or have received little or no prenatal care during a prior pregnancy need to be screened early in pregnancy.

Coombs' Test

The coombs' test detects the presence of antibodies in maternal serum (indirect Coombs) or detects if antibodies are attached to the infant's red blood cells (direct Coombs). A woman with Rh-negativity is tested early in pregnancy and is retested several times during the pregnancy. If she is sensitised already (has Rh D antibodies), her antibody titer is checked frequently. An increase in the titre indicates that the process is continuing and the foetus will be in jeopardy unless intervention occurs.

Passive Immunisation

Passive immunisation is performed to prevent iso-immunisation of the Rh-negative woman who bears an Rh-positive foetus. A serum concentrate containing pooled anti-Rh D antibodies (immune Globulin) is administered after a potential "insult" or infusion of foetal blood into the maternal system. These extrinsic antibodies (not the mother's) will "recognise" the antigen (RhD) and begin the destruction of the foreign foetal cells. The maternal system then is protected from receiving an imprint, a code to make such antibodies again. The woman must be reimmunised each time a foetal or maternal transfusion occurs, after an abortion of any kind, after amniocentesis, and within 48 to 72 hours of a live birth or stillbirth (especially after a caesarean birth). Currently, each woman also receives Rho(D) immune globulin at 28 weeks. It may also be given a 34 weeks of gestation to protect the mother and foetus.

Dosages of immune globulin may vary according to the estimate of foetal transfusion. This may be confirmed by maternal blood testing by use of the Foetaldex or Kleihauer-Berke test to determine the presence and amount of foetal red blood cells. The woman's blood is cross-matched with the dose, and the immune globulin is given by deep intramuscular injection using the Z-track method. There should be no side effects. The woman is given complete information about her condition and the injection and takes home a card with the date of immunisation. Administration of Rho (D) immune globulin is a standard of care, and omission by neglect or error constitutes malpractice.

If a woman has a positive Coombs titer, it is too late to prevent isoimmunisation. A positive indirect Coombs result means that her body is already reducing antibodies against the foetal Rh factor.

ABO Incompatibility

So far no procedure exists for preventing ABO incompatibility. There are no blood or amniotic fluid tests to distinguish between naturally present A or B agglutinins (antibodies) in an O mother's serum and an increased titre resulting from introduction of foetal red blood cells with A or bantigens. Fortunately ABO incompatibility usually is less severe because maternal natural antibodies are weaker in haemolytic effect than are Rh antibodies. No special testing is performed before birth.

Genetic inheritance of one factor from each parent leads to six possible genotyes in the ABO blood groups:

Homozygous	*Heterozygous*
OO	AO
AA	BO
BB	AB

Table 4.7: Typing of Rh groups

Group	CDE Typing
Positive	
Rh 1	D
Rh 2	C
Rh 3	E
Negative	
Rh 4	C
Rh 5	e

The antibody in the serum depends on the antigen in the red cell. For example, if a person has typs B antigen, anti-A antibodies are in the serum (Table 4.8).

This problem is more frequent in the type O mother because she already possesses A and B agglutinins (that is, anti-A and anti-B antibodies), which may cross the placental barrier and interact with the A or B factors in the erythrocytes of the foetus. Interestingly, when Rh and ABO incompatibility exists, anti-A or anti-B antibodies in the maternal serum usually suppress her production of Rh Antibodies.

ABO may account for about two-thirds of the maternal isoimmunisation that leads to neonatal problems, but the effects are less severe. Three combinations are possible:

Mother	*Infant*
O	A, B, or AB
A	B
B	A

Problems occur most frequently with an O mother and an A infant, less commonly with the O mother and B infant, and very rarely in the other combinations.

New borns who are affected by either Rh or ABO incompatibility will show evidence of problems by a positive direct Coomb's test result and will have jaundice in the first 3 days of life.

In every case of an Rh-negative woman's care during pregnancy, birth, and recovery the following measures must be ensured:

1. Check mother's blood type and Rh factor on clinic laboratory reports.
2. With Rh-negative status, alert midwife or physician; flag chart to note Coomb's test administration and results.
3. If invasive procedure is performed during pregnancy (amniocentesis) chronic villus sampling), ensure that immunoglobulin is given on schedule.
4. After abortion at any week, ensure that immunoglobulin is given on schedule.
5. Alert labour and postpartal nursing staff to Woman's Rh and Coombs' titre status.

ASSESSMENT OF PHYSIOLOGICAL CHANGES IN PREGNANCY

The goal of maternity care is a healthy pregnancy with a physically safe and emotionally satisfying outcome for mother, infant and family. Consistent health supervision and surveillance are of upmost importance in achieving this outcome. However, may maternal adaptations are unfamiliar to pregnant women and their families. Helping the pregnant woman recognise the relationship between her physical status and the plan for her care assist her in making decisions and encourages her to participate in her own care.

Noticeable physical changes occur throughout pregnancy, especially in the skin, breasts, abdomen and pelvis. Less noticeable changes occur in other body systems, including the cardiovascular system, gastrointestinal genitourinary, respiratory and musculoskeletal system. Physical examination of the pregnant woman is similar to examination of other people and requires only occasional modification of technique.

The recognition of a normal events in pregnancy demands a clear understanding of the normal process of maternal adaptation. In all mammalian species, there are extensive biochemical, physiological and structural changes during pregnancy and puerperium.

From a teleological point of view, there are two main reason for these changes.

- To provide a suitable environment for the nutrition, growth and development of the foetus
- To prepare the mother for the process of parturition and subsequent support of the newborn infant.

Prenatal assessment involves periodic check-ups throughout pregnancy. Although the frequency of professional examinations depends on the person, the following schedule for clinical visits is generally recommended.

- First 28 weeks : every 3 to 4 weeks
- Last 12 weeks : every 1 or 2 weeks.

At each prenatal visits, the following aspects of maternal and foetal health are evaluated.

- Weight
- Blood pressure
- Glucose and protein in the urine.

Fluid retention (oedema)
- The height of the fundus
- The position of the foetus (leopold's manoeuvres)
- Foetal heart sounds.

Other evaluations are conducted as needed, and includes the following:
- A complete head-to-toe physical examination at first prenatal visions
- Pelvic examinations at the first prenatal visit and during the last trimester
- Evaluation and measurement of the bony pelvis at the first prenatal visit and again at 32 to 36 weeks
- Specific examinations indicated by the condition of the mother of the foetus, such as abdominal ultrasound, amniocentesis, or antibody titres.

Signs and Symptoms of Pregnancy

Pregnancy is confirmed on the basis of characteristic subjective symptoms, physical signs and laboratory values. Signs and symptoms are grouped into categories called Presumptive signs, probable signs and positive signs.

1. Presumptive signs of pregnancy include symptoms reported by the woman such as:
   - Amenorrhoea 10 days or more past the date, the period was expected to begin, the time of occurrence (gestational age) is usually 4th week. The other possible causes will be ruled out for amenorrhea will include stress, vigorous exercises, early menopause, endocrine problems and malnutrition
   - Morning sickness, nausea or vomiting persisting 3 weeks or more (4 to 14 weeks) past the missed period
   - Tingling, soreness, or heaviness of the breasts will be experienced by the woman between 3-4 weeks
   - Urinary frequency will start between 6-12 weeks of the gestational age
   - Fatigue around 12 week
   - Quickening, i.e. maternal perception of foetal movement usually occurs between 16 and 20 weeks of gestation.
2. Probable signs of pregnancy include many physical examination findings:
   - Uterine enlargement
   - Hegar's sign: Softening of uterine isthmus 6 to 8 weeks palpated during manual exam
   - Piskacek's sign: Asymmetrical enlargement of one uterine cornua
   - Chadwick's sign: Bluish pigmentation of the vagina and cervix at 6-8 week of gestation (Time of occurrence). Violet colour of vaginal muscus membrane, that is visible from approximately the fourth week of pregnancy caused by increased vascularity
   - Goodell sign: Softening of the cervix, a probable sign of pregnancy occurring during 5th week
   - Internal ballottement of the uterus at 16-28 week: Ballottement is a diagnostic technique using palpation: a floating foetus, when tapped pushed, moves away and then returns to touch the examiner's hand
   - Braxton Hicks contractions at 16th week. This sign is mild, intermittent, painless, uterine contractions that occur during pregnancy; occur more frequently as pregnancy advances but do not represent the true labour, however this should be distinguished from preterm labour
   - Urine or serum that is positive for human chorionic gonadotropin (hCG).
3. Positive signs of pregnancy confirm the presence of foetus and include auscultation of a foetal heartbeat, palpation of foetal movement and identification of foetal parts by X-ray or ultrasound.
   - 5-6th week (GA): Visualization of the foetus by real-time ultrasound examination.
   - 16th week: Visualization of the foetus by X-ray study
   - 6th week: Foetal heart tones detected by ultrasound examination.
   - 8-17th week: Foetal heart tones detected by Doppler ultrasound stethoscope.
   - 17-19th week: Foetal heart tones detected by foetal stethoscope
   - 19-22 week: Foetal movement palpated
   - Late pregnancy: Foetal movement visible.

Integumentary Changes during Pregnancy

Skin changes during pregnancy are common and include changes in colour and pigmentation, moisture, thickness, turgor, and vascularity. The degree in which these changes occur varies from woman to woman. Some women become alarmed by the changes and need to be reassured about why the changes occur, when they will occur and how long they will last.

Alteration in hormonal balance and mechanical stretching are responsible for several changes in the integumentary system during pregnancy which include the following and which will be examined by inspection and palpation.

Colour and pigmentation

a. Month 2 through term: a generalized hyper-pigmentation develops, especially over the bony prominences and breast nipples and areola hyperpigmentation is stimulated by the anterior pituitary hormone melanotropin, which is increased during pregnancy. Darkening the nipples areolae, axillae, and vulva occurs at approximately the 16th week of gestation. Facial melasma, also called "cholasma" or "mask of pregnancy" is a blotchy, brownish hyperpigmentation of the skin over the cheeks, nose, and forehead especially in dark-complexioned pregnant women. Cholasma caused by normal pregnancy usually fades after birth.
b. Week 16 through term, the "LINEA NIGRA" is a pigmented brownish line extending from the symphysis pubis to the top of the fundus in the midline this line is known as the LINEA ALBA before the hormone induced pigmentation. In primigravida, the extension of the linea nigra, beginning in the third month, keeps pace with the rising side of the fundus; in multigravidas the entire line often appears earlier than the third month. Not at all pregnant woman develops linea nigra.

Changes in the colour and pigmentation the pigmentation of the skin during pregnancy are associated with an increased blood level of melanocyte stimulating hormone. The resulting hyperpigmentation is benign, although, body image may be altered.

Moisture increased blood supply to the skin leads to increased perspiration is secondary to an increased output of the exocrine gands.

Thickness: Gum hypertrophy may occur secondary to the proliferation of blood vessels in the oral mucosa. An epulis (gingival granuloma gravidarum) is a red, raised nodule on the gums that bleeds easily. This lesion may develop around the third month and usually continues to enlarge as pregnancy progresses. It is usually managed by avoiding trauma to the gums (e.g., using a soft tooth brush). An epulis usually regresses spontaneously after birth.

Turgor and mobility: Localized oedema or ankle oedema may occur secondary to an increase in venous pressure in the lower extremities. This is usually not considered pathological. General oedema may be caused by sodium retention and water retention secondary to elevated levels of steroid hormones.

Vascular alterations: Angiomas are commonly referred to as 'Vascular Spiders". They are tiny, star-shaped or bronchea, slightly raised and pulsating endarterioles usually found on the neck, thorax, face, and arms. They occur as a result of elevated levels of circulating oestrogen. These are secondary to the effects of oestrogen and usually insignificant except for possible effects on body image. These spiders are bluish in colour and do not blanch with pressure. Vascular spiders appear during the second to the fifth month of pregnancy. The spiders usually disappear after birth.

Pinkish-red, diffuse mottling or well-defined blotches are seen over the palmar surfaces of the hands during pregnancy also called "Palmar erythema: are related primarily to increased oestrogen levels.

Skin lesions: Striae gravidarum or streth marks especially over breasts, abdomen and thighs caused by stretching of the skin as weight is gained and the foetus grows, which appear in pregnant women during the second half of pregnancy. This may also be caused by action of adrenocorticosteroid. Striae reflect seperation within the underlying connective (collagen) tissue of the skin. These slightly depressed streaks tend to occur over areas of maximum stretch (i.e, abdomen, thighs, and breasts). The stretching sometimes causes a sensation that resembles itching. The tendency to develop striae may be familial. After birth they usually fade, although they never disappear completely. Colour of striae varies depending on the pregnant woman's skin colour. The striae appear pinkish on a woman with light skin and are lighter than surrounding skin in dark-skinned woman. In the multipara, in addition to the striae of the present pregnancy of listening silvery lines (in light-skinned woman), for purpish lines (In dark-skinned women) are commonly seen. These represent scars of striac from previous pregnancies.

Nail and hairs: Nail growth may be accelerated. Some women may notice thinning and softening of the nails. Oilyskin and acne vulgaris may occur during pregnancy. For some women the skin clears and look radiant. Hirsutism, the excessive growth of hair or growth of hair in unusual places is commonly reported. An increase infine hair growth may occur but tends to disappear after pregnancy. However, growth of coarse of bristly hair does not usually disappear after pregnancy.

Breast Changes during Pregnancy

The breast contains 10-20 lactiferous ducts, which branch into a series of ducts and ductules terminating in multiple clusters of milk-secreting alveoli. The alveoli surrounded by band-like myoepithelial cells which squeeze milk into the duct. The ducts and alveoli are surrounded by fat cells, connective tissue, blood vessels, and lymph ducts. The ducts grow under the stimulus of high oestrogen levels, and the alveoli develop as a result of the action of progesterone and prolacting. From 3-4 months onwards, a thick, glossy protein rich fluid known as colostrum can be expressed from the breast. Prolactin stimulates the cells of the alveoli to secrete milk by inducing the production of enzymes needed to pregnancy by the peripheral action of oestrogen and progesterone, but shortly after delivery the sudden fall in these hormones enable prolactin to act in an uninhibited manner on the breast, and hence lactation begins. Suckling stimulates the release of both prolactin and oxytocin via neurological pathways between the nipple and the hypothalamus and oxytocin stimulates contraction of the myoepithelial cells and hence ejection of milk.

Breast changes are normal during pregnancy and includes changes in size, shape, colour, vascularity and tissue quality. If the mother intends to breast-feed, here understanding and feelings about breasfeeding should be explored during the third trimester. The nipples should also be examined to see if they are everted and therefore suitable for breastfeeding. If the nipples are inverted, the mother should be shown how to roll the nipple to promote eversion. Nurse should determine to use with a rough, dry wash cloth. This prepares the nipples to better withstand the infant's suckling. Breast-self examination should be practiced during pregnancy (Fig. 4.7A to J).

Examination of Breast during Pregnancy

Size and shape: Month 2 through term the breasts and nipple enlargement accompanies the increase in glandular and ductal tissue occurring because of hormonal influences. During the second and third trimesters, growth of the mammary glands accounts for the progressive breast enlargement, Fullness, heightened sensitivity, tingling and heaviness of the breasts begins in the early weeks of gestation in response to increased levels of estrogen and progesterone. Breast sensitivity varies from mild tingling to sharp pain.

Skin colour: Hyperpigmentation of the nipples and areolae are secondary to increased levels of melanocyte-stimulating hormone. Nipples and areoles become more pigmented; secondary pinkish areola develop, extending beyond the primary areolae; and nipples become more erectile.

Vascularity: Venous engorgements of the breasts causes the breasts to appear larger, caused by the venous pressure increases of pregnancy. The richer blood supply causes the vessels beneath the skin to dilate. Once barely noticeable, the blood vessels becomes visible, often appearing in an intertwining blue network beneath the surface of the skin. Venous congestion in the breasts is more obvious in primigravidas.

Tissue quality: Increased nodularity—The breasts may feel generally lympty as glandular and ductal tissue becomes more prevalent during pregnancy. Other breast lumps should be considered and ruled out. Hypertrophy of the sebaceous (oil) glands embedded in the primary areola.

Montgomery tubercle: May be seen around the nipple. These sebaceous glands may have a protective role in that they keep the nipples lubricated for breastfeeding.

Lesions: Striae gravidarum or stretch marks may appear at the outer aspects of the breasts, secondary to skin stretching as the breasts enlarge.

Discharge: Week 16 through term, colostrum may be excretion from the nipples. Colostrum is secreted from the mammary glands. During second and third trimesters mammary glands accounts for the progressive breast enlargement. The high levels of luteal and placental hormones in pregnancy promote proliferation of the lactiferous ducts and lobule-alveolar tissue. So palpation of the breast reveals a generalized coarse nodularity and as a result the tissue becomes softer and looser.

Although development of the mammary glands is functionally complete, by mid pregnancy, lactation is inhibited until a drop in oestrogen level occurs after the birth. A thin, clear, viscous secretory material (Precolostrum) can be found in the acini cells by the third month of gestation colostrum, the creamy, white/yellowish to orange premilk fluid may be expressed from the nipple as early as 16 weeks of gestation.

Abdominal Changes during Pregnancy

The abdomen is evaluated at regular intervals during pregnancy to determine foetal growth and development, gestational age, foetal position, and foetal lie. Abdominal alterations may also be noted during pregnancy, and include changes in size and contour, abdominal movement, peristalisis, vascular sounds and muscle tone.

Examination Techniques

Measuring fundal height: The term 'Fundus' refers to the body of the uterus. During pregnancy, the height of the fundus is measured at each prenatal visit to evaluate foetal growth. The height of the fundus correlates with gestational age (Fig. 4.2). Before 13 weeks of gestational age, the height of the fundus is evaluated by bimanual pelvic examination. After 13 weeks the fundus is palpable with one had over the abdomen. With the woman supine, place your (Nurse's) fingers over the abdomen (as shown in figure 4.3).

Start to palpate from above the point where your (Nurse) expect the fundus to be palpable, then progressive-lypalpate downward. When you (nurse) note a change in tissue consistency from soft to firm, you (nurse) have palpated the fundus. Estimate and record the distance between the symphysis pubis and the fundus in centimeters.

When the fundus expands above the umbilicus, the height of the fundus may be measured with a tape measure. Place the end of the tape measure at the top of the symphysis pubis and measure the distance in centimeters to the height of the fundus. (Fig. 4.4). Slight measurement variations may occur with different examiners. Nevertheless progressive increases in fundal height should be noted throughout pregnancy.

Foetal heart auscultation: Foetal heart tones are an indicator of the health of the foetus throughout pregnancy beginning about 10 weeks when heart sounds are first detected by Doppler flow devices. After 16 weeks, heart tones may be detected by the fetoscope. Normal foetal heart rates between 120 and 160 beats per minute.

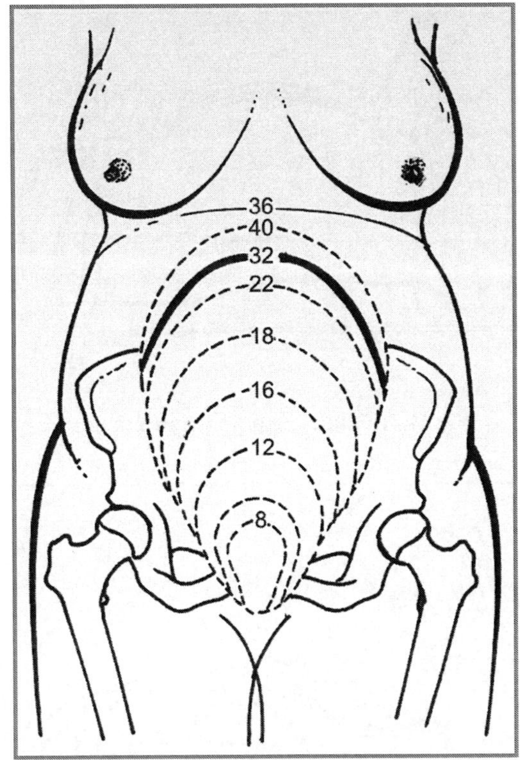

Fig. 4.2: Fundal height and gestational age

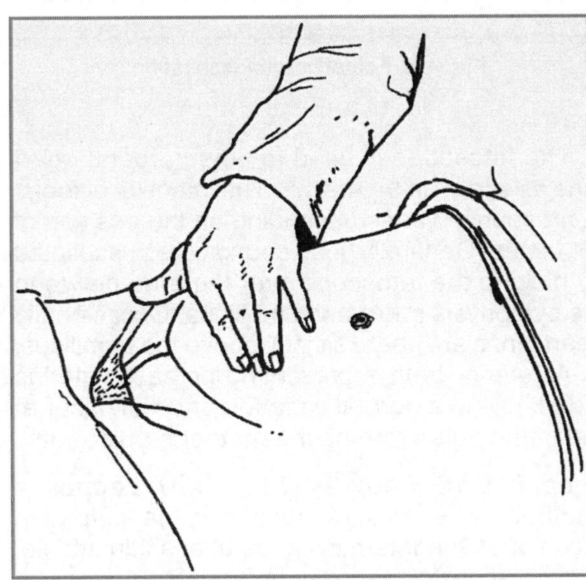

Fig. 4.3: Fundal height palpation

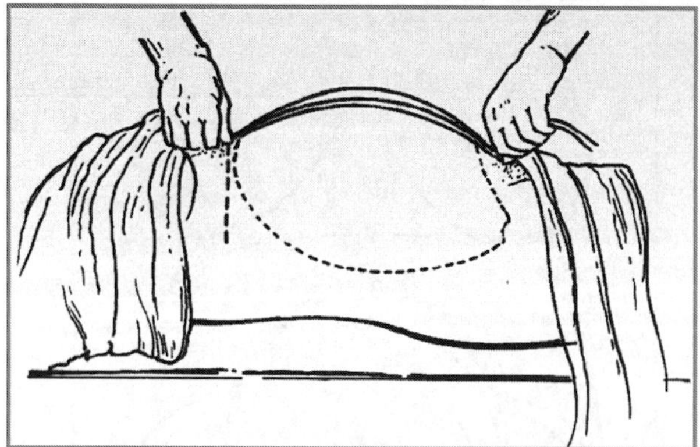

Fig. 4.4: Fundal height measurement

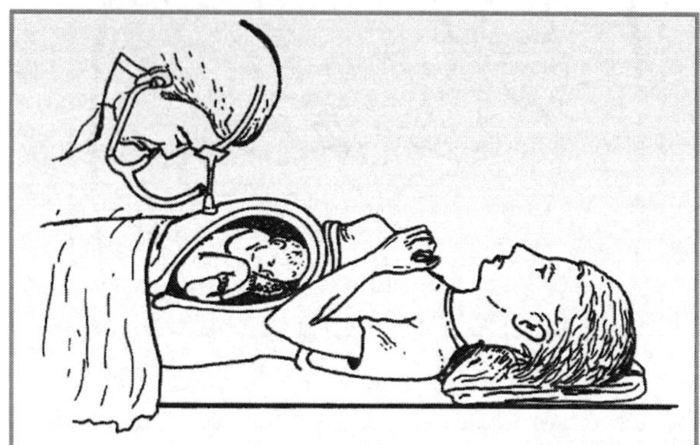

Fig. 4.5: Foetal heart auscultation

The fetoscope is used to detect, foetal heart tone as shown in Figure 4.5. The intensity of foetal heart sounds varies depending on the position of the foetus. Generally heart sounds are auscultated by placing the fetoscope over the area between the symphysis pubis and umbilicus. Occasionally heart tones are heard slightly above the umbilicus.

An uterine bruit, representing increased uterine blood flow is a normal variation and will occur at the same pulse rate as the mother's pulse rate.

Leopold's manoeuvres (Table 4.4): Leopald's manoeuvres consist of four abdominal palpation techniques for determining foetal position and lie. They are performed routinely after 26 week of gestation when the foetal part are more discernable (see Table 4.9 and Figs 4.6A to D).

Leopold's manoeuvres are performed while the mother is supine on the examining table. Tensing of the abdominal muscles may be minimized by slightly flexing the knees and supporting them with pillow.

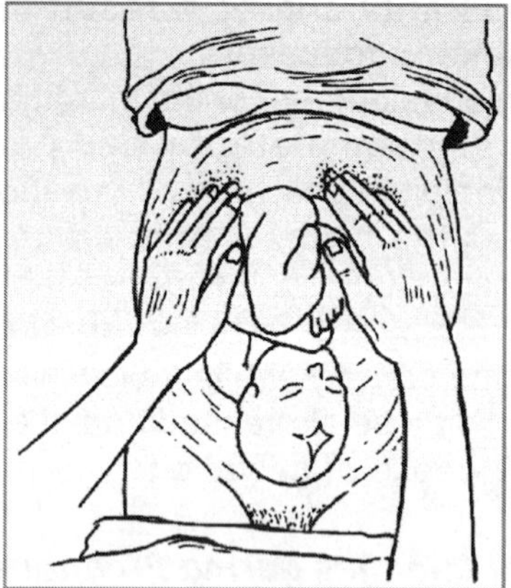

Fig. 4.6 A : First Leopold's sign: Fundal palpation

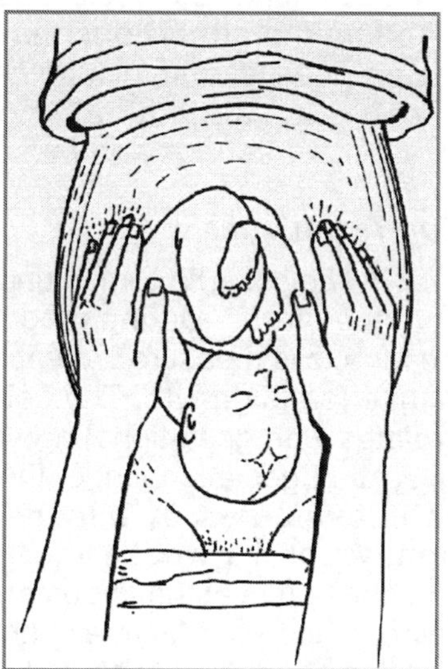

Fig. 4.6 B: Second Leopold's manoeuvre: Lateral palpation

Table 4.8: ABO antigen placement

Type antigen	in red cell	antibodies in plasma
O	None	Anti-A, anti-B
A	A	Anti-B
B	B	Anti-A
AB	A and B	None

Begin with fundal palpation to determine what foetal part occupies the fundus. Stand beside the woman facing her head. Place both hands on top of the fundus and palpate to determine which foetal part present (Fig. 4.6A). The buttocks of the foetus will feel soft and lightly irregular with limited

Table 4.9: Nursing action and rationale of Leopold's manoeuvres

Nursing action	Rationale
1. Instruct the woman to empty her bladder and to lie on her back on the examination bed with her knees bent	An empty bladder contributes to the woman's comfort during the examination. The bent-knee position relaxes the abdominal muscles, facilitating palpation of the foetal parts
2. Provide a wedge under the woman's right or left hip to maintain a slight lateral tilt	A wedge under the woman's hip displaces the uterus sufficiently to prevent compression of the maternal blood vessels and subsequent supine hypotension
3. With warm hands, perform each manoeuvre systematically using gentle but firm motions. Stand by the woman's side, facing her head for the first three manoeuvres	Warm hands help prevent tightening of the abdominal muscles and promote the woman's comfort. Position facilitates the case and accuracy of performing the procedure
First Manoeuvre	
4. Palpate the uterine fundus with both hands to identify the foetal part (either the breech or the head) and the fetal lie	Determines whether the foetal presentation is cephalic (breech in fundus) or breech (head in fundus).The breech is softer, broader, less uniform, and less movable than the head. Also determines whether the foetal lie is longitudinal, transverse, or oblique
Second Manoeuvre	
5. Move your hands to the sides of the abdomen to locate the Fetal back. With one hand in place to steady the uterus, use the other hand to palpate the opposite side of the uterus with firm, circular motions to identify either a smooth fetal back or knobby small parts, such as knees or feet. Repeat the manoeuvre, but palpate the opposite side of the uterus to confirm your findings	Determines the position of the foetus in relation to the uterus
Third Manoeuvre	
6. With the thumb and fingers of one hand, gently grasp the lower portion of the abdomen just above the symphysis pubis to hold the presenting part (the part nearest the cervix). Attempt to move the presenting part side to side between your thumb and fingers to determine whether the part is the head (hard and smooth) or the breech (soft and irregular) and whether it is floating above the pelvis, dipping into pelvis, or engaged (immobile) in the pelvis	Confirms data on presentation of fetus from frist manoeuvre. Provides information about the level of descent of the presenting part in the pelvis
Fourth Manoeuvre	
7. To do the fourth manoeuvre, turn and face the woman's feet. Place the plamar surface of your hands on each side of the abdomen. Move your hands down the sides of the abdomen towards the symphysis pubis, palpating with your fingertips for resistance on either side, to locate the cephalic prominence. One of your hands will continue, unimpeded, toward the symphysis pubis. Your other hand will feel resistance because it has come upon the cephalic prominence. If you first feel resistance on the side opposite the foetal back, the cephalic prominence is the foetal brow (forehead); this indicates that the fetal head is well flexed. If you first feel resistance on the same side as the foetal back, the cephalic prominence is the occiput; this indicates that the foetal head is not well floxod. Note whether the head is free and floating or flexed and engaged.	The manoeuvre is easier to perform if you are facing the woman's feet. It provides information about foetal attitude (flexion versus extension of the head) and engagement (descent of the head into the pelvis)
8. Throughout the examination, ask yourself: • What part am I feeling? • What is the presentation of the foetus? • What is the position of the foetus? • How large is the foetus? • Is there more than one foetus?	Questions provide guidance for interpreting information
9. When listening to foetal heart tones after completing the Leopold manoeuvres, note the location of the foetal heart tones. Compare that information with your assessment from the examination. If there is a possible conflict between the information gained from the Leopold manoeuvres and that gained from listening to foetal heart tones, perform Leopold's manoeuvres again	Because the location of foetal heart tones varies according to the position of the baby, noting the location is a way to verify the accuracy of fetal position as determined through Leopold manoeuvres

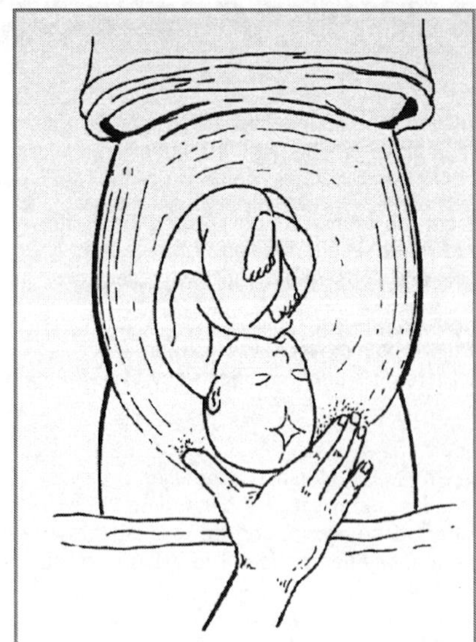

Fig. 4.6C: Third Leopold's manoeuvre: Pawlik palpation

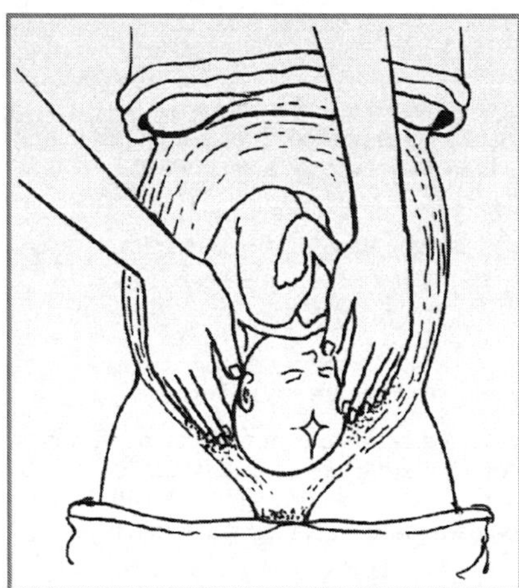

Fig. 4.6D: Fourth Leopold's manoeuvre: Deep pelvic palpation

side-to-side mobility. The head will feel firm, hard and round and be more freely movable.

Next, determine the position of the supine by *lateral palpation*. Move your (nurse's) hands from the fundus to the sides of the abdomen. Support one side of the foetus with one hand while using your (nurse's/examiner's) other hand to palpate the opposite sides of the uterus. Then palpate the other side of the abdomen in a similar fashion (Fig. 4.6D). The foetal spine will feel bony and continuous, whereas limbs will feel irregular or nodular.

The third manoeuvre called *Pawlike palpation*, determines what foetal part lies over the pelvic inlet. Place your (nurse 8s/examiner's) right hand

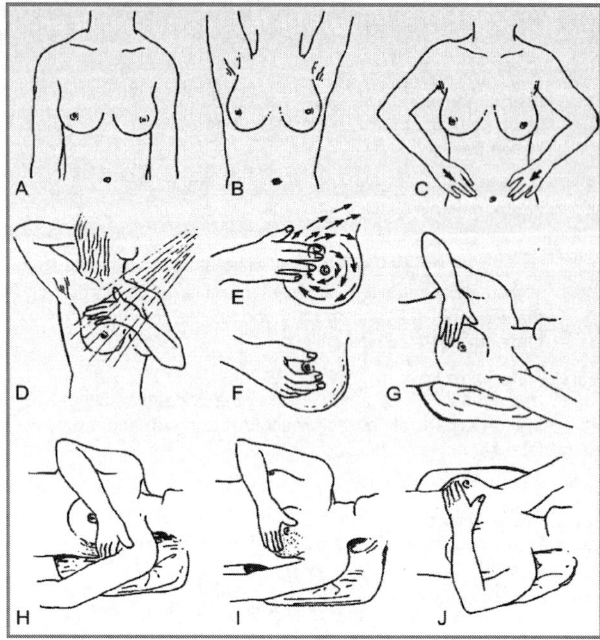

Figs 4.7A to J: Self-examination of female breasts and axillae, accomplished by observation and palpation. Various positions are assumed while standing in front of a mirror. **A.** Relax the arms at the sides. Lean forward, **B.** Raise the arms high overhead. Press the arms behind the head, **C.** Place the hands on the hips and firmly press inward to flex the chest muscles, **D.** In the shower, examine the breast contours, **E.** Method of palpating the breast. Use the fingers to press gently in small circular motions around an imaginary clock face (begin at 12 o'Clock). Move outward, an inch at a time, **F.** Finally squeeze the nipple gently between thumb and index finger, **G to I**: Palpate the breast while lying down: **G.** Position to palpate inner breast, **H.** Position to examine the axilla, **I.** Position to examine the outer breast, **J.** Repeat the entire process for opposite breast and axilla

Just above the symphysis pubis. Then grasp the skin firmly between your thumb and third finger (Fig. 4.6C). A non-engaged head is palpable as a moveable round, hard, smooth mass of the head is engaged. You may feel a shoulder as a bony non-moveable nodule.

Leopold's Manoeuvres (Table 4.9)

Purpose: To provide information about foetal presentation, position, presenting part, lie, attitude, and descent. Can aid in location of foetal heart tones, assessment of foetal size, and determination of single versus multiple gestation. Performed in latter part of second trimester or third trimester, after foetus has become large enough for outline to be felt through abdominal wall.

Equipment

- Flat examination bed.

Finally, perform *deep pelvic palpation* to determine the position of the head (cephalic prominence) change position to face the woman's feet. Place both hands over the neck of the uterus just above the pelvic inlet. Ask the woman to inhale deeply and exhale slowly. During exhalation, apply pressure to each side of the uterine neck. If the presenting part in engaged, one hand will descend further than the other. Cephalic prominence refers to the part of the foetal head preventing hand descent. If the head is flexed, prominence of the forehead is most likely. If the head is extended, the occiput will be prominent.

The following findings will be noted during examination of the abdomen of pregnant:

1. *Size and countour*: There is progressive increase in fundal height associated with foetal growth.
2. *Movement and peristalsis*: After six months, there will be occasional abdominal movement, i.e. foetal movement. There will be reduced peristalsis secondary to relaxation of the muscle of the large intestine.
3. *Respiratory movements*: After 7 months, thoracic breathing replaces abdominal breathing. The breathing pattern changes as diaphragm is displaced by the growing fundus.
4. *Vascular sounds*: After 10 weeks, foetal heart sounds detectabel by Doppler and after 16 weeks, heart sound detectable by fetoscope. It Indicates foetal growth.
5. *Muscle tone*: There will be decreased muscle tone secondary to separation of the rectus abdominal muscle by the expanding uterus.

Genital and Pelvic Changes during Pregnancy

Changes in the genitals and pelvis are noted throughout pregnancy and includes alteration in the appearance of the genitals, vagina, cervix and changes in the consistency of the cervix and uterus. Some of these alterations may help establish the confirmation of pregnancy and others are monitored as indicators of normal foetal growth and development. Generally, the pelvic examination is conducted in the same manner for pregnant and non-pregnant women. Special variations in the technique of bimanual plapation may be required to elicit pregnancy signs. For example isthmus. This change is detected by bimanual pelvic palpation. Place two fingers of the vaginal examining hand in the anterior vaginal fornix in front of the cervix. Use the abdominal palpating hand to compress the uterus slightly above the symphyis pubis so that the isthmus is trapped between both hands.

Following findings will be considered during genital and pelvic examination:

1. *Genital pigmentation*: May note hyperpigmentation of labia and/or vulva. Hyperpigmentation is secondary to increased levels of melanocytes stimulating hormone during pregnancy.
2. *Vaginal discharge*: There may be moderate to profuse thick, clear, odourless mucus present from 6 weeks through term. Discharge is associated with the increased vascularity of vagina. Leucorrhoea may be noted and represents discharge secondary to hypertrophical cervical glands.
3. *Vaginal walls*: Rugae become more pronounces cause by an increase in vaginal vascularity. Vaginal tissue becomes more oedematous. Vaginal skin develops a bluish pigmentation (Chadwicks sign).
4. *Cervix*:
   - By 6 to 8 weeks, the cervix has bluish pigmentation (Chadwick's sign) secondary to increase vascularity and venous congestion
   - By 5 to 6 weeks, the cervix softens (Goodell's sign)-secondary to increased vascularity.
5. *Uterus:*
   - After 6 weeks, Piskacek's sign appears (asymmetrical uterine enlargement). It is related to rapid uterine enlargement at site of ovum implantation
   - After 6 to 8 weeks, Hegar's signs appears (softening of the uterine isthums)- secondary to increased vascularity
   - After 6 weeks, McDonald's sign appears (cervix and uterus may be flexed at junction during bimanual palpation)- secondary to increased vascularity
   - After 16 weeks uterine bollottement is possible.

Other Physical Changes during Pregnancy

Posture

- Increased lumbar lordosis. The expanding uterus contributes to the lumbar lordosis
- Increased dorsal kyphosis and cervical lordosis. These changes represent compensation for lumbar lordosis and are necessary to maintain the centre of gravity.

Gait: Waddling gait- secondary to postural alterations.

Weight: Progressive weight gain: Optional weight gain is 24 to 28 pounds (kg). It is secondary to foetal growth, maternal fat storage, and maternal water retention.

Vital signs

- Heart rate may increase slightly above baseline. This may be secondary to increased blood volume and increased oxygen consumption.
- Systolic blood pressure usually unchanged, diastolic may decrease slightly. A decreased peripheral vascular resistance alters the diastolic blood pressure.
- Respiratory rate may increase secondary to increased oxygen consumption.

Heart sounds: A physiologic systolic murmur (grade II/IV) may be heard during the third trimester. Which results from increased blood flow secondary to an increased blood volume.

Hair: Loss or straightening of scalp hair: increased facial or abdominal hair growth. This may be secondary to increased amounts of androgens and corticotrophic harmones.

NURSING MANAGEMENT OF FIRST TRIMESTER

Assessment

Ideally the woman receives continuous care for health promotion before conception and in between pregnancies. Beginning with the initial visit, when the woman seeks health care because she suspects she is pregnant, the process of assessment is then continued throughout the prenatal period. Assessment techniques include the interview, physical examination, and laboratory tests.

A checklist of care needs spanning pregnancy is a valuable tool and provides the team of health care providers with a communication tool to prevent gaps in the care and identify areas of repeated concern for pregnant woman. When the checklist is shared with pregnant women, this can provide reassurance to them and their families because they can then see from the items on the list that their concerns are common in many pregnancies. Reading the checklist also reminds women of otherwise forgotten data. A checklist for the first trimester is given below:

First-Trimester Checklist

- Diagnosis and expected date of birth
- Schedule and events of visits
- Counselling for self-care
- Birth plan
- Adaptations/discomforts
  - — Breast Changes
    - – Urinary frequency
    - – Nausea and vomiting
    - – Nasal stuffiness and epistaxis
    - – Gingivitis and epulis
    - – Leucorrhoea
    - – Fatigue
    - – Psychosocial responses and family dynamics
    - – Exercise and rest
    - – Relaxation
    - – Nutrition
    - – Sexuality
- Cultural variation
- Warning signs of potential complications
- Resources
  - — Education
  - — Dental Evaluation
  - — Medical service
  - — Social service
  - — Emergency room
- Diagnostic tests
  - — Specify
- Other.

Interview

The therapeutic relationship between the nurse and the woman is established during the initial assessment interview. It is a time for planned, purposeful communication that focuses on specific content. The data collected are two types: the woman's subjective appraisal of her health status and the nurse's objective observations. During the interview the nurse observes the woman's affect, posture, body language, skin colour, and other physical and emotional signs. These are important observations. The initial evaluation includes a comprehensive health history emphasizing the current pregnancy, previous pregnancies, the family, a physical. Assessment, diagnostic testing, and an overall risk assessment. A prenatal history form is the best way of documenting the woman's history at the initial visit.

Often the client is accompanied by one or more family members. The nurse also needs to build a relationship with these people as part of the social context of the client. In addition, family members help recall and validate information related to the client's health. With the client's permission, those accompanying her can be included in the initial prenatal interview, and the observations and information about the woman's family form part of the interivew. For example, if the woman is accompanied by small children, the nurse can ask about her plans for child care during the time of labour and birth.

The interview provides information about the woman's biopsychosocial status as well. Although the format for interviewing and recording the woman's health history may differ, the type of information obtained is universal.

The Reason for Seeking Care

The reason given by the woman for requesting care is quoted verbatim in the record, for example, "I think I am pregnant" or "My legs get so swollen I can hardly walk." This statement does not constitute a diagnosis, because the woman's condition needs to be confirmed by the health care provides before any care is instituted. The purpose of recording the chief reason for a visit in the woman's own words is that it alerts other personnel to the "priority of need" as soon by the woman.

Current Pregnancy

The presumptive signs of pregnancy or results of a home pregnancy test usually prompt a woman to seek care. A review of symptoms, she is experiencing, and the way that she is coping with them, helps establish a data base for the development of a plan of care.

Obstetric/Gynaecologic History

Data are gathered on the woman's age at menarche, menstrual history, and contraceptive history; the nature of any infertility or gynaecologic conditions (for example, fibroids); her history any sexually transmitted diseases (STDs); her sexual history; and the history of all her pregnancies, including the present pregnancy, and their outcomes. The date of the last Papanicolaou test end the result are noted. The date of her LMP is obtained to establish the EDB.

Medical History

The medical history includes those medical or surgical conditions that may affect the pregnancy or that may be affected by the pregnancy. For example, a pregnant woman who has diabetes or epilepsy will require spacial care. Because most woman are anxious during the initial interview, the nurse's referance to cues, such as a Medic-Alert bracelet, will prompt the woman to explain allergies, chronic diseases, or medications being taken (for example, cortisone, insulin, or anticonvulsants).

The nature of previous surgical procedures should also be described. If a woman has undergone uterine surgery or extensive repair of the pelvic floor, this may necessitate caesarean birth; appendectom rules out appendicitis as a cause of lower right quadrant pain; spinal surgery may contraindicate the use of spinal or epidural anaesthesia. Any injury involving the pelvis is noted.

Often women who have chronic or handicapping conditions forget to mention during the initial assessment because they have become so adapted to them. Special shoes or a limp may indicate the existence of a pelvic structural defect, which is an important consideration in pregnant women. The nurse who observes these special characteristics and can inquire about them sensitively can obtain individualised data that will provide the basis for a comprehensive nursing care plan. Observations are provide the basis for a comprehensive nursing care plan. Observations are vital components of the interview process because they prompt the nurse and woman to focus on the specific needs of the woman and her family.

Nutritional History

The woman's nutritional history is an important component of the prenatal history because her nutritional status has a direct effect on the growth and development of the foetus. A dietary assessment can reveal special diet practices, food allergies, eating behaviours, and other factors related to her nutritional status. Pregnant women are usually motivated to learn nutrition generated by this assessment.

Drug Use

A woman's past and present use of legal (over the counter (OTC), prescription, ceffine alcohol, nicotine) and illegal (marijuana, cocaine, heroin) drugs needs to be assessed because many substances cross the placenta and may therefore harm the developing foetus. Periodic urine toxicology screening tests are often recommended during the pregnancies of women who have a history of illegal drug use.

Family History

The family history provides information about the woman's immediate family, including parents, siblings and children. This helps identify familial or genetic disorders or conditions that could affect the present health status of the woman or her foetus.

Social and Experimental History

Situational factors such as the family ethnic and cultural background and socioeconomic status are determined during the social and experiential history taking. The woman's perception of this pregnancy is explored by asking her such questions as the following; Is this pregnancy wanted or not, planned or not? Is the woman/couple pleased, displeased, accepting, or nonaccepting? Is the pregnancy "hers" or "theirs"? What problems may arise because of the pregnancy; financial career, and living accommodations? The family support system is determined by asking her such questions as the following: What primary support is available to her? Are changes needed to promote adequate support? What are the existing relationships among the mother, father/partner, siblings, and in – laws? What preparations are being made for her care and that of depending family members during labour and for the care of the infant after birth. Is community support needed, for example, financial or educational? What are the woman's /couple's ideas about childbearing, their expectations of the infant's behaviour, and their outlook on life and the female role? Other such questions that need to be asked include: What does the woman/couple think it will be like to have a baby in the home? How is her/their life going to change by having a baby? What plans does having a baby interrupt? During interviews throughout the pregnancy the nurse should remain alert to the appearance of potential parenting problems, such as depression, lack of family's support, and inadequate living conditions. The nurse needs to assess what the woman's/couple's attitude toward health care is, particularly during childbearing, what she/they expect of the health care provider; and what their view of the relationship between the woman couple and nurse.

Coping mechanisms and patterns of interacting are also identified. Early in the pregnancy the nurse should determine the woman's couple's knowledge of pregnancy, material changes, foetal growth, care of self, and care of the newborn, including feeding. It is important to ask about attitudes toward unmedicated or medicated childbirth and about her/their knowledge of the avaliability of parenting skills classes. Before planning for nursing care the nurse needs information about the woman's / couple's decision-making abilities and living habits, personal hygiene, clothing). Common stressors during childbearing that have been identified includs the baby's welfare, labour and birth process, behaviours of the newborn, woman's relationship with the baby's father, changes in body image and physical symptoms.

Attitude concerning the range of acceptable sexual behaviour during pregnancy should also be explored by asking questions such as the following; What has your family (partner, friends) told you about sex during pregnancy? The woman's sexual self-concept is given more emphasis by asking questions such as the following? How do you feel about the changes in your appearance? How does your partner feel about your body now? Do maternity clothes make pregnant women attractive?

All women should be assessed for a history or risk of physical abuse, particularly because the likelihood of abuse can increase during pregnancy. Although visual cues from the woman's appearance or behaviour may suggest the possibility, if questioning is limited to those women who fit the supposed profile of the battered woman, many women will be missed.

Review of Systems

During this portion of the interview, the woman is asked to identify and describe preexisting or concurrent problems with any of the body systems and her mental status is assessed. The woman is question or pain. Pregnancy affects, and affected by, all bodysystems, therefore information on the present status of the body systems is important in planning care. For each sign or symptom described, the following additional date; should be obtained; body location, quality quantity, chronology setting, aggravating or alleviating factors, and associated manifestations.

Birth Plan

The woman's preparation for the childbirth experience is also assessed. If she planning to attend childbirth/parent education classes (with or without her partner) during the first trimester? Is the couple considering formulating a birth plan? Attendance at childbirth-parent education classes and the development of a birth plan may vary with the client's culture, usual means of camping (classes and reading material or other), and feelings about the role of the health care providers. Some women may come with a form of birth plan; for example, having experienced the birth of an ill or preterm infant, the woman anticipating a second birth may prefer to give birth only at a tertiary care centre with a neonatal intensive care unit. A highly dependent woman may allow the health care team to make decisions about birth plans, assuming that the decision of the professionals is the wisest. A more independent, assertive woman may seek health care that conforms to her philosophy of care and her beliefs and knowledge; she wants her wishes honoured during pregnancy, labour and birth, and the postpartum period.

Women with a Disability

Women with serious and handicapping physical or emotional disorders—the deaf, blind, depressed, physically disabled, mentally retarded, brain injured—must all be respected and the assessment approach adapted to their needs. Women who are emotionally restricted may not be able to give an effective history, but they must be respected, and the history should be obtained from them the extent possible. Their points of view and attitudes matter. Still, whenever necessary, the woman's family, other health professionals involved in her care, and her record must be consulted to get complete information. Each woman must be fully respected and involved to the limit of her emotional and cognitive capacities or physical handicap.

Physical Examination

The initial physical examination provides the baseline data for changing subsequent changes. The examiner needs to determine the woman's needs for basic information regarding the structure of the genital organs and provide this information if necessary to demonstrate the equipment that may be used during the examination, and explain the procedure itself. This interaction requires an unhurried, sensitive, and gentle approach rendered with a matter-of-fact attitude.

The physical examination begins with the assessment of the woman's vital signs, height and weight, and blood pressure. Because the bladder must be empty before a pelvic examination can be done, the urine spacimen is obtained at this time.

Each examiner has developed a routine way of performing the physical examination: most choose the head-to- toe progression. Others choose a systems approach. The comprehensiveness of the examination varies by examiner. Heart and lung sounds are evaluated. The skin is assessed for pigmentation changes, rashes, and oedema. The distribution, amount, and quality of body hair is of particular importance because these findings reflect a woman's nutritionals status, endocrine function, and general emphasis on hygiene. The thyroid gland is assessed carefully as are the breasts and abdomen. The arms and legs are assessed for swelling and varicosities. The pelvic examination is usually performed last. The typical basic examination is usually completed without much difficulty for the healthy woman. During the examination, the examiner needs to remain alert to cues given by the woman that give direction to the assessment and indicate possible problems.

Thyroid gland: The thyroid gland is the largest endocrine gland in the body and the only one accessible to direct physical examination because the effects of thyroid activity are also widespread, the assessment of thyroid function or possible dysfunction involves more than observation and palpation of the thyroid gland. The metabolic rates and rhythms, including menstrual regularity in the woman of child bearing age, are governed by the thyroid gland and need to be evaluated. The woman's behaviour and appearance and the status of her skin, eyes, hair and cardiovascular system are also important indications of thyroid function. Several findings (for example, enlargement, coarse and gritty consistency, nodules) require further evaluation.

Breasts: The physical examination includes an examination of the breasts, primarily to establish a data base of normal findings. However, at all times the practitioner needs to be alert to the possibility of carcinoma. Early detection of potential malignancies has been and continues to be the single most important factor in the successful treatment of this disease. Because professional assessment is done only periodically, each woman is advised to perform a breast self-examination (BSE) on a monthly basis. However, because of changes in breast tissue during pregnancy and lactation the BSE findings are not as reliable during these times. It used to be recommended that women with inverted or flat nipples who wished to breastfeed needed to be identified so that early interventions could be implemented. Recent studies have shown, however, that the techniques used yield to no useful benefit.

Abdomen: The examination of the abdomen is done carefully and systematically. The general condition of the skin is assessed, this includes its colour; the nature of rashes, lesions, or scars; whether there are striae or dilated veins; its turgor; its texture; and the hair distribution. The contour and symmetry of the abdomen and the presence of hernias are also noted. Bowel sounds are auscultated. Any abdominal masses are assessed by palpation.

Pelvic examination (Table 4.10)*:* When a woman makes an appointment for a pelvic examination, she is told to refrain from sexual intercourse, douching (NOTE: douching is not recommended during pregnancy), or using vaginal medications for the 24 hours before the appointment because these can cloud the nature of secretions, marking insertion of the vaginal speculum more difficult.

For the examination, the woman is assisted into a lithotomy position (lying supine with the hips and knees flexed and the thigs abducted and drawn upward toward the chest.

External inspection: The examiner sits at the foot of the table for the inspection of the external genitals and for the speculum examination. In good lighting, the external genitals (the clitoris, labia and perineum) are inspected for sexual maturity. There may be healed scars after child birth or other trauma.

External palpation: The examiner then palpates the external genitalia, all the time keeping the woman informed about the procedure. For example, before touching the genital area, the examiner says, “I am going to touch you now.” The examiner wears gloves for this portion of the assessment. In addition to the routine assessments normally done during this part of the examination, particular attention needs to be paid to the perineum, the area between the vagina and anus. It is assessed for the presence of scars from old lacerations or episiotomies and for thinning, fistulas, masses, lesions, and inflammation. The anus is assessed for the presence of haemorrhoids or haemorrhoidal tags and for the integrity of the anal sphincter. Occasionally, after a vaginal birth that involved lacerations extending into the anal sphincter, the muscle-may not have been repaired correctly, for example, the examiner will see a “dimple” over two ends of separated muscle and the “wink” relax is incomplete.

Assisting with Pelvic Examination (Table 4.10)

Purpose: To help the woman feel at ease throughout the examination and to assist the woman’s health care provider as needed. The woman’s health care provider performs the examination at the first prenatal visit and again toward the end of pregnancy unless otherwise indicated. The first examination is performed to detect any pelvic abnormalities that would influence pregnancy, labour, or birth; to assess uterine size and pelvic size and shape; and to collect cytologic specimens. The later examination is done to assess cervical readiness for labour, as well as foetal descent into the pelvic cavity, and to obtain cultures if necessary.

Equipment

- Sterile gloves
- Vaginal speculum
- Water-soluble lubricant
- Materials for PAP smear and cultures, including biohazard bag and labels for cultures
- Other culture media for additional specimens
- Mirror
- Light
- Sheet
- Examination table with stirrups.

If the anal sphincter was not repaired correctly, the woman may have a history of incontinence. The anal area is also assessed for lesions, masses abscesses, and tumours. If there is a history of sexually transmitted disease the

Table 4.10: Nursing action and rationale of assisting with pelvic examination

Nursing action	*Rationale*
1. Greet the woman warmly and make her feel at ease. Instruct her to empty her bladder and to undress from the waist down. Give her a sheet to place around her and ask her to sit on the end of the table	Feeling that the nurse is interested and concerned about her decreases the woman's apprehension and anxiety. An empty bladder promotes comfort during the examination and helps assure accurate assessment of the uterus during the bimanual examination. A sheet helps decrease the woman's self-cousciousness by providing privacy
2. Explain the purpose of the pelvic examination. Describe the procedure and what the woman will feel. Show her the equipment that will be used	Knowledge of the procedure decreases apprehension and fear
3. Assist the woman into the lithotomy position for the examination, making her as comfortable as possible. If the foetus is large enough to compress maternal blood vessels, place a wedge under the woman's right or left hip to maintain a a slight lateral tilt. Elevate her head and shoulders slightly. Her arms should rest either at her side or on her breast. Position her buttocks at the bottom of the table. Place her feet in the stirrups, with her legs wide apart. Drape the sheet over her from the waist down	Correct positioning enhances the health care provider's ability to perform the examination and increases the woman's ability to relax during the examination. Placing a wedge under the woman's hip displaces the uterus sufficiently to prevent compression of maternal blood vessels and subsequent supine hypotension. The sheet provides privacy and helps decrease the woman's self-consciousness
4. When the examination begins, encourage the woman to remain relaxed. Show her how to do slow-paced breathing. Involve her in the procedure as much as she wishes. For example, offer her a mirror if she would like to observe the procedure. Inform the woman about what to expect at each point of the examination (inspection of external genitalia, speculum examination, bimanual examination, and assessment of the bony pelvis).Instruct her to bear down as the speculum is being inserted	Relaxation and slow-paced breathing enable the woman to minimize discomfort. Involvement in the procedure promotes learning. A mirror enables her to learn about Her own anatomy during the examination. Bearing down helps relax pelvic floor muscles, open the vaginal orifice, and decrease intravaginal pressure
5. Assist the woman's health care provider with the examination as needed. Before handling specimens, wash hands and put on gloves. Prepare specimens for transfer to the laboratory	Washing hands, wearing gloves, and correct handling of specimens help prevent cross-contamination and infection
6. Assist the woman to a sitting position, assuring that she remains covered with the sheet. Offer her a towel to wipe lubricant from the perineal area. Provide privacy as she dresses. Ask whether she has any questions before she leaves	Assistance in moving to a sitting position is sometimes needed because lying supine may cause postural hypotension. Wiping off lubricant and vaginal secretions makes the woman feel more comfortable. Providing privacy whenever possible helps decrease self-consciousness. Giving the woman an opportunity to ask more question after the examination helps promote learning and decrease anxiety

examiner may want to obtain a culture specimen from the anal canal at this time. Throughout the genital examination the examiner notes whether any odor that may indicate an infection or poor hygiene is discernible.

Speculum Examination and Internal Examination

A speculum is inserted so that the vagina and cervix can be visualised and specimens collected.

Collection of specimens: The collection of specimens for cytologic examination is an important part of the gynaecologic examination because this allows infection to be diagnosed. A culture specimen is obtained to screen women for gonorrheal infection that could affect the woman, her foetus, and her partner. This is routinely tested for at the first prenatal visit and again toward the end of pregnancy (week 36). A initial pelvic examination, a specimen for viral culture is obtained from the lesion, and this is done at repeated intervals thereafter. An abnormal Papanicolaou smear result may be caused by infection with herpes simplex virus type 2 or human papilloma virus (HPV).

Bimanual palpation: A bimanual examination is done in the same way as it is during a routine examination in a nonpregnant woman. The examiner will find that the vagina enlarges and supporting structures are more relaxed as pregnancy advances. Whenever the examination is performed, the tone of the pelvic musculature and the need for and the woman's knowledge of kegel's exercises are assessed. Particular attention is paid to the size of the uterus because this is an indication of the timing of gestation. Pelvic measurements are often done at this time. The nurse present during the examination can coach the woman in broathing and relaxation techniques at this time, as needed.

Laboratory tests: The laboratory data yielded by the examination of these specimens add important information concerning the symptoms of pregnancy and the woman's health status. Such information is used for making nursing and medical diagnoses.

Specimens are collected at the initial visit so that the cause of any abnormal findings can be treated (See Tables 4.11 and 4.12). Tined or purified protein derivative of tuberculin (PPD) tests are administrated to assess for exposure to tuberculosis. The woman is tested for hepatitis B surface antigen (HBsAg) and hepatitis B surface antibody (HBsAb). During the pelvic examination, cervical and vaginal smears are obtained for cytologic studies and for diagnosis of infection (for example, chlamydia, gonorrhoea). Blood is drawn for a variety of tests; VDRL test for syphilis; complete blood cell count (CBC) with haematocrit, haemoglobin, and differential values, tests for blood type and Rh factor; antibody screen (Kell, Duffy, rubella, toxoplasmosis, and anti Rh); test for sickle cell anaemia; and measurement of the folacin level, when indicated. Urine is tested for glucose (diabetes), protein (pregnancy-induced hypertension); and nitrites and leucocytes (urinary tract infection); culture and sensitivity tests are ordered as necessary. Testing for antibody to the human immunodeficiency virus (HIV) is strongly recommended for all pregnant women.

The finding of risk factors during pregnancy may indicate the need to repeat some tests at other times. For example, exposure to tuberculosis or an STD would necessitate repeat testing.

Testing Urine with Urinary Dipstick

Purpose

To detect the presence of substances in the urine that indicate a potential problem requiring further investigation. To identify trends by comparing current specimen results with those collected previously. Performed at each prenatal visit throughout pregnancy.

Equipment

- Fresh urine specimen
- Dipsticks
- Gloves.

Foetal Development

Toward the end of the first trimester before the uterus is an abdominal organ, the foetal heart tones (FHT) can be heard with an ultrasound fetoscope or an ultrasound stethoscope. To hear the FHT the instrument is placed in the midline just anterior to the symphysis pubis and firm pressure applied. The woman and her family should be offered the opportunity to listen to the FHTs.

Table 4.11: Test and results of blood test during pregnancy

Test	*Results and comments*
Complete blood cell count	
Hemoglobin	Measured as g/dl. May drop to 11.5 g/dl later in Pregnancy because of increase of plasma in ratio to RBCs
Hematocrit	Volume of RBCs in 100 ml blood, measured in a Percentage, 33 per cent is lowest acceptable level.
Mean corpuscular volume	Average volume of individual RBC, below average indicates some types of anaemia.
Blood cell count haemodilution	Neutrophils (50 %), lymphocytes (21 %-35%), Monocytes, (4%) basophils (3%), eosinophils (2.7%). Total count is 7000-10,000/mm^3. Rises to 18,000 by late pregnancy in preparation for the healing process after birth.
RBC count	Number of RBCs in each microliter of blood. In pregnancy, haemodilution level may drop to 3.75 million/mm^3
Haemoglobin electrophoresis.	Determines sicke cell trait.
Glucose	
Hemoglobin A_{lc}	Less than 3.5% is normal, if over, indicates Hypeglycaemia within 6 weeks used to identify diabetic problems.
1-hr 50-g glucose load test	Less than 3.5% is normal if over, indicates Hyperglycaemia within 6 weeks used to identify diabetic problems. Load at 28 weeks; if 1-hr level is under 135, it is normal. If over, then glucose tolerance testing is done.
Blood type (ABO)	Check partner's blood type and potential for incompatibility.
Rh factor	Indirect Coombs' test should remain negative.
Coombs' test	Retested at 28 weeks in Rh-negative woman.
Infection	
Rubella titre	Less than 1:8—immunize after birth. If titer more Than 1:128 in early pregnancy, repeat test.
STD: serum	
Venereal Disease Research Leboratory, (VDRL) or fluorescent treponemal antibody absorption (FTA-ABS) test	False positive results may occur with VDRL. FTA-ABS specific for antireponemal antibodies. Repeat VDRL, at 32 weeks.
STD: vaginal and cervical smear Gonorrhoea	Gram stain or enzyme-linked immunosobent assay (ELISA) test; repeat at 28 weeks
Chlamydia	Direct examination of smear on slide
Gram-positive streptococcus	Direct slide examination
Hepatitis B surface antigen	Hepatitis B virus-infected infant can be treated if mother is dagnosed early
Skin tests: Tine, Mantoux	X-ray examination performed after positive finding
Tuberculosis	Screen for tuberculosis
Skin tests: Tine, Mantoux	X-ray examination performed after positive finding
Urine	
Glucose, ketones Albumin Cells: leucocyte, red blood cells, bacteria casts Specific gravity	Urinalysis performed during each visit. Catch clean midstream specimen for culture if cells present

Table 4.12: Nursing action and rationale of testing urine with urinary dipstick

Nursing action	*Rationale*
1. Ask woman to collect urine midstream in a clean specimen cup	The chance of contamination or inaccurate test result is reduced by obtaining a fresh midstream urine specimen in a clean cup
2. With gloved hands, pull a dipstick from the bottle and check the date on the bottle that indicates when it was opened	The shelf life of on open bottle of urinary dipsticks is 30 days
3. Dip the stick into the urine specimen until all the coloured tabs are wet	An accurate result is obtained only if all the colored tabs are immersed in the specimen.
4. Wait sufficient time (according to directions on the bottle) for the colours on the stick to change	Waiting a sufficient amount of time is essential for obtaining on accurate result.
5. Compare the colours on the stick to the colour chart on the bottle	The colour chart on the bottle indicates how to interpret the colours on the stick. The presence of glucose, protein, ketones, or nitrites in the urine could indicate a potential problem
6. Remove gloves, wash hands, and record your findings	Removing gloves and washing hands prevent cross-contamination. Recording findings enables the nurse to compare result from previous appointments and look for trends

The foetal development at 13 weeks are as follows:

- Differentiation of tissues is complete as period of organogenesis ends
- Foetus has human appearance
- Foetus's sex is distinguishable externally
- Skeleton is ossifying
- Tooth buds are forming
- Respiratory activity is evident
- Insuline is being secreated (since eighth week)
- Kidneys are secreating urine
- Intestine is returning to abdomen
- Head is one-third of total length
- Length: 9 cm (3½ in)
- Weight: 15 g (½ oz¼).

Foetus is less susceptibel to malformation caused by teratogenic agents after 8 to 10 weeks gestation.

Signs of Potential Problems

The interview, physical examination and laboratory tests may yield findings suggesting the existence of complications. Thus, when the data base is complete the woman's risk status and need for referral for specialized care or further evaluation can be determined. A variety of assessment tools have been developed to assess the degree of risk.

Table 4.13: Signs of potential complications

First trimester Signs/Symptoms	*Possible causes*
Severe vomiting	Hyperemesis gravidarum (see Chapter)
Chills fever	Infection
Burning on urination	Infection
Diarrhoea	Infection
Abdominal cramping, vaginal bleeding	Spontaneous abortion, miscarriage

During pregnancy, warning signs (signs of potential complications, (Table 4.13) may also appear. The woman and her family need to be made aware of these signs so that they can then promptly seek appropriate interventions.

Nursing Diagnoses

Each woman and her family will exhibit a unique set of responses to pregnancy. To attend to these responses, the nurse begins by formulating appropriate nursing diagnoses. The following are examples of diagnosis that may be formulated after an analysis of assessment findings during the first trimester.

- Anxiety related to:
  - Concern about herself.
  - Physical change with pregnancy.
  - Her (or other's) feelings about the pregnancy.
- Pain related to:
  - Early discomforts of pregnancy.
- Altered family processes related to:
  - Family's response to diagnosis of pregnancy.
- Anxiety related to knowledge deficit:
  - Maternal and familial adaptations to pregnancy
  - Maternal and familial adaptations to EDB
- Altered nutrition, less than body requirements, related to:
  - Morning sickness.
- Altered sexuality patterns related to:
  - Discomforts of early pregnancy.

Planning/Objectives

Planning care for clients during the first trimester is based on the findings revealed by the biopsychosocial assessment of the woman and her family. A plan is developed for each woman that relates specifically to clinical and nursing problems. The information given in this chapter is general: that is, not all women will experience all the problems discussed or require all facets of the care described. The nurse selects those aspects of care relevant to the woman and her family based on client-centered expected outcomes pertaining to physiologic and psychosocial care, and include that the woman (and family when appropriate) will do the following:

- Demonstrate pertinent knowledge of the adaptation of the maternal body to a developing foetus as a basis for understanding the rationale and necessity for various modes of care.
- Use knowledge of self-care for meeting nutritional needs and sexual needs, performing activities of daily living, and dealing with the discomforts of pregnancy.
- Identify and report symptoms that indicate deviations from the normal.
- Actively participate in her care during the first trimester.

Plan of Care and Implementation

The nurse-client relationship is critical in setting the tone for further interaction. The technique of listening with an attentive expression, touching and using eye contact have their place, as does recognizing the woman's feelings and her right to express these feelings the intervention may occur in various formal or informal settings. The clinical home visits, or telephone conversations all provide opportunities for contact and can be used effectively for the purpose. Some times women repeatedly seek information about a particular problem. At other times, there may be another underlying problem the women is hesitant to breach. The nurse needs to be as true in identifying such unvoiced needs and can help the woman by asking for a client generated solution and a subsequent report of its effectiveness.

In supporting a client the nurse must remember the both the nurse and the women are contributing to the relationship. The nurse has to accept the woman's responses as a factor in trying to be of help.

The nurse also needs to accept that the woman must be a willing partner in a purely voluntary relationship. As such, the relationship can be refused or terminated any time by the pregnant woman or her family.

Supportive care involves developing, augmenting, or changing the mechanisms used by women and their families in coping with stress. The nurse tries to promote active participation by the people in the solution of their own problems. The nurse can help a woman gather pertinent informtion, explore alternative actions, decide on a course of action, and assume responsibility for the outcomes. These outcomes may be any or all of the following: living with a problem as it is, easing the effects of a problem so that it can be accepted more readily or eliminating the problem by effecting change.

At other times a successful outcome can be documented readily. For example, a woman who early in her pregnancy had predicted a severe depressive state in the postbirth period was elated when such a state did not materialize. She remarked to the nurse who had provided support during the pregnancy and birth. "You're the best nerve medicine I've ever had."

Education for Self-care

Health maintenance is an important aspect of prenatal care, and the participation of the client in the care ensures the prompt reporting of possible problems. A client's assumption of responsibility for health maintenance is promoted by her understanding of the maternal adaptations to the growth of the unborn child and a readiness to learn. Nurses can provide women with the information they need for self-care and compliance with health care measures. Before developing a plan of care, however, the nurse also needs to determine whether the woman observes cultural, ethnic, religious or other practices that can affect health.

The expectant mother needs an overview of the prenatal care planned and information about many other subjects. During the initial health assessment the woman may indicate a need to learn about self-care activities such as, ways to prevent urinary tract infection, maintain good hygiene and nutrition, and perform kegel's exercises.

Prevention of Urinary Tract Infection

Urinary tract infections are common in pregnancy, but they may be asymptomatic. Women should know, however, to inform their health care provider if blood or pain on urination occurs. Whether symptomatic or not, these infections pose a risk to the mother and foetus, and thus the prevention and treatment of these infection are essential. In addition, the nurse must assess the woman's understanding and use of good handwashing techniques before and after urinating and whether she knows to wipe from front to back. Soft, absorbent toilet tissue, preferably white and unscented, should be used, because harsh, scented, or printed toilet paper may case irritation. Bubble bath or other bath oils should be avoided because these may be irritating to the urethra. Woman should wear underpants and panty hose with a cotton crotch and avoid wearing tight fitting slacks or jeans for long periods because anything that allows a blood-up of heat and moisture in the genital area may foster the growth of bacteria.

Some women do not consume enough fluid and food. After discovering her food preferences, the nurse should advise the woman to drink 2 or 3 quarts (8 to 12 glasses) of liquid a day to maintain an adequate fluid intake that ensures frequent urination and not limit fluids to reduce the frequency of urination. Women need to to know that if urine looks dark (concentrated) they need to increase their fluid intake. Cranberry juice may be suggested because cranberry juice is more acidic than other fluids and by lowering the pH of the urinary tract makes it less hospitable to bacteria. The consumption of yogurt and acidophilus milk may also help prevent urinary tract and vaginal infections.

The nurse should review with the woman healthy urination practices. Women should be told not to ignore the urge to urinate, because holding urine lengthens the time bacteria are in the bladder and thus allows them to multiply. Women should plan ahead when they are faced with situations that may require them to delay urination (for example, a long car ride). They should always urinate before going to bed at night. Bacteria also can be introduced during intercourse. Therefore, women are advised to urinate before and after intercourse, then drink a large glass of water to promote additional urination. The nurse can be reasonably assured that the teaching has been effective if a urinary tract infection does not develop.

Kegel's Exercises

Kegel's exercises (exercises for the pelvic floor) strengthen the muscles around the reproductive organs and improve muscle tone. Many women are not aware of the muscles of the pelvic floor (See Figs 4.8A to C). Until it is pointed out that these are the muscles used during urination and sexual intercourse and therefore can be consciously controlled. In as much as the muscles of the pelvic floor encircle the outlet through which the baby must pass, it is important that they be exercised, because an exercised muscle can tie stretch and contract readily at the time of birth.

Kegel's exercises should also be done immediately after giving birth to help the pelvic floor muscles return to normal functioning. They can then strengthen these muscles and improve muscle tone. If practised on a regular basis, the exercises can help prevent a prolapsed uterus and stress ncontinence from occurring later in life.

Several ways of performing Kegel's exercises have been described. One method that can be taught to the woman is described in teaching guidelines.

Teaching Guidelines

Kegel's Exercises

The exercise: The muscles that stop the flow of urine are the pubococcygeal muscles. Doing

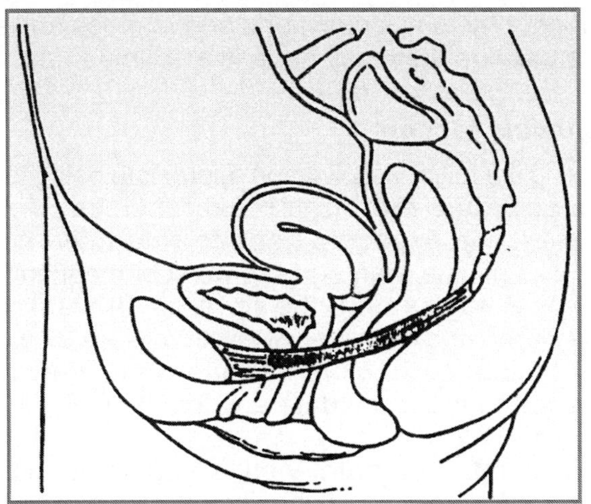

Fig. 4.8A: Proper position and good tone of the pubococcygeal muscle provide support of the pelvic organs

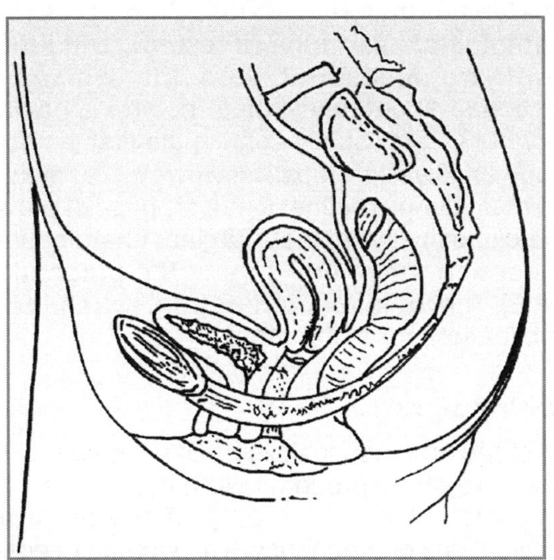

Fig. 4.8B: Incorrect position and poor tone of the pubococcygeal muscle can result in prolapse of the pelvic organs

Kegel's exercises during urination helps the woman know whether she is doing them correctly. If she can stop the stream of urine, her tone is good.

After a woman has located the correct muscles, she is taught that Kegel's exercises can be done in the following ways:

1. *Slowly*: Tighten the muscle, hold it for the count of three and relax it.
2. *Quickly*: Tighten the muscle and relax it as rapidly as possible.
3. *Push out, Pull in*: Pull up the entire pelvic floor.

The Kegel muscle, also known as the pubococcygeal muscle, serves as the major muscle of support for the pelvic floor. The Kegel muscle is like a hammock that attaches in the front at the symphysis pubis and in the back at the coccyx.

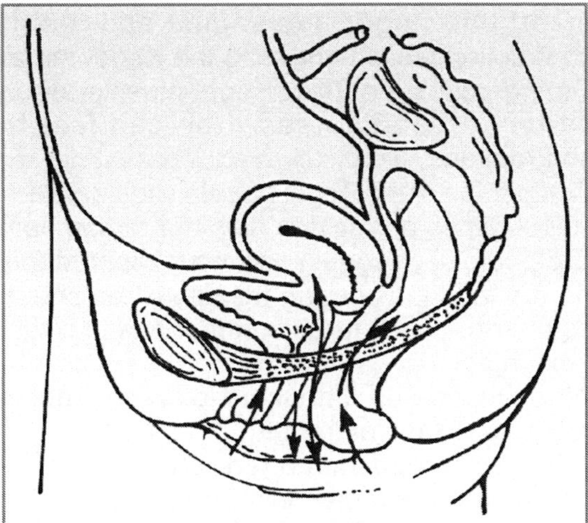

Fig. 4.8C: Contraction and release of the pubococcygeal muscle (Kegel exercises) can improve muscle tone, thereby providing better support for the pelvic organs

The Kegel muscle provides support for the uterus, bladder, rectum, and vagina. Proper position and good tone of the Kegel muscle prevent prolapse of these pelvic organs and also prevent stress incontinence. At the time of birth, the Kegel muscle is more elastic and stretches more readily if it has been exercised. When the Kegel muscle is in good tone, it provides support to the vaginal walls, contributing to increased sexual enjoyment during coitus.

The Kegel muscle is exercised by contracting and releasing it; two forms of the exercise can be done:

1. *Contract-release*: When contracting the muscle, tighten around the urethra, vagina, and rectum—as if trying to prevent urination. Pull the hammock of muscle up into the pelvis; when releasing the muscle, relax the hammock and feel it sag.
2. *Elevator:* Contract the Kegel muscle gradually in six steps, as if taking an ascending elevator to the sixth floor of a building; release the Kegel muscle slowly six levels until completely relaxed at the first floor.

The following checks can be made to ensure correct performance of the exercise:

- When voiding, begin flow of urine, then contract the Kegel muscle to stop flow of urine midstream

- Insert one finger into vagina and feel for contraction while tightening the Kegel muscle
- During coitus, contract Kegel muscle around partner's penis to see if he can feel the contraction.

Contraction of the Kegel muscle should be done 50 to 100 times per day; to help her remember to do the exercise, suggest that your client identify some routine times during the day when she will remember to do 10 to 20 contractions at a time. For example:

- Whenever doing a household chore, such as washing dishes or ironing
- Whenever stopped at a red light
- Whenever a commercial comes on TV
- Whenever standing in a line, such as at the bank or grocery store.

The nurse can be reasonably assured that the teach in has been effective if the woman reports an increased ability to control urine flow and greater muscular control during sexual intercourse.

Additional Teaching

Other subjects about which clients need information include diet, exercise sleep, bowel habits, smoking, alcohol ingestion, medication usage, and sexual relations. It is impossible to impart at one visit all the information the women and her family may need at the time her pregnancy is diagnosed. She can be given printed information at this time, such as material prepared by her health care provider, published pamphlets, or a list of books about pregnancy intended for lay people. However, the health care provider should have read all the latter materials carefully to be certain they supply the kind of information desired.

Proper nutrition is an important factor in the maintenance of maternal health during pregnancy and the provision of adequate nutrients for embryonic and foetal development. Assessing a woman's nutritional status and nutrition during pregnancy or interviews them to assess their knowledge of these topics. Nurses can refer women to a registered dietitian if a need is revealed during the nursing assessment.

Formal classes in childbirth and parenthood education have proved successful for some women and families. "Early bird "classes provide fundamental information that meets the needs of most expectant parents during the first trimester. Giving the expectant mother or her family the opportunity to ask questions and express anxieties or fears they may have is also important.

Schedule for Care

During the initial visit, women appreciate being told the schedule for return prenatal visits. Most women can expect to need to return every 4 weeks until the twenty-eighth week of pregnancy, every 2 weeks until the thirty sixth week of pregnancy and then every week from week 37 until the time of birth. More frequent visits may be needed to accommodate a woman's individual needs.

The initial prenatal visit is usually lengthy because the examination is comprehensive. The examination at subsequent visits is usually more focused and includes assessment and evaluation of foetal and maternal status. Blood pressure, weight, foetal heart tone (if tested), and fundal height are measured, and the woman is questioned about any symptoms she is having. Laboratory tests usually done in the first trimester include urinalysis by dipstick. However, screening for protein during routine urinalysis has not proved to be clinically beneficial. Vaginal examinations are not performed until late in the pregnancy, unless there is an indication, such as a complication, for doing them.

Warning Signs

One of the first responsibilities of people involved in the care of the pregnant woman is to alert her to the signs and symptoms of the potential complications of pregnancy. The woman needs to know the way and to whom to report such warnings signs when a person is stressed by a disturbing symptom, it is difficult to remember specifics. Therefore the woman and her family are better served if they are given a printed form listing the signs and symptoms that justify an investigation and the telephone numbers to call with questions or in an emergency.

Discomforts of Pregnancy

Women pregnant for the first time are confronted with symptoms that would be considered abnormal in the non-pregnant state. Much of the prenatal care requested by such women is prompted by the need for explanations of the causes of the discomforts and for advice on ways to relieve the

Table 4.14: Problems related to maternal adaptation during the first trimester

Problems	*Physiology*	*Education for self-care*
Breast changes, new sensations: pain, tingling	Hypertrophy of mammary glandular tissue and increased vascularization, pigmentation, and size and prominence of nipples and areolae caused by hormonal stimulation	Wear supportive maternity bras with pads to absorb discharge, may be worn at night; wash with warm water and keep dry, breast tenderness may interfere with sexual expression/foreplay but is temporary
Urgency and frequency of urination	Vascular engorgement and altered bladder function caused by hormones; bladder capacity reduced by enlarging uterus and foetal presenting part	Perform Kegel's exercises, limit fluid intake before bed time; wear perineal pad; report pain or burning sensation to primary health care provider
Languor and malaise fatigue (early pregnancy, usually)	Unexplained; may be caused by increasing levels of oestrogen, progesterone, and hCG or by elevated BBT; psychologic response to pregnancy and its required physical/psychologic adaptations	Rest as needed, eat well-balanced diet to prevent anaemia
Nausea and vomiting, morning sickness—occurs in 50 to 75% of pregnant women; starts between Ist and 2nd missed periods and lasts until about fourth missed period; may occur any time during day if mother does not have symptoms, expectant father may; maybe accompanied by bad taste in mouth.	Cause unknown; may result from hormonal changes, possibly hCG; may be partly emotional, reflecting pride in, ambivalence about or rejection of pregnant state	Avoid empty or overloaded stomach maintain good posture—give stomach ample room, stop or decrease smoking; eat dry carbohydrate on awakening; remain in bed until feeling subsides, or alternate dry carbohydrates. 1 hour with fluids such as hot herbal decaffeinated tea, milk or clear coffee the next hour until feeling subsides; eat five to six small meals per day avoid fried, odorous spicy, greasy, or gas forming foods; consult primary health care provider if intractable vomiting occurs
Pyalism (excessive salivation) may occur starting 2 to 3 weeks after first missed period	Possibly caused by elevated oestrogen levels; may be related to reluctance to swallow because of nausea.	Use astringent mouth wash; chew gum
Gingivits and epulis (hyperemia, hyper -trophy, bleeding, tenderness); condition will disappear sponta -neously 1 to 2 months after delivery	Increased vascularity and proliferation of connective tissue from oestrogen stimulation	Eat well-balanced diet with adequate protein and fresh fruits and vegetables brush teeth gently and observe good dental hygiene, avoid infection
Nasal stuffiness; epistaxis (nose bleed)	Hyperemia of mucus membranes related to high oestrogen levels	Use humidifier, avoid trauma normal saline nose drops or spray may be used
Leucorrhoea; often noted throughout pregnancy	Hormonally stimulated cervix becomes hypertrophic and hyperactive, producing abundant amount of mucus	Not preventable do not douche; wear perineal pads; perform hygienic practices such as wiping front to back; report to primary health care provider if accompanied by pruritis, foul odour, or change in character or colour
Psychosocial dynamics, mood swings, mixed feelings	Hormonal and metabolic adaptations, feelings about female role, sexuality, timing of pregnancy, and resultant changes in life and lifestyle	Participate in pregnancy support group; communicate concerns to partner, family and others, required referral for supportive services if needed (financial assistance).

discomforts. Information about the physiology and prevention of and self-care for discomforts experienced during the first trimester is given in Table 4.14.

Nurses can do much to allay a first time mother's anxiety about such symptoms by telling her about them in advance, using terminology that the woman (or couple) can understand. Such women who understand the physical discomforts of pregnancy are less able to become very anxious about their health. In addition, understanding the rationale for treatment promotes their participation in their care.

Employment

Many women continue to work outside the home during pregnancy whether the expectant mother can work and for how long depends on the physical activity involved, industrial hazards she may be exposed to and medical or obstetric complications that may occur. A prime consideration is for her to avoid being in a foetotoxic environment (for example, chemical dust particles or gases such as inhalation anaesthesia).

Physical Activity

Many women exercise regularly and strenuously in the nonpregnant state, and they are then concerned about losing their physical fitness during pregnancy when such activity must be decreased. On the other hand, woman who have led sedentary lifestyles need to start engaging in physical activity of very low intensity and advance the activity levels gradually. A number of researchers have recommended moderate exercise during pregnancy. It has been recommended that aerobic activty that does not cause the maternal heart rate to exceed 140 beats/min. Any activities continued to the point of exhaustion or fatigue compromise uterine perfusion and foetoplacental oxygenation. If the woman is accustomed to jogging, she may continue to do so, however, she should not reach the point of fatigue. Heat stress may also endanger the foetus.

As gestation advances, the woman's centre of gravity changes, her bony pelvic support loosens, her co-ordination usually decreases, and she notices a sense of awkwardness that may cause her to lose her balance and fall, injuring her self. Individually taught exercise has also been shown to lower the back pain common in pregnant women.

Exercises such as those shown are taught at prenatal classes or by the nurse in the clinic or the physician's office. Such exercises promote comfort and help prepare the woman for labour. Other topics for discussion and demonstration are correct posture and the way to lift and move objects safely to counteract the awkwardness and prevent the discomfort experienced starting in the second trimester of pregnancy.

Dental Health

Dental care during pregnancy is especially important because nausea during pregnancy may lead to poor oral hygiene, allowing dental caries to develop. No physiologic alteration during gestation can cause dental caries, however. Because calcium and phosphorous in the teeth are fixed in enamel, the old age "for every child a tooth" is not true.

There is no scientific evidence that filling teeth or even dental extraction involving the administration of local or nitrous oxide-oxygen anaesthesia precipitates abortion or premature labour. Antibacterial therapy should be considered for sepsis, however, especially in pregnant women, who have had rheumatic heart disease or nephritis. Emergency dental surgery is not contraindicated during pregnancy. However, the risks and benefits of dental surgery need to be explained to the mother.

Medication

Although much has been learned in recent years about foetal drug toxicity, the possible teratogenicity of many drugs, prescription and OTC, is still unknown. This is especially true for new medications and combinations of durgs. Moreover, certain subclinical errors or deficiencies in intermediate metabolism in the foetus may cause an otherwise harmless drug to converted into a hazardous one. The greatest danger of drug-caused developmental defects in the foetus extends from the time of fertilization through the first trimester, a time when the woman may not realize she is pregnant. Self-treatment must be discouraged. The use of all drugs, including OTC medications and vitamins, should be limited and a careful record kept of all therapeutic agents used.

Immunizations

There has been some concern over the safety of various immunization techniques during pregnancy. Immunization with live or attenuated live viruses is contraindicated during pregnancy because of its potential teratogenicity. Live virus vaccines include those for measles (rubeola and rubella). Chickenpox and mumps, as well as the Sabin's (oral) poliomyelitis vaccine. Vaccines consisting of killed viruses may be used. Those that may be administered during pregnancy include tetanus, diphtheria, recombinant hepatitis B and rabies vaccines.

Alcohol, Cigarette Smoke, and Other Substances

A safe level of alcohol consumption during pregnancy has not yet been established. Although the consumption of occasional alcoholic beverages may not be harmful to the mother or her developing embryo or foetus, complete abstinence is strongly advised. Maternal alcoholism is associated with high rates of spontaneous abortion, and the risk for spontaneous abortion in the first trimester is dose related (three or more drinks one day).

Cigarette smoking or continued exposure to a smoke filled environement (even if the mother does not smoke) is associated with foetal growth restriction and an increase in perinatal and infant morbidity and mortality. Exposure to nicotine has been shown to have a negative effect on the growth of the foetus. Smoking is also associated with an increased frequency of preterm labour, premature rupture of membranes (PROM), abruption placentae, placenta previa, and foetal death resulting possibly from decreased placental perfusion. Laboratory studies have revealed that smoking causes foetal hypoxia. All pregnant women who smoke should be strongly encouraged to quit or at least cut down. Pregnant women need to be told about the negative effects of even second hand smoke on the foetus. Research has shown that early intervention may be effective in helping the woman cut down or quit smoking. Most studies of human pregnancy have revealed no association between caffeine consumption and birth defects or low birth weight. Because other effects are unknown, however, pregnant women are advised to limit their caffeine intake.

Any drug or environmental agent that can get into the pregnant woman is bloodstream has the potential to cross the placenta and harm the foetus.

Childbirth/Parent Education Classes

In a typical preparation for parenthood program is recognized that expectant parents and their families have different interests and need different information as the pregnancy progresses. Consequently such programs are designed to meet the informational needs of parents during the three major stages of pregnancy and after birth—first-trimester classes, second-trimester classes, third-trimester classes, and postpartum ("fourth-trimester") classes.

First-trimester ("earlybird") classes provide fundamental information and focus on the following topics: (1) early foetal development, (2) physiologic and emotional changes that occur early in pregnancy, (3) human sexuality, (4) birth settings and types of health care providers, (5) rest, exercise, and measures for relieving common discomforts, (6) the nutritional needs of the mother and foetus, and (7) the development of a birth plan. Environmental and workplace hazards have become important concerns in recent years, so even though pregnancy is considered a normal process, exercises, warning signs, drugs and selfmedication are now topics of interest and concern.

Support systems that are available during pregnancy and after birth are discussed throughout the series of classes. Such support systems can help parents function independently and effectively. During all the classes, participants are welcome to openly express their feelings and concerns about any aspect of pregnancy, birth, and parenting.

For those who do attend such classes, extensive preparation is possible but not all pregnant women and support people attend formal classes to prepare for child birth. The reasons for this vary and include previous experience with childbirth; employment; inaccessibility because of time; cultural, ethnic or religious orientation; cost; lack of knowledge regarding choices in childbirth/parent education classes; and lack of readiness. Therefore, clinicians need to provide this information as needed and encourage participation.

Birth Plan

The birth plan is a natural evolution of the contemporary wellness-oriented lifestyle. It is a tool by which parents can explore their childbirth options and choose those that are most important to them. Many parents already indicate some of their preferences by the type of health care provider and birth setting (hospital, freestanding birth centre or home) they have chosen. Some pregnant women enlist the services of a health care provider only after an interview and a tour of the birth facility. Others do not give conscious thought to the conduct of their pregnancies, the labour and birth process, recovery, and early parenthood. These women may need help with decision-making. After confirmation of pregnancy, couples tend to focus on the reality of their situation and their emotional responses. However, it is acceptable for the nurse to initiate a discussion of a birth plan during the first and second prenatal visits. Some maternity clinics provide printed material describing available options and giving answers to frequently asked questions. In addition tours of the birth setting are offered by almost all facilities that provide perinatal services.

Client's expectations must be reasonable and in keeping with the resources available in the community. The nurse can provide couples with pertinent information so that they can make informed decisions, alerting them to various options and the advantages and consequences of each.

The nurse needs to assess client's readiness to learn and avoid overloading them with information. Some health care providers provide birth plan lists. A discussion of the printed list can serve as a means of getting couples to start thinking about, discussing, and identifying what is personally important to them. However, it is important to remember that some options may only be appropriate for low-risk women. The options of women with a high-risk pregnancy or those in whom complications develop during labour may be severely limited.

Topics for discussion and decision-making may include any or all of the following:

- *Partner's participation*: Attend prenatal visits? Childbirth/parent education classes? Present during labour? During birth? During caesarean birth?
- *Birth setting*: Hospital delivery room or birthing room (if available) A birthing centre? Home?
- *Labour management*: Would you like to walk around during labour? Use rocking chair? use a shower? Have a perineal shave or enema (if they are still done routinely at that particular setting)? Consider an electronic foetal monitor? Be interested in having music or dimmed lighting? Have older children or other people present? Is telemetry monitoring available? Consider stimulation of labour? Consider medication—what kind?
- *Birth*: Have you considered the various positions for birth—side lying? On hands and knees, kneeling, or squatting? Use a birthing bed or delivery table? will you be photographing, video-taping, or recording any of the labour or birth, who would you like to be present—partner, older siblings, other family members, or friends, what are your feelings about forceps? episiotomies? Will your partner want to cut the umbilical cord?

Other relevant topics might best be brought up during the second trimester the pregnant woman and her partner and between the couple and health care providers. An early introduction to the idea of a birth plan allows the couple time to think about events or situations that could make their childbearing experience more meaningful and those they would prefer to avoid. The nurse-client discussion of the birth plan needs to take place in an accepting atmosphere in which the clients can see themselves as unique and yet normal.

Sexual Counselling during Pregnancy

The sexual counselling of expectant couples includes countering misinformation, providing reassurance of normality, and suggesting alternative behaviours. The uniqueness of each couple is considered within a biopsychosocial framework (Fig. 4.9).

Sexuality in first trimester of pregnancy

- Be aware that maternal physiologic changes, such as breast enlargement nausea, fatigue, abdominal changes, perineal enlargement, leucorrhoea, pelvic vasocongestion, and orgasmic responses, may affect sexuality and sexual expression.
- Discuss responses to pregnancy with your partner.

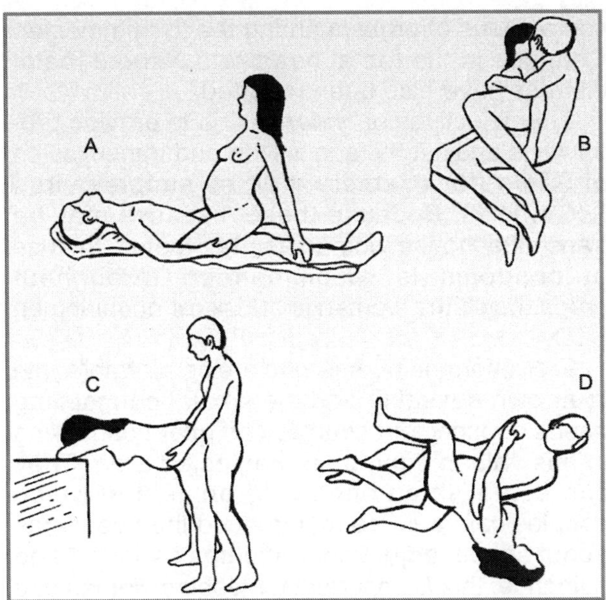

Fig. 4.9: Positions for sexual intercourse during pregnancy. **A.** Female superior, **B.** Side by side, **C.** Rear entry, **D.** Facing each other

- Keep in mind that cultural prescriptions (dos) and prescriptions may affect your responses.
- Although your libido may be depressed during the first semester, it increases during the second trimester.
- Discuss and explore with your partner:
  - Alternative behaviours (for example, mutual masturbation, foot massage, duddling)
  - Alternative positions (for example, female superior, side-lying) for sexual intercourse.
- Intercourse is safe as long as it is not uncomfortable. There is no correlation between intercourse and spontaneous abortion but observe the following precautions:
  - Abstain from intercourse if you experience uterine cramping or vaginal bleeding; report event to your primary health care provider as soon as possible.
  - Abstain from intercourse (or any activity that results in orgasm) if you have a history of cervical incompetence, until it is corrected.
  - Continue to use "safer sex "behavioures. The partners of women at high risk for acquiring or transmitting sexually transmitted diseases are encouraged to use condoms during sexual inter-course throughout her pregnancy.

Counselling couples concerning sexual adjustments that may be made during pregnancy demands self assessment on the part of the nurse, as well as a knowledge of the physical, social, and emotional responses to sex during pregnancy. Not all maternity nurses are comfortable dealing with the sexual concerns of their clients. Therefore, those nurses who are aware of their personal strengths and limitations in dealing with sexual content are better prepared to make referrals if necessary.

Many women merely need permission to be sexual during pregnancy. Many other women, however, need to be given information about the physiological changes that occur during pregnancy and have the myths associated with sex during pregnancy dispelled. Such tasks are within the purview of the nurse and should be an integral component of the health care rendered.

Some couples need to be referred for sex therapy or family therapy. Couples with long standing problems with sexual dysfunction that are intensified by pregnancy are candidates for sex therapy. Whenever a sexual problem is a symptom of a more serious relationship problem, the couple would benefit from family therapy.

Obtaining a history: The couple's sexual history provides a basis for counselling, but history-taking is also an ongoing process. The couple's receptivity to changes in attitudes, body image, partner relationships, and physical status are relevant topics throughout pregnancy. Whenever changes occur, unexpected problems may arise that require intervention. The history reveals the client's knowledge of female anatomy and physiology and her attitudes about sex during pregnancy, as well as her perceptions of the pregnancy, the health status of the couple, and the quality of their relationship. An understanding of the couple subjective experience provides the direction and focus for sexual counselling.

Countering Misinformation

Many myths and much of the misinformation related to sex and pregnancy are masked by seemingly unrelated issues. For example, a question about the baby's ability to hear and see *in utero* may be prompted by questions about the baby being an observer of lovemaking. The counsellor must be extremely sensitive to the questions behind such questions when counselling in this highly charged emotional area.

Suggesting Alternative Behaviours

At this time research has not proved conclusively that coitus and orgasm are contraindicated at any time during pregnancy for the obstetrically and medically healthy women. However, a history of more than one spontaneous abortion or a threatened abortion in the first trimester; impending miscarriage in the second trimester; and premature rupture of membranes, bleeding or abdominal pain during the third trimester warrant precaution when it comes to coitus and orgasm.

Solitary and mutual masturbation and oral-genital intercourse may be used by couples as alternatives to penile-vaginal intercourse. Partners who enjoy cunnilingus may full "turned off" by the normal increase inthe amount of odour of vaginal discharge during pregnancy. Couples who practice cunnilingus should be cautioned against the blowing of air into the vagina particularly during the last few weeks of pregnancy when the cervix may be slightly open. An air embolism can occur if air is forced between the uterine wall and the foetal membranes and enters the maternal vascular system through the placenta.

Showing the woman or couple pictures of possible variations of coital position is often helpful. The female-superior, side by side, and rear entry positions are possible alternative positions to the traditional male-superior position. The woman as tride (superior position) allows her to control the angle and depth of penile penetration, as well as to protect her breasts and abdomen. The side-by-side position is the preferred one, especially during the third trimester, because it requires less energy and places less pressure on the pregnant abdomen (Fig. 4.9).

Multiparous women sometimes experience severe breast tenderness in the first trimester. A coital position that avoids direct pressure on the woman's breasts and decreased breast fondling during love play can be recommended to such women. The woman should also be reassured that this condition is normal and temporary.

Some women complain of lower abdominal cramping and backache after orgasm during the first and third trimesters. A back rub can often relieve some of the discomfort and provide a pleasant experience. A tonic uterine contraction, often lasting up to a minute, replaces the rhythmic contractions of orgasm during the third trimester. Changes in the foetal heart rate without foetal distress have also been reported.

The objectives of "safer sex" is to provide prophylaxis against the acquisition and transmission of STDs (for example, herpes simplex virus (HSV, HIV). Because these diseases may be transmitted to the woman and her foetus, the use of condoms is recommended throughout pregnancy if the woman is at risk for acquiring an STD.

Well informed nurses who are comfortable with their own sexuality and the sexual counselling needs of expectant couples can offer counselling in this valuable but often neglected area. They can establish an open environment in which couples can feel free to introduce their concerns about sexual adjustment and seek support and guidance. this is important for lesbian women and their partners, as well as for women partnered by men.

Cultural Variations in Prenatal Care

Prenatal care as we know it is a phenomenon of western medicine. In the western biomedical model of care, women are encouraged to seek prenatal care as early as possible in their pregnancy by visiting a physician, nurse-midwife, or office or clinic. Such visits are usually routine and as already mentioned follow a systemic sequence, with the initial visit followed by monthly, then bimonthly, then weekly visits. Monitoring weight and blood pressure; testing blood and urine; teaching specific information about diet, rest, and activity and preparing for childbirth are common components of prenatal care. This model is not only unfamiliar but commonly seems strange to many groups.

Many cultural variations in prenatal care exist. Even if the prenatal care described is familiar to a woman, some practices may conflict with the beliefs and practices of a subculture group to which she belongs. Because of these and other factors, such as lack of transportation, and poor communication on the part of health care providers, women from many such groups do not participate in the prenatal care system. Such behaviour may be misinterpreted by nurses as uncaring, lazy or ignorant.

A concern for modesty is also a deterrent to the seeking of prenatal care for many women. For some women exposing body parts, espcially to a man is considered a major violation of their modesty. For many women, invasive procedures, such as a vaginal examination, may be so threatening that they cannot be discussed, even with their own husbands. Thus, many women prefer a female to a male health care provider. Too often, health care providers assume women lose this modesty during pregnancy and labour, but actually most women value and appreciate efforts to maintain their modesty.

For numerous cultural groups a physician is deemed appropriate only in times of illness, and because pregnancy is considered a normal process and the woman is in a state of health, the services of a physician are considered in appropriate. Even if problems with pregnancy do develop from the stand point of western medicine, they may not be perceived as problems but considered normal by members of these cultural groups.

Although pregnancy is considered normal by many certain practices are expected of women of all cultural to ensure a good outcome. Cultural prescriptions tell women what to do, and prescriptions establish taboos. The purposes of these practices are to prevent maternal illness resulting from a pregnancy-induced imbalanced state and to protect the vulnerable foetus. Prescriptions regulate the woman's emotional response, clothing, activity and rest, sexual activity, and dietary practices.

Emotional response: Virtually all cultures emphasize the importance of maintaining a socially harmonious and agreeable and environment for a pregnant woman. An absence of stress is important in ensuring a successful outcome for the mother and baby. Harmony with other people must be fostered, and visits from extended family members may be required to demonstrate pleasant and noncontroversial relationships. If discord exists in a relationship, it is usually dealt with in culturally prescribed ways.

Besides prescriptions regarding food, other prescriptions involve imitative magic. Many Indians believe pregnant women should not witness an eclipse of the moon because it may cause a cleft palate in the infant. They also believe that exposure to an earthquake may precipitate preterm birth, miscarriage, or even a breech presentation. In some cultures, a pregnant woman must not ridicule someone with an affliction for fear her child might be born withthe same handicap. A mother should not hate a person least her child resemble that person, and dental work should not be done because it may cause a baby to have a "harelip." A widely held folk belief in many cultures is that the pregnant woman should refrain from raising her arms above her head and tying knots so that the umbilical cord does not wrap around the baby's neck or knot. Other cultures believe placing a knife under the bed of a labouring woman will "cut" or pain.

Clothing: Although most cultural groups do not prescribe specific clothing to be worn during pregnancy, modesty is an expectation of many. Some women of the wear a cord beneath the breast and knotted over the umbilicus. This cord, is thought to prevent morning sickness and ensure a safe birth. Amulets, medals, and beads may also be worn to ward off evil spirits.

Physical activity and rest: Norms that regulate the physical activity mother during pregnancy vary tremendously. Many groups, encourage women to be active, to walk and to engage in normal although not strenuous activities to ensure that the baby is healthy and not too large. On the other hand, other culture believe that any activity is dangerous, and others willingly take over the work of the pregnant woman. Some believe that this activity protects the mother and child. The mother is encouraged simply to produce the succeeding generation. If health care providers do not know of this belief, they could misintepret this behaviour as laziness or noncompliance with the desired prenatal health care regimen. Again, it is important for the nurse to find out the way each pregnant woman views activity and rest.

Sexual activity: In most cultures, sexual activity is not prohibited until the end of pregnancy. Many view sexual activity as necessary to keep the birth canal lubricated. On the other hand, some may have definite prescriptions against sexual intercourse, requiring abstinence throughout the pregnancy because it is thought that sexual intercourse may harm the mother and foetus.

Diet: Nutritional information given by health care providers may also be a source of conflict for many cultural groups, but such a conflict commonly is not known by the health care providers unless they understand the dietary belief and practices of the particular people for whom they are caring. For example, Muslims must eat meat slaughtered in accordance with Muslim law. If this is not possible, they will accept Kosher or vegetarian foods. Many cultures permit pregnant women to eat only warm food.

Evaluation: Maternal and foetal expected outcomes are continuously evaluated according to measurable, established criteria. The clinical findings that represent: normal responses are presented as plans and expected outcomes in the nursing care plan for each woman. These criteria are used as a basis for selecting the appropriate nursing actions as well as evaluating their effectiveness (plan of care), and include that the woman (and family when appropriate) have achieved the following:

- Lists maternal adaptations to pregnancy
- Lists nutritional and self-care measures
- Knows the warning signs and whom to report them to if they occur
- Become active participants in her care during the first trimester.

Home Care for Pregnancy—Exercise Tips for Pregnant Women

Consult your health care provider: When you know or suspect you are pregnant discuss your medical obstetric history, your current exercise regimen, and the exercises you would like to continue throughout pregnancy.

Seek help: In determining an exercise routine that is well within your limit of tolerance, especially if you have not been exercising regularly.

Consider decreasing weight-bearing exercises (Jogging, running) and concentrating on non-weight bearing activities such as swimming, cycling or stretching. If you are a runner, starting in your seventh month, you may wish to walk instead.

Avoid risky activities: Such as surfing, mountain, climbing, skydiving, and racquet ball because such activities that require precise balance and coordination may be dangerous. Avoid activities that require holding your breath and bearing down (Valsalva's manoeuvre). Jerky, bouncy motions also should be avoided.

Exercise regularly: At least three times a week,—To improve muscle tone and increase or maintain your stamina. If you do exercises sporadically, this may put undue strain on your muscles. Limit activity to shorter intervals. Exercise for 10 to 15 minutes, rest for 2 or 3 minutes, than exercise for another 10 to 15 minutes.

Decrease your exercise level: As your pregnancy progresses. The normal alterations of advancing pregnancy, such as decreased cardiac reserve increased respiratory effort, may produce physiologic stress if you exercise strenuously for a long time.

Take your pulse: Every 10 to 15 minutes while you are exercising. If it is more than 140 beats/min, slow down until it returns to a maximum of 90 beats, min, you should be able to converse easily while exercising. If you cannot you need to slow down.

Avoid becoming overheated: For extended periods of time. It is best not to exercise for more than 35 minutes, especially in hot, humid weather. As your body temperature rises, the heat is transmitted to your foetus. Prolonged or repeated elevation of foetal temperature may result in birth defects, especially during the first 3 months. Your temperature should not exceed 38° C (100.4°F).

Avoid the use of hot tubs and saunas: Warm up and stretching exercises prepare your joints for more strenuous exercise and lessen the likelihood of strain or injury to your joints. After the fourth month of gestation you should not perform exercise flame on your back.

A cool-down period: Of mild activity involving your lets after an exercise period will help bring your respiration, heart, and metabolic rates back to normal and prevent the pooling of blood in the exercised muscles.

Rest for 10 minutes after exercising: Lying on your left side. As the uterus grows, it puts pressure on a major vein on the right side of your abdomen which carries blood to your heart. Lying on your left side removes the pressure and promotes return circulation from your extremities and muscles to your heart, thereby increasing blood flow to your placenta and foetus. You should rise gradually from the floor to prevent dizziness or fainting (orthostatic hypotension).

Drink two or three (8-ounce) glasses of water: After you exercise to replace the body fluids lost through perspiration. While exercising, drink water whenever you feel the need.

Increase your caloric intake: To replace the calories burned during exercise and provide the extra energy needs of pregnancy. (Pregnancy alone requires an additional 300 kcal/day.) Choose such high-protein for as fish, milk, cheese, eggs or meat.

Take your time: This is not the time to be competitive or train for activities requiring long endurance.

Wear supportive bra: Your increased breast weight may cause changes in posture and put pressure on the ulnar nerve.

Wear supportive shoes: As your uterus grows, your centre of gravity shi and you compensate for this by arching your back. These natural change may make you feel off balance and more likely to fall.

Stop exercising immediately: If you experience shortness of breath, dizziness, numbness, tingling, pain of any kind, more than four uterine contraction per hour, decreased foetal activity, or vaginal bleeding, and contact your health care provider.

NURSING MANAGEMENT OF SECOND TRIMESTER

The second trimester spans weeks 14 through 26 of pregnancy. By this trimester the pregnancy usually has been verified the woman and her family have had time to adjust to the idea of pregnancy, and she has come in for the intial visit and possibly a follow-up visit. For many women the discomforts common to the first trimester are resolving, but it is still too early for them to focus on labour and birth.

Most women have no major problems. For them, a common pattern for return visits in scheduled. Through-out the second trimester, monthly visits are sufficient, although additional visits may be scheduled should the need arise.

Ideally a trusting relationship has already been established among the pregnant woman and her family, the nurse, and other health care providers. The nursing plan of care has been initiated, and changes brought to light by the ongoing evaluation are being addressed. As in the case during the first trimester, health promotion and the prevention of complications remain the focus of nursing care. However, the continued growth and developement of the mother and her foetus and the family unit require that certain changes in nursing management be made during the second trimester. Maternal assessment and foetal assessment can be performed as described below:

Maternal Assessment

Interview: Follow-up visits are less intensive than the initial prenatal visit. At each of these follow-up visits, the woman is asked to summarize relevant events that have occurred since the previous visit. She is asked about her general emotional and physiologic well-being, complaints or problems, or questions she may have. Personal and family needs are also identified and explored.

Because the woman's emotional state has an impact on her general well-being and on that of her family, her and her family's emotional well-being is assessed at each visit. Emotional changes are common during pregnancy, and, therefore, it is reasonable for the nurse to ask whether the woman has experienced any mood swings, reactions to changes in her body image, bad dreams or worries. Positive feelings (her own and those of her family) are also noted. The reactions of family members to the pregnancy and the woman's emotional changes are recorded.

How the woman is progressing through the developmental tasks of pregnancy is also assessed. By the beginning of the second trimester, most women have accepted the biologic fact of pregnancy. Usually by the fifth month, pregnant women are experiencing a growing awareness of the child as a separate being, distinct from themselves; women can say, "I am going to have a baby". With quickening, she turns her attention inward (becomes introspective) to her pregnancy and toward her relationships with others (for example, her mother, partner).

The success or failure of self-care measures is discussed, and the woman's learning needs and readiness for learning are assessed. The nurse inquires about her participation in childbirth education classes. Did the woman (with or without her partner) attend early birth classes during the first trimester? If so, what questions does she have? Is she planning to attend second-trimester classes? If a birth plan is being formulated, what questions does she have and how far have she and her partner come in its development?

A checklist of care needs during the secured trimester of pregnancy is a valuable tool. This checklist provides the team of health care provides with a communication tool to prevent gaps in care and identify areas of concern for clients. A sample checklist for the second trimester is given below:

- Schedule of visits and events
- Maternal assessment
- Foetal growth and development
- Diagnostic tests
  - Specify
  - Counselling for self-care
  - Birth plan
  - Adaptations/discomforts
  - Skin changes
  - Palpitations
  - Faintness
  - Gastrointestinal diseases
  - Varicosities
  - Neuromuscular and skeletal disease.
- Safety (seat belts with shoulder harness and head rest)
- Exercise and rest
- Relaxation
- Nutrition
- Alcohol and other substances.
- Sexuality
- Personal hygiene
- Warning signs of potential complications
- Other.

Physical examination: Revelation is a constant aspect of a pregnant woman's care. Each woman reacts differently to pregnancy. As a result, careful monitoring of the pregnancy and her reactions to care is vital. The data base is updated at each time of contact with the pregnant woman. Physiologic changes are documented as the pregnancy progresses because this makes it possible for any deviations from normal progress to be identified.

At each visit, pulse and respiration are measured; blood pressure (same arm with woman sitting) is taken; her weight is determined and whether the weight gain (or loss) is compatible with the overall plan for weight gain is evaluated; urinalysis is performed; and the presence and degree of edema are noted. Abdominal inspection and palpation and measurement of fundal height are aspects of the examination at each visit; these are discussed in more detail in the following section. While assessing the pregnant woman's abdomen with the woman in the lithotomy position, the nurse must watch for the occurance of supine hypotension, and intervene as given below:

Supine Hypotension

Signs/Symptoms

- Pallor,
- Dizziness, faintness, breathlessness
- Tachycardia
- Nausea
- Clammy (damp, cool) skin; sweating.

Interventions

Position woman on her side until her signs and symptoms subside and vital signs stabilize within normal limits.

When a woman is lying in this position the weight of abdominal contents may compress the vena cava and aorta, causing a drop in blood pressure. If the woman cannot tolerate the lithotomy position, the genital examination can be done with the woman in the lateral position.

The findings revealed during the interview and physical examination reflect the status of maternal adaptations. When any of the findings are suspicious, an in-depth examination is performed.

Careful interpretation of blood pressure is important in the risk factor analysis of all pregnant women. Blood pressure is evaluated on the basis of absolute values and the length of gestation and is interpreted in the light of modifying factors. An absolute systolic blood pressure of 140 mmHg or more and diastolic blood pressur of 90 mmHg or more indicate the existence of hypertension. A rise in the systolic blood pressure of 30 mmHg more than the baseline pressure or in the diastolic blood pressure of 15 mmHg more than the baseline pressure is also a significant finding regardless of whether the absolute values are less than 140/90 mmHg. For example, if a woman's blood pressure normally is 105/60 mmHg, a change of 120/75 mmHg indicates a heightened risk for hypertension. The blood pressure decreases slightly in midpregnancy then returns to baseline by term. An increase in the systolic blood pressure is a better indicator of the risk for pregnancy induced hypertension (PIH) than is an increase in the diastolic pressure.

In assessing blood pressure the nurse needs to always keep in mind that an increase in blood pressure could indicate the onset of either PIH or the HELP syndrome (Haemolysis, elevated liver enzymes, and low platelet count). Either of these could result in devastating consequences for the women or her foetus.

Laboratory tests: The number of routine laboratory tests done during the second trimester is limited. A clean-catch urine specimen is obtained to test for glucose (to assess for diabetes), protein (to assess for PIH), and nitrites and leucocytes (to assess for infection). Urine specimens for culture and sensitivity, as well as blood samples, are obtained only if signs and symptoms warrant. A hematocrit determination is done at each visit in some offices. A blood specimen is obtained at 16 weeks to determine the alpha-fetoprotein level.

The multiple-marker, or triple-screen, test is being used to detect Down's syndrome. Done between 16 and 18 week's gestation,it measures the maternal serum level of alpha-fetoprotein (MSAFP), human chorionic gonadotropin (hCG) and unconjugated oestriol (UE3). Adjusted values are combined to yield the risk for Down's syndrome. Low levels may be associated with Down's syndrome and other chromosomal abnormalities.

Signs of potential problems: The mother is monitored continuously for signs and symptoms of potential complications. Persistent and excessive vomiting may inidicate the development of hyperemesis gravidarum. Uterine cramping and vaginal bleeding are signs of threatened abortion. Chills and fever are symptoms of infection. The cause of hypertension may be investigated. Discharge from the vagina may be amniotic fluid or associated with infection signs of Potential complications are as follows:

Signs of Potential Complications

Second and Third Trimesters

Sign/Symptom	Possible causes
Persistent, severe vomiting	Hyperemesis gravidarum
Amniotic fluid discharge from vagina	Premature rupture of membranes
Vaginal bleeding, severe abdominal pain	Miscarriage, placental separate
Chills, fever, burning on urination, diarrhoea	Infection
Change in foetal movements; absence of foetal movement after quickening any unusual changes in pattern or amount	Foetal jeopardy or intrauterine foetal death
Uterine contractions	Preterm labour
Visual disturbances, blurring, double vision or spots	Hypertensive conditions, PIH
Swelling of face or fingers and over sacrum	Hypertensive conditions, PIH
Headache: severe, frequent, or continuous	Hypertensive conditions, PIH
Muscular irritability or convulsions PIH	Hypertensive conditions,
Epigastric pain (perceived as severe stomach ache)	Hypertensive conditions, PIH
Glucosuria, positive glucose tolerance test result	Gestational diabetes mellitus

Foetal Assessment

Fundal height: During the second trimester the uterus becomes an abdominal organ. Measurement of the height of the uterus above the symphysis pubis is used as one indicator of foetal growth progress. The measurement also provides a gross estimate of the duration of pregnancy. In addition, it may aid in the identification of high-risk factors. A stable or decreased fundal height may indicate the pressure of intrauterine growth restriction excessive increase could indicate the presence of multifoetal gestation or hydramnios.

A paper tape measure or a pelvimeter may be used to measure fundal height. To increase the reliability of the measurement, the same person could examine the pregnant woman at each of her prenatal visits, but often this is not possible and different clinicians see the woman at prenatal visits. All clinicians who examine a particular pregnant woman should be consistent in their measurement technique. Ideally a protocol should be established for the health care setting in which the measurement technique is explicitly set forth and the women's position on the examining table, the measuring device, and method of measurement used are specified. Conditions under which the measurements are taken can also be described in the woman records, including whether the bladder was empty and whether the uterus was relaxed or contracted at the time of measurement.

Various positions for the measurement of the fundal height have been described in the literature. The women can be supine, have her head elevated, have her knees flexed, or have both her head elevated and knees flexed. Studies have shown that the measurements obtained with the woman in the various positions differ, making it even more important to standard size the fundal height measurement technique.

Placement of the tape measure can also vary. The tape can be placed in the middle of the woman's abdomen and the measurement made from the upper border of the symphysis pubis to the upper border of the fundus with the tape measure held in contact with the skin for the entire length of the uterus. In another measurement technique, the upper curve of the fundus is not included in the measurement. Instead, one end of the tape measure is held at the upper border of the symphysis pubis with one hand and the other hand is placed at the upper border of the fundus. The tape is placed between the middle and index fingers of the other hand and the point when these fingers intercept the tape measure is taken as the measurement.

During the second and third trimesters (weeks 18 to 30), the height of the fundus in centimeters is approximately the same as the number of weeks of gestation if the woman's bladder is empty at the time of measurement.

Gestational age: In an uncomplicated pregnancy, foetal gestational age is estimated after the duration of pregnancy and the expected date of birth (EDB) are determined. Foetal gestational age is determined from the menstrual history, contraceptive history, pregnancy test result, and the following findings obtained during the clinical evaluation:

- First uterine size estimate: date, size
- Foetal heart (FH) first heard: date, Doppler stethoscope, fetoscope
- Date of quickening
- Current fundal height, estimated foetal weight (FFW)
- Current week of gestation
- Ultrasound date, week of gestation, biparietal diameter (BPD)
- Reliability of dates
- See Table 4.15.

Quickening (* feeling of life) refers to the mother's first perception of foetal movement. It usually occurs between the sixteenth and twenteeth weeks of gestation.

In some centers, ultrasonography is performed routinely in all pregnant women, and this allows a more exact estimation of gestational age cannot give a precise date for her last menstrual period (LMP) or if the size of the uterus does not conform the stated date of the LMP. The efficacy of the routine use of sonography is low-risk pregnancies has not been documented to be associated with improved foetal outcome, however.

Health status: The assessment of foetal health status includes consideration of foetal movement, the foetal heart rate (FHR) and rhythm and abnormal maternal or foetal symptoms.

The mother is instructed to note the extent and timing of foetal movements and to report immediately if the pattern changes or if movement ceases. Regular movement has been found to be a reliable determinant of foetal health. The FHR is checked on routine visits once it has been heard. Early in the second trimester the heart beat may be heard with the Doppler stethoscope. To detect the heart beat before the foetus can be palpated by Leopald's manoeuvres the scope is moved around the abdomen until the heart beat is heard. Each nurse developes a set pattern for searching the abdomen for the heart beat; for example, she may start first in the midline about 2 to 3 cm (1 in) above the symphysis, then move to the left lower quadrant, and so on. The heart beat is counted and the quality and rhythm noted. Later in the second trimester the FHR can be determined with the fetoscope or Planard's stethoscope. A normal rate and rhythm are other good indicators of foetal health. Once the heart beat is noted, its absence is cause for immediate investigation.

The second trimester is a period of rapid growth. Foetal development during this time is summarized are as follows:

Foetal development at 26 weeks

- Viable at 24 weeks
- Foetal movements are obvious
- Foetal heart beat is readily heard
- Scalp hair, eyebrows, and eyelashes have formed, and fine downy lanugo and vernix cover the skin
- Eyelids are still fused
- Skin is red, shiny and thin
- Face is wrinkled, giving an "old man appearance"
- Length is 30 cm (12 in)
- Weight is 600 g (1½ lb)
- Uterus is at or just above level of umbilicus.

The foetus is considered to achieve viability at 20 weeks gestation or when it weighs 500 g rated if any maternal or foetal complication arise (for example, maternal hypertension, intrauterine

Table 4.15: Evaluation the unborn infant using gestational age (GA)	
Age	
Important for medical legal considerations, legal considerations, e.g. dating of prospective abortion (or elective ceasarean birth) An indirect, unreliable assessment of maturity	1. Date of first day of last normal menstrual period (Nagele' srule:count back 3 months, add 7 days to determine delivery date). 2. Fundal height [(assumes normal foetal growth). 3. Appearance of foetal heart tone at 10 to 12 weeks maturity using "Doppler" fetoscope. 4. Ultrasound measurements (trans-abdominal or transvaginal) a. Size of amnioic sac/uterine cavity. b. Foetal crown to rumplength. c. Biparietal diameters, abdominal or thoracic circumferences during the second trimester for greatest accuracy. 5. Amniotic fluid analysis (amniocentesis) a. Bilirubin levels during pregnancy uncomplicated by maternal-foetal blood incompatibilities usually reach peak at 16 to 30 weeks, then fall, disappearing by 36 weeks. b. Creatinine levels rise as foetal urine increases: unreliable if maternal-foetal complications occur. c. L/B ratio usually 2 at 35 weeks, but appearance of normal levels may be accelerated or retarded by maternal-foetal disorders
Maturity	
Various body system development may be monitored, but overall foetal maturity difficult to ascertain	1. Amniotic fluid analysis (amniocentesis) a. L/s ratio usually rises to 2 or more when lungs have matured, other biochemical tests (e.g., amount of saturated fats) increase reliability of lung maturation evaluation in complex obstetric cases. b. Positive form of shak test usually rules out lung immaturity. c. Fatty cell recovery percentage—19 w reliability. d. Creatinine levels may assist in assessment of renal maturity.
Well-being	
Indications of some specific defects, as well as clues of general foetal wellbeing possible, but not all problems identifiable	1. Ultrasound measurements a. Evaluation of foetal presentation; multiple pregnancy b. Detection of some structural abnormalities, e.g. central nervous system and genito - urinary anomalies c. Localization of placenta; diagnosis of placenta previa d. Identification of excessive or diminished amniotic fluid volume; related to possible fetal abnormalities or jeopardy. e. Motion picture (real-time techniques) may confirm foetal death. 2. Amniotic fluid analysis (amniocentesis). a. Chromosomal studies may reveal the following: 1. Foetal abnormalities in chromosome number and gross structure (e.g., Down's syndrome) 2. Sex of infant to help evaluate probability of sex-linked genetic disorders (e.g., Duchenne's muscular dystrophy, classic haemophilia) b. Biochemical studies may reveal the following 1. Anencephaly-myelomeningocele, based on level of alpha fetroprotein 2. A number of metabolic and blood diseases (e.g., thalassaemia) 3. Meconium-stained amniotic fluid; possible foetal oxygen lack (hypoxia) 4. Foetal movement—usually reassuring if not exaggerated 5. Foetal heart rate and contraction monitoring—external or internal. a. Helps identify episodes of hypoxia resulting from uteroplacental insufficiency or cord compression during labour b. Positive oxytocin challenge test or nipple stimulation contraction stress test may predict foetal jeopardy in true labour

growth restriction (IUGR), premature rupture of membranes (PROM), irregular or absent FHR, or absence of foetal movements after quickening).

Careful, precise, and concise recording of client responses and laboratory results contributes to the continuous supervision vital to ensuring the well-being of the mother and foetus.

Nursing diagnoses: Each woman is affected differently by pregnancy, and careful monitoring of the pregnancy and her responses to care are of utmost importance. Nursing diagnoses commonly encountered during the second trimester may include the following:

- Body image disturbance related to
  - Anatomic and physiologic changes of pregnancy.
- Alteration in health maintenance related to
  - Knowledge deficit regarding self-care measures.
  - Rest and relaxation
  - Personal hygiene (increased perspiration, oily skin, leucorrhoea).
- Pain related to
  - Discomforts of pregnancy
- Risk for injury related to
  - Nonuse of safety measures and head rest in automobiles.
  - Exposure to harmful chemicals
- Altered family processes related to
  - Lack of understanding of second-trimester changes
  - Change in sexual relationship or partner support.
- Anxiety related to:
  - Discomforts of pregnancy
  - Changing family dynamics
  - Foetal well-being.

The planning of care for women during the second trimester of pregnancy is guided by the nursing diagnoses. To the extent possible, the woman participates in developing an individualized plan that relates specifically to her needs. The information in this chapter is general; not all women will experience all the problems discussed or require all the facets of care described. The expected outcomes pertaining to physiologic and psychosocial care are similar to those for the first trimester and may include the woman/family doing the following:

- Verbalize understanding of maternal adaptations and foetal development during the second trimester.
- Describe self-care measures.
- List symptoms that indicate deviations from normal progress and the protocols for reporting them.
- Be active participants in her care during the second trimester.
- Continue to develop a birth plan.
- Describe continued confidence in her case.

Plan of Care and Implementation

The supportive and therapeutic nurse client relationship grows as the nurse implements the nursing process during the second trimester. The nausea often experienced in the first trimester has resolved, nutrition counselling is offered at each visit, and the woman is complimented on her progress, as appropriate. Women experience several new discomforts or changes as maternal adaptations continue into the second trimester. Women who have given birth before tend to manifest some pregnancy related discomforts earlier than first time mothers do. It is impossible to clearly distinguish the problems and changes by trimester, but the benefit of discussion, they have been distinguished in this way (Table 4.16).

Reinforcement of counselling about sexuality and the dangers of exposure to alcohol, cigarette smoke, and other substances if provided as necessary. It must be remembered that alcohol abuse during pregnancy is the leading cause of mental retardation. It is also associated with an increased risk of spontaneous abortion. Because the safe amount of alcohol that may be consumed during pregnancy without causing harm to the foetus has not been established it is, therefore prudent to advise pregnant women to abstain completely.

Women who are prepared for the possibility of experiencing emotional changes are more likely to feel reassured that they are not unusual or unnatural if they should occur and that it is acceptable to talk about their reactions. As pregnancy progresses, women become more open about their feelings toward themselves and others. Active listening and explanations by the nurse can help reassure women that their experiences are normal. If a psychologic disturbance is severe, however referral for appropriate treatment may be necessary.

Clothing: Comfortable, loose clothing is best. Washable fabrics (for example, absorbent cottons)

Table 4.16: Problems related to maternal adaptations to pregnancy in the second trimester

Discomfort	*Physiology*	*Education on self-care*
Pigmentation deepens acne, oily skin	Melanocyte-stimulating hormone (from anterior pituitary)	Not preventable; usually resolves during puerperium
Spider nevi (telangiectasia) appear over neck, thorax, face, and arms during second or third trimesters	Focal networks of dilated arterioles (end-arteries) from increased concentration of oestrogens	Not preventable, they fade slowly during late puerperium; rarely disappear completely
Palmar erythema occurs in 50% of pregnant women; may accompany spider nevi	Diffuse reddish mottling over palms and suffused skin over thenar eminences and fingertips may be caused by or genetic predisposition or hyperestro -genism.	Not preventable; condition will fade within 1 week after giving birth
Pruritus (noninflammatory)	Unknown cause; various types as follows; non-popular; closely aggregated pruritic papules	Keep fingernails short and clean; contact primary health care provider for diagnosis of cause
	Increased excretory function of skin and stretching of skin possible factors	Not preventable; symptomatic Keri baths, mild sedation
		Distraction, tepid baths with sodium bicarbonate or oatmeal added to water lotions and oils; change of soaps or reduction in use of soap, loose clothing.
Palpitations	Unknown; should not be accompanied by persistent cardiac irregularity	Not preventable; contact primary health care provider if accompanied by symptoms of cardiac decompensation
Supine hypotension (vena cava syndrome) and bradycardia	Induced by pressure of gravid uterus on ascending vena cava when woman is supine; reduces uterine-placental and renal perfusion	Side-lying position or semisitting posture with knees slightly flexed
Faintness and, rarely syncope (orthostatic hypotension) may persist throughout pregnancy	Vasomotor lability or postural hypotension from hormones; in late pregnancy may be caused by venous stasis in lower extremities	Moderate exercise, deep breathing, vigorous leg movement; avoid sudden changes in position and warm crowded areas; move slowly and deliberately keep environment cool; avoid hypoglycaemia by eating 5 to 6 small meals per day; wear elastic hose; sit as necessary; if symptoms are serious contact primary health care provider
Food cravings	Cause unknown; cravings determined by culture or geographic area	Not preventable; satisfy craving unless it interferes with well-balanced diet; report unusual cravings to primary health care provider.
Heartburn (pyrosis or acid indigestion); burning sensation, occasionally with burning and rogurg -itation of a little sour -testing fluid	Progesterone shows or tract motility and digestion, reverses peristalsis, relaxes cardiac sphincter, and delays emptying time of stomach; stomach displaced upward and compressed by enlarging uterus	Limit or avoid gas-producing or fatty foods and large meals; maintain good posture; sip milk for temporary relief; hot herbal tea, chewing gum; primary health care provider may prescribed anti-acid between meals, contact primary health care provider for persistent symptoms
Constipation	GI tract motility slowed because of progesterone, resulting in increased resorption of water and drying of stool; intestines compressed by enlarging uterus; predisposition to constipation because of oral iron supplementation	Drink six glasses of water per day; include roughage in diet; moderate exercise maintain regular schedule; for bowel movement; use relaxation techniques and deep breathing; do not take stool softener, laxatives, mineral oil, other drugs, or enemas without first consulting primary health care provider

Contd...

Contd...

Discomfort	*Physiology*	*Education on self-care*
Flatulence with bloating and belching	Reduced GI motility because of hormones, allowing time for bacterial action that produces gas; swallowing air	Chew foods slowly and thoroughly; avoid gas producing foods fatty foods, large meals, exercise; maintain regular bowel habits
Varicose vein (varicosities); may be associated with aching legs and tenderness; may be present in legs and vulva; haemorrhoids are varicosities in the perianal area	Hereditary predisposition; relaxations of smooth muscle walls of veins because of hormones causing tortuous dilated veins in legs and pelvic vasocongestion; condition aggravated by enlarging uterus, gravity, and bearing down for bowel movements; thrombi from leg varices rare but may be produced by haemorrhoids	Avoid obesity, lengthy standing or sitting constrictive clothing, and constipation and bearing down with bowel movements; moderate exercise rest with legs and hips elevated; wear support stockins; thrombosed haemorrhoid may be evacuated; relieve swelling and pain with warm sitz baths local application of astringent compresses.
Leucorrhoea; often noted throughout pregnancy	Hormonally stimulated cervix become hypertrophic and and hyperactive, producing abundant amount of mucus	Not preventable; do not douche maintain good hygiene, wear perineal pads; report to primary health care provider if accompanied by pruritus, foul odour, or change in character or colour.
Headaches (through week 26)	Emotional tension (more common than vascular migraine headache eye strain (refractory errors); vascular engorgements and congestion of sinuses resulting from hormone stimulation	Conscious relaxation; contact primary health care provider for constant "splitting" headache to assess for PIH
Carpal-tunnel syndrome involves thumb, second and third fingers, lateral side of little finger)	Compression of median nerve resulting from changes in surrounding tissues; pain, numbness, tingling, burning; loss of skilled movements (typing); dropping of objects	Not preventable; elevate aftected arms splinting of affected hand may help; regressive after pregnancy; surgery is curative
Periodic numbness, tingling of fingers (acrodysesthesia) Occuring 5% of pregnant women	Brachial plexus traction, syndrome resulting from drooping of shoulders, during pregnancy (occurs espacially at night and early morning	Maintain good posture; wear supportive maternity bra; condition will disappear if lifting and carrying baby does not aggravate it
Round ligament pain (tenderness)	Stretching of ligament caused by enlarging uterus	Not preventable; rest; maintain good body mechanics to avoid overstretching ligament relieve cramping by squatting or bringing knees to chest
Joint pain, backache and pelvic pressure hypermobility of joints	Relaxation of symphyseal and sacroiliac joints because of hormones, resulting in unstable pelvis; exaggerated lumbar and cervicothoracic curves caused by change in centre of gravity resulting from enlarging abdomen	Maintain good posture and body mechanics; avoid fatigue wear low low-healed shoes; conscious relaxation; sleep on firm mattress; apply local heat or ice; get back rubs; do pelvis rock exercise; rest; condition will disappear 6 to 8 weeks after birth

are often preferred. Maternity clothes may be purchased new or found at thrift shops or garage sales in good condition because they rarely wear out. Tight bras and belts, stretch pants, garters, tight top knee socks, panty girdles, and other constrictive clothing should be avoided because tight clothing over the perineum encourages vaginitis and miliaria (heat rash) and impaired circulation in the leg can cause varicosities.

Comfortable shees that provide firm support and promote good posture and balance are also advisable. Very high heels and platform shoes are not recommended because of the woman's changed centre of gravity, which can cause her to lose her balance. In addition, in the third trimester the woman's pelvis tilts forward and her lumbar curve increase. The resulting leg aches and cramps are only aggravated by nonsupportive shoes.

Posture and body mechanics: Many maternal adaptations predispose the woman to suffering backache and incurring possible injury. The pregnant woman's centre of gravity changes, pelvic joints soften and relax, and stress is placed on abdominal musculature as pregnancy progresses. Poor posture and body mechanics contribute to the acquire a kinesthetic sense for good body posture. The activities described in the client self-care (Table 4.17) can also promote greater physical comfort.

Bathing and swimmings: Tub bathing is permitted even in late pregnancy because water does not enter the vagina unless it is under pressure. However, tub bathing is usually contraindicate after rupture of the membrane. Baths and warm showers can be therapeutic because they relax tense, tired muscles, help counter insomnia, and make the pregnant woman fell fresh. However, physical maneuverability poses a problem (increased risk of falling) late in pregnancy. Swimming is also permitted during normal pregnancy, although diving is discouraged because of possible injury.

Physical activity: Physical activity promotes a feeling of well-being in the pregnant woman. It

Table 4.17: Client self-care

Posture and body mechanics	
To Prevent or relieve backache	*To restrict the lumbar curve*
Do pelvic tilts • Pelvic tilt (rock) on hand and knees and while sitting in straight-back chair • Pelvic tilt (rock) in standing position against a wall or lying on floor • Perform abdominal muscle contractions during pelvic tilt while standing, lying, or sitting to help strangthen rectus abdominis muscle • Use good body mechanics • Use leg muscles to reach objects on or near floor. Bend at the knees, not the back. Knees are bent to lower body to squatting position Feet are kept 12 to 18 in apart to provide a solid base to maintain balance • Lift with the legs. To lift nearby object (young child), one foot is placed slightly in front of the other and kept flat as woman lowers herself onto one knee. She lifts the weight holding it close to her body and never higher than the chest. To stand up or sit down, one leg is placed slightly behind the other as she raises or lowers herself	For prolonged standing (for example, ironing, out-of home employment), place one food on low foot stool or box; change position often Move car seat forward so that knees are bent and higher than hips. If needed, use a small pillow to support low back are sit in chairs low enough to allow both feet to be placed on floor and or preferably with knees higher than hips To prevent round ligament pair and strain on abdominal muscle

improves circulation, promotes relaxation and counteracts boredom, as it does in the nonpregnant woman. Detailed exercise tips for pregnancy are realy presented. A way of doing Kegel's exercises to strengthen the muscles around the reproducive organs and improve muscle tone is described. Exercises that help relieve the low back pain that often arises during the second trimester because of the increased weight of the foetus are demonstrated.

Rest and relaxation: The pregnant woman is encouraged to plan regular rest periods, particular as pregnancy advances. The side lying position recommend because it promote uterine perfusion and fetoplacental oxygeation by eliminating pressure on the ascending vena cava and descending aorta, which can lead to supine hypotension. During shorter periods, the woman can assume the position to promote venous drainage from the legs and relieve leg oedema and varicose veins. The mother should also be shown the way to rise slowly from a sidely in position to prevent placing strain on the back and to minimize the ortstatic hypotension caused by changes in position common in the latter of pregnancy. To stretch and rest back muscles at home or work, following show the woman the way to do the following exercises.

Stand behind a chair: Support and balance self using the back of the chair squat for 30 seconds. Repeat six times, several times day as needed.

While sitting in a chair, lower head to knees for 30 seconds. Raise hold up. Repeat six times, several times per day, as needed.

Conscious relaxation: Is the process of releasing tension from the mind and body through conscious effort and practice. The ability to relax consciously and intentionally can be beneficial for the following reasons.

It can relieve the normal discomforts related to pregnancy.

It can reduce stress and therefore diminish pain perception during the childbearing cycle.

It can heighten self-awareness and trust in own ability to control one's responses and functions.

It can help the client cope with stress in everyday life-situations whether she is pregnant or not.

The techniques for conscious relaxation are numerous and varied. The guidelines given in the client self-care can be used by anyone.

The client self-care: Conscious relaxation are as follows:

Preparation: Loosen clothing, assume a comfortable sitting or side-lying position with all parts of body well supported with pillows.

Beginning: Allow self to feel warm and comfortable. In hale and exhale slowly, and imagine peaceful relaxation coming over each part of the body, starting with the neck and working down to the toss. Often people who learn conscious relaxation speak of feeling relaxed even if some discomfort is present.

Maintenance: Use imagery (fantasy or daydream) to maintain the state of relaxation. Using active imagery, imagine yourself moving or doing some activity and experiencing its sensations. Using passive imagery imagine yourself watching a scene, such as a lovely sunset.

Awakening: Return to the wakeful state gradually. Slowly begin to take in stimuli from the surrounding environment.

Further retention and development of the skill: Practice regularly for some periods each day, for example, at the same hour for 10 to 15 minutes each day, to feel refreshed, revitalized, and invigorated.

Employment of pregnant women has been shown to have no adverse effects on pregnancy outcomes. Job discrimination that is based strictly on pregnancy is illegal.

Activities that depend on a good sense of balance should be discouraged, however, especially during the latter half of pregnancy. Commonly, excessive fatigue is the deciding factor in the termination of employment. Women in sedentary jobs need to walk around at intervals to counter the usual sluggish circulation in the legs that can cause varices and thrombophlebitis to develop. They should neither sit nor stand in one position for long periods and they should avoid crossing their legs at the knees because these foster such conditions. The pregnant woman's chair should provide adequate back support. Use of a footstool can prevent pressure on veins, relieve strainon varicosities and minimize swelling of feet.

Travel: Travel is not contraindicated in low-risk pregnant women, but those with high-risk pregnancies are advised to avoid long-distance travel after foetal viability has been reached so as to avert the economic and psychologic consequences of giving birth to a preterm infant far from home. Travel to areas when medical care is poor, water is untreated, or malaria is prevalent should be avoided if possible. Another thing to be borne in mind by women contemplating foreign travel is that may health insurance carriers do not cover a birth in a foreign setting or even hospitalization for preterm labour.

Pregnant women who travel for long distances should schedule periods of activity and rest. While sitting, the woman can practice deep breathing foot circling, and alternately contracting and relaxing different muscle groups. She should avoid becoming fatigued. Although travel in itself is not a cause of adverse outcomes such as spontaneous abortion or preterm labour, certain precautions are recommended while travelling in a car. Some women do not use automobile restraints. A woman who does not wear automobile restraints risks injury to herself and her foetus. Maternal death as a result of injury is the most common cause of foetal death. The next most common cause is placental separation. This occurs because body contours change in reaction to the force of a collision. The uterus as a muscular organ can adapt its shape to that of the body, but the placenta is not resilient, so that at the impact of collision placental separation can occur. A combination lap belt and shoulder harness is the most affective automobile restraint and both should be used. The lap belt should be worn low across the pelvic bones.

The 8 per cent humidity at which the cabins of commercial airlines are maintained may result in some water loss; hydration (with water) should, therefore, be maintained under these conditions, sitting in the cramped seat of an airliner for prolonged periods may increase the risk of superficial and deep thrombophlebitis. A pregnant woman is encouraged to take a 15-minute walk around the aircraft during each hour of travel to minimize this risk. A seat in the nonsmoking section of flights on which smoking is permitted is advised to prevent her carboxy-hemoglobin levels from becoming elevated.

Warning signs and symptoms: The nurse can reinforce teaching about the warning signs and symptoms of potential complications by inquiring about whether there have been any such problems in the time since the last visit. A printed list to be placed by the telephone along with the telephone number to call, is helpful for quick referral. The woman is reminded about the way to describe what is happening, for example, "I can't keep anything down" or "I lost a teaspoonful of blood".

Childbirth education classes: Childbirth education classes are available in some communities to meet the needs of parents during the second trimester. Second-trimester classes emphasize the woman's participation in self-care and provide information about preparation for breast-feeding and formula feeding; basic hygiene; common complaints and simple, safe remedies, continued foetal development; infant health; parenting; and the updating and refining of the birth plan. Discussion of concerns may touch on topics such as birth choices including labour and birth positions labour, delivery, recovery and postpartum (LDRP) rooms, medications to stimulate labour; and episiotomy. These topics are usually discussed more extensively in the third-trimester classes when labour and birth are closer. Support systems that expectant parents can use are also discussed. Open discussion of feelings and concerns is encouraged. If the expectant parents have not yet begun to think about a birth plan, they are encouraged to do so at this time.

Birth plan: During the second trimester, the nurse can answer questions and discuss concerns that arise during the formulation of the birth plan. However, clients need to be reminded that no birth plan can be guaranteed and alternative plans need to be considered. For example, if a caesarean birth proves necessary, does the woman want her partner to be present during the procedure? Does she want to hold the baby immediately after birth (if the baby's and mother's conditions warrant it? Such alter-native plans serve to reduce disappointment. Following are some questions the mother or couple, need to consider with regard to various aspects of the birth:

- *Immediately after birth*: Do you want to hold the baby right away? To breastfeed immediately?
- *New born care*: What about cirmcision for your baby (if male)? Will the baby be breastfed or bottlefed?
- *Postpartum care*: What kind of care do you anticipate - LDRP, mother-baby coupling, "request" coupling (newborn cared for in nursery while mother rests)? How long does your insurance company or employes allow you to

stay? Would you like to attend self-care classes or prefer to get such information from videotapes? On which subjects?

If older siblings are to be included in the labour and birth process, this needs to be reviewed and cleared with the physician or nurse-midwife as well as with the staff at the birth setting. This should be done long before the EDB so that the stress this type of negotiation could engender during labour can be avoided. Some facilities require that a sibling present at a birth specify who will be responsible for the sibling during labour and birth, since this is a requirement at many facilities.

Evaluation: Continuous evaluation of the effectiveness of interventions is essential to the management of the pregnant woman and her family's care during the second trimester. Evaluation is based on the degree to which expected outcomes have been achieved.

- The pregnant woman and her family have verbalized an understanding of the maternal physical and psychosocial adaptations and foetal development that are taking place.
- Questions or concerns of the woman and her family have been addressed.
- To the degree they have desired, the woman and her family have participated in prenatal care during the second trimester.

NURSING MANAGEMENT OF THIRD TRIMESTER

In the third trimester the quiet period of the second trimester gives way to an active period in which there is more emphasis on the practical realities of expectant parenthood. Parental attachment to the foetus grows in the third trimester, a period spanning weeks 27 to 40. Mixed among the daydreams about the "coming baby" however, are parental anxieties concerning possible mental and physical defects in the child. The expectant mother's attention turns to thoughts of a safe passage (an eventful birth process) for herself and her child. Fears of pain and mutilation and concerns about her behaviour and possible loss of control during labour are important issues.

In addition, physical discomforts and foetal movements often interrupt the expectant mother's rest. Most women experience dyspnoea, the return of urinary frequency, backache, constipation, and varicosities late in pregnancy. Increased bulkiness and awkwardess effect her ability to perform activities of daily living, and comfortable positions are more difficult to achieve. Increasingly she becomes more impatient to "get this over with"

Many expectant fathers or partners become more involved with the pregnancy at this time. As already mentioned, increased activity and energy to create and achieve characterize this phase. However, the style of involvement differ according to their perception of the male and fathering roles within their social groups. Men begin to redefine their relationship to the foetus and themselves as fathers. Role-playing through daydreaming is common. The expectant father or partner feels some of the same concerns as the expectant mother. Often however, he may not confide these concerns to anyone.

Expectant families approaching childbirth have many needs beyond those of just the mother and couple. Siblings and grand parents must be considered, too. Clearly the nurse is in a pivotal position within the team of health care providers to assist parents and families with these needs during the third trimester, and the schedule of care reflects this increased need. Starting with week 28, maternity visits are scheduled every 2 weeks until week 36, and then every week until birth. The educate the mother regarding selfcare and safety (Table 4.18).

Assessment

During the third trimester, current family situations and their effect on the mother are assessed, for example, siblings and grandparents responses to the pregnancy and the coming child. In addition, the following questions are addressed:

- What anticipatory planning is in progress concerning new parenting responsibilities, sibling rivalry, recuperation from pregnancy and birth and fertility management?
- What successes or frustrations with diet, rest and relaxation, sexuality and emotional support is the mother experiencing?
- What is the mother's understanding of her family's needs in relation to the pregnancy and the unborn child?
- How well prepared are the parents for coping with an emergency? That is, does the mother know the warning signs, understand what they represent, and the way and to whom to report them?

Table 4.18: Self-care: Safety during pregnancy

Physical adaptations to your pregnancy involve relaxation of the joints, an altered centre of gravity, faintness, and discomforts. Because problem with coordination and balance are common, you should follow these guidelines:

- Use good body mechanics.
- Use safety features on tools or vehicles; these include safety seat belts, shoulder harnesses, head rests, goggles, and helmets, as specified.
- Avoid engaging in activities requiring coordination, balance and concentration.
- Take rest periods and reschedule daily activities to meet rest and relaxation needs.
- Embryonic and foetal development is vulnerable to environmental teratogens. Many potentially dangerous chemicals are present in the home, yard, and workplace. These consist of cleaning agents, paints, sprays, herbicides, and pesticides. The soil and water supply may also be unsafe. Therefore, you should follow these guidelines:
- Read all labels for ingredients and proper use of the product.
- Ensure adequate ventilation with "clean" air.
- Dispose of wastes appropriately.
- Wear gloves when handling chemicals.
- Change job assignments or workplace as necessary.
- Avoid being in high attitudes (not including pressurized aircraft) which could jeopardize oxygen intake.

- Does the mother know the signs of preterm and term labour?
- What is the mother's understanding of the labour process and expectations of herself and others during labour, does she know what to bring to the hospital or birthing centre?
- If she is having a home birth have all the necessary supplies been obtained?
- What plans have the mother and her family made for labour?
- What anxieties are the mother or her family experiencing regarding labour or the unborn child?
- What does the mother wish to know about the control or discomfort during labour?
- Is the mother (and her partner or support person) planning to attend any parent education classes?
- Does the mother have questions about foetal development and methods to assess foetal wellbeing?

A checklist for the third-trimester assessment should be used to ensure that all the important areas are addressed as given below:

- Schedule and events of visits
- Counseling for self-care
- Adaptations/discomforts
- Dyspnea
- Insomnia
- Psychosocial responses and family dynamics
- Gingivitis and epulis
- Urinary frequency
- Perineal discomfort and pressure
- Braxton Hicks contractions
- Leg cramps
- Ankle Edema
- Safety (balance)
- Exercise and rest
- Relaxation
- Nutrition
- Sexuality
- Warning signs of potential complications
- Warning signs-preterm labour
- Foetal growth and development
- Preparation for baby
- Feeding method
- Nipple preparation
- Preparation for labour
- Recognition: false versus true
- Prenatal classes
- Control of discomfort
- Hospital tour
- Provision for other family members
- Preparation for home coming
- Diagnostic tests
- Specify
- Other.

Maternal Assessment

Interview: The first question asked by the health care provider at a woman's third-trimester interview is intended to identify her main concern of the moment. Focusing on the woman takes advantage of her readiness to learn and affirms the health care provider's interest in the woman as a person.

Based on the woman's expressed needs, her status to date, and the general needs of most women in late pregnancy, the nurse's knowledge and clinical judgment guide the content and direction of the interview.

The nurse determines whether the woman has attended second-trimester parent education classes. If so, she should ask what questions and concerns arose as a result of these classes that may need to be addressed. Does the couple plan to attend third-trimester parent education classes? Has the birth plan been developed with realistic expectations? Is the plan feasible and flexible?

A review of the woman's physical systems is appropriate at each meeting and any suspicious signs or symptoms assessed in depth. Discomforts reflecting adaptations to pregnancy are identified. Special inquiries are made about possible infections (for example, genitourinary tract, respiratory tract). The woman's knowledge self-care measures is assessed, as well as the success of these and prescribed therapy. The psychosocial responses of the woman, partner, and family to the pregnancy and approaching parenthood are also assessed.

Physical examination: During the third trimester physical examination, temperature, pulse, blood pressure, respirations and weight are assessed and noted as are the presence, location and degree of edema. Any suspicious signs and symptoms revealed during the interview are evaluated. The gestational age is also confirmed. Fundal height continues to be measured, and Leopold's Manoeuvres are performed to determine foetal position. Risk assessment continues throughoug the third trimester.

One of the greatest risks to the woman and her foetus is pregnancy-induced hypertension (PIH). In some studies the findings yielded by the roll-over test have been shown to be somewhat pretictive of PIH after the twentieth week of gestation. Instructions on the way to perform the roll-over test are as follows:

Roll-over test

Administered at 28 to 32 weeks' gestation.

- Woman is placed inleft lateral recumbent position
- Blood pressure is monitored until stable-usually about 15 minutes
- Roll woman to supine position and measure blood pressure
- Measure blood pressure again in 5 minutes
- An increase in the diastolic blood pressure exceeding 20 mmHg is considered positive.

Significance

- If negative, chance are less than 1 in 100 that pre-eclampsia will develop in the woman
- If positive, the risk of a hypertensive problem is increased close monitoring of the third trimester may be indicated.

Assessing Pitting Oedema, Deep Tendon Reflexes and Clonus

Purpose An increasing degree of oedema or hyper-reflexia can indicate pre-eclampsia or, in a known case of pre-eclampsia, a worsening of the condition. Oedema is assessed routinely at each prenatal visit after 20 weeks' gestation. For women with increasing oedema or risk factors for pre-eclampsia, the evaluation of deep tendon reflexes (DTRs) and clonus is added to this routine assessment (Table 4.19).

Equipment

- Reflex hammer or a reasonable substitute, such as the edge of a stethoscope bell, the fingertips, or the sides of the fingers (Fig. 4.10).

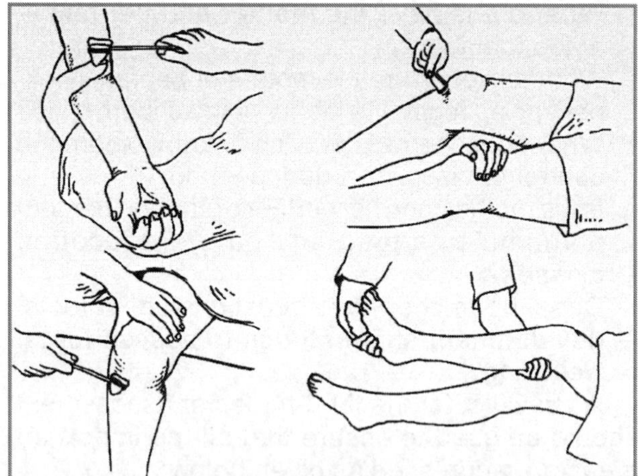

Fig. 4.10: Assessment of the deep tendon reflexes is essential to determine whether the woman is receiving too much or too little magnesium sulfate and to identify the woman likely to have a convulsion

Laboratory tests: At each visit, urine is tested for glucose (to assess for diabetes), protein (to assess for PIH) and nitrties and leucocytes (to assess for infection). A urine culture and sensitivity test is done as necessary. Hematocrit

Table 4.19: Assessing pitting oedema, deep tendon reflexes, and clonus

Purpose	*Equipment*
An increasing degree of oedema or hyperreflexia can indicate pre-eclampsia or, in a known case of pre-eclampsia, a worsening of the condition. Oedema is assessed routinely at each prenatal visit after 20 weeks gestation. For women with increasing oedema or risk factors for preeclampsia, the evaluation of deep tendon reflexes (DTRs) and clonus is added to this routine assessment.	• Reflex hammer or a reasonable substitute, such as the edge of a stethoscope bell, the fingergips, or the sides of the fingers.
Nursing action	*Rationale*
Assessing pitting oedema	
1. Ask the woman and/or family members if the woman's face or hands appear swollen.	Nonpitting oedema may be found in the patient's fingers, face, and eyelids. It may be best recognized by the woman or family members who are familiar with her normal appearance.
2. Inspect the woman's face, extremities, and sacral area for signs of pitting oedema.	A thorough physical assessment of the woman for oedema is important for differentiating dependent oedema, which occurs in normal pregnancy, from generalized pitting oedema, which may be associated with preeclampsia
3. Press each area firmly with the thumb or index finger for several seconds and release Evaluate the extensiveness of the oedema, the depth of the depression, and the length of time it takes to clear	This technique helps the nurse determine the presence and degree of pitting oedema. Pitting oedema leaves a depression after finger pressure has been applied to an affected area
4. Grade the pitting edema according to the following scale: 1+ = Minimal oedema of the lower extremities 2+ = Marked oedema of the lower extremities 3+ = Oedema of the lower extremities, face, and hands 4+ = Generalised, massive oedema	An increasing degree of oedema may indicate a worsening condition. The use of a standardized scale lends objectivity and consistency to assessments among health care providers.
5. Record your findings. Compare your findings with those previously recorded	By recording and comparing findings, trends demonstrating a worsening of or an improvement in the condition can be seen
Assessing deep tendon reflexes and clonus	
1. Explain the procedure for assessing DTRs to the woman. Position her so that her arms and legs are flexed or semiflexed and her muscles are relaxed	Understanding her role in the procedure increases the woman's ability to keep her muscles relaxed. Relaxation of muscles is required in order to elicit the DTR response successfully
2. Locate the tendon and the corresponding muscle of the reflex to be tested. For example, prior to assessing the patellar reflex (knee jerk), locate the ligamentum patellae tendon at the base of the patella. Before eliciting the biceps reflex, flex the woman's elbow and place your thumb across the tendon in the antecubital space	Identifying the correct tendon is essential to eliciting a reflex response

Contd...

Contd...

Nursing action	*Rationale*
3. Tap the tendon directly using the reflex hammer or, in the case of the biceps reflex, firmly tap your thumb, which is pressing on the tendon	The reflex response occurs when the tendon is briskly tapped. The tendon stimulates the corresponding muscle to contract and the body part to move or jerk (normal response)
4. Rate the reflex response according to the following scale: 0 = Absent 1+ = Diminished 2+ = Normal 3+ = Brisk 4+ = Hyperactive	Rating helps the nurse evaluate the status of the woman's reflex responses. The use of a standardized scale lends objectivity and consistency to assess -ments among health care providers. Absent or diminished reflexes are on abnormal finding and may be seen with magnesium toxicity. Brisk or hyperactive reflexes may indicate central nervous system irritability (as in pre-eclampsia) and require physician follow-up
5. Repeat the procedure if you are unable to elicit the reflex or to confirm the response as absent or diminished. To confirm absent or diminished reflexes, instruct the woman to contract a group of muscles different from those being evaluated. For example, while testing reflexes in the lower extremities, ask the woman to interlock her fingers and pull her arms outward, contracting the muscles in her arms	Confirmation of absent or diminished reflexes is essential for an accurate assessment. By having the woman concentrate on muscles other than those being evaluated, a more accurate result may be elicited
6. Assess each reflex symmetrically, comparing the reflex response on one side with the reflex response on the other side.	The reflex response for a tendon should be the same on both the right and left sides
7. When checking for clonus, explain the procedure to the woman first Position the woman so that her knee is semiflexed. Support her leg by placing one hand or your arm under her knee	Understanding the procedure improves cooperation Relaxation of muscles is required to assess for the presence of clonus
8. Using your other hand, sharply dorsiflex the woman's foot, maintaining slight pressure on her foot after dorsiflexion. Release her foot and observe its movement	Clonus (foot jerks rapidly) is an abnormal neurologic finding that may be elicited when a muscle is sharply stretched and the stretch is maintained in either flexion or extension. The absence of clonus (foot simply returns to its normal position) is a normal finding
9. Count the beats of clonus present as you observe for rhythmic contraction and relaxation of the gastrocnemius and soleus muscles	Clonus is evaluated by counting the number of times the muscle contracts and relaxes after it has been sharply stretched (e.g., "three beats")
10. Record your findings. Compare your findings with those recorded previously	By recording and comparing findings, you can see a trend in a worsening or an improving condition

is determined by the finger stick method at each visit in some facilities. The following blood tests are repeated as necessary: RPR/VDRI, test for syphilis, complete blood cell count with hematocrit hemoglobin, and differential values; antibody screen (rubella, toxoplasmosis, anti-Rh, HIV, sickle cell; and level of folacin then indicated). If not done earlier in pregnancy, a glucose screen is performed in women over 25 years of age. A glucose challenge is usually done between 24 and 28 weeks gestation. Cervical and vaginal smears are repeated at 32 weeks or as necessary to examine for chlamydia organisms, group streptococcal infection, gonorrhea, and herpes simplex virus types 1 and 2.

Signs of Potential Problems

The nurse is constantly on the alert for potential problems, such as the following:

- Haemorrhagic condition—vaginal bleeding, severe abdominal pain

- Hypertensive conditions
  - Visual disturbances—blurring, double vision, or spots before the eyes.
  - Swelling of face or fingers and over sacrum
  - Headaches—severe, frequent, or continuous
  - Muscular irritability or convulsions
  - Epigastric pain (perceived as severe stomach ache)
- Infections—positive laboratory test results.
  - Chills, fever.
  - Burning on urination, frequency and aching back and side.
  - Diarrhoea
- Diabetes mellitus; glucosuria, positive glucose tolerance test result
- Fluid discharge from vagina—amniotic fluid.
- Signs of preterm labour.

Foetal Assessment

Foetal health status is evaluated at each visit. Beginning at the thirty-second week, the foetal presentation, position, and station (engagement) is assessed weekly, with the aid of Leopold's manoeuvre. This period of rapid foetal growth is summarized as follows:

- Foetal Development at 40 Weeks
- Nutrients and maternal immunoglobulins are stored
- Subcutaneous fat is deposited.
- Dramatic storage of iron nitrogen, and calcium.
- In male; testes are within well-wrinkled scrotum.
- In female: labia are well developed and cover vestibule.
- Lanugo has been shed, except for shoulders, generally.
- Body contours are plump.
- Decreased vernix.
- Scalp hair is 2 to 3 cm (1 in) long
- Cartilage in nose and ears is well developed.
- Foetus is 45 to 55 cm (18 to 22 in) long.
- Foetus weighs 3400 g (7½ 1b) (average)
- Fundal height is below xiphold after lightening.

Fundal height is also measured at each visit using the method described earlier. The uterine measurements and the size (weight) of the foetus are compared with the supposed duration of pregnancy. Although some clinicians can estimate foetal weights with unbelievable accuracy, such estimations are generally inconsistent and unreliable. However, the accuracy of foetal weight estimation is improved by ultrasound determination of the biparietal diameter (BPD). Possible intrauterine foetal growth restriction (IUGR) a multifoetal pregnancy, or an inaccurate estimated date of birth (EDB) may be disclosed by ultrasound imaging.

The mother is also asked to describe the nature of the foetal movements and to report any warning signs that may have occurred, such as rupture of membranes or absent or decreased foetal movement.

Nursing Diagnosis

Each woman and her family respond to and are affected by pregnancy in different ways. Careful moniotring of the pregnancy and the woman's responses to care, are there one of the utmost importance. The following are representative nursing diagnoses that may be formulated in the third trimester resulting from the database of the characteristics of a so called normal pregnancy.

- Impaired individual coping related to knowledge deficit regarding:
  - Assessment for risks such as preterm labour.
  - Recognizing onset of true versus false labour.
  - Self-care measures.
  - Emergency arrangements.
- Altered family processes related to
  - Inadequate understanding of third trimester changes and needs.
  - Increased concern about labour.
  - Insomnia or sleep deficit.
- Sleep pattern disturbance related to
  - Discomforts of late pregnancy.
  - Anxiety about approaching labour.
  - Activity intolerance related to increased weight and change in center of gravity.
  - Anxiety.
  - Sleep disturbances.

Planning

The planning of care for women and families during the third trimester is guided by the nursing diagnoses identified and the findings yielded from a comprehensive view of the expectant family. To the extent possible, a plan is developed mutually with the woman and individualized, so that it specifically addresses the woman's needs and the needs of her family. The expected outcomes for the third trimester are similar to those for the first and second trimesters and may include the woman/family doing the following:

- Be able to provide pertinent information concerning maternal adaptations and foetal development as a basis for understanding the management of care during the third trimester
- Be able to describe self-care measures
- List symptoms that indicate deviations from normal and the protocols for reporting them
- List signs of preterm labour and the protocols for reporting them
- List the difference between true and false labour
- Be active participants in her care during the third trimester
- Finalize her birth plan
- Voice continued confidence in her care.

Plan of Care and Implementation

Social support: Esteem, affection, trust, concern, consideration of cultural and religious responses, and listening are all components of the motional support given the pregnant woman and her family. The woman's satisfaction with her relationships and support, her feeling of competence, and her sense of being in control are important issues to be addressed in the third trimester. A discussion of the unborn child's responses to stimuli, such as sound, light, maternal posture, and tension, as well as the child patterns for sleeping and waking can be helpful. Also discussed are emotional tensions that can arise related to the childbirth experience, such as those stemming from fear of pain, loss of control, and possible birth of child before reaching hospital; anxieties about the recognized responsibilities and tasks of parenthood; mutualparental concerns about the safety of the mother and unborn child; mutual parental concerns about siblings and their acceptance of the new baby; mutual parental concerns about social and economic responsibilities, and mutual parental concerns arising from conflicts in cultural, religious or personal value systems.

The father's or partner's commitment to the pregnancy, the couple's relationship, and their concerns about sexuality and sexual expression care merge as issues for many expectant parents. An important support measure is to validate the normality of their responses (if they fall within normal limits). Validation, feedback and social comparison. Characterize the support given.

Providing the mother and father to be an opportunity to discuss their concerns, providing a listening ear, and validating the normality of their responses can meet their needs to varying degrees. Nurses must also recognize that men feel more vulnerable during their partner's pregnancy. Female partners may also have these feelings. Anticipatory guidance and health promotion strategies can help partners cope with their concerns. Nursing intervention may either directly help them deal with much concerns in the event that such intimate feelings are confided or do so indirectly through the education of the mothers. Health care providers can stimulate and encourage open dialogue between the couple.

The birth plan is finalized during the third trimester. When the plan is ready, it can be written out, signed by the woman and primary health care provider, and added to the prenatal record. The intent of this is to decrease the possibility of a conflict arising with staff members over, for example, the use of drugs to relieve pain. A pleasant, relaxed atmosphere does much to help encourage expectant parents to ask questions and verbalize their anxieties and fears without worrying about possible disapproval. Thoughtful answers that reflect the nurse's caring attitude can be reassuring. However, women should not feel pressured either to attend parent education classes or to prepare a birth plan.

Immune system support: Rh sensitization may occur during pregnancy in the woman who is Rh negative. Rh immunoglobulin (RhIG) is administered at about 28 weeks gestation in women found to have the Rh (D) or Rh variant (D^{o}) with a negative Coomb's test result. This helps prevent the formation of maternal antibodies to foetal Rh-positive cells. In all pregnant women who are not sensitized and who undergo amniocentesis, RhIG is also administered at the time of the procedure.

One way to immunize newborn infants is to vaccinate mothers late in pregnancy, thus in effect, vaccinating babies before they are born. The babies are immunized through the passage of protective antibodies from the mother to the foetus. Hypothetically, newborns could be protected from haemophilus influenzae type B, which can cause a lethal infection resulting from meningitis or pneumonia; infection with this bacterium is a leading killer of children. Researchers are now investigating whether a whole variety of infections could be prevented in this way; this includes whooping cough, and infection with group B streptococcus, pneumococcus, *Escherichia coli* and pseudomonas.

During the third trimester, some woman are retested for sexually transmitted diseases (STDs) such as syphilis, gonorrhea, group B streptococcus, and chlamydia.

Teaching for self-care: Not only do some new discomforts arise in the third trimester, but others experienced in the first trimester (for example, fatigue) can also recur. Older pregnant women may experience an aggravation of varicose veins or severe backache resulting from the postural changes produced by the heavy pendulous abdomen and relaxed joints. Such symptoms can be frightening and uncomfortable.

The physiology and prevention of and the self-care measures for relieving several of the problems are summarized in Table 4.20.

Preparation for feeding the newborn: Pregnant women are usually eagar to discuss their plans for feeding the newborn. Breast milk is the food of choice, in part because breastfeeding is associated with a decreased incidence of perinatal morbidity and mortality. However, a deep-seated aversion to breast feeding on the part of the mother or partner, the mother's need for certain medications, and certain medical complications, such as active tuberculosis, newly diagnosed breast cancer, and hepatitis C are contra-indications to breastfeeding. Although hepatitis B antigen-positive women receive the hepatitis B vaccine and hepatitis B immunoglobulin (HBIG) immediately after birth, HIV infected women in countries where infant mortility exceeds 50 per cent as the result of diarrhoea and other infectious diseases (excluding AIDS) are advised to breastfeed. In developed countries, women who are HIV positive are discouraged from nursing because the risk of HIV transmission outweighs the risk of the infant dying from another cause.

The woman and her partner are encouraged to decide which method of feeding is suitable for them. Once the couple has been given information about the advantages and disadvantages of bottle feeding and breastfeeding, they are then in a position to make an informed choice. Health care provider need only to support their decisions.

The pinch test is done to determine whether the nipple is everted or inverted. The nurse shows the woman the way to perform the pinch test. It involves having the woman place her thumb and forefinger on or areola and gently press inward. This will cause her nipple to stand erect or invert. Most niples will stand erect.

It used to be recommended that women with flat or inverted nipples do Hoffman's exercises to break the adhesions causing the nipple to invert but recent studies have shown that this does not work and that it may in fact precipitate uterine contractions. The use of breast shells by women with flat or inverted nipples is still recommended. They work by exerting a continuous, gentle pressure around the areola that pushes the nipple through a central opening in the inner shield. Breast shells should be worn for 1 to 2 hours daily during the last trimester of pregnancy. They should be worn for gradually increased length of time. However, interestingly a study conducted revealed that women who wear breast shells or who do nipple-rolling exercises (now contraindicated in all cases) are less likely to breastfeed than women, who are not treated for inverted nipples. Breast stimulation is especially not recommended in women at risk for preterm labour. Therefore, the decision to recommend the use of breast shells to women with flat or inverted nipples must be made judiciously. Continuous support and guidance must be given to the woman as part of the nursing care plan.

The woman is taught to cleanse the nipples with warm water to keep the ducts from being blocked with dried colostrum. Soap, ointments, alcohol, and tinctures should not be applied because they remove protective oils that keep the nipples supply. The use of these substances may cause the nipples to crack during early lactation.

The woman who plans to breastfeed should purchase a nursing bra that will accommodate her increased breast size during the last few months of pregnancy and during lactation. If her breasts are very heavy, or if the woman feels uncomfortable with the weight unsupported, the bra can be worn day and night.

Review of Warning Signs

The nurse needs to answer questions honestly as they arise during pregnancy. Because it is often difficult for the woman to know, then to report

Table 4.20: Problems related to maternal adaptations during the third trimester

Problem	*Physiology*	*Education for selfcare*
Shortness of breath and dyspnea occur in 6% of pregnant women	Expansion of diaphragm limited by enlarging uterus; diaphragm is elevated about 4 cm (1½ in); some relief occur after lightening	Maintain good posture; sleep with extra pillows avoid overloading stomach; stop smoking; if symptoms worsen, consult health care provider to rule out anemia, emphyaema, and asthma.
Insomnia (Later weeks of pregnancy	Fetal movements, muscular cramping, urinary frequency, shortness of breath, or other discomforts	Perform conscious relaxation; have partner perform back massage or effleurage support body parts with pillows; drink warm milk or take warm shower before retiring.
Psychosocial responses food swings mixed feelings increased anxiety	Hormonal and metabolic adaptations, feelings about impending labor birth, and parenthood	Seek reassurance and support from partner and nurse; improve communication with partner and nurse improve communication with partner, family and others
Gingivitis and epulis (hyperemia, hyper -trophy bleeding, tenderness); condition will disappear spontaneously 1 to 2 months after birth	Increased vascularity and proliferation of connective tissue resulting from estrogen stimulation	Eat well-balanced diet with adequate intake of protein, fresh fruits, and vegetables, gentle brushing and good dental hygiene avoid infection
Urinary frequency and urgency return	Vascular engorgement and altered bladder function caused by hormones; bladder capacity reduced by enlarging uterus and fetal presenting part	Perform Kegel's exercises; limit fluid intake before bedtime; wear perneal pad; consult health care provider if pain or burning sensation occurs
Perineal discomfort and pressure	Pressure from enlarging uterus, especially when standing or walking multifetal gestation	Rest, perform conscious relaxation, and maintain good posture consult health care provider for assessment and treatment if pain is present: assess for onset of labour
Braxton-Hicks contractions	Intensification of uterine contractions in preparation for work of labor	Rest, change position, practice breathing techniques when contractions are bothersome; effleurage; assess for onset of labor
Leg cramps (gastroenomius spasm), especially when reclining	Enlarging uterus compresses nerves supplying lower extremities reduced diffusable serum calcium level or elevated serum phosphorus level, aggravating factors, fatigue, poor peripheral circulation, pointing toes when stretching legs or when walking drinking more than 1L of milk per day	Have health care provider rule out blood clot, if clot ruled out use massage and heat over affected muscle; dorsiflex foot until spasm cases stand on cold surface; initiate oral supplementation with calcium carbonate or calcium lactate tablets, take aluminium hydroxide gel (1 oz) with each meal to remove phosphorus by absorbing it
Ankle edema (nonpitting) to lower extremities	Edema aggravated by prolonged standing, sitting, poor posture, lack of exercise, constrictive clothing (e.g., garters), or by hot weather	Maintain ample fluid intake for natural diuretic effect; put on support stocking before arising rest periodically with legs and hips elevated moderately, consult health care provider if generalized edema develops; diuretics are contraindicated

signs and symptoms, however, she should be encouraged to refer to a printed list of warning signs and to listen to her body. Education regarding client self care as given below:

Client Self-Care during III Trimester

How to recognize preterm labour: Because the onset of preterm labour is subtle and often hard to recognize, it is important to know how to feel your abdomen for uterine contractions. You can feel for contractions in the following way. While lying down place your fingertips on the top of your uterus. A contraction is the periodic tightening or hardening of your uterus. If your uterus is contracting, you will actually feel your abdomen get tight or hard and then feel it relax or soften when the contraction is over.

If you think you are having any of the other signs and symptoms or preterm labour, empty your bladder, drink three to four glasses of water for hydration, liedown tilted toward your side, and place a pillow at your back for support.

Check for contractions for 1 hour. To tell how often contractions are occurring, check the minutes that elapse from the beginning of one contraction to the beginning of the next.

It is normal to have some uterine contractions throughout the day. These usually occur when a woman changes positions. These usually irregular and mild contractions are called braxtonhicks contractions. They help with uterine tone and uteroplacental perfusion.

It is not normal to have frequent uterine contractions (every 10 minutes or more often for 1 hour).

Contractions of labour are regular, frequent and hard. They also may be felt as a tightening of the abdomen or a backache. This type of contractions causes the cervix to efface and dilate.

Tell your primary health care provider clinic, or labour and birth unit or go to the hospital, if any or the following signs occur:

- You have uterine contractions every 10 minutes or more often for 1 hour or;
- You have any of the other signs and symptoms for 1 hour or;
- You have any bloody spotting or leaking of fluid from your vagina.

It is often difficult to identify preterm labour. Accurate diagnosis requires assessment by the health care provider, usually in the hospital or clinic.

Post these instructions where they can be seen by everyone in the family.

If the woman senses that "something is wrong, "she should notify her health care provider. Several signs and symptoms need to be discussed more extensively with her. These include vaginal bleeding, alteration in foetal movements. Symptoms of PIH, rupture of membranes, and preterm labour.

If vaginal bleeding occurs in the third trimester, it is important to rule out the growing spotting that can occur 48 hours after a vaginal examination and the "show" of pinkish mucus. The woman should immediately telephone her primary health care provider for instructions if the bleeding is other than one of these types.

Should the woman notice a cessation, noticeable lessening, or acceleation in the foetal movements, she should know to call her primary health care provider for advice. The foetal movements, she should know to call her primary health care provider for advice. The foetal movement alterations noticed by the mother have been shown to be an accurate gauge of foetal well-being.

If oedema of the hands and around the eyes, severe headaches, visual changes, or feelings of jitteriness appear, this is cause for immediate evaluation for hypertension. Severe PIH can lead to increased maternal and foetal morbidity and mortality.

A gush or trickle of clear watery discharge that appears to come from the vagina may indicate rupture of membranes. However, the woman must usually be evaluated at the clinic or hospital to establish the diagnosis.

Recognizing preterm labour: Teaching each mother-to-be recognize preterm labour is necessary. Preterm labour is that which occurs after the twentieth week but before the thirty seventh week of pregnancy. It is a condition in which uterine contractions cause the cervix to open earlier than normal, and it can result in preterm birth. Although certain factors, such as multifoetal pregnancy, may increase a woman's chances of going into preterm labour, the specific cause, or causes, are not known. If the woman knows the warning signs and symptoms of preterm labour and seeks care early enough, should they occur, it may be possible to prevent a preterm birth.

Prebirth preparation: Not all expectant mothers and support people attend formal classes in preparation for childbirth. For those who do attend, extensive preparation is possible. However many do not take advantage of classes for a variety of reasons—employment; inaccessibility because of time; cultural, ethnic, or religious orientation, cost, lack of knowledge regrading choices in prenatal education classes or lack of readiness. For these women, clinicians need to provide information that includes the following:

- Process of labour; admission, examination, care in labour.
- Plans to get to hospital (when to go and where); care of other children.
- Methods to control pain (for example, analgesia and anesthesia, breathing and relaxing techniques).
- Supplies to have in a suitcase already packed for the trip to the hospital or birthing centre; personal items for grooming, items for labour as desired (for example, warm socks, focal point), supportive bra, slippers.
- Responsibilities of the partner, family member, or friend who will be supporting the woman during labour and birth.
- Emergency arrangements (for example, precipitous birth).

A nurse needs to be ready to teach the woman when she is ready to learn, as shown by the following example of one nurse's experience:

I tried to teach her about relaxation and breathing techniques during her pregnancy, but she was not interested. When she phoned to tell me she was at the hospital in labour, she said "What was all that stuff you were saying about breathing?" In between the next few contractions, I repeated the crucial points.

Even if the woman of couple have attended parent education classes, the nurse should review the following topics to further ensure their preparation for child-birth:

- Symptoms of impending labour and the information to report
- Breathing and relaxation techniques
- Involvement of partner
- Plans to get to hospital
- Plans during labour, terminology involved, and what care to expect
- Preparation for baby
- Preparation of grandparents and siblings.

The symptoms of impending labour will include:
Uterine contractions: The woman is instructed to report the frequency, duration and intensity of uterine contractions. True labour is characterized by an increase in frequency, strength and duration of contractions. In true labour an increase in activity intensifies these symptoms. If the woman is in false labour an increase in activity usually causes the symptoms to diminish. Nulliparas are usually counseled to remain at home until contractions are regular and 5 minutes apart. Parous women are counselled to remain at home until contractions are regular and 10 minutes apart, if the woman lives more than 20 minutes from the hospital or has a history rapid labours, these instructions are modified accordingly.

Rupture of the membranes—Fluid may leak slowly or may gush.

Bloody show—The show is scant, pink, and sticky (contains mucus).

If a hospital birth is planned, often the woman must preregister at the hospital of choice. Most hospitals now provide pamphlets containing information such as where to report when labour begins and the policies pertaining to visitors and visiting hours. Many facilities also conduct tours.

Counselling is provided to relieve emotional tensions, which often relate directly to the childbirth experience (for example, anxiety about pain or possible birth of the child before reaching the hospital). Nursing strategies include providing the woman with an opportunity to discuss her specific fears or anxieties, helping her make definite plans concerning what she will do when labour starts, repeating instructions willingly and aranging for her to have "sharing sessions" with mothers who have recently given birth. If possible, involve the partners in this preparation for the birth and arrange to have them participate in a supportive way during labour and birth. These techniques may be effective in preventing or minimizing anxiety.

Most partners of women who are approaching labour may have their anxieties allayed through intervention rendered before the event. Fantasies can be replaced by knowledge gained through activities such as the following:

- A hospital tour so that they can see the labour or birthing room and waiting areas.
- A demonstration of ways to help and comfort the woman during labour.
- A brief review of what to expect from the whom during labour.

- A description of what to expect of the staff during the woman's labour.

A realistic discussion of all the known factors surrounding the birth process helps the father or partner problem solve more rationally and plan for the event. Such discussions are ego strengthening because they help the father or partner focus his or her energies toward more appropriate coping strategies by easing anxieties about the unknown. Today many partners elect to participate actively during labour and the birth of the child. However, because of personal or cultural concepts, some partners neither wish nor intend to participate. The important object is that each partner aggressive on the other's roles. For nurses to advocate any changes, in these roles, may cause confusion or feelings of guilt.

Sibling and grand parent preparations are also available.

Evaluation: Evaluation is a continuous process. The effectiveness of each intervention is evaluated and an alternate intervention implemented as necessary. If there is any change in the woman's condition or a concern arises, the nursing care plan must be readjusted accordingly. The extent to which the expected outcomes for the mother couple or foetus are achieved is continuously evaluated.

Multifoetal pregnancy: A multifoetal pregnancy places the mother and foetuses at risk. The maternal blood volume is increased, resulting in an increased strain on the maternal cardiovascular system. Anaemia often develops because of a greater demand for iron by the foetuses. Marked uterine distension and increased pressure on the adjacent viscera and pelvic vasculature also occur, multifoetal pregnancies and diastasis of the two recti abdominal muscles (in the midline) may occur. Placenta previa develops more commonly in multifoetal pregnancies because of the large size or placement of the placentas. Premature separation of the placenta may occur before the second and any subsequent foetuses are born.

Twin pregnancies often end in prematurity. Spontaneous rupture of membranes before term is common. Congenital malformation are twice as common in monozygotic twins as in singletons, though there is no increase in the incidence of congenital anomalies in dizygotic twins. In addition, two vessel cords—that is, cords with a single umbilical artery—occur more often in twins than in singletons, but this abnormality is most common in monozygotic twins. However, the most serious problem for the fetus is the local shunting of blood between placentas (twin-to-twin transfusion), causing the recipient twin to be larger and the donor twin to be small, pallid dehydrated, malnourished and hypovolemic. However, congenital heart failure may develop in the larger twin during the first 24 hours after birth.

The clinical diagnosis of multifoetal pregnancy is accurate in about 90 per cent of cases. The likelihood of a multifoetal pregnancy is increased if any one or a combination of the following factors is revealed durig a careful assessment:

- History of dizygous twins inthe female lineage
- Use of fertility drugs
- More rapid uterine growth for time in pregnancy
- Hydramnios
- The palpation of an excessive number of small or large parts
- Asynchronous foetal heartbeats or more than one foetal electrocardiographic tracing
- Ultrasonographic evidence of more than one foetus.

Prenatal care: The prenatal care given women with multifoetal pregnancies includes changes in the pattern of care and modifications in other aspects such as the amount of weight gained and the diet observed. The prenatal visits of these mothers are scheduled at least every 2 weeks in the second trimester and weekly there after. No specific recommendation for weight gain for women with multifoetal pregnancies has been made. In twin gestations, reports of gains of 20 kg (44 lbs) have been associated with positive outcomes. Iron and vitamin supplementation is desirable. Attempts are made to prevent pre-eclampsia and eclampsia, which occur more frequently during multifoetal pregnancies, and vaginitis, if they cannot be prevented, they are treated.

The considerable uterine distension involved can cause the backache commonly experienced by pregnant women to be even worse. Elastic stockings are maternity tights may be worn to control leg varicosities. If there are risk factors for preterm birth (for example, premature dilatation of the cervix), abstinence from orgasm and nipple stimulation during the last trimester is commended to help avert preterm labour. Some practitioners recommend bed rest beginning at 20 weeks in women carrying twins to prevent preterm labour. Other practitioners question the value of prolonged bedrest. If bedrest is recommended, the mother needs to assume left lateral position to promote increased placental perfusion. If birth is delayed until after the thirty—sixth week, the risk of morbidity and mortality for the neonates decreases.

Psychosocial adjustment: The diagnosis of a twin pregnancy can come as a shock to many expectant parents, and they may need additional support and education to help them cope with the changes they face. The mother will need nutrition counselling so that she gains more weight than that needed for a singleton birth, counseling that maternal adaptations will probably be more uncomfortable, and information about the possibility of a preterm birth.

The degree to which parents are overwhelmed is dramatized by the following actual story. A young couple had known they were to become parents of twins since an early sonogram had revealed the presence of two gestational sacs. They had adjusted to the idea and were looking forward to twins. At birth, however, a third baby was born. The father became irate accused the physician of negligence in not diagnosing triplets, and threatened to sue her. The couple needed additional support during their initial adjustment period.

The additional newborns will likely palce a strain on finances, space workload, and the mother's and family's coping capability. Lifestyle changes may be necessary. Parents will need assistance in making realistic plans for the care of the babies, for example, whether to breastfeed and whether to raise them as "alike" or as separate persons. Parents should be referred to national organizations such as Parents of Twins, Mothers of Multiples, and the La League for further support.

Child Birth Education

Preparation for birth takes several forms. Because couples may not have a supportive extended family from which to learn, child birth education assumes increased importance. Nursing interventions can change perceptions of the childbirth experience, even for an unprepared couple. It is important, therefore that the nurse understands the support and teaching role in child birth education.

The objectives of childbirth education are as follows:

Objectives of childbirth education:

- To minimize anxieties, correct misconceptions, and reduce fear by providing factual information about pregnancy, labour and recovery
- To reach neuromuscular and respiratory skills to facilitate coping during labour
- To provide a framework of reference for the pregnant couple in which they may place their responses and concerns
- To create a setting within which parents may effectively use verbal and nonverbal communication
- To develop a relaxed, open group atmosphere conductive to learning and growing in self awareness
- To promote informed consumerism.

The content must be relevant no easily understood, with enough detail to give the couple an accurate and realistic picture of labour. Effective learning will take place if self esteem is enhanced and anxiety is lessened by a positive approach.

Another goal of the educator is to create informed and assertive consumers. Too often the couple has been passive in the childbirth experience, allowing health care providers to do almost anything without questioning them. There still are many degrees of acceptance by those in the medical profession of the couple's involvement in the childbirth process; not all physicians welcome it. A couple should be encouraged to consult with their chosen physician about possible approaches and together make a tentative birth plan for labour, including potential use of analgesia or anaesthesia.

Birth plans: Helping couples create meaningful birth plans means a careful and reasoned exploration of traditional and nontraditional approaches to birth. The nurse must not place unreasonable expectations on the couple and must know the community and the likelihood of newer methods being used in local settings. Birth plans help the woman formulate a realistic view of the approaching events and can provide continuity in care when several health care persons are involved.

Partner's skills: As the couple perfects neuromuscular and respiratory skills, childbirth educators provide opportunities for exploration of feelings, involving partners in nonthreatening ways. From the very first session the partner is introduced as the chief supporter and coach, and as the class progresses, his importance in the process is emphasized. However, the educator should be sure to indicate that the coach can be someone other than the father and that women without partners are encouraged to choose a close friend or relative for that role.

In a more general way, childbirth educators encourage mutual respect for the roles of father and mother during the childbirth experience and foster the concept of birth as family experience. Through this learning experience the partners become independent and cooperative and increase their self-esteem. Locus of control is not taken from them as they learn to manage a stressful situation. The result of childbirth preparation extends beyond the specific techniques used during labour. The family can be strengthened and emotional readiness for parenthood enhanced.

Content of Classes

Introductory class During the first class (Table 4.21) group interaction is facilitated by making introductions that should be limited to simple information, including name, parity, due date, community, and hospital, describing occupations might divide the group along socioeconomic lines.

The educator makes general comments about the purpose of the course, presents realistic goals, and introduces basic concepts. Parents need to understand that they can establish their own goals as the class evolves.

Because the class is still a collection of persons and not yet a group couples respons more readily to concrete and factual details. Pertinent information about conception and the trimesters of pregnancy is enhanced by the use of visual aids. Discussion of foetal developments and maternal changes reinforces the reality of the baby. The use of words such as "Now your baby's heart can be heard" helps the couple to identify their baby, particularly if it is their first. Comments such as "Many women feel very tired at the point"or "you may feel the need to talk over each detail" enhance maternal self-awareness.

Introducing physical condition exercises is appropriate to this first class. Couples are anxious to do something. These exercises increase the woman's sense of well-being and physical comfort during pregnancy. They are directed not toward the development of muscular strength but toward improvement of circulation, ventilation, body

Table 4.21: Sample class outline

Introductory class
- Introduce self and class participants
- Discuss basic purpose and goals of the course
- Present common terms
- Discuss highlights of conception, fetal development, maternal reactions, and physical changes.
- Teach physical conditioning exercises and rationale:
- Tailor press
- Tailor stretch
- Tailor reach
- Pelvic tilt
- Bent-leg lift.
- Perineal Control (Kegel exercise).
- Teach basics of controlled relaxation:
- Achieving comfort
- Facilitating relaxation
- Self-detection of tension and relaxation
- Coach's detection of tension and relaxation
- Role of touching and stroking to enhance relaxation
- Use of precise verbalcues.

Intermediate classes
- Practice relaxation techniques
- Introduce and develop the medianism of labor
- Discuss related maternal reactions and emotional responses to the mechanism of labour
- Teach various labour techniques in which the couple needs to become proficient
- Integration of controlled relaxation
- Rationale for respiratory techniques
- Rhythmic chest breathing; slow and modified rates
- Shallow chest breathing; combined with rhythmic chest breathing (modified rate) and rhythmic pattern of shallow breaching and short belows
- Open-glottis pushing
- Recognizing, preventing, and dealing with hyperventilation
- Expulsion techniques; overdoming fear of pushing, integrating controlled relaxation (especially prineal), using abdominal muscles effectively in directing pushing effort, correcting position to enhance the effort.

Managing back labor
- Develop the couple's confidence and self-awareness
- Introduce couples to community resources (e.g. baby care classes, visiting nurse services, family planning services)
- Acquaint couples with local hospital facilities and policies.

Concluding class
- Complete review of mechanism of labor, maternal reactions, labor techniques and partner's role
- *Discuss immediate postpartum period*
- Physical recuperation
- Emotional responses
- Emotional needs
- Hospital faciltities; recovery area, postpartum unit, nursery.

Discuss newborn
- Appearance at birth
- Care of infant in delivery room
- Characteristics of newborn during first few days
- Need for mother's physical contact
- Feeding, if pertinent to class needs.

Discuss postpartum period at home
- Physical changes
- Emotional needs and responses
- Simple exercises to improve muscle tone and sense of well-being
- Partner's needs and role.

The Instructor uses visual aids, demonstration, questions and discussion, group participation, role playing, and tours in the class.

awareness, and posture. Exercise videotapes for pregnancy are available.

Controlled relaxation is the foundation on which all other techniques are applied. As the woman begins to develop awareness of bodily change, she learns how to be comfortable, to detect tension in her body, and to facilitate relaxation. Her partner begins to learn to detect tension in her by touch and observation. Together they concentrate on achieving the active vs passive relaxation-necessary for control during labour. The partner is encouraged to touch and stroke her in ways to enhance relaxation and rest. Stroking always accompanies the verbal cue "relax" so that stroking itself soon becomes a signal for relaxation. Although jet hydrotherapy is not offered by many birth units, it too apears to helpful.

Managing pain: Childbirth education allows the woman alternatives to pharmacologic means to lessen pain. Pain is modified or inhibited when the person is able to have a specific focus of attention; when anxiety, fatigue and muscle tension are reduced, and when there is an increase of controlled sensory input.

As strategies, the woman may use light stroking (effleurage) by the coach or herself to creat organized, controlled sensory input to relieve local irritability. When concentrating on the sensation at the skin, she may be able to disregard the more diffuse sensation from the pain fibres of the uterus or cervix. When the woman performs alternate activities such as breathing in specific patterns or relaxing in learned ways, she may further modify pain transmission. Mental rehearsal and imagery activate concentration and improve performance.

The woman is encouraged to respond to labour in a variety of ways. She may assume several positions, breaths as she is comfortable doing and ask for assistance. It should be emphasized that the coach and staff members are available to assist her.

Intermediate classes: Building on the information and report of the introductory class, subsequent classes are expanded in a logical progression. Content is carefully structured to the interest of the couples, who need a clear understanding of what happens, how the woman will feel and react, how she can cope during each phase, and how her partner can support and direct her efforts.

In teaching the second stage, for instance, the instructor needs to be alert to the anxiety about and fear of giving birth. Attitudes toward sexuality fear for safety, misconceptions and inaccurate information contribute, to these fears of pain and injury held by both partner and woman. The couple must gain an accurate.

Breathing techniques: To enhance relaxation and remove the focus away from the contraction, breathing rhythms can be altered. Breathing normally is automatic, we do not think about breaths at all. To learn new techniques takes practice and interest in self-help. Starting with Dick-read, child-birth education has taught various patterns for use during labour stages. Classic Lamaze's technique has been modified by most teachers of psychoprophylaxis and includes the following basic aspects:

1. *Chest* breathing is said to diminish diaphragmatic interference on the uterine fundus and is used through-out. The woman feels as though she is breathing higher and higher in the chest as she progressed with the techniques.
2. A deep breath initiates and concludes each contraction. Also, the deep breath clears carbon dioxide and increases oxygen levels. This is an important signal for the woman and her coach. She has learned to relax consciously as she exhales this breath. These beginning and ending breaths make each contraction a single entity, as opposed to the sense of endless contractions.
3. *A focal point* increases the woman's concentration and diminishes distraction. It serves to direct her attention to dealing with the contraction constructively. The point of focus may change from time to time.
4. Verbal and nonverbal cues are used to indicate when the woman will use a breathing technique (e.g., "contraction begins—contraction ends"). At times these cues may be used by the coach during labour if the woman has become drowsy, tired, or uncertain about the actual onset of each contraction.
5. A comfortable position is important for effective relaxation and efficient respiration. The supine position will interfere with the progress of labour and cause undesirable intra-abdominal pressure on the large blood vessels. The woman is encouraged to use a tailor sitting, side-lying, or a more upright position in the bed or chair.

These techniques may be practiced in front of a mirror or with the partner timing the "practice" contraction. The couple should inform the nurse at the start of labour which sequences of breathing they have been practicing.

- *Early phase*: The first respiratory pattern the woman will use is rhythmic chest breathing at the slow rate of about eight breaths per minute. She inhales through the nose and exhales through the mouth; exhalation is stressed and slightly prolonged. In rhythm with the breathing, she can apply a circular stroke over the abdominal area, using her fingertrips. Stroking may be done with one or both hands or by her coach. This type of breathing is continued as long as it is effective.
  With the advance of dilation as the phase progresses, the woman also may need to progress in breathing activity. She modifies the rhythm chest breathing by increasing the rate to 16 or 20 breaths per minute, continuing rhythmic stroking.
- *Active phase:* To deal with the intensity, the woman progresses to a combined pattern of modified rhythmic chest breathing and shallow chest breathing. She matches the increment and decrement with the rhythmic chest breathing pattern; she uses the lighter, faster shallow breathing for the acme. Rhythmic stroking is continued if she finds it soothing. As contractions demand, she may use shallow breathing for the entire contraction, permitting greater flexibility in rate and depth. When using this technique, she breathes lightly and evenly, inhaling and exhaling through her slightly opened mouth. The rate is just fast enough to ensure respiratory exchange (as opposed to simply moving tidal air) with minimal effort and depth of respirations.
- *Transition phase*: To handle this difficult period, a woman must use specific strategies. She uses a rhythmic pattern of shallow chest breathing with short puffs, which requires concentration and promotes a sense of control. The sequence usually is three or two breaths or one shallow breath, alternating with a puff. These patterns are altered in response to the intensity of each contractions. The pattern of one shallow breath and one fuff is particularly useful in controlling intense peaks, sensations of [pressure, or the urge to push.
- *Expulsion phase*: Technique focuses on controlled relaxation and voluntary bearing down. Recent research and studies have made it clear that expulsion techniques should avoid sustained breath holding. The woman learns to use her oblique abdominal muscles and a fixed diaphragm to bear down. By pushing as though she is going to quickly empty her bladder, she will direct her efforts through the vagina and not the rectum. Conscious release of the perineum reduces resistance to the head. Correct positioning into a shape, whether semisitting or upright, will allow her to favorably influence the axis of the birth canal. The position of her body and legs influence the relaxation of the perineum, further reducing resistance to the baby's head as it emerges.

The woman learns to push during the peak of each contractions, permitting the contraction to build by taking two deep breaths. Then she is encouraged to bear down repeatedly, tuning in to her body.

To sustain the work, to increase the efficiency of that effort and the efficiency of her ventilation, and to avoid Valsalva's manoeuvre, she learns to use a series of breaths, holding for a moment to start the push and then bearing down vigorously as she exhales slowly; this is open glottis pushing. She can say a word such as "push" or "out" or grunt to control the release of air as she maintains her pushing efforts. She may alternately hold her breath and bear down without the controlled exhalation as long as she avoids sustained breath holding.

Valsalva's manoeuvre: Holding breath and bearing down for more than 5 or 6 seconds is associated with a lowering in maternal blood pressure and a decrease in placental circulation. Like a domino effect, foetal pH and oxygen pressure (pO2) decrease and carbon dioxide pressure (pCO2) and foetal heart rate increase. Thus bearing down should be brief, accompanied by open glottis pushing with air release. Although this technique has been known since 1980, many units continue to ins that the woman do forceful sustained pushing during the second stage of labour. Here is an area for nurse advocacy for the health of the labouring woman.

Caesarean birth preparation: When Caesarean birth is expected, couples may attend classes that omit te emphasis on self-help during labour. Although preparation details may differ, basics remain the same. Following lists topics that are helpful to the couple:

- Reason for, safety, and risks of caesarean birth
- Couple's understanding or these reasons or their prior experiences
- Potential of vaginal birth after caesarean delivery
- Policies regarding cesareans, differing facilities, and costs
- Preparation before admission and procedures on admission
- Anesthesia choices and recovery process
- Couple's understanding of their choices
- Role of physician, anaesthesiologist, nurse
- Signs of labour onset and what to do if early
- Actual caesarean procedure (films)
- Support role of partner before and after birth
- Parent-infant contact opportunities
- Recovery process, intravenous lines, catheters, pain management, fluids, food
- Relaxation responses that help—breathing, imagery
- Involution patterns and recovery expectations
- Discharge timing and choices
- Home care opportunities
- Managing at home
- Infant feeding choices, lactation support
- Neonatal care in delivery area, pattern of care in hospital
- Expected emotional response, integration of experience
- Possibilities of a caeserean support group.

Not all women take advantage of such classes, and the nurse will care for women who are unprepared or did not expect a caesarean birth. In these cases the list inbox will be useful for teaching.

Concluding class: The couple's proficiency in technique and knowledge of labour must be reviewed and evaluated in the concluding class. The instructor can introduce material pertinent to the postpartum period. Couples need a basic awareness of the physical changes and emotional and social adjustments of the recover period. They also need to be prepared for the unfinished" quesities of the newborn, as well as its demands and needs. First-time parents need to be aware that they will not suddenly transformed into the romanticized image of parenthood but will grow into their new role.

Many primigravidas are unprepared for various aspects of physical recovery. A brief discussion of what to expect aids understanding of the physiology of the recovery period and provides a few practical suggestion for dealing with this recuperative period.

Because couples share in excitement and learning, new friendship start. The childbirth educator often offers to hold a "reunion" at able time in the future.

ADAPTATION TO PREGNANCY

People learn how to be mothers or fathers from their own parents. Memories of their parent's behaviour and attitude lead them to develop ideas about what a parent is or should be. Once formed, these ideas are extremely difficult to change. If parent-child relationships were loving. Individuals are likely to become loving parents. If relationships were full of distrust and abuse, these patterns are also likely to be repeated in the next generation.

Because parents are role models, children at play often mimic parents acts. As children mature, play is replaced by a more inward rehearsal. The adolescent dreams of future roles and rehearses them in the mind. In adulthood, this process occurs through a series of images. During times of change, particularly when a major change in life-style is anticipated, a person imagines himself or herself in the situation. For example, an expectant mother imagines herself rocking her baby, or an expectant father pictures himself comforting a crying child.

Motivations for pregnancy vary widely. The couple may want to prove their ability to reproduce or to achieve adult status. They may be fulfilling the cultural expectation that "everyone" wants children or may wish to fulfill their parents' wish for a grandchild. A woman may desire to again experience the closeness of the mother-child relationship or to strengthen ties with her partner. More positively, having a child may be viewed as a new beginning, an enriching life experience leading to feelings of creativity and competence. The woman may be reaching the age when she feels that "it's now or never," that she must soon decide to have a baby or risk the inability to conceive or carry the baby to term. However, when the time comes, transition to first-time parenthood is abrupt, the new parents often feel unprepared for the reality of the responsibility.

Developmental Tasks During Pregnancy

Many developmental tasks occur during the psychologic transition from nonparent to parent. This transition parallels and is stimulated by the development of the child within the womb.

During the early weeks, the expectant mother tests the reality of the pregnancy. Even after she has confirmation through tests, she looks for affirmation in other signs and symptoms. These symptoms reassure her that the pregnancy is real.

First-trimester

On woman's first pregnancy, first-trimester needs very care. A first pregnancy is like any other first experience. The expectant mother feels curiosity and concern about the changes ahead. Even the most carefully planned educational programme does not fully relieve the anxiety.

Although the woman may have chosen to become pregnant, there is always an ambivalence until the idea of being pregnant becomes a reality and an acceptance of the growing foetus integration or incorporation, take place.

Acceptance: The expectant parents conscious or unconscious motivation and eagerness for pregnancy change the normal degree of ambivalence about anticipated life changes pregnancy causes. For the first-time mother, the infant is a final step away from the girl she once was. She must give up her image of herself as a childless person before she can accept her pregnant self. Some women experience considerable nostalgia for the person they once were, feeling unready for the "mother person" they will become. This is often expressed in dreams and images of younger days.

Occasionally, unresolved ambivalence can interfere with acceptance of pregnancy. Inconvenient social circumstances such as being young and single may cause the expectant mother to deny the existence of the pregnancy. A disintegrating relationship with the expectant father can cause anger, which may lead to maternal rejection of the foetus.

The following dimensions (Lederman, 1984) should be considered when assessing the woman's acceptance of the pregnancy:

1. *The desire for pregnancy and/or infant*: In Lederman's study, some women wanted an infant but disliked being pregnant. In less healthy case some loved the warm feelings related to being pregnant but could not look ahead to actually nurturing an infant. However, resolution of negative feelings usually occurred by the third-trimester.
2. *Amount of happiness or unhappiness*: For some women in the study, emotional gratification came from feelings of biologic fulfilment and from their conscious desire for a child despite mood swings and emotional ability. In women with a history of depression, however, the pregnancy tended to trigger recurrence. Low self-esteem greatly increased fears related to labour and/or the ability to mother the newborn.
3. *Discomfort during pregnancy*: The amount of discomfort experienced during pregnancy varies considerably from woman-to-woman. When discomfort seems intensified and markedly prolonged, it may indicate a problem with acceptance of the pregnant state.
4. *Acceptance of body changes*: In our society, the media have promoted the idea that the skinny body is the model for beauty. Many women fear viewed as "fat" and feel relieved when they look obviously pregnant. Such women look forward to wearing maternity clothing and may choose to wear it early in the pregnancy. New views expressed in the media may change perceptions.
5. *Amount of unresolved ambivalence*: Most women accept pregnancy by the beginning of the third-trimester. To assess how well the woman is accomplished this task, discuss her feelings about the infant and help her express how she sees herself as a new mother. Some mothers accept pregnancy, but are still unable to imagine themselves as mothers. Women, which receive little or no psychologic support may have particular difficulty.

As a nurse, there is a need to assess the degree of interference with the woman's acceptance process. For example, ambivalence in natural if a woman must give up a rewarding career or if financial considerations mean that the timing of the pregnancy is poor. These feelings do not mean that the woman has rejected pregnancy; her attitude of happiness or unhappiness is a far more accurate indication of her state of mind. She is in the period of pregnancy validation, a necessary developmental phase of pregnancy.

Concerns: Most pregnant women are concerned during the first-trimester with the changes in their room own bodies and how these changes will affect their lives. Some of their expressed concerns have to do with the following:

1. Normal symptoms of pregnancy ("Should I worry? Am I normal? What shall I do?")
2. Changes in life-style that will result from the pregnancy ("I wonder how pregnancy will make me different.")
3. Changes in relationship with the partner ("How will he accept this pregnancy? How will it change our sexual responses?"
4. Medical care—the sequences and reasons for visits ("How can I get help between visits?")

The woman may appear to be very self-concerned. Because she probably will not be able to focus on instructions concerning future events such as labour, delivery, child care, or contraception, such topics are best discussed in later visits.

Practical concerns may centre around finances, especially if the new infant's arrival will mean curtailment of the woman's income, or about the expenses of having and raising a child. Women, may worry about loss of freedom, increased dependency, or other changes in relationships. Although these concerns are most evident in the first pregnancy, relationships also shift and change with later children.

Signs of difficulty: Signs of difficulty in first-trimester tasks may be demonstrated as exaggerated discomforts such as severe nausea, sleeplessness, and fatigue. In addition, she may have unresolved anger, feel depressed, and be hostile towards her partner. Interventions may assist her to resolve these conflicts.

Second-trimester

By the end of the first-trimester, discomforts from physiologic changes have usually disappeared. The expectant mother settle down and her concerns begin to shift from her own bodily changes to the growing infant, separate from herself, or foetal differentiation, is normally completed by the end of the trimester.

Infant as non-self: Beginning with quickening the parents thoughts turn inward to the separateness of the child. The infant is part of them but is distinct and familiar; however, they can't guess how he or she will look, Physical sensations, which at first are described as light, flettering, and exciting, may later seem disruptive. Women complain, "he never leaves me alone; always giving me a thump when I want to sleep. This period has been called foetal embodiment, a developmental task of the second-trimester.

Visualization: Through visualization, the woman imagines that her child is like and becomes acquainted with it, as she notices what disturbs and what soothes it. For instance, most foetuses react to loud music, such as rock music with strong movement, yet quiet down and are soothed by smooth, lilting melodies. An expectant mother may experiment with and note reactions to rhythmic sensations such as when she leans against the spinning dryer or when she rules firmly in a particular spot. Many "play" with the foetus by pushing against a protruding spot and waiting to be kicked in return.

When the expectant mother has a sonogram early in pregnancy, she can actually see her child moving about within her. Women frequently report that this was the first time they experienced the feeling that another person was really there. Encourage the mother to ask for an ultrasound "photo" of her infant to help her picture the child and develop feelings for it.

Dreams: Fears often arise as an expectant mother begins to accept this separateness. Low self-esteem intensifies the women's fear that her child will not be perfect. This fear does not diminish with later pregnancies, even when the first infant was healthy. This woman may believe that she could not possibly be lucky again after her first infant was "perfect."

These are often fears expressed in dreams. A theme common in dreams is the monster-child, devouring from within, or the woulf-child suckling at the breast. These themes may indicate that the woman feels ambivalence and feat towards the unknown "other" or that she will be so consumed by the coming infant that she will never regain her sense of self.

Emotional separateness: Emotional separation between self and the infant is a total stranger and are surprised that the infant may have reactions different from their own. For example, the expectant mother may be fond of rock music and be amazed to find that her unborn child is clearly restless when it is played. For women who have not completed the process of individuation (adolescents, for example), this realization is especially difficult.

Maternal role attainment: The newly pregnant woman begins to "put on" her new role in the first-trimester. She looks for role models who have had this experience. Rubin (1984) calls this activity *replication*, copying behaviours in other pregnant women or successful mothers. The pregnant woman then plays these roles and tries the various ways of interaction. During the second-trimester, the process moves a step further to *internalization*, when the woman lingers over images of herself in various situations. Using imagery, she begins adapting to the future.

In the third-trimester, as the woman's focus shifts to look forward to the end of pregnancy discomforts, the foetus may be a threat and cause anxiety. Role assumption behaviours, now focus on evaluation and criticism of others, including her own mother. She is *differentiating* herself from others to become the kind of mother she imagines.

Relationship with her own mother: The need of expectant mothers to get reacquainted with their own parents is universal. Expectant parents relieves past and present relationships with their parents in their mind and try to come to terms with them.

If her own mother is available, the expectant mother may attempt to get closer to her. If there are still unresolved issues of separations and power between them, she may exclude her mother from participation. Rivalry between the expectant mother and her mother may cause friction in everything from naming the infant to whether or not the new grandmother will be invited to come to help out when the baby comes home.

If her own mother is unavailable, the woman may try to be friend another motherly person to serve as her alternate maternal role model. This person may be a friend with children whom the expectant mother admire and wishes to emulate.

Concerns: In general, in the second-trimester, the mother is interested in protecting the health of the infant, and her concerns will reflect her awareness of its needs. The general concerns are as follows:

1. Nutritional intake (am I gaining too much? too little?)
2. Amount of exercise, travel (what restrictions are necessary?)
3. Progression of foetal growth (how big is the baby this month?)
4. Warning signs of problems.
5. Changing body image (how reflected in clothes, hygiene, hair, skin).
6. Changes in sexual desires (concern about restrictions and misconception.

Signs of difficulty: Signs of difficulty with second-trimester tasks may include continuing angery and depression because of lack of acceptance. Physical complaints and a focus on her own concerns rather than thoughts of the foetus may indicate problems. Clues to difficulty in parenting may become evident in self involvement or in regression to more childish behaviour.

Third-trimester

Separation and birth: In the final weeks the mother's tank is to prepare for the end of the pregnancy and for the birth itself. As the mother looks forward to the birth, she may again feel considerable ambivalence. She must prepare for *letting* go of the pregnancy and all its warm feelings of fusion and creativity, or *foetal separation*. Conscious or unconscious fears of mutilation, death, or abandonment often surface at this time. Anticipatory anxiety is considered in this phase to be normal and healthy. As the birth nears, the over-riding concern is how to cope with the stresses of labour and delivery and whether there will be a safe passage. As the work on structuring a mental image of what labour and birth will be like, man couples seek out other new parents for advice and questioning and listen to their stories of how they dealt with their birth experiances.

Increasing dependency needs: During pregnancy, dependency needs increase and reach a peak in the third-trimester, labour, and the early nurturing period after birth. The expectant mother needs to be nurtured to store reserves for the time when she is nurturing the infant. This is not limited to the first-pregnancy, only to expectant women. Men, also feel heightened need to have someone dependable to care for them, particularly because the expactant mother becomes more introspective with advancing pregnancy and perhaps withdraws some of the "mothering" attention she usually gets from her.

By becoming a parent, a person is no longer the child in the relationship with parents. As a parent, a person becomes the provider rather than the recipient. In this sense, becoming a parent for the first time means that the new parents can never return to childhood.

Childhood education: Many couples seek childbirth classes to make them feel prepared. In these classes, expectant parents learn the facts and techniques of childbirth but also receive support.

The woman is eager to learn any methods and techniques to relieve discomforts and to assist her during the later part of pregnancy and labour. She well use exercises and practice breathing in these weeks. Counselling continues on an individual basis and may now include preparation for infant's arrival and care. In the third-trimester, information for recovery, self-care, and infant care should be presented because early discharge does not allow adequate time to teach these things.

Concerns: Expectant mother needs in the third-trimester are expressed in approximately the same ways despite differences in background, educational, level and experience. A woman focuses on the infant, the process of labour, and her own changing physical condition and emotions. Even multiparas have questions about the difference in labour and delivery with each infant. Concerns expressed in this trimester tend to pertain to the following:

1. The infant's well-being (questions on birth defects, signs of foetal well-being, how birth affects the infant, affects of medication and anesthesia)
2. The costs of having an infant (fees, having to stop work, expenses for equipment).
3. The process of labour and delivery (pain, fears, misconceptions, when to go to the hospital).
4. Family (how other children will accept the infant, how to plan for them during hospitalization, how her partner will respond to the infant).

The changing contours of the woman's body become more prominent; backaches, legaches, lower abdominal pressure, ligament pain, fatigue, extraweight, cause her to be impatient for labour to begin (Table 4.22).

"Nesting" Some women are superstitious about buying anything for the infant before its birth; to do so might risk death or injury to the child they have been told. Nurse may acknowledge that some hold this belief but should turn the conversation to the equipment that will be needed by the new infant, even though purchasing will begin later. The father or grandparents may have this task during her hospitalization, but the mother will want to know how to plan. The only important fact to emphasize is that planning should be done before taking the infant home. Mothers who have limited apartment space or income will usually welcome suggestions on how to economize. All women feel the "nesting" impulse, an urge to prepare for the infant.

Signs of difficulty: Signs of difficulty in the third-trimester include a continuing high-level of anxiety about herself, labour, or the discomforts of pregnancy. If the woman neglects health practices or cannot prepare for or focus on the needs of the coming infant, she may be indicating that she cannot adjust to what is happening in her body.

Expectant Father's tasks: Like his mate, the expectant father must make the psychologic shift from his idea of himself as a man or boy without children to that of a *man with a child*, a father. The case with which he is able to do this is related to his readiness for the pregnancy and the amount of ambivalence he has experienced. That readiness is related to the men's sense of financial security, of stability in the couple relationship, and of readiness to end the childrens state within the couple's relationship. Although his experience lacks the immediacy of the expectant mother's role shift, it follows a similar pattern.

In the beginning tests confirm the pregnancy, and couples tell their significant family and friends. This early phase is called the announcement phase and does not last long. After this period, many men pull away psychologically and may distance themselves and avoid discussion of the coming infant, postponing emotional investment. The father's acceptance frequently lag behind the mother's. Until he is able to imagine that he will actually be a father and have a real child to raise, the whole process may not have an impact. He may involve himself in other pursuits for long periods of time, "for getting" about the pregnancy. This is the avoidance phase of acceptance.

Table 4.22: Maternal tasks, concerns and problems

Tasks	*Concerns*	*Problems*
First Trimester		
To acknowledge pregnancy	Normality of symptoms, future changes in lifestyle	Exaggerated discomforts such as nausea, sleeplessness
To begin to work through conflicts with own mother to begin to develop own mothering role	Changes in relationship with partner.	Excessive need for reassurance that she is pregnant.
Pregnancy validation acceptance	Cost of care, how to manage Normality of ambivalence.	Anger, rejection of idea of pregnancy. Depression, crying, extreme mood swings. Distance from sexual partner.
Second Trimester		
To regard foetus as a reality, foetal embodiment. To manage shifts in dependency from the role of daughter to the role of mother. To continue working through conflicts with own parents. To use mimicry, role playing, imagery to help herself to assume the role of mother.	Nutritional intake. Changing body image Changing lifestyle, sexual needs. Progression of foetal growth. Warning signs of problems	Lack of acceptance of pregnancy. Depression, anger, anxiety continue. Numerous physical complaints, focus on own concerns. Indications of no family support. Indications of inability to plan ahead.
Third Trimester		
To view foetus as a separate individual to be "let go" through birth To accept physical, psychologic changes. To prepare for entering To prepare for labour, birth, and accept the risk of "safe passage"	Infant's well-being, factors affecting labour and birth. Anxiety over possibility of deformed baby. Expenses Process of labour, delivery Acceptance of infant by other children Present discomforts	High level of anxiety about self, labour. Continued nonacceptance of pregnancy. Behaviour that neglects health practices. Lack of support from family or spouse. Lack of preparation for or focus on needs of new infant.

As the expectant father adjusts to the reality of the situation, his partner experiences her own increased need for support and reassurance. Sensing his withdrawal, she may attempt to involve him more closely. Frequently he withdraws even more. Disagreement between marital partners are common, and the expectant mother feels that his lack of enthusiasm is a lack of caring. The expectant father feels pressured to organize himself and his priorities around the pregnancy. He may desire a moratorium on pregnancy talk, having trouble with its reality.

In research findings, the transition from the avoidance phase takes place near the start of the third trimester and in many cases is quite abrupt. For some men, emotional investment is triggered by the physical reality of the infant of notice the obvious changes in his partner's body, feeling foetal movements, or by actually becoming involved in preparations. He suddenly realizes that he will be the father of the child, and he begins to define himself as a father through imagine making. Like his partner, he begins to imagine himself as a father, remembering how he was fathered and accepting or rejecting that role. Other relationships are examined (for example, his parents as grandparent) He seeks friendship with others who have children and tends to drift away from those who do not. Jordan (1990) calls this "Labouring for relevance" as the father works through phases to become ready for parenting.

He and his partner must also work out the degree of involvement he will have in childbirth and later in parenting the child. This decision needs to be made by both partners. If a couple's expectations differ, they need to reach a compromise before the birth, or unmet expectations may lead to conflict or rejection.

Somatic symptoms: Couvade The father's adjustment may include a migrating series of health symptoms and complaints, termed couvade. It is thought that this demonstrates a positive level of identification with the pregnant partner. It also been found that men who experienced symptoms scored higher on scales measuring paternal role preparation than men who reported to symptoms. Because paternal bonding begins during the pregnancy, this finding seems logical. One father's experience is recorded below:

One father left the scene of the birth of his first child, to cry alone. He shared with me his deep sadness that he could not also bear a child. He also continued to be a very nurturing father.

A recent study identified 39 symptoms reported by the men in the survey. These symptoms included intestinal gas pains, nausea, hunger and weight gain, restlessness, sleeping difficulties, and bad dreams. These symptoms may persist into the early postbirth period.

COPING DURING PREGNANCY

Most women do well with support. Others find pregnancy an additional stress that puts them off balance. With an understanding of the normality of body changes, the woman may enjoy her progress. If she is uniformed, she may resent or be fearful of what is happening. If she looks forward to and recognizes the steps of pregnancy, she will feel pride and enjoyment. If she is stressed, her changing body responses may cause anger and frustration.

Any inhibition of the mother's progress through the developmental steps may result in anxiety or conflict that further hinders her ability to form an image of her maternal self. Such impediments can arise from low self-esteem, Lack of a maternal role model, or conflicts between the mother-self and career-self roles. If the woman is very young or is older, or when medical or social problems occur, maternal role attainment may be more troublesome.

Low self-esteem makes it difficult for the expectant mother to visualize herself in labour or as a competent mother. Her poor selfimage projects itself onto her idea of what kind of parent she will be. She will need strong support and reinforcement for her abilities.

Nursing Management

Assessment

Nurse may use the questions to elicit information regarding family and individual situations that may precipitate stress during pregnancy. Often when questions focus on what the woman really needs or is concerned about, the presenting need is far from what the nurse assumes it to be. Always listen first, before giving instructions or advice.

Nurse can determine whether the woman has positive role models by asking her who she will talk with about her pregnancy. Find out if the woman is socially isolated (even within a marriage) by asking her how she spends time with friends or family.

Nursing Diagnosis

Whenever a nurse work with expectant parents the following should be considered:

- Altered role performance related to adaptations to the pregnancy
- Family coping: potential for growth related to anticipation of parenting
- Ineffective coping compromised by inadequate family support or disengagement
- Situational low self-esteem related to prior life experiences or level of support during pregnancy.

Planning/Objectives

Consider these example of objectives to direct patient care.

- Seeks assistance from appropriate resources and referrals
- Verbalizes changes that are taking place
- Seeks involvement of the partner in the care process
- Father participates in care and preparation for birth
- Increases understanding of self as a future parent
- Works on problem resolution.

Nursing Interventions

Nurse must be perceptive to identify some of the subtle indications of problems and need to recognize the importance of psychosocial adaptation in planning care during pregnancy and recovery. The following examples of questions that may elicit the woman's perception of her life events:

1. What do you think caused your problem?
2. Why do you think it started when it did?
3. What do you think the problem does to you? To your infant?
4. How do you think you can resolve this problem?

5. Can you express the anxiety that comes from this problem?

The woman will often articulate a different emphasis than the health care professional would have expected. The cultural differences play a significant part in the emphasis placed on the meaning of the problem. If you note a depressed effect or lack of grooming, further assess for more severe problems and make appropriate referrals.

Plans to help the mother, become more active in her own self-care can be as simple as reinforcing her ability to make appropriate choices. To do this, you will have to allow her to make choices about her care and to give her the responsibility of carrying them out. Self-care means that you must treat the expectant parents as adults, even when they are adolesents.

In addition, refer to social service any woman with stressed life circumstances or economic problems that interfere with adequate nutrition, housing, or future care of the infant and herself.

Evaluation

Sample questions to evaluate if the mother reached outcomes are listed below:

- Did the partners seek to learn about pregnancy and parenting?
- How was her partner planning to be involved?
- Were clinic appointments kept and outside resources used?
- Did she indicate adequate social support?
- Has she received and followed through on referrals for unresolved problems.

SEXUAL RESPONSES DURING PREGNANCY

Woman's Responses

In the course of prenatal counselling, a woman may express anxiety about sexuality during pregnancy. She may allude to particular problems. Even if she does not, Nurse should approach the subject in a nonthreatening way, either individually or in prenatal classes. A number of women react positively to their changing body image, feeling less restricted in their sexual expression. Some experience a sense of fulfillment when pregnant or feel more attractive than before. For these women, there may be heightened interest in sexual activity. Other women feel less desirable and awkward and because of discomforts, express less interest in sexual activity.

For many couples, sexual responses may differe between the women and her partner. She may be more interested, or less interested. Interest levels also change as the pregnancy progresses. Research studies have shown that each trimester may have a different set of responses. Regardless of which responses are expressed, most women indicate an increased need to be nurtured and held closely.

Partner's Responses

Although many men have no change in sexual desires because of pregnancy, some feel an increased closeness, intimacy and eroticism. Certain men express a fear of harming the woman or foetus or have questions about whether intercourse is "right" when the woman is pregnant. They may have fantasies about the foetus or about being inadequate to satisfy the woman's increased desires. Other men may withdraw or seek a sexual outlet outside the partnership.

Changes during Phases of the Sexual Response

Cycle

When pregnancy responses are placed within each phase of the sexual cycle, the difference may be seen more clearly.

Desire

Changes in body image may increase or decrease sexual interest. A women may be more tense or relaxed. If she enjoys her body changes, there will be increased interest in more frequent intercourse. Any pregnancy discomforts reduce desire.

Excitement

The phase of physiologic excitement includes vasocongestion of vaginal and labial tissues and clitoral enlargement. Pregnancy increases lubrication and vasocongestion, and excitement may come more quickly. Breasts, too, are already enlarged and may be tender or even sore. Sexual excitement makes nipples erect and may bring discomfort for some; breasts may be a new focus in sex-play because all women have enlargement. In some cases the woman may be increasingly uncomfortable with the enlargment, whereas her partner finds it stimulating.

Plateau and Orgasm

The vaginal tract becomes engorged during pregnancy. Because muscle tension and venous engorgement increase, many women experience orgasm quickly and may have several during sexual activity. Some women describe orgasm as "fulminating". Mild uterine contractions during orgasm do not appear to harm the foetus.

Resolution

The period of decrease in tissue engorgement and relaxation is often changed. Vasocongestion does not diminish quickly. Some women have continuing discomfort and take longer to relax.

Nursing Management

Assessment

When working with different ethnic groups, nurse should seek information about any cultural sexual taboos during pregnancy and recovery. By seeking this information from each client, nurse can avoid stereotyping and plan care-based on individual needs.

Nursing Diagnosis

There are only a few possible diagnoses to use for this concern, depending on whether the problems expressed are related to the partner or to the woman, or stem from a medical complication during pregnancy.

- Altered sexuality patterns related to differing responses to pregnancy.
- Individual coping stressed by changes demanded by complications of pregnancy.
- High-risk for sexually transmitted infection depending on partner's status.

Planning/Objectives

- Expresses feelings regarding sexual responses during pregnancy.
- Incorporates anticipatory guidance.
- Protects herself from sexually transmitted diseases (STDs)

Nursing Interventions

The most effective intervention for sexual problems expressed by the client during pregnancy is *anticipatory guidance*. On the basis of current understanding of the physiologic changes of pregnancy, the following may be taught regarding sexual activity during pregnancy:

1. There is little potential for injury.
   a. The foetus is not injured by normal coitus becauses it is cushioned by amniotic fluid and protected by the cervix and uterus.
   b. In the last few weeks, after the foetal head has descended into the pelvic canal, a woman may find deep thrusting uncomfortable.
2. There is little potential for harm by stimulating uterine contractions.
   a. Miscarriage in the first-three months is rarely caused by coitus. Almost all reasons for spontaneous abortion are intrinsic, related to genetic causes or poor developement of the embryo.
   b. If there is threatened abortion, abstinence is suggested until it is clear that the pregnancy will continue.
   c. Prostaglandins in semen may stimulate mild uterine contraction, especially a few days before labour begins. For this reason, women who have threatened premature labour onset or third-trimester bleeding should abstain from a number of weeks (determined by their condition) before their due date. Conversely, if the infant is overdue, some encourage the couple to have intercourse in hope of stimulating labour. One study recommends that condoms should be used with coitus occurring during the last month to prevent potential infection or stimulation of labour.
3. STDs and infection have adverse effects on the foetus:
   a. STDs should be taken very seriously. Both partners should be treated if an infection is dignosed. Inform the woman how to seek personal protection.
   b. Women with new partners or multiple partners must insist that partners use a condom for protection. Women whose partners are at risk should always insist on condom use, but may be able to do so.
4. Air must never be blown in to the vegina during sex play because there is a rare chance of death due to air embolism. Because of partial dilation of the cervix, air forcibly blown may enter the uterus and through the placenta find a way into maternal circulation.

5. Variations in sexual interest are normal and reflect physiologic changes:
   a. *First-trimester*: Because of increased blood supply to vaginal tissue and the enlarging uterus, some women have a more total orgasmic response. Nulliparas may have a decreased response, often because of discomforts and fatigues, Multiparas often find relief in not needing contraception.
   b. *Second-trimester*: There is an increase in eroticism and orgasmic response noted by all women. Most women indicate increased interest. The enlarging uterus begins to require changes in position for coitus including side to side, rear entry, and woman-superior, for instance.
   c. *Third-trimester*: As the due date approaches the frequency of intercourse is reduced for all women. Fatigue and discomfort play a part but women may also be worried about arbitrary instructions by health professionals. It is common to hear "6 weeks before and 6 weeks after as the period of abstinence. Such instruction should no longer be provided.

Evaluation

Evaluation questions that may be asked to determine progress towards the outcomes include the following:
- Did the couple/ woman ask appropriate questions and indicate understanding of the effects of pregnancy on sexuality?
- Did she state that the used precautions to protect against STDs?
- Did a medical condition during pregnancy cause stress between partners?
- Were they able to resolve these problems?

Increased Psychosocial Risk

When the parent-child relationship is healthy, the child learns to socialize with others from parents and becomes an adult who can complete the developmental and pregnancy related tasks in preparation for becoming a parent who can form bonds to her or his own children.

People in urban societies move away from the family of origin: extended kinship groups may not exist. Parents often raise their children without the support of a group. Without an extended family on which to depend, the *parent-child relationship is absolutely crucial to the child's psychologic growth*. Today's new mother may have only her own family as a role model or may come from a single-parent family; as a result, her problem is compounded.

Women at either extreme of reproductive age—the older, mature gravida and the adolescent gravida—are at increased psychosocial risk. These risks vary with a correspond to developmental states.

Mature Gravidas

The pregnant woman over 35 years faces unique problems. The primigravida in this age category has generally decided to postpone child bearing until her carreer is well established. Although the child may be wanted and anticipated, she will often have much ambivalence and concern about how motherhood will affect her life-style and how it will affect her relationship with the father of the baby. She might be a single woman deciding to have a child on her own, perhaps even by artificial insemination or *in vitro* fertilization. She might be having a child later in her childbearing years because of remarriage or by "accident." This child may be much desired or unwelcome. Nurse need to ascertain this information because the woman's and her family's responses are closely tied to their feelings.

Developmental Stage

Women over 35 years are generally in the developmental stage of *intimacy vs isolation*, which is described by Erikson (1963) as the time in which The young adult, emergive from the search for and the insistence on identity, is eager and willing to fuse his identity with that of others. He is ready for intimacy, that is the capacity to commit himself to concrete affiliations and partnerships and to develop the ethical strength to abide by such commitments even though they may call for significant sacrifices and compromises.

The woman over 40 years may have entered the life stage of *generativity vs stagnation* defined by Erikson (1963) as "primarily the concern in establishing and guiding the next generation.

Concern is accentuated in women who realize that the time in which to have a baby is running out, often referred to as hearing the "biological clock" ticking louder. Even women who have other children may feel the desire to have another before it is too late.

It may seem that these women are the best prepared psychologically for the demands of pregnancy and parenthood because their lives are stable. This readiness intensifies their need for nursing care. They are heavily invested in these pregnancies because of the need to have the first, the only, or the last child or because they have decided to carry and deliver and unplanned pregnancy because it may be their last chance. When something goes wrong or threatens to go wrong, there may be guilt and sorrow.

Genetic Concerns

Genetic concerns complicate the psychosocial needs of these women and their families. The decision to undergo genetic testing is not always easy. Some women are certain that they would abort a genetically defective foetus; others are equally resolute that they would not. Others agonize over what they would do. These additional concerns are superimposed on normal on normal worries. This phenomenon, called the tentative pregnancy, occurs when women are unsure whether they are mothers or "carriers of a defective foetus." They are concerned because there is higher ratio of Down's syndrome and other autosomal trisomies.

Chorionic villus sampling shortens the waiting period for genetic diagnosis. Even so, a considerable amount of anxiety is generated. Geneticounsellors can furnish the client with statistics that can put risks into perspective and aid in the decision to undergo or to forego genetic testiing.

Issues of Control

Issues particularly important are control and past coping behaviours. Many women have been successful in their careers by manipulating situations to their advantage. When faced with a situation in which they are not in control and must trust others, severs, anxiety develops. Their past coping behaviours will not be effective, and this will intensify their anxiety. They feel unable to take care of themselvels and often have little experience in relying on others during times of need. The educational level of the client must be considered when recommending literature.

An important part of anticipatory guidance is letting the client know that her old ways of dealing with situations need to change during the pregnancy. A newborn disrupts its parents' life-style tremendously and the client needs to begin to consider this during pregnancy.

Reassurance

In the past, many studies grouped genetic defects with all other problems for the older woman. In fact, some research shows a better outcome when the mother is older. There is a reduced risk of preterm birth, infant mortality, and sudden infant death syndrome. It is important to distinguish between women delaying childbirth to have the first child and women who have had several children before age of 35 years. For the latter group of women, there is an increased rate of twins and triplets.

For women having a first pregnancy later in life, fear about the infant's health and survival often becomes the dominant feeling. This may be the "last egg in the basket" and this very much valued. As a result, cesarean birth is chosen more often by obstetricians, and indicated an overcautious approach to birth problems. None theless, the woman approaching a first birth in her later reproductive years may be encouraged by the positive findings of greater satisfaction with motherhood and greater commitment to parenting.

ADOLESCENT GRAVIDA

The adolescent mother and her family create a particularly difficult problem. The needs can be so extensive that care will be fragmented and ineffective unless an inter-disciplinary team approach coordinates the school, social, and health care services.

Incidence of Adolescent Pregnancy

The scope of adolescent pregnancy is enormous. The mean age of menarche around of 12 years. Forty two percent of girls and 64 per cent of young boys are sexually active by age 18.

A family's reaction to teenage pregnancy varies considerably. In certain ethnic and cultural groups, teenage parenting is common. Indeed, the girl's mother may have been a teenage parent herself. In these cases, the situation is not a crisis. In other families, major problems result.

Developmental Stage

The developmental stage of adolescence is described as identity vs role confusion, Erikson speaks about the essence of the crisis of adolescence, including the dramatic body changes and drives, and the need to be accepted to conform and to be someone. Teenagers role models are their peers and television and movie personalities, not their parents, older sibings or teachers.

Need for Sex Education

Adolescents lack knowledge about their bodies and bodily changes. Many parents find it difficult to talk with their children about maturation, sex, birth control, and parenting. Parents may not understand that this information is vital and that it must be given early. Furstenbert (1980) found that although 59 per cent of mothers frequently talked to their daughters about sex, most of the messages were "not to get mixed up with boys" and "not to do anything she would be sorry for later." This is hardly the information teenagers require. On the other hand, 50 per cent of birth control used contraception at least occasionally.

Need for Family Planning

The pregnancy rate among teenagers is so high because only one in three sexually active teens always uses contraceptives. Only about half of these use the most effective methods. The most common reasons given by teenagers for not using contraception are (1) they do not feel they will get pregnant and (2) they did not anticipate having intercourse. In Piaget's cognitive framework, adolescents are in the transition from the phase of concrete operations to the phase of formal operations, which is usually not reached until adulthood. In formal operations, the individual can think abstractly, consider alternatives, and recognize the consequences of behaviour. Until the adolescent reaches this stage, she will be likely to take risks without considering consequences.

On the average, teenagers wait almost one year to attend a family planning clinics after initiating intercourse. Half of all teenage pregnancies occur in the first 6 months after initiation of intercourse and 20 per cent in the first month alone.

Experience in other countries where teenage sexual activity is just as prevalent shows that the rate of pregnancy can be reduced by making effective contraception readily available. High-quality sex education programmes have been found to be useful only if accompanied by provision of supplies. Programmes designed to reach out to sexually inexperienced teenagers to inform them about contraceptive methods and where to obtain them are most effective.

While the national debate continues over where and by whom sex education programmes should be taught, research is clear; we must begin early and be specific. Teenagers are at risk not only for pregnancy but also for STDs including HIV infection. It is unlikely that the State will soon develop policies to encourage early sex education programmes even though the urgency of the rates of HIV infection and of teenage pregnancy demand it. The media has begun to modify its approach to sexuality because of the risk of HIV infection, but there is still much to be done. The emphasis needs to be on responsible sexuality, including abstinence, as well as on contraception.

As nurses, role is two fold; nurse must care for adolescent parents and support their parents and teachers in efforts to communicate about responsible sexual behaviour before pregnancy occurs and after its termination, either by abortion or delivery. Parents and teachers need education also. The fears that are talking about sex encourage earlier sexual activity are unfounded in communities are reduced and healthy attitudes towards childbearing and childrearing are acquired.

Influences

Some teenagers, either consciously or subconsciously, want to have babies because their friends have them, or because they want something they can succeed in doing, something to love, or something to make them feel important or special. Some teenagers want to keep their boyfriends and fear that refusing to have sex will drive them away. Some want to gain attention from their parents. These are all adolescent ways of expressing basic needs for belonging, love and self-esteem.

Denial of Pregnancy

Many adolescents do not expect to become pregnant. They may deny it until the signs are so obvious they can no longer be ignored by family members. It is common for teenagers to diet and wear constricting clothes to hide their condition and to succeed in hiding the pregnancy until it is quite advanced, sometimes until delivery. The levels of denial in some teenagers and their families can be quite high. Nurse must be especially concerned about a teenager who arrives in labour and delivery, claiming she did not know that she was pregnant. She may have been brought in by her family, with whom she was living, who also claim they were unaware of it. This may truly be denial of way for her family to hide their embarrassment about the pregnancy on the delay in care. Nevertheless, the ability of the family to care for the infant in these cases requires further assessment by the interdisciplinary team members.

Adolescent Fathers

The adolescent father is often neglected in these situations. Some families are angry and upset and will ostracize him. At other times, both families pool their financial, physical and emotional resources to support the young parents as they care for their infant. Some young men are not involved by their own choice, but others may distance themselves because they assume that they do not have a role to play or they are not needed by their partner for support. They may fear that they will be forced to marry and provide financial support before they are capable of doing so, or be "saddled" with 20 years of child support payments. These young men are in the same developmental stage as the young women. "Teenage fathers have many problems. They are young; are capable of sexual reproduction, but not considered adults; are cognitively and psychologically immature: possess few legal rights and are out of life cycle synchrony with their peers.

Adolescent fathers are less likely to receive a high school diploma or general education diploma by age 20. Fathering a child as an adolescent is associated with reduced levels of education in general. Lower educational levels limit career choices and earning potential. Adequate wages for male employment have been found to be important in determining the success of early marriage.

Problems with Economic Support

Adolescent parents are rarely able to support themselves and their children. Optimally, the family should be involved early. Detailed arrangements must be worked out, and allowing enough time before delivery makes the crisis less overwhelming. Building on and supplementing family resources and only substituting for families when absolutely necessary is believed to be the most effective way to help adolescents and their infants.

Women who become parents as teenagers are less likely to complete their education or to be employed, especially if they are younger than 17 years. Availability of child care, especially by family members, is a crucial factor in the mothers returning to school.

Women who become parents as teenagers are more likely to be welfare dependent, especially those who are very young at the birth of their first child. They are more likely to have large families especially if they get married. They are also less likely to be happily married.

After the first child, 80 per cent of teenage mothers state that they plan to wait at least? years before having another child, In Furstenberc's study less than half did. He found some had already reached or exceeded the number of children they ever wanted within 5 years. Those who returned to school had a lower rate of recurrent, early pregnancy.

Parenting success: Adolescents generally have unrealistic expectations of the abilities and needs of an infant. Responsibilities of parenting may be difficult, Sacrificing personal pleasure for the needs of another is a developmental growth task not usually completed by this age. There is evidence that the majority of teenage parents do well with proper intervention. Teenage mothers have been observed to have adequate maternal warmth and physical interaction. Many, however, do not talk much to their infants.

These findings indicate a need for more parenting education as well as assessment for potential problems. Child abuse is not more common, as some have thought. The presence of a supportive extended family is an assential factor in development of good parenting skills.

Choices: Today, a pregnant woman has three choices; to abort, to have the child and place it for foster care or adoption, or to have the child and raise it. Adolescent parents have the same choices, but may need to be guided through the decision-making process. In some areas legal requirements for a waiting period before elective abortion and parental notification affect these choices. Some teenagers have sought confirmation of pregnancy and then chosen abortion without involving family members. They tend to be older and more goal directed. Others tell their parents or a relative and enlist their support. The way in which the situation is handled depends on the teenager's relationship with the father of the child and his family, and their cultural and ethnic backgrounds and beliefs. These and other variables may interact in a variety of ways. More teenagers are intending to raise their children with the help of ways. More teenagers are intending to raise their children with the help of grand-mothers or aunts than in previous decades.

Nursing Management

Nursing Diagnoses

These diagnoses may be selected to be included in a complete nursing care plan for the pregnant adolescent or the more mature gravida.

- Ineffective individual coping related to developmental level, situation in which pregnancy occurs
- Coping, family potential for growth related to responses to adolescent or mature pregnant woman.

Planning/Objectives

- Recognizes potential for growth in the situation
- Chooses to obtain pre-natal care
- Follows through on referrals
- Seeks support for expressed needs
- Recognizes foetal needs for a healthy start.

Nursing Interventions

Nurse must first gain an understanding of the teenager's situation when she comes in for the visit. She has chosen to come in for the visit. She has chosen to come in, which reflects a big decision for her. She may be afraid to tell her parents and may need assistance, or, she may have been brought in by her mother, and the dynamics between them will reveal much about the situation. She and her family may need a variety of assistance programmes such as, public assistance, or general social service. Unless you learn this at the first encounter, the young woman may be lost ot follow-up. Do not wait for her to volunteer information. It is important to engage her trust, a difficult task because an adolescent may not trust easily and may have difficulty, relating to authority figures. The adolescent fears breach of confidentiality. A climate of strict confidentiality is vital is all nursing situations, but is crucial for adolescents. For these reasons, care is best given in a setting that has providers who specialize in adolescent health care.

Respond to the adolescent's needs rather than to her behaviour. For example when asked how her mother feels about the pregnancy, a teenager may state "Fine" When probed further, she may get angry and respond, "why do you care perhaps she is afraid to tell you that she has not told her mother or that her mother is insisting that she have an abortion. Respond to the need; do not react. For example, state, "Lots of pregnant girls of your age have real problems when they tell their parents or are even afraid to tell them. Let us talk about that.". In this way, she is given the opportunity to talk to a provider who shows caring and understanding.

Because she may not want her parents to know where she is going and is concerned that you will call them, a teenager may not give correct information. She may not be able to secure the insurance information on her own. Ability to pay or provide insurance information should also become a barrier in provision of care of adolescents.

Identify the girl's readiness to use referrals. Ask her to write down sequence of what has been planned together, because tension will prevent her remembering what to do. Follow through with telephone contact if she skips appointments—if her family is aware of her condition. If she still does not tell them early in the pregnancy, ask her for a way to establish contact. Keep gently urging full disclosure of the family, because it will become evident in a very short time that she is pregnant. Help her identify othersources of support in her extended family circle.

The key is to keep the teen parent in the health care system and to keep her in school, since there appear to be no adverse effects on the mothers and infants, if quality care is provided, such care becomes of prime importance. In the most effective settings, the supportive primary nurse adds the new client to her case load and follows through the pregnancy with her. The impersonal nature of large clinics is counter productive for the adolescent mother.

Peer support groups in schools for pregnant adolescents or in clinics are helpful in preparing teens to cope with the demands and sacrifices of parenting. Educational programmes and literature should be geared to teens. Providers must like working with teens and understand their unique problems and responses. The teen's father needs to be involved as much as possible. He should be invited to clinic visits and parenting classes and assisted to see his role in providing physical and emotional support for his partner and his child.

The nurse by her own attitude will influcence how well the teen follows through on care.

Evaluation

The results of comprehensive care for a teenage mother would show some of the following:
- Stated she learned a great deal about herself and problem solving.
- Followed through on referrals and obtaining assistance.
- Involved father of child in planning and in care of infant.
- Followed guidelines for nutrition and self-care during the pregnancy.
- Attended school and parenting classes.

ATTACHMENT AND BONDING

Background of Bonding Theory

As early as 1952, scientists wrote about imprinting behaviour in birds and other animals and described a critical period during which attachments between the mother and her young must be formed. Separation during this critical time resulted in rejection of the young. Researchers observed that human mothers separated for long periods of time from premature or sick infants often had difficulty in accepting them when the emergency was over; this observation led researchers to wonder whether there was a time for attachment in humans.

Researcher demonstrated that this period exists in the first few hours after birth. They noted that close physical contact between an infant and its mother set in motion an intricate set of reciprocal actions whereby each stimulated and rewarded the other. Based on their research on animals and humans, they hypothesized that around the time of delivery, hormonal stimulation prepared the mother to receive and respond to her newborn. If this opportunity were missed, the mother-infant pair never bonded.

Humans give birth throughout the year and bear young that are wholly dependent for an extended period, requiring a relationship that is specific, stable and enduring. Strong feelings of protectiveness and caring are evoked in human mothers even after their children have reached adulthood and may have been separated from them for years. Further more, unlike maternal behaviour in animals, maternal behaviour in humans must be flexible, adapting to the circumstances and the developmental level of the child.

Researcher also studied the effects of early skin-to-skin contact on later mothering behaviour. In their study, a group of poor, inner city mothers who had 1 hour of contact immediately with their newborns and 5 hours of contact each day in the hospital were compared with a control group who received traditional, more isolated contact, only during four hourly feeding periods. These early-contact mothers showed differences in maternal behaviour, including holding infants more affectionately and showing more concern for them three months and one year later.

Early and unlimited access to the infant is desirable because it enhances the mother's feeling of competence and self-esteem but the early studies are flawed. Although the study group of earlycontact mothers showed positive changes in expected behaviour patterns, the effects of the extra attention by nurses and others given to this group were not taken into account. Moreover, existing differences in temperament of mothers and infants were not considered. Later studies failed to demonstrate any lasting differences.

Changes in maternity care now allow extended contact between parents and infants. If a baby is high-risk or ill and separated from its parents in the ICU, the parents may be anxious about "Nursing" bonding. The nurse can be very helpful by assuring them that although the early recovery period is the ideal time for attachment to take place, it is not the only time. The mother who began attachment with visualization early in pregnancy is unlikely to be seriously hindered if initial interaction with her newborn must be deferred. Hormonal stimulation may contribute to the attachment, but social and cultural components play a far more influential role.

Encouraging Attachment and Bonding during Pregnancy

Around the fourth month of pregnancy the expectant mother becomes increasingly aware of her foetus as a separate individual through

Table 4.23: Nursing care plan of childbearing families related to potential or actual stress caused by cultural diversity

Problem	*Reason objective*	*Nurses intervention*	*Rationale*
Communication, impaired verbal related to language barriers	Woman will have an opportunity to share information and stages she understands what is explained to her	1. Arrange for a family or staff member interpreter as needed	1. Interpreter can provide support for woman and help lessen her anxieties; poor communication can result in time delays, errors, and misunderstanding of intent
		2. Clearly define instructions in woman's language of origin	2. A shared language is necessary for communication to take place
		3. Provide written instructions in woman's language wherever possible	3. Written instruction can be reviewed at less stressful time by client; in some cases it is necessary to determine if person can read
		4. Explain the use and purpose of all instruments and equipment, along with the effects or possible effects on the mother and fetus	4. Education of family lessens anxiety and provides family with sense of control
		5. Provide opportunities for clarification and questions	5. Learning takes time; repetition of important material promotes learning; nurse can determine woman's understanding of information and clarify misconceptions
Family coping; compromised related to isolation, different customs, attitudes, or beliefs	Family members will state that they feel welcome and safe in the environment provided	1. Encourage prenatal classes and a visit to the maternity unit before delivery	1. Families who have clear, accurate information can better participate in labor and delivery; viewing the delivery setting before using it decreases anxiety about the unknown
		2. Inform families about routines, visiting hours, significant persons who can assist in labor and delivery, and location of newborn after delivery	2. Families have different expectations of the health-care system; they may hesitate to ask questions because of shyness or fear of "losing face"
		3. Determine and respect practices and values of family and incorporate them into nursing care plans as much as possible	3. Clarification of culturally specific values and practices will avoid misunderstanding and conflict with the nurse's value system; nursing care plans promote, organization of care and communication among staff members

movement and begins to develop feelings for it. Before this time, her feelings for it were for an abstract notion of what "a baby" is like. From the time of quickening onward, she becomes acquainted with her infant by identifying foetal parts, and by nothing its response to changes in its environment such as when she is anxious or taking a warm shower or is listening to loud or soothing music. The more she becomes familiar with her infant's responses to her actions the more she feels, she "knows" the infant before birth. The fact that mothers form an attachment to their unborn foetuses is indicated by their grief when their infants are stillborn.

Nurse can encourage pre-natal attachment while perform usual care-giving tasks. Ask the woman what she calls her infant; it can be the name that will be put on the birth certificate or an affectionate nickname such as "the lump" or "Thumpet". This name helps her to personalize the infant within. Help her to examine behaviours to identify "who the infant is like" in her or her partner's family. When the woman complains "This baby is always moving, "ask, "who in your family is like that?" Encourage her to pay attention to foetal activity and to note what behaviour on her part seems to influence the infant to move or kick.

An ability to identify foetal parts can be encouraged by guiding the pregnant mother's hands to identify the hard, round head; the long, curved back; the softness of the rump; the fleeting movements and a surprisingly large number of prods from heels, toes, knees, shoulders, elbows, and hands. She can be urged to soothe and quiet her baby by massaging, stroking or rocking.

Nurse can also use a Doppler that amplifies foetal heart tones during pre-natal visits to help parents identify its various sounds; the hoof beat rhythm of the foetal heart tones; the slower, more measured rate of the mother's heartbeat; the swooshing sound as the blood rushes through the umbilical cord; and the gurgling of the mother's intestines. Time spent in this way gives the parents a feeling of increased knowledge and reduced uncertainty.

When a sonogram has been done, this can also be used as an aid for discussion on attachment. Some women report that they felt that the infant was real for the first time when they saw its features in the sonogram. The literature has shown that women who are concerned for the infant's survival often fear attachment. However, women who have experienced threatened miscarriage or similar problems often express positive feelings for their infants after viewing the sonogram. Encourage parents to request a copy of their infant's "picture".

By the end of the third-trimester a strong attachment should have formed for the infant. If the mother demonstrates obvious negative behaviours during later pregnancy, closely observe post delivery interactions. Phases of bonding occur throughout pregnancy and parenting. The process goes through phases of acquaintance, with cues of acceptance being exchanged, to attachment, with affectional exchanges when parents and the infant are in close contact. These exchanges are more positive than negative. Nursing interventions during pre-natal care can be very supportive of the young family. Nursing interventions during pre-natal care can be very supportive of the young family. Remember, in most family-infant groupings bonding will occur a positive, loving relationship that will be able to endure over time and distance.

CULTURAL DIVERSITY

Child bearing families have cultural diversity, which may lead to stress. The nursing care plan of stress caused by cultural diversity are as given in Table 4.23.

C H A P T E R

5 Assessment and Management of Intranatal Period

INTRODUCTION

Intranatal care begins with the onset of labour and after delivery which includes the examination of the mother and baby to confirm both are in good condition. The aims of good intranatal care are:

- Thorough asepsis.
- Delivery with minimum injury to the infant and mother.
- Readiness to deal with complications such as prolonged labour. APH, convulsions, malpresentations, prolapsed cord, etc.
- Care of the baby at delivery resuscitation, care of the cord, care of the eyes, etc.

During late pregnancy, the woman and foetus prepare for the labour process. The foetus has grown and developed in preparation for extrauterine life. The woman has under one various physiological adaptations during pregnancy, that prepare her for birth and motherhood. Labour and birth represent the end of pregnancy, the beginning of extrauterine life for the newborn and a charge in the lives of the family.

Labour is the process, whereby, the products of conception are expelled from the uterus after the 24th week of gestation:

- Normal labour or eutocia is the process of expulsion per vaginum of a mature live foetus presented by vertex followed by the placenta and membranes spontaneously without any complication or delay.
- Premature labour is defined as labour occurring before the 36th week of gestation.
- Prolonged labour is defined as labour lasting in excess of 24 hours in primigravida and 16 hours in a multigravida.

FACTORS AFFECTING LABOUR

Labour is the process by which the uterus expels or attempts to expel the foetus, placenta and amniotic sac. It is accomplished by rhythmic contraction of the uterus. Anatomic landmarks of the uterus important during labour. Pressure against cervix created by the foetus and amniotic sac results in effacement and dilations of the cervix which allow passage of the foetus from the uterus through the cervix and birth canal and into the extrauterine environment. To accomplish this process, at least five factors affect the process of labour and birth. These are easily remembered as the five 'P's.

1. P-Powers are the contractions of the uterus.
2. P-Passage way (birth canal) in the bony pelvis, cervix, vagina and introitus.
3. P-Passengers are the foetus, amniotic sac, umbilical cord, and placental.
4. P-Position of the mother.
5. P-Psychological response of the mother

And other factors such as place of birth preparation, type of care provider and procedure implemented are also important.

Normal labour requires that the powers be sufficient to expel the foetus, that the passage be of adequate size to allow descent and expulsion of the foetus and that the passengers be of average size and in positions to allow negotiation of the passage during labour.

1. THE POWERS

The uterus provides the force necessary to expel the foetus. Effective contraction of the uterus leads to changes in the cervix necessary for delivery.

Uterine contractions: Normally the uterus begins to contract effectively 280 days after the last menstrual period (LMP) or 266 gestational days after ovulation and fertilization. However, irregularities in the menstrual cycle make precise calculation of gestational age difficult. Amniotic fluid studies and ultrasonography can be used to more accurate determine gestational age of the foetus and the estimated date of birth (EDB, or EDD).

Contractions supply the involuntary or primary power for birth. During the last stage of labour the woman must add, by pushing down, the voluntary or secondary powers to complete the birth.

The muscles have a unique structure that provides the ability to contract from the fundus down and in a mesh like fashion, to constrict the numerous blood vessels that cross the muscle to enter the placenta. The lower uterine segment in contract, is stretched by the pressure of the foetus and fluids and does not rhythmically contract in the same way. This allows the foetus to descend smoothly.

After birth the empty uterus rapidly reduces its size by contraction. The myometrium thickens and the fundus moves, within a few minutes, from just under the diaphragm to below the umbilicus.

Uterine muscle becomes increasingly sensitive to oxytocin as birth approaches. Largely blocked during pregnancy by hormonal action, oxytocin levels rise slightly as labour approaches. Prostaglandins also affect contractions; increased amounts have been found in amniotic fluid as labour nears. Finally there are pace-makers in the myometrium; groups of these pacemakers trigger rhythmic contractions.

Uterine contractions originate in the fundus, the location of the highest concentration of muscle cells. The contraction then spreads into the lower segment. The contractility of the uterus increases as pregnancy progresses. Mils contractions occur in frequently throughout pregnancy. These contractions, which do not change the cervix are short in duration and occur irregularly. During the last month of gestation, they increase in frequency and may occur every 10 to 20 minutes. They can be palpated by an observer but usually are not experienced as discomfort by the mother. If measured by a dynamometer, they rarely exceed 20 mmHg or last longer than 60 to 80 seconds. During late pregnancy these contraction patterns, which also are known as Braxton-Hicks Contractions may be misunderstood for preterm labour.

Effective contractions provide the powers with which to efface and dilate the cervix and then, with maternal pushing efforts, expel the foetus and placenta. Each contraction has three parts: an increment (increasing intensity). an acme (peak), and a decrement (decreasing intensity). The increment is steep and rapid, whereas the decrement is more prolonged and gradual. The contraction is a bell-shaped curve, with a steeper slope during increment. A relaxation phase (decrement) lasts for two-thirds of contraction. Resting tone (lowest intramniotic pressure between contractions) amounts to 10 mmHg. The area above 10 mmHg is considered an active pressure area. Pain threshold is intrauterine pressure above which contraction is painful, about 10 to 15 mmHg over resting tone. As labour progresses, the tonus or resting tone may begin to rise.

The degree of relaxation between contractions is very important because it allows the foetus and uterine muscles to recover from the stress of the contractions. During the interval or resting phase the uterus and placenta refill with blood, allowing for the exchange of oxygen, carbon dioxide, and nutrients at the placenta. A uterus does not relax sufficiently between contractions when there are hypertonic contractions. This contraction pattern is abnormal and may result in foetal hypoxia or a rapid, uncontrolled delivery. If the uterus is unable to contract strongly enough to be effective, it is in hypotonic labour. Abnormally slow or non-progressive labour pattern is called dystocia. If the uterus is incapable of the necessary powers to allow progress of labour, the result is a prolonged labour phase caused by uterine dysfunction.

Contractions may be monitored by palpation of the fundus, by external monitoring, or by internal pressure catheter. Contractions must be assessed for frequency, intensity and duration frequency is the time from the beginning of one contraction to the beginning of the next, usually recorded in minutes. Strength or intensity is the force of the contraction and is recorded as mild, moderate, or strong. Duration is the time from the beginning to the end of contraction, usually recorded in seconds. The nurse uses this information when the woman is in active labour and assess contractions to identify a pattern of effective contractions.

Although external monitoring gives only an approximation, contractions are recorded as mild, moderate, or strong contractions by palpation or by monitor readings as follows:

By Palpation	*By Internal Monitor*
Mild Under	40 mmHg
Moderate	40-70 mmHg.
Strong	Over 70 mmHg.

Cervical changes: Effective contractions lead to progressive changes in the cervix. With each contraction the cervix draws slowly and progressively up into the lower uterine segment. This shortening and thinning of the cervix is called effacement. The force of the contractions, with the pressure of the presenting part and amniotic sac, causes cervical dilatation (opening). There is a difference in primigravid and multigravid effacement and dilation can occur at the same time.

The cervix itself must be ready for labour. Normally it is firm, resembling the consistency of the tip of one's nose. For labour to be effective, it must be soft or "ripe" partially dilated and effaced, and tipped forward or anteriorly in the vagina. These changes normally occur during the weeks before the onset of labour.

The progress of effacement and dilation is assessed by internal vaginal examination. These examinations should be performed only as needed. Strict asepsis must be maintained to avoid introduction of bacteria into the birth canal.

2. THE PASSAGE WAY

The passage way, or birth canal is composed of the mother's rigid bony pelvis and the soft tissues of the cervix, pelvic floor vagina, and introitus (the external opening to the vagina). Although the soft tissues, particularly the muscular layer of the pelvic floor, contribute to vaginal birth of the foetus, the maternal pelvis plays far greater role in the labour process because the foetus must successfully accommodate itself to this relatively rigid passage way. Therefore, size and shape of the pelvis must be determined before childbirth begins.

Pelvis: Pelvis is the bony ring through which body weight is distributed to the lower extremities. It consists of the sacrum, coccyx and two innominate bones. The innominate bones are joined to the sacrum by the sac folliac joints, the sacrum and coccyx joined by the sacrococcygeal joint, and innominate bones are joined together in front of by the symphysis pubis. Anatomic land marks important during assessment of the adequacy of the pelvis are the ischial spines and the ischial tuberosities. There appears to be very little flexibility in pelvic joints; however, because ligaments are made more stretchable by relaxin, some flexibility in the pelvis possible during pregnancy and birth.

The pelvis is divided into the true or false section at linea terminalis. The false pelvis although essential to support abdominal organs, is of no obstetric significance. The true pelvis is the bony birth passage. By a vaginal delivery, this passage must be adequate size and shape to allow the movement of the foetus.

Passage: Each pelvis is classified according to the shape of the inlet. The gynecoid pelvis (the classic female type) is ideal for birth. The platypelloid (the flat type) shape allows the foetus to enter only occipit traverse position because the anteroposterior diameter is too short. The android pelvis resembling the male pelvis, forces the foetal head to engage in an occiput posterior (OP) position because of cephalo-pelvis disproportion (lack of fit). The antropoid shape resembling the pelvis of anthropoid ape tends to result in an OP position. These positions usually result in long labour and delivery with forceps or require caesarean birth.

The pelvis is divided into the inlet plane, midpelvic plane and outlet. The inlet plane is assessed by the diagonal conjugate, obstetric conjugate and conjugate vera. The diagonal conjugate is the most significant measurement and measured during vaginal examination by placing the tip of the middle finger on the sacral promontory and then marking where the symphysis pubis touches the index finger. If the measurement is atleast 11.5 cm the pelvic inlet is of adequate size.

The middle pelvic plane can be assessed by X-ray examination. The planes of greatest and least pelvic dimension reflects this plane.

Inadequacies may be suspected if the ischial spines are prominent if the pelvic side walls are narrow, or if the curve of the sacrum is shallow. The interspinous diameter (usually 10 cm) is smallest diameter which the foetus must accommodate. The sacrum, coccyx and ischial spine can be palpated by the examinner's fingers. The coccyx should be movable.

The plane of outlet is assessed by measurement of the transverse diameter, the distance between the ischial tuberosities. A measurement of 8 cm or greater in considered adequate. The pubic arch must allow passage of the foetal head as it extends during birth. The angle of the arch should be at least 90 degrees.

Soft tissues: The soft tissues of the passage way include the distensible lower uterine segment, cervix, pelvic floor muscles, vagina and introitus. Before labour begins, the uterus is composed of the uterine body (corpus) and cervix (neck). After labour has begun, uterine contractions cause the uterine body to have a thick and muscular upper segment and a thin walled passive, muscular lower segment. A physiologic retraction ring separates the two segments. The lower uterine segment gradually distends to accommodate the intrauterine contents as the wall of the upper segment thickens and its accommodating capacity is reduced. The contractions of the uterine body thus expert downward pressure on the foetus, pushing it against the cervix.

The cervix effaces (thins) and dilates (opens) sufficiently to allow the first foetal portion to descend into the vagina. As the foetus descends the cervix is actually down upward and over the first portion.

The pelvic floor is a muscular layer that separates the pelvic cavity above from the perineal space below. This structure helps the foetus rotate anteriorly as it passes through the birth canal. As noted earlier, the soft tissues of the vagina develop throughout pregnancy until at term the vagina can dilate to accommodate the foetus and permit passage of the foetus to the external world.

3. THE PASSENGERS

The passengers are the foetus and the placenta. Various foetal factors, including lie, attitude, presentation, position, and station are assessed during labour.

The foetus: To negotiate the maternal passageway, the foetus must fit through the bony pelvis. The foetal head is the largest, least compressible, and most common presenting part. It consists of seven bony plates separated by suture lines. These bony plates, which are soft and not totally ossified, may change position slightly, resulting in molding. Molding allows the foetal head to adopt to the shape of the bony pelvis.

The presenting diameter of the foetal head varies greatly, depending on the degree of its flexion or extension. Ideally the head should be flexed, chin on the chest; thus the smallest diameter, the suboccipito-bregmatic, comes first.

Lie: Lie is the relationship of the long axis of the foetus to the long axis of the mother. Until the ninth month the foetus has had room to move in the uterus and has taken a variety of positions. During the last few weeks of pregnancy as the foetus approaches the maximum size and the amount of amniotic fluid decreases, the lie becomes stabilized. In 99 per cent of pregnancies at term the foetus exhibits a longitudinal lie. The infant in a longitudinal lie. If the focus is sideways, the lie is transverse.

Attitude: Attitude refers to the position of foetal body parts in relation to themselves. The foetus commonly assumes the "foetal position", with the back curled, head flexed, and legs folded on the abdomen. The arms are at the sides or are flexed and crossing the chest.

Presentation: Presentation refers to that portion of the foetus coming first to the pelvic inlet. There are three major presentations, vertex, breech and shoulder. The incidence of these presentations is 95 per cent of vertex, 3.5 per cent breach, and 0.5 per cent shoulder. The presentation determines the presenting part, the part of the foetus closest to the cervix, and that can be felt by the examining finger during vaginal examination. Presentations other than vertex may result in prolonged labour or a caesarean delivery.

4. POSITION

Position refers to the relationship between a point of reference on the presenting part and the four quadrants of the maternal pelvis. The point of reference in a cephalic presentations is the occiput, in a face presentation, the chin (mentum), and in a breech presentation, the sacrum. The foetus is commonly in the left occiput transverse (LOT) position at engagement and rotates to left occiput anterior (LOA) as it descends through the pelvis. This means that the occiput of the foetus is directed toward the mother's left abdominal surface as the foetus descends through the birth canal. Figure 5.1 shows the foetus in an LOA

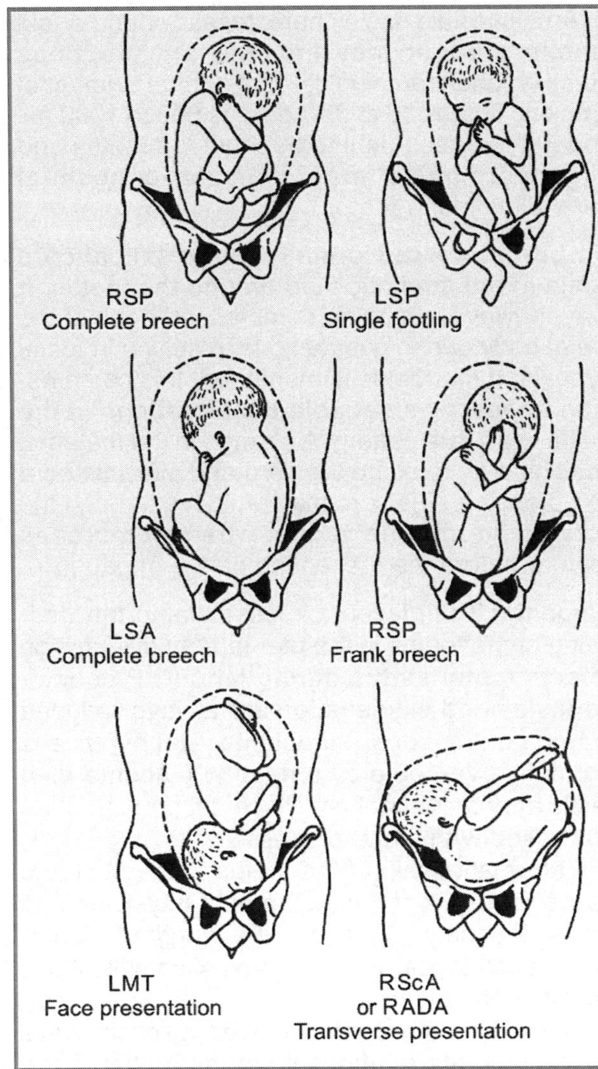

Fig. 5.1: Various presentations and positions

position. There are six possible positions for each of the presentations, which are demonstrated on the pelvic model (Table 5.1).

Foetal position and presentation can be assessed by abdominal palpation, vaginal examination and ultrasonography. Figure 5.2 indicates the suture lines that would be palpated vaginally with a foetus in an LOA position. Figure 5.3 illustrates other positions of the foetal head. Abdominal palpation is performed by using leopold's maneuvers. Any variation in position, lie, or presentation can adversely affect the progress of labour. More attention has been directed toward changing position of the foetus by maternal positioning. An occiput transferse (OT)

Table 5.1: Possible variations in position

Presenting Part	*Foetal Point of Reference*	*Material Relationship*
Vertex	Occiput (O)	Anterior or posterior (A or P)
Face	Mentum (M)	
Brow	Brow (B)	Right or left side (R or L)
Buttocks (breech)	Sacrum (S)	
Feet	Sacrum (S)	Transverse (T)
Shoulder	Scapula (Sc)	

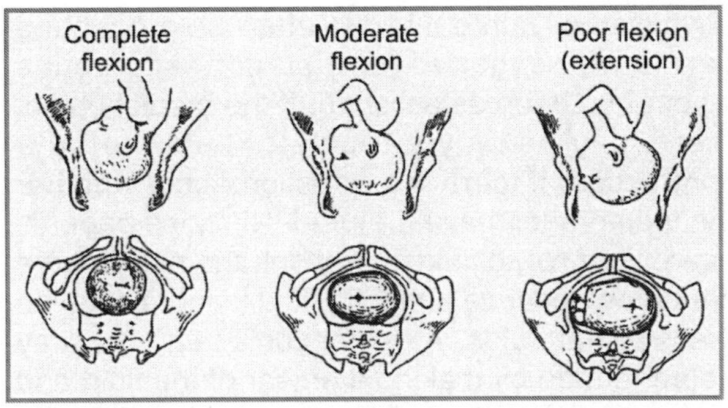

Complete flexion — Moderate flexion — Poor flexion (extension)

Fig. 5.2: Head diameters in various degrees of flexion. Complete flexion, moderate flexion, poor flexion (extension)

or occiput posterior (OP) position can be influenced by maternal positioning; standing, kneeling, leaning on hands and knees, or using the lateral Sims position may help to attain an occiput anterior (OA) position. There is a trend towards increased use of the external version (turning) to change breech presentations to vertex and thus facilitate vaginal delivery (see malposition) (Fig. 5.1).

Station: Station refers to the relationship of the presenting part to the ischial spines of the pelvic midplane when the presenting part is at the level of the ischial spines, it is said to be at a station; this is engagement. Levels above the spines are designated in centimeters by negative values, –1, –2, –3. Levels below the spines are designated in centimeters by negative positive values, +1, +2, +3, +4, down to the pelvic floor. A presenting part that does not descend to 0 station is called floating. If during labour the presenting part fails to descend a caesarean birth will be necessary.

Station is important when determining and comparing the rate of descent with normal rates.

An arrest of descent can be detected, which usually indicates cephalopelvic disproportion (CPD). If stations do not progress, operative birth is chosen.

Amniotic fluid: Membranes, of the amniotic sac, normally remain intact until middle or late labour. The surrounding fluid will equalize pressures on all parts of the foetus. A pocket of fluid the forewaters, cushions the presenting part and is considered a protection from the pressures exerted by the cervix and uterine muscle.

The amniotic sac or membranes may rupture spontaneously (SROM) before or during labour or be artificially ruptured (AROM or ARM) by a physician or nurse midwife after the presenting part is well engaged (at 0 station) and active labour has been established. If the break is high, there may be only a trickle of fluid during a contraction. If there is a question about whether the membranes have ruptured. Nitrazine paper is used. If amniotic fluid is present, the paper turns dark blue because amniotic fluid is more alkaline that vaginal fluids. A microscopic test also may be performed by making a smear of the fluid and then observing for ferning, a fern-like crystallization of sodium chloride.

When membranes rupture, the foetal heart rate should be checked. If the rupture is accompanied by a gush of fluid and the head is not well engaged, the umbilical cord may be washed downward and be compressed between the presenting part and the cervix. If the membranes are ruptured artificially (ARM or AROM) by the physician, the foetal heart beat should be checked before and after the procedure.

The amniotic fluid should be observed for colour, odour, and amount. Normally it is a clear, strew colour, with flecks of vernix caseosa, the creamy substance on the foetal skin. If it is a brownish-green, it indicates the presence of meconium caused by a relaxation of the foetal and aback sphincter. Note the colour and consistency of the fluid that contains meconium to determine whether it is thick or thin, dark or light green, or looks "old" or "new". Meconium-stained fluid at the introitus is considered normal in a breech presentation because of pressure on the baby's abdomen, which causes stooling. If the fluid is yellow, it indicates the presence of bilirubin. If any blood is present, it usually indicates haemorrhage (very rare).

Amniotic fluid has a characteristic odour. A foul smelling odour may indicate an infectious process, chorioamnionitis. The normal amount of amniotic fluid at 36 to 38 weeks is 800 to 1000 ml. and it decreases until term polyhydromnios and oligohydramnios may indicate congenital anomalies in the foetus.

Umbilical cord: Normally the umbilical cord floats in the amniotic fluid around the foetus. It may, however, become compressed against the foetal body during contractions, resulting in foetal hypoxia. If the foetus is monitored, this compression appears as variable decelerations in the foetal heart rate pattern. A change in the maternal position may relocate the cord and alleviate cord compression. The cord may prolapse through the cervix and into the vagina when membranes rupture before the presenting part is engaged.

Placenta: The placenta is essential to the well-being of the foetus in the uterus. Any dysfunction affects foetal status during labour. Placental perfusion and oxygenation are always reduced during contractions. Transient foetal hypoxia is normally overcome by a healthy placenta as it refills after a contraction. Placental problems are discussed with foetal distress.

The relationship of the foetus to the obstetric passage way is of interest to both physician and nurse. It usually influences the length of labour, preparation for delivery, and type of complications possibly encountered.

Some common words are used in special ways to describe the relationship of the foetus to the obstetric passage. For example, in maternal health care, one often refers to the following terms: lie, presentation, attitude, position, station, engagement, effacement and show.

Lie and presentation: The lie of an infant means the relationship of the long axis of the foetus to the long axis of the uterus. If the length of the foetus is parallel with the length of the uterus, the lie may be called "longitudinal". However, if the foetus lies crosswise in the uterus, the term transverse lie may be used.

Many times the term presentation is used synonymously with the phrase presenting part, the part of the baby that is coming or attempting to pass through the pelvic canal first. Headfirst placement is referred to as a cephalic presentation. Feet or buttocks presented first is termed breech. Presentation is usually determined by abdominal palpation and rectal, vaginal or ultrasonic examinations.

A breech birth is to be avoided, if possible, because it typically involves a greater risk to the infant. Today, an increasing number of obstetricians are attempting to turn selected breech presentations into cephalic. This is done by external manipulation, called version. Version is being used more frequently than has been the case in several years because of the simultaneous availability of electronic FHR monitoring continuous real-time sonograms, and medications (tocolytics) that help relax the uterus. The use of these tools has substantially increased the safety and success of versions and offers another alternative to abdominal or caesarean delivery. However, a version may be contraindicated for a number of reasons, e.g. if a condition also exists that would already call for a caesarean birth (an abnormally positioned placenta), if more than one baby occupies the uterus, or if the infant is exceptionally large.

Attitude: The attitude refers to the degree of flexion of the body, head (Fig. 5.2) and extremities of the foetus. The normal attitude is complete flexion. A well-flexed head presents the smallest cephalic diameter fewer mechanical problems in descent and delivery. This chin-chest posture makes possible the vertex delivery desired.

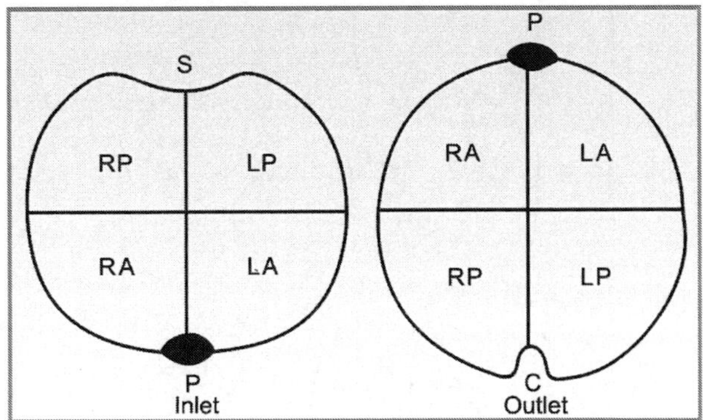

Fig. 5.3: Maternal pelvic quadrants, C—coccyx; P—pubic bones; S—sacrum

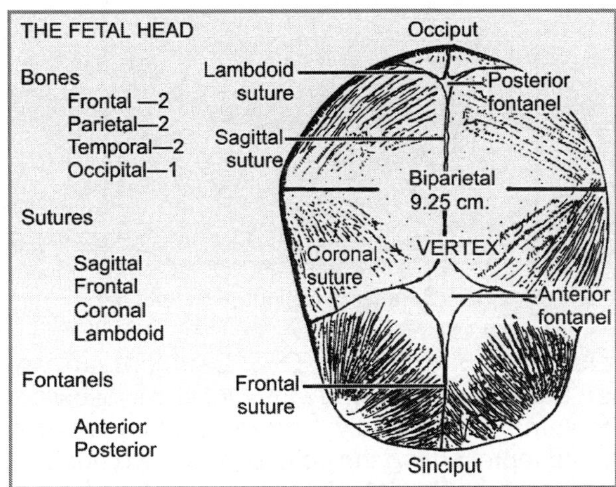

Fig. 5.4: Foetal head—physician's map

Position

The position is technically the relationship of a certain point of reference on the presenting part of the foetus to the pelvic quadrants of the mother. It gives more detailed information about foetal progress because the presenting part turns to adopt to the shape and size of the various parts of the birth canal. The maternal pelvic quadrants are identified as right and left posterior and right and left anterior (Fig. 5.3). The pelvic quadrants never change location. Sometimes the quadrants are seen from "below", that is, as they appear to the physician in front of the delivery table ready to receive the baby. Sometimes they are viewed from "above", from the vantage point of the unborn child entering the pelvis. The point of reference, of course, varies according to the presenting part discussed and the amount of flexion present. In the event of a well-flexed cephalic or vertex presentation the point of reference employes is the occipital bone, or occiput. It is the most accessible bone to identify in rectal or vaginal examination. The vault of the foetal skull is made up of three paired bones and one single bone separated by tough softer membranous seams, or sutures. It is fairly easy to follow these sutures with a gloved finger after sufficient cervical dilatation has occurred and to determine the placement of the occiput. The sutures tracay, and occiput is found between the top shafts of the Y behind the triangular posterior fontanel (Fig. 5.4).

To simplify reference to the various positions, the descriptive phrase usually begins with either right or left (of the mother's pelvis), followed by the point of reference used (on the foetus) and the adjectives anterior, posterior, or transverse (referring again to the part of the mother's pelvis towards which a particular point on the foetus is directed). Thus the most common vertex position

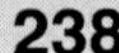

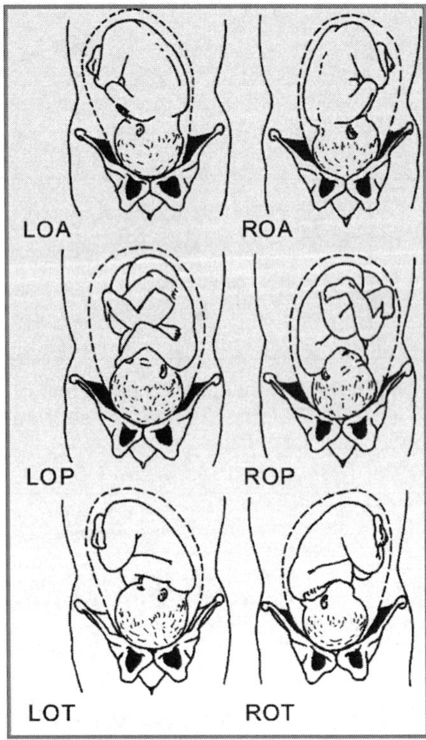

Fig. 5.5: Cephalic positions—vertex type

is left occiput anterior (LOA). Each presenting part has the possibility of eight positions following the same pattern. Only the middle initial or code letters representing the point of reference need to be changed (Fig. 5.5). For example,

1. Right occiput anterior ROA
2. Left occiput anterior LOA
3. Right occiput posterior ROP
4. Left occiput posterior LOP
5. Right occiput transferse ROT
6. Left occiput transverse LOT
7. Occiput at sacrum OS
   Occiput posterior OP
8. Occiput at the pubis
   Occiput anterior OA

Note that a transverse position is not the same thing as a transverse presentation, or lie. The letter "O" is usually employed only in the case of well-flexed or median vertex presentations. In the rare case of cephalic presentations demonstrating more deflexion, other points of reference must be sought, because the occiput is no longer available or meaningful to the examiner. In a brow presentation, the letter "F" for fronto is used, referring to the area of the anterior fontanel. Brow presentations are usually slow and difficult because of the increased diameter of the skull trying to force its way through the passage way. This presentation may require a caesarean birth. In instances of full extension of the head that results in a face presentation, the letter "M" for mentum, or chin, is used. Now a days, face presentations are rarely delivered vaginally because of a significant risk of injury to the infant's cervical spine (Fig. 5.5).

Breech presentations employ the sacrum or coccyx as a point of reference and the code letter "S" (Fig. 5.1). Characteristically, three types are described. A complete, or full breech involves the flexion of the foetus's legs, usually tailor fasion so that the buttocks and feet appear at the vaginal opening almost simultaneously. A frank or single breech occurs when the thighs are flexed on the abdomen with the extended legs against the trunk and the feet against the face (foot in the mouth posture). The term incomplete breech may indicate the initial appearance of either the feet or knees. The presentation of one or both feet is labelled a single or double footling, respectively. Frank breech is commonly encountered. Breech birth is associated with a higher perinatal mortality.

A transverse lie, sometimes called a shoulder presentation, usually involves the scapula or its upper lip, the acromion; for reference "Sc" or "A" is the code. The foetus lying crosswise in the uterus may be positioned with his back towards the front or back of his mother. The foetus's scapula posteriorly located, indicates the position of his back. Sometimes the terms dorso-anterior or dorso-posterior may be used to clarify this foetal position. A foetus whose shoulder and head occupy the right side of the mother's pelvis and whose back is towards her front is in the right acromildorso anterior position (RADA). This is an impossible presentation for normal birth.

Station and engagement: Another measurement related to the location of the foetus in the passage way is station, which is the relationship of the presenting part of the ischial spines of the pelvis. When the presenting part is at the level of the ischial spines, it is considered engaged, and the station is said to be 0. If the presentation is above the ischial spines, it is considered high, and the station is said to be –1, –2, etc. an estimate of its location in centimeters above the ischial spines. If the presenting part is below the ischial spines, the station is coded as +1, +2, etc. making an estimate in centimeters. (A centimeter is a little less then ½ inch) A plus station is considered low.

Effacement of dilatation (dilatation): One should not forget that frequent and progressively stronger uterine contractions creat the shortening and thinning (effacement) and dilatation (or dilation) of the cervix) to an opening approximately 10 cm (about 4 inches) in diameter. It should be noted that effacement may occur "silently" as the result of unobtrusive Braxton-Hicks contractions before the onset of more definitive, vigorous labour. Limited cervical dilatation (approximately 1 to 3 cm) may also take place before the onset of more definitive vigorous labour. Limited cervical dilatation (approximately 1 to 3 cm) may also take place before the onset of the formal labour period. The disappearance, or effacement of the cervical canal as its walls move upward to become part of the lower uterine segment is expressed in percent. Primiparas (nulliparas) usually undergo 100 per cent effacement before dilatation (Fig. 5.6). The cervix of a multipara typically undergoes effacement and dilatation at the same time.

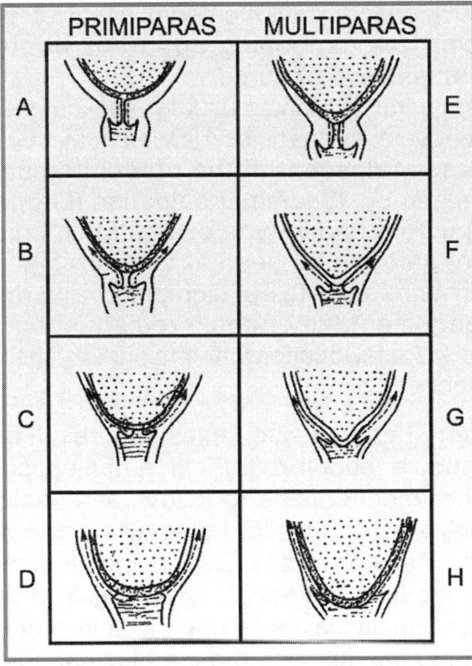

Fig. 5.6: The columns above compare the typical progress of cervical effacement and dilatation demonstrated by women in labour during their first viable pregnancies compared with that of women in labour with their second or consecutive pregnancies. A and E show long cervix. Multiparas usually have a relaxed cervical canal. B and F, Effacement or shortening of cervix begins. C and G, Cervix thins in primiparas but little dilatation occurs. Effacement and dilatation are simultaneous in multiparas. D and H, Effacement and dilatation are complete

Show: Dilatation of the cervix is usually accompanied by what is called show. During pregnancy, the mucus producing glands of the cervix have formed a deposit in the cervical canal that protects the interior of the uterus from infection. When the cervix begins to dilate, this mucus plug is discharged. As the cervix continues to dilate, small capillaries in the cervix break and stain the mucus with blood. The faster the cervix dilates and the closer it is to complete dilatation, the more abundant and red will be the "show". However show should not assume the proportions or characteristics of frank bleeding or contain clots.

After complete dilatation both abdominal and uterine muscles contract to push the foetus through the pelvic canal. The mother has no control over the contractions of her uterus, they are under involuntary control. However once dilatation is complete, she may push with her abdominal muscles when her uterus contracts so that the foetus can descend in the pelvic canal.

Thus to determine the progress of the foetus, the physician is interested in the presentation, the body part that comes first; the position, the relationship of the presenting part to the pelvic quadrants; and the station, the depth of the presenting part in the pelvic canal. If these are known plus the relative size and shape of the pelvis and foetus, the condition of the soft-tissue uterine exit called the cervix, and the quality and frequency of the uterine contractions, the physician has a good basis to evaluate the progress of the labour and the mechanisms involves.

This external rotation occurs as the shoulders engage and descent in manoeuvres similar to those of the head. As noted earlier, the anterior shoulder descends first. When it reaches the outlet, it rotates to the midline and is delivered from under the pubic arch. The posterior shoulder is guided over the perineum until it is free of the vaginal introitus.

Expulsion: Expulsion or birth of the rest of the baby occurs as the anterior shoulder moves just under the symphysis pubis. The posterior shoulder should be delivered carefully to prevent perineal bearing, and then the anterior shoulder and the rest of the body should follow easily.

After birth of the shoulders, the head and shoulders are lifted up toward the mother's pubic bone and the trunk of the baby is born by flexing it laterally in the direction of the symphysis pubis.

When the baby has completely emerged, birth is complete and the second stage of labour ends.

To accomplish these manoeuvres, proper co-ordination of the passengers, passage and powers must exist. If the presenting part is too large or the lie is transverse, engorgement cannot occur. If the position is occipito posterior the head does not apply equal pressure on the cervix and labour is slowed. If contractions are too weak or irregular, the force does not propal the foetus through the pelvis. If the pelvis is too small, the foetus cannot negotiate the passage.

MECHANISM OF LABOUR

Female pelvis has varied contours and diameters at different levels and the presenting part of the passenger is large in proportion to the passage. Therefore vaginal birth to occur, the foetus must adopt to the birth canal during the descent. The turns and other adjustment necessary in the human birth process are termed as "mechanism of labour". To negotiate the bony pelvis the foetus must go through the mechanism of labour or the cardinal movements. The seven cardinal movements of the mechanism of labour that occur in a vertex presentation are engagement, descent, flexion, internal rotation, extension, external rotation (restitution) and finally by birth expulsion. Although these movements are discussed separately in actuality a combination of movements occurs simultaneously. For example engagement involves both descent and flexion.

Engagement: First, the presenting part must be engaged, or descent to enter the true pelvis. When the biparietal diameter of the head passes the pelvic inlet (Fig. 5.3). In most nulliparous pregnancies, this occurs before the onset of active labour because the firmer abdominal muscles direct the presenting part into the pelvis. In multiparous pregnancies in which the abdominal musculature is more relaxed, the head often remains freely movable above the pelvic brim until labour is established.

The head usually engages in the pelvis in a synclitic position. One that is parallel to the antero-posterior plane of the pelvis. Frequently asynclitism occurs (the head is deflected anteriorly or posteriorly in the pelvis), which can facilitate descent because the head is being positioned to accommodate to the pelvic cavity. However, extreme asynclitism can cause cephalo-pelvic disproportion, even in a normal size pelvis, because the head is positioned so that it cannot descend.

Descent: Descent refers to the progress of the presenting part through the pelvis. Descent depends on at least four forces:

- Pressure exerted by the amniotic fluid
- Direct pressure exerted by the contracting fundus on the foetus
- Force of the contraction of the maternal diaphragm and abdominal muscles in the second stage of labour and
- Extension and straightening of the foetal body.

The effect of these forces are modified by the size and shape of the maternal pelvic planes and the size of the foetal head and its capacity to mold.

The degree of descent is measured by the station of the presenting part. There is little descent which occurs during the latent phases of the first stage of labour. Descent acceleration in the active phase when the cervix has dilated to 5 to 7 cm. It is especially apparent when the membranes have ruptured.

In the primi descent is usually slow but steady; in subsequent pregnancies, descent may be rapid. Progress in descent of the presenting part is determined by abdominal palpation (Leopold's manoeuvres) and vagina examination unit the present part can be seen at the introitus. This descent is referred to as 'Lightening' and results in engagement. Lay people remark about this change in foetal location with the phrase "the baby has dropped."

Flexion: The head also flexes as a result of the resistance encountered. Flexion must occur for the other mechanisms to follow, and flexion is maintained until the last step when the head extends. As soon as the descending head meets resistance from the cervix, pelvic wall, or pelvic floor, it normally flexes so that the chin is brought into closer contact with the foetal chest. Flexion permits the smaller suboccipitobregmatic diameter (9 cm) rather than the larger diameter to present to the outlet.

Internal rotation: Next the head, to pass the ischial spines, must rotate 45 degrees to right or left from that transverse position. The outlet is widest in the anteroposterior diameter, however. Therefore, for the foetus to exit, the head must rotate. Internal rotation begins at the level of the ischial spines but is not completed until the presenting part reaches the lower pelvis. As the occiput rotates anteriorly, the face rotates posteriorly. With each contraction the foetal head is guided by the bony pelvis and the muscles of the pelvic floor. Eventually, occiput will be in the midline beneath the pubic arch. The head is almost always rotated by the time it reaches the pelvic floor. Both the Levator ani muscles and the bony pelvis are important for achieving anterior rotation. When the part has rotated, the foetus is said to be LOA, ROA, LOP, ROP, LOT or ROT position (Fig. 5.5).

Extension: The head then extends under the symphysis. Extension allows it to negotiate the pelvic arch. It is this point that the infant's scalp or buttocks are seen at the vaginal opening. When the foetal head reaches the perineum for birth, it is deflected anteriorly by the perineum. The occiput passes under the lower border of the symphysis pubis first, then the head emerges by extension; first the occiput, then the face, finally the chin. The maximum distension of the perineum and introitus is followed rapidly by final expulsion of the head, a process that is known as "*crowning*".

Restitution and external rotation: After the head is born, it rotates briefly to the position it occupied when it was engaged in the inlet. This movement is termed as "restitution". The 45-degree turn realigns the infant's head with her or his back and shoulders. This head can then be seen to rotate further. External rotation involves two movements. After the head is delivered, it turns to realign with the shoulders, which are still in the transverse diameter of the pelvic inlet. The movement also involves the rotation of the shoulders to an anteroposterior position so that they may emerge from the vaginal opening.

PROCESS OF LABOUR/PHYSIOLOGY OF LABOUR

Labour is the process of moving foetus, placenta and membranes out of the uterus and through the birth canal. Various changes take place in the woman's reproductive system in the days and weeks before labour begins. Labour itself can be discussed in terms of the mechanism involved in the process and the stages the woman moves through.

Normally, the onset of labour is the anticipated climax of 9 months of constructive waiting. Under normal conditions, each day has better prepared the foetus to make the transition from intrauterine to extrauterine existence smoothly, without undue strain. As the time of labour and birth approaches, the pregnant woman should be instructed when to call the physician/or health care provider and come to the hospital.

Signs Preceding Labour/Signs of Impending Labour

Several signs and symptoms usually precede the onset of true labour the progressive opening of the cervix and expulsion of the baby and placenta. At the end of a full-term pregnancy the mother is willing to relinquish her lively and bulky border; however, she also has feelings of anxiety, as she considers the actual period labour and birth. Signs preceding labour are:

- Lightening.
- Return of urinary frequency.
- Backache.
- Stronger Braxton-Hicks contractions.
- Increase in contraction rate to more than 4-5 hour; contraction rate intensifies with walking.
- Weight loss 0.5 to 1.5 kg.
- Surge of energy.
- Feeling of heaviness in pelvis.
- Cervical ripening.
- Ruptured membrane.
- Increased vaginal mucus; expelling the thick strand of blood-stinged mucus (Bloody show).
- Diarrhoea (May be).

Lightening: In the first time pregnancies the uterus sinks downward and forward approximately 2 weeks before term, when the foetus's presenting part (usually the foetal head) descends into true pelvis. As the foetus drops into the true pelvis (a process called lightening) and the presenting part "becomes engaged" (the largest diameter of the presenting part passes the pelvic brim), women feel less congested, able to breathe more freely with less pressure on her diaphragm.

Primigravidas are expected to experience lightening and engagement before true labour begins. In a multi-gravida, lightening may not take place until after uterine contractions are established and true labour is in progress.

Frequent urination: After lightening, there is more bladder pressure as a result of the shift and consequently a return of urinary frequency and woman may feel need to urinate frequently.

Backache: The woman may complain of persistent low backache and sacroiliac distress as a result of relaxation of the pelvic joints. She may identify irregular, strong, frequent, uterine contractions.

Uterine contractions: The uterus contracts and relaxes intermittently all during pregnancy, but its contractions are usually mild and not detected by the mother-to-be. However in the last few weeks of waiting, these uterine contractions may become annoying and contrary to what some experts declare, may be painful. The most discouraging aspects about these contractions of late pregnancy is that they often rehearse for the real thing. They do not serve to dilate the cervix progressively and, therefore, called "false labour".

The characteristics of false labour contrasted with true labour contractions include the following:

- The duration of the contractions remain about the same, not becoming appreciably longer or more intensive as do true contractions.
- The period between contractions remain long and irregular. True contractions are regular, with a gradually decreasing interval.
- Pressure or pain is felt primarily in the abdomen rather than in the small of the back.
- Walking can be tolerated during the contraction. In fact, walking may help relieve discomfort, whereas true labour contraction may be intensified by ambulation.
- Show, or the appearance of a mucoid vaginal discharge tinged with blood is absent in false labour, but usually present in true labour.
- On rectal examination or more commonly vaginal examination, the cervix is usually found to be very long and closed in false labour but is effacing or dilating in true labour.

Weight loss: The loss of weight (0.5 to 1.5 kg) caused by water loss resulting from electrolyte shifts that in turn are produced by changes in oestrogen and progesterone levels.

Surge of energy: Many women experience a phenomenal "burst of energy" just before going into labour and want to clean the whole house and put everything in order.

Bloody show: The vaginal mucus becomes more profuse in response to the extreme congestion of the vaginal mucus membranes. Brownish or blood tinged cervical mucus (bloody show) may be passed. It indicates dilation of the cervix and equated with the onset of effective but early labour.

Cervical ripening: The cervix becomes soft (ripens) and partially effaced and may begin to dilate. The membranes may rupture spontaneous.

In addition, less commonly, some women experience diarrhoea, nausea, vomiting and indigestion.

Onset of Labour

Labour onset is thought to be a combination of a number factors working together. The following factors are as follows:

- Genetic factors have a role, perhaps influencing hormonal levels and pattern of labour
- An increase in availability of oestrogen and decrease in availability of progesterone in the myometrium is present (progesterone suppresses uterine contractions). Oestrogene fosters gap junctions, prostaglandin production. Some oestrogen originates in the foetal adrenals so that foetal adrenals activity helps to trigger labour onset.
- PGE2 (Prostaglandin) contributes to cervical changes and PGF2 to contractions and formation of gap junctions. These prostaglandin increase calcium ion flow in the cells, which will strengthen contractions. Prostaglandins come from placenta, foetal membranes and the uterus. The effect of prostaglandin may be seen in the fact that antiprostaglandin agents such as aspirin and indomethacin will delay labour onset.
- Oxytocin receptors increase 100 to 200 times by term. Thus oxytocin effectively stimulates labour in full-term pregnancy but has less effect earlier.
- Relaxin is present throughout pregnancy and probably works with progesterone to block uterine activity. Its role during labour is unclear but may be involved with connective tissue charges.
- Uterine distention contributes in some way.

Stages of Labour

Labour is considered 'normal' when the woman is at or near term, no complications exist, a single foetus presents by vertex and labour is completed within 24 hours. The course of normal labour which is remarkably constant consists of:

- Regular progression of uterine contractions.
- Effacement and progressive dilation of the cervix, and
- Progress in descent of the presenting part. Labour has been classically divided into three stages. Now a fourth stage has been identified.
  i. Stage 1—From the onset of regular labour contractions beginning with effacement and dilation of the cervix to complete dilation 10 cm.
  ii. Stage 2—From complete dilation to the birth of the baby.
  iii. Stage 3—From birth of the baby to the expulsions of the placenta and membrane.
  iv. Stage 4—Normally above a 2-hour period of transition, stabilization and initial recovery from childbirth (see Table 5.2).

First Stage

The first stage of labour is considered to last from the onset of regular uterine contractions to full dilatium of the cervix. The onset of labour is often difficult to establish because the woman may be admitted to the labour unit just before birth and beginning of labour may be only an estimate. The first stage is much longer than the second and third combined. Great variability is the rule, however depending on the factors already discussed. Full dilation may occur in less than 1 hour in some stages.

The vertical side of the graph indicates the cervical dilatation 0 to 10 centimeters and the horizontal side indicates the number of hours in labour. The length of labour is much shorter for multiparas, accounting for the variance in the curves.

Two main phases are described: a relatively show-moving, flt first section called the latent phase, involving cervical softening, effacement, and early dilatation (it traces the period extending from onset of labour until more rapid dilatation manifests itself at a approximately 2 to 3 cm) and a second section, the active phase, which is indicated by the sudden upswing and steep ascent of the tracing, ending with a brief rounding at the apex. This active phase of dilatation has in turn been divided into this phases: (1) the acceleration phase is the curve upward from the latent phase that first identifies cervical dilatation has increased in tempo; (2) the phase of maximum slope is the steepest part of the tracing; and (3) the deceleration phase is the rounding of the apex, which represents a slowing of the dilatation just before the client is completely dilated. Existence of the deceleration phase has been disputed, and it has often been characterized as short or absent in multiparas.

It is difficult at times to determine when the latent phase begins, since effacement and early cervical dilatation are "silent." or false labour may confuse the issue. The patient's labour graph is usually begun when a nullipara's (primipara's) contractions are experienced at regular 3 to 5-minute intervals or when a multipara attains regular contractions at 5 to 10-minute intervals.

Although the conditions of the mother and the foetus is considered more important than the meticulous observation of a clock for the passage of time periods, analysis by comparison of the cervical dilatation of a maternity patient to the appropriate curve developed by Dr Friedman may be helpful in identifying problems affecting labour. Using this standard, a labour is considered prolonged if:

1. The latent phase lasts
   a. 14 hours or more for nulliparas.
   b. 20 hours or more for nulliparas.
2. The rate of maximum slope is
   a. 1.5 cm/hr or less for multiparas.
   b. 1.2 cm/hr or less for multiparas.
3. The maximum slope shows no progress in dilatation for 2 hours or more (secondary arrest- the most damaging dilatation pattern).
4. The deceleration phase lasts
   a. More than 1 hour for multiparas.
   b. More than 3 hours for nulliparas.

These abnormalities are shown in these conditions exist, the physician may decide to:

1. Intensify maternal and infant assessment.
2. Use sedation for the mother.
3. Stimulate uterine contractions with oxytocic medication.
4. Prepare for caesarean birth.

Second Stage

Changes in station or descent, Friedman's (1985) study of the rate of descent of the foetus through the pelvic canal also produces a curve that is divided almost the same way as the dilatation curve. It is sometimes superimposed on the dilatation graph to show that the phase of

Table 5.2: Stages and phases of labour

Stage	Characteristics	Nursing intervention
First Stage (Stage of Dilation)	Average duration: nullipara, 8-10 hr; multipara, 6-8 hr; onset of labour until full dilation of cervix	
Latent Phase	Onset of labour until about 4 cm of cervical dilation Cervix effaces almost completely in the nullipara; may remain thick in the multipara Contractions mild and infrequent at first; gradually increase to moderate intensity, about every 5 min Woman is usually relatively comfortable Woman is sociable and excited, although somewhat anxious	Orient woman and her partner to the labour area Review parent's birth plan, if they have made one; ask if they have any specific requests about how labour and birth are conducted Monitor foetus by intermittent auscultation or with foetal monitoring (continuous or intermittent) Monitor woman's vital signs (temperature every 4 hr, or every 2 hr after membranes rupture); assess pulse, respirations, and blood pressure hourly Teach or review coping skills, such as breathing techniques Encourage walking if there is no contraindication sign permits Initiate procedures such as laboratory examinations, shave prep, and enaema
Active Phase	Cervix dilates from 5 to 7 cm; effacement is completed Membranes may rupture Contraction intensify until about 3 min apart, duration 45 sec or longer; intensity is moderate to firm Woman concentrates inwardly, although still cooperative May need analgesia or epidural anaesthesia during this phase	Continue foetal and maternal assessments Observe amniotic fluid for colour, quantity, and odour when the membranes rupture Provide general comfort measures, such as attention to her environment, hygiene Encourage changes of position about every half hour; avoid the supine position Watch for bladder distention Assist the woman to use breathing and relaxation techniques Provide reassurance, praise, and support for both the labouring woman and her partner
Transition Phase	Cervix dilates from 8 to 10 cm Intense contractions, firm, 2-3 min apart; duration of some may be as long as 90 sec Woman becomes uncooperative and irritable	Continue maternal and foetal assessments Continue comfort measures, but do not disturb the woman unnecessarily Reassure woman and her partner that this is a short, intense phase and that she will regain control
Second Stage (Stage of Expulsion)	Average duration: nullipara, 1.5 hr; multipara, 20-45 min Cervix fully dilated (10 cm) Rectal pressure as foetus descends results in urge to push with contractions; women with epidural anaesthesia may not have characteristic urge to push Contractions are still intense but may be slightly less so than in transition phase	Continue comfort measures, reassurance, support, maternal and foetal assessments Observe for perineal bulging and crowning of the foetal head Coach woman in effective pushing techniques; advise her to exhale while pushing or hold her breath for no longer than 5-6 sec Make final preparations for birth (multiparas are prepared earlier than nulliparas)

Contd...

Contd...

Stage	*Characteristics*	*Nursing intervention*
Third Stage (Placental Stage)	Average duration: 5-10 min; up to 30 min Woman may feel a slight cramp when placenta detaches Uterus must contract firmly to control bleeding Woman is fatigued and excited; wants to see baby	Give medications as ordered and as appropriate within scope of practice Observe for blood loss Give initial care to the infant, focusing on respirations and temperature maintenance
Fourth Stage (Immediate Postbirth Recovery)	First 1-4 hr after birth Uterus should remain firmly contracted, about halfway between the woman's umbilicus and symphysis pubis Bleeding (lochia rubra) should staturate no more than one pad per hour Afterpains (uterine cramping) may occur	Assess woman's temperature at beginning of recovery period Assess pulse, respirations, blood pressure every 15 min the first hour, every 30 min the second hour, then hourly Assess uterine fundus for firmness, height, and deviation from the midline with each blood pressure check; massage if not firm Have woman try to urinate if bleeding is excessive or if the uterus is high or not in the midline of the abdomen; catheterize her if she cannot urinate Provide analgesia if needed; place ice compresses to her perineum as needed

maximum slope for cervical dilatation normally corresponds to the phase of acceleration for descent.

Descent abnormalities occur alone or in conjunction with problems in dilatation. Descent is considered to be abnormally slow or arrested if:

1. During the maximum slope the rate is:
   a. 2 cm/hr or less for multiparas.
   b. 1 cm/hr or less for nulliparas.
2. During descent labour progress is stopped for 1 hour or more.

If problems in descent occur, re-evaluation of foetal presentation and position and the adequacy of the maternal pelvis is made. Changes in labour posture or activity of the mother may be helpful, for example, squatting. Oxytocics may be ordered or a caesarean birth scheduled.

Note: Too rapid descent of precipitate labour (not to be confused with precipitate delivery, which means a birth without adequate preparation) can also be a problem. Too rapid descent is usually defined as a labour of less than 3 hours, which may be accompanied by maternal uterine and perineal lacerations, lowered foetal oxygenation, and infant birth injury (especially cerebral haemorrhage).

The Friedman curve is not universally employed to monitor labour progression, but it is a useful concept and tool that has added specific terminology to the analysis of childbirth.

A wise nurse or physician makes no specific predictions regarding the length of the stages of labour. However Table 5.3 may be useful in estimating possible time intervals.

Labour lengths for both primiparas and multiparas have decreased in the last generation.

The second stage of labour lasts from the time of the cervix is fully dilated to the birth of the foetus. The major function of the second stage of the labour is 'descent'. The second stage takes an average of 20 minutes for a multiparous woman and 50 minutes for a nulliparous woman. Labour upto 2 hours has been considered within the normal range for the second stage, but there can

Table 5.3: Usual duration of the stages of labour

	First stage	*Second stage*	*Third stage*
Primiparas (nulliparas)	10 to 12 hours	30 monutes to 2 hours	5 to 20 minutes (often aided by oxytocins or manual pressure)
Multiparas	6 to 8 hours	20 minutes to 1½ hours	5 to 20 minutes (often aided by oxytocics or manual pressure)

be significant variations. For example, a woman who has received epidural analgesia may take upto 3 hours.

The normal limits of descent to guide recognition of early problems. This guide is for normal presentations uncomplicated by malposition or other problems. For the nullipara whose birth canal has not been previously distended, the foetus can be expected to descend at least 1.5 cm/hr but in most doses at 3 cm/hour. In the multipara, the foetus usually progresses faster than 2.1 cm/hr and most often at about 5 cm/hr. The average duration of second stage for the multipara is 30 minutes to 1 hour and 1 to 2 hours for the multipara. This second stage usually does not exceed 3 hours.

Simkin and Ancheta (2000) describe the latent and active phases of the second stage labour. The latent phase is a period that begins around the time of complete dilation of the uterus when the contractions are weak or not noticeable and the woman is not feeling the urge to push, is resting or is exerting only small bearing-down efforts with contractions. The active phase is a period when contractions resume and the woman in making strong bearing-down efforts and the foetal station is advancing.

To accomplish descent, the resistance of the vaginal canal must be overcome. The pelvic floor composed chiefly the levator ani muscles and fasciae, must be displaced downward and outward by foetal head. The resistance if variable and can be evaluated during vaginal examination. The folds (rugae) of the vagina from a lining membrane for the canal. The fascial layers are thinned as they stretch, making vaginal tissue susceptible to tears. The client must add voluntary expulsive efforts during contractions to achieve the pressure needed for this process.

Third Stage of Labour

The third stage of labour is characterized by the separation of the placenta and its expulsion. Third stage of labour lasts from the birth of the foetus until the placenta is delivered. The placenta normally separates with the third or fourth strong uterine contractions after the infant has been born. Immediately after the birth of the infant, then uterus should contract firmly around the placenta. The site of placental attachment becomes smaller than the placenta, causing separation, descent, and expulsion of the placenta and membranes. In most instances, by 1 to 5 minutes after delivery, there will be indications that the placenta has separated and moved into the lower segment of vagina.

- The uterus becomes smaller and spherical.
- There is slight gush of blood from the vagina.
- The umbilical cord lengthens by several inches.
- The uterus may rise in the abdomen because the separated placenta displaces it upward.
- The duration of third stage may be as short as 3 to 5 minutes although upto 1 hour is considered within normal limits. The risk of haemorrhage increases as the length of third stage increases.

Fourth Stage of Labour

The fourth stage of labour arbitrarily lasts approximately 2 hours after delivery of the placenta. It is the period of immediate recovery, when homeostasis is re-established. It serves as an important period of observation for complications such as abnormal bleeding.

The third and fourth stages of labour are probably the most dangerous for the mother because of haemorrhages which most often occur during this time. To lessen blood loss, oxytocins, medication that help contract the uterus, may be administered. The medications used will depend on the phase of delivery that their action desired, the condition of the client, the anaesthesia used and personal preference of the attending physician obstratician.

MANAGEMENT OF NORMAL LABOUR

Pain Management

Pregnant women commonly worry about the pain they will experience during labour and birth and how they will react to deal with that pain. A variety of child birth preparation methods can help the woman or couple cope with the discomfort of labour. The interventions selected depend on the situation and the preference of both the woman and her health care or provider nurse midwife.

The discomfort experienced during labour has two origins. During the first stage, of labour, uterine contractions cause cervical dilation and effacement, and uterine ischaemia results from compressions of the arteries supplying to myometrium. Pain impulses during the first stage of labour are transmitted via T11and T12 spinal nerve segment and accessory lower thoracic and upper lumbar sympathetic nerves. These nerves originate in the uterine body and cervix. The discomfort from the cervical changes and uterine ischaemia is visceral pain. It is located over the lower portion of the abdomen and radiates to the lumbar area of the back and down the thighs. The woman usually experiences discomfort only during contraction and is free of pain between contractions.

During the second stage of labour, the stage of expulsion of the baby, the woman experiences perineal or somatic pain. Perineal discomfort results from stretching of perineal tissues to allow passage of the foetus and from traction on the peritoneum and uterocervical supports during contractions. Discomfort also can be produced by expulsive forces or by pressure exerted by the presenting part on the bladder, bowel, or other sensitive pelvic structures. Pain impulses during the second stage of labour are transmitted via the S1 to S4 spinal nerve segments and the parasympathetic system.

Pain experienced during the third stage of labour and the after pains of the early postpartum period are uterine, similar to the pain experienced early in the first stage of labour. Pain may be local, with cramping, and a tearing or bursting sensation caused by distention and laceration of the cervix, vagina, or perineal tissues. This description is commonly perceived as intense burning sensation as the tissue stretches. Pain also may be referred pain in which discomfort originating in the abdominal viscera is felt in the back, flanks or thighs.

A woman's pain during childbirth is unique to each woman and is influenced by a variety of factors. These factors include culture, anxiety and fear, previous birth experience, child birth preparation and support.

- It has been identified culture in one of the factors influencing pain response. As nurses care for women and families from a variety of cultural backgrounds, they must have knowledge and understanding of how culture mediates pain. An understanding of the beliefs, values and practices of various cultures helps the nurse provide appropriately culture-sensitive care.
- Excessive anxiety and fear causes more catecholamine secretion, which increases the stimuli to the brain from the pelvis because of decrease blood flow and increased muscle tension, which in turn magnifies pain.
- Woman who have had a difficult and painful previous birth experience, anxiety and fear from this past experience may lead to increased pain.
- The gate control theory of pain helps explain the way hypnosis and pain relief techniques taught in child birth preparations classes work to relieve pain during labour.
- Providing comfort measures and supporting with pharmacological and nonpharmacological measures also relieves pain.

Methods of Pain Relief

The physiologic origin of labour pain has not been adequately explained. It results partly from intermittent muscular contractions of the fundus of stretching of muscle fibres of the cervix, lower uterine segment, and vagina. The amount of painful stimuli produced is also influenced by the individual patient's pelvic anatomy, the size and flexion of her baby's head, the strength, duration, and frequency of her uterine contractions, and the presence or absence of certain obstetric deviations or complications.

Within the last few years it has been found that a person's pain threshold also may be significantly altered by the level of available endorphins, morphine like hormonal substances in the body. These special proteins appear to interfere with the transmissions of pain-producing impulses to the brain or the brain's sensitivity, to those impulses. The endorphin level falls in the presence of anxiety, tension, fatigue, or extended negative stimuli. This phenomenon may offer a physiologic basis for the observation that a woman's perception of pain and her resulting behaviour are greatly influenced by her interpretation of what is occurring, the training she has received, her cultural background, and the emotional support she gains from those about her.

Therefore, methods of pain relief during labour and birth involve more than the administration of drugs; they also include ways available to help the patient understand the process of childbirth and to cooperate consciously with what her body is trying to accomplish. Usually a clean, calm, quiet attractive environment, attention to techniques of relaxation, application of counter pressure to the mother's back, possible position changes, close supervision and encouragement from a concerned nursing staff and physician and the companionship of those she loves greatly decrease the need for administration of analgesic and anaesthetic medications. Methods of relief depend on the patient's special needs and wishes, the availability of desired agents or equipment and the expertise and willingness to utilise them. Incorporated in their selection also should be the important considerations of risk versus benefit and financial constraints.

Key Vocabulary

Five words are defined before a discussion of pain relieving drugs or procedures is attempted.

Amnesic A technique or medication that causes memory loss of varying degrees.

Analgesic A technique or medication that reduces or eliminates pain.

Anaesthetic A technique or medication that partially or completely eliminates sensation or feeling. It may be a nerve blocking type (local or regional anaesthesia) or a sleep producing type (general anaesthesia).

Hypnotic A technique or medication that causes sleep.

Sedative or tranquilzer A technique or medication that relieves anxiety and quiets the patient.

Obstetric analgesia (first and second stages of labour) The prescription and administration of analgesic drugs during the first stage of labour must be carefully considered and performed. Actually, the physician is caring of two patients. It must be realized that all analgesics may have a hypnotic effect not only on the mother but also on her foetus. Dosage and time of administration must be calculated so that the baby will not be too sleep the time of birth to breathe on his own. Before birth, sleepiness of the foetus is not crucial because he does not have to breathe; he gets all his oxygen from his mother. But after birth, this oxygen supply is no longer available. Failure to breathe or respiratory depression, results in a condition known as asphyxia neonatorum. If a premature birth is expected, the mother is encouraged to continue her labour with a minimum amount of analgesia because the premature infant does not detoxify drugs well and may exhibit respiratory depression at birth. Some antagonistic medications for example, naloxone hydrochloride (Narean) are now available to counteract the depressant action of drugs containing narcotics on the newborn infant's respiratory system. Naloxone is very effective, although its dose may need to be repeated. It has no known detrimental action in newborns except where used to treat addicted newborns. Then it may precipitate acute withdrawal symptoms.

Another consideration in the administration of drugs during the first stage of labour is the possible effect of the medication on the progress of the labour. Given too soon during the latent phase, many analgesics may unnecessarily slow down or even stop contractions. Most physicians do not wish to give any drug before active labour has been established or approximately 4 cm of cervical dilatation has been achieved. Many patients will not need medication before or even after this dilatation has been reached.

Analgesics, hypnotics and amnesics; effects and side effects: An analgesic commonly used in labour is the narcotic meperidine (Demerol). This drug is frequently given in combination with a tranqulizer such as hydroxyzine (Atarax or Vistaril) or promethazine (Phergan). These combinations are more effective because they increase the analgesic effect and counteract the nausea often associated with the narcotic.

Intermittent inhalation analgesia used in the latter portion of the first and during most of the second stage of labour has had considerable popularity in certain areas of the world. The patient breathes anaesthetic gases through a mask or a mouth piece. When these gases are properly administered in low concentrations, the patient does not become unconscious but benefits from a real reduction in discomfort. Nitrous oxide may be self administered by the patient using a specially designed dispenser, or it may be administered by an anaesthesiologist or nurse-anaesthetist using an anaesthesia machine. It is important that such analgesia not become anaesthetic in depth, since regurgitation and aspiration can become a real and deadly complication. Instructions for the use of various types of gases and equipment must be carefully followed. Inhalation analgesia usually does not provide sufficient relief for the entire second stage of labour. Often its analgesic effects are augmented by a pudendal block or infiltrations of the perineum with a local anaesthetic.

Obstetric anaesthesia (first, second and third stages of labour) Anaesthesia is the province of a trained physician, anaesthesiologist, or nurse-anaesthetist. Nurses should not attempt to function in this area without skilled advanced training. Administration of anaesthesia is not a nursing function.

General anaesthesia In obstetrics a general anaesthetic may be inhaled or administered intravenously. General anaesthesia in obstetrics is used less often than formerly for normal births. This is because regional anaesthetics are safer and parental participations in the birth process is being emphasized.

Special Considerations

When a general anaesthetic is planned, it is important to know when the labour started and how recently the patient has eaten, because a real danger of aspiration, obstruction of the airway (asphyxiation) and pneumonia exists. The patient should be given nothing by mouth unless it is ordered, because during labour digestion stops and recent means may remain in the stomach. Even if a woman in labour has not eaten recently, her highly acidic gastric secretions may still pose the threat of acid aspiration pneumonitis (Mendelson's syndrome). To counteract this possibility some physicians order oral administration of 15 to 30 ml of an antacid such as sodium citrate every 3 hours during labour, and most order one dose just before a scheduled caesarean birth. Chilling the liquid antacid may increase its acceptance. In case of vomiting, the patient's head should be turned to the side or, if possible, she should be placed on her side. Chewing gum or dentures are removed from the mouth before administration of anaesthetic.

Some anaesthetic gases used in the past were either flammable (either, chloroform) or explosive (cyclopropane). Now, other effective gases are available that do not present safety hazards, and older anaesthetic gas products have been essentially phased out or banned. This has eliminated the need to be concerned with the build up of static electricity in personnel and other safe guards against explosion, and has facilitated and noise should also be avoided at the time of emergence.

Because all anaesthetics cross the placenta and, if given in sufficient concentration, produce symptoms in the child, they should not be started too far in advance of the expected birth. When the condition of the foetus requires emergency caesarean birth or when rapid uterine relaxation is need for various obstetric manoeuvres, general anaesthesia may be favoured. It does not cause the maternal hypotension that sometimes accompanies regional conductive anaesthetics and may be administered rapidly with good results. Usually general anesthesia is induced by an intravenous injection of a sleep dose of thiopental (Pentothal) and a paralyzing dose of succinylcholine (Anectine). This is followed by rapid placement of a curved endotracheal tube into the trachea. The nurse may be asked to help at this time by pushing on the cricoid cartilage of the larynx (just below the "Adam's apple"). This helps close off the oesophagus. Both circoid pressure and endotracheal intubation help prevent aspiration. The anaesthesia is then maintained with nitrous help prevent aspiration. The anaesthesia is then maintained with nitrous oxide, oxygen, a muscle relaxant, and perhaps halothane. Once the baby is delivered, a narcotic and a tranquilzer are usually given intravenously to complete the anaesthetic. Oxygen must always be mixed with gas anaesthetics to supply the body needs of the mother and her unborn child.

Thiopental (Pentothal) produces a rapid induction by intravenous injection. If thiopental is given for only brief periods, the brain of the foetus is bypassed and little neonatal depression is seen.

Nitrous oxide (*laughing gas*) sis often given for analgesic effect in the period of expulsion during contractions. Administered in low concentrations, it relieves the mother's pain but still allows her to bear down with her contractions. When nitrous oxide is used as an anaesthetic, care is needed to prevent maternal respiratory and neonatal depression. Nitrous oxide may support combustion but is nonexplosive.

Halcerane (Flucthane) and isoflurane (Flrane) are anaesthetic gases that are useful in producing rapid uterine relaxation when needed. In low concentrations they can be used to decrease awareness during the early stages of operative deliveries if a light general anaesthetic is desired). Both anaesthetic gases can cause uterine haemorrhage and hypotension if concentrations become too high.

Ketamine hydrochoride (Ketaject) given by intravenous injection, produces rapid anaesthesic and is used primarily for emergencies in obstetric anaesthesia. It is useful when blood pressure needs to be low. It should not be used with hypertensive patients and may be associated with dream like episodes and hallucinations. Reduced stimulation during emergence is recommended.

Regional (Conductive) anaesthesia Regional or conductive anaesthetics have become popular in recent years.

Subarachnoid block The use of a subarachnoid block, commonly called a spin 1 or saddle, has been particularly successful for vaginal deliveries. The patient is supported in a sitting position on the edge of the delivery table or lies on her side with her curved back facing the physician. Next, a thin sterile spinal needle (with or without a larger introducing needle) is inserted between the vertebrae at about the level of the iliac crests. Its tip is placed in the subarachnoid space below the spinal cord identified by the appearance of cerebrospinal fluid dripping from the needle's hub. Between contractions an anaesthetic that is heavier than the cerebrospinal fluid such as lidocaine (Xylocaine) is injected into the subarachnoid space. The patient is then positioned on her back with her uterus displaced to her left side. Her head and shoulders are elevated and her legs are placed in stirrups.

Classically a saddle block is supposed to affect only those areas of the body that would be touched by a saddle if a person were riding horse. In practice the anaesthesia is more extensive. Low spinal anaesthesia commonly numbs the abdominal and pelvic areas below the umbilicus, affecting the abdomen, perineum, legs, and feet. It takes effect immediately and gains maximum potency in 3 to 5 minutes. How long it lasts (1 to 3 hours) depends on the medication used. For caesarean birth a subarachnoid block that is designed to go higher (up to the nipples) is frequent used. Because of vertebral abnormalities, or past back surgery not all women can have spinal anaesthetics. A very few women are allergic to the type of medications usually injected. Sometimes lack of time or qualified medical personnel precludes the use of this type of anaesthetic.

Much has been said about the aftereffects of subarchnoid anaesthesia. The so-called spinal headache is a complication often feared by patients. Actually the incidence of spinal headache has been estimated as less than 5 per cent and it is decreasing. The use of an intravenous infusion to promote better hydration of the patient and the use of only small-box needles to cut down on the possibility of crebrospinal fluid leakage has reduced the incidence of postdelivery spinal headaches. It is debatable whether keeping the patient flat during the post delivery period is helpful. Subarachnoid block anaesthesia does entail certain other inconveniences, however. The mother must sit quietly while the procedure is carried out. This is difficult to do during the second stage of labour, even with the support of an understanding nurse. Subarachnoid block anaesthesia does not stop contractions, but the patient does not feel them. The patient may find it difficult to push properly, and usually outlet forceps are used. Occasionally, a patient's blood pressure may drop, possibly affecting the baby's oxygen supply, or the patient may have trouble breathing because of a high level of anaesthesia. In the immediate postpartum period, the patient may find it more difficult to void spontaneously.

Many practitioners believe that the positive aspects of subarachnoid anaesthesia outweigh the negative aspects. The baby is not in danger of being put to sleep and of having a difficult time breathing at birth because of the anaesthetic. The mother is awake. She may see her baby being born. She can hear his first cry a real thrill. The regional anaesthetics are safer than gas anaesthetics for obstetric patients. Nausea and vomiting during and after use of regional anaesthetics are minimal. The patient is awake and less likely to choke or aspirate, even if she vomits.

Recently very thin catheters capable of passing through a spinal needle have become available. They allow continuous administration of a spinal anaesthetic. In certain situations, the procedure may offer the benefits of more versatility, less side effects, and more safety than the "single shot" spinal or the continuous epidural anaesthetic discussed below.

Epidural Anaesthesia Techniques

Other types of regional anaesthetics are available. In considerable vogue, some time ago was continuous caudal anaesthesia, or one-shot caudal. This technique introduced local anaesthetic agents in to the sacral canal, where significant nerves travel outside the meninges or spinal cord coverings. It is rarely used today.

Another kind of regional anaesthesia, less difficult to administer than caudal is called a *lumbar epidural block*. The drug is injected into the epidural space, usually between the second and third or the third and fourth lumbar vertebrae, while the mother lies on her side or is supported in a sitting position. Following careful identification of the desired location, a nylon or plastic catheter is threaded through the needle at the insertion site and the needle is removed. The catheter is conscientiously secured in position with tape. After a small test dose, cautions instillation of the anaesthetic is begun. Currently bupivacaine (Marcaine), 2-chloroprocaine (Nesacaine), and lidocaine (Xylocaine) are the most frequently used local anaesthetics.

The patient should be informed about what she may experience during the initiation of the epidural. She may detect a burning or staining sensation at the site of the injection of the local anesthesia before the insertion of the needle and cannula, local pressure during insertion, and a "crazy bone feeling in her leg, hip or back if the flexible catheter touches a nerve as it advances into the epidural space. During the 5 minute period after the test dose is injected, she should be observes for the appearance of hypotension and questioned regarding lower extremity sensory changes and loss of ability to move her legs. These symptoms may indicate unwanted penetration through the duramater into the subarachnoid space. This is to be avoided, since the larger amounts of anaesthetic routinely used during epidural techniques could cause dangerously high anaesthesia, compromising respiration and oxygen supply. A dural puncture could also predispose the mother to spinal headache.

Another complication that can occur is the rare unintentional injection of the anaesthetic into a blood vessel. The patient may indicate ringing in the ears, light-headedness, circumoral tingling or numbness, and the sudden recognition of a metallic taste. Convulsions may follow, at which time, the patient is placed in a side position, the airway is preserved, and oxygen is given. Diazepam (Valium) or thiopental sodium (Pentothyal) may be administered to stop the seizure.

When epidural dosage is administered during labour, the patient may remain on her side with her head slightly raised, or she may be placed in a modified supine position with a firm wedge-shaped pillow under her right hip so that her uterus is tilted to the left. These postures are assured to help control the level of anaesthesia obtained and to prevent the weight of the uterus from compressing the maternal aorta and vena cava. When the compression of these vessels interferes with the circulation of the blood in the mother and eventually deprives the foetus of oxygen, the resulting signs and symptoms have been called the aortacaval or supine hypotensive syndrome. One must always be alert for developing maternal hypotension. As epidural block may also cause hypotension by blocking certain sympathetic nerve fibres in the epidural space.

The anaesthetic may be infused through the catheter in small continuous amounts using an infusion pump or given intermittently when the analgesic action lessens. Usually pain relief begins within 3 to 5 minutes after injection, and full effect is obtained in 8 to 15 minutes. According to one study, about 85 per cent of the women receiving epidurals are free of pain, 12 per cent experience partial relief, and a remaining 3 per cent do not benefit at all. Many women will still confirm sensations of abdominal or perineal pressure and note weakness or numbness in their legs. Because of the loss of normal pelvic sensation together with routine intravenous hydration, many are prone to urinary distention. They should be asked to empty their bladders before the epidural is begun and should be watched carefully for difficulty in voiding. The patient may need to be catheterized. For a caesarean birth, the effects of an epidural block may be extended by injecting more local anaesthetic until the level of numbness is felt up to the nipple line.

Contraindications to using an epidural anaesthesia include current anticoagulant therapy, a history or presence of haemorrhage or shock, septicemia or local infection in the area of the proposed injection, and various spinal problems.

Epidural techniques can be used to good advantage in the latter part of the first stage of labour and continued into the second and third stages. The patient is typically alert and comfortable. Those women wishing medication during their labours are usually enthusiastic regarding the method. However, epidural anaesthesia requires the supervision of an anaesthesiologist, special apparates, and continuous maternal-foetal monitoring and support by the nurse. It is very important to detect signs of maternal hypotension and to evaluate the duration and quality of uterine contraction progress in labour, and foetal heart rate response. The mother's urge and ability to push may be impaired, and forceps deliveries are more common than in patients who have received no anaesthesia before delivery.

It is now becoming a fairly common practice in some hospitals to inject narcotics along with local anaesthetics in to the subarachnoid (spinal) or epidural spaces to manage pain during both vaginal and caesarean births and to provide postoperative pain control. One technique uses long-lasting morphine (Duramorph) and/or other shorter acting narcotics such as fentanyl (Sublimaze). It can provide very effective analgesia. However side effects such as itching, nausea and vomiting occur frequently when narcotics are used in this way. Urinary retention also may occasionally result. The major concern is a rare but potentially foetal complication delayed respiratory depression. Because of the possibility of this problem when narcotics are injected into the subarachnoid or epidural spaces, the respiratory patterns of the patient must be carefully monitored over an extended period. Protocols for special observation and care should be in place.

Local Anaesthesia and Nerve Blocks

Pudendal Block

Local anaesthesia by direct infiltration of the perineal tissues or infiltration of those nerves that, serve to relay sensation initiated in the perineal area to the brain, is probably the safest anaesthesia for both mother and baby available today. A popular technique called pudendal block stops sensory impulses from the pudendal nerve by infiltration of a local anaesthetic into specific areas with a long needle. With its use, an episotomy may be performed. It may be used satisfactorily in conjunction with nitrous oxide. However, some women do not experience the relief they desire.

Paracervical Block

Another type of analgesic technique is called a para-cervical block. It features injections of local anaesthetic into the lateral fornices of the vagina at the junction of the vaginal wall and the partially dilated cervix. Although it may relieve discomfort from contractions, the technique in most instances is not sufficient to meet the total needs of most patients during delivery. Even more important, the paracervical block has been associated with episodes of foetal bradycardia and a few foetal deaths. For all these reasons, this type of block is infrequently undertaken today.

Education for Childbirth

Most, in the hospital setting, were given types and doses of drugs designed to relieve pain, which also produced at least partial amnesia of the event. These medications too often were associated with the birth of infants whose respirations were depressed at birth.

Modern trends in obstetric favour a more alert patient during labour who is able to participate with dignity in her experience of childbirth. To this end greater effects have been made to educate the woman for her role, both psychologically and physically. Many different courses have been instituted to teach helpful techniques in posture, breathing, and relaxation, as well as to impart basic information about labour and birth to the expectant mother. Husbands or chosen companions are encouraged to attend the sessions to understand and aid their partners.

English obstetrician Dr Grantly Dick-Read probably popularized the term "natural childbirth" in his book childbirth without fear. In his writings and lectures he stressed that much of the fear pregnant women feel is caused by a lack of knowledge of what is really happening and an ensuring feeling of helplessness. He declared that fear builds tension and that tension eventually produces pain. Because of the much of his effort was spent in educating the future mother and prescribing exercise to condition her body for labour and birth.

French obstetrician Fernand Lamaze became intrigued with the labour and delivery techniques based on Pavlov's theories of conditioned response that he had observed during a visit to the Soviet Union. When he returned to Paris, he introduced psychoprophylactic concepts into his practice to prepare his patients for their maternity experiences and to assist them in conscious rewarding participation in the birth of their children. Much of what Dr Lamaze emphasized was also stressed by Dr Read. However, the relaxation taught by Dr Lamaze is based on the principle that a high level of concentrated cerebral activity can inhibit the reception of other stimuli. That is, the mind (psycho) could be induced to prevent (prophylaxis) the reception of unpleasant and painful sensations. The patient is educated (conditioned) to respond neuromuscularly to specific verbal cues. Intense preoccupation with certain muscular tension and release patterns, respiratory movements, and massage may help attain these goals. A specially prepared labour coach, sometimes called a monitrice, may be assigned to assist and support the patient in her efforts to utilize her training.

Frequently, the husband or chosen companion of the expectant mother fills the role of labour coach. The coach and the labour-delivery room staff should work as a team for the realization of a constructive, dignified aware, satisfying parturition. The attending nurses should be calm, cheerful, and knowledgeable concerning the aims of the techniques employed. The methods used may differ, but it is helpful if the nurses acquaire themselves with the different types of programs that may be available in their communities and the ways in which expectant mothers have been taught.

Today, many childbirth educators are emphasizing the need for increased flexibility and individualization in the labour techniques offered to their clients. In this broader teaching perspective more consideration is given to the wide range of normal physiologic responses found in women, their varying cultural backgrounds, and different personalities. These considerations affect their perception and tolerance of pain and the selection of coping skills and has led to the support of more types of maternal behavior during labour. This broad teaching perspective relieves a certain rigidity (reflected especially in past teaching of certain respiratory patterns to coincide with contractions), which was helpful to some, but not to all.

Women trained for labour need nursing support and encouragement from a nurse who will enhance their efforts help evaluate and aid relaxation; render sacral support or pressure as directed; share information regarding progress in labour; and be sincerely complimentary of the idealism and efforts manifested by the patients and their partners. In addition, the nurse should render the other nursing care services and observation that all labouring women require. Occasionally symptoms of hyperventilation may be associated with some of the rapid-breathing techniques used. The patient may complain of tingling hands and feet, which causes annoyance or loss of concentration. Slowing respirations or breathing into a paper bag helps relieve these problems. Symptoms related to hyperventilation are not frequent because rapidbreaching patterns have been modified to include slower acceleration and deceleration periods and shallower respirations.

The absence of all forms of drug induced analgesia or anaesthesia is not a prerequisite of either the Read or Lamaze method, although this interpretation has been made. However, some women do not use any analgesic or anaesthetic drugs. With the greater availability of epidural anaesthesiain, more women are currently using the various nonmedical techniques learned in classes during early labour and completing their labour and birth experience with epidural anaesthesia.

Those who have evaluated psychoprophylactic techniques (used them or cared for patients who were prepared as recommended) generally believe that they are of real value. The breathing and relaxation exercises, patterned light massage (effleurage), visual focal point or imagery, and mental and physical conditioning that such team efforts involve represent helpful tools that many mothers can profitably employes that they face the task of childbirth. If a labouring woman decides to use other alternatives (such as analgesia, tranquillizers, or anaesthetics), she should not feel herself to be a failure or guilty of betraying a concept. She is not a competitor in a contest. She is a participant in an experience

The main problem in using psychoprophylactic techniques seems to be in securing enough time and personnel to prepare the woman adequately. She may find it difficult to attend instruction classes. Many people do not agree that these methods of caring for the childbearing woman are truly natural childbirth. They look on them as intensive education and preparation for childbirth. Some women respond very well to the conditioning offered. Others have personal histories or personality structures that make constructive participation in psycho-prophylactic labour and birth, such as Read, Lamaze, and others have recommended, difficult or impossible. These methods are advised only for those undergoing a normal labour and birth. For patients seeking a sympathetic practitioner and undertaking the preparation involved, such management of labour and birth can bring many enduring rewards, not the least of which is a characteristically noisy, vigorous new member of the family.

Hypnosis and Acupuncture

No discussion of obstetric analgesia and anaesthesia can be undertaken without mentioning hypnosis and acupuncture. Hypnosis, an intense altered stage of receptive concentration, is greatly enhanced by high motivation. The psychoprophylactic method of preparation for childbirth incorporates certain aspects of this technique. The ability to obtain a trance like state can be measured by use of the hypnotic induction profile. A trance may be induced by another person or self-induced. Training for this type of pain relief has been typically time consuming and expensive. The use of group sessions has made hypnosis more accessible. However, it still has not become a popular form of pain control for maternity patients.

The use of acupuncture for vaginal deliveries has received mixed reviews found that acupuncture associated with electric stimulation (electroacupuncture) in the dorsolumbar and lumbosacral areas may eliminate painful sensation during labour. It also has been proposed that acupuncture releases endorphins (morphine like compounds) from the pituitary gland and midbrain. Surely these forms of pain relief and control are worthy.

No perfect means of pain relief applicable to all women and situations has been found. But physicians have at their disposal many agents of worth that, when used judiciously and backed up by good nursing care, will assist the patient tremendously.

NURSING CARE DURING LABOUR AND BIRTH (TABLES 5.4 AND 5.5)

After admission is completed, unless birth is imminent, a prolonged period of waiting and observation ensues in which the physical and emotional support of the woman and preparation for the birth are paramount. Usually presence of her mother, husband or chosen companion at the bedside is a source of support. Often the husband or companion may have been trained to be the woman's labour coach and, as such, is extremely important in sustaining the morale and comfort of the parturient. If such viaitation is not supportive or if it appears to anatgonize or upset the patient, such observations should be reported to the concerned nurse or doctor.

FIRST STAGE OF LABOUR

The first stage of labour begins with the onset of regular uterine contractions and end with complete cervical effacement and dilation. Labour care begins when the woman reports one or more of the following:

- Onset of progressive, regular uterine contractions that increase in frequency, strength and duration.
- Blood-tinged vaginal discharge (bloody or pink show) indicating that the mucus plug (operculum) has passed.
- Fluid discharge from the vagina representing the spontaneous rupture of membranes (SROM, SRM).

The first stage of labour consists of three phases: the latent phase (0 to 3 cm dilation), the active phase (4 to 7 cm dilation) and the transition phase (8 to 10 cm of dilation). Most nulliparous women seek admission to the hospital in the latent phase because they have not experienced labour before and are unsure of the "right" time to come in. Multiparous women usually do not come to the hospital until they are in the active phase.

Nurses should involve the labouring woman as a partner in formulating an individualized plan of care that preserves the woman's sense of control facilitates her participation in her own childbirth experiences, and enhances her self-esteem and level of satisfaction. Women often have lingering impressions of their childbirth experience. Care givers who are supportive, respectful, encouraging, kind, patient, professional and comforting, help these women to remember their childbirth experience in positive terms.

The woman in latent phase (early labour) is characteristically alert, talkative, and nervous. She is generally eager to cooperate with the heal care providers in attendance and respond readily

Table 5.4: Nursing care plan for the woman in uncomplicated labour

Problem/Objective	*Nursing Interventions*	*Rationale*
Nursing Diagnosis: Anxiety related to unfamiliarity with hospital birth environment		
• Woman will express reduced anxiety after interventions • Woman will have a relaxed body posture and facial expression after interventions	1. Greet woman and her partner/ family warmly on arrival, and escort them to the assigned birthing room	1. Makes family feel welcome and that staff will be considerate of their needs and desires
	2. Briefly orient woman/couple to birthing room; place call signal within easy reach and tell her how to use it; explain any equipment that is used, including its purpose and how it will fell and sound	2. Teaching helps decrease anxiety related to the unknown and increases a sense of personal control over the situation
	3. Talk with woman/couple about what they expect of the birth experience; for example, ask who they plan on having present at (or immediately after) birth and type of medications or anaesthesia anticipated about their desires	3. Enables nursing staff to help woman/couple achieve their expected experience more closely, which promotes their satisfaction; even if all their expectations are not met, they will probably be less anxious. It they believe staff cares
Nursing Diagnosis: Altered comfort related to effect of uterine contractions and pressure from foetal descent		
• Woman will state that she is able to manage and tolerate the discomfort of labour	1. Encourage woman to assume any position she finds comfortable, other that supine	1. Promotes comfort; supine position can reduce placental blood flow and compromise foetal oxygenation
	2. Assist woman to assume specific positions for special situations in labour: a. Upright positions (sitting, walking, standing) facilitate foetal pressure against cervix, favouring effacement, dilation, and descent b. Back labour may be lessened by sitting or standing while leaning forward or by hands-and-knees position because they shift foetal head away from mother's back c. Squatting can increase the pelvic diameters slightly, straighten the pelvic curve, and promote foetal descent by gravity	2. Many women are not aware that position can significantly improve comfort during labour; position can also facilitate normal processes of labour. Although any position except supine is usually acceptable, these positions may be more comfortable for the mother in the situations described
	3. Adjust temperature with a fan if woman is hot, or a warm blanket if she is cool; have her wear socks if her feet are cold	3. Environmental comfort promotes relaxation, which decreases pain perception and increases pain tolerance
	4. Change disposable underpads when they become wet or soiled; use a folded towel between her legs if a large quantity of amniotic fluid is draining	4. Hygienic measures promote comfort and make the environment less favourable for growth of microorganisms
	5. Give woman ice chips, Popsicles, hard candy, or fruit juices as permitted; if she must remain NPO, use lemon-glycerin swabs to moisten her mouth; a wet wash cloth can also be used	5. Relieves discomfort of a dry mouth; fruit juices, hard candies, and Popsicles also provide some calories for energy

Table 5.5: Nursing care plan for the woman needing pain management during labour

Problem/Objective	*Nursing Interventions*	*Rationale*
(1) Nursing Diagnosis: Pain related to uterine contractions and descent of foetus in pelvis		
• Woman will relate that her discomfort is manageable during labour using techniques learned in prepared childbirth classes • Woman will have a relaxed facial and body appearance between contractions	1. Assess for presence and character of pain continuously during labour: a. Statement of pain (assess nature of pain, such as location, intensity, whether intermittent or constant) b. Crying, moaning during and/or between contractions c. Tense, guarded body posture or thrashing with contractions d. "Mask of pain" facial expression	1. These are common verbal and nonverbal signs of pain; assessment enables nurse to identify whether pain is normal for woman's labour status; assessment also helps nurse identify best interventions for pain relief (nonpharmacologic and/or pharmacologic measures); evaluating nonverbal and verbal communication helps nurse evaluate need for pain relief in women who may not directly communicate their need for pain relief or who do not speak prevailing language
	2. Provide general comfort measures, such as a. Adjust the room temperature and light level for comfort b. Reduce irritants, such as wet underpads c. Provide ice chips, Popsicles, or juices to relieve dry mouth, if medical orders permit d. Avoid bumping her bed	2. These general measures reduce outside irritants that make it harder for woman to use prepared childbirth techniques; they are also a source of discomfort themselves
	3. Encourage woman to assume positions she finds most comfortable, other than the supine	3. Position changes promote comfort and help foetus adapt to size and shape of woman's pelvis; supine position can result in supine hypotensive syndrome which may reduce placental blood flow and foetal oxygenation
	4. Observe for a full bladder every 1-2 hr, or more often if the woman receives large amounts of PO or IV fluids	4. A full bladder is a source of discomfort and can prolong labour by inhibiting foetal descent; it may cause pain that persists after epidural anesthesia is begun
	5. Promote use of prepared childbirth techniques, including labour partner as appropriate: a. Do not stand in front of her focal point b. Offer a back rub or firm sacral pressure; ask the best location and amount of pressure; use baby powder to prevent skin irritation c. Encourage woman to switch to more complex patterns only when simpler ones are no longer effective	5. These are examples of how to assist woman and her partner in using methods they learned most effectively; use of nonpharmacologic pain relief techniques avoids problems associated with pharmacologic interventons and supplements an drug therapy used; they also give woman and partner a sense of control and mastery, which enhances perception of birth as a positive experience
Nursing Diagnosis: Pain related to uterine contractions and descent of foetus in pelvis.		
	d. Breathe along with woman if she has trouble maintaining patterns; make eye contact	
	6. If woman has signs of hyperventilation (dizziness, numbness or tingling sensations, spasms of the hands and feet), have her breathe into her cupped hands, a small bag, or a washcloth placed over her mouth and nose; or instruct her to hold her breath briefly	6. Hyperventilation often occurs when woman uses rapid breathing patterns because she exhales to much carbon dioxide; these measures help her conserve carbon dioxide and rebreathe it to correct excess loss

Contd...

Contd...

Problem/Objective	*Nursing Interventions*	*Rationale*
	7. Tell woman and her partner when labour progresses; for example, if she is pushing and her baby's head becomes visible, let her see or feel it tolerate pain	7. Labour does not last forever; knowing that her efforts are having desired results gives her courage to continue and helps her
(2) Nursing Diagnosis: Knowledge deficit: procedures and expected effects of epidural block.		
• After explanations, woman will state that she understands what will happen during and after epidural block is begun	1. Explain what to expect as the epidural block is begun (reinforcing explanations of anaesthesiologist or nurse-anaesthetist): a. An IV will be started and she will receive fluids to offset the tendency of her blood pressure to fall b. Foetus will be monitored by electronic foetal monitoring c. Nurse-anaesthetist or anaesthesiologist will position her; she should remain still in this position d. A small plastic catheter will be taped to her back to allow constant infusion of medication (or reinjection, depending on the anaesthesia clinician's preference) e. Her blood pressure will be checked every 5 min when block is first begun	1. This list reflects a common sequence of events for starting an epidural block; anaesthesia clinician explains the procedure and expected effects; nurse reinforces explanations as needed; knowledge reduces anxiety and fear of the unknown; if woman understands that these procedures are a normal part of epidural block anaesthesia, she is less likely to interpret them as abnormal
	2. Explain that she will lie relatively flat for a short period but that a small pillow will be placed under her right hip. After she is numb, she should regularly turn from side to side	2. These methods allow even dispersion of anaesthetic drug to prevent a one-sided block; pillow under hip avoids supine hypotensive syndrome
	3. Explain that she will feel less pain but that she may still feel pressure; she may be able to move her legs normally or she may not be able to move them variation in effects, she is less likely to interpret them as abnormal or as evidence that block is not working	3. Helps woman understand that epidural block is not expected to completely eliminate pain; leg movement is affected in varying amounts; if she understands
(3) Nursing Diagnosis: High risk for injury related to loss of sensation		
• Woman will not have an injury, such as muscle strain or fall, during the time her epidural is in effect Foetus will not be born in uncontrolled delivery	1. Keep woman in bed while block is in effect; check for movement and sensation before ambulating after birth; ambulate cautiously, with an assistant, after her sensation returns	1. Woman is likely to fall if she does not have sensation and full control over her movements; there is considerable variation in time required for sensation and movement to return
	2. Observe for signs that birth may be near: a. Increase in bloody show b. Statement of pressure or need to push (may not be present, depending on individual response to block) c. Bulging of the perineum or appearance of head	2. Loss of sensation varies considerably among women; with her pain relieved, woman's labour may progress more rapidly than expected; these are signs associated with imminent birth that should be evaluated by the experienced nurse, nurse-midwife, or physician

to a calm, cheerful nurse, who seems genuinely interested in her welfare. Her contractions are not very frequent or intensive, and show is not remarkable, she will probably appreciate being up and around for a while and not automatically confined to her bed just because she has been admitted to the hospital. It has be found that when she does rest in bed, there is less interference with maternal and foetal circulation, increased urinary function and greater uterine efficiency, if she reclines on her side. However, it is true that a number of nursing observations and procedures (manual FHR monitoring and checking the dilation or perineum) may be more easily carried out if the patient turns to the supine position intermittently. Later, in labour during transition and while the mother pushing a semi sitting position may be preferred. However, other postures, upright or squatting, may be used in some settings (Table 5.5).

Assessment begins at the first contact of the woman whether by telephone or in person. The m anner in which the nurse communicates with the woman during this first contact can set the tone of positive birth experience. A caring attitude by the nurse encourages the woman to verbalize her questions and concerns. The nurse should ask and see the copies of records maintained by the mother. Then certain factors are assessed and initially to determine whether the woman is in true labour and should come to hospital for further assessment or admission.

The nurse should describe the measures to the woman and her family and can use to enhance the progress of labour, reduce anxiety and maintain comfort. The woman is encouraged to ambulate and asked to adjust her oral intake according to the preferences of her primary health care provider. A warm shower can be relaxing for the woman is early labour. However warm baths should be avoided until the cervix is approximately 5 cm dilated, because water immersion in early labour could prolong this labour process and increase the use of oxytocin to stimulate uterine contractions and epidura analgesia for pain reduction. Soothing back, foot and hand massage or a wam drink preferred liquids such as tea or milk can help the woman to rest and even to sleep, especially if false labour or early labour is occurring at night. Diversional activities such as walking, reading, watching, TV, doing needle work, or talking with friends can reduce the perception of early discomfort, help the time pass and reduce anxiety.

When the woman arrives at the perinatal unit, assessment in the top priority. The nurse first performs screening assessment, using the technique of interview and physical assessment and reviews labouratory findings to determine the health status of the woman and her foetus and the progress of her labour and concerned physician or nurse is notified. Because first impressions are important, the woman and her family are welcomed by name and introduced to staff members who will be involved in their care. If the woman wishes, her partner is included in the assessment and admission process.

As part of the admission process, the nurse orients the woman and her family to the layout and operation of the unit and the features of their room. The nurse may assist in obtaining the required consents for the care of the woman and her newborn are to receive. The nurse can minimise the woman's anxiety by explaining terms commonly used during labour. The woman's interest and response guide the depth and breath of these explanations.

Admission forms can provide guidances for the acquisition of important assessment information when a woman in labour is being evaluated or admitted. Additional sources of data include:

- The prenatal record;
- The physical examination to determine baseline physiologic parameters (general system assessment, vital signs, Leopold manoeuvres, FHR, uterine contractions, vaginal examination);
- Laboratory and diagnostic test results; (urine, blood amniotic, infection);
- Expressed psychosocial and cultural factors; and
- Clinical evaluation of labour status.

If the patient is going to be supine position in the bed for an appreciable length of time, the head of the bed should be elevated approximately 30 degrees to prevent circulating and respiratory disturbances. She should conserve her physical and nervous energy for the more demanding period of labour to come. Her temperature, pulse and respiration should be documented at least every 4 hours and more often if individual history or indications warrant it. Blood pressure should be recorded routinely every hour. Foetal heart tones should be checked at 30 minutes intervals or less during the first stage of labour and with increasing frequency as labour progresses. The amount and character of any show or amniotic drainage, if present, should be noted. At times, question of whether the bag of waters has broken may exist. It is important to try to determine the time of its rupture, since the possibility of uterine infection after rupture becomes greater as the hours go by before birth. Such a situation may be detrimental to both mother and child. To find out whether any vaginal leakage in amniotic fluid, the nurse (before any antiseptic or lubricant other than water is used on the perineal area may gently insert a sterile applicator or gloved finger into the vaginal canal to be moistened by the fluid present. It is then passed against a strip of phenaphthazine (nitrazine paper). If paper turns blue indicate alkaline drainage, the moisture is probably amniotic fluid—it is uncontaminated by blood. A yellow or acidic reaction usually indicates urine.

Rupture of the Membranes (Spontaneous)

If the bag of water breaks at any time while the patient is in the labour area (if not ruptured before admission). She should be instructed not to get out of bed or sit up completely. The nurse inspects the perineum for signs of a prolonged cord or, in the case of advanced labour, evaluates signs of the advance of the presenting part (bulging perineum, appearance of the foetal scalp) and the amount and colour of the amniotic fluid.

Normal fluid is very light yellow. If there is any meconium (infant stool) in the fluid, staining it a brownish—yellow to gray-black, it should be reported immediately. Meconium-stained amniotic fluid during cephalic presentations is considered a sign of foetal distress-the response of the foetus to oxygen lack. Such staining during a breech presentation is usually not considered significant, since the pressure exerted on a breech during its passage through the pelvic canal may cause the discharge of meconium, and no real foetal distress may be involved. The appearance of red-tinged amniotic drainage, old, dark blood, bright red, frank bleeding, or blood clots at any time during labour should also be reported. Foetal heart tones should be checked immediately after the rupture of the membrane to try to detect possible cord prolapse and compression. The fact that the bag of waters appears to have ruptured should be reported to the charge nurse immediately. Contractions should be frequently evaluated, depending on the progress the patient seems to be making.

Evaluation of Progress

Rectal or Vaginal Examinations

Proof of the labour progress may be gained through rectal or vaginal examinations. Vaginal examinations have been increasingly employed because of the greater accuracy and helpfulness of the information obtained and the lack of infectious complications observed when they are performed appropriately. (In most maternity departments, the rectal examination has been abandoned). Pelvic examinations should be kept to a minimum because of the discomfort to the patient and the possibility of introduction of infection. Student nurses are not routinely taught the techniques of rectal or vaginal examinations. To instruct all students in the techniques would be useless because unless these techniques are practiced frequently, the ability to interpret what is felt is never learned or is easily lost. In addition, the patient would have the discomfort of duplicate examinations.

The patient is usually supine with head elevated slightly for either rectal or vaginal examination. The attending nurse prepares and assist the patient and helps her to relax during the examinations. If a rectal approach is to be used, only clean gloves and lubricant are needed. If a vaginal examination is desired, preparatory procedures differ from institution-to-institution and physician-to-physician. In some instances, the patient is cleansed and draped as for delivery, and the physician may scrub his hands with a brush before putting on sterile gloves. In other hospitals the preparation may not be so elabourate. However, certain principles should always be observed. The vulva should be cleansed. A sterile examining glove should be used. A sterile lubricant and disinfectant per physician's order should be poured over the gloved fingers not to touch anything but the actual vaginal canal so that organisms from anal or other areas are not introduced into the canal. Usually it helps if the patient drops her knees toward the outside and breathes deeply through her open mouth during the digital examination. Holding the nurse's hand seems to give some patients great comfort, too.

After the examinations, the patient's perineal area should be cleansed of any remaining lubricant or antiseptic, and dried and she should be encouraged and reassured. A vaginal examination can reveal information not detected by a rectal examination because the cervix and presenting part are felt directly by the fingers and not through rectovaginal wall. It may help greatly in the determination of the type of presentation the position, and the condition of the bag of waters. Pelvic evaluations should not be performed routinely if abnormal vaginal bleeding is observed because such examinations may increase blood loss.

Rupture of the Membrane (Artificial)

At times, in an effort to induce or to apply an internal monitor lead, the physician artificially ruptures the membranes during a vaginal examination. This is done however, only under certain conditions. The cervix should be effaced, and some dilatation must be present. The head should be engaged. The physician originally uses a sterile instrument with a small claw like end, such as an all is, Iowa, or special plastic hook. The membranes are ruptured between contractions, and the fluid flow is controlled to avoid the cord being swept out of place by a sudden gush of "water". Prolapse of the cord and its subsequent pinching between the presenting part and the bony pelvis is a serious complication for which one must watch. As always, immediately after the membranes have ruptured, the foetal heart rate should be checked to determine any distress of the foetus.

The actual rupture of the big causes no pain because there are no nerves in the membranes, but the pressure exerted to perform the vaginal examination and to position the instrument may cause some discomfort. The patient should be encouraged especially during this period. If rupture of the membranes is anticipated at the time of a vaginal examination, the patient should be placed on several bed-protecting pads to catch the drainage. Some advocate placing the patient on a bedpan; however, the patient's discomfort is usually increased in such a position. The approximate amount (small, moderate, or large) of fluid expelled and its colour should be noted and recorded. Remember, the appearance of meconium in the amniotic fluid during a head presentation is interpreted as a sign of foetal distress. After the examination the patient should be made as comfortable as possible. The excess lubricant should be wiped from the vulva, using good technique (wiping from front to back with no return of a used sponge to the vaginal region). Dry protective bed pads should be in place. If the presenting part of the baby is tight against the cervix and the physician so orders, the labouring mother may be allowed to ambulate.

Intensified Labour: Characteristics and Care

As labour progresses, more frequent and intensive contractions are experienced. More and more, the woman's attention is focused on meeting the demands of these contractions on her physical and psychologic resources. If she has had training in relaxation and breathing techniques, these usually are of great aid. Some abdominal and high chest breathing exercises are described in the chapter. If a labouring patient has had no previous training in these techniques, she may still benefit from some simple instruction in abdominal breathing. This usually eases the discomfort significantly. Rapid breathing techniques can also be taught; but if the woman is unfamiliar with the method, she is likely to hyperventilate, and the normal proportion of oxygen to carbon dioxide in the blood will be upset. She may feel light-headed, and her fingers may begin to tingle. Such side effects should be avoided. If they appear, it may help if she breathes into a paper bag or places the sheet momentarily over the nose. The patient should be especially encouraged, and signs of her progress and condition should be frequently shared with family members.

Probably the most difficult period of labour is that called transition, lasting approximately from 8 to 10 cm dilatation. The labouring patient is now fatigued and usually discouraged. She wonders if she is ever going to have her baby and worries about her performance when she does. Her contractions may be irregular, at times seeming to come "one right after another". Nausea and vomiting are common.

SECOND STAGE OF LABOUR

The second stage of labour is the stage in which the infant is born. This stage begins with full cervical dilation (10 cm) and complex effacement

(100 per cent) and ends with the baby's birth. The bearing down efforts (BDE) facilitate achievement of the expected outcome of a spontaneous uncomplicated vaginal birth.

The second stage comprises three phases. Latent, descent and transition. These phases are characterized by maternal and verbal behaviors, uterine activity, the urge to bear down and foetal descent.

The Latent Phase

The latent phase is a period of rest and relative calm (i.e. labouring down). The woman is quick and often relaxes with her eyes closed between contractions. The urge to bear down is not well established and is experienced primarily during the acme of a contraction. Allowing a woman to rest during this phase, and waiting until the urge to push intensifies (delayed pushing), has been found to reduce maternal fatigue, conserve energy for bearing down efforts and provide optimal maternal and foetal outcomes.

The Descent Phase

The descent phase is characterized by strong urges to bear down as the ferguson reflex is activated when the presenting part presses on the release of oxytocin from the posterior pituitary gland, which provokes stronger expulsive uterine contractions. The woman becomes more focussed on bearing down efforts (BDE) which becomes rhythmic. She changes positions frequently to find a more comfortable pushing positions. The woman often announces the onset of contractions and becomes more vocal as she bears down.

The Transition Phase

In this phase, the presenting part is on the perineum and bearing down efforts are most effective for promoting birth. The woman may be more verbal about pain, may scream and swear, and may act out of control. The nurse encourages the woman to 'listen' to her body as she progresses through phases of the second stage of labour. When a woman listens to her body to tell her when to bear down, she is using an internal locus of control and often feels more satisfied. With her efforts to give birth to her baby. Her sense of self-esteem and accomplishment is enhanced and her efforts become more effective. The woman's trust in her own body and her ability to give birth to her baby should be fostered.

The only certain objective sign that the second stage of labour has be found is the inability to feel the cervix during vaginal examination, indicating that the cervix is fully dilated and effaced. Other signs suggest that onset of the second stage include the following:

- Sudden appearance of perspiration on upper lip
- An episode of vomiting
- Increased bloody show
- Shaking of extremities
- Increased restlessness, verbalization that 'I can't go on'
- Involuntary bearing down efforts.

These signs commonly appear at the time the cervix reaches full dilation (except women with epidural block).

The duration of the second stage of labour influenced by several factors, such as the effectiveness of the primary and secondary powers of the labour; the type and amount of analgesia or anaesthesia used; the physical and emotional condition, position, activity level, and parity of the labouring woman; and the nature and source of support the woman receives.

Care of the Second Stage of Labour

During this period the patient needs to be evaluated frequently concerning the possibility of the onset of the second stage of labour, the period of expulsion. The physician and other delivery room personnel should be kept informed of the patient's progress. The second stage will orginally be heralded by (1) an increase in show, (2) an involuntary urge to push or bear down with each contraction as the presenting part escapes the uterus and descends. (3) the foetal heart tone usually being heard just above the pubic bone in head presentations and (4) late signs, including the bulging of the perineum, the dilatation of the anus, and the appearance of caput, or the foetal scalp. It is fervently hoped that a multipara will be adequately prepared for the actual birth before these last signs manifest themselves. Usually, multiparas are transferred to the delivery room at about 8 cm dilatation to avoid a last-minute race. However, women bearing their first babies are often not transferred to the delivery room proper before these last signs appear, since the period between complete dilatation and the birth of the infant may be relatively protracted for a primipara. One reason the 'birthing room' concept is popular is that it avoids transfers of patient from one room to another for different stages of labour. Such transfers can be quite difficult at times.

Most hospitals in the developed countries now allow fathers of the expectant mother's chosen companion in the delivery room, especially those who have attended child birth education classes. The excitement and wonder of the occasion are appropriately shared with these significant persons. The father sits at the head of the delivery table, encouraging the mother in her efforts and watching with her the progress of the birth together appears to creat a "natural high" that they never forget. However, the father or companion will have previously agreed to leave in the event of problems when his presence is thought to compromise the best interests of the mother. Not all men want to see their children born, but for those who do, it seems to be a memorable, positive experience.

Pushing

Although she may wish to do so, a woman usually should not be urged by the nurse to bear down or push before complete dilation of the cervix is determined. To do so could cause greater fatigue for the mother, greater stain on the foetus, and possible swelling and injury to the cervix. After complete dilatation and preparations for the birth are made, pushing is usually recommended. Most women are relieved by pushing and cooperate well in following instructions if they are not confused by too many instructors.

Preparation of the Delivery Room

Before the second stage of labour is reached, the delivery room should be prepared for the actual birth of the baby. The responsibility of its preparation may be that of a trained vocational nurse. Hers is an important responsibility. To execute it correctly she must have a clear concept of he principles of sterile technique, know where supplies are kept, and know the patient's special needs and the attending physician's desires. She should have some idea when the room will be needed so that she can plan her work. The actual preparation of the delivery room will vary in different maternity services, but the basic needs to be met and the principles employed will be the same.

Practice of Aseptic Techniques

The practice of asepsis is not really difficult if the appropriate equipment and supplies are available and if conscientious, knowledgeable persons are involved in their use and care. It is however a serious responsibility that involves evaluation of the area environment, including the nurses dress and personal health problems that may threaten the safety of the patient. Four simple rules sums up aseptic technique:

1. Know what is sterile.
2. Know what is not sterile.
3. Keep the two apart.
4. Remedy contamination immediately.

Using Transfer Forceps

The use of transfer forceps, or "pick ups" in the handling of sterile supplies is as safe as the techniques employed for their care. Because wet forceps often become contaminated, their use has all but disappeared. When used, any wet forceps should be held so that the grasping ends are pointed downward. If wet forceps are used, care should be taken not to touch the ends of the instrument on any exposed inner side of the holding canister. The area above the level of solution cannot be considered sterile because of prolonged exposure to the air. In some areas a fresh, dry, sterile canister and forceps may be used for each birth setup. Transfer forceps should not be held below the level of the waist or above the shoulder. Today, the nurse commonly wears sterile gloves to set up the delivery supply table.

General Considerations

Review the methods of unwrapping and placing supplies. When approaching a sterile field to add sterile supplies, take care to avoid accidentally brushing or touching the area. When passing a sterile field, keep a safe distance away and, if possible face the field. Never turn your back on a sterile area. Avoid turning your back on a sterile area. Avoid turning your back toward an associate who is gowned in a sterile manner.

If contamination of a sterile area does occur, the event must be immediately reported. It is no terrible sin to contaminate. It is dangerous and irresponsible to contaminate a sterile field, to know it, and to nothing about it when something can be done. No one at the time may see the lapse of asepsis, but ultimately the patient may suffer the results. The medical-nursing team should be glad to have breaks in technique or inadvertent contamination called to their attention so that they may correct the situation.

Delivery Room Set Up

Purpose The purpose of this procedure is three fold:

1. To provide an aseptic field for the anticipated birth and subsequent newborn and maternal care.
2. To ensure the convenient placement and operation of all necessary articles to promote safely, speed, and confidence on the part of the staff on behalf on the physical and emotional care of the mother and child.
3. To aid in the necessary legal and statistical recording of the event

Set Up

1. Personal preparation
   a. Secure information:
      - Which physician (for glove size, etc).
      - Which delivery room.
      - Type of anaesthesia to be used, if any anticipated.
      - Special problems involving the patient (Rh-negative, preeclampsia, varicosities of the extremities etc).
      - Approximate time the room is needed.

   b. Put on mask. Be sure all your hair is covered by a cap.
   c. Wash hands.
   d. Review in your mind the principles of sterile technique.
2. Open necessary sterile packs. Check outside tapes on packs for proof of sterilization if this type of tape is used. Check dates on packs to avoid outdated materials. Usually included are:
   a. The basic dolivery pack with drapes and materials used on the patient or for the delivery.
   b. The instrument pack (unless instruments are taken directly from a sterilizer).
   c. The brain-st pack, used to provide a sterile basin for the placenta gloved hands, or cleansing the patient.
   d. The perineal preparation tray may provide:
      - Acleansing solution
      - Sterile gauze sponges
      - Sterile gloves or sponge sticks
      - An antiseptic for the skin after the cleansing of the area (this is not always used).

   e. The anaesthesia supplies (if appropriate)
   f. Any indicated obstetric forceps are usually placed conveniently (still wrapped) in the room until called for, except piper forceps used in breach deliveries for the aftercoming head. Piper forceps are used unwrapped previously and placed on the supply table.
3. Check infant care equipment and supplies (warmer, suction, oxygen and bulb syringe, blankets, nurses gown and examination gloves).
4. At the time of birth the necessary records are brought into the room for completion, and the identification procedure for mother and child are carried out.

Precautions

As soon as the head emerges, the nose and mouth are cleared of mucus and amniotic fluid to prevent aspiration when the infant first breathes. The physician feels for the cord. If it is wrapped around the neck, an attempt is made to slip it over the head. If this cannot be done, it is clamped and cut. Usually the anterior shoulder advances to the pubic arch, which acts as a pivot. Then the posterior shoulder moves forward over the perineum. The anterior shoulder will be lodged just at the upper vaginal opening, and while watching the perineum carefully and applying steady pressure, the nurse-midwife delivers the posterior shoulder. The rest of the body slips out easily.

There are differences of opinion regarding whether the cord should be cut before or after draining the residual volume of blood to the foetus. The prevailing opinion is that this extra blood increases the likelihood of hyperbilirubinemia in the neonatal period. Therefore the baby is held at the level of the perineum until cord pulsation has ceased or the cord is clamped in two places and cut between the clamps. A baby held too high above the perineum may transfuse blood back into the placenta and be anaemic with a low blood volume during the recovery period.

The irritability, discouragement, and agitation that marked the final hour of the first stage disappear at full dilation and the beginning of the woman's cooperative efforts. It is important that the woman be prepared for the sensations that accompany expulsion so she can put them in proper perspective. These include distension of the vaginal tissue (increasing pressure on the perineum), rectal pressure, and absence of the perception of the contraction itself with the pushing effort.

The father's encouragement to sustain the immense pushing efforts very important. Although she becomes oblivious to peripheral activity, she was susceptible to confusion if conflicting directions are given or several people attempt to direct her. The unprepared woman may completely lose control. She may utter loud screams at the peak of the contraction. She frequently is unable to follow directions unless they are simple and repeated.

The father's presence at the birth can be a profound experience for the new parents and makes them aware of parenthood as a mutually shared effort. The partner remains at the woman's side, speaking directly into her ear, if needed. He has learned the correct pushing technique to encourage her efforts. During practice and in delivery, use cue words such as breathe-in, out; in, out; hold (your breath); Relax (key areas, such as jaw, mouth and perineum, pass out (use the abdominal muscles; push out through the vagina, while releasing air and grunting).

Repeat the sequence several times for each contraction and slowly count to help her sustain pushing for up to 6 to 8 seconds at a time. Between contractions, encourage her to relax by speaking in soothing tones, stroking, or using a cool cloth.

The woman will appreciate anything to increase her comfort, such as wiping her face, giving her ice chips or adjusting the birthing bed to a higher position. It is impossible to push effectively when lying supine.

During the second phase, the coach may also assist in placing a warm wet towel over the perineum to relax the tissues, or an ice compress may be placed over the clitoris during crowning to reduce the pain.

By recognizing the mother's progress through the phases of the second stage and changing interventions as needed, the nurse backs up the father or coach. It is important to control the number of people giving directions to the woman. Too many voices confuse her. Only one person should take the lead, with turns taken by another. The woman should not be left alone to push. If the second phase lasts more than an hours, the coach will be fatigued and needs comfort, too, with explanations.

One cannot push in the supine position. The birthing bed has many settings or the woman may assume a hands and knees posture, especially if the foetus is in a posterior position (see Fig. 5.7B). Squatting is the usual birthing position for women in many developing countries. It opens the passage as widely as possible. In Europe, many births are in the side-lying position. Pushing can be done effectively in this position; the upper knee may be held by the coach. The side-lying position may slow descent but appears to relax the perineum, thereby reducing the need for an episiotomy.

Positioning for the third phase had been routinely in the lithotomy position, with the legs higher than the trunk and head. This is incorrect and should be altered to a moderate semi-Fowler's position, with the knees and legs lower than the heart. When the legs are put high into the leg holders, approximately 2000 ml of blood are auto-transfused into the central system, increasing cardiac workload. Since BDEs also affect cardiac function, a woman with hypertension or cardiac problems will be compromised by such a position. (if haemorrhage occurs, the head may of course be lowered). With a birthing bed it is possible to adjust the legs in a number of positions.

Throughout the second stage, the foetus is monitored, with observation every 10 minutes as a standard of care. This must be continued until birth. In units where the woman is moved to a delivery room, this means using a portable deptone to obtain FHR, which must then be documented correctly.

SUMMARY OF NURSING RESPONSIBILITIES

1. Assess the phases of the second stage, changing comfort measured as indicated.
2. Observe foetal responses every 10 minutes and notify occurance of any adverse changes. Be alert to the emergence of end-stage variables, document findings.
3. Position the woman for effective BDEs
4. Support the coach in giving verbal instructions to push or rest.
5. Maintain safe environment.
6. Protect self and staff with universal precautions for body fluids.
7. Maintaining hygiene and fluids and encourage voiding, catheterize of bladder in full and mother is unable to void.
8. Prepare birth equipment.

9. Explain each step of the activities's position, monitoring, and preparation of birth.
10. Evaluate the woman's response to intervention.
11. Assist physician or nurse midwife during birth.
12. Fill in all records of the birth and condition of the body.

Transfer and Immediate Predelivery Care

The transfer of the patient to the delivery room should be as smooth as possible. If the patient has a strong desire to push and it is not appropriate activity at the time, she should be advised to pant through her open mouth. Care should be taken in the transfer of the patient. She can usually help considerably in the move to the delivery table if the staff is able to wait until a contraction is not present. It is imperative that observation and recording of maternal pulse and blood pressure as well as FHR patterns continue in a consistent manner (at least every 15 minutes) after the patient has been transferred to the delivery room, whether a vaginal or caesarean birth is expected.

While the patient is being prepared in the delivery room, the physician may be dressing and scrubbing of the administration of the spinal anaesthesia, fused, or for the delivery itself. Many obstetric units currently have anaesthesiologists on staff to assist with deliveries. The circulating nurse uncovers the sterile table and basin set and turns on the necessary lights, if no spinal anaesthesia is used, the physician generally advises the staff when the patient should be placed in dorsal lithotomy position with her legs in supports, if this position is used.

Positioning (Fig. 5.7 and Table 5.6)

Ideally, two nurses assist in lithotomy positioning, although it can be accomplished by one. To prevent strain on the patient's back, both legs

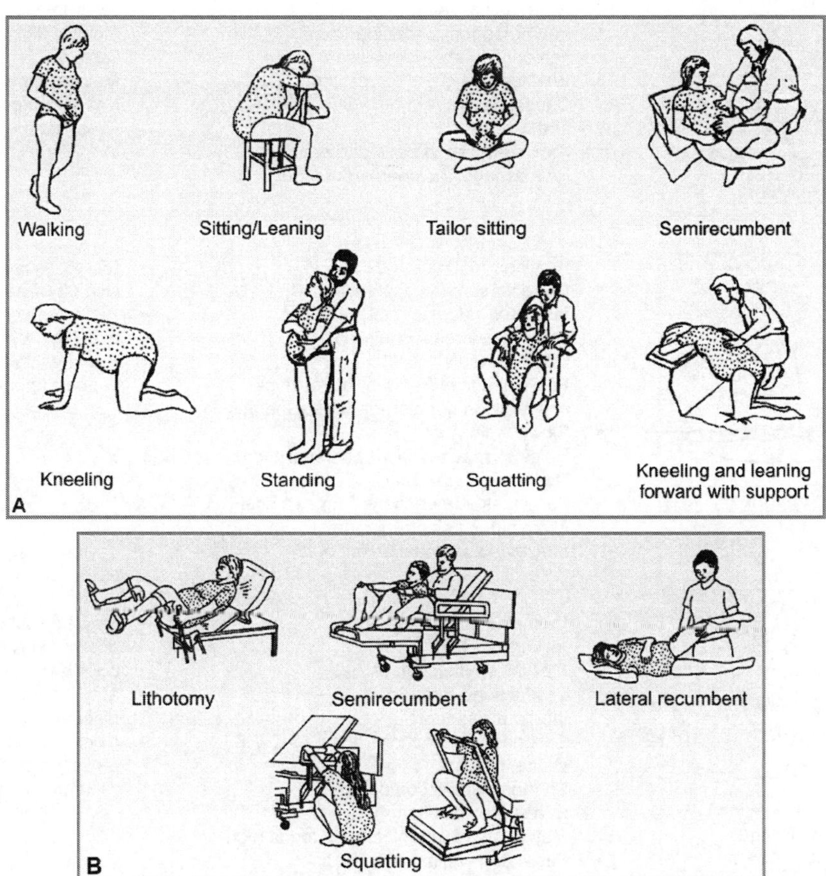

Figs 5.7A and B: Positions for labour and birth. A, Positions for labour. B, Positions for giving birth

Table 5.6: Advantages and disadvantage of various positions for labour and birth (Figs 5.8A to I)

Position	*Advantages*	*Disadvantages*
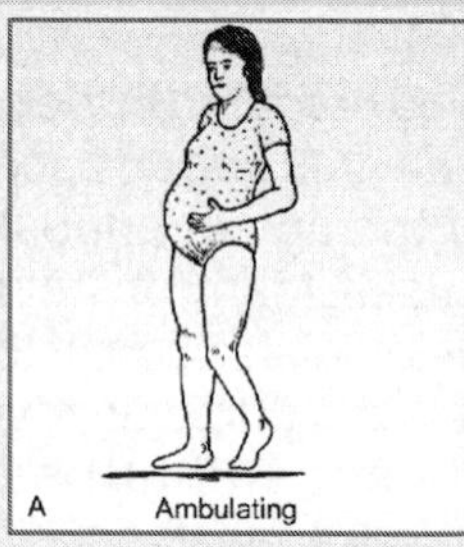 A Ambulating	• Utilizes gravity; applies presenting part against cervix • Places foetus in alignment with pelvis; facilitates descent • Enhances effect of contractions and decreases pain • May decrease length of labour • Decreases foetal heart variable decelerations • Relieves backache	• May be tiring • Telemetry required for continuous electronic foetal monitoring • Not possible with regional anesthesia
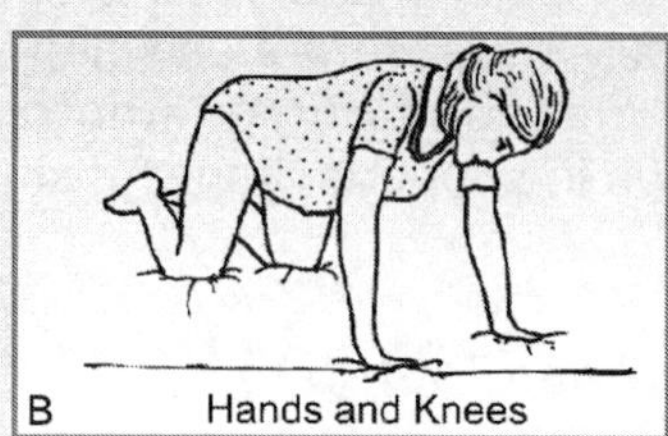 B Hands and Knees	• Simulates rotation of foetus from posterior to anterior position • Relieves backache • Relieves rectal pressure • Facilitates pelvic rocking and pelvic mobility • Eliminates weight on inferior vena cava and decreases foetal distress • Relieves pressure on cord if prolapsed • Facilitates delivery, especially in cases of shoulder dystocia, breech position, or persistent occiput posterior position	• May be tiring; causes wrist fatigue • May be embarrassing • External electronic foetal monitor difficult to keep in place • Not possible with regional anesthesia
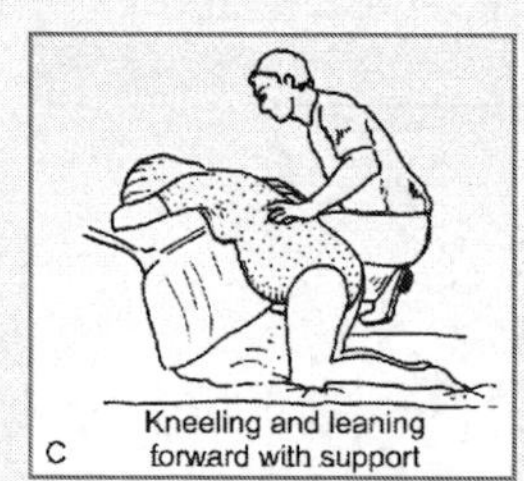 C Kneeling and leaning forward with support	• Relieves backache • Facilitates foetal rotation from posterior to anterior position • Enables use of pelvic rocking • Causes less strain on wrists and hands • Allows access to back and sacrum for massage and counterpressure	• External electronic foetal monitor difficult to keep in place • May be tiring • Not possible with regional anesthesia
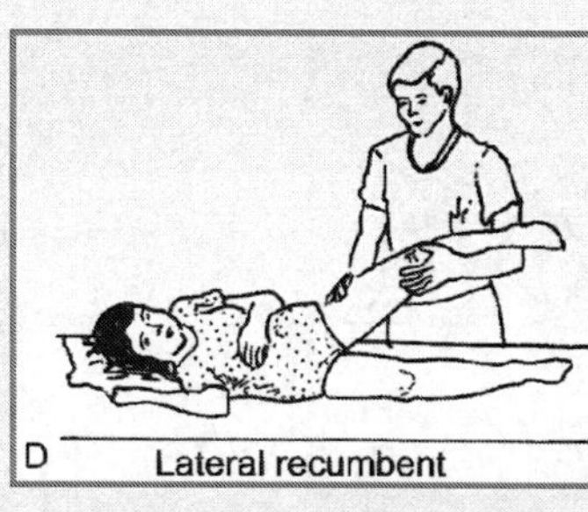 D Lateral recumbent	• Provides rest; comfortable • Corrects supine hypotension; facilitates fetoplacental perfusion • Helps to decrease maternal blood pressure • Facilitates less frequent but stronger contractions compared with supine position • Slows rapid labour • Helps to rotate occiput posterior foetus • Decreases back pain • Facilitates interventions (e.g., vaginal examination, electronic foetal monitoring, regional anesthesia)	• More effective if alternated with other positions • Not as effective for expulsive efforts • Requires that someone support upper leg for delivery
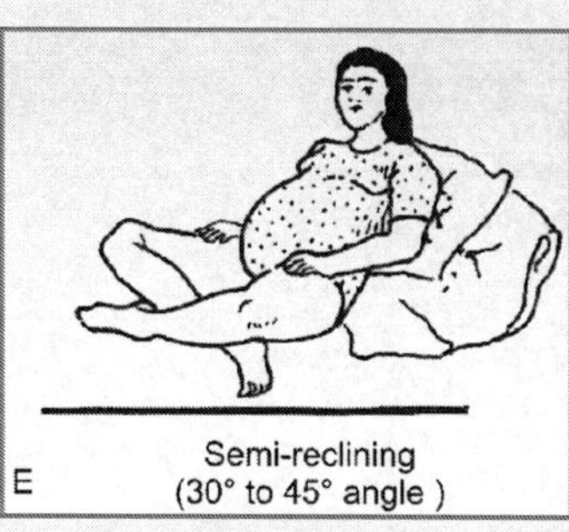 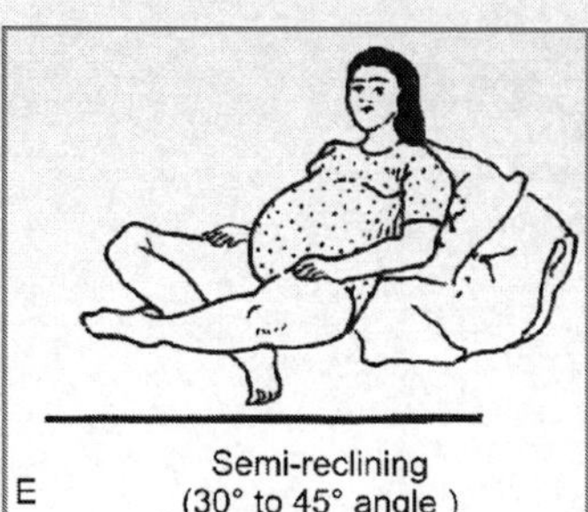 E Semi-reclining (30° to 45° angle)	• Promotes comfort; good resting position • Maximizes direction of contractions force to facilitate descent • Enhances contractions compared with supine position • Shortens labour compared with supine position • May be used with electronic foetal monitor • Facilitates vaginal examination	• May slow labour if not alternated with other positions • May increase back discomfort • Contractions not as intense as with standing or lateral recumbent positions

Contd...

Contd...

Position	*Advantages*	*Disadvantages*
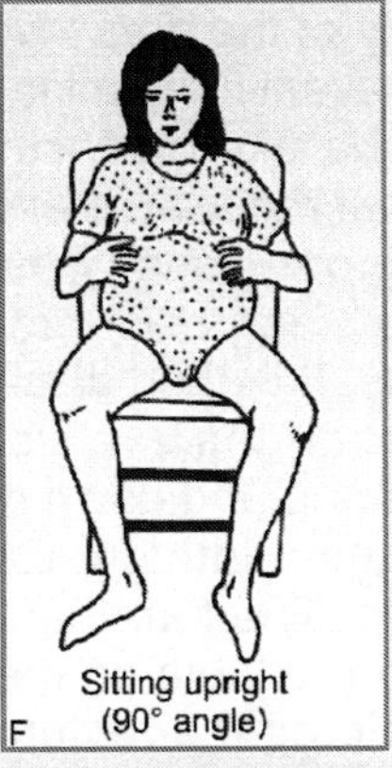 F Sitting upright (90° angle)	• Decreases back pain; comfortable • Utilizes gravity • Avoids supine hypotensive syndrome • Shortens labour compared with supine position • May use with electronic foetal monitor • Shortens second-stage labour; increases pelvic diameter • Enhances interaction with partner • Allows access to back and sacrum for massage and counterpressure when leaning forward	• Contractions not as intense as with standing or lateral recumbent positions • May slow labour if not alternated with other positions • May increase suprapubic pain • May cause edema of vulva or cervix
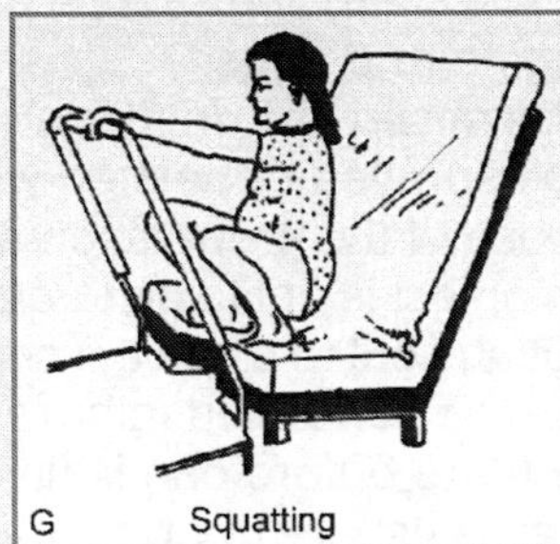 G Squatting	• Utilizes gravity • Increases pelvic diameters • Relieves backache • Facilitates pushing efforts in second-stage; Increases intra-abdominal pressure • Promotes foetal descent and rotation; may shorten second stage • Enhances interaction between woman, labour partner, and birth attendant	• May impede descent before engagement • May be uncomfortable; tiring • May be embarrassing • May increase risk of uterine prolapse with strenuous bearing down • May increase perineal and cervical edema or lacerations • May increase blood loss
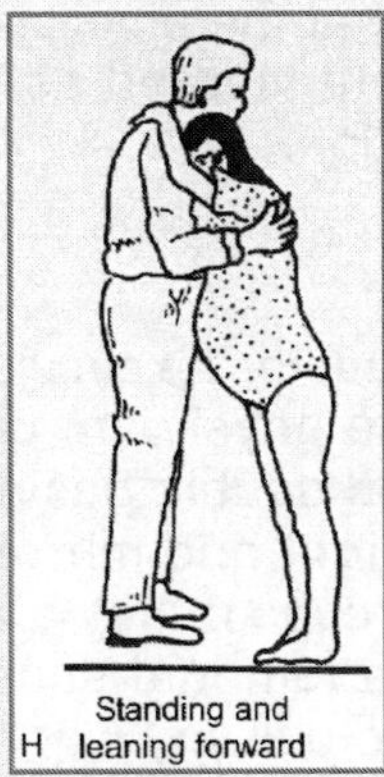 H Standing and leaning forward	• Utilizes gravity; applies presenting part against cervix • Places foetus in alignment with pelvis; facilitates descent • Enhances effect of contractions and decreases pain • Promotes comfort; decreases backache because foetus moves forward • May decrease length of labour • Facilitates rest during contractions • May be used with electronic foetal monitor	• May be tiring • Not possible with regional anesthesia • May be difficult to keep external electronic foetal monitor in place • Needs two supporters if used in second-stage
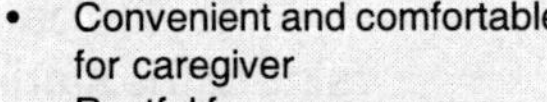 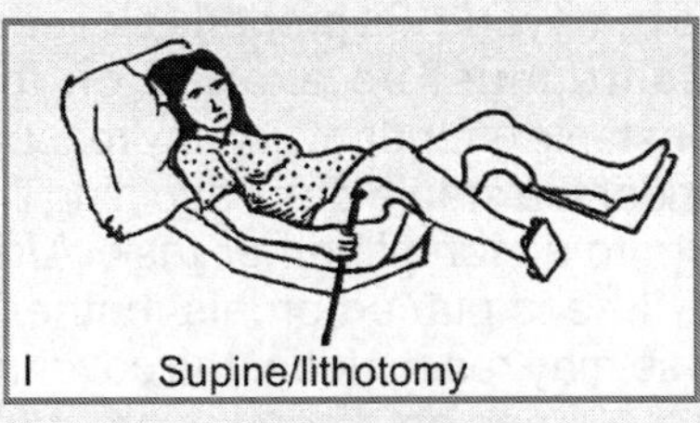 I Supine/lithotomy	• Convenient and comfortable for caregiver • Restful for some women • Facilitates foetal monitoring and vaginal examination • Facilitates interventions (foetal heart rate, forceps, episiotomy, repair of lacerations) • Facilitates maintenance of asepsis • Facilitates comfort and security for legs for some women through stirrups • Decreases ability to push	• Supine hypotensive syndrome • Increases back discomfort • Contractions less efficient, more painful, and longer in duration • Women may feel psychologically vulnerable or dependent • Decreases maternal participation during birth • Stirrups can promote blood clots or discomfort in legs • Risk of aspiration if woman vomits

Figs 5.8A to I

should be raised or lowered at the same time. Coaching her to bend her knees as her legs are raised helps. If crutch or stirrup type leg supports are used, the supports must be fitted to the patient, not the patient fitted to the supports most delivery tables have some method of dividing in half, temporarily eliminating the foot portion of the table to allow the buttocks to hand over the end of the upper part of the table and the physician to stand directly in front of the perineum. As soon as the patient's legs are adequately secured in the preferable position.

This is called "dropping" or "breaking" the table.

Giving birth in lithotomy position is not an anatomic necessity it is the position that is associated with the use of spinal or general anaesthesia and is the most familiar to many physicians. In England, a modified side position is often used. In some cultures the mother gives birth in a squatting position. In parts of Europe a modified Fowler's position is typically used, with flexion and abduction of the lower extremities. These last two postures allow gravity to aid the mother in her efforts to push the baby to the outside world. Special adjustable combination labour-delivery beds or chairs are now available that assist the mother to maintain a more physiologic birth position.

Sterile Perineal Preparation (Fig. 5.9)

As soon as the table is 'dropped', the circulating nurse cleanses the abdomen, thighs, and complete perineal area with a soap or antiseptic solution. This procedure is the so called sterile prep. Again, it is carried out in different ways in different institutions. It may involve sterile gloving or the use of sterile forceps or sponge sticks. The principles are the same; to help prevent infection and to increase the visibility of the area involved. In performing the prep to prevent contamination of the birth canal, care should be taken to ensure that no sponge is used in the anal rectal area and then returned to the vulvar region. Usually the first sponge is used to cleanse side to side from the pubic bone to the umbilicus. It is then discarded. The second and third sponges are used in cleansing the thighs with an up and down motion from the labia majora to the midthigh. Each is discarded directly after use. The fourth and fifth sponges are used to clean the labia on the right and left of the vagina, avoiding the rectum, and then discarded. The last cleansing sponge passes directly over the vagina and anus.

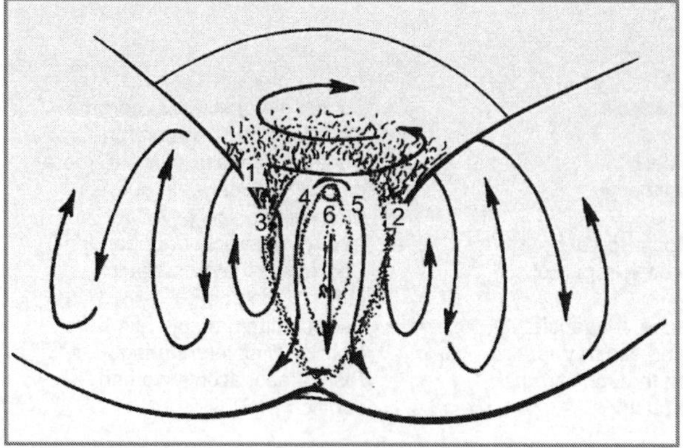

Fig. 5.9: Perineal scrub preparation, which is done just before birth. Numbers and arrows indicate the order and direction of each stroke

The patient may be rinsed and dried in a similar manner and perhaps sprayed or painted with an antiseptic. The purpose of the preparation should be kept in mind. The object is not to go through so many prescribed motions but to clean the skin. On the other hand, it must be performed rather swiftly, or the baby may be there before one is finished. The gowned physician is usually ready to drape for delivery as soon as the nurse is finished. Care must be taken to see that the physicians hands and gown are not contaminated as the nurse completes the preparation.

Draping

During the draping procedure, the circulating nurse provides a stool for the physician, pushes the sterile supply table and double basin rack into position, adjusts the light and mirror (if being used), unwraps the forceps if they are desired, secures any needed additional supplies, and begins her record of the delivery.

After the patient is draped, no part of the exposed side of the sterilelinen (or paper) covering the patient should be touched by anyone not properly glovedor gowned. If pressure must be exerted on the abdomen by a "nonsterile attendant" for any reason, she must reach under the sterile drap, avoiding the exposed perineum to accomplish her task. After the baby is born, if he is placed on his mother's abdomen, the nurse may reach under the covering drape and, using the drape as a hand guard, hold on to an infant arm or leg to help give support while his airway is aspirated or the cord is tied. Babies can be very slippery.

Delivery

Forceps and Episiotomies (Figs 5.10A to E)

After the sterile preparation and draping are complete, First the mother's bladder needs to be emptied or a special urine specimen is necessary, the physician will perform a catheterization before the birth of the baby. But the procedure is no longer as common before delivery as it once was.

At times, especially if the mother is bearing her first baby, the physician may use outlet forceps to lift out the baby's head. Judicious application of these forceps may shorten the second stage of labour considerably if the mother is finding it difficult to push effectively or the baby's or mother's condition makes more rapid delivery advisable. However, the use of outlet forceps just to save time is questionable. Forceps are usually applied in conjunction with a planned incision of the perineum to enlarge the vaginal opening called an episiotomy.

An episiotomy may be performed without the use of forceps. It is done to prevent lacerations or damage to the perineum, to avoid possible prolonged pressure on the infant's head, and to has ten delivery. There are two main types of episotomies: (1) the midline or median, which features an incision from the vaginal opening straight down toward but not extending into the anus, and (2) the mediolateral, which begins at the midline above the anus but angles to the left or right. The midline type is said to be easier to repair and more comfortable for the mother but occasionally it may extend during the birth, tearing the anal sphincter. The mediolateral type of episiotomy is designed to prevent this complication but is considered more difficult to repair and usually is more painful during the postpartum period. The routine use of outlet forceps and/or episiotomy is controversial and has stirred considerable debate. The birth of many babies does not involve the use of either forceps or episiotomy.

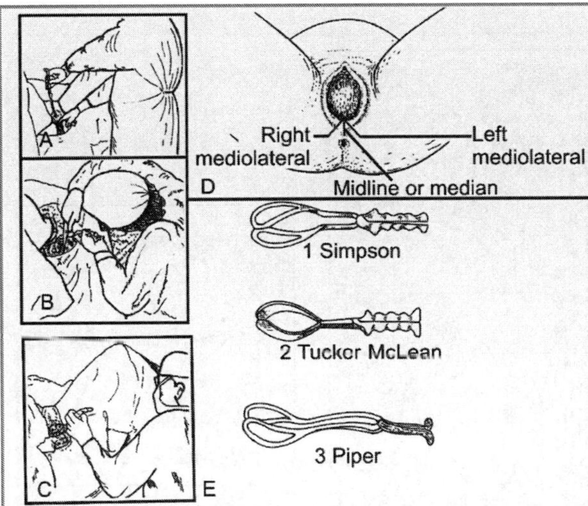

Figs 5.10A to E: A, Insertion of one forceps blade. B, Midline episiotomy (one blade of the forceps has been inserted). C, Use of outlet forceps. D, Various types of episiotomies. E, Three kinds of obstetrical forceps: 1. Simpson; 2. Tucker-McLean; 3. Piper (sometimes employed to deliver after-coming head of breech presentation)

Rather rarely, other types of forceps may be used to achieve progress at delivery associated with head rotation or midforceps application. High forceps (historically applied before engagement has taken place) are never recommended in modern obstetrics.

Delivery Mechanisms (Figs 5.11 to 5.13)

If forceps are not used for the complete delivery of the head, it may be delivered manually between contractions by slow gentle extension. If the mother is able, she may be asked to bear down between contractions to facilitate the actual passage of the head from the vaginal canal. After the head is delivered, the physician cheeks to see whether the umbilical cord is wound around the baby's neck. If it is, it must be slipped over the baby's head or clamped and cut to avoid strangulation or excessive pulling. Even before the entire body of the baby is delivered, the mouth may be aspirated to clear the airway. To deliver the shoulders, the physician usually turns the baby's head to the side so that the occiput lines up with his back. The physician may then gently but firmly pull down to deliver the top (anterior) shoulder and then gently pull up to deliver the bottom (posterior) shoulder.

Scarcely before one realizes it, all of the baby has been born. Further aspiration of the airway may be necessary. Usually the infant cries very soon after birth. His umbilical cord is clamped in two places and cut between the clamps. He is then handed to the nurse for further care in a way that protects the physician's gloves from contamination and makes a safe transfer. Increasingly, the baby is being given to the mother or father to hold soon after birth. Mother-infant skin-to-skin contact is believed to promote attachment and assists in maintaining the baby's body temperature.

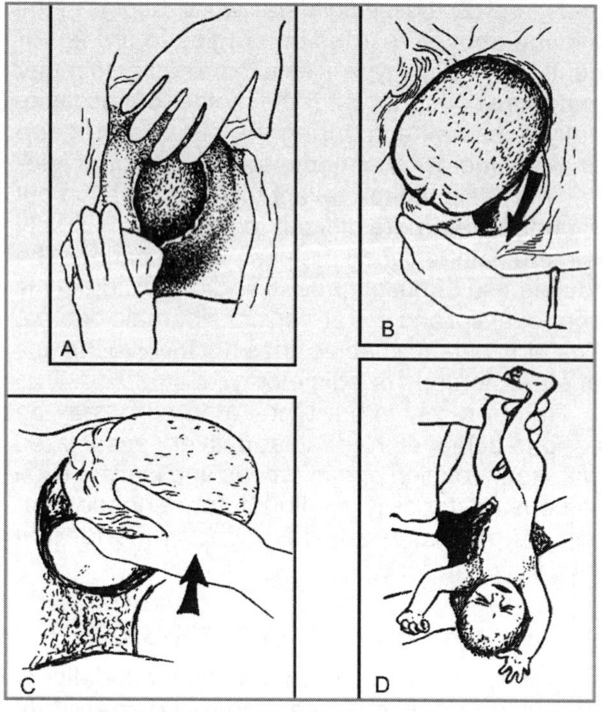

Figs 5.11A to D: Vaginal birth of a foetus in a vertex presentation. A, The foetal head is crowning. An episiotomy has been done to enlarge the vaginal opening. B, Birth of the foetal head and restitution as the head realigns with the shoulders. C, The foetal head has externally rotated, the anterior shoulder has been brought under the mother's symphysis pubis, and the posterior shoulder is now being brought over her perineum. D, The physician or nurse-midwife firmly grasps the baby as it slips from the mother's vagina

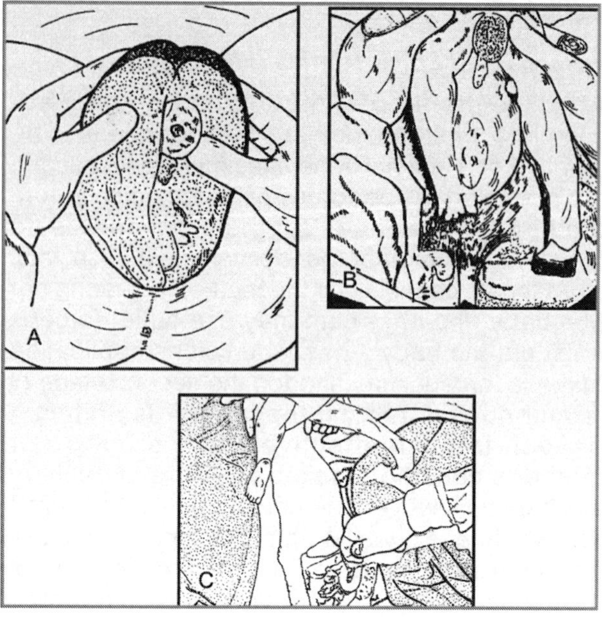

Figs 5.12A to C: Delivery of a male foetus in a frank breech presentation. A, The foetal outtocks and legs emerge. B, The foetal legs, abdomen, and most of the chest have emerged. Note that the foetus's umbilical cord is now out and can be compressed between the foetal head and the mother's pelvis. Thus, the head must be delivered quickly. C, An assistant holds the foetal legs while the obstetrician assists birth of the foetal head with forceps

The Baby

Immediate Care

The nurse caring for the newborn infant should wear a clean overgown. Freshly washed hands should be covered by disposable gloves until all fluid is removed from the baby's skin. To avoid the metabolic problems brought on by cold stress, the first step in the management of the newborn infant is to prevent the loss of body heat. This can be an especially critical factor in a newborn who needs resuscitation. Heat loss is prevented by placing the infant under a radiant heat source and quickly drying him. These two steps, which should be done for all infants following delivery, require only few seconds to accomplish and can prevent the infant from becoming cold stressed as a result of evaporative, convective, and radiant heat losses. Even healthy term infants are limited in their ability to produce heat when exposed to a cold

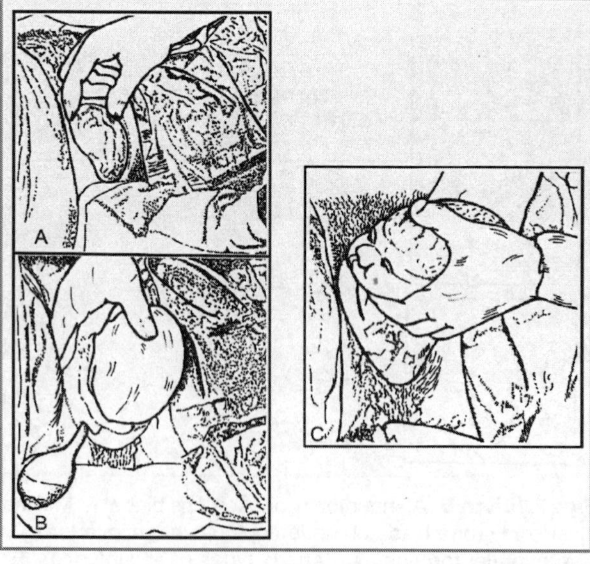

Figs 5.13A to C: Delivery sequence LOA, Crowning. B, Delivery of head and clearing of airway, mouth, then nose. C, Delivery of posterior shoulder

environment, especially during the first 12 hours of life.

An overhead radiant heater allows access to and full visualization of the infant. Do not cover the infant because this prevents the radiant heat waves from reaching the skin. Place the infant under the warmer and using a warm towel or blanket gently and quickly dry the head and body to remove the amniotic fluid and prevent evaporative heat loss. The stimulation that this activity provides may initiate or help maintain aspiration. Remove the wet towel or blanket from the bed.

Many adjustments must be made in the newborn's body to fit him for his new environment. He should be placed on his side and carefully and frequently observed. The nurse must provide warmth (usually in the form of an incubator, heated blanket, or a radiant infant warmer), observe his colour and breathing pattern, and attach the identification approved by the hospital. During the same period of time, she usually performs the prophylaxis prescribed to prevent gonorrheal infection of the eyes (although some neonatologists state that it may be safely delayed up to an hour after birth when that time is desired to enhance the maternal-infant attachment process and early breastfeeding). It prescribed an instillation of 1 per cent silver nitrate (AgNO3) solution, erythromycin 0.5 per cent in single use tubes, or sterile ophthalmic ointment containing tetracycline 1 per cent into the newborn's eyes for the prevention of ocular gonorrheal infection. Many hospitals have been using erythromycin, which has been thought to be more effective against chlamydial infection and does not cause the eye irritation associated with the application of less constantly silver nitrate. However, reports of a recent large research study indicates that erythromycin may not be significantly more effective than silver nitrate in preventing chlamydial infection. Saline or water irrigations following the instillation of AgNO3 unfortunately do not reduce the incidence of chemical conjunctivitis and may curtail the efficacy of the solution.

Apgar Evaluation

If the Apgar method of evaluating the newborn infant is used, the infant should also be scored for heart rate, respiratory effort, muscle tone, reflex irritability, and colour, 1 and 5 minutes after birth. This scoring may be done by the physician, anaesthesiologist, or nurse; but the nurse is thought by some to be the more "impartial" and available "observer, especially for the 5 minutes evaluation. The Apgar score is used in follow-up studies of the child and is reviewed in many research inquiries. Infants receiving a score of 7 to 10 are considered vigorous. Scores of 1 to 6 denote mild to moderate depression whereas 0 to 3 indicates severe depression. The highest score that can be given is 10. Dr Apgar believed that few newborn infants conscientiously scored deserve a first rating totaling 10. She believed that few babies are completely pink, 1 minute after birth (Table 5.7).

Table 5.7: Modified Apgar scoring chart to evaluate newborn status 1 and 5 minutes after birth

New name	*Traditional sign*	*0*	*1*	*2*
A Appearance	Colour	Blue, pale	Body pink Extremities blue	Completely pink
P Pulse	Heart rate	Absent	Slow (below 100)	Over 100
G Grimace	Reflex response (e.g. to catheter in nostril)	No response	Grimace	Cry, cough or sneeze
A Activity	Muscle tone	Flaccid	Some flexion of extremities	Actual motion
R Respiratory effort	Respiratory effort	Absent	Slow, irregular	Good, crying
Total score:	1 min	Severely depressed Moderately depressed	0 to 3 4 to 6	
	5 min	Vigorous	7 to 10	

The birth experience and immediate treatment of the newborn have been critiqued provocatively by the French obstetrician Frederick Leboyer in his book and film, Birth without violence. His call for more consideration of the sensory needs of the newborn seems to be legitimate, although his methods have stirred much comment. For normal births he stresses the following: a quiet, dimmed atmosphere, support for the infant's spine, maternal-child skin-to-skin contact, an intact umbilical cord until pulsation has ceased, newborn body message, and a gentle body temperature water bath followed by warm wrapping and breastfeeding. Objections most often voiced regarding his techniques involve the dimmed environment, which may inhibit an adequate ability, to observe, and the additional time and space that is needed to carry out his recommendations in busy maternity services. Most labour-delivery units will use this technique if parents request it. Cord infection is not increased.

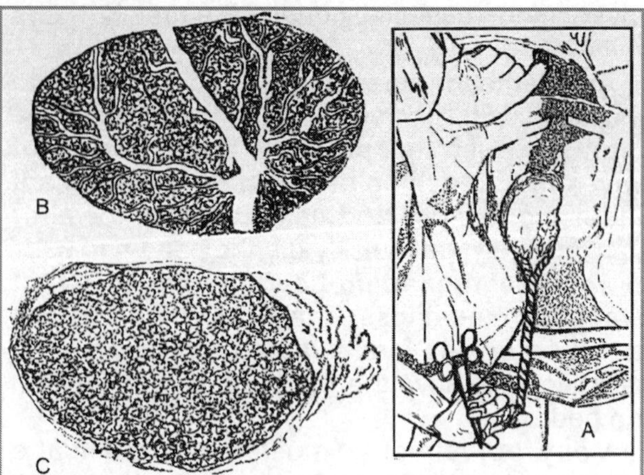

Figs 5.14A to C: A, Delivery of placenta (afterbirth). B, Maternal side showing cotyledons and membranes pulled to one side. The cord attaches on opposite side. If this side appears first at outlet, placenta is said to have separated by Duncan's mechanism. C, Foetal side showing insertion of cord. If this side appears first at outlet, placenta separation is by Schultz's mechanism

THIRD STAGE OF LABOUR

The third stage of labour lasts from the birth of the baby until the separation and expulsion of the placenta. The goal in the management of the third stage of labour is the prompt separation and expulsion of the placenta, achieved in the easiest, safest manner.

Delivery of Placenta (Figs 5.14 and 5.15)

The placenta is attached to the decidual layer of the basal plates thin endometrium by numerous fibrous anchor villi. After birth of the foetus, strong uterine contractions occur that cause the placental site to sink markedly. This causes the anchor villi to the placental site to sink markedly. This causes the anchor villi to break and the placenta to separate from its attachments. Normally, the first few strong contractions that occur 5 to 7 minutes after the baby's birth cause the placenta to be sheared away from the basal plate. A placenta cannot detach itself from a flaccid (relaxed) uterus because the placental size is not reduced in size. After it has been separated from the uterine wall, the placenta may be delivering through the bearing down efforts of the mother if she is awake, or it may be expressed by the physician. This must be done very carefully and only when the placenta has separated and the fundus is firm. Otherwise, the grave complications of haemorrhage or inversion, a turning inside-out of the uterus may occur.

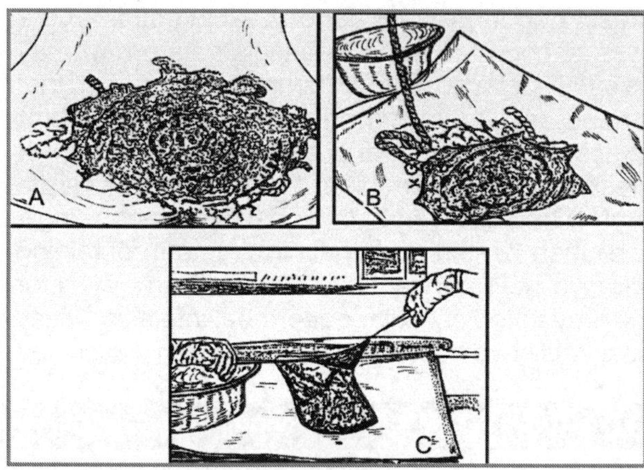

Figs 5.15A to C: The placenta after delivery. A, Maternal side (Duncan delivery). B, Foetal side (Schultze delivery). C, The amniotic sac, which housed the foetus during intrauterine life

Placental separation is indicated by the following signs:

- The rising of the uterus to or above the umbilicus.
- A firmly contracting fundus.
- A change in the uterus from a dicoid to a globular ovoid shape and the placenta moves into the lower uterine segment (the rounding out and firming up of the fundus).

- A sudden gush of dark blood from the introitus (small gush of blood to the exterior).
- Apparent lengthening of the umbilical cord as the placenta descends to the introitus (the lengthening of the umbilical cord outside the vulva).
- The finding of vaginal fullness (the placenta) on vaginal or rectal examination or of foetal membranes at the introitus.

The placenta, after completing its intricate life-sustaining function, separate from the wall of the uterus after it contracts. The uterus is now considerably smaller, assumes globular shape. The placenta is expelled on the mother pushes for the last time. The physician or nurse may ask her to bear down to deliver the placenta if she is anaesthesized, fundal pressure may be exerted. Controlled cord traction may be used to facilitate delivery after separation occurred. Cord traction and fundal pressure must be performed with great care to avoid inversion of the uterus and avulsion of the cord. Expectant management allows the placenta to separate spontaneously. It may involve the use of gravity or nipple stimulation to facilitate separation expulsion. Active management facilitates placental separation and expulsion with administration of oxytocics after birth of foetus, early clamping and cutting off the umbilical cord, and application of controlled traction on the cord.

After the placenta is delivered, it must be inspected to be certain that no segments of membranes have been left in the uterus. Medications such as oxytocin and lactated ringers may be routinely given intravenously in hospitals after delivery of the placenta to help uterine contractions and decrease the risk of haemorrhage. However, nipple stimulations or breastfeeding adequately stimulates oxytocin release from the posterior pituitary for normal births.

Tho placenta is a unique and valuable organ even after delivery. In some hospitals, placentas that have not become contaminated with stool or were not born of women whose pregnancies were complicated by infectious diseases, fever, or premature rupture of the membrane are saved and later processed by a pharmaceutical concern to extract immunoglobulin they contain. The cords of these placentas have also been evaluated and processed to provide vascular grafts to patients with circulation problems.

Immediate Postpartum Care

Most acute injuries and lacerations of the perineum, vagina, uterus and their support tissues occur during childbirth. Some injuries to the supporting tissues, whether they were acute or nonacute and whether they were repaired or not, may lead to gynaecologic problems later in life, e.g. pelvic relaxation, uterine prolapse, cystocele and rectocele.

After the delivery of placenta, any perineal repair can be made. Generally if an anaesthetic was used for a delivery, the same one can be employed. Sometimes a local anaesthetics is administered. If this is used, the physician will need a syringe (usually) some infiltration needles and the local anaesthetic of choice, as well as the usual materials involved in the perineal repair. A seat and good light should be provided.

In spite of precautions lacerations or episiotomy extensions occasionally occur. Some maternal tissues tear more easily them others. Very large babies or unusual positions are a special threat to the perineum. Lacerations of the perineum are defined in terms of its depth.

- *First degree*: Lacerations that extends through the skin and structures superficial to muscles.
- *Second degree*: Laceration which extends through muscles of the perineal body.
- *Third degree*: Laceration that continues through the anal sphincter muscle.
- *Fourth degree*: Lacerations that also involves the anterior rectal wall.

As stated above, first-degree lacerations involving a tear in the mucous membrane and skin only, are fairly common and usually of no permanent consequence. Second degree lacerations include a tear into the muscles of the perineal block but exclude the rectal sphincter. Adequately repaired, they usually heal well with little problem. However, third degree lacerations include a tear into the muscles of the perineal block but exclude the rectal sphincter. Adequately repaired, they usually heal well with little problem. However, third degree lacerations which by definition involve the circular anal sphincter muscle, are more difficult to repair and may result in permanent damage to the perineum and sphincter (review the anatomy of the pelvic floor). Fourth-degree lacerations also involve the rectovaginal wall. To avoid third-and fourth degree lacerations or episiotomy extensions, that are uncontrolled and more difficult to repair, some physicians are purposely cutting the rectum when the perineum is endangered. Lacerations may involve areas other than the true perineum. Tears of the labia, interior vaginal wall and cervix, are not uncommon. All there areas should be inspected for such tears after a birth.

If repair is nonexistent, inadequate or improper, the patient is soon a possible candidate for haemorrhage, haematoma, and infection. As weeks and years pass, certain pelvic displacements and malfunctions may show themselves. The woman may be troubled with urinary or faecal incontinence or she may suffer from a sagging of the pelvic musculature. When the tissue wall between the bladder and the vagina becomes abnormally relaxed, usually because of previous injury, the bladder drops out of place and pushes the anterior vaginal wall backward. The resulting abnormal condition is called a cystocele. A similar hernia-like abnormality involving the rectovaginal wall and falling forward of the rectum is known as a rectocele. Small rectoceles or cystoceles are usually asymptomatic and are to surgically repaired. Large abnormalities of this type however may cause complaints such as "dragging sensations" in the pelvis and conditions such as stress incontinence, urinary retention and cystitis in the case of cystocele or constipation and haemorrhoids in the case of rectocele. A vaginal repair of these difficulties, or colporrhaphy, may be performed. If both a bladder nad a rectal prolapse are surgically treated, the procedure is often called an A and P (anterior posterior) repair. Prolapse, or a falling out of place of the uterus, often accompanies these other displacements. Occasionally abnormal canals or tracts between two body cavities or a body cavity and exterior develop as a result of obstetric injury. These tracts, most often found are termed fistulas and are difficult to eliminate. An adequate early repair of any obstetric injuries to the birth canal or its supports is important to continuing good health.

After birth the baby is shown or given to the mother. The infant may remain with her and her husband or companion for a more extended period designed to promote attachment, or he may be taken to the nursery, with his birth records after only a short interval. If the mother is not alert, definite arrangements should be made for her to see the infant later as soon as she is able.

With the termination of any repair and the cleansing of the perineum, the head and foot of the delivery table are against realigned and the patient's legs removed from the stirrups or supports. Before the perineal pads are attached, if an episiotomy or laceration has occurred an ice pack may be ordered and applied to the patient's perineum to help prevent swelling and discomfort. The perineal pads are attached, and a warm, clean hospital gown replaces the one worn by the patient during the birth. She is covered by a warm blanket.

In some maternity services any initial preparation of the breasts of nursing mothers is done at this time also. Some mothers nurse their babies while still on the delivery table or in the delivery room if the baby is in good condition and free of excessive mucus and the new mother is alert and so wishes. The nursing of a baby directly following delivery of the placenta has a physiologic basis, since stimulation of the breasts causes the uterus to contract and helps prevent blood loss when other means of control are not available (something to remember in a disaster situation). The early establishment of an intimate motherchild relationship involving touch and nourishment is also considered one way to promote positive maternal emotions or maternal attachment. For some mothers who are not troubled by the relative lack of privacy and are not too tired, this opportunity may be cherished.

Observation

Throughout this early postpartum period, often called the fourth stage of labour, the patient is being observed for excessive bleeding and the respirations observed. The uterus is palpated frequently determined and the respirations observed. The uterus is palpated frequently to discover any relaxation of the fundus. If an intravenous infusion is in place (often used in conjunction with spinal anaesthesia) it is carefully watched for rate of administration and possible infiltration. Many of these infusions contain an oxytocic and should not be given rapidly. Great care should be exercised to ensure that the needle is not dislodged during the transfer of the patient from the delivery table. Several hands may be needed for this project if the patient has an intravenous infusion and is temporarily unable to use her legs properly because of the lingering effects of spinal anaesthesia. However, the staff may be fortunate in having a mechanical aid for the patient transfer. The new mother may remain in the delivery room suite for a specified time for close observation near equipment that may be needed, or she may be transferred to a special postpartum recovery room. At the time of her various changes in location, special attention should be given to the transfer of her personal belongings. Family members should see her as soon after the birth as is appropriate.

Alternative Childbirth Arrangements

The labour-delivery procedures just described could be called a "modified traditional" hospital maternity experience, although different hospitals incorporate their own variations. Within the last few years, a growing number of couples have wished to investigate alternatives to birth in traditional hospital settings. Several reasons are given for their search for other childbirth arrangements. They include a desire for a more relaxed, "personal" atmosphere and more flexibility in the types of care offered with the possible presence of other family members and friends (including, in some instances, sibling observation of the event); a perceived inhospital attitude that childbirth is an abnormal or pathologic process; a wish for a birth with less medical intervention (for example, obligatory foetal monitoring, administration of drugs, artificial rupture of the bag of waters, routine transfer from the labour area to a "delivery room" episiotomy, and forceps application); an expressed need to have the newborn near at hand; disappointment in the organization or lack of fooming-in accommodations; concern over possible infant contact with "hospital germs", lack of rest; and the high cost of hospitalization.

It is important that hospital administrators, physicians, and nurses examine and evaluate these reasons. Consumer discontent may be valid and un-necessary in many instances. The rationale of some hospital routines may be questioned. The alternatives that some families have chosen may not sufficiently recognize that, although childbirth is a physiologic process, it can be complicated by unexpected considerations that call for decisions based on professional expertise and experience.

Alternative to so called traditional hospital birth vary in availability and safety. Some parents have decided to give birth at home. The birth attendant may be a physician, certified nurse midwife lay-midwife, friend or father. The legality and proficiency of the attendant differ depending on locale and circumstances. They cite the small but important percentage (5% to 10%) of mothers and infants who, although not considered high risk, develop problems during the labour birth period. They are concerned about professional backup in the event that they cannot attend the birth and about the threat of malpractice judgements. They are also influenced by the accessibility of hospital facilities and perinatal centers.

Another method of meeting the objections to traditional childbirth is the use of a birthing room or an alternative birth center (APC), which is part of or near a hospital or clinic where emergency equipment and staff are available if needed. It is typically designed to care for uncomplicated births in a home like setting. The room serves for labour, birth and early postpartum care. Such centres have liberal visitation policies and usually discharge the mother and baby several hours after birth, Early follow up nursing visits are made to the home. Most of these centers have been in operation a relatively short time. They may use nurse-midwives as well as Physicians to monitor the labour and assist at the birth.

Still another alternative in maternity services suggested is Single Room Maternity care, currently being called the "wave of the 90s."

- The long used traditional hospital labour and delivery unit is based on the surgical transfer model with mother being moved from room to room, often during the most critical biologic or psychologic moments of the birth experience. In contrast, Single Room Maternity Care provides for the labour, birth, recovery and initial postpartum care in one location. Mother, baby and her support person stay in one or at the most, two rooms during the entire hospital stay. This concept combines the science and safety of modern medicine, the knowledge of the care givers, and the needs of the family into one package.

LDR (Labour, Delivery, Recovery)

The mother is admitted to a birthing suite and remains there for her labour, delivery and recovery. The rooms often are decorated much like hotel rooms but all necessary medical equipment is readily available. Although alternative birthing rooms were never completely successful, they did prove that good outcomes are still possible in less than sterile environments.

Now hospitals are able to meet consumer demand for more "humanized services" in a medically safe environment with the initiation of Single Room Maternity Care.

Following recovery, the mother and her infant are moved to a Mother-Baby Unit, where the goal is to enable one nurse to care for the mother and baby together. There are many advantages to this type of nursing care. It encourages both parents to get to know their baby and begin functioning as a family unit under the guidance of skilled maternity personnel. Nursing is less fragmented. Assessments, treatments, and teaching are more easily coordinated when one nurse knows the status of both patients. It decreases chances for error, minimizing the number of people receiving a report on each patient. The risk of infection can also be decreased when mother and baby remain together.

LDRP (Labour, Delivery, Recovery, Postpartum)

LDRP is essentially the same as the LDR except that the mother is not required to move to another unit following recovery, but continues to be cared for in the same room.

Unlike other alternative birth options no "screening out" is needed for this system. Because the mother and her baby are in a hospital setting with all available equipment and personnel, all women who are having vaginal deliveries can be taken care of in the Single Room Care System.

It will be extremely interesting to observe how maternity care services will be structured in another 10 years. Certainly they are undergoing a period of intense scrutiny, evaluation and change. Families are so diverse in their expectations, desires, and needs; perhaps a "cafeteria of options" (without sacrificing valuable maternal and neonatal safeguards) can be developed to provide true family centered maternity care.

SPECIAL SITUATIONS

There are some special situations that occasionally arise in the labour delivery sequence.

Precipitate Delivery

First to be considered is "precipitate delivery". This means a birth that occurs with such speed and in such a situation that proper preparation and medical supervision of the event are lacking. A multipara with a relaxed perineal floor may have an extremely short period of expulsion. Two or three powerful contractions may cause the baby to appear. In this instance the nurse may be the only one at the bedside or delivery table to assist the patient. In no instance should she leave the patient alone. If it is obvious that the baby would be born before the delivery room is reached (for example, the patient has had three children and the head is almost delivered), the nurse should do the best she can with what she has at hand. The call light should be turned on.

Birth of the Head

There is seldom time for washing and putting on gloves in a precipitate delivery, although this could be ideal. The baby's head should not be forcibly held back, since this may cause foetal distress and aspiration, but it is important to maintain flexion of the foetal head to avoid trauma to maternal periurethral and perineal tissue. This restraint can usually be achieved by allowing the baby to emerge slowly against a guiding hand placed on the top of the advancing head. The fingers of the nurse should not enter the vagina. If the bag of waters is not broken, it must be pinched or torn to release the fluid and protect the baby from aspiration. The actual delivery of the head should be accomplished between contractions, with the mother panting or lightly bearing down. As soon as the head is born, the nurse should wipe off his face and, if possible, suction the baby's mouth and nose. She should also check to determine whether the cord is around the neck. If it is she should slip it over the head or shoulders to prevent choking. Rarely it may be too tight to slip over with the fingers. If this happens, it is hoped that sterile clamps and scissors are available in the labour room or that a staff member has answered the light and brought the emergency pack containing the clamps and scissors necessary to cut the cord. The mother should be firmly instructed to pant through her open mouth and not push during this interval.

External Rotation and Expulsion

After the head is delivered, the face wiped, suction employed, and the location of the cord determined, frequently the rest of the child's body emerges without further assistance. However, if there seems to be no further progress and the back of the head has not already turned toward the mother's thigh, it can be turned in the direction of least resistance to line up with the child's back. There is no need to hurry. Next the head should gently but firmly be directed downward to deliver the top shoulder. After the top shoulder is expelled, the baby is lifted up toward the pubic bone to release the bottom shoulder. The rest of the child is delivered without any particular problem. Before the birth of the baby, it is sometimes helpful if the mother's hips can be elevated (or the foot portion of the table lowered a few inches) by another person to give more support and the gentle up-and-down manoeuvre described a and to help keep the baby's face free of vaginal and anal drainage.

Immediate Care of the Baby

As soon as possible, the infant's airway should be cleared. If a suction bulb is available, it is usually quite effective. The baby should not lie and a puddle of amniotic fluid where aspiration can take place. Baby's body should be supported on the nurse's hand and arm at the level of the mother's uterus and tilted to "drain" without any tension being placed on the umbilical cord. After the airway is clear, he may be gently stimulated to cry, if necessary, and placed on his side-head slightly lower than its body on his body on his mother's abdomen. (Most of these babies cry immediately). Baby should be wrapped in a towel or blanket for warmth. There is no haste to cut the cord or, for that matter to deliver the placenta. The cord can wait until proper sterile equipment is available. The nurse should wait for delivery of the placenta unless professional aid is very long in arriving or excessive bleeding occurs. However, if no professional help is forthcoming, if the signs of separation of the placenta have occurred, if the uterus is firm, and if the mother experiences a return of contractions, she may be asked to bear down to deliver the placenta. It should be supported as it is expelled so that the membranes are not torn. It should be saved for later evaluation by a physician. Usually the physician, who in the meantime has been contacted by the staff, completes the delivery of the placenta and repairs any lacerations.

A calm, reassuring manner on the part of the nurse (even if she does not really feel calm) is helpful to the mother and all concerned. Usually no great permanent harm results from a precipitate delivery, but every effort should be made to prevent its occurrence. All patients should be evaluated frequently for progress during labour. Signs of the approach of the second stage of labour should not be ignored. In such births the advantages of antisepsis and asepsis are largely lost, and there is greater danger or injury to the maternal tissues, of aspiration and injury to the baby, and embarrassment for the patient, not to mention the nurse.

Induction of Labour

At times in the labour suite there may be admitted a pregnant woman who has come on appointment to have her labour artificially initiated or induced.

Indications for an induction of labour may include: (1) A problem with erythroblastosis foetalis (isoimmunization), (2) prolonged rupture of the membranes after 37 weeks' gestation without spontaneous onset of contractions, (3) increasing symptoms of preeclampsia, (4) Postmaturity (baby definitely late in arriving), (5) maternal diabetes mellitus, or (6) foetal death without labour onset. Induction planned for the convenience of the patient or the physician is seldom considered a valid reason.

Methods and Care

Candidates for induction of labour must be selected care fully, since it is not a procedure totally without risk to the mother and baby. Today, labour is most often induced by intravenous administration of the synthetic pituitary hormone oxytocin (Pitocin or Syntocinon). Unless the cervix is ready, labour will not occur. The cervix must at least be partially effaced and soft and pliable. One method used fairly often today to prepare or "ripen" a cervix to make it more likely to respond to oxytocin is the application of prostaglandin E2 gel alone may initiate labour.

If the membranes are artificially ruptured and labour does not begin within 24 hours, the increased possibility of introducing infection must be faced. Posterior pituitary hormone is powerful and can cause violent uterine contractions that can lead to premature detachment of the placenta, uterine rupture, and foetal hypoxia. For this reason oxytocin (usually 10 units per 1,000 ml of Ringer's solution) should be given only in small amounts per infusion pump. Another liter of fluid without oxytocin should be included in the IV setup (piggyback) allowing the nurse to discontinue the uterine stimulation if necessary while still maintaining access to the vein. The labour of the induction patient should be electronically monitored. A strip showing the FHR pattern before introduction of the oxytocin should be obtained and electronically monitored. During induction, it is usually recommended that the FHR, the maternal blood pressure and pulse, and the frequency and duration of any contractions, as well as the quality of the uterine relaxation period, be assessed and documented every 15 minutes. Uterine contractions lasting more than 60 seconds or occurring more than every 2½ to 3 minutes exaggerated uterine tone and poor relaxation and signs of FHR abnormalities usually indicate that the infusion of oxytocin for induction need to be determined and followed. The physician should be readily available in the event of problems.

Caesarean Birth

With the decreasing risk involved in the performance of caesarean birth (removal of the child through incisions in the abdominal and uterine walls), the operation is used more frequently in modern obstetrics. Many hospitals were reporting that approximately 20 per cent of their births were by caesarean. The rise in caesarean births has been attributed to (1) a more aggressive approach to poor progress in labour, (2) an increased tendency to use caesarean for breech birth delivery, (3) a rise in repeat caesarean patient, and (4) the medical malpractice climate. Electronic foetal monitoring may be a factor, especially when first introduced to an obstetric service.

The most common reason for caesarean birth has been a previous caesarean birth. However, some physicians now are less reluctant to consider a trial labour and vaginal birth if the reasons for the former caesarean birth do not persist, if the mother so wishes, and if the previous uterine incision was not vertical in direction. Others think that the possibility of uterine rupture is too great.

Needless to say, a mother entering the hospital for a repeat caesarean is usually not enduring the stress of an unexpected surgery hastily arranged, because of the appearance of an obstetric complication. However sometimes women who are admitted to the labour area suddenly demonstrate symptoms that suggest the emergency use of the procedure; conditions such as abruptio placentae, placenta previa, foetal-pelvic disproportion abnormal presentations prolapsed cord, uterine inertia (failure of the uterus to contract sufficiently to continue progress in labour), or signs of foetal distress. Conditions that indicate acute foetal distress or maternal jeopardy demand the prompt and rapid preparation of the patient once the condition has been discovered and the course of action determined. A patient scheduled for an emergency caesarean delivery is subjected to many procedures in a few minutes. Everything should be done as calmly and quickly as possible. The patient's morale should be supported because, if she is alert, she will probably be frightened.

Preparation for Caesarean Birth

The following procedures are routinely carried out:

1. Signing of the operative permit by the patient or responsible party.
2. An abdominal perineal preparation, which starts at the nipple line and includes the entire abdomen from side to side as well as the perineal area visible when the legs are parallel.
3. Insertion of an indwelling catheter sometimes done in surgery after anaesthesia.
4. Blood type and crossmatch and haemoglobin determination.
5. Removal of any hairpins or hard objects from the hair; application of a surgical cap; removal of cosmetics, any extra jewelry, glasses, contact lenses, etc. to be given to the family, taping of wedding and engagement rings to the fingers without impeding circulation.
6. Removal and safe keeping of any dentures.
7. Preoperative medications as ordered.
8. Removal of nail polish so that nailbeds may be checked for cyanosis is infrequently requested now because of the increasing availability of the oximeter, the vogue of artificial nails, and the recognition that nail cyanosis is a relatively late sign of poor oxygenation.

The patient is given nothing by mouth from the time Caesarean birth is contemplated, if this restriction has not been instituted previously. If not already in progress, an intravenous infusion is started.

Patients may be transferred to an operating room suite for surgery or a delivery room may be prepared for the procedure. During all the busy preparations, any family members present should not be forgotten, and provision should be made for them to wait in as much mental and physical comfort as possible. Some hospitals permit the fathers to stay with the mothers during the section if general anaesthesia is not used. In many are classes are now available to parents anticipating or interested in caesarean birth.

Breech Presentation

A breech presentation is another situation that may be part of labour delivery experience. Approximately 3 per cent of all births are breech. There is currently renewed interest in trying to change a breech presentation to that of cephalic.

Although a breech presentation would probably not be considered an abnormality, it involves more risk to the infant than a cephalic birth, and the mother is likely to have a longer and more tiring labour. As a rule there is greater possibility of prolapse of the umbilical cord during breech labour, and during the delivery of the baby it may be compressed against the pelvic outlet. The baby may try to take a breath before his head has been born and aspirate tenacious vaginal secretion. Occasionally trouble is encountered in the extraction of the arms. Sometimes an unexpectedly large head may cause concern, and cerebral damage may occur. Although few maternity services today routinely provide a sterile scrub nurse in the delivery room, many physicians appreciate and request the help of such a nurse at the time of breech birth. Such an attendant usually helps support the baby's body or may, when instructed, apply fundal pressure when it comes time for the delivery of the head. A special type of forceps called Piper's forceps applied to the aftercoming head, may be used at the time of a breech birth. It should always be on the sterile supply table when a breech birth is anticipated. The head is often delivered so that the baby almost seems to do a guided half some result over the mother's abdomen. A rather deep episiotomy is custo-mary in breech births. The baby may have edematous or bruised genitalia. Today the physician may elect to perform a caesarean birth because of the increased foetal mortality and morbidity (10 to 15%) of a vaginally delivered breech. However, many of these breech births involve premature infants-another factor to consider when evaluating.

Twins or Multiple Births

Twins are another interesting occurrence in an obstetrics. They occur about once in every 90 pregnancies. There are two types of twins-fraternal and identical. Fraternal twins are the result of two simultaneous pregnancies developing from the fertilization of two separate ova by two distinct spermatozoa. They do not resemble one another any more than siblings resemble one another. They may be of the same or of opposite sexes. The placental circulation of each foetus is separate, although the adjoining placentas may be fused. Each foetus develops within its own amniotic and chorionic sac.

Identical twins result from the division of one fertilized ovum into two identical halves that develop into two similar individuals of the same sex. The placental circulation is shared by the attachment of two umbilical cords. Each infant is encased in a separate amniotic sac but shares the chorionic sac with his twin. Fraternal twins are more common than identical. Approximately 54 per cent of twins are premature, and the risk of intracranial haemorrhage, developmental respiratory distress syndrome, and other neonatal difficulties is high. Mortality for a second born twin is about three times higher than it is for the first born sibling, probably because of a greater incidence of malpresentations. Thus the nursery should be alerted when a twin birth is anticipated. Occasionally such an event is not anticipated, and the family, physician, and nurse are surprised to receive a "bonus baby".

When twinning is expected, two sets of identification should be ready with double newborn record sheets. Two sterile baby receiving blankets, two cord clamps, and two aspirator bulbs should be available. In almost one half of all twin births, both infants are cephalic presentations, but any combination of presentations and positions may exist. Occasionally the babie's relative positions cause problems in their birth. Mothers of twins are more likely to suffer from preeclampsia and placenta previa and, because of the greater distention of the uterus, are more often victims of postpartum haemorrhage.

The nurse's experience in the labour delivery room area can be a highly satisfying, rewarding type of nursing. If skilled in human relations and the observations and procedural techniques necessary to care for her patients, she can play an indispensable, gratifying role in a crucial period in a family's life. The alert student in this area can learn much and gain an appreciation of and reverence for life that she will never forget.

FOURTH STAGE OF LABOUR

The first hour after delivery is a critical period for the mother. The blood vessels and myometrium are inter-twined in such a way that natural ligatures are created when the uterus contracts. Observations every 15 minutes must be made to see that firm contraction of the fundus is maintained to prevent haemorrhage. The uterus is palpated to assess the degree of contraction. The fundus should be firm, at the level of the umbilicus or below, and in the midline. The perineal pad and bed pad are observed for lochia, colour, clots and amount. Normally the lochia is bright red and may contain small clots. The amount should not saturate more than one pad in an hour. The perineum and episiotomy (enlargement of the vaginal opening), if present, should be inspected for haematomas and swelling. An ice pack should be routinel applied to the perineum to decrease swelling and alleviate discomfort.

During the hour after placenta delivery, the physician or midwife repairs the episiotomy and any lacerations that may be present, using a local anaesthetic. The mother's general condition is observed, particularly in regard to bleeding. The placenta is examined to ensure that it was delivered intact.

The major complication of the fourth stage is haemorrhage. Hemorrhage from the placental site is controlled by contraction of the uterus. Anything interfering with the normal contraction of the uterus, including a full bladder, may result in haemorrhage. Displacement of the uterus upward or laterally indicates a full bladder. The client should be encouraged to void and if unable to do so may have to be catheterized. If the fundus is not firmly contracted (boggy) it may be gently massaged until it becomes firm. The presence of a well contracted uterus, but with large clots and excessive bleeding, may indicate soft tissue lacerations caused by the trauma of delivery or retained placental fragments. If lacerations are suspected, the client may need to be returned to the delivery room for inspection and repair of the lacerations. If retained placental fragments or membranes are suspected, they must be manually removed. Pain management can be carried out by relaxing and breathing technique.

Intrapartal Foetal Assessment

During the birth process the foetus is passive and wholly dependent on its environment for survival. Simultaneous measurement of foetal heart rate and uterine contractions allows detection of the foetus unable to with stand the stress of labour.

Foetal heart rate monitoring is now commonly man dated during active labour in most hospital birth units. Some units require that the client be monitored constantly after admission. Factor a that require continuous monitoring are a premature or postmature foetus, abnormal foetal heart rate, tracing or labour pattern, early rupture of membranes, meconium-stained fluid, and chronic problems such as diabetes or hypertension.

The purposes of timing obstetric contractions (uterine contraction) is:

- To help evaluate the efforts of the uterus to dilate the cervix and expel the baby and to aid in determining the progress of labour.
- To detect any abnormalities such as lack of uterine relaxation, which may reveal the onset of complications.
- To help detect foetal distress by simultaneous observation of contraction and foetal heart rate patterns. When internal or external electronic manoeuvres are used.
- To reassure the patient and her family by nurses presence and interest and at the same time, to helper better sauger her labour by:
  a. Encouraging her and listening.
  b. Rubbing her back or providing sacral support as desired.
  c. Helping with relaxation, breathing, or pushing techniques as needed.
  d. Moistening her lips and offering oral hygiene.
  e. Changing pillow cases and replacing bed pads.
  f. Watching for signs of the patient's changing needs (for example, the beginning of the second stage of labour).
  g. Assisting the selected labour coach to meet the patient's needs.

Procedure

1. Before going to the bedside, if possible, learn the following about each patient:

a. Number of pregnancies, viable births, living children.
b. Marital status and any special arrangements for the baby.
c. Whether she has attended childbirth education classes, specific requests regarding labour/birth.
d. Any special complications or problems anticipated.

2. The fact that you (nurse) are feeling her uterus, as it contracts and relaxes under the abdominal wall, to help measure her progress in labour should be explained unless he has previously had contractions timed.
3. Your (nurses) hands should be clean and not too cold.
4. In the past many labour nurses have been told not to consider the world "pain" as a synonym for the contraction of the uterus because not all concentrations are painful and "its use may interfere with positive maternal conditioning for childbirth." Although the term contraction may have more neutral or constructing connotation, realistic minded childbirth educators are now cautiously reincorporating the "p-word" into their professional vocabulary. At present, both words are being heard at the bedside spoken by both patient and nurse.
5. If the pregnancy is full term, the fundus, where the strongest muscular contraction can be felt, will be located about four finger widths above the umbilicus. The nurse's hand should rest lightly there to best detect the uterine contractions.
6. When the uterus contracts, it gradually becomes hard. The degree of hardness is called the intensity of a contraction. As the uterus contracts and the uterine muscle fibres shorten, the uterus may be seen or felt to rise in the abdominal cavity. It then gradually relaxes. The time that the uterus is discernibly firm or tight is called the contraction's duration. Usually contractions are easier to feel on multiparas than on primiparas because of the differences in abdominal muscle tone.
7. The term interval in the timing of contractions is used a bit differently from what is sometimes supposed. The nurse times from the beginning of one contraction to the beginning of the following contraction when using manual assessment.
8. The time between contractions is called the Relaxation Time—a period equally as important as the interval or duration. If the relaxatioin time is very short or non-existent, the baby may suffer from lack of oxygen. A continuously contracted, hard uterus may be symptom of abruption placentae. Between contractions the fingers should be able to depress the abdominal wall, a sensation similar to depressing a foam rubber pillow.
9. The contraction and relaxation periods and the interval have often be diagrammed. The straight line represents complete relaxation, and the curved line the actual tone of the uterine musculature.
10. Usually a relationship exists between the duration and frequency of uterine contractions and the dilatation of the cervix.
11. Recording of observations of contractions would include duration, interval and intensity as well as possible patient tolerance. For example "Contractions 5 minutes for 35 seconds, mild in character. Using abdominal breathing effectively."
12. When electronic monitors are used, instructions for individual models must be consulted. Both external and internal contraction monitor are available. When traced electronically, the frequency of contractions is often stated, as the time elapsed between contraction peaks. Monitor strips are evaluated at least every 30 minutes and more frequently during labour induction or active labour or if possible signs of foetal distress occur.

Danger signals-report (Table 5.8) Contraction duration more than 2 minutes of intensity >100 mm Hg measured by internal monitor.
Relaxation period less than 30 seconds.
Poor relaxation quality (intrauterine resting tone > 20 mm Hg).

Foetal Heart Rate (FHR) Monitoring

Purpose

1. To help the presence of foetal life at the time of admission.
2. To detect possible foetal distress.

Equipment Needed

Foetal heart rate monitoring may be performed using varied equipment ranging from fairly simple

Table 5.8: Common uterine contraction and dilatation relationships and possible danger signals

Cervical dilatation	Contraction	
	Duration	Interval
1. Fingertip to 2 cm	20 to 30 seconds	6-8 minutes
2. 2 cm to 4 cm	30 to 35 seconds	5-6 minutes
3. 4 cm to 6 cm	40 to 50 seconds	4-5 minutes
4. 6 cm to 8 cm	45 to 60 seconds	3-4 minutes
5. 8 cm to 10 cm	50-90 seconds	2-3 minutes.

(Most difficult periods fatigue, nausea, vomit tends to be irregular, intensive contractions, "transition")

hand held fetoscopes to rather complex devices capable of continuous electronic sensitivity and simultaneous visual and printed records. At this writing there is a revival or interest in the study and use of foetal heart monitoring employing frequent intermittent auscultation.

The following section discusses the use of "manual" fetoscopes as well as basic principles of simultaneous foetal heart and contraction monitoring.

Manually Held Monitors

Manually held monitors used intermittently

1. The Leffscope—a stethoscope with a large, heavily weighed bell.
2. The De Lee-Holl is head scope.
3. An ordinary stethoscope equipped with rubber bands to prevent the sound distortion that results when the bell is handled directly.
4. Various "lubricated" ultrasonic fetoscopes, which may amplify the FHR held in the examiner's hand against the abdominal wall.

Procedure

1. Explain that you (nurse) are checking the baby by listening to his heart beat.
2. Listen to the FHR immediately following a contraction or better yet, if your patient will allow you, listen during, as well as immediately following the contraction to hear the heart beat adequately. This may enable you to detect late deceleration of the heartbeat-a condition thought to be related to foetal distress resulting from uteroplacental insufficiency. However the pressure exterted on the abdominal wall during a contraction by the manual fetoscope (especially, 1, 2 or 3) may be uncomfortable and annoying to mothers and not easily tolerated by many. For this reason, a monitor attached to the mother may be at times more helpful than manually held types, and listening immediately following a contraction will probably the more frequent observation pattern used. Listen for 30 to 60 seconds, if possible. Multiply as necessary to obtain the rate for 1 minute. Every separate beat heard should be counted. It usually sounds lie a little watch. At first much concentration will be needed to hear it.
3. Be sure that friction noises from the fingers or the abdominal surface do not distort the sounds. Keep your fingers off the bell. Press firmly on the abdominal wall.
4. The area where the FHR may be heard best is related to the following:
   a. *Presentation*: In head first (cephalic) prestations the FHR is found in the lower abdominal quadrants, below the umbilicus. In breech presentations the FHR is usually found at the level of the umbilicus above.
   b. *Position*: If the back of the infant is toward the mother's left (LOA or LOP position) the FHR will probably be heard best on the mother's left. If it points to her right, the FHR will most frequently be heard best on her right. Just because an FHR can be heard in more than one place does not necessarily mean that more than one baby is involved. However, you may want to check by having another nurse listen simultaneously, using a finger-wagging technique to be sure that the pattern heard in both areas is the same.
   c. *Station*: As internal rotation and descent occur, the location of the FHR changes, swinging gradually from the right or left quadrants to the midline and dropping until immediately before birth it is found just above the pubic bone.
5. It is recommended that the FHR be taken at 30 minute intervals in the first stage of labour. In the presence of risk factors, the FHR must be monitored every 15 minutes. FHR assessment must always be documented with time indications on an official record. The mother should be told at the time of admittance that a frequent check of the FHR is routine. Early in labour she or her partner may enjoy listening once, too. In the second stage of labour, the FHR of low risk patients should be evaluated every 15 minutes. Higher risk patients should be evaluated every 5 minutes during this period.

6. Normal FHR is usually considered to be 120 to 160 beats per minute (bpm) Rates outside this range or a rise or fall of 30 bpm from the usual level of the FHR, noted between contractions (even if still remaining within the normal range), should be reported to the supervising nurse.

   Rates determined between contractions consistently higher than 160 are showing a 30 bpm baseline increase (foetal tachycardia) may be associated with a variety of problems (for example, materna fever, foetal hypoxia, and prematurity). Consistent FHR of less than 120 bpm or showing 30 bpm baseline decrease (foetal bradycardia) not associated with contraction patterns may signal maternal hypotension. A rate that is too rapid or especially too slow may be a sign of foetal distress. A foetal heart rate under 100 bpm usually sign of foetal distress. A foetal heart rate under 100 bpm usually signals definite distress. However, even though the heart rate with or without the pressure of a contraction may at no time leave the normal range, significant periods of deceleration or slowing may occur undetected unless the labour is continuously monitored. Certain patterns of deceleration may indicate foetal distress. Precise periods of FHR deceleration are difficult to determine with intermittent monitoring techniques, and, therefore, continuous monitoring technology has been developed.
7. Other sounds may be heard in the mother's abdomen as well. Do not mistake them for the foetal heartbeat.
   a. The maternal pulse may be heard. The nurse should guard against reporting the maternal pulse as the FHR by feeling the mother's radial pulse at the same time as she is listening with a fetoscope. They should be different rhythms and rates.
   b. The increased sound of the pulsation of the uterine arteries can sometimes be identified. Identification of this "sh" sound with the same rhythm as the maternal pulse does not guarantee that the foetus is alive. Sometimes the FHR can be heard at the same time in the background. Move the fetoscope about 2.5 cm (1 inch) to hear the FHR better.
   c. Rarely a sort of soft whistling sound occurring at the same rate as the foetal heart rate can be heard. This has been called the Funic Souffle, or cord whistle. Some think it is caused by a compression of the cord. Its presence indicates foetal life.
   d. Many labouring mothers are hungry, so the nurse may hear peristalsia.

Monitors attached to a mother or foetus for extended or continuous use:

1. External sensors attached to the maternal abdomen to detect the mechanical energy of the foetal heartbeat. These may produce instantaneous visual or audible signals, and when appropriately equipped, they may produce permanent written records. They may be used early in labour before significant cervical dilatation or rupture of the bag of waters. They are simple to use, and there has been no known foetal injury related to their use. However, the position of the sensors may need frequent attention as labour becomes more advanced and accuracy of the recording becomes more difficult to obtain. These FHR sensors may be combined with an externally placed diaphragm that is capable of recording the frequency of uterine contractions when held in place with abdominal strapping.

   Examples are:
   a. Small amplifying microphones (phonocardiography) used for antipartum monitoring.
   b. Ultrasonic or Dopper-type instruments that produce characteristic reflected sound waves, which are usually more clear.
2. Foetal electrode radiography to detect the electrical energy associated with foetal heart beat.
   a. Indirect foetal electrocardiography is possible with electrodes attached to the abdominal wall. It can be used well in early labour, but considerable "electrical noise" may be generated with patient movement during advanced labour and the recording obtained is inferior to that of direct monitoring.
   b. Direct foetal electrocardiography requires ruptured membranes. 1 to 2 cm of cervical dilatation, and a presenting part no higher than 2 station. A physician or specially trained obstetric nurse attaches the electrode vaginally to the presenting part (scalp or buttock), penetrating the epidermis by a tiny metal spiral or clip. Infection and soft tissue injury are possibilities but have not been significant problems.

3. Uterine contraction patterns interpreted by pressure exerted on a catheter inserted cervically into the uterus just beyond the parietal diameter of the foetal head may be viewed and recorded concurrently with the FHR.

Concepts Regarding Monitor Strip Patterns

Baseline FHR zThe rate determined either before labour begins or during labour in a 10 minute interval exclusive of any periodic changes. Baseline rate is usually 120 to 160 beats per minute. A certain amount of beat-to-beat spacing variation is considered to be an indication of a well-developed, healthy, autonomic nervous control system. It is best evaluated by internal electrodes monitors. Baseline variability of less than 5 beats per minute may be a sign of foetal jeopardy, particularly when lack of variability is found in conjunction with periods of late deceleration of the foetal heart. However, reduced variability may also be produced by the administration of certain analgesic or sedative drugs to the other. Reduced long-term variability may also be found during 20 to 30 minute intervals of so-called foetal sleep or inactivity.

Foetal cardiac deceleration Three types of periodic foetal cardiac decelerations according to their sequential relationships to uterine contractions, have been described and may be detected by continuous monitoring devices.

a. Early foetal cardiac decelerations start at the onset of a contraction and occur only at the same time as the contraction. This pattern is probably due to head compression and increase in the intracranial pressure of the infant. As far as is known, the pattern is harmless. It does not call for an intervention on the part of the obstetric team.
b. Late deceleration patterns are characterized by a slowing of the foetal heart after the peak, or acme, of the uterine contraction and by a delayed return to baseline and a regular waveform reflecting the uterine contraction. They may be found first within the normal FHR range of 120 to 160 beats per minute. As foetal distress increases, the range and frequency of the FHR deceleration increase. This pattern is frequently associated with uterine hyperactivity caused by oxytocin administration, maternal hypotension, or various high-risk pregnancies obstetric interventions to decrease or eliminate foetal distress include stopping any oxytocin administration, providing oxygen by mask or cannula to the mother at 6 to 8 L/min. turning the mother to either side, and possible foetal scalp stimulation.
c. Variable deceleration patterns characterized by a periodic, unpredictable slowing of the FHR that show neither a consistent sequential relationship to the uterine contractions nor a regular repetitive range or duration. The deceleration typically traces a steep-sided V or U. This type of pattern is considered to be the result of umbilical cord compression. Changes in maternal posture, to either side, oxygen administration to the mother, and possible vaginal examination are recommended interventions. A prolonged Trendelenberg position may not be appropriate in some cases, especially if the mother is receiving epidural anaesthesia. Other means of decompressing a cord should be sought.

If either late or variable decelerations persist for 30 minutes after the above interventions have been carried out, the physician may consider operative termination of the labour.

Foetal cardiac acceleration Periodic accelerations of the FHR are usually considered benign. They are often initiated by foetal movement, uterine contractions, or even maternal abdominal contractions. Indeed, accelerations of the foetal heart rate with foetal movement indicate foetal well-being and serve as the basis of the so called nonstress test. However, repetitious accelerations associated with contractions may occasionally precede the development of progressive late deceleration patterns. For this reason, they should be carefully observed.

Nurses Role in FHR Monitoring

The nurse should develop a system of interpretation that provides a comfortable approach, for example, starting with observation of the foetal heart tracing and then interpreting the maternal tracing before putting the two together. The monitor pen records the foetal heart rate on the upper tracings with graph paper. Note the marking on the tracing paper.

The nurse looks first on the foetal tracing when there are no uterine contractions. These are called 'baseline changes'. The 1 'baseline foetal heart rate' is the average rate during a 10-month segment that exclude periodic or episodic changes, periods marked variability, and segments of the baseline that differ by more than 25 beats/per minute. The normal range at term is 110 to 160 beats per minute.

Tachycardia

Tachycardia is a baseline FHR above 16 beats/mm. It can be considered an early sign of foetal hypoxia and can result from maternal or foetal infection, such as prolonged rupture of membranes with amnionitis, from maternal hyperthyroidism or foetal anaemia or in response to drugs, such as atrophine, hydroxyzine (vistaril), turbulence, or street drugs such as cocaine or methamphetamines.

The cause tachycardia may be sympathetic stimulation related to breathing movements or pressure applied to foetal parts other than the head, mild foetal asphyxia, maternal drug use, intrauterine infections, maternal temperature elevations and foetal auditory stimulations. A rising baseline during labour signals concern because an elevation of more than 20 beats/min. indicates beginning tachycardia even though the actual number may be in the normal range. Often, for instance, this mild tachycardia begins before signs of elevated maternal temperature.

Persistent tachycardia in absence of periodic changes does not appear serious in terms of neonatal outcome, tachycardia is non reassuring sign when associated with late deceleration, severe variable decelerations, or absence of variability.

The nursing intervention will be depending on cause for reduce maternal fever with antipyretics as ordered and cooling measures; oxygen at 8 to 10 L/min per face mask may be of some value; carryout health care providers: orders based on alleviating cause.

Bradycardia

Bradycardia is a baseline FHR below 110 beats/min. It can be considered later sign of foetal hyposia and is known to occur before foetal demise. Bradycardia can result from placental transfer of drugs such as propranolol, anaesthetics for epidural, spinal, caudal, and prudential blocks, prolonged compression of the umbilical cord, maternal hypothermia, maternal hypotension, prolonged maternal hypoglycaemia, Maternal supine hypotensive syndrome caused by uterine pressure (the weight of the gravid uterus) on the vena cava, interferes with the return of blood flow to the maternal heart, which then reduces maternal cardiac output and blood pressure.

If the umbilical cord is occluded or the placenta is compressed during uterine contractions, foetal baro-receptors react to the increase in foetal arterial blood pressure and cause foetal bradycardia. Increased intra-cranial pressure (which may develop late in labour) interruption of blood supply) or direct pressure to branches of the vagus nerve also can cause bradycardia. Asphyxia and acidosis are other causes of bradycardia.

Bradycardia with moderate variability and absence of periodic changes is not a sign of foetus compromise, if FHR remains above 80 beats per minute; bradycardia caused by hypoxia is a nonreassuring sign when associated with loss of variability and late deceleration.

Nursing intervention is dependent on cause. Intervention not warranted in foetus with heart block diagnosed by ECG; oxygen at 8 to 10 L/min per face mask may be of some value; Carry out health care providers orders based on alleviating cause; Scalp stimulation may be performed to determine whether or not the foetus has the ability to compensate physiologically for stress (FHR will accelerate).

Variability

The interaction between sympathetic and parasympathetic stimulation causes quickening and slowing of the foetal heart rate. This change can occur from one beat to the next, causing 'beat to beat variability". These changes indicate foetal well being. The baseline variability is the irregularity of the entire foetal heart rate bracing. It is important to look for baseline changes in rate or variability that have occurred during 10 minutes of tracing.

Variability of the FHR can be described as irregular, fluctuations in the baseline FHR of 2 cycles per minute or greater variability has been described as short term (beat-to-beat) or long term (rhythmic waves) or cycles from baseline) Currently there is no distinction between these two, but identified four ranges of variability. These are based on visualization of the amplitude in the peak to through segment in beats permanent and include the following:

- Absence or undetected variability.
- Minimal variability (greater than undetected not more than 5 beats/min).
- Moderate variability (6 to 25 beats/min)
- Marked variability (greater than 25 beats/min). Absence of or undetected variability is considered nonreassuring.

Increased variability results from early mild hypoxia, caused by foetal stimulation (by uterine palpation, uterine contractions, foetal activity, maternal activity, street drugs). The significance of marked variability is earliest FHR sign of mild hypoxaemia. Nursing intervention of increased variability will include:

- Observe FHR tracing carefully for any nonreassuring patterns including decreasing variability and late decelerations
- If using external mode of monitoring consider using internal mode (spiral electrode) for a more accurate tracing.

Decreased variability can result from foetal hypoxaemia and acidosis and narcotics (meperidine, alpha prodine, morphin, pentazocine) barbiturates (secobarbitol, pentobarbitol, ambobarbital), tranquilizer (diazepam) ataractics (promethazine, propiomazine, hydroxizine, promazine), parasympatholytics (atrophine) general anesthetics, prematurity (Less than 24 wk), foetal sleep cycles, congenital abnormalities, foetal cardia arrhythmias also causes decreased variability. It may be benign when associated with periodic foetal sleep states, which last 20 to 30 minutes, if caused by drugs, variability usually increases as drugs are excreted.

Decreased variability considered nonreassuring if caused by hypoxia/asphyxia, occurring, with late deceleration decreased variability associated with foetal acidosis and low Apgar scores.

Nursing interventions are dependent on cause, intervention not warranted if associated with foetal sleep states or temporarily associated with foetal sleep states or temporarily associated with CNS depressant. Nurse can consider performing external stimulation or scalp stimulation during a vaginal examination to elicit an acceleration of FHR or return to average variability. And consider application of internal mode (spiral electrode) assist health care provider with foetal blood sampling for pH if ordered; prepare for birth if so indicated by the primary health care provider or nurse.

Periodic Changes

Changes from baseline patterns in FHR are categorized as periodic or episodic. Periodic changes are those that occur with uterine contractions. These patterns include accelerations and decelerations.

Acceleration of the FHR is defined as a visually apparent abrupt increase in FHR above the baseline rate. FHR accelerations usually are associated with foetal movement. There are transient elevations that may rise 5 to 15 beats/min from the baseline, stay elevated. For several seconds to minutes, and then return to the baseline rate. Accelerations indicate that cardiac control center in the medulla is functional; the rise in heart rate seen in foetal movement is similar to a rise after physical activity. Acceleration, with foetal activity may be less varied in the premature foetus. The presence of accelerations with foetal movement is a reassuring sign and the basis of the nonstress test. Acceleration are caused by dominance of the sympathetic nervous response and are usually encountered with breech presentations. Acceleration of FHR that are episodic occur during foetal movement and are indications of foetal well being.

Deceleration may be benign or non-reassuring is caused by dominance of parasympathetic response. FHR decelerations may indicate foetal distress or may not be significant. Decelerations are classified as early, late and variables or types I, II, III respectively. The differences in the three are related to their shape and timing in relation to uterine contractions.

Early decelerations result from a vagal response to head compression often after rupture of membranes or during the second stage of labour. It is normal and usually benign finding. This deceleration is characterized by a uniform shape and on early onset corresponding to the rise in intra-amniotic pressure as the uterus contracts. When present, it usually occurs during the first stage of labour when the cervix is dilated 4 to 7 cm. Early decelerations sometimes are seen during second stage when the woman in pushing.

Late deceleration of the FHR is a visually apparent gradual increase in and return to baseline

FHR associated with uterine contractions. Persistent and repetitive late decelerations usually indicate the presence of foetal hypoxemia stemming from insufficient placental perfusion. It is caused by the maternal supine hypotensive syndrome, which can be correctable by positioning. Late deceleration caused by uteroplacental insufficiency can result from uterine hyperstimulation with oxytocin, pregnancy-induced hypertension. Post-date or post-term pregnancy, amnionitis, small for gestrational age foetus, maternal diabetes, placenta previa, abruptio placentas, conduction anaesthetics, maternal cardiac disease, and maternal anaemia. Late decelerations indicate foetal distress.

Variable deceleration is a visual abrupt decrease in FHR below baseline. The decrease is usually more than 15 beats/min. lasts at least 15 seconds and usually returns to baseline in less than 2 minutes from time to onset. Variable decelerations occur any time during the uterine contracting phase and are caused by compression of the umbilical cord, which inhibits flow to the foetal system if encountered during second stage of labour as a result of umbilical cord compression during foetal descent. Variable decelerations are also associated with neonatal depressions only when cord compression is severe or prolonged (e.g. tight nuchal cord, short cord, knot in cord, prolapsed cord).

Foetal distress The foetus sends a signal that its environment is lacking nutrients or oxygen this reaction is foetal distress. Foetal distress may be chronic, occurring during the course of pregnancy, or become acute, usually occurring during labour but also when the woman is deprived of oxygen (with poorly administered anesthesia or a bleeding complication). The classic description of a distressed foetus included abnormalities of the heart rate and meconium in the amniotic fluid. These signs are now recognized as later signs of deepening distress. Foetal monitoring capabilities and foetal blood sampling have made early diagnosis more precise.

The stresses of labour and delivery may leave the infant poorly equipped for the major adjustments that must be made. The following risk factors require close follow-up:

1. Rupture of membranes more than 12 to 24 hours before birth or maternal hyperhermia.
2. Anything that might reduce maternal blood pressure and, therefore, diminish blood supply to the placental circulation, including a drug reaction, reaction to conduction anaesthesia, supine hypotension, or haemorrhage.
3. Any indication of hypertonic or ineffective contractions.
4. Any foetal response outside of normal ranges.
5. Occlusion of the cord by any cause.

Foetal Responses to Hypoxia

Foetal distress is a sign of increasingly poor tolerance to the stress of labour. This stress is imposed by contractions, during which the blood flow to the placenta is basically stopped. If there is sufficient reserve in the foetus, the 60 to 90 second period without "new oxygen" is not harmful and the foetus recovers quickly in the rest period when oxygen freely circulates to the maternal foetal placental transfer points.

Remember good foetal oxygenation is shown by a foetal heart rate between 120 to 160 beats/min. and not more than 20 points change in baseline rate during labour, while maintaining good beat-to-beat variability. During any contraction the foetus will demonstrate the ability to maintain its normal heart rate. When distress occurs, the heart rate well change in the following ways. Decelerations occur from baseline: these may be brief, with a slow recovery, or they may persist in bradycardia. Loss of normal long and short-term variability in heart rate (a flat rate) often is accompanied by increasing tachycardia. Without intervention the foetus in distress will become increasingly acidotic and when born may be slow to recover, may be injured by asphysia, or may die.

Meconium

In utero meconium passage is seen only after 34 weeks of gestation and, therefore, is considered a maturational sign. Although it often accompanies foetal hypoxia, term infants may pass meconium without having been asphysiated. A baby in breech position usually passes meconium during the descent phase. Hypoxic stress may cause the diving reflex, with shunting of blood away from the gastro-intestinal tract and toward vital organs such as the brain and heart. Dilation of the anal sphincter and peristalsis follows:

About 11 to 22 per cent of all babies have meconium in the amniotic fluid at birth. Not all of these infants will be distressed at birth. Meconium is a sign. Not a cause, of foetal distress. The visually black faeces are full of bilirubin, which when diluted have a strong yellow-green colour. The concentration of meconium is directly related to the volume of amniotic fluid. Assessment of the characteristics of meconium-stained fluid is critical because thick meconium is more likely to cause respiratory problems in the newborn. The readings are subjective unless a "meconium crit" is performed. Amniotic fluid is collected and spin in a centrifuge, and readings are obtained as for hematocrit readings.

< 4 g/dl ml = Thin = dilute brownish fluid.

4-9 g/dl ml = Moderate: yellowish brown fluid, not clear.

> 9 g/dl ml = Thick : pea-soup consistency.

If an asphyxiated foetus takes deep gasping breaths before birth, stimulated by hypoxia, the meconium-stained fluid can be aspirated into the lower portion of the lung and, it is thick, can partly obstruct airways. Meconium aspiration syndrome (MAS) may lead to further cardiorespiratory problems.

Asphyxia

Asphyxia is the metabolic state of hypoxia, hypercapnia, and acidosis. The cycle of events leading to foetal asphyxia begins with the lack of oxygen (O2) and excess build-up of carbon dioxide (CO2) gradient between mother and foetus is greatly affected by alterations in placental perfusion, exchange across the placenta, or maternal hypoxemia. Respiratory acidosis begins first as CO2 increases. As oxygen levels fall, further energy production converts from aerobic to anaerobic paths, causing lactic acid to accumulate. The result is a mixed respiratory and metabolic acidosis. Further management of labour varies with the progress of labour and other foetal or maternal condition. Operative delivery will be arranged quickly to prevent further damage in an asphyxiated infant.

Whenever a foetus is distressed, the physician is obligated to check pH from the foetal scalp and make a decision regarding method of birth. A pH value must be obtained from the cord blood as well.

Cord pH values should be obtained on every new born who has been subjected to extra labour stress and had any difficulty maintaining into normal heart rate, on every baby of a high-risk pregnancy, and every infant with an Apgar score below 7 at 1 minute. Blood should be obtained from the umbilical artery, which is more difficult to puncture because arteries are smaller, but the blood here gives a truer picture of the newborn's status. The cord arterial pH is 0.05 to 0.07 below that of the umbilical vein pH.

Lactate Levels

Lactate is a result of anaerobic metabolism; first CO2 rises, then O2 levels fall. Lactate is thought to build up after CO2 levels rise and to be more damaging. The pH levels are the result of combined elevated lactate and hypercapnia. A new dry strip test similar to Dextrostix has been developed to assess foetal or cord blood lactate levels. Testing lactate levels may be used along with the pH to decide on the depth of the asphyxia in the foetus or newborn.

Foetal Scalp Blood Sampling (Procedure)

Another technique for diagnosis of foetal distress was needed when it was found that sometimes with variable or late deceleratins the foetus was indeed not acidotic. Analysis of foetal blood for pH reveals whether the foetus is acidotic. Blood can be obtained by making a small puncture in the foetal scalp (or breech). The amniotic membranes must already be ruptured and the cervix partially dilated. Indications for foetal blood pH measurements are as follows:

1. Severe late or variable decelerations with poor return to baseline.
2. Poor beat-to-beat variability bradycardia, or tachycardia.
3. Thick meconium with oligohydramnios.

Uteroplacental Insufficiency (UPI)

Late decelerations (type II) are deceptively subtle. The form is similar to that of the early decelerations; smooth and U-shaped. However, the timing is different. A late deceleration starts when the contraction is at its height, peaks when the contraction is almost over, and does not return to baseline until well after the contraction has ended. It resolves late. Again, the foetal heart rate most often stays within the normal range. Late decelerations are caused by UPI which may occur in the following instances:

1. Complicated pregnancies in which placental abnormalities such as infractions or calcifications are present.
2. Labour patterns with intense contractions occurring less than 2 minutes apart.
3. Hypertonic contractions lasting more than 90 seconds in active labour and 120 seconds during the transition phase.
4. Maternal hypotension from vena cava syndrome.
5. Epidural or general anaesthesia that decreases blood pressure and uteroplacental perfusion.

It is common to see late decelerations, a rising baseline rate, and decreased baseline variability together because hypoxia depresses the cardiac control centre in the medulla. The presence of late decelerations is always ominous and necessitates immediate investigations about the cause and appropriate interventions to increase foetal oxygenation.

Interventions for Late Decelerations

When signs of distress related to uteroplacental insufficiency appear, assessment must reveal the possible causes. Because blood supply may be affected on the maternal or foetal side, the examiner looks first for the most common causes:

- Maternal hypotension, with or without low blood volume, which may be caused by:
  - Venacaval compression
  - Dilation of lower extremity vessels after epidural or spinal anaesthesia
  - Bleeding, hidden or overt, that depletes blood volume
- Hypertonic uterine contractions from excessive response to oxytocin or naturally hypertonic contractions in later labour.
- Poor placental perfusion related to placental abnormality such as preeclampsia, hypertension, diabetes, premature separation of placenta or inadequate placental size that causes intrauterine growth retardation (IUGR) or birth defects.

On the basis of the signs, interventions must be directed in correct causes, beginning with the least complicated interventions and observing responses of the foetal heart.

1. Change position in bed; vena caval compression by the heavy uterus can occur in lithotomy, supine, semi-Fowler's and a slight right or left lateral tilt. Turn her completely to the left or rightside. Sometimes sitting up or getting on hands and knees can be helpful.
2. Increase main line Ringer's lactate solution if the problem could be a low blood volume related to anesthesia or bleeding. Be sure to note exactly when and how much fluid is given during the period.
3. At the same time, observe the monitor and the character of the contractions are they hypertonic for the stage of labour? Is oxytocin infusing a secondary line? If contractions are strong and oxytocin is infexing turn off the intravenous (IV) pump to stop the flow.
4. Begin, according to protocol, oxygen by mask set at 8 to 10 l/min. Women are mouth breabhers during labour, thus nasal oxygen freely, believing that it does not change the uptake significantly).
5. Check maternal blood pressure and pulse to correlate with recent activities such as regional anaesthesia and examinations.
6. Notify the physician or nurse midwife of the incident and results of interventions. Document time of notification and response on chart and monitor strip. If late decelerations do not improve as a result of interventions, the physician or nurse midwife must check foetal pH levels and plans may begin for caesarean "rescue" operation.

Variable Decelerations

Cord Compressions

Variable deceleration (type III) look different from early and late decelerations and often look different from each other. The foetal heart rate decreases sharply, stays down for a variable number of seconds, and then usually returns to baseline as sharply as it descended.

Occlusion of the unbillical cord first causes the heart rate to increases; the foetus with normal placental oxygen reserve compensates with tachycardia. As the occlusion progresses, it interrupts blood flow through the umbilical arteries, causing an increase in paripheral resistance. Stimulation of foetal carotid sinus and aortic arch baroreceptors follows; parasympathetic fibres then cause the foetal heart rate to decrease.

Although an occasional variable deceleration is benigh, repetitive decelerations are serious and indicate a foetus who may become increasingly hypoxic and acidotic. A late component may start to appear, during which variable decelerations fail to return to baseline until after the contraction has ended. There may be loss of baseline variability as the foetal cardiac control centre is depressed further. The rule of 60's is used to determine ominous cord compression.

Second Stage Variables

Variables often are seen toward the end of labour after rupture of membranes, when cord compresion accompanies foetal descentand expulsion. Then they are called end-stage variables. About 90% of the labour patterns show variable decelerations in the second stage. Some are significant; most are not. If, however, variable have begun in the first stage, they may become progressively worse. To note the various patterns seen in the second stage of labour when head compression plus descent may be aggravated by the expulsive pushing efforts of the mother.

Types 0 to 1	Are considered normal because the baseline is maintained between contractions.
Type 2	Shows progressive bradycardia added to cord compression and is an ominous sign.
Type 3	Is ominous because the peaks you see are really accelerations above a bradycardic baseline; the infant will enter a state of severe acidosis rapidly.
Type 4	Show a normal heart rate, which followed by a rapidly falling bradycardia and loss of beat-to-beat variability, and is very serious.

Causes

Variable decelerations are a result of compression of the umbilical cord and may be caused by a number of precipitating events.

1. Cord is caught between foetus and uterine wall.
2. Cord around foetal neck, arm, shoulder, or other part is being pulled tightly as foetus descends in labour (nuchal cord).
3. There is a knot in the cord that is tightened during labour.
4. Occult (hidden) or frank (obvious) prolapse of the cord occurs through the cervix.
5. There is pressure on cord because of insufficient amniotic fluid (coligohydramnios).
6. Foetus is growth retarded and has a deficient amount of Wharton's jelly to cushion the cord.

Long or Short Cord

Knots or loops in the cord occur if the cord is excessively long (>100 cm). During labour these knots may be pulled tighter or if looped around the neck (nuchal cord), the cord becomes stretched and narrowed as the foetus goes through descent.

A short cord (< 32 cm) also is likely to show signs of traction, with narrowed umbilical vessels during the descent. End-stage variables result from these type of changes, as well as from pressure against all parts of the cord during the second stage. Remember, if recovery to baseline occurs after the contraction, the foetus is not considered in jeopardy with variable decelerations. If, however, the patterns are accompanied by a late component or continuing bradycardia with no recovery and poor beat-to beat variability, the foetus requires rescue and intervention must be prompt.

Cord Prolapse

When the cord lies beside the presenting part or below it, the pressure of the head or buttock will pinch off circulation *cord prolapse* will result in varying degrees of cord compression (CC) and variable decelerations or in complete loss or heart rate. Complete CC occurs most frequently with premature rupture of membranes when the foetal presenting part not engaged or when there is a footing or complete breech presentation. Fifteen per cent of cord prolapse cases occur at home with rupture of membranes, and these carry a high-risk of foetal death. First there is a change in foetal heart rate and a lack of foetal movements. A vaginal inspection might show the bluish shiny cord protruding through the cervix.

Interventions for Variable Decelerations

Prevention is important. When artificial rupture of membranes (AROM) occurs, the fluid should be released very slowly and the vaginal area inspected at once. Monitoring should continue before and after the procedure.

If variable changes begin, position change must be tried first to relieve pressure.

1. Use the lateral sims position first. Rotate to the other side if no effect is achieved. If the cord

is not through the vagina, it may be between the internal os and the head.

2. Then a knee-chest position may help to move the foetus off the cervix. Because this position is difficult to assume during labour, a modified Trendelenburg position can be tried.
3. If the cord is prolapsed and visible in the vagina, the only recourse is to put on a sterile glove and manually push the presenting part off the cord so that circulation can continue while preparations are made for emergency caesarean delivery.
4. Some units report that inserting a Foleys catheter and instilling 500 ml. into the bladder while holding the foetal head off the cord will push the foetus up in the uterus and relieve pressure long enough for surgery. Of course the surgeon would not use a low incision near the distended bladder.
5. Continue monitoring with FECG clip (position may prevent obtaining a contraction pattern).
6. Use appropriate interventions for late decelerations also; administer oxygen by mask and stop oxytocin flow.

If prolapse is not the cause of variable decelerations, a simple position change, as noted in the preceding list, may solve the problem. Should the baseline return to normal and the decelerations improve, no further action may be required. As labour progresses, however, these variables may recur.

Amnioinfusion (Procedure)

When there is less amniotic fluid than normal, the cord may be compressed for normal volumes. If variable decelerations are not improved by other interventions, amnioinfusion instilling a warmed sterile normal saline solution into the uterine cavity by catheter; can have a beneficial effect. In one series it reduced the rate of caesarean deliveries from 22 to 3% in those with distress from variable decelerations. Usually the physician and nurse work together in this procedure.

Preparation for amnioinfusion must be accomplished quickly once the need arises. The woman needs a careful explanation of the procedure and its objectives. In addition, many units ask the woman to sign an informed consent.

The purpose of managing foetal nonreassuring responses at any level is support placental perfusion to the foetus. Thus, if one pictures the flow directions, the rationale for these corrective intervention will be logical. The procedures, which involve , which involve more one nurse, must be performed rapidly. Therefore, it is helpful to think of steps as simultaneous.

The nurse also will be checking the foetal heart rate for improvements. If an internal electrode has not yet been placed, it should be accomplished as soon as possible. At the same time the woman needs explanations about what is occurring and why so that she may co-operate.

SUMMARY OF PATTERNS

Reassuring Patterns

Provide information that indicates the adequacy of foetal oxygenation and perfusion. The baseline rate is considered normal between 120 and 160 beats/min. Remember that baseline variability can be truly assessed only during internal monitoring: an average of 6 to 10 beats/min. is considered normal. Normal periodic changes include accelerations with foetal movements and early decelerations during the later phrases of labour. The nurse's intervetion for reassuring patterns is to continue observation.

Questionable Patterns

Signal possible alterations in foetal oxygenation or perfusion. The baseline rate may be near the upper or lower limits of normal. Mild bradycardia (100 to 120 beats/min) may be normal if no other problems are present and the baseline heart rate has not changed significantly. *Mild Tachycardia* may be related to prematurity, foetal arrhythmias, perinatal infection, chronic or mild foetal hypoxia, maternal or foetal anaemia, maternal fever, anxiety or hyperthyroidism, or administration of beta-sympathomimetic or parasympatholytic drugs to the client.

Increased Baseline Variability

Increased baseline variability (over 25 beats/min) is associated with maternal and foetal movements but may be an early sign of foetal malposition or cephalopelvic disproportion (CPD). Finally, *Variable* decelerations may be considered questionable patterns, if the foetal heart rate drops no lower than 80 beats/min for less than 30 seconds, variability remains normal and there is no late component or significant change in baseline rate.

Ominous patterns indicate significant alterations in foetal oxygenation or perfusion; these usually are mixed or show several configurations *Bradycardia* is especially worrysome when associated with late decelerations, variable decelerations, or loss of variability. Decreased baseline variability (less than 3 to 5 beats/in) may be related to maternal drug administration (meperidine and other analgesics, magesium sulfate), foetal sleep, prematurity, anomalies of the central nervous system, or foetal tachycardia or hypoxia. Decreased variability is always a warning sign if not explained by medications or foetal sleep-wake patterns.

NURSING RESPONSIBILITIES DURING FOETAL MONITORING

The nurse is the primary manager of foetal monitoring. Skill in interpretation of patterns and regulating equipment is expected. Hospital units must educate and evaluate the nurse's competency in recognition of broderline and ominous foetal heart rate patterns. Nurses also need to take initiative and seek out continuing education in this area. The rate of lawsuits that involve use or misuses of the foetal monitor reinforces the nurse's need to know the documentation requirements.

Documentation to Avoid Liability

One half of the recent malpractice claims in the United States involved the use or misuse of electronic foetal monitoring (EFM). Cases include failure to monitor in labour and just before birth or failure to respond correctly to the tracing results, especially to perform a caesarean delivery to interrupt foetal distress. Failure to monitor or respond correctly indeed may not have happened, but someone neglected to write down the findings. It should be kept in mind that according to legal statute, "If it is not written, it was not done". The importance of documentation is heightened because cases may come to court 5 to 10 years later; no one can remember details for so long. Thus, nurses must take special care in documenting observations. There is a bedside flow sheet for noting the usual points, vital signs, contraction characteristics, amniotic fluid status, and vaginal examinations and findings about cervix status and station, as well as foetal heart rate and reactivity. Treatments, medications, and anesthesia also are noted in written form in several places. In careful recording, most of this information also will be noted on the monitor strip but in an abbreviated recording, most of this information also will be noted on the monitor strip but in an abbreviated fashion. Table 5.9 shows information required on the strip. Legally the strip should be able to stand alone as a record of the foetal response to labour. The nurse already known that this in true about the client's chart, and the strip is an important part of the chart.

Table 5.9: Correct documentation for foetal strip and maternal chart

Nurse/Physician activity	*Client activity*
Vaginal examinations and result	Change of position
Artificial rupture of membranes	Spontaneous rupture of membranes (SROM)
IV Therapy	Bedpan use
Oxytocin rate	Vomiting
Other medication dose/rate	Oral intake
External/Internal transducer change	Pushing
Epidural	Vital signs
Oxygen begun/ended	
Procedures	

Each unit has a protocol for foetal monitoring management. On newer monitors, automatic entries are printed on the strip and times are printed with each entry. Otherwise, the nurse must remember to include the time for an entry. The bedside chart and the strip nead to show evidence of at least one entry every 30 minutes, even if just an initial on the strip of a client who is in an early phase.

If there is artifact and a poor FHR signal, that also should be noted. Sometimes it is difficult to obtain an adequate external foetal heart reading for an obese patient. Contraction characteristics, as well as variability and periodic changes, that appear on the strip must be described on the flow sheet. In this legal climate, documentation is essential to the practice of "defensive nursing". It is also important to list times of physician notification and response. When the physician does not respond promptly, nursing actions should be included. The nurse who notes inadequate physician response or intervention is legally required to report to a superior nurse supervisor or attending physician to obtain satisfactory follow-up. A number of nurses have been involved in lawsuits because they did not follow through in securing adequate help for the foetus in distress.

Nursing Diagnoses

Although nursing diagnoses are not formulated in this emergency, think through which would apply:

1. Fear related to setting, lack of preparation, loss of control.
2. High risk for altered tissue integrity and infection related to trauma of birth.
3. High risk for altered maternal-foetal perfusion related to rapid birth.
4. Ineffective thermoregulation related to environmental temperature.
5. High risk for altered oxygenation of newborn if adequate assistance is not available.

Objectives

1. Woman is cooperative and responsive to nursing assistance.
2. Completes uneventful birth of a viable infant.
3. Infant exhibits consistent body temperature between 97° and 98° F.

Nursing Interventions

In making a decision about the timing of birth, determine your options. Evaluate the location. Enlist someone to get help, someone to control a potential crowd, and someone to get equipment. Suggested types of equipment are listed below:

For cleansing the mother	:	Water with dishwashing liquid, or wipe down with underclothes
For padding or protection	:	Newspapers (unused), during delivery when in a public space, large plastic bags, old sheets, towels, shower curtain
To clear infant's airway	:	Ear bulb syringe,meat bastign syringe, and manual milking of nose and throat
For the cord (if no help available)	:	Strong yarn, new razor blade, scissors or knife (flame sterilized) (only if no help to be available)
To warm the body	:	Mother's clothes, skin-to-skin contact, blanket, towel, sheet, clean newspapers, padded box
To feed the baby if no help available	:	Milk powder, bottle, nipple (if not breast-feeding)
Fluids for the mother	:	Any available

Follow Figures 5.16 and 5.17 to note the hand positions for the delivery of the head and shoulders.

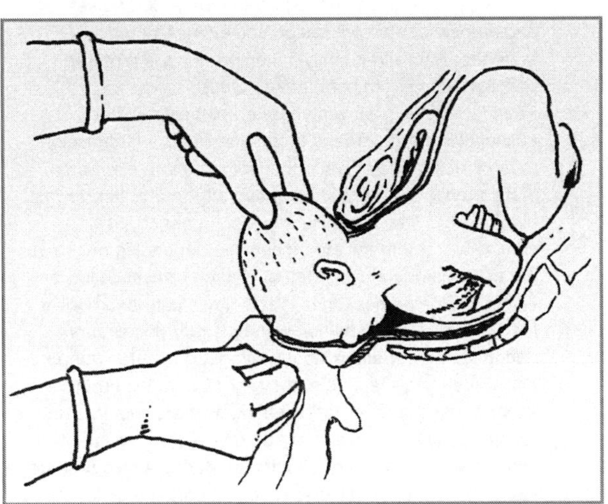

Fig. 5.16: Assistance may be needed if head does not extend smoothly (Ritgen's manoeuvre). Exert hand pressure downward on occiput with forward pressure applied to obstetric perineum, just between vaginal and anal openings Feel for chin, and exert forward pressure on it through perineal tissue. For emergency delivery, use article of mother's clothing (cleanest material available) because skin will be slippery

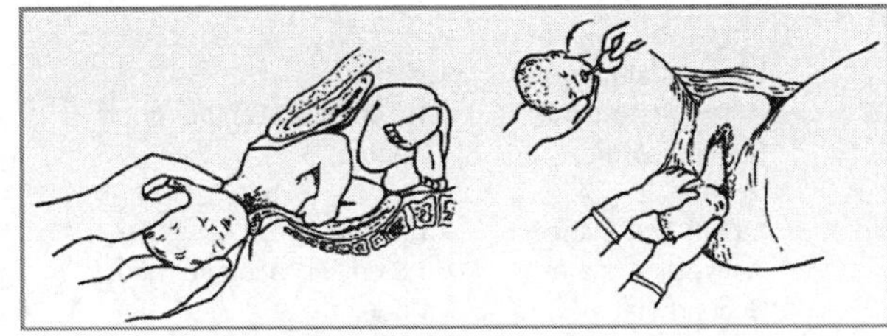

Fig. 5.17: Baby's head is gently directed downward it help in partial delivery of anterior (upper) shoulder to "park" it under the symphysis pubis. Then proceed with delivery of lower shoulder by pulling up on the head

PROCEDURES USED DURING LABOUR AND BIRTH (TABLES 5.10 TO 5.19)

Monitoring women during labour and in the immediate postpartum period (Table 5.10).

Table 5.10: Monitoring women during labour and immediate postpartum

Nursing action	*Rationale*
Monitoring During Labour 1. Assess the following parameters during the first and second stages of labour at regular intervals:	
• *Vital signs*. Assess and record blood pressure on admission and at least hourly during the active phase of labour (more frequently if blood pressure is elevated). Assess and record termperature, pulse, and respirations on admission and every 4 hours thereafter (more frequently if membranes are ruptured or if deviations from normal are noted)	An ongoing evaluation of maternal and foetal status during labour ensures that deviations from normal findings are identified and appropriate nursing actions are implemented
• *Foetal well-being*. To verify foetal well-being, either auscultate and record the foetal heart rate on admission to the birthing unit or place the woman on an electronic foetal monitor for 20 to 30 minutes after admission to the birthing unit. After the initial monitoring period, use continuous or intermittent monitoring, depending on the maternal-foetal risk, status. Whether auscultation or electronic foetal monitoring is used, evaluate and record foetal heart rate for low-risk women every 60 minutes during latent first-stage labour, every 30 minutes during active first-stage labour, and every 15 minutes during second-stage labour. For high-risk, women, evaluate and record foetal heart rate every 30 minutes during latent first-stage labour, every 15 minutes during active first-stage labour, and every 5 minutes during second-stage labour	
• *Uterine activity*. Assess and record the frequency, duration, and intensity of uterine contractions every 30 to 60 minutes by direct palpation or through interpretation of electronic foetal monitoring strips. Assess and record the uterine resting tone between contractions by direct palpation	
• *Labour progress*. Perform a vaginal examination to assess cervical effacement and dilatation, foetal position and station, and status of membranes. Record your findings. Determine whether duration of labour exceeds the normal limits: *Primigravida* Latent first stage > 20 hours Active first stage < 1.2 cm dilatation per hour Second stage > 2 hours *Multipara* Latent first stage > 14 hours Active first state < 1.5 cm dilatation per hour Second stage > 1 hour	
• *Intake and output*. Assess the women's intake to ensure adequate hydration. Initiate intravenous fluid administration as needed or before administration of epidural anesthesia. Encourage the woman to empty her bladder frequently labour, as a distended bladder can impede the descent of the foetal presenting part and slow labour progress. Catheterize the woman with bladder fullness and inability to void due to epidural anesthesia. Evaluate other output measures including vomiting and diarrhoea	

Contd...

Contd...

Nursing action	*Rationale*
2. Evaluate the following psychosocial parameters throughout the labour process: • Support system • Level of understanding of the labour process and procedures related to the care of a woman in labour • Effectiveness of coping strategies of deal with the labour process and the pain of labour	The psychosocial assessment provides the basis for education of the patient, anticipatory guidance, and provision of supportive care including both pharmacologic and nonpharmacologic measures
Monitoring in the Immediate Postpartum Period (First Hour After Birth)	
1. Assess and record the following parameters every 15 minutes and more frequently if deviations from normal are noted: • Blood pressure, pulse, and respirations. In the absence of complications, they will return to prelabour values within the first hour postpartum • *Uterus*. Palpate the uterus to assess its height, position, and consistency. Place one hand just above the symphysis pubis and apply gentle downward pressure to support the lower segment of the uterus. Place the other hand on the uterine fundus. The uterine fundus should be at the level of the umbilicus or slightly below it and in the midline of the abdomen. The uterus should be firm rather than boggy. If the uterus is boggy, initiate uterine massage of stimulate the uterus to contract • *Lochia*. Assess the colour (lochia rubra), the amount (scant, small, moderate, heavey), and whether odour is fleshy (normal) or foul smelling (indicative of infection). Assess lochial flow; report continuous trickle of bright red blood (abnormal) to health care provider, Note presence of clots; report numerous large clots (abnormal) to health care provider	An ongoing evaluation of maternal status in the immediate postpartum period ensures the identification of potential problems and the prompt initiation of nursing actions
2. Assess the following parameters at least once during the immediate postpartum period and more frequently if deviations from normal more frequently if deviations from normal are noted: • Temperature. The temperature may remain slightly elevated. Notify health care provider if temperature is greater than 2ºF above normal (indicative of infection) • Perineum. Using a flashlight or penlight, inspect the perineum using the REEDA scale. Evaluate redness, oedema, and ecchymosis. Confirm that episiotomy or laceration repair is intact and without drainage. Assess for the presence of haematomas and haemorrhoids. Assess the woman's perception of perineal discomfort or pain • Bladder fullness. Assess bladder fullness directly by suprapubic palpation or indirectly by fundal location (the fundus is displaced above the umbilicus and to the right by a full bladder). Assess the woman's ability to void spontaneously and the need for catheterization • Breasts. Assess status of the nipples. Assist breastfeeding mothers with correct positioning of the infant and latching on techniques • Extremities. Assess the women's reactivity after anaesthesia by evalusting her ability to move her lower extremities	An ongoing evaluation of maternal status in the immediate postpartum period ensures the identification of potential problems and the prompt initiation of nursing actions

Table 5.11: Auscultating FHR during labour

Nursing action	Rationale
1. Explain the procedure to the woman and her partner, including the reason for and the frequency of the procedure	Helps to decrease anexiety and improve compliance with the procedure
2. Instruct the woman to lie on her back on the bed, with a pillow under her head. Place a wedge under her right or left hip to maintain a slight lateral tilt during the procedure. Lower the head on the bad so that it is flat	Proper position facilitates location of foetal heart tones. A wedge under the woman's hip displaces the uterus sufficiently to prevent compression of maternal blood vessels and subsequent supine hypotension
3. Perform Leopold manoeuvres to locate the foetal back	Foetal heart tones are best heard through the foetal back. As the foetus changes position during labour, the location of foetal heart tones also changes
4. If you are using the Doppler stethoscope, turn it on and gently tap the auscultating end, listening for a resultant sound. Put a small amount of conducting gel onto the Doppler stethoscope	To ascertain whether the Doppler stethoscope is in working order. The gel enhances the conduction of sound
5. If you are using a fetoscope, place the metal band on your head with the diaphragm extending out from your forehead	The metal bond adds bone conduction to facilitate transmission of the sound
6. With firm pressure, place the Doppler stethoscope or bell of the foetoscope on the appropriate quadrant of the woman's abdomen	The heart tones of a foetus in the cephalic presentation are generally heard over one of the two lower quadrants of the maternal abdomen. As labour progresses and the foetus descends into the pelvic cavity, the foetal heart tones may be found midline in the lower abdomen. The position of the baby determines where the heart tones are best heard
7. Listen for foetal heart tones and differentiate them from other sounds	The foetal heart has a characteristic sound similar to that of a galloping horse; count only one beat for each double rhythm. In contrast, blood moving through the uterine vessels or umbilical card has a soft`swooshing" sound
8. Compare the rate of what you are hearing through the fetoscopy or Doppler stethoscope with the rate of the maternal heart by palpating the woman's readial pulse	To confirm that you have located the foetal heart tone rather than the maternal pulse
9. Determine the baseline rate by counting the number of beats for 30 to 60 seconds between contractions. Determine foetal response to the stress of contractions by listening for deceleration or acceleration of the foetal heart rate during a uterine contraction and for 30 seconds thereafter	A normal baseline foetal heart rate for a full-term foetus is between 120 and 160 beats per minute and is counted between contractions. An acceleration is usually associated with a healthy foetus; a deceleration could indicate foetal stress
10. Auscultate foetal heart rate at regular intervals	Current guidelines for frequency of foetal heart rate auscultation during labour are as follows: Low-risk / High-risk First stage Latent: Every 60 minutes / Every 30 minutes Active: Every 30 minutes / Every 15 minutes Second stage: Every 15 minutes / Every 5 minutes
11. Wipe off the women's abdomen and the tip of the Doppler stethoscope with a clean, dry cloth	Prevents the gel from getting onto the women's clothing
12. Record the baseline rate, rhythm, and foetal response to uterine contractions. Nursing interventions in response to nonreassuring findings must also be documented.	Repeated findings provide information on foetal status and well-being. If nonreassuring findings are noted, the nurse is obligated to intervence appropriately and place the patient on an electtronic fetai monitor to better detect subtle changes in the foetal heart rate

Table 5.12: Vaginal examination during labour

Nursing action	*Rationale*
1. Prepare the woman for examination by explaining the procedure and describing the sensations to expect	Anticipatory guidance decreases the woman's anxiety and facilitates cooperation during the examination
2. Lower the head of the bed. Position the women so that her knees are flexed. Ask her to separate her legs. Place a wedge under the woman's right or left hip to maintain a slight lateral tilt during the procedure	Proper position allows the health care provider's easier access to the cervix and enhances the woman's ability to relax during the procedure. A wedge is used in the supine position to prevent compression of the maternal blood vessels and subsequent supine hypotension
3 Wash your hands and apply one glove to the examining hand using sterile technique. Using the other hand, apply sterile lubricant to index and middle fingers of gloved hand	The use of sterile technique decreases the possibility of introducing organisms that may lead to maternal or foetal infection. Lubricant reduces friction between the gloved hand and the vaginal wall during the procedure
4. Instruct the woman to relax and to begin slow, rhythmic breathing	Slow, rhythmic breathing may facilitate the women's relaxation and comfort during the examination.
5. Gently insert the index and middle fingers into the vagina until they the cervix. The fingers may initially be directed with the palmar surface downward and then rotated upward curl the last two fingers inward. Either tuck the thumb in with the last two fingers or keep it above the symphysis pubis	Directing the palmar surface initially downward enhances the woman's comfort because the posterior surface of the vaginal wall is less sensitive than the anterior surface. Tucking in the thumb or keeping it above the symphysis pubis prevents obscuring the women's genitalia or irritating the clitoris during the examination
6. Assess the following parameters: • Cervical position • Cervical consistency • Cervical effacement • Cervical dilatation • Presenting part • Foetal position as determined by the foetal suture lines and position of the fontanelles (in cephalic presentations) in relation to the maternal public bone • Foetal station as determined by the presenting part in relation to the ischial spines of the pelvis • Status of membranes	These assessments are the basis for determining labour progress and the relationship of the foetus to the maternal pelvis
7. To determine dilation accurately, proceed as follows: • After inserting fingers into the cervix, determine the *internal os* of the cervix by curling tip of index finger over upper edge of cervix	It is important to determine the internal os of cervix for accurate measurement
• Measure the number of fingers of dilatation within the internal os of the cervix by counting across the presenting part with your index finger	Dilatation proceeds from 0 to 10 cm. You need to know the size of your index fingertip in centimeters. One finger usually equals 1.5 to 2 cm, depending on size of the individual
• Measure the number of fingers of cervix on each side of the cervical opening with your index finger and subtract from 10 cm using the procedure again	This number is used to assess the accuracy of your measurement of dilataion and should equal the centimeters of dilatation. If it does not, repeat measurement of dilation
8. To determine the position of the foetal head, proceed as follows: • Locate the posterior fontanelle by gently palpating the foetal head. Distinguish the posterior fontanelle, which is triangle shapped, from tho anterior fontanelle, which is diamond-shaped • Determine the relationship of the posterior fontanelle to the maternal pubic bone. If the posterior fontanelle is located just under the maternal public bone, the foetal position is anterior. If the posterior fontanelle is located toward the back of the maternal pelvis, the foetal position is posterior	The position of the foetal head provides valuable information about the expected progress of labour
9. After the examination, explain the examination results to the woman and her partner, place a clean pad under the woman's buttocks if needed, and help her to a position of comfort	Measures to keep the couple involved and keep the woman comfortable enhance the labour experience
10. Remove gloves and wash your hands	Prevents cross-contamination

Contd...

Contd...

Nursing action			*Rationale*
11. Record vaginal examination findings on the foetal monitor tracing and on the labour flow record as follows:			Recording these results allows comparisons to assess labor progress
Cervix	Position	Posterior or anterior	
	Consistency	Firm or soft	
	Effacement	0 to 100%	
	Dilatation	0 to 10 cm	
Presenting part	Cephalic, breech, shoulder, compound		
Foetal position	Left, right,anterior, or posterior		
Station	-5/5 (floating) to + 5/5 (crowning)		
Membranes	Intact, bulging, or ruptured spontancously or artificially		

Purpose

To determine that maternal-foetal status is within normal limits during labour and that maternal status is within normal limits in the immediate postpartum period; to intervene when deviations from normal are noted.

Equipment

- Thermometer
- Blood pressure cuff
- Stethoscope
- Electronic foetal monitor or fetoscope
- Flashlight or penlight

Auscultating Foetal Heart Rate During Labour (Fig. 5.18)

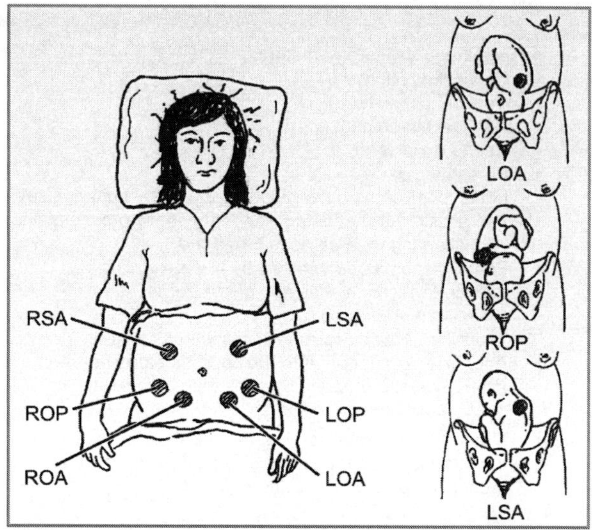

Fig. 5.18: Ausculating foetal heart rate during labour

Purpose

The foetal heart rate is auscultated on admission to the labour suite and at regular intervals throughout labour to assess foetal status and well-being. Frequent assessments detect changes in the foetal heart rate and presence of accelerations and decelerations, all indicators of how well the foetus is tolerating labour.

Equipment

- Listening device, such as a fetoscope or doppler ultrasound stethoscope
- Ultrasonic gel.

Vaginal Examination During Labour (Fig. 5.19)

Purpose

Vaginal examinations during labour are performed only when indicated to evaluate labour progress. Performed with use of sterile technique, a vaginal examination during labour can provide information on cervical position, consistency, effacement, and dilatation; foetal presentation, position, and station; and status of membranes.

Equipment

- Sterile glove
- Sterile lubricant

Table 5.13: Identifying the newborn

Nursing action	*Rationale*
In-hospital Delivery	
1. Prepare equipment and ascertain that the numbers on the identification bracelets match	Matching the numbers ensures that the correct infant is always given to the correct parent
2. At delivery, record necessary information on the bracelet inserts (e.g., mother's name, date and time of birth, sex of baby, and medical record number)	Recording the appropriate information at delivery further ensures accurate matching of parent and infant
3. Apply bracelets according to hospital policy. Usually, one bracelet goes around the mother's wrist, one around the baby's ankle and wrist, and the last to a person designated by the mother. When applying the bracelet to the body, keep your finger under the bracelet while closing the clasp	Bracelets on the mother and partner that match the ones on the infant allow either person to take or accept the infant from the nursery. Bracelets on the infant should be snug but not too tight. Leaving a gap the width of a finger between the baby and the bracelet allows adequate circulation to the baby's foot or hand while also ensuring that the bracelet is snug enough to stay on the baby
4 Explain the purpose of the identification bracelets to the parents and instruct them not to remove the bracelets until the baby is discharged from the hospital	Understanding the reason for the bracelets improves parents compliance with the procedure
5. Record the identification bracelet number on the delivery record with the name of the person who applied the bracelets	In case a question arises, the identification bracelet number and the name of the person applied the bracelets can be found on this legal document.
6. If footprints are required, wipe the sole of the baby's foot clean	The footprint will be more distinct if the foot is clear of vernix, blood, or meconium
7. Place the sole of the newborn's foot on the ink pad so that the entire sole is covered	A print of the infant's entire sole is essential for identification purposes.
8. Place one hand against the back of the footprint document to provide a firm surface and press the baby's foot onto the paper in the designated spot, being careful not to smudge the print. Repeat with her other foot	A clear print in which the lines of the foot can be deciphered is essential for identification purposes.
Out-of Hospital Delivery	
1. Before mother and baby are separated, open blanket and identify sex of infant with parents	Clarifies any misconception that may have happened in the confusion during an emergency birth
2. Follow procedure for in-hospital delivery	The same precautions should be taken regardless of where delivery has occurred
On Postpartum Unit	
1. When handing the infant to the new mother in her room or in the nursery, visually confirm that the numbers and names on the identification bracelets match each time	Ensures that the correct infant is always given to the correct mother
2. If someone other than the mother picks up the baby from the nursery or wishes to accept the baby in the hospital room, check to see that this person is wearing an identification bracelet and that the information on the bracelet matches that of the baby's each time	Ensures that the correct infant is given to the correct individual
3 Document this process on the newborn's recored	If a question arises, documentation that this procedure was followed is available
4. When picking up the infant from the mother's room or on return of the infant to the nursery by a parent, positively identify the newborn again	Ensure that the infant received into the nursery is the correct infant
5 At the time of discharge from the hospital, check to see that the names and numbers on the identification bracelets match	Ensure accurate matching of baby and parents at time of discharge

Table 5.14: Maternal foetal transport

Nursing Action	*Rationale*
1. Assess the woman's condition to ensure that she is stable for transport	Patients in stable condition before transport are less likely to require emergency intervention enroute.
2. Communicate with family and physician. It is the responsibility of the referring physician to discuss with the receiving physician the status of the woman's condition and to ascertain whether room is available at the receiving hospital. Physicians should also discuss the risks and benefits of transport with the woman and her family. Withness informed consent:	Anticipatory guidance improves the efficiency of the transport and helps to lessen the family's fears and anxieties concerning maternal foetal transport. Include the following information as you prepare the family for transport
• Mode of transportation • Personnel involved in transport • Basic discussion of anticipated care at tertiary care centre • Information on family visiting and necessary phone numbers	Witnessing information consent is necessary because the form is a legal document
3. Plan for the transport.Obtain estimated times for transport arrival at the referring hospital, departure, and arrival at the receiving hospital. Discuss equipment and personnel needed. Photocopy the woman's chart for the receiving hospital. Also send the consent for transport and other pertinent documents such as sonograms and foetal monitor tracings	Planning needs ahead of time prevents delays during which the woman's condition could change. The receiving hospital needs all information regarding the patient's diagnosis, care and medications received, and current status. This helps ensure the development of an appropriate plan of care at the receiving hospital
4. When the transport team arrives, provide them with an up-to-date report on the women's status, including maternal vital signs, foetal heart rate, uterine contraction status,medication schedule, and other information relevant to patient diagnosis. Assist in transfer to the stretcher. Document in the woman's chart that a verbal report was given, and record the time of arrival and departure of the team. Ensure that the woman's personal belongings accompany her on transport	Up-to-date information on the status of the women helps the transport learn anticipate problems taht might occur on route. Thses transfer forms become part of the permanent record
5. Call the receiving hospital when the transport team leaves	This provides the receiving hospital with an estimated time of patient arrival

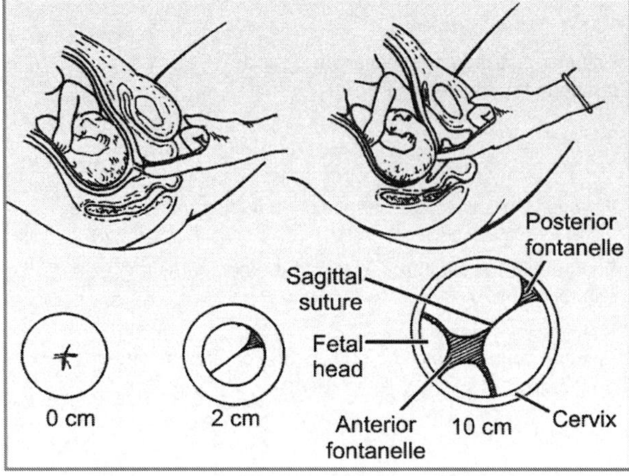

Fig. 5.19: Vaginal examination during labour

Identifying the Newborn

Purpose

To establish accurate identification of the newborn and to ensure that each newborn is given to the right mother, The initial identification of the newborn should always be done before mother and newborn are separated.

Equipment

- Set of four identification bracelets with inserts
- Pen
- Disposable ink pads
- Footprint document

Table 5.15: Assisting with amniotomy

	Nursing Action	*Rationale*
1.	Prepare the woman for aminotomy by explaining the procedure, including the reason it is being done, and describing the sensations to expect	Anticipatory guidance will decrease the women's anxiety and facilitate cooperation during the procedure
2.	Lower the head of the bed. Position the woman so that her knees are flexed. Ask her to separate her legs and relax them. Place pads under the woman's buttocks to absorb the amniotic fluid after amniotomy. Place a wedge under the woman's right or left hip to maintain a slight lateral tilt during the procedure	Proper positioning allows the health care provider easier access to the cervix and enhances the women's ability to relax. A wedge is used when the woman is in the supine position to prevent compression of the maternal blood vessels and subsequent supine hypotension. Foetal well-being must be confirmed before and after amniotomy
3.	Check the foetal heart rate by Doppler or apply the external foetal monitor ultrasound transducer	
4.	Assist the woman's health care provider by applying sterile lubricant to his or her gloved hand and opening the sterile pack-age containing the Amnihook	Lubricant decreases friction between the gloved hand and vaginal wall during the procedure. Sterile technique is essential during amniotomy to prevent potential contamination and decrease the risks of maternal and foetal infection
5.	Instruct the women to relax the pelvic floor muscles and to begin slow, rhythmic breathing	Relaxation of the pelvic floor muscles and slow, rhythmic breathing make performance of the procedure easier and contribute to the woman's relaxation and comfort during the procedure
6.	Place one hand on the uterine fundus and apply gentle downward pressure to maintain contact between the foetal head and the cervix while the woman's health care provider inserts and Amnihook into the vagina next to the examining fingers during a vaginal examination. The health care provider uses the tip of the Amnihook to puncture the amniotic sac, allowing the amniotic fluid to be released	The risk of prolapsed cord after aminiotomy will be decreased if the foetal head is engaged and well applied to the cervix
7.	Evaluate the colour, amount, and odour of amniotic fluid present after amniotomy. Note whether the amniotic fluid is bloody	The colour, amount, and odour of aminiotic fluid observed after amniotomy can correlate with foetal well-being. Absent, decreased, or increased amount of amniotic fluid may indicate foetal stress. (Normal amniotic fluid volume is approximately 1000 ml. The position of the presenting part against the cervix will affect the amount of fluid expelled). The amniotic fluid should be clear or slightly cloudy and should have no odour. Meconium-stained amniotic fluid (dark green or brown in colour) may indicate foetal stress and place the infant at risk for meconium aspiration. Foul-smelling amniotic fluid may indicate a complication
8.	Evaluate foetal heart rate after amniotomy	Foetal well-being must be confirmed after amniotomy to assess foetal tolerance to the procedure
9.	Change the underpad and help the woman to a comfortable position	A dry underpad enhances maternal comfort
10.	Record your findings	Information regarding the status of membranes and the amount, colour, and odour of amniotic fluid is important when assessing foetal well-being and labour progress and in planning for delivery
11.	Record maternal temperature every 2 hours	A rise in maternal temperature might indicate an intrauterine infection (chorioamnionitis)

Table 5.16: Induction of labour by oxytocin infusion

Nursing action	*Rationale*
1. Explain the procedure for oxytocin induction of labour to the woman and her partner. Include the following points in your discussion: • Rationale for oxytocin induction of labour • Expected maternal response to oxytocin • Nursing care during oxytocin infusion (frequency of assessment of vital signs, uterine contractions, and foetal heart rate; adjustments in oxytocin flow rate; comfort measures)	An explanation of the procedure for the induction of labour reduces the woman's anxiety and promotes her compliance
2. Place the woman on the foetal monitor to assess foetal well-being and to establish a baseline for uterine activity. A minimum of 20 minutes of foetal monitoring before induction of labour is essential. Do not start the oxytocin infusion if nonreassuring foetal heart rate patterns are identified	A baseline of foetal well-being and uterine activity must be established before induction so that the nurse will recognize complications associated with oxytocin administration, such as uterine hyperstimulation and foetal distress
3. Establish a primary intravenous line for the infusion of a physiologic electrolyte solution without oxytocin	A primary intra-venous line is essential to maintain the intra-venous infusion when the oxytocin infusion is stopped
4. Prepare oxytocin solution according to hospital policy or as follows: Add 10 units of oxytocin to 1000 ml of lactated Ringer's solution or other physiologic electrolyte solution. Make sure the oxytocin solution is labelled	Hospital protocols may vary as to oxytocin concetrations used and dosing regiment
5. Attach intravenous tubing to the oxytocin solution. Set up an intravenous infusion pump with the oxytocin solution according to the manufacturer's guidelines	An intra-venous infusion pump must be used during oxytocin induction to ensure that accurate volume and dosage of oxytocin are administered to the woman
6. Connect a secondary line containing the oxytocin infusion as close as possible to the primary venipuncture site	An oxytocin intusion is connected as close as passible to the primary venipuncture site to avoid administering a bolus dose of oxytocin, which would occur if the oxytocin were piggybacked distal to the venipuncture site and the primary line infusion rate were increased
7. Start oxytocin infusion according to hospital protocol or physician's written order.	The initial dose of oxytocin is usually 0.5 to 1.0 mU/min
8. Assess and record the woman's blood pressure and uterine contractions and the foetal heart rate before each increase in oxytocin dosage. Assess and record maternal intake and output	During oxytocin administration, accurate monitoring of uterine contraction frequency, duration, and intensity and uterine resting tone is essential to evaluate the effect of each oxytocin dosage level and determine the need to increase the infusion rate. An ongoing assessment of the woman's fluid balance (intake and output) is necessary since oxytocin has an antidiuretic effect.
9. Increase the dosage of oxytocin gradully by 1 to 2 mU/min at the dosing interval specified by hospital policy or physician's written orders until and effective labour pattern is established	Different oxytocin protocols have been studies and suggest that acceptable dosing intervals may vary from 15 to 60 minutes
10. Disconinue the oxytocin infusion and notify a physician if maternal or foetal complications develop, including uterine hyperstimulation (contractions closer than every 2 minutes), hypertonic uterine contractions (contraction duration greater than 90 seconds), elevated uterine resting tone (resting tone greater than 20 mm Hg), or nonreassuring foetal heart rate patterns	Since the half-life of oxytocin is very short (1 to 6 minutes), stopping an oxytocin infusion may quickly reverse the effects of excessive uterine activity and improve foetal oxygenation.
11. Initiate additional nursing interventions as necessary, including: • Positioning the patient on her left side • Increasing the primary intravenous fluid rate • Initiating oxygen via a face mask • Administering (in some case) a tocolytic agent, such as terbutaline, to half excessive uterine activity	Nursing interventions to improve uteroplacental perfusion and foetal oxygenation are indicated when foetal stress results from excessive uterine activity

Table 5.17: Preparation for caesarean birth

Nursing action	Rationale
1. Complete a thorough nursing history, which includes an assessment of pregnancy, medical and familial risk factors. Perform a physical assessment, including vital signs, foetal heart rate, uterine contraction status, and labour progress	An assessment for risk factors and for information on the current status of mother and fetus prepares the term for possible complications
2. Withness the woman signing a consent form for the caesarean birth	Physicians are responsible for explaining medical procedures they willp perform. The nurse's signature as witness on the consent form means that the individual who signed the form is that individual and that the nurse was present when the individual signed the form
3. Briefly discusss the caesarean delivery process, including transport to the delivery room, what to expect during the procedure, the role of the partner, and the return to the recovery area. Tailor teaching to address the specific concerns of the woman and her partner	Anticipatory guidance helps ease anxiety
4. Start or maintain an intravenous infusion preferably with a large-bore, 18-gauge needle	Intravenous solutions hydrate the woman and allow intravenous access for medications and , if needed, blood transfusion
5. Obtain laboratory tests ordered by the physician. These will include at least a complete blood count, platelet count, electrolytes, and type and crossmatch for potential blood replacement. If there are high-risk factors, other tests may be ordered, such as clotting studies. Inform the physician of the results	The physician must know before surgery of any abnormal laboratory values. Certain disease processes as evidenced by abnormal laboratory values could cause problems during the procedure. Laboratory values obtained before surgery are useful for comparison with those obtained in the postoperative period
6. Shave the abdominal area	Depending or hospital policy and the type of incision, the area shaved may extend from the nipple line to the labia. Shaving decreases the risk of contamination at the incision site
7. Administer antacid 15 to 30 minutes before the birth	Antacids decrease the acidity of gastric contents and reduce the complications associated with possible aspiration
8. Assist with regional anaesthesia by properly positioning the woman and giving her moral support. In emergency situations in which the woman does not already have regional anaesthesia in place, general anaesthesia is used	Proper positioning of the woman facilitates regional anaesthesia insertion and provides an opportunity to answer questions and reduce anxiety. General anaesthesia, although more hazardous, works more quickly than regional anaesthesia and expedites delivery in emergency situations
9. Insert a Foley's catheter. Bladder distention during surgery and enables collection of urine so that the nurse can evaluate urinary output and assess for haematuria	An indwelling urinary catheter prevents
10. Position the woman on the delivery table. Place a wedge under her right or left hip to maintain a slight lateral tilt. Check the foetal heart rate	Placing a wedge under the hip help maintain placental perfusion. The foetus should be monitored just before the abdominal preparation to ascertain foetal status.
11. Prepare the woman's abdomen for surgery according to hospital policy	Scrubbing the maternal abdoment reduces the number of microoganisms on the skin's surface
12. Close and tie the gowns of the physicians and scrub nurse; check suction, baby warmer, and other delivery room equipment for proper functioning. Fill basins with sterile water and normal saline and perform initial instrument, sponge, and sharpcounts. (Note: Sharps are the suture needles and the blades that are put on the incision knives). Call nursery staff before surgery. Call neonatal or paediatric medical staff according to hospital policy	The gowns of sterile personnel should be closed and tied by unsterile personnel. All emergency equipment must be in working order before the start of the procedure in case complications arise during surgery. Basins are used to soak instruments and wet sponges during surgery. A count of instruments, sharps, and sponges is made before, during, and after surgery to make sure all the accounted for. Calling nursery staff before surgary alerts them to the impending birth. Calling neonatal or paediatric medical staff enable them to be present in case the baby has problems.
13. Prepare necessary paperwork, such as identification bracelets, delivery record, operative record, and preoperative checklists	Documentation of nursing actions is reuired to show that care was taken to ensure a safe environment for mother and foetus

Table 5.18: External electronic foetal monitoring

Nursing action	*Rationale*
1. Explain the purpose and function of external electronic foetal monitoring to the woman and her partner. Assure them that while she is being monitored, the woman will still be able to change positions, stand, and walk in the room if the foetal heart pattern allows	An explanation of the purpose and function of external electronic foetal monitoring and assurance that it will not limit her mobility will reduce the patient's anxiety and promote her cooperation
2. Turn on the monitor and press the TEST button. Confirm that the paper speed switch on the back of the monitor is set at 3 cm per minute	A correct function tèst ensures that the internal circuity is calibrated properly and that data obtained during labour are accurate. Setting the paper speed at 3 cm per minute increases the health care provider's ability to interpret the total monitor strip accurately
3. Record complete patient identification information at the beginning of the monitor strip. Record date and time monitoring is started on the foetal monitoring tracing. Enter the name and credentials of the nurse placing the patient on the foetal monitor	The foetal monitor tracing is a legal part of the patient's medical record and should include patient identification and ongoing documentation of the patient's status and care provided during the monitoring period.
4. Perform Leopold's manoeuvres to determine foetal position and the location of the foetal back	Foetal heart tones are best heard when the ultrasound transducer is placed over the foetal back As labour progresses and the foetus descends lower in the pelvix cavity, the ultrasound transducer will need to be moved downward and toward the women's abdomen
5. Place monitor belts under the woman's back so that they are flat against her skin. Position the woman in a semi-Fowler or lateral tilt position	Belts that are smooth against the back are more comfortable and easily adjusted to maintain steady contact between the transducers and the abdomen. The supine position is avoided to prevent compression of maternal blood vessels and potential supine hypotension
6. Connect the ultrasound transducer and the tocotransducer to the foetal monitor. Apply ultrasound gel to the ultrasound transducer. Adjust the volume	Ultrasound gel is needed to improve conduction
7. Confirm the presence of foetal heart tones with a fetoscopy or stethocope (see Procedure before applying the ultrasound transducer)	The electronic monitor reliably detects and records pulse-like sounds; however, it cannot discriminate between pulse-like sounds of similar rate and intensity. Confirming the presence of foetal heart tones with a fetoscope or stethoscope before appoying the ultrasound transducer helps ensure that the source of the pulse detected by the electronic monitor is the foetal heart. If any doubt about the presence or foetal heart tones arises during external electronic foetal monitoring, recondfirm the foetal heart rate with fetoscope or stethoscope before relying exclusively on the machinery
8. Place the ultrasound transducer on the maternal abdomen over the foetal back. Move the transducer until clear, audible foetal heart tones are heard and the signal light is flashing steadily. Secure the ultrasound device in place with the belt. Confirm that the foetal heart rate is different from the maternal pulse rate by palpating the maternal radial pulse while listening to the rate on the monitor	A clear heart rate is needed to obtain a foetal monitor strip that is interpretable, that is, without gaps of information. Maternal heart rate may be recorded if the ultrasound transducer is improperly positioned or in the event of a foetal demise.
9. Place the tocotransducer on the fundus of the uterus so that the pressure-sensitive button is flush against the maternal abdomen. Secure the transducer in place with the belt. Set baseline utering activity according to the foetal monitor manufacturer's guidelines	Since normal uterine contractions originate in the fundus, the fundal region is the best place to position the tocotransducer. When properly positioned, the pressure-sensitive tocotransducer senses changes in the tonus of the maternal abdomen to identify the frequency and duration of contractions. Since it is an external device, if cannot measure the true intensity of contractions
10. Evaluate the quality of the tracing to determine whether it is adequate for interpretation. If it is not, reposition the transducers until an interpretable tracing is obtained	It is the responsibility of the nurse placing the woman on the electronic foetal monitor to obtain a tracing that can be interpreted as reassuring or nonreassuring
11. Explain to the woman and her partner what the foetal monitor shows. The top portion depicts the foetal heart rate pattern; the lower half shows contraction frequency and duration	Explaining the patterns recorded on the monitor promotes the patient's understanding of foetal status during labour

Contd...

Contd...

Nursing action	Rationale
12. Evaluate the tracing the baseline rate; long-term variablility; accelerations and decelerations; and uterine contraction frequency, duration, and return to resting tonus between contractions	A systematic review of this information allows the nurse to assess foetal tolerance to labour and to intervene in a timely manner if indicated. The standard of care delineating the frequency of these evaluations is as follows: *Low-Risk* / *High-Risk* First Stage Latent: Every 60 minutes / Every 30 minutes Active: Every 30 minutes / Every 15 minutes Second Stage: Every 15 minutes / Every 5 minutes
13. Record data at the intervals specified in step 11	In case the foetal moniotr strip becomes separated from the chart, all data and physician/nursing interventions are recorded in the woman's chart as well. Possible findings are: • Baseline foetal heart rate — Between 120 and 160 bpm is normal • Long-term variability — Decreased, average, or increased • Accelerations — Present and are 15 beats above the baseline for 15 seconds • Decelerations — May be early, late, or variable type • Uterine contractions — Duration and frequency vary depending on stage of labour but should always return to resting tone between contractions

Table 5.19: Administration of RhoGAM and other blood products

Nursing action	Rationale
Rho(D) Immune Globulin Administration	
1. Review mother's and baby's charts to identify whther RhIG should be administered	Administration of RhIG (currently available as RhoGAM, 300 ug dose, and as Mic-RhoGAM, 50 mg dose) is indicated when it is known or suspected that foetal red blood cells have entered the circulation of an Rh-negative, unsensitized mother. This can occur during pregnancy or delivery, during adminocentesis or chorionic villus sampling procedures, during an abortion, during foetal surgery, or after an incident of abdominal trauma such as a fall or motor vehicle accident. The Rh-negative, unsensitized mother should receive an RhIG injection under any of the following circumstances: • After an incident of exposure risk that occurs before 28 weeks' gestation • At 28 weeks' gestation (prophylactic administration) • Within 72 hours of delivery if her baby is Rh positive A negative indirect Coombs test provides evidence that sensitization of the mother has not already occurred
2. Provide the woman with a complete explanation of the procedure, its purpose and its effect on future pregnancies and blood transfusions. Determine that the woman has had no previous adverse reactions to preparations of immune globulin. If required by hospital protocol, have the woman sign a consent form. globulin preparation. A signed consent form indicates that the woman acknowledges she has been informad of the risk	Understanding the reason for the procedure helps ease the patient's anxiety. Understanding the importance of taking immune globulin with each pregnancy can affect the type of care the woman seeks in future pregnancies. Identifying previous reactions enables the nurse to inform the physician of adverse reactions to an immune
3. Obtain correct preparation and dosage of RhIG, which is usually stored in the blood bank or pharmacy. Confirm lot number, crossmatch, and patient's identity before administration	Verifying that the blood product is correct for the patient before its administration is essential to decreasing the occurrence of adverse reactions

Contd...

Contd...

Nursing action	*Rationale*
4. Administer injection intramuscularly within 72 hours of exposure risk. If administering a minidose (usually 50 mg), use the deltoid muscle; if administering a full dose (usually 300 mg), use the gluteus medius muscle of other deep muscle site	The maximum amount of time from exposure to successful immunization that has been established is 72 hours
5. Record procedure according to hospital protocol	Recording procedure provides written documentation in a permanent, legal record that RhIG was given
Food Product Administration	
1. obtain patient's transfusion history and explain procedure. Instruct patient regarding the symptoms of an adverse reaction and the importance of reporting these symptoms. Have patient sign a consent form if required before the transfusion	An explanation of the procedure and expected sensations helps case the patient's anxiety. Inform the physician if patient has a history of an adverse reaction to a blood transfusion. A signed consent form indicates that the patient acknowledges having been informed of the risk.
2. Select or start an IV infusion with a large-gauge catheter, such as an 18-gauge catheter for an adult	A catheter smaller than 18-gauge can haemolyze RBCs
3. Obtain blood product from the blood bank just before use by following hospital protocol kept at room temperature for more than 30 minutes usually may not be returned to the blood bank because they are potentially unsafe	Strict guidelines regarding this step vary among institutions. Unopened blood products
4. Identify the blood product and the patient with another registered nurse. To do this: • Compare the name and identification number on the patient's wristband with the name and number on the blood bag and order slip • Double-check the patient's blood group and Rh type, the donor's blood group and Rh type, unit serial number, the bag's expiration date, and the type and number of blood components ordered • Inspect the bag for air bubbles, leaks, and discolouration	Adverse reactions to blood transfusions often result from failure to identify the blood product or the patient properly.
5. Take baseline vital signs	A deviation from the baseline assessment can indicate a transfusion reaction
6. Prime the Y-type filtered blood administration tubing with normal saline solution. Never add medications to the blood or blood tubing. Wearing gloves, insert the spike of the administration set straight into the port of the blood bag	Dextrose solutions cause haemolysis of the RBCs, and loctated Ringer's solution, which has calcium, could cause clotting. Keeping the blood and blood tubing free of medications helps prevent confusion over the cause of any transfusion reactions that might occur. Inserting the spike straight into the port allows the blood to flow freely from the bag
7. Start the transfusion slowly (approximately 2 mL/min). Fill the filter with blood, and monitor the patient closely for the first 15 minutes of the transfusion. Observe for chills, flushing, low back pain, itching, dyspnoea, rash, hives, and other signs of a transfusion reaction	If the patient has an adverse reaction, only a small amount of the blood product will have infused. If a reaction occurs, stop the infusion, keep the vein open with normal saline, and call the physician and blood bank. Follow hospital protocol
8. If the patient has no adverse reaction within the first 15 minutes, increase the rate to what the physician ordered. Ideally, the blood should be transfused in 2 hours. Continue to monitor the patient and take vital signs at least every 30 minutes	Red blood cells begin to deteriorate after 2 hours at room temperature. A pressure bag around the blood bag may help maintain the prescribed rate. Monitoring the patient throughout the transfusion is necessary because adverse reactions can be slow and subtle
9. When the transfusion is complete, flush the IV line with normal saline. If another unit is ordered, follow the same procedure, omit ting steps 1 and 2	Using a new blood administration set with each unit of blood ordered helps prevent confusion over the cause of any transfusion reactions that might occur. A new blood administration set also allows blood products to transfuse more quickly because of the new filter in the tubing
10. Complete the following required paperwork: • Signatures of the two persons who identified the blood product and the patient • The blood product administered • Patient's baseline vital signs • Time the transfusion was started and time it was completed • Total volume of fluid transfused • Patient's response to the transfusion • Any nursing action taken in response to an adverse reaction	Written documentation of the procedure becomes part of the patient's permanent record and can be referred to in case of questions

Maternal-Foetal Transport

Purpose

A maternal-foetal transport to a tertiary care centre is indicated when the condition of either the women or the foetus warrants more intensive evaluation or intervention than can be provided where the women is currently hospitalized. when the birth of a compromised neonate is possible, a maternal-foetal transport prevents the transport of a sick newborn soon after birth. Adequate communication and information are imperative for effective maternal-foetal transport.

Equipment

- Consent form
- Copy of mother's chart
- Transfer form.

Assisting with Amniotomy (Fig. 5.20)

Purpose

Amniotomy (artificial rupture of membranes) is performed to induce or augment labour, to insert an internal foetal electrode or an intrauterine pressure catheter for electronic foetal monitoring, or to obtain a foetal scalp blood sample.

Equipment

- Electronic foetal monitor or Doppler ultrasound stethoscope
- Sterile gloves

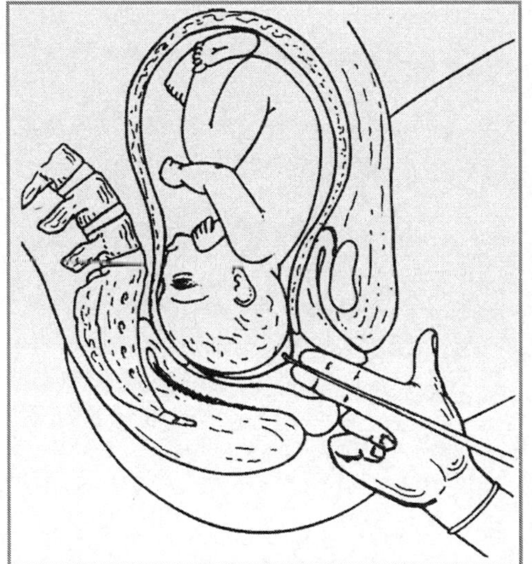

Fig. 5.20: Amnihook rupture the membranes

- Sterile lubricant
- Amnihook
- Absorbent underpads.

Induction of Labour by Oxytocin Infusion

Purpose (Table 5.16)

To stimulate the onset of uterine contractions in order to facilitate progressive cervical effacement and dilatation and descent of the foetus. The decision to initiate labour using oxytocin is made only after risk factors, cervical readiness, and foetal maturity are evaluated.

Equipment

- Electronic foetal monitor for continuous monitoring of foetal heart rate and uterine activity.
- Oxytocin (Pitocin)
- Infusion pump

Preparation for Caesarean Birth

Purpose (Table 5.17)

To prepare the woman for the delivery of the baby through abdominal and uterine incisions when maternal factors, foetal factors, or both make vaginal delivery unsafe. To assist the physician and other surgical staff as needed.

Equipment

- Consent form
- Shave prep tray
- Antacid
- Caps
- Abdominal preparation tray
- Shoe covers
- Warm blankets
- Foley catheter
- Intravenous infusion with 18-gauge needle
- Foetal heart monitoring device
- Surgical mask
- Sterile water and saline.

External Electronic Foetal Monitoring (Table 5.18)

Purpose

An external electronic foetal monitor is used when the health of the mother and foetus warrants intensive monitoring or when it is mandated by hospital policy. An external electronic monitor allows the health care provider to assess foetal tolerance to labour by evaluating subtle changes in baseline foetal heart rate, variability, and the presence of accelerations or decelerations. The external electronic foetal monitor also measures uterine contraction frequency and duration, but it is not a reliable indicator of uterine contraction intensity.

Equipment

- Electronic foetal heart monitor
- Ultrasound transducer
- Tocotransducer
- Ultrasound gel
- Belts to hold transducers in place.

Administration of Rho (D) Immune Globulin (RhoGAM or Mic-RhoGAM) and Other Blood Products (See Table 5.19)

Purpose

Administration of Rho(D) Immune globulin (RhIG) is indicated to prevent an Rh-negative mother from developing antibodies to the red blood cells of an Rh-positive foetus. Administration of blood products replaces fluid and blood lost after a maternal haemorrhage.

Equipment

- Requisition slip for blood
- Blood product
- Blood administration set with filter
- Intravenous (IV) bag of normal saline
- Patent IV site with a large-gauge catheter
- Blood documentation form
- Gloves
- Patient's chart
- Thermometer and sphygmomanometer
- Pressure bag
- Vial of RhIG
- Diluent
- Syringe with needle
- Alcohol pad.

CHAPTER 6

Assessment and Management of Postnatal Period

INTRODUCTION

The postnatal period is usually considered the interval extending from the birth of the baby until 6 weeks after. It is the 6 weeks interval between the birth of the newborn and the return of the reproductive organs to their normal nonpregnant state. This interval is characterized by the development of lactation and the return of the reproductive organs to their approximate pre-pregnant positions. Of course, some mothers not wishing to or unable to nurse their babies, do not experience the full development of lactation. The return of the reproductive organs to the non-pregnant state is called the process of "*involution.*" The postpartal days are numbered starting with first day after birth. This period is sometimes referred to as the "*Puerperium*" or 'Fourth Trimester' of pregnancy.

The physiologic changes that occur during the reversal of the process of pregnancy, though distinctive are normal. Dramatic changes begin to occur in a woman's body systems as soon as a baby is born; the process that occurred during pregnancy are reversed. Some systems undergo only minimal reversal, whereas others undergo extensive changes. For example, more pregnancy and involutional changes occur in the cardiovascular and reproductive systems than in the respiratory system. Within 6 weeks the woman's body will revert to her prepregnant physical status.

With the new mother and family view's this period may be as positive or negative time, depends in part on the nurturing received during the hospital stay. The nurse can do much to influence the new mother through the teaching and caring, she receives and through affirmation of her parenting skills and abilities.

To provide care during the recovery period that is beneficial to the mother, her infant and her family, the nurse must synthesize knowledge of maternal anatomy, and physiology of recovery period, the newborn's physical and behavioural characteristics, infant care activities and family response to the birth of the infant.

PHYSIOLOGICAL CHANGES IN POSTNATAL INVOLUTION OF REPRODUCTIVE ORGANS

Involution is the process whereby the pelvic reproductive organs, particularly the uterus, return to their pre-pregnant size and position. This period also has been referred to as the recovery, postpartum, postnatal or postdelivery period, or the puerperium. All women who deliver an infant must pass through this recovery period.

The recovery period usually is considered to last from immediately after the delivery to the sixth week (42 days). After delivery the woman is cared for in the postpartum unit until discharged and is instructed to return in 6 to 8 weeks to her physician or clinic for a checkup. By this time most of her pelvic organs have returned to their pre-pregnant position and approximate pre-pregnant size. Many women, however, do not feel recovered from pregnancy and birth in 6 to 8 weeks and may require a longer period.

Uterus

At delivery the woman's uterus weighs approximately 1000 g (2.2 pounds), and by the end of puerperium, it will have returned to its pre-pregnant weight of 60 g (2 ounces). The uterus can return to its pre-pregnant weight and shape because muscle cell size increased during pregnancy although the number of cells remained basically the same. During recovery the protein cytoplasm of the muscle fibres undergoes catabolic or autolytic changes that cause a reduction in cell size. The products of this process are carried off in the urine as nitrogenous waste.

Immediately after delivery, the very hard, round contracted uterus lies midway between the symphysis pubis and the umbilicus. Within hours of delivery, it rises to the level of the umbilicus or slightly above it. The uterus begins its descent into the pelvic cavity on the first postpartum day. It diminishes rapidly in size, weight, and position until the tenth day, when it may be palpated at or below the level of the symphysis pubis. Throughout the postpartum period the firm and contracted uterus should be found in the midline.

Because uterine blood vessels and the uterine muscles are inter twined, a tourniquet action prevents bleeding or haemorrhage from the open blood vessels at the placental site when the uterus contracts. After delivery the uterus contracts on its own unless there is interference; for example, placental fragments keep the uterus from contracting. Occasionally, because of overdistension from multiple gestation, a large foetus, or an exhausted uterine muscle, a uterus may contract poorly.

Uterine Atony

Failure of the uterus to remain firmly contracted, can lead to postpartum haemorrhage.

A full bladder is a major cause of uterine atony. Because of change in intra-abdominal pressure after delivery and volume of intravenous (IV) fluids the bladder becomes easily distended, pushing the uterus up and to the side generally the right. The uterus must be able to contract to stop the bleeding from the placental site, therefore, a soft, "boggy" uterus, out of the midline and above the umbilicus, is a strong indicator that the bladder is full.

Lochia

After delivery the decidual lining of the uterus sloughs off as lochia. This discharge contains blood, decidual tissue, epithelial cells from the vagina, mucus, bacteria, and occasionally fragments of membranes and small clots. Its odour is flexhy but not offensive (as menstrual discharge can be).

The lochia, which is red and bloody during the first stage, is called *Lochia rubra* (rubra meaning red). This phase lasts 1 to 3 days and initially may contain a few small blood clots. The next stage is termed *lochia serosa*; it lasts 5 to 7 days, is *seros anguineous*, and is reddish pink to brown. The third and final stage is called *Lochia alba*. It is white (primarily because of leucocytes) and lasts 1 to 3 weeks. The colour of lochia indicates healing of the placental site. By 6 weeks the placental site usually has healed from the inner epithelial surface outward as the necrotic area covering the placental site sloughs off and is replaced with new, healthy cells. This process prevents placental scarring. Otherwise, after a few pregnancies the inside lining of the uterus would be full of scar tissue, making it unsuitable for further implantation. Table 6.1 lists lochial characteristics.

Table 6.1: Lochial characteristics

	Rubra	*Serosa*	*Alba*
Colour	Bright red, bloody	Pink-brown	Creamy-white
Clots	Small clots	No clots	No clots
Odour	Slightly "flexhy"	No odour	No odour or stale body odour
Length	1-3 days	5-7 days	1-3 wk

Return of Menses

The exact mechanism responsible for resumption of the menstrual cycle is not fully understood. With the drop in oestrogen and progesterone levels after placental separation, however, the menstrual cycle is re-established. In general, it takes longer for nursing mothers than non-nursing mothers to resume their cycles. The speed with which a woman resumes menses depends on whether she is breastfeeding, if she is feeding at night, and if she is relying completely on breastfeeding or merely supplementing her infant's diet. Cycles can begin in lactating mothers as early as 8 weeks or as late as 14 months after delivery. If the mother is breastfeeding and not supplementing the infant's diet, menses may resume 4 to 8 months.

The cycle may begin in the non-lactating mother as early as the fourth to sixth week, although the average time is 6 to 8 weeks. Menses resumes in most non-lactating mothers by the third month. The first menstrual cycle usually is anovulatory; in other words menstruation occurs before the body produces and expels mature ova. A few cycles may pass before menses resume their pre-pregnant rhythm and length. Precautions against conception, however should always be taken.

Cervix

Whereas the upper part of the uterus after delivery is firm, hard and contracted, the lower uterine segment and cervix remain loose, thin and stretched. The cervix also may appear oedematous and bruised from the delivery and may have some tears or lacerations. It will admit the entire hand for several hours, making manual examination of the uterus possible. By the first postpartum day, however, the cervix has sufficiently narrowed and regained its normal consistency to admit only two fingers. The parous cervix does not (will never again) look like the nonparous cervix. The external os, which previously resembled a dimple now resembles a slit or smile, and any lacerations to the cervix during delivery may lead scar tissue.

Vaginal Canal

The vaginal canal has been stretched to accommodate the delivery of the foetus and placenta. The external vaginal orifice or introitus appear jagged and irregular in shape after delivery. Tears may occur as a result of delivery, particularly if it was very rapid or uncontrolled. Occasionally, haematoma may develop as a result of descent and delivery. The usual places for the development of haematomas are the introitus, vaginal wall at the ischial spins, and the episiotomy site. Any woman who complains of severe or excessive perineal pain or sensitivity should be carefully assessed for haematomas.

In a few weeks the introitus will be sufficiently healed for resumption of sexual relations, although the vagina may be dry until hormonal balance is restored.

Perineum

After delivery the muscles of the floor of the perineum are stretched, swollen, and often bruised. Some tears may be extensive, invading the deeper levator ani muscles. The type of episiotomy will be noted in the client's record.

During pushing and the delivery of the foetal head, the straining and pressure on the lower bowel often cause the extrusion of internal haemorrhoids. After delivery, however, they reduce in size and can be manually reinserted into the rectum. Haemorrhoids present during the pregnancy also shrink. Surgical reduction after delivery rarely is necessary.

Ovaries

The ovaries have been inactive during the last two trimesters of the pregnancy. Because of the drop in the placental hormone level, however, the body gradually resumes its prepregnancy menstrual cycle.

Breasts

Depending on whether the mother decides to breastfeed or bottlefeed, the breast responds accordingly. If she determines to breastfeed, the stimulation of the baby's sucking will relase prolactin, causing the breast to produce milk. As the blood and lympth surge into the breast in anticipation of milk production, the breast enlarge and swell, becoming very firm and warm around the third postpartum day.

If there is no stimulation by the infant, the breasts, which had been prepared for breast-feeding during pregnancy, will recede in size back to their prepregnancy state. Non-nursing mothers also experience fullness and engorgement. *Let down reflex is triggered by the infant's sucking*

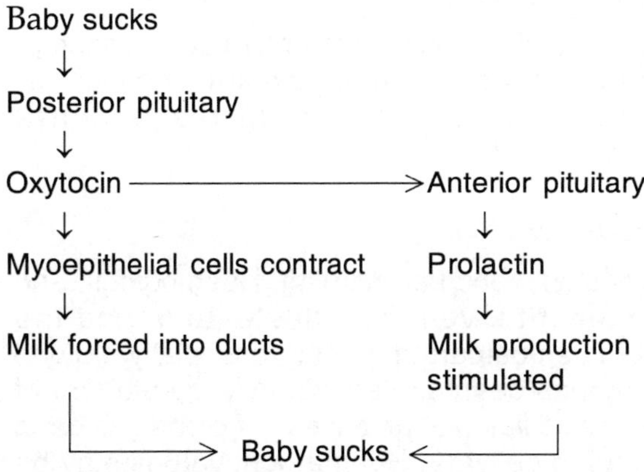

Cardiovascular Function

Some of the most dramatic changes in the puerperium occur in the cardiovascular system. During pregnancy the blood volume increases by 30 to 50% over the prepregnancy volume. After delivery, however, there is no need for excess blood volume, and drastic shifts occur in body fluids. During birth and placental delivery, however there is no need for excess blood volume, and drastic shifts occur in body fluids. During birth and placental delivery, the woman loses approximately 300 to 500 ml of blood (up to 1000 ml during caesarean birth). This loss depletes a portion of the additional fluid.

The blood from the pelvic region returns to the general circulation and the extracellular fluids that accumulated during pregnancy return to the circulating blood for excretion. Additional fluid will be lost through diuresis and diaphoresis.

Heart Rate and Blood Pressure

During pregnancy the heart rate increases upto 15 beats/min over the pregnancy baseline, and the stroke volume increases to handle the increased blood volume. After delivery, however, the heart rate decelarate at times reaching as low as 40 to 60 beats/min. Therefore, if an increase in pulse rate is noted, a secondary cause, such as haemorrhage, infection, thrombosis, anxiety, or excitement related to the delivery should be explored.

During labour the blood pressure may fluctuate; it may rise during contractions or when the woman pushes or experiences pain. It also may fall because of supine hypotensive syndrome, regional anaesthesia, or haemorrhage. It should, however, return to normal after delivery, unless complications such as pregnancy-induced hypertension (PIH) have occurred.

Although the delivery may have been uncomplicated, orthostatic hypotension may occur because of fluid shift and decreased intra-abdominal pressure.

Blood Values

Haemoglobin and haematocrit. Haemoglobin and haematocrit levels may fluctuate during the immediate postpartum period, especially if blood volume has been diluted with a large amount of intravenous fluids or an excess of blood has been lost during delivery. Haematocrit values may be altered from prenatal blood values, depending on several factors, including the following:

- The amount of intravenous fluids received during the intrapartum period
- The amount of blood loss at the time of delivery
- The amount of perspiration during labour and delivery
- An elevated temperature during delivery
- Fluid shift from extravascular tissues to the general circulation.

After the first day, the fluid shift from extravascular tissues into the vascular compartment may depress the haematocrit level because of this dilution. If levels dropped on the first postpartum day, a repeat evaluation is obtained. If the client lost a considerable amount of blood during delivery, labouratory values should be periodically checked at the same time every day because haemoglobin and haematocrit levels tend to fluctuate during the day being slightly higher in the morning than in the afternoon.

White Blood Cells

The normal white blood cells count when the woman is not pregnant is between 5,000 and 8,000/mm3. The count rises during late pregnancy and labour and can reach levels of 18,000/mm3. This count is within normal limits for pregnancy and immediate recover levels fall quickly to 6,000 to 10,000/mm3 and to normal levels by 4 to 7 days. Therefore persistent elevation indicates infection.

An increase in the granulocytes, particularly neutrophills (which are polymorphonuclear (PMN) cells) causes the increase in white blood cells. Neutrophils, which normally constitute more than half of the white blood cell profile, increase in the body in response to inflammation, pain, anxiety, stress, and labour and delivery; protect against invading organisms, engulfing them through phagocytosis; and debride the decidual tissues of dead cells during the healing process.

Red Blood Cells

The red blood cell count actually increases during pregnancy, but because of a greater increase in plasma volume, these values appear to drop slightly. During recovery the red blood cell count gradually returns to pregnancy blood values.

Platelets and Fibrin

Platelet and fibrin levels are elevated during recovery and may contribute to formation of a thrombus.

Respiratory Function

After delivery and during recovery the respiratory rate should not noticeably change. However, the respiratory system should be assessed regularly during the immediate recovery period. Because the enlarged uterus no longer presses upward on the diaphragm, women find breathing easier. If, however, the woman received inhalation or general anaesthesia, extra precautions should be instituted because of the possibility of vomiting, with aspiration or congestion. Lung sounds should be assessed by auscultation.

Renal Function

The hormones (particularly progesterone) that caused ureter dilation are no longer present. Dilated ureters require a longer period than the rest of the urinary tract structures to return to the prepregnancy conditions. The enlarged uterus no longer compresses the bladder, causing frequency. Instead, as a result of decreased intra-abdominal pressure and relaxed abdominal muscles, the capacity of the bladder increases. It may fill to 1,000 or 1,500 ml without discomfort.

Retention of urine may result because of stretching of the perineal floor, with accompanying bruising and oedema of the trigone and urethral meatus. During labour and delivery, the foetus places pressure on the bladder, particularly if it is full. Regional anaesthesia may temporarily diminish sensations from the bladder, contributing to urinary retention. Because a full bladder can lead to a relaxed uterus and subsequent haemorrhage, the nurse must assess the bladder regularly during the recovery period and encourage and assist the client to void.

Body water in the extravascular spaces and excess blood volume from the pregnancy are eliminated rapidly. By the second postpartum day, diuresis and polyuria occur. Up to 3 L or urine are eliminated daily for a few days. This physiologic condition should be explained to the client. Within a week, she will return to her prepregnancy voiding pattern because diuresis diminishes and the muscle tone of the bladder returns.

Glycosuria, primarily caused by the presence of lactose, may occur during the puerperium. Also, as a result of catabolic changes taking place in the uterus, nitrogenous waste may appear in urine. These are physiologic changes during involution.

Gastrointestinal Function

After the delivery of the placenta and cessation of placental hormones, the gastrointestinal tract begins to refer to its prepregnancy peristaltic and digestive activities. After delivery, women generally are hungry or thirsty and want to eat or drink something light (e.g. juice, toast, or tea). The type of analgesia or anaesthesia and the delivery route influence when the client may have her first oral intake. Many units wait 1 hour to monitor recovery and then provide fluids ad lib. No woman should be given oral fluids or food until she has recovered from general anaesthesia. After initial adjustment, however she may request extra portions of food, by discharge, most women have regained their usual appetite.

Most recovering women do not have a bowel movement until a few days after delivery. The reasons are varied. The woman may have had diarrhoea at the onset of labour and no food intake for upto 24 hours (or more). An enema may have been given during early labour. Fear of pain with the episiotomy while straining for a bowel movement poses a barrier. Painful haemorrhoids also may delay the first bowel movement. Because so many women experience this delay, it has become standard practice in many hospitals to order stool softeners the first few days after delivery. If a woman has not had a bowel movement by the third day, an enema or suppository may be prescribed. The speed with which her bowels become regulated will depend on her daily activities, diet (adequate roughage and fluid), activity (including exercises), and schedule.

Weight Loss and Nutrition

Although diuresis and diaphoresis provide mechanisms for reduction of body water, fat deposits intended for lactation remains. If the mother breastfeeds, these deposits are slowly metabolized in the first 3 to 5 months and she should lose weight gradually. If she bottlefeeds, these fat deposits must be lost by calorie reduction and exercise.

The recovery diet should follow the same guidelines as the pregnancy diet, with a gradual reduction of dairy products from four to two servings (if not breastfeeding) and a gradual reduction of protein foods from three to two servings. Avoiding concentrated sweets facilitates weight reduction. Severe caloric restriction cannot provide sufficient nutritional supply to replace calcium, iron, protein, or vitamin stores that may have been reduced during pregnancy. When oral contraceptives are used, additional nutrients such as folic acid, vitamin B6 and to a lesser extent, riboflavin, thiamine, and ascorbic acid appear to be indicated.

Integumentary Function

After delivery the changes that occurred in the skin of the pregnant woman begin to recede. The hormone particularly the melanocyte stimulating hormone that caused pigmentational changes, have been eliminated. Not all changes will completely disappear. The striae gravidarum or stetch marks, for example, will turn a silvery colour and fade, but many women have them indefinitely. The linea nigra and the darkened areola fade, but in some women faint traces remain. Melasma disappears unless excessive pigmentation occurred.

Palmar erythema because of increased circulation and oestrogenic influence also subsides. Accelerated hair and nail growth slows down. Many women complain after delivery that their hair falls out "by the handful."

Actually hair growth has entered a resting phase, and the additional hair that grew during pregnancy is just being shed. In a few months, hair and nail growth will return to prepregnancy patterns. Spider nevi also recede during the postpartum period and urticarial rashes usually subside.

Musculoskeletal Function

Immediately after delivery the woman may be fatigued or even exhausted. The labour positioning and pushing techniques may leave arms, neck shoulders, and perinial muscles sore and aching.

Under the influence of relaxin the pelvic joints, particularly the symphysis pubis, may separate slightly during labour and delivery. After birth the ligaments and cartilage begin to ease back into the prepregnancy position; as a result, some women feel pain and discomfort in this area. Eventually this pain, described as a "pinching" subsides. A few women have severe pain and difficulty in walking for a short time.

During pregnancy, labour, or delivery some women may experience a separation of the vertical, central abdominal muscle group (the rectus abdominis muscles). This is called diastasis recti abdominis (diastasis meaning separation). If this occurs before or during delivery, pushing may become difficult or impossible because these muscles help to push the baby through the birth canal. In general, no particular treatment is indicated for this condition, but restoration of the muscles may be prolonged. The abdominal wall is somewhat relaxed for all women in the first few weeks of puerperium.

Shivering

Many clients experience transient trembling after delivery. Several theories concerning this shivering have been proposed. These include exhaustion from the strenuous activities of labour and delivery, the sudden decrease in intra-abdominal pressure, the sudden and complete withdrawal of placental hormones, and reaction to the small transfusions of foetal blood or amniotic fluid that may have entered maternal circulation during placental separation. The cool environment of labour rooms and room temperature, IV fluids are a major cause of chilling. This trembling and chill usually are not associated with an elevation of temperature.

Exercise

After delivery the client gradually may resume exercising in the same way she exercised during the prenatal period. She should be cautioned not to exercise too strenuously at first but to pace her activities. Frequent walking is one of the best exercises; when women were confined to bed for extended periods after delivery, many complications such as hypostatic pneumonia, thromboses, and emboli occurred. For this reason, encourage ambulation and exercise soon after delivery. In addition, Kegel's exercises for perineal muscles are continued into the recovery period.

Endocrine Function

Placental hormones are abruptly reduced at delivery. Oestrogen and progesterone no longer after the blood vessels, ureters, intestinal tract, and reproductive tract. It takes several weeks, however, for all these structures to regain muscle tone and proper function. Full restoration of normal bowel functioning may take a few weeks, and urinary tract changes may require a month.

After delivery, prolactin production is taken over entirely by the anterior pituitary gland. The impetus for prolacting excretion is nipple stimulation. Otherwise the hormone is not secreted.

Stimulation of the breast during breastfeeding also induces the release of oxytocin, which causes the milk to be released from the breasts by the action known as the let-down reflex. At the same time, oxytocin causes strong contractions of the uterus, the afterbirth pains.

Other endocrine glands—the thyroid and adrenal glands and the pancreas—return to their prepregnancy size and activity within a few weeks of delivery.

Infection

The skin is the first line of defense against infection. Any break in that barrier by surgery or trauma can result in pathogenic invasion. Signs of infections may be subjective, for example, a woman's complaint of severe, unexpected pain, malaise, or chills. Often the signs are objective, such the presence of fever or abnormal tissue. If any discharge occurs, always, send a specimen for a culture and sensitivity test and notify the physician for follow-up care. Antibiotics should not be administered until the culture is obtained but may be administered before results are received. Culture and sensitivity results are necessary for the definitive diagnosis of an infection.

Fever

An elevation of temperature in the first 24 hours after delivery may be caused by dehydration, excitement, fatigue, chilling, and blood loss. The temperature may be as high as 38°C (100.4°F) which is within normal limits. If the temperature remains elevated after the first day, however the cause must be found and treated. Infection should be considered, especially if here is a history of premature rupture of the membranes, haemorrhage, a long or traumatic labour and delivery, or a preexisting infection. A through assessment of the woman's condition provides data about the sources of the problem.

Most often, low grade fever accompanies engorgement of the breasts. The infant is not separated from the mother then she has a fever, unless specifically directed by the physician. Because the infant and mother usually have the same bacterial and viral agents, nothing is usually gained by isolation.

PSYCHOSOCIAL ADJUSTMENTS

Bonding

Postpartum can be viewed as a time of transition from non-parenthood to parenthood. Parent-infant attachment that leads to the bonding depends in part on the infant's responsiveness. The baby's response reinforces the parents and encourages them to continue interaction. The result is a stable bond between the infant and parents that will endure despite any separations bond formation is an outgrowth of reciprocal attachment stimulus-response and affectional ties that help form a coordinated, constructive social relationship. The nurse can only infer that bonding is progressing satisfactorily through observation of attachment behaviour (i.e. behaviours that serve to maintain contact and demonstrate affection towards the baby). Examples of this behaviour include kissing, fondling and cuddling and holding the infant in the enface position to maintain eye contact.

Maternal Developmental Tasks

There are several stages or phases that the new mother goes through during recovery, these include taking in, taking hold, and letting go. After the delivery, the mother is exhausted and needs rest and sleep. During the first or second day, she will be taking in all the experiences of labour and delivery and may become introspective and comtemplative. She may asks questions regarding the labour and delivery experience and worry about her condition and her infant. Her physical needs and deficits of nourishment, rest, and comfort must be met by a caring nursing staff; then the new mother will be able to care for the needs of her baby. Taking hold describes the period when the mother attends to the infant's care needs, the role changes to come, and her own recovery needs. During this phase women usually are eager to learn how to care for themselves and their infant.

During recovery the mother also must let go and view the infant as a separate person. Some women have difficulty accomplishing this task, and if it is not resolved, psychologic problems could ensure. A mother may have great difficulty letting others assist with care of the infant, for example, or an overprotective mother may not allow herself to go out if a baby-sitter is needed. She still is attached to the child because she views it as an extension of herself. Because this behaviour is not evident in the hospital stay the clinic nurse or paediatric staff members could identify this unresolved task. Occasionally, professional psychologic help may be necessary.

Self-esteem Needs

All persons need self-esteem; it underlies personal satisfaction and effective functioning. It is the extent to which an individual believes herself to be capable, worthy, successful, and significant. Self-esteem depends on maintenance of control over self and achievement of expectations. In adulthood, individual expectations are affected by demands from the common group, society or culture and experienced as roles. During pregnancy, these roles take on new meaning, and emphasis is placed on responsibilities toward the growing child. Studies show that women set psychologic tasks to carry out, especially during labour and delivery. The role performance was selected as a leading concern of women after birth. the congruence or lack of congruence between the idealized self and the actual self-determines feelings of self-worth and self-esteem. Childbirth is a crisis event, an emotional milestone. The woman, already in a state of disequilibrium, is vulnerable to self-criticism from others. A woman who has planned for and expects to give birth in a controlled situation with her partner feels disappointment, anger, sadness, guilt, and failure when she is unable to achieve this goal.

In today's society, in which a great emphasis is placed on active participation in and control over life experiences, many couples disire the 'deal' childbirth experience, which includes a prepared and well controlled labour and delivery, sharing with the baby's father, and no medication. When a woman who planned birth without medication and with minimal assistance experiences a labour that deviates from normal and then requires medication, anaesthesia, or forceps or cesarean delivery, she often feels that she has failed. The outcome may be some degree of shame and decreased self-esteem.

The husband is undoubtedly the most important influence in the woman's self-satisfaction. His reactions to her performance greatly affect her self-esteem, and if she senses disappointment from him because he was unable to participate or be present at his child's birth, she feels less "successful."

Potential for Mood Changes

The first few days after delivery—even up to 10 or 14 days—could be considered a period of "normal" crisis and disequilibrium, especially for the first-time mother. It is a time of transition, readjustment, reappraisal of roles, added responsibility, excitement, fatigue and recovery from pregnancy labour, and delivery. Relationships are strained. It rarely is a time of peace and tranquility because the new family attempts to establish boundaries, functions, schedules and roles.

Many new mothers (and even new fathers) experience "the blues "on postpartum depression. *POSTPARTUM DEPRESSION* can be divided into the following categories, depending on the severity of symptoms manifested by the mother—whether she has "postpartum blues" or postpartum psychosis. The baby blues, or third-day blues, is considered to be a normal mils, transient mood disturbance lasting a few days or more. Changes in mood coincide with the drop in the hormones estrogen and progesterone, which reach their lowest level on those days.

Other causes of postpartum blues in addition to the drop in hormone levels have been suggested, these include lack of sleep during the first months of recovery, the demand of additional responsibilities, and discomforts of infection or pain. Several studies have examined the reasons for postpartum blues according to maternal responses. Some of the reasons given by mothers included worries about the baby, difficulties involving breastfeeding, home sickness, and pain, but many could give no reason for their depressed feelings.

Postpartum depressed feelings are characterized by one or more of the symptoms. Depending on the source cited, the incidence of postpartum blues ranges between 50% and 70%.

The symptoms of postpartum depression are as follows:

- Irritability
- Restlessness
- Crying spells
- Sleeplessness
- Anger directed at family members including the infant
- Anxiety
- Inability to concentrate
- Moodiness.

Postpartum Psychosis

The severe form of postpartum depression is postpartum psychosis or puerperal psychosis. The depression is characterized by acute psychotic behaviour characteristic of affective, schizophrenic or organic disorders. It manifests suddenly sometime within the first 2 weeks of delivery. It occurs in approximately one or two of every thousand mothers. Clients at risk include women with a history of psychiatric disorders, primigravidas, and women displaying anxiety and neuroticism during pregnancy. Postpartum psychosis probably results from a combination of factors. As with the postpartum blues, the leading causative factor is the drop in the level of the hormones estrogen and progesterone. Other factors are the change in roles added responsibilities and hostilities toward family (baby, husband, other children), and physical problems such as infection and sleep cycle disturbances.

As with any psychiatric disorder, the actions of the client are exaggerated. For example, the mother experiencing postpartum blues may express irritability, moodiness, and hostility but to the degree that the mother developing a psychosis might. The exaggerated and often prolonged periods of irritability, hostility, labile behaviour, ineffective coping mechanisms, withdrawal, and inappropriate responses to the baby, herself or her family should indicate that she is experiencing more than just postpartum blues. The health and well being of the baby and the mother must be safeguarded in this instance. Professional help, not merely emotional support, comfort, and encouragement is needed. When hospitalization is required, every attempt should be made to keep the mother-infant relationship intact while caring for both parties.

Education seems to prevent or reduce the incidence of postpartum depression. The best results were obtained when the husband attended classes, when resources (personal and social) are mobilized in the early puerperium, and outside interests are maintained. Women need to be prepared for childbirth and the transition to motherhood roles, and families need to be prepared and assisted in making the transition from hospital to home. Rooming in, is a way of introducing the mother and father to their new responsibilities and roles while under the supervision of professional care givers.

Implications of Early Discharge

Usually, a woman was hospitalized for 7 days after birth. Recovery was called confinement. Over the years, however, health care personal have realized that early return to normal activities is the best course for uncomplicated births. Today, going home in 24 hours is not unusual, and a 2 to 7 day stay for vaginal birth and 4 to 8 days of caesarean birth is a diagnosis related group (DRG) standard.

Early discharge limits the time the woman has to listen, to learn, and to practice self-care. Consequently nurses begin discharge teaching at the first postpartum check—reinforcing, expanding and evaluating its effectiveness until the woman goes home. Written instructions assume new importance. Because there are too many impressions in these first few hours after birth, the woman may not remember instructions. Many units follow-up by a telephone call in the next day to see how the parents are managing. Such follow-up is especially appreciated by the parents.

NURSING MANAGEMENT POSTNATAL MOTHER (NORMAL)

Whether the woman has had a spontaneous vaginal delivery, assisted delivery, or a surgical delivery, certain aspects of care are universal.

The woman in recovery is a person at risk; she is vulnerable in many ways. Physical stability must be ensured and a positive client-nurse relationship established so she can be assisted in her developmental tasks of parenting and maintaining self-esteem.

Assessment

The transfer from the labour and delivery area does not end the recovery process. The critical phase of recovery necessitates accurate observations, nursing history, and physical assessment to allow formulation of appropriate nursing diagnoses and an effective plan of care.

Initial Observations

First impressions of a client provide the nurse with a good idea of how she is recovering from childbirth. Establishing physical stability is critical. Two factors easily noted are general appearance and presence of pain. The client's colour reflects circulation and perfusion. Observe her for pallor, flushing, or cyanosis and note general responsiveness. Is she extremely fatigued, unusually quiet, or very excitable or anxious? Does she look comfortable, or Is she in distress?

An intravenous line still may be in place when a woman is admitted to the postpartum unit, and its patency must be ensured. Note the type of solution, any medications added, amount left in the bag, and the rate of flow and assess the insertion site for irritation or infiltration. If the woman has had surgery a Foley's catheter will be in place. If she is at risk for phlebitis, there may be an alternating pressure device or elastic stockings on her legs; check for placement of the sleeves and wrappings and for the functioning of the pump.

In addition to physical findings, the nurse notes whether the client is alone or accompanied, and if so, by whom. Is support evidenced, does the mother speak about the baby or is she very concerned over her own welfare?

Although far from thorough, this initial admission assessment gives basic information and can provide direction for possible problems and areas for further investigation.

Physical Assessment

As soon as possible after admission to the postpartum unit, the woman's stability is determined, which provides a base for further evaluation. The following facts are checked:

Vital signs: Take pulse, respiration, and blood pressure to assess normal blood volume and recovery. Temperature is taken to ensure that the woman is not dehydrated and to rule out infection.

Involution: For vaginal delivery, check the fundus level and tone to determine adequate uterine contraction and descent. For caesarean delivery, check the dressing, including its condition and presence of bleeding.

Abdomen: Check for distention, softness or firmness, rigidity and tenderness. Check also for the presence or absence of bowel sounds after general anaesthesia or caesarean delivery.

Bladder: Palpate for emptiness or fullness and distention. Observe whether a Foley's catheter is in place.

Breasts: Determine whether they are soft or firm or tender or nontender; ask the mother if she is planning to breast-feed.

Perianal area: Observe the perineal pad for amount and colour of lochial discharge, noting unusual odour or presence of clots; check for intact sutures along the line of episiotomy; any bleeding, oedema, ecchymosis, or pain, and observe the anus for repaired laceration or haemorrhoids.

With initial physical assessment completed, the nurse can determine whether the woman can be left comfortably and safely, which will provide time to complete data collection.

Nursing History

Depending on the institution, information can be obtained from a history taken on admission to labour and delivery or a second interview during the postpartum period. Necessary background data include the following:

1. Type and time of delivery.
2. Anaesthesia and medications received during labour and delivery.
3. Present gravidity and parity; blood type and Rh factor.
4. Status of baby.
5. Chosen method of feeding the baby.
6. Significant past medical and surgical history.
7. Allergies, including medication, food, and environ-mental conditions.
8. Medications taken on a regular basis.
9. Diet, including medical, religious or cultural limitations.
10. Social, occupational and economic factors that may affect the woman's recovery and parenting.
11. General educational background for this experience, including prepared childbirth.
12. Classes attended.
13. Home situations that will affect recovery and parenting, including whether she will have help with the baby or need to climb stairs after a difficult or surgical delivery.

Chart Review

The final source of pertinent data is the chart itself. Use it to verify any previously obtained information and obtain additional facts about the labour and delivery, before planning care. Check the physician's orders in terms of activity, diet medications, intravenous infusions, orders and any special treatments or procedures. The antepartum chart usually contains laboratory data, including the woman's blood type and Rh factor, serologic tests and rubella titre.

Nursing Diagnoses

The nurse identifies specific selfcare needs or deficits appropriate to each postpartum woman and formulates nursing diagnoses that focus on the woman's problems. These diagnoses will be the basis for the plan of care that should reflect her physical, emotional, and developmental needs.

Some nursing diagnoses are universal to every woman, regardless of type of delivery. These include the following:

1. High risk for fluid volume deficit related to uterine atony, retained placental fragments, or bleeding.
2. High risk for infection (uterine, perineal, incisional) related to type of birth.
3. Pain related to type of incision.
4. Knowledge deficit regarding parenting, hygiene, or recovery process related to prior experience.
5. Constipation related to anaesthesia, diet, medication or pain.
6. Urinary retention related to periurethral oedema from delivery.

In other instances the type of delivery or other special circumstances necessitate formulation of diagnoses to meet specific needs. After a complicated birth or caesarean delivery, a woman may exhibit needs related to the following diagnoses:

1. Altered tissue perfusion (phlebitis) related to immobility.
2. Situational low self-esteem related to childbirth difficulties.
3. Altered parenting related to disappointment or discomfort.

It is interesting to note that the nurse and client may focus on different problems. It saves time for the nurse and the new mother to sit down and discuss priorities. A study by Tribotti et al (1988) found significant variations in concerns, which changed day by day during recovery. The five nursing diagnoses recovering women most frequently selected in the early period were as follows:

1. Alteration in comfort (pain)
2. Potential for growth (family coping)
3. Alteration in body fluids (fluid volume excess or deficit).
4. Impaired physical mobility.
5. Sleep pattern disturbance.

These women focussed on their bodily changes at first. After caesarean birth these physical changes assumed an even greater importance. By 25 to 72 hours after birth, women were concerned about altered sleep patterns and facing the future. By 73 to 96 hours after birth, many more diagnoses were selected by the participants (an average of 9 each).

Planning

Because of the short stay, the nurse usually will be able to evaluate only short-term achievement during the short hospital stay. Therefore outcomes need to be brief, with referral for problems that cannot be quickly resolved. Reasonable expectations include the following outcomes:

1. Fluid balance restored as evidenced by stable vital signs lochial flow and hydration.
2. No signs of infection during recovery.
3. Re-establishement of normal elimination patterns.
4. Comfort achieved.
5. Attachment begins with signs of bonding.
6. Performs self-care appropriately.
7. Demonstrates basic infant care and feeding techniques.
8. Apparent availability of family support.
9. Talks about birth experience and evidences positive self-esteem.

Nursing Interventions

Preparation and Transfer

The basic care of the postpartum patient is an extension of the care given in the delivery or birthing room after childbirth. If the concept of continued care in one setting is followed the patient may labour, give birth, and receive her postpartum nursing care in the same room. However, many maternity services include a special postpartum recovery room where a new mother is closely observed and cared for during the first 2 to 4 hours after birth or until her condition is considered stabilized. The patient who is transferred to a postpartum area is put in a unit previously prepared for her. The bed is turned down, and bed protectors are placed to catch extra vaginal drainage. Near at hand are a sphygmomanometer, stethoscope, and individual unit equipment, such as towel and wash cloth set, wash and emesis basins, soap, bedpan, back care lotion, breast and perineal pads, perineal irrigation equipment, and newspapers or paper bags for discarding pads. If the patient has an intravenous infusion, support for the bottle also is needed.

The transfer of the patient from the stretcher to the bed may required two or three persons, depending on her condition and the equipment available. When planning to move her, it is important to know the type of delivery (vaginal or abdominal) experienced, the kind of anaesthesia employed, if any, and the status of her recovery. Women who have delivered in an LDR (Labour, Delivery, Recovery) setting may be transferred by wheelchair. Before the delivery room nurse leaves the area, checks the patient's fundus and vaginal flow to determine whether the uterus is firm and raises side rals, if appropriate. When transferring records, she makes sure that any pertinent information concerning the patient, her delivery, and the status of her infant is related to the postpartum charge. The patient's personal effects are carefully transferred so that nothing is lost in the move. The description of care that follows relates particularly to the patient who delivered vaginally.

Immediate Postpartum or Recovery Period

The postpartum nurse checks and records the mother's pulse, respirations and blood pressure at least every 15 minutes during the first hour and thereafter until her condition is stable. During this same period, the mother's temperature should be recorded once. The nurse must also check and appropriately document:

1. Consistency and location of the fundus every 15 min.
2. Type and amount of vaginal discharge (lochia) and the appearance of the perineum every 15 min.
3. Signs and symptoms of distention of the urinary bladder every 15 min (intake and output ahould be recorded carefully during this period).
4. Rate of flow and condition any of/infusion present and amount and type of medication.
5. General condition of the patient; colour, feel of her skin (warm or cold, dry or clammy), level of consciousness (drowzy) apprehensive (unresponsive) and presence of nausea or vomiting.
6. Emotional status: depression, any special complaints (pain) or requests (need to see husband and infant, interactions with infant, family, and friends).
7. Recovery from anaesthesia, if any (return of motion, sensation, or consciousness).
8. Nutritional and fluid status.

Observation for Signs of Haemorrhage

Blood pressure, pulse, and general condition: Occasionally the blood pressure is elevated at the time of transfer. This condition may be the result of the excitement of the birth and seeing the baby. It may be related to the type of oxytocic the patient received or is still receiving by intravenous infusion. It may be a sign of preeclampsia or may be caused by the presence of pain or urinary retention. It is important to know the patient's baseline vital signs and what they have been since the birth. Blood pressures over 130 mmHg systolic or 90 mmHg diastolic should be reported to the charge nurse.

The mother's blood pressure may be low. Any pressure of 100 mmHg systolic or below should definitely be reported. Other pressures that are higher but not hypertensive compared with the patients baseline and that continue to fall should be reported for evaluation. Many patients with a systolic reading of 90 mmHg or below are going into circulatory collapse or shock. Such a falling blood pressure is accompanied by an initially rising pulse. However, if the patient continues into shock, pulse will gradually slow, weaken and have a thready quality. Abnormal dilated pupils, pale, cyanotic, or clammy skin, apprehension, and unconsciousness are also signs of shock.

Some postpartum patients have a relatively slow pulse, but it is of good and is not associated with other signs of shock. This pulse rate (usually) in the 60s is not significant.

Lochia: The attending nurse is also interested in the amount and character of vaginal drainage, or lochia. As she examines the patient drainage, she must check under the patient's hips because much of the drainage may not be on the perineal pad but may seek lower dependent areas.

Immediately after birth, the lochia should be moderate in quantity and dark or bright red—a quality called RUBRA. (About 2 days later the lochia changes to pinkish-brown called SEROSA). The fresh drainage normally has a fleshy but not foul odour. The presence of clots should be reported. The patient usually wears two perineal pads (peripads) that must be changed once or, at most, twice during her first 2 hours postpartum. These should always be removed and applied from front to avoid bacillary contamination of the perineum.

Accurate visual assessment of the amount of locial flow is often difficult. Estimating the amount by measurement of the stain on the peripad may be complicated by the different types of pads used and how often they are changed. However, saturation of one peripad within 1 hour is usually considered heavy drainage. When estimating blood loss and its significance, the nurse must also consider the size and condition of the patient.

Fundus: The first consideration related to blood loss is the condition of the uterus. Is the fundus firm and contracted? Is it at or below the umbilicus? If a fundus is large, soft, or boggy (seems to contain excess blood), it should be gently massaged with a circular motion until firm while one hand is held against the top of the pubic bone to prevent the uterus from being inverted or prolapsed. If clots are suspected, once the fundus is firm it may be gently grasped and positioned in the middle of the abdomen. Pressure is then exerted in the direction of the pelvic canal to push out the clots that were emptied from the uterus into the lower uterine segment and vagina during the massage. The uterus can be overstimulated by excessive mani-pulation, leading to the relaxation and possible haemorr-hage. Students should not attempt to express clots alone until instructed individually, in the event of excessive vaginal bleeding, massage is the first measure employed to control vaginal haemorrhage.

It is surprising how quickly the uterus responds to simple massage in most cases. The nurse can easily feel the uterine muscles tighten. This tightening of the uterine muscle to make a firm fundus is essential. It pinches off the large vessels that brought blood to and from the placental sinuses before the placenta separated and was delivered. A nursing baby will also stimulate the uterine muscles to contract.

Postpartum haemorrhage: When the uterus does not contract or remain contracted, the presence of placental fragments in the uterus is suspected (Fig. 6.2). If bleeding continues to be excessive and the uterus remains firm a cause other than uterine relaxation must be sought to explain the blood loss. Excessive bleeding may develop because of a previously undetected cervical or vaginal laceration or a defective suture or repair. An abnormally bleeding patient may be returned to the delivery room for inspection of the uterus and vaginal canal (Figs 6.3 and 6.4). In some cases a dilatation and curettege of the uterus or the insertion of vaginal canal. In some cases a dilatation and curettage of the uterus or the insertion of vaginal or more rarely, uterine packing is undertaken. If no lacerations or abnormal tissue retention is evident, treatment is usually confined to the administration of additional oxytocines, such as cytocin, synthetic injection (pitocin, syntocinon), ergot, or its modification, methylergonovine (Methergine). Such treatment combats the lethargy of the uterine muscles known as uterine inertia. Blood transfusion may be required. Patients who have had many children, multiple or frequent pregnancies, large babies long or induce labour, uterine dystocia, or pre-eclamsias should be essentially observes the uterine inertia.

Management of Women with Early Postpartum Haemorrhage (Tables 6.2 to 6.4)

All the women must be assessed for early postpartum haemorrhage (PPH). The presence of certain risk factors, however, puts some women at higher risk for this complication. Identification of risk factors before delivery is a key component of the nursing role, as is prompt diagnosis and intervention postpartum.

Equipment

- Blood pressure recording device
- Peripads
- Underpads
- Gloves
- Gram scale to weigh pads
- Intravenous access with 18-gauge catheter
- Oxygen source with face mask
- Foley catheter
- Light source.

The location and consistency of the fundus are important. A high soft fundus suggests uterine

Table 6.2: Nursing care for women with early postpartum haemorrhage

Nursing action	*Rationale*
1. Anticipate PPH from the woman's history and intrapartum course	Numerous risk factors place a woman at increased risk for PPH, including uterine overdistention, precipitous or prolonged labour, medications that relax the myometrium, and high parity
2. Obtain and record the woman's blood pressure and pulse at least every 15 minutes for the first hour after delivery, then every 30 minutes for the next hour. Notify the physician if the woman is tachycardic or hypotensive	Overt hypotension and signs of shock associated with PPH will not be seen until the woman has lost almost one third of her blood volume (1500 to 2000 ml). Tachycardia and orthostatic blood pressure changes will be observed before overt hypotension
3. Evaluate the amount of vaginal bleeding every 15 minutes for the first hour after delivery, then every 30 minutes for the next hour. The terms scant, small, moderate, and large (as defined here) can be used to describe the amount of blood loss after delivery: Scant — Peripad blood stain <2 inches (<10 ml) within 1 hour Small — Peripad blood stain >2 inches <4 inches (10 to 25 ml) within1 hour Moderate — Peripad blood stain > 4 inches but < 6 inches (25 to 50 ml) within 1 hour Large — Peripad blood stain > 6 inches to saturated peripad (50 to 80 ml) within 1 hour; a saturated peripad holds approximately 80 ml of blood	PPH is most likely to occur during the first hour after delivery of the placenta. Blood loss may be more accurately quantified by weighing peripads: 1 g = 1 ml of blood
4. Assess for uterine atony at least every 15 minutes for the first hour after delivery, then every 30 minutes for the next hour. If the uterus is soft or difficult to locate, begin external uterine massage. (Place one hand above the symphysis pubis to support the uterus and prevent uterine inversion; use the other hand to massage the uterine fundus). Note the passage of blood clots	Dark red vaginal bleeding with clots and a soft, boggy uterus usually accompany uterine atony or retained placental fragments. External uterine massage usually stimulates the uterus to contract. If external uterine massage is ineffective, the physician might choose to initiate bimanual compression
5. If the uterus remains soft after external uterine massage or if the fundus is located above the umbilicus, evaluate the woman for bladder fullness. Ask her to void to empty her bladder. If she is unable to void, catheterize according to the physician's order	A full bladder interferes with uterine contraction in the postpartum period
6. Administer pharmacologic agents used in the treatment of uterine atony according to the physician's orders	Oxytocin, the ergot alkaloids (Methergine and Ergotrate), and prostaglandins are used in the treatment of uterine atony. Each agent differs in mode of administration and potential side effects
7. If vaginal bleeding continues despite a well-contracted uterus and an empty bladder, notify the physician or certified nurse-midwife to examine the woman for the presence of a perineal, vaginal, or cervical laceration	A continuous trickle of bright red blood, despite a well-contracted uterus, can indicate a laceration of the lower genital tract.
8. Initiate intravenous fluid replacement and obtain laboratory studies as ordered by the physician. Administer blood products as needed	A comparison of the postpartum haemoglobin level and haematocrit with values of the sample drawn on admission can help estimate the severity of the blood loss. Rapid infusion of intravenous fluids or blood products with one or more large-bore catheters is used to correct hypovolemia and to replace the blood loss associated with PPH
9. If the woman's condition warrants, administer oxygen by face mask. Insert a Foley catheter. Position the woman with her legs elevated at a 30-degree angle	Supplemental oxygen is administered to increase oxygen to peripheral tissues. A Foley catheter monitors urine output, which reflects intravascular volume status. Positioning the patient as described facilitates venous return and promotes oxygenation of vital organs
10. Prepare the woman and her partner for uterine exploration or surgical intervention as indicated. Transfer the woman to the operative area	Surgical measures used to control PPH include repair of laceration, evacuation of haematomas,ligation of uterine arteries, and hysterectomy. Preparing the woman by answering her questions and explaining the medical and nursing interventions helps alleviate her fears and decrease tension

Table 6.3: Nursing care plan for the woman with postpartum haemorrhage

Problem/Objective	*Nursing interventions*	*Rationale*
Nursing Diagnosis 1. High-risk for altered tissue perfusion related to excessive blood loss secondary to uterine atony or birth injury	1. Identify whether woman has added risk factors for postpartum haemorrhage	1. Women who have risk factors should be assessed more frequently than those who do not; usual protocols may not be frequent enough for woman at increased risk for haemorrhage
• Woman's blood pressure and pulse will be within 10% of her values when she wasadmitted	2. According to facility protocol, or more often if risk factors are present, assess woman's • Fundus for height, firmness, and position • Lochia for colour, quantity, and clots; count pads and degree of saturation (weigh pads for greatest accuracy) • Blood pressure, pulse and respiratory rates	2. The fundus must be firm to compress bleeding vessels at the placenta site; bladder distention interferes with uterine contraction and causes the fundus to be high and displaced to one side; rising pulse rate is often first sign of inadequate blood volume; rising pulse and falling blood pressure also occur; most blood lost after birth is visible rather than concealed—observing lochia provides an estimate of actual blood loss
• Woman will not have signs or symptoms of hypovolemic shock	3. Observe for less obvious signs of bleeding: • Constant trickle of brighter red blood with a firm fundus • Severe, poorly relieved pain, especially if accompanied by changes in the vital signs or shock signs and symptoms	3. Most postpartum haemorrhage is caused by atony, which has dramatic blood loss; however, blood loss from a laceration or haematoma can be significant, even though it is less obvious
	4. Observe for other signs and symptoms symptoms of hypovolemic shock	4. Excessive blood loss can result in hypovolemic shock
	5. If signs of haemorrhage are noted, take appropriate actions, according to probable cause for haemorrhage: • Uterine atony: Massage uterus until firm—do not overmassage; expel blood from uterine cavity when uterus is firm; have breastfeeding woman nurse baby; notify registered nurse and/or physician or nurse-midwife for orders and medication if uterus does not become firm and stay firm • Lacerations: Notify registered nurse and/or physician/nurse-midwife to examine woman • Haematoma: Notify registered nurse and/or physician or nurse-midwife to examine woman; apply cold pack to small haematomas on the vulva	5. Haemorrhage can cause death of a new mother if not promptly corrected; most minor episodes of uterine atony are easily corrected with fundal and massage and infant suckling; if the uterus does not remain firm, physician or nurse-midwife physician or nurse midwife examines woman to identify and correct cause of bleeding; oxytocin (Pitocin) infusions are often ordered to contract uterus—other drugs, such as methyl ergonovine (Methergine) or prostaglandin, may be needed; overmassage of uterus can tire it, possibly resulting in inability to contract Trauma such as laceration or haematoma may require repair by physician or nurse-midwife; small haematomas on vulva can be limited by cold applications because they reduce blood flow to area; cold applications also numb area and make woman more comfortable

Contd...

Contd...

Problem/Objective	*Nursing interventions*	*Rationale*
Nursing Diagnosis		
2. High risk for injury (falls) related to anaemia secondary to blood loss • Woman will not fall or have other injury while in birth facility	1. Caution woman not to get out of bed without help until her condition has stabilized 2. When helping woman out of bed, partially elevate head of bed, then help her slowly rise to a sitting position on the side of the bed 3. Before she stands or walks, have her sit on side of bed for a few minutes; have her rotate her feet and ankles and move her legs as she sits on bed 4. Remain with woman when she walks; after she is stable and has been up several times, a family member can walk with her 5. If woman feels faint, have her sit down immediately; if she faints, gently lower her to floor	1. While lying in bed, woman may not realize that she is likely to be dizzy or lightheaded when she ambulates 2. Blood loss reduces amount of circulating blood volume; woman may not have enough volume to maintain circulation to all parts of her body if she changes position quickly 3. Gradual changes of position reduce risk that she will fall because her circulatory system adapts to the changes; moving her feet and legs prevents blood from pooling in her lower extremities 4. Someone accompanying woman can prevent her from falling if she becomes dizzy or faint 5. Prevents injury due to a fall if woman does faint

bleeding; a high, firm fundus more often indicates urinary retention. A distended bladder, located just below the uterus, causes the fundus to rise (usually to one side and most often to the right). This is an important cause of postpartal haemorrhage. After the completion of the third stage of a normal full-term labour, the fundus should be found below or possibly just at the umbilicus. Any higher position is suspected.

The position of the fundus is usually coded by counting finger widths above or below the umbilicus in the following manner. If the fundus (which usually feels somewhat like a large cantaloupe through the abdominal wall) is two finger widths above the level of the umbilicus, it is recorded as +2. If it is locate done finger width below the level of the umbilicus, but usually nurses write "umbilicus." A typical record of the condition of the fundus would be "Fundus: firm -2 midline." On the first postpartal day the fundus is usually felt at the umbilicus or below at -1 or even -2 position. The location of the fundus may be influenced by the size of the patient's baby, the condition of her uterine muscles the content of the urinary bladder and abnormal conditions such as retained placental fragment and the development of uterine infection. Normally the uterus undergoes involution at the rate of about one finger width a day. At the end of 10 days, it is usually down behind the pubic bone again and not palpable (Figs 6.1A and B).

Multiparas often complain of "aftercramps" caused by the contraction of the uterus in the process of involution. They are most often bothered by cramping than are primiparas, who usually possess better muscle tone. Nursing mothers may experience more aftercramps because of the stimulation of the uterus during the process of nursing. Mild analgesics usually relieve the discomfort.

Observations for Signs of Urinary Distension

The most common cause of a high fundus is a full bladder. Even if a woman is catheterized just before birth, she may have a full bladder fairly soon after admittance to the post-partum area, especially if she is receiving or has had intravenous infusions. Catheterization just before birth, which was once routine, is now relatively infrequent.

Other signs of urinary distension are a puffy area just above the pubic bone, complaints by the

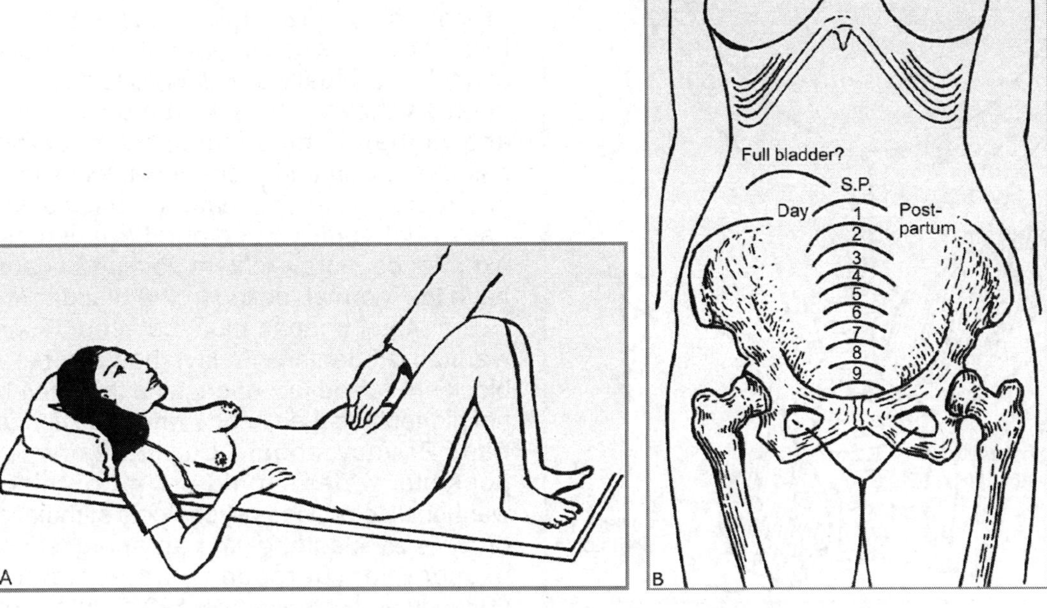

Figs 6.1A and B: Involution of uterus, showing various positions of fundus, SP, Level just after separation of placenta from uterine wall before its delivery

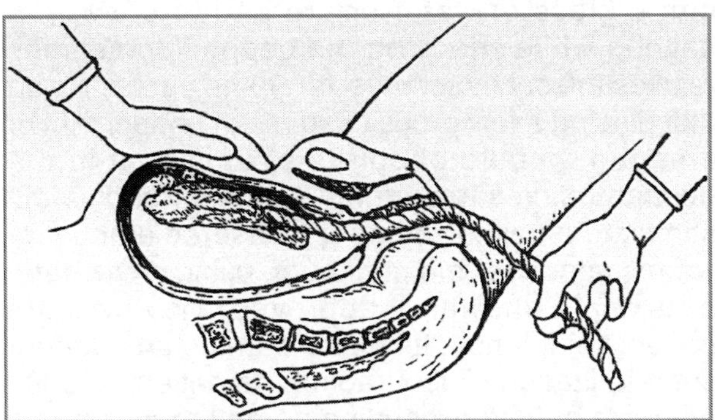

Fig. 6.2: Primary postpartum haemorrhage may occur in the presence of a retained placenta

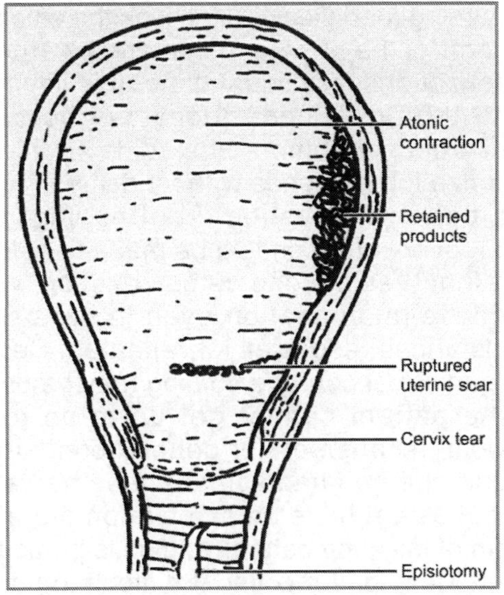

Fig. 6.3: Causes of postpartum haemorrhage

patient that she feels, she should void but cannot or the voiding or small amounts, less than 200 ml. This is called dribbling and usually indicates a full bladder that can contract only partially to release limited bladder tone and may lead to the development of residual urine, an amount that routinely remains in the bladder and is not voided. Residual urine is an excellent medium for bacterial multiplication. A distended bladder may also interfere with the normal contraction of the uterus and predispose the patient to haemorrhage. The condition can be painful and add to after cramping experienced by some patients.

Encouraging Voiding

Voidings of postpartum patients are usually measured until two voidings of over 300 ml are recorded and a fundus check after the voidings indicates that the patient is emptying her bladder wall. Thereafter patients are encouraged to void every 3 to 4 hours and to report any associated

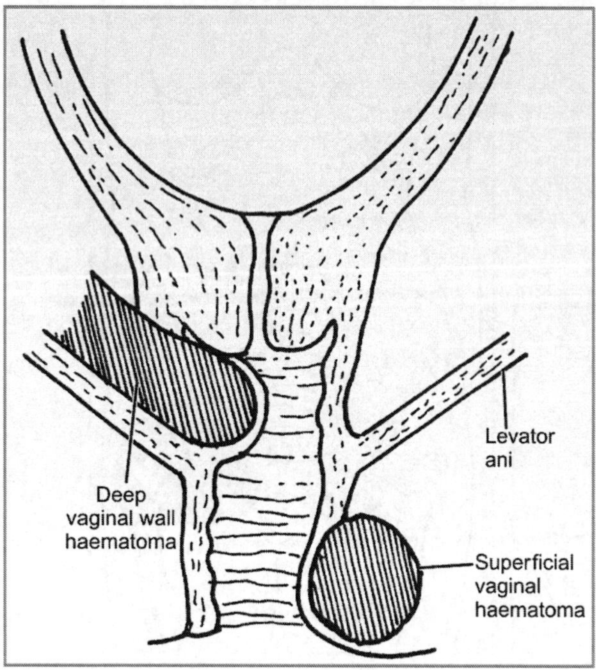

Fig. 6.4: The sites of vaginal wall haematomas

pain, burning, or difficulty. To check the efficiency of a bladder, the physician sometimes orders a catheterization for residual urine. It is important that all the equipment necessary be at the patient's bedside before she voids so that the catheterization proceeds without delay.

If a patient is suspected of having a full bladder, every effort should be made to help her void without resorting to catheterization, which may cause inflammation even in the best of circumstances, especially if repeated. Several techniques to encourage voiding may be useful.

If the patient cannot get up to go to the bathroom because of her general condition or because she has had spinal anaesthesia and does not as yet have an ambulation order, the problem of initiating natural voiding is particularly difficult. Many patients find it difficult to use the bed. The time that physicians allow their patients to ambulate postpartum differs widely. Patients who have received subarachnoid spinal (saddle block) anaesthesia may be confined to bed, flat or with only one pillow for 8 to 12 hours after the birth. The restriction of ambulation and posture is chiefly to prevent the leakage of spinal fluid through the puncture site in the dura, causing a decrease of fluid and pressure related to the onset of "spinal headache". New mothers who have had epidural anaesthesia usually may ambulate with assistance when the anaesthetic has "worn off." The often feel dizzy the first time they sit up in bed. Those rare patients who have had a general anaesthetic usually are allowed to rise with aid as soon as they wish. Sometimes if a physician knows that a choice must be made between catheterization and probable success in voiding, he orders earlier ambulation. Patients who have had saddle block or epidural anaesthesia also experience more problem voiding because they have lost normal feeling in the bladder area.

If a metal bedpan must be used, it should be warmed. Patients who have had a subarachnoid block are raised just enough so that their hips are not higher than their heads while positioned on the pan. Privacy should be maintained, and if possible, water should be left running into a washbowl to provide psychologic stimulation. If an order is available, giving an analgesic such as oxycodone (Sercodan) or acetaminophen (Tylenol) and codeine about 20 minutes before the bedpan is offered often solves the problem. Having the patient blow bubbles through a straw into a glass of water or pretend to blow up a balloon while she is on the bedpan sometimes relaxes the sphincter muscle. Some nurses report that placing a few drops of spirits of peppermint or an open ampule of spirits of ammonia in the bedpan relaxes the urinary sphincter and safely stimulate a void. Pouring a measured amount of warm water over the perineum, using a sitz bath, or taking a shower, if approved, may help the patient void. If not , it helps clean the area before catheterization. Encouraging the patient to drink amounts of fluid exceeding normal requirements before she voids usually adds to rather than relieves the problem and is not recommended.

The height of the fundus should always be determined after voiding or catheterization to evaluate, by change in the position of the fundus, the efficiency of the emptying process and other possible problems with fundal relaxation.

Catheterization Technique

If none of the preceding methods brings bout the desired result, catheterization must be carried out. The nurse should know whether a specimen should be saved for laboratory analysis. The technique of catheterization and the materials used differ from hospital to hospital. The following instructions are general to make allowances for the different setups used, but they include principles that should be understood as well as review information for the student.

Individual differences of opinion still exist regarding how much urine should be removed from the bladder during the catheterization of a postpartum patient. The most common practice is to empty the bladder completely but slowly, even after more than 700 to 1,000 ml of urine is obtained. Although there could be a mild sympathetic response of slightly lowered blood pressure when more than 1,000 ml is removed, this could result from decreased maternal anxiety caused by the pressure of a full bladder. Lowered blood pressure has not been found to be significant in this type of patient. If urine remains in the bladder, the problems that may be encountered usually outweigh any mild sympathetic response.

Catheterization Postpartum Area

Use hospital procedures, bearing the following principles in mind:

1. Check the physician's order regarding catheterization.
2. Explain in simple terms what is going to be done for the patient and that she will feel better as a result of the procedure.
3. Provide privacy and lighting.
4. Get sufficient exposure to identify the urethral meatus, but be gentle.
5. Some of the newly delivered "saddle" patients have little feeling in the area others are very sensitive.
6. Once a nurse's hand has touched the patient, the hand is contaminated.
7. Sometimes holding the labia back with a cotton ball under one supporting finger helps maintain the position.
8. Technically, if the labia close after the crucial area has been washed with antiseptic, the area must be rewashed, since it has been contaminated by the enfolding tissue; thus it is important to maintain the labia in the drawback position.
9. The female urethra is about 1½ inches long. No more than 4 inches of the catheter should be inserted, to avoid bladder puncture. If obstruction is encoun-tered, the catheter should never be forced. There may be an abnormality of the canal (presence of a tumour, stricture, etc), or the meatus may not be properly identified.
10. A slight downward incline of the catheter may aid insertion as are urethral canal slopes downward when the patient is in dorsal recumbent position.
11. Always measure the amount of urine obtained and record it. Note also the colour of the urine. Note whether a catheter was left in place and if specimen was obtained and sent to the laboratory.
12. Assure the patient that the inability to void is usually temporary.

Emotional Status

The patient's emotional status can be as early indication of psychologic or physical problems. Also, this is an important time for the patient to begin the development of maternity, which supplies her with the emotional energy needed for feeling that here infant occupies an important part of her life. This is a time for developing bonds of affection. The postpartal woman must have met her own needs so that she may meet those of her baby. She must control her own body before she can best undertake the mothering tasks ahead.

The labour experience is often one of the most demanding periods for a woman. To use it strictly in her life, she will need to talk about it and relive it.

During all recovery care certain critical elements must be observed and adherence is assumed in good nursing practice.

The Critical Elements: Maternity Care

- Use latex gloves when there is contact with blood or other body fluids. Universal precau-tions are considered an essential part of maternity care.
- Explain before and after a procedure.
- Encourage participation in self-care.
- Provide privacy by pulling curtains and draping appropriately.
- Support parents during hospital stay.

Involution check: The postpartum "check" is first performed on the woman's admission to recovery, whether in a labour-delivery-recovery (LDR), a labour delivery-recovery and postrecovery (LDRP), or post-partum unit. At regular intervals in the next days it is repeated. During the first hour, uterine and lochial checks are performed every 15 minutes and then every 1 to 2 hours to the next 4 hours. If all signs show expected progress, checking is decreased to every 8 hours until the woman is discharged.

Fundus check: An assessment of the uterus is performed after vaginal and caesarean birth (Figs 6.5 and 6.6).

Palpate the abdomen to locate the fundus or top of the uterus by pressing in and down with the side of the palm (Fig.6.6). Describe the descent by measurements in *fingerbreadths* from the umbilicus (one finger-breadth measures 1 cm).

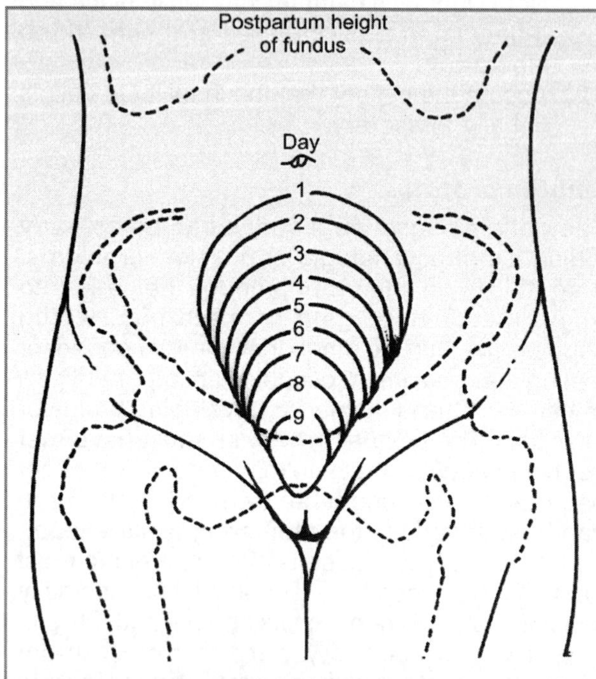

Fig. 6.5: Uterine involution showing changes in the height of the fundus

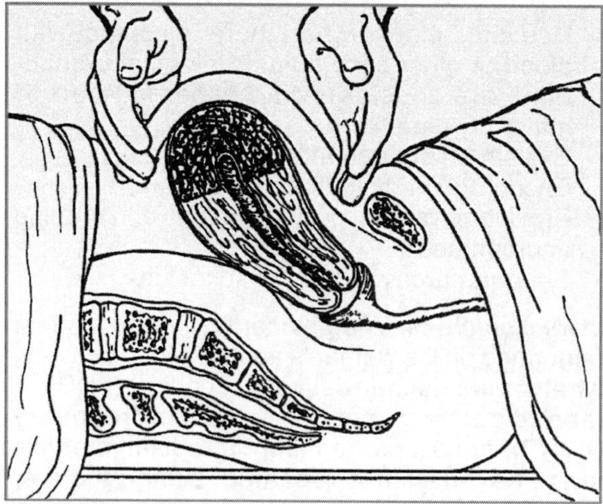

Fig. 6.6: When massaging the fundus, the nurse keeps one hand firmly on the lower uterus, just above the symphysis pubis. The uterus is massaged in a firm, circular motion. After the uterus becomes firm, the nurse pushes downward, toward the outlet, to expel accumulated blood

In the surgical birth, palpation generally may be omitted when there is a vertical incision to avoid pressure on tissue and incision lines. Checks are part of protocol. Perform them gently, approaching from the sides to the midline for a woman with a low segment incision.

PROCEDURE FOR ASSESSING AND MASSAGING THE UTERINE FUNDUS

Materials

Unsterile gloves are worn. Offer perineal care and provide a clean pad. Explain the procedure before beginning.

Method

1. Identify the need for fundal massag. In most cases, the uterus will be soft and higher than the umbilicus.
2. Have the woman empty her bladder, because a distended bladder raises and displaces the uterus.
3. Place the woman in a supine position with the knees slightly flexed. Lower the perineal pad to observe lochia as the fundus is palpated.
4. Place the outer edge of nondominant hand just above the symphysis pubis, and press downward slightly to anchor the lower uterus.
5. Locate and massage the uterine fundus with the flat portion of the fingers of the dominant hand in a firm circular motion.
6. When the uterus is firm, gently push downward on the fundus, toward the vaginal outlet, to expel blood and clots that have accumulated inside the uterus. Keep the other hand on the lower uterus to avoid inverting the organ.
7. Measure the number of fingerbreaths at which the fundus is felt either above or below the umbilicus.
8. Document the consistency and location of the fundus. For example, "FF 2 U" means the fundus is firm and two fingerbreaths below the umbilicus.
9. Notify registered nurse if the uterus does not become firm or if the fundus becomes boggy when massage has stopped.

The uterus should be firm in consistency, comparable to a grapes fruit. A fundus that is hard to find or one that is soft or boggy signifies inadequate contraction and haemorrhage could occur. If the fundus is firm at the midline and at the expected level and if lochia is the appropriate colour and amount, the nurse accurately documents these data. If, however the fundus is soft or boggy, gentle massage is applied by rotating the cuped hand over the fundus until it feels firm. Vigorous massage or kneading should be avoided because it may over-stimulate the uterus and cause it to become more fatigued and thus decrease contractility.

While palpating the fundus, inspect the perineal pad and bed pad. Lochia may be increased as "old" clots or lochia pooling in the vagina is expelled by pressure. On the other hand, a boggy or relaxed fundus may indicate excessive bleeding. Note if the fundus becomes firm, and measure the amount of blood on the pads after palpation. The fundus should be located in the midline. If it is to the side, the bladder is assessed for distension, which is the usual cause of an atonic uterus. After the bladder is emptied, the location and finances are determined again.

During discharge explain the procedure and why it is important for the fundus to be firm. Show the woman how to palpate the fundus, and teach her how to massage it to improve uterine contractility in the first few days.

Lochia

Lochia is observed for amount and colour. The terms rubra, serosa and alba describe if the flow is bright red, pinkish brown (serosanguineous), or whitish. Describing amount is more difficult. The terms *scant*, *moderate*, and *heavy* (large) describe the amount. Descriptions are based on the number of pads used in 1 hour and the saturation of the pad. Ask the woman who might have discarded a pad to describe the flow in terms of usual menstrual amounts. In the initial recovery period, lochial flow is normal if no more than two pads are saturated within the first hour (the bed pads should be checked as well). As involution continues, the flow decreases to one pad per 2 to 4 hours in the next 8 hours and then will be comparable to menstrual flow.

Objective evaluation of flow is important in cases of abnormal amounts. A "flow chart" is kept and amounts charted. Remember that for every 500 ml blood lost, the haemotocrit will fall 3 to 4% and haemoglobin 1.0 to 1.5 gm/dL. A more standardized approach measures the size of the lochial stain or the weight of the pad. Absorbency of the pad will affect measurements; the type of pad in use in each unit should be tested. It has determined that for one pad type, scant lochia was a stain less than 2 inches long with a volume of less than 10 ml. A large lochial flow was seen on a pad with greater than a 6 inch stain and with more than 50 ml volume. (Weight of 1 g of blood equals approximately 1 ml of blood).

In addition to noting amount and colour, characteristics are evaluated to determine whether they are appropriate for the time of recovery. Any change in pattern or unusual characteristic should be noted. If the fundus is firm, and there is too much lochia, the physician should be notified. Constant trickling of oxygenated blood (brighter red) may mean an unrepaired arterial laceration or a clotting defect. Assessment of lochia is important for the woman after caesarean delivery. It is common to see a gush of lochia when the woman gets out of bed for the first time. Fluid has collected in the vagina during sleep. Reassure her and provide an extra disposable bed pad to catch the "drip" until she gets to the bathroom.

When lochial flow is excessive or suddenly increases, check for a change in the client's activity level (e.g. excess straining, lifting, or walking). If a fundal check and uterine massage do not produce a firm fundus, oxytocic agents such as methylergonovine maleate (Methergine) may be indicated. If unusual lochial colour or odour is found, obtain a specimen for a culture and sensitivity test, check vital signs and notify the physician for medical follow-up care.

During discharge describe the usual sequence of lochial changes. Instruct the woman in the warning signs, resumption of heavy bleeding after lochia serosa begins, clots passed in the lochia, or any unusual of unpleasant odour to the flow.

Oxytocic Use During Recovery

To stop excessive blood flow after birth, oxytocin doses of 10 to 20 units (U) may be given intramuscularly (IM) or in an IV solution of 1000 ml Ringer's lactate to run at 125 ml. If the bag has less than 500 ml at the time of recovery begins, a new bag of fluid should be started to prevent too concentrated an infusion.

The main side effect is an antidiuretic effect (a partner hormone from the posterior pituitary is vasopressin, an antidiuretic hormone). Therefore during an infusion with oxytocin the total fluid intake must be carefully watched and checked hourly with output. Repeatedly, it has been noted that doses over 20 U/1000 ml fluid in 8 hours result in oliguria. When the solution is changed to an isotonic, plain solution, diuresis immediately begins to occur. Water intoxication also has resulted if the dose has been given in large amounts of IV solution. Signs are elevated BP and headache.

Ergot Derivatives

Two members of the oxytocic family may be used after birth for bleeding. Ergonovine maleate (Ergotrate) 0.2 mg may be given orally or intramuscularly. The half-life is 3 to 4 hours; thus the drug is never given before the baby is born. Because the uterus is capable of contracting without any drug, intervention should not be excessive. When there is frank haemorrhage uncontrolled by oxytocin, ergonovine maleate or methylergonovine maleate (Methergine) may be given. Both drugs have a hypertensive effect and are administered only if the maternal blood pressure is in the normal range. Ergonovine maleate particularly causes systemic and pulmonary hypertension and is, therefore, much less commonly used today.

Infection (Table 6.4)

A perineum that has undergone the trauma of an episiotomy or a laceration is at risk for infection from the proximity of faecal material and the potential growth medium that lochial bleeding provides. Once infected, the tissue allows pathogens to travel into the vagina and even to the uterus itself.

Visual inspection of the perineum for signs of infection is important. Elevated temperature and complaints of severe pain are clues that an infection may be developing. An abdominal incision should be examined carefully, after the initial dressing is removed.

The abdomen is palpated for distention or rigidity, and an involutional check is performed to rule out complications. The incision is inspected for signs of bleeding, haematoma, or infection. The woman should be assisted to turn to a more comfortable position, such as side lying, to decrease tension on the sutures.

If the client becomes febrile, the incision is reassessed. If infection occurs, warm soaks or irrigations with peroxide and saline may be indicated, with frequent sterile dressing changes. Support of the client during this time is vital; the treatment should be explained, and she needs help to cope with another interruption of the childbirth experience; this problem also may affect her self-esteem.

Perineal Care

Perineal hygiene is essential in preventing infections. The client is instructed to use lavage each time she voids or defecates, first cleansing with the aseptic solution if used by protocol and then with plain warm tap water to rise. Teach her to cleanse at the front, moving toward the anus to prevent the spread faecal organisms to the vaginal area. Soft wipes instead of regular toilet tissue should be provided, and the client should use a front-to-back single tissue wiping technique.

During discharge beginning with the first perineal care after birth, explain how to perform the correct technique. She should continue perineal care until the perineum heals and lochia ceases. It should be emphasized that perineal pads should be applied that perineal pads should be applied and removed in a front-to-back direction. Hand washing before and after is reinforced as essential in prevention of infection. Suggest that the woman inspect her perineum and episiotomy by means of a mirror. A woman may feel uncomfortable handling her own genitalia because of personal or cultural factors. Providing a mirror may help to assess the perineum.

Output

Bladder distention is assessed with each involutional check, and output records are kept during the first 24 hours. When the woman ambulates on her own to use the bathroom independently, provide a pan that will fit under the seat and instruct her to report voiding so volume may be measured. She should be taught always to fill the bottles to the same level so the amount of water used in the lavage may be subtracted from the total urine output.

Early specimens always are mixed with lochia. A clear-voided specimen must be obtained if there are any questions regarding urine colour and clarity, if there is cloudiness or unusual colour, if

Table 6.4: Nursing care plan for the woman with postpartum infection

Problem/Objective	Nursing interventions	Rationale
Nursing Diagnosis		
1. High risk for infection related to loss of skin integrity (caesarean incision) and increased risk factors (prolonged labour)	1. Use handwashing when providing care; teach woman personal hygiene measures, such as handwashing, perineal care, regular changes of perineal pads	1. Limits transfer of infectious organisms between clients and from one area of the body to another, regular pad changes also reduce amount of time organisms have to multiply in its warm, dark, and moist environment
• Woman will not have signs of infection, as evidenced by oral temperature below 38°C (100.4°F) and normal progression of lochia that does not have a foul odour	2. Assess vital signs every 4 hr, or more frequently if signs of infection are present	2. An elevated temperature and pulse are signs of infection; if they occur, woman should be assessed for other signs and symptoms of infection
	3. Assess lochia for amount, colour, and odour with vital signs	3. Endometritis is more common if a woman has a caesarean birth and is evidenced by foul-smelling lochia that may be increased or decreased; it is sometimes brown
	4. Assess uterus for height, firmness, and descent	4. Endometritis is characterized by an enlarged, tender uterus
	5. Assess for cramping or other pain	5. Prolonged cramping may occur with endometritis; a wound infection may be painful
	6. Assess the wound each shift for redness, oedema, discharge, and intactness	6. A wound infection is characterized by signs of inflammation; suture line may separate if there is infection in the area
	7. Assess for signs and symptoms of urinary tract infection. Encourage high fluid intake (3 liters/day)	7. Identifies possible presence of urinary tract infection so that it can be reported to the physician; fluid intake regularly flushes microorganisms from bladder and reduces chance that they will infect urinary tract
Nursing Diagnosis		
2. High risk for altered nutrition, less than body requirements, related to increased demand for nutrients secondary	1. Determine foods woman usually eats	1. Identifies her preferences and areas of nutrient adequacy or inadequacy; nurse can build on her preferences and dislikes
• After teaching, woman will verbalize foods that provide nutrients she needs for healing	2. Teach sources of foods high in protein, vitamin C, and iron: • Protein: eggs, meats, cheeses, milk, legumes, combinations of grain foods • Vitamin C: citrus fruits and juices, strawberries, cantaloupe, tomatoes, broccoli, peppers, cabbage • Iron: meats, enriched cereals and breads, dark-green leafy vegetables, dried beans and fruits	2. Protein and vitamin C are necessary for healing; anaemia, which is usually related to iron deficiency, can be corrected by high-iron foods; vitamin C also improves body's ability to use iron
	3. Reinforce physician's orders about vitamin supplements	3. Many physicians have woman take remainder of her prenatal vitamins to be certain she has adequate nutrients

Contd....

Contd....

Problem/Objective	*Nursing interventions*	*Rationale*
	4. If woman is breastfeeding, incorporate diet recommendations for nursing mother into teaching.	4. Nursing mother requires added nutrients to meet her own needs for healing and restoration, plus enough to make breast milk
	5. Have woman restate appropriate foods to meet her nutritional needs after teaching her	5. Identifies is she learned and identifies need for further teaching
	6. Refer to social services for financial assistance, such as the Women, Infants, and Children (WIC) program for food supplementation	6. Helps overcome financial barriers to obtaining adequate food

the client becomes febrile, or if there are signs of dysuria or frequency. A specimen is sent for culture and sensitivity testing and the physician notified for medical follow-up care. The only way to obtain a clear, sterile specimen is by means of straight catheterization.

If the woman is unable to void, increase fluid intake and ambulation. Running Tap water, using a sitz bath to relieve oedema and relax the sphincter, and applying ice to the suprapubic area are aids to urination.

There will be a standing order to relieve distension by straight catheterization once. After that, the physician is notified and an indwelling Foley catheter is inserted and attached to a closed gravity drainage system. Although the general rule is to allow no more than 800 ml of urine to drain at one time, this is not as critical in the postpartum woman, who has been able to withstand increased intra-abdominal pressures from a gravid uterus and a full bladder and has already experienced a sudden decrease in pressure with delivery. Therefore slowly drain the initial 800 ml, leave the catheter in position, and clamp for a few minutes. Continue draining until the bladder is completely emptied.

Constipation

Constipation also is a potential problem. The intestinal musculature, already relaxed by progesterone, responds further to anaesthesia and analgesia and becomes more sluggish. In addition, fear of pain from a perineal laceration, episiotomy or haemorrhoids and the inconvenience of sharing bathroom facilities my inhibit normal bowel movement. Change in diet and activity also plays a part.

The abdomen is visually inspected for distention, palpated for firmness or rigidity, and auscultated for the presence of bowel sounds, especially after surgical delivery. The woman is asked if she is able to pass flatus rectally or feels the urge to defecate. Encourage her to increase fluid intake and recommend ambulation to enhance peristalsis. Stool softeners and laxatives are administered as ordered. If these measures fail, an enema or suppository may be needed.

Pain

Any complaint of pain requires a nursing response. Because pain is subjective, assess the level of pain by asking for a description on a numerical scale, with the lowest number indicating absence of discomfort. Observe the woman's pain behaviours as well. Location and kind of pain are determines sharp, burning, throbbing, aching. Precipitating factors are identified. Pain unrelieved by standard interventions usually indicates complications, and the physician is notified for follow-up.

Contractions

Strong contractions of the involuting uterus are called afterbirth pain. Cramping is increased when the uterus has been distended, for example, with very large infant or a multiple pregnancy. For the first hours after birth an infusion that contains oxytocin to improve muscle contraction may be used. Breastfeeding contributes to these cramping pains because sucking stimulates oxytocin release from the pituitary. Reassure the woman that uterine contractions are a normal part of recovery from childbirth and that they last for only a few days. She can lie prone with a small pillow or rolled towel under the middle of her abdomen. The cramping may worsen initially because of pressure on the uterus, but she should soon notice relief.

Incisional Pain: Episiotomy

Most women who have had an episiotomy or vaginal lacerations will experience some degree of pain during immediate recovery after the local anaesthetic effect wears off. Assess any changes in the suture line by putting on a pair of gloves and using a light to inspect the perineum. Observe also for haemorrhoids, anal fissures, and unrepaired surface vaginal tears. The external labia are carefully observed during the inspection, and note if touching the area elicits more pain. The acronym REEDA describes findings:

- Redness, inflammation around wound
- Oedema of surrounding tissues.
- Ecchymosis around area (includes evaluation for haematoma).
- Discharge from wound.
- Approximation of skin surfaces.

Inspection ensures an accurate description.

During discharge, nurse should teach techniques of sitting can decrease pain. Instruct to tighten the buttocks and perineum before sitting to alleviate pulling on the area. Encourage her to take rest periods in bed with her feed elevated. The use of Kegel's exercises to increase blood circulation to the area and to tighten perineal muscles can be reinforce. The woman should be able to demonstrate these comfort measures before discharge.

Abdominal Incision Pain

The low, transverse, "bikini" incision usually is less painful than a vertical incision. Some pain, however is related to an incision. A distended abdomen will cause pressure on suture lines and increase pain sensation.

The woman is taught to support the incision while moving and to splint by holing her hand or a pillow over the incision during deep breathing and coughing. A binder may be ordered to provide extra support for an obese woman or during recovery from caesarean birth. It should be applied when the client is supine or in a low Fowler's position.

Women with an abdominal incision should learn postoperative self assessment, checking wound, REEDA and noting temperature elevation or localized, unresolving pain.

Pain Management

Although most patients are able to describe discomfort it is important to make a systematic assessment of the presence, cause, type, and location of pain. Perhaps, nursing measures such as emptying the bladder, comfort and cleansing procedures, or positioning, will ease the discomfort. Application of cold or heat, as ordered, may be indicated. And of course, analysis will be used when needed. The success of every measure in relieving pain must be evaluated and documented.

Pharmacologic management after caesarean birth has improved in the last few years. Long-acting epidural narcoting analgesia will last upto 24 hours. If this is not available, meperidine (Demerol, Pethidine) is given at doses of 75 to 100 mg. depending on body weight, administered IM every 3 to 4 hours. Patient-controlled analgesia (PCA) is used in some centers. An IV solution containing a narcotic is inserted as a secondary line into the mainline setup. Programmed by pump to deliver small bolus injections, this arrangement shows a woman to have the dose as she needs it. Safety features built into the pump prevent accidental overdose, and a record is kept of the number of doses infused. The stepdown is to percocet or percodan and then usually oral acetaminophen as needed, 600 to 900 mg every 4 hours. By the third or fourth day a woman should be mainly free from pain except for soreness on moving, and acetaminophen may keep her comfortable.

Cold compresses are applied as soon after birth as possible and for the first 24 hours to prevent and decrease oedema and to diminish local sensation. Commercial cold packs may be used, or an examination glove can be filled with crushed ice tied shut, and wrapped in a paper washcloth. Never apply cold packs directly against skin without a barrier in between. Cold packs should be left in place only for about 20 minutes and removed for a period before reapplications. Sustained vasoconstriction from cold can cause tissue damage and is not advisable.

After cold is used in the first period, warm, moist heat is offered by providing the woman with her own sitz bath kit. She is taught to fill it with comfortable warm water, place on the toilet seat, and sit in it. Adding warm water to keep the desired temperature. Provide topical analgesic creams or ointments or pads such as Tucks.

Breast Discomfort

At delivery the breasts, which are soft and not tender, secrete colostrum. Milk flow will occur about the third or fourth day. Sudden breast fullness and firmness or engorgement precede this milk flow. For nonlactating engorgement show the woman how to use ice packs to decrease fullness and pain and emphasize that these packs should never be placed directly on the skin but wrapped in a washcloth to prevent tissue burns. Discourage expression of milk manually or by pump. Although expression may seem to give relief initially, it actually stimulates milk production and causes the discomfort to last longer. The woman should be advised to wear a well fitting brassiere at all times.

If a woman asks for medication to "dry up" the milk, explain that medications usually are not given. Some physicians prescribe antilactation drugs, most commonly, bromocriptine mesilate (Parlodel). However, engorgement may recur after medication is discontinued. Therefore all women need to know how to care for engorgement.

Activity

Rest The amount of energy expended during labour and birth leaves the new mother in great need of rest. Often women fall asleep during a quiet recovery. Others are so excited that they find it impossible to relax and sleep. After the initial period of elation and stimulation, encourage the woman to use relaxation techniques to calm herself. Although sleep may not seem very important to the new mother, she will become fatigued if she does not set regular times of rest. Fatigue adversely affects milk production, interferes with learning, can participate depression, and can lower her self-esteem.

Care should be planned so that the new mother can rest while she is in the recovery unit. If the baby is rooming in (LDRP) encourage the partner in helping her rest. Discuss with her the ways she can get rest in the home situation, for example, limiting visitors, at first, encoura-ging helpers to do the nonbaby care tasks, and disconnecting helpers to do the nonbaby care tasks, and disconnecting the telephone during feeding or nap times. She will miss sleep at night, so she should plan to nap when the baby does. The nurse can emphasize to the partner the importance of rest while encouraging him to assist with baby and mother care.

Exercise: After delivery the client may gradually resume exercising in the same way she exercised during the prenatal period (Fig. 6.7). She should be cautioned not to exercise too strenuously at first but to pace her activities. Frequent walking is one of the best exercises; when women were confined to bed for extended periods after delivery, many complications such as hypostatic pneumonia,

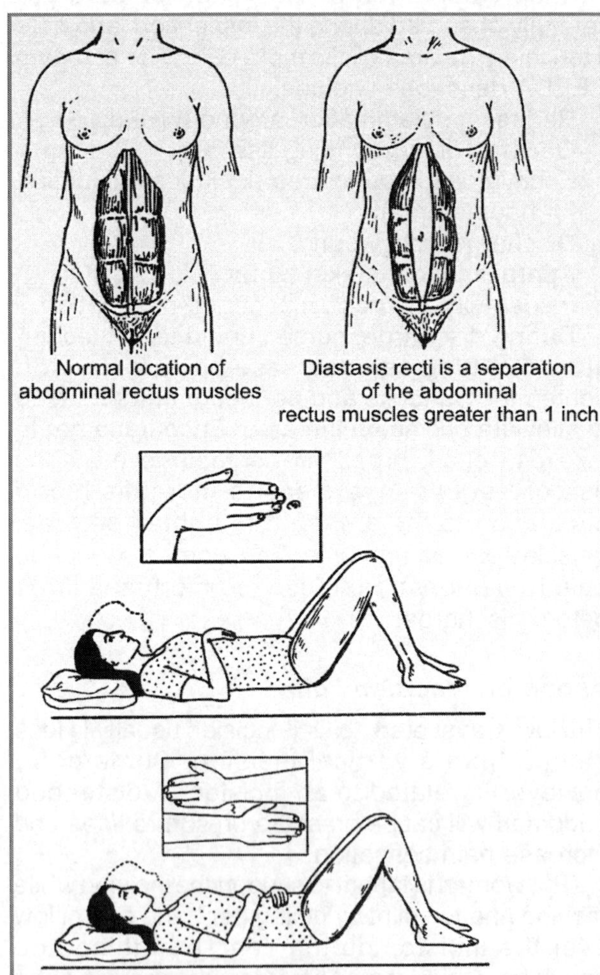

Fig. 6.7: The postpartum woman needs to check for diastasis recti before beginning an exercise program. If the rectus muscles are separated by more than 2 inches, she will need to do exercises to correct the problem so that the separation does not increase

thromboses, and emboli occurred. For this reason, ambulation and exercise are encouraged soon after delivery. In addition, Kegel's exercises for perineal muscles should be continued into the recovery period.

Gentle isometric stretching exercises may begin after birth. For the next few days, abdominal strengthening exercises, such as arm and leg lifts, and flexing to touch the chin to the chest start the process of returning to the woman's pre-pregnant condition. Sit-ups are delayed for a few weeks (Guidelines for exercise during the post-partum period and (Figs 6.8A to H) demonstrates typical exercises to regain contours) are as given below:

Sexuality and Contraception

Sexual intercourse usually is restricted until the perineum (in a vaginal delivery) and uterus have completely healed. Traditionally healing was considered accomplished by 6 weeks, but it is probably adequate at 2 to 4 weeks. After that time generally no physical contraindication to the resumption of normal sexual activities is indicated. Often, however, fear of pain from an episiotomy or laceration, discomfort from breast stimulation in the nursing mothers or abdominal tenderness after a cesarean delivery may inhibit new parents.

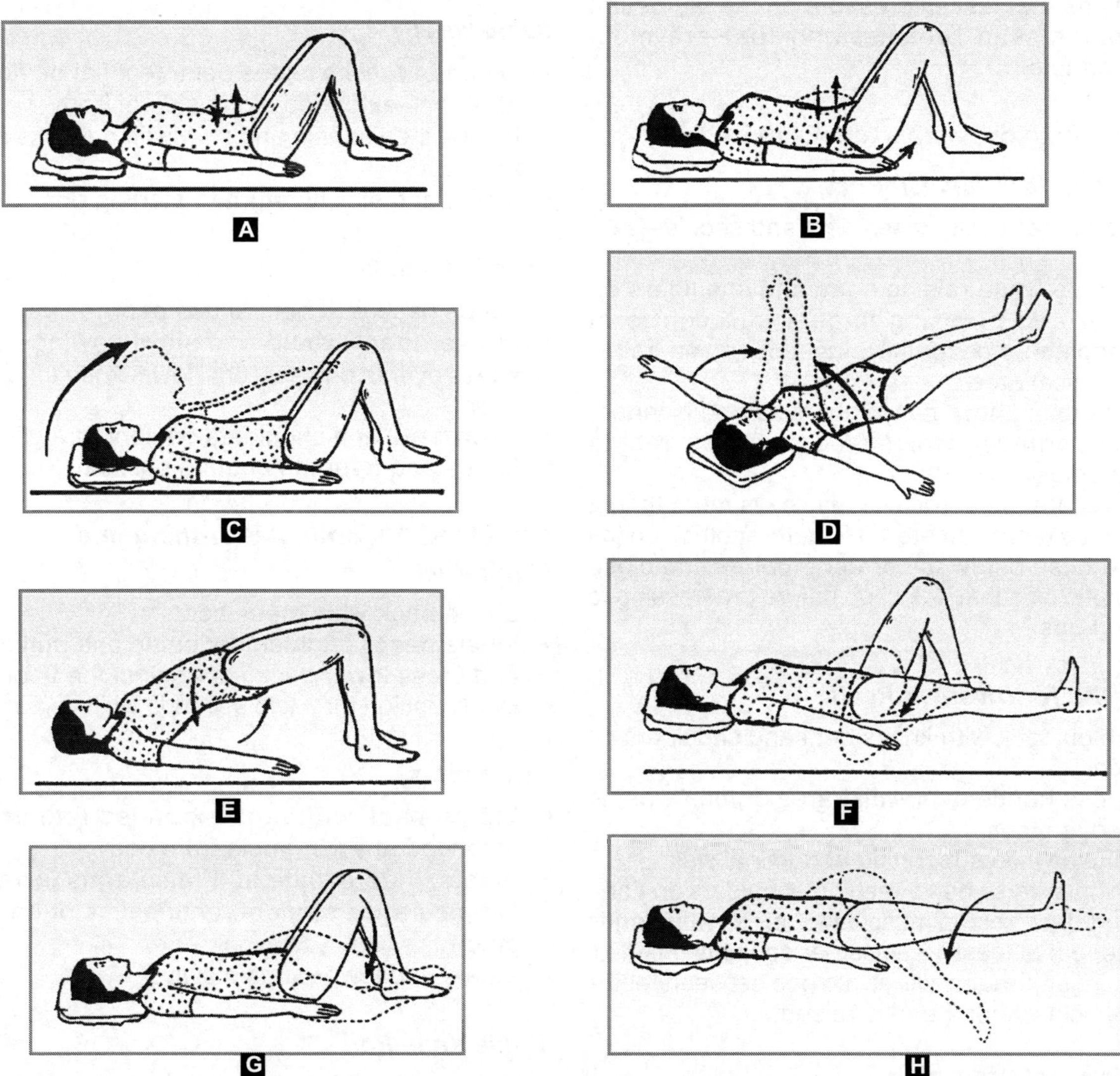

Figs 6.8A to H: A postpartum exercise program is important to both the physical and emotional well-being of the new mother

The topic of sexual relations is introduced as early as possible in the postpartum period and before discharge the couple's expectations and understanding of potential problems are assessed. The nurse discusses methods of relieving discomfort during intercourse, such as the use of water-soluble lubricants or plain vegetable oil to decrease perineal trauma and vaginal dryness. The mother needs to be reassured that it is normal to experience strong contractions during organs. The nursing mother should be told that stimulation of full breasts may be uncomfortable, may cause some leaking, and will be less bother-some if "planned" after a feeding rather than before. The couple should be encouraged to try various positions that lessen pressure on the perineum, abdomen, and breasts, and that are most comfortable.

Guidelines for Postpartum Exercise

Checking for Diastasis Recti

- Lie on back with knees bent and shoulders on floor
- Exhale while raising head and shoulders off floor and pressing fingers into centre of abdomen, horizontally, just above and below umbilical area
- Determine how many fingers can be inserted, horizontally, into space between rectus muscles
- If separation of rectus muscles is more than 2 inches (approximately 3 fingerbreadths), do the exercise below to correct problem and close gap to less than 2 inches before progressing to curl-ups

Exercise for Diastasis Recti

- Lie on back with knees bent and shoulders on floor
- Cross hands over waist area so one wrist is above other
- Inhale while supporting abdominal wall
- Exhale, raise head keeping shoulders on floor, and draw rectus muscles together with hands
- Repeat at least 12 times per day until only 1 or 2 fingerbreadths will fit into gap between rectus muscles when head is raised.

Abdominal Breathing

- Lie on back with knees bent
- Inhale deeply through nose, keeping rib cage as stationary as possible while allowing abdominal muscles to expand
- Exhale slowly through mouth and tighten abdominal muscles.

Straight Curl-UPS

- Lie on back with knees bent
- Inhale, then exhale while bringing head and shoulder forward off the floor and reaching toward knees
- Curl-up only as far as possible while keeping waist on floor
- Inhale and slowly uncurl.

Buttocks Lift

- Lie on back with knees bent, feet flat on floor, and arms extended along side of body
- Inhale, then exhale and slowly lift buttocks and arch back
- Inhale and slowly return to starting position.

Double Knee Roll

- Lie on back with both knees bent
- Inhale, then exhale and slowly swing both knees over to one side until lower knee touches floor
- Keep head and shoulders on floor at all times
- Inhale and return to starting position.

Combined Abdominal Breathing and Pelvic Rock

- Lie on back with knees bent
- Inhale deeply, tighten abdomen and buttocks and press lower back flat against the floor
- Hold position for 3 to 5 seconds while exhaling.

Arm Raises

- Lie on back with legs extended and arms extended at a 90° angle from body
- Inhale, then exhale and raise arms inward, keeping arms straight, until palms of hands touch
- Inhale and lower arms slowly.

Single Knee Roll

- Lie on back with one leg straight and other leg bent at knee

- Inhale, then exhale and slowly swing leg with knee bent over other leg until knee touches floor
- Keep head and shoulders on floor at all times
- Inhale and return to starting position.

Leg Roll

- Lie on back with legs extended
- Inhale, then exhale and lift one leg and roll it over other leg to touch floor
- Keep shoulders on floor and leg extended
- Repeat exercise with other leg.

The couple also should be encouraged to express their feelings about another pregnancy and how they plan to prevent it. Facts about the return of menstruation and ovulation are reviewed. The parents may be worried about another pregnancy but unsure of the appropriate method of family planning. Because birth control often is planned around the menstrual cycle, the woman should understand that she may not have her first menses for 4 to 6 weeks if she is not nursing and for as long as 4 months if she is not supplementing breastfeeding.

Condoms with foam or gel are useful when lactating. The breastfeeding mother should not use combined oral contraceptives because lactation hormones and the milk supply may be affected. Because the cervix and vagina are enlarged after delivery, an old diaphragm may not fit properly and, therefore, will be ineffective and must be refitted. Natural family planning, which involves interpretation of the cycle and mucous secretions is not always possible until hormone levels have stabilized and several cycles have occurred. The only contraceptive choice in the immediate postpartum period may be the use of a condom with foam or gel, doubling the amount until involution is complete.

Special Care after Caesarean Birth

Although child birth is the main factor in planning care for all postpartum women, the mother who has had a caesarean birth has special needs related to her surgery and will require additional nursing considerations. After surgical birth the woman requires affirmation to reinforce her confidence and feelings of self worth.

The stress of childbirth is worsened when a woman is unprepared for a surgical procedure, additional anxiety, pain and frustration, or loss of self-esteem result. In the recovery period, some women state that they have little memory of the details of the surgical birth, especially if it was unexpected or an emergency. The nurse can arrange a time to review the experience with the new mother with questions such as the following:

- Tell me what you understand about what happened during surgery.
- Did you feel that you had unanswered questions?
- What could have the nurses done to make things easier for you?

Listen to the woman's feelings about her experience and encourage her to recount her perceptions and express excitement, pride, sadness, regret anger, or disappointment. There may be elements of the grieving process as she copes with the perceived loss of an active birthing experience. In the recovery period, the nurse emphasizes the woman's individuality and ability as a new mother. As she talks about her caesarean delivery the focus should be on achievement and the birth of her baby.

Postpartum "blues" are seen more often after surgical delivery because she is hospitalized longer than other mothers. The nurse assesses for excessive reactions and refers her for counselling if her coping mechanisms do not appear adequate. Follow-up care by telephone or home care visits is planned, and the mother is prepared for the fatigue and discomforts the new mother often feels at home and on her own with the new infant.

A father who needs to discuss his experience. The nurse offers understanding of the disappointment or even anger that he may feel and encourages communication with his partner to foster mutual support. Emphasize with his partner to foster mutual support, Emphasize the importance of his role as successful father, especially if the mother is unable to fully participate in infant care because of pain or limited mobility.

Complicated births often result in compromised infants who require special care in a neonatal intensive care unit (NICU). To the new parents this causes additional stress and a sense of loss because of fear for their baby's well-being and interruption of the normal bonding process. Encourage and assist them to visit the nursery to see, touch and participate as much as possible in care of their baby. If this is not possible, act as liaison between the parents and the NICU nurses to relay information about the infant's condition and progress.

Respiratory Needs

Discomfort from a surgical incision, especially a classic or vertical incision, and abdominal distention interfere with the mother's normal respiratory pattern. To prevent increased abdominal pressure, she avoids deep breaths and coughing, which result in decreased tidal volume, decreased air exchange, and accumulation of bronchial secretions. Complications that can arise are atelectasis and pneumonia.

As soon as possible, explain pulmonary exercises, assisting the woman to as high a Fowler's position as she can tolerate and offer her a pillow to hold across her abdomen while she coughs. Gentle pressure supports the abdominal musculature, decreasing pain and relieving anxiety that "the stitches will rip."

"Ladder" breathing or "huffing" before coughing is useful and an incentive spirometer will be ordered. These devices encourage deep breathing by having the client use her breaths to make a ball or gauge move. The deeper the breath, the more the ball rises, and the client can see results and work at her own pace, increasing respirations gradually as tolerated.

Pain medication is offered before begining respiratory therapy, with the explanation that it will help the woman with the activity. After an IM injection the wait is 15 minutes and after oral analgesics half a hour to allow for adequate absorption and action. Auscultate the lung fields before and after treatment to assess patency and air flow.

Recovery from Anesthesia

During the initial assessment the type and duration of anaesthesia are noted. Some womem will be groggy and confuse as they awaken from general anaesthesia. They may have been in labour a long time before the decision for caesarean birth was decided, and fatigue will be a major factor in their recovery. When an epidural has been planned for and understood, women may have a very smooth recovery period. Other women after regional block anaesthesia feel heaviness in the legs and have difficulty when first out of bed. The newly recovering woman should never get up alone and should sit on the side of the bed for a period to prevent orthostatic hypotension.

Circulation

After a complicated or surgical birth, ambulation may be difficult. When muscular activity is decreased or absent, venous return is decreased and stasis may occur. A state of increased viscosity from fluid losses and the temporary elevation in clotting factors in the immediate period have already occurred; these factors predispose the woman to the formation of phlebitis and thromboembolism.

The initial assessment reveals a history of or risk for thrombophlebitis or varicose veins. If complications require bed rest for even 1 or 2 days, preventive care includes isometric exercises and active range or motion. Be alert for complaints of pain in the legs; examine extremities for warmth, redness, and swelling, and assess for Homan's sign.

Obviously, the best prophylactic treatment plan calls for helping the woman walk as soon as possible.

For the client unable to ambulate early, leg movement, isometric exercises, and turning are encouraged. Anti-embolism stockings are applied to give support to the vein walls and thus aid blood flow. After caesarean or complicated deliveries, the woman may enter the unit with a counter pressure mechanical pump. The pump, connected to bandages or plastic sleeves over thrombo-embolic disease (TED) stockings, provides intermittent inflation to apply pressure needed to assist venous return. The nurse checks the settings, verifies the functioning of the system, and reassures the woman about the sensations she may experience.

Isometric exercises are initiated during early recovery. The woman can elevate her legs at home when sitting and avoid crossing her legs while lying or sitting. Describe the signs of phlebitis and emphasize the need to report any evidence to the physician.

Delayed Peristalsis

Intestinal peristalsis can be decreased by the action of anaesthetics, analgesics, altered food intake, and change in activity level. After a caesarean delivery, for example, it may take 24 hours for motility in the small intestine to resume and 3 to 5 days for complete function in the large intestine to return. Air and the breakdown of old materials in the colon produce flatulence and distension and thus pain and incisional discomfort because of increased pressure.

Small sips of water and ice chips may be allowed until bowel sounds are heard, and then the ordered diet is advanced slowly. The woman avoids iced and carbonated drinks that may increase flatulence. Early and frequent ambulation is encouraged to stimulate normal peristalsis. If a medication such as simethicone is ordered prophylactically, the client is instructed to chew the tablets thoroughly before swallowing.

Gas pains generally occur on the third postoperative day. The woman is advised to lie on her right side and to turn frequently to facilitate passing gas. The nurse may place a rectal tube to decompress the lower bowel or administer a Harris flush (return-flow enema) as ordered. The use of analgesics that further slow peristalsis is discouraged.

Evaluating outcomes within the short stay for birth must be directed toward the preparation for going home.

1. Have vital signs stabilized? Is involution pattern normal?
2. Can she demonstrate accurate self-assessment and care.
3. Does she exhibit confidence and competence in infant care?
4. Are there needs for referral?
5. Can she describe infant needs for nutrition, rest, sleep, activity, and safety? Have the parents obtained a car seat for going home?
6. Has she received follow-up literature and instructions in all areas of self-care including family planning?

CONTINUING CARE IN POSTPARTUM

Good aseptic technique during all procedures in the postpartum area is needed because, within the uterine cavity, easily accessible to micro-organisms from the exterior, is an open "wound" the former place of placental attachment. This diminishing but still easily infected area is well supplied with veins and arteries. It provides an ideal entry into the general body circulation and the possibility of septicaemia. Infection is still a threat if nurses are not enlightened and conscientious in their techniques.

Perineal Care

During the last 50 years postpartum perineal cleansing has been given in countless ways in maternity services across the nation. Techniques have ranged from the use of separate sterile irrigation setups by a masked nurse each time the procedure was needed to teaching the mother which way to wipe with a clean wash cloth. The acceptance of a technique should be based on its safety, adequacy, simplicity, expence, and aesthetic satisfaction for all concerned. The principles involved in perineal care should be the same whether it is done by the nurse or the patient herself.

Perineal cleansing is performed to prevent infection, eliminate odour, observe the area and lochial flow, and ease the patient. Any equipment used by one patient should be absolutely clean and should not be used by another. Reusable equipment should be sterilized between patients. Client should be taught in cleansing the perineum and in removing and applying perineal pads so that soil cannot be introduced to the vulva. This means, for both nurse and patient, wiping from front to back once only with each cleansing surface that is next to the perineum.

At least once each shift the perineum of the patient who gave birth vaginally should be observed for signs of trauma. A haematoma in the area may develop slowly. Sufficient light should be provided to see the area clearly. The perineal pad should be changed each time the toilet is used. Some maternity services issue plastic squeeze bottles for antiseptic solution or warm tap water plus cellulose wipes to each mother for self-care. Water temperature should be tested on the thigh or wrist to promote comfort and prevent burns. Other services issue pitchers and furnish appropriate solutions. Still others provide individually wrapped, moist towel impregnated with rapid-drying antiseptic. The use of a clean wash cloth when showering is appropriate, with the mother using only the front-to-back-motion.

In most instances, the mother is taught perineal cleansing for use after each trip to the bathroom. This should be continued at least twice a day until the lochial flow has stopped. If a bed rest regiment is necessary, the patient may be placed on a bedpan and warm water poured over her perineum, taking care to avoid entering the birth canal with the water. Then she may be patted dry front to back with clean tissue.

For patients who have episiotomies or laceration repairs, perineal care usually involves more than just cleansing. Many hospitals provide an antiseptic, analgesic benzocaine perineal spray such as Dermoplast. The physician may also order sitz baths to increase circulation and ease discomfort in the perineum. Maternity services may also offer a perineal lamp ("Perilight") several times a day for 20 minute intervals to improve circulation, promote healing, and ease discomfort. Lamps and sitzbaths are usually not offered until 12 hours after birth. If given too early, they may stimulate additional healing. This consideration may mean that many mothers will be discharged before any such treatments are received. When perineal lamps are used, care must be taken that they are no less than 18 inches of blondes, redheads, and other fairskinned women should always be draped before the lamp is used. This is a good time to observe the perineum.

Patients with standard episiotomies and first- and second degree lacerations usually respond well to the combination of cleansing heat lamp or sitz bath, and analgesic spray. However, at first many such women still would prefer to stand rather than sit. Advising the mother to tense her buttocks and touch in her pelvis before sitting down often lessens the pull and discomfort of the perineum.

Other local analgesics may also be ordered, such as dibucaine (Nupercainal) ointment and witchhazel compresses such as Tucks.

Mothers with third-degree perineal laceration (extending into the rectal sphincter) may need more help. Great caution must be exercised in giving patients who have such problems any type of enema, suppository, or cathartic if they are ordered. If the anterior rectal wall has also been torn (fourth-degree laceration) even more care is needed. Oral and topical analgesics may be ordered.

Occasionally, swelling of the perineal tissues is likely in a certain patient. An order for the application of cold compresses or ice packs may be written. An ice pack should be wrapped with clean, waterproof material and a fairly thin, absorbent outer layer and intermittently applied directly to the perineum. It may be held in place by its own attachments or by an encircling sanitary pad. Various commercial clean and sterile perineal ice packs are now available. They need to be fairly comfortable periods. If no such pads are available to the nurse, she may fill a rubber glove with cracked ice and water, close it tightly, and wrap it in a light, changed often. The perineal area should be observed frequently for developing haematoma or increased swelling. Application of ice is usually limited to the first 24 hours, when it is most effective in preventing oedema.

Ambulation

As previously stated, the ambulation of the postpartum patient is determined by the orders of the attending physician and depends on the type of anaesthetic given during delivery and the general condition of the patient. Early judicious ambulation of postpartum patients lessens the incidence of respiratory, circulatory, and urinary problems, prevents constipation, and promotes the rapid return of strength. When the patient is first allowed, out of bed, the nurse should not leave her along. These patients often become dizzy and faint. If the patient does become fait, she should be eased onto a chair her bed, or even gently to the floor. She should never be left alone. If she is on a chair, the nurse can support her while she lowers her head to her knees. No matter how many days postpartum, the nurse should always evaluate her ambulating patient.

The first time the postpartum patient gets up, she may experience a sudden, temporary gush of vaginal discharge. If it is dark red, it is probably not significant. It reflects the patient's change inposture after being recumbent for several hours when the uterine drainage was not as efficient. However, the patient should be evaluated for shock.

Bathing and Breast Care

Although a postpartum bed bath for patients who have delivered vaginally is not routinely done in all hospitals, cleanliness, comfort, and observation for infection must be prime considerations for the newly delivered mother. The postpartum patient is likely to perspire heavily. It is one way in which the body rids itself of excess fluids. A bed bath or shower should be offered in a timely manner.

If a bed bath is to be done, special attention should be given to the two areas that are easily infected the breasts and the perineum, which leads to the internal reproductive tract. If the patient delivered by caesarean, the incision line would constitute a third area susceptible to infection.

Postpartum Bathing Procedure

Whether the mother is to shower or to have a bed bath, she should be instructed in care of her breasts. Usually, only clear water is used in washing the breasts. Soap may have a drying effect and cause cracked nipples.

1. Wash in a circular manner from the nipple outward.
2. Dry the area carefully; if the mother is nursing, exposure of her nipples to air for short periods, (15 minutes) will help maintain healthy tissue.
3. Apply brassiere: All patients should have some type of adequate breast support and breast pads if needed.
4. Be sure the brassiere is large enough. The breasts should not be pushed down against the chest wall. The should be elevated and lifted toward the opposite shoulder.

While giving a bed bath, do not massage or rub the mother's feet or legs vigorously because of the danger of emboli. Perineal care is done as a separate procedure following the bath. At this time the principles of perineal self-care may be taught.

A brief description of the anatomy of the breast permits a greates understanding of the basics of breast care, the technique of nursing an infant, and the principles involved in pumping the breasts.

The breasts, or mammary glands, are divided into segments,or lobes which in turn are divided into lobules (smaller lobes). These contain the actual milk-producing glands known as *acini*, or alveoli. The breasts are richly supplied with blood vessels, lymphatics, and nerves.

Each segment of the breast radiates from the central coloured portion, known as the areola, which in turn rings the sensitive erectile tissue known as nipple. Milk ducts from the acini travel toward the areola and open out onto the surface of the nipples. Usually each nipple has 15 to 20 such openings.

As each major milk duct approaches the areola, it widens temporarily, forming a small reservoir, or sinus. When the baby begins sucking, oxytocin from the posterior pituitary is released. Its action stimulates the contraction of muscles around the milk ducts, allowing the milk to flow into the sinus to be readily available to the baby. The physiologic response is called the let down reflex. It may be accompanied by a tingling or shivering sensation. It occurs in both breasts, even though the baby is only nursing at one. The oxytocin also stimulates the uterine muscles to contract, thus lessening the possibility of haemorrhage and increasing the rapidity of involution. When a mother pumps her breasts manually, she obtain the best flow if she first presses the breast tissue back with her thumb and fingers and then squeezes the breast. Properly holding the breast with one hand during nursing not only allows the baby to breathe more comfortably but also encourages secretion of milk.

Breast Engorgement

Breast engorgement may occur about the third day postpartum and is often regarded by mothers as the result of the milk "coming in". However, the tenderness and swelling do not result entirely from the presence of more milk. Engorgement results, for the most part, from the increased venous and lymphatic congestion in the breast tissue.

Engorgement may be avoided or lessened by breast massage techniques and manual expression of colostrum during the prenatal period. It also will be greatly reduced or eliminated by frequent early (on-demand) feedings of the newborn. With engorgement the breasts may feel hard and nodular. People have called this "caked breasts", this uncomfortable and painful condition is sometimes eased for nursing mothers by the manual extraction of a small amount of milk. Good breast support worn continuously, warm, moist compresses, a warm shower, or the use of an oxytocin nasal spray prescribed to enhance the let down reflex and the flow of milk may be helpful. Analgesic drugs may also be prescribed to relieve the pain. Many medications can pass through the milk to the nursing infant with varying effects. A nursing mother should always check with her physician before taking medication.

Nonnursing mothers may be made more comfortable by snug breast binders, supportive bras, the application of ice "caps" to the breasts, and analgesics. The prescription of oral oestrogenic compounds, such as stilbestrol and chlorotrianisene, to suppress lactation is now infrequent and not recommended. The incidence of painful engorgement experienced by nonnursing mothers who did not receive such medications is low, and other means of treating the discomfort are preferable. Research indicates that a causal relationship may exist between the later development of endometrial cancer and the use of such substances. An increased occurrence of thrombo-emboli following the use of oestrogens, especially after caesarean birth, has been reported; therefore informed patient consent is required before oestrogens are given.

A nonhormonal drug, bromocriptine mesilate (Parlodel), which suppresses lactation by preventing the secretion of prolactin, is sometime prescribed. However, it has been associated with sudden episodes of hypotension, nausea and vomiting and other side effects.

Many physicians believe that the best therapies available relieve the discomfort of the nonnursing mother are the mechanical aids previously described plus the "tincture of time".

Pumping the Breasts

When the order is given for a mother's breasts to be pumped, it is usually done to maintain or encourage her milk supply. This procedure is not advised routinely to relieve engorgement in nonnursing mothers, because emptying the breasts stimulates more milk production.

A mother may pump her breasts manually as described or use a hand or electric pump. Whatever method is used, she should be supported comfortably in a sitting or side position with her hands and breasts freshly washed. Any equipment that touches her breasts should be sterilized before use. If the milk is saved for the baby, it should be collected in a sterile container, using aseptic technique. The mother should be instructed on how to empty her breasts using the method that is ordered preferred. If the electric breast pump is used, the nurse must make sure that the suction is not to great. It should be increased gradually. A record of the amount of milk obtained should be kept in the patient's chart. Mothers sometimes are distressed by the colour of their milk. They should be assured that although human breast milk looks more bluish than cow's milk, it is perfectly suited for the baby colostrum, the first secretion from the breast, is most creamy or orange in appearance.

Learning Infant Feeding

Formula Feeding

Emphasis today is placed on breastfeeding, and the nursing mother receives encouragement, support, and assistance. The woman who chooses to bottle feed has many needs as she begins caring for and satisfying her baby. If there is an apparent lack of understanding about how to do it, a young mother will become quickly frustrated if her baby does not resond to her efforts or is unsatisfied after a tense feeding time.

The mother is encouraged to ask questions and express concerns. Is she comfortable holding, offering the bottle to and bubbling the baby? The nurse stresses the importance of cuddling and eye contact during the feeding and observes for signs of attachment in her feeding behaviours. It should be reinforced that the method of feedig is not as important as the mother's and baby's satisfaction with the experience.

It is important not to appear judgmental of the woman who does not wish to nurse or she becomes frustrated with infant feeding. Those with low self-esteem often feel the baby "does not like me" if the infant is sleepy at feeding time or slow to such. The new mother needs positive reinforcement for her ability to decide how she wishes to feed her child and to learn the best ways to do so.

Benefits of Breastfeeding

In recent decades the popularity of bottle-feeding over breastfeeding has led to a gap in knowledge. Mothers and grand mothers cannot instruct their daughters in the art of breastfeeding, although there is increasing awareness that it is good for the baby.

Breastfeeding provides a unique bonding experience for mother and child. It stimulates most of the senses, and close body contact allows the baby to recognize its mother's small. The baby also can feel and hear the sound of her heartbeat, which is similar to the intrauterine environment.

Breastfeeding can and should be a satisfying experience for both mother and baby. The nurse needs to be prepared to support the decision to breastfeed. By acknowledging anxiety and frustration, offering needed assistance and direction, and praising successes the nurse aids in Empowering the new mother to overcome the possible difficulties that will be encountered in the first few weeks.

The scientific approach to breastfeeding is a relatively new field one that is constantly evolving. Thus some older theories and protocols such as limiting time one the breast at first, must be unlearned so that an improved approach may be used. It often is difficult to make changes in policy or in habits. By introducing new findings with confidence, the nurse can assist in improving care for breastfeeding women.

Before going home, the woman must have a basic understanding of the mechanism of lactation, She needs to know self-care, including breastcare, adequate nutrition, fluids and rest, and sources of support from other women.

I. Immunologic Benefits

Human milk is a biochemically unique substance perfectly adopted to the infant's needs. Colostrum is available to the baby for the first 2 to 3 days of life. It contains antibodies, depending on the maternal titres of antibodies, against organisms such as Staphylococcus, Salmonella, poliovirus, influenza virus, *Bordetella pertussis*, *Escherichia coli* and others. The newborn has immature antibody response until about 6 weeks of age. Without the protection of the antibody system the baby is vulnerable. In addition, before the system functions well in the gastrointestinal tract, large molecules of protein can reach the intestinal tissues of the formula fed baby and be absorbed into the intestinal tissues of the formula fed baby and be absorbed into the circulation, producing an immune response and predisposing the baby to an allergy to cow's milk. It has been estimated that 5 to 6% of all infants are sensitive to cow's milk. This allergy can cause eczema, vomiting, diarrhoea, diaper rash, and upper respiratory tract infections.

In the breastfeeding baby, however, the intestine is coated with immunoglobulins that were in the colostrum. Human milk has low allergenicity and contains a factor that promotes growth of *Lactobacillus bifidus*, which produces lactic and acetic acids in the gastrointestinal tract. These acids turn the stool acidic and provide additional protcction against the growth of enteric infections. The formulated baby has a more alkaline stool that does not have the same protective effect.

II. Nutritional Benefits

Breastmilk contains a proper amount of nutrients for an infant. There is a lower solute load and more unsaturated fatty acids. Proteins and fats are more easily digested, and carbohydrate content is appropriate for growth. When an infant is breastfed, problems caused by poor sanitation, lack of refrigeration, ignorance, or illiteracy are avoided. Finally for the baby, adequate protein intake is available even in a diet deficient environment.

III. Maternal Physiologic Benefits

Breastfeeding benefits not only the infant. There are also physiologic benefits for the mother. Nipple sucking by the breastfeeding infant stimulates the release of oxytocin from the posterior pituitary, which in turn causes the uterus to contract. Each time the infant nurses, the uterus contracts, hastening the descent of the uterus back into the pelvic cavity. The contraction of the uterus also reduces the possibility of postpartum haemorrhage, which can result from a relaxed uterus.

Breastfeeding requires the expenditure of a great deal of energy by the mother to produce milk, thereby helping the mother loss weight and return to her prepregnancy weight sooner.

Maternal Nutrition During Lactation

The nutritional status of the mother has no direct relation to the nutritional quality of breast milk instead, if nutritional intake is inadequate, there will be less MI but its quality remains stable. A lack of fluid intake also leads to reduced production of milk.

Human milk is very different from cow's milk in composition, all formulas must be modified to be as similar as possible to human milk (Table 6.5).

Table 6.5: Contrast between human and cow's milk concentrations

	Human	*Cow*
Calories	Higher	Lower
Protein	Lower	Higher
Fat	Higher	Lower
Carbohydrates	Higher	Lower
Calcium	Lower	Much higher
Phosphorus	Lower	Higher
Iron	Low	Only trace
Sodium	Lower	Higher
Potassium	Lower	Higher
Vitamin A	Higher	Lower.

A remarkable characteristic of human milk is its variation in concentration during the day. In addition, fore milk (available at the start of feeding) varies from hind milk (available at the end). Hind milk contains four to five times more fat than fore milk.

Levels of protein fat and carbohydrates are in the following ranges:

Protein	0.6-1.5 g/dl.
Fat	2.1-3.3 g/dl.
Carbohydrates	6.9-7.2 g/dl (lactose)
Water	87-95%.

Calories: During the first 2 weeks, an average of 600 to 650 ml/day is produced. As the baby matures, production rises to about 950 to 1000 ml/day. The mother uses 30 calories for every 30 ml of milk produced (there are 20 calories in 30 ml of breast milk). Stored maternal fat provides an extra 100 to 150 kcal per day for milk production in these first 3 months. There are, at first, the woman should add 500 calories to her baseline prepregnancy diet. After her weight has returned to its former level, she needs to take in about 750 calories over baseline (more if she is undernourished) to maintain caloric requirements for lactation.

Protein: Lactation requires an increase in protein of 15 to 20 g over baseline. During lactation the woman takes the same milk requirements (4 cups of whole milk), while will provide all the extra calories, protein and calcium can be used. The nurse should encourage her to include alternative sources in her diet.

A thin or malnourished woman may use extra milk to supply her increased protein and calcium intake. Protein needs may pose a problem for vegetarians. Many vegetarians allow protein increases when they understand the importance of the increase.

Other nutrients: Consumption of citrus fruits, vegetable oils, and green vegetables satisfies the increased need for ascorbic acid, iron, vitamin E, and folic acid. Dark-green and yellow vegetables provide vitamin A. The breast-feeding mother may continue to take prenatal vitamins.

Fluid intake: Because the lactating woman produces 900 ml or more of milk, she should receive at least that amount of extra fluid through her normal intake. The importance of fluids to a new mother should be stressed (see Table 6.6 for fluid and nutritional recommendations).

Table 6.6: Nutritional and fluid intake during lactation

Foot	*Amount for adult*
Milk	4 cups (5-6 cups for teenager)
Meat/meat substitutes	2 servings
Vegetables	2-3 servings
Fruits	2-3 servings
Breads	6 servings
Fluids	6-8 cups in addition to milk (noncaffeinated and water)

Precautions

A mother often asks whether she should omit any foods. There is no physiologic basis for avoiding certain foods, such as curry, garlic, or chocolate. Foods tolerated by the mother generally are tolerated by the baby. If there is a question about a food, the health care provider may advise omitting it on a trial basis.

Alcohol, too is secreted in milk. Empiric data indicate that a small glass of wine or a light beer is unlikely to affect the nursing baby and in a tired mother may assist the let-down reflex by increasing relaxation. Excess alcohol, however, may inhibit milk ejection. Larger quantity of alcohol have a dose response effect.

Smoking should be curtailed or eliminated during lactation. Passive smoking has been recognized as a major health problem, especially for young infants because of rapid absorption through the lungs. Smoking also reduces the volume of milk produced by affecting the release of prolactin and oxytocin.

Caffeine in large quantities can cause the mother and infant to be jittery, wakeful, and irritable. Caffeinated beverages (coffee, tea, soda) should be limited to two servings a day.

Preparation of Breasts

No special preparation of breasts is necessary. There is no need to toughen the nipples by rubbing, rolling or applying alcohol. In fact, these measures can irritate, injure, and dry the tissue. In addition, nipple stimulation may cause increased contractions during the last trimester. Colostrum that may ooze from the nipples in the last trimester may be washed away or rubbed into the nipple as a lubricant. Manual expression of colostrum is not necessary.

Breast size and nipple size vary widely and are not important to breastfeeding. The woman should be reassured that milk supply depends on breast mass but on the alveoli in the breast. Small, flat nipples are not a problem if the infant can latch on. To assess this, the woman can press the thumb and index finger in to the breast behind the nipple, if the fingers can grasp the nipple, the baby will be able to do so. Nipple that appear inverted often respond to pressure on the areola while the areola occasionally may be used. Only rarely do inverted nipples prevent lactation. Care must be taken not to allow too great a pressure that could immure the tissue.

Initiation of Feeding

Breastfeeding should be initiated as soon as possible after delivery. After the placenta is delivered and the mother is comfortable, the baby can be put to the breast for a few minutes. The infant may nurse enthusiastically of may just lick the nipple and not suck at all; however, this skin-to-skin contact is an intense bonding experience for a woman and her child. The mother and baby should not become chilled. A radiant warmer, if available, can be placed over the delivery table or in the recovery room.

Positions for Nursing

Common positions are the "Madonna hold" with the baby cradled in an arm the "football hold" in which the mother's arm supports the baby's head and back and the infant's body and legs are to the side and behind the mother, or side lying with the mother and infant facing each other. Side lying may be most comfortable for the woman who has had an episiotomy or a surgical birth.

Latching on, the ability of the baby to grasp the nipple, is the single most important aspect of breastfeeding. Regardless of position the baby must be lined up with the mother's body so that the head is directly in front of the breast and the nipple within easy reach. Pillows can be used to obtain this position. If necessary, the mother supports her breast with four fingers under and the thumb on top. Neigther the baby's head nor the breast should be moved to the side, or the neck will be extended, hyperextended, or turned, interfering with swallowing and also creating traction on the nipple tissue. With correct positioning the nipple is simply guided to the baby's open mouth for latching on.

Sucking and Swallowing

The sucking reflex is developed by week 34 of gestation, although small infants may become easily fatigued. Because sucking involves compression of the nipple and areola between the tongue and palate, the mouth must be open enough and the tongue positioned at the bottom of the mouth along the gum. The mouth must cover the nipple and at least 1 inch off the areola as well. This amount of breast tissue must be within the mouth that the laciferous sinuses can be compressed.

Swallowing is assessed after the first attempts at latching on. Swallowing should be quiet and rhythmic, quicker at first and slowing as the ejection of milk increases. Sucking or smacking noises or milk dribbling from the lips indicates incorrect attachment. The baby should be repositioned.

Timing of Feedings

Hungry babies should be fed on demand, usually even 2 to 3 hours at first. This means that newborns have feedings 8 to 10 times a day. The method of assessing intake is to examine the voiding and stooling pattern. If the baby wets clear urine and has soft, often pasty yellow stools, intake usually is sufficient. Hospital routines have interfered with lactation when babies were brought to the mothers every 4 hours. With rooming in the woman is free to observe signs of hunger and to respond. When the baby is sleepy or seems disinterested at first, gentle stimulation, unwrapping, or talking may awaken the infant to eat. To feed well, breastfed infants must be awake and interested.

Length of feeding sessions no longer is limited. Traditionally women were told to limit early feedings to 2 to 3 minutes on a side, building up time gradually. Because it takes at least 5 minutes of sucking to trigger the let down reflex in first-time mothers, limiting the time is self-defeating. The nipples will not become sore if the baby is correctly positioned and, therefore, not "chewing on the nipple". Instead the mother learns to recognize signs of satisfaction in the infant-slowing down in sucking and swallowing and finally falling asleep.

The mother who has had a caesarean birth or is very tired will need help in changing sides during feeding. Pillows can make both comfortable and perhaps a raised side rail can be used as a handle for turning.

Bubbling

Bubbling or burping the baby should be performed before the feeding to eliminate air in the stomach that might displace milk or cause it to bespit up. Often the baby has been crying or sucking the first and swallows air this way. If the baby sucks correctly, less air is swallowed. Usually women find it easiest to bubble the baby halfway through the feeding, while changing sides, or when the infant appears to slow down. Small amounts of undigested milk may be regurgitated (spit up) with the bubble. This is different from vomiting of partially digested milk.

Supplemental Feedings

Supplemental feedings adversely affect the establishment of the mother's milk supply. Therefore newborns should not be given supplemental feedings of glucose water or formula unless indicated by the medical condition of the mother or baby. In some states, with holding of supplementation for breastfeeding infants is mandated by state health policies. Early supplementation also may cause "nipple confusion" and result in the baby's refusal to breastfeed. Mothers are strongly encouraged in the initial establishment period of 2 to 3 weeks to only breastfeed until the milk supply is stable.

Variations for Multiple Births

A mother who breastfeeds twins will find that she has enough milk. Two babies sucking provide a tremendous stimulus to the breasts and milk production increases accordingly. The mother will need to greatly increase her fluid and caloric intake and be particularly aware of her own nutritional needs. Twins can be fed at the same time or alternative. If fed together, the mother will need initial help in positioning the babies.

Breastfeeding twins can be easier to manage than bottle-feeding them. Once a routine is established, nursing the two together can actually be simpler because both are satisfied at the same time. Many variations all of course possible. A number of mothers use both breast and formula, feeding the hungriest first on the breast then giving a bottle to the next. Some mothers change in the middle of the feeding, one hand giving a bottle to one while breastfeeding the other because it is awkward to feed both at the breast at the same time.

Caesarean Birth

Initially, breastfeeding can be more difficult after a cesarean delivery. With regional anaesthesia the mother should be encouraged to nurse as soon as she feels able, within several hours of delivery. After general anaesthesia the mother and baby will be groggy and, in the baby's case this grogginess may last several days. The nurse will need to spend time waking the baby up and geeting the mother into a comfortable position, she will probably be most comfortable in a side-lying position. She needs help in switching the baby from one breast to the other. Leaving the bed rails up can give her something on which to hold as she turns over.

Common Problems

Discomfort: Breast fullness The two human mammary glands are designed to provide enough milk to feed more than one infant. Because most women to provide enough milk to feed more than one infant. Because most women have only one baby at a time, there is an overabundance of milk, especially in the first 10 days. When the milk "comes in" about the third postpartum day, fullness occurs. Lactation specialists now differentiate between fullness and its more severe state, engorgement. Nurses often still refer to this first fullness as engorgement. Breasts are full, heavy, and uncomfortable. The mother usually can alleviate this fullness by nursing the baby frequently (q 2 to 3 hours) to empty the breasts, wearing a supporting brassiere, and applying warm compresses before feeding. Because milk supply works on a demand basis, once lactation has been established, the amount produced will decrease to the amount the growing baby needs.

Engorgement: Engorged breasts will look swollen and shiny. They feel hot, heavy, hard, or lumpy and may leak a little milk. The nipple recedes into the engorged breast, making it harder for the baby to latch on. The mother will complain of tenderness and pain in the breasts and nipples.

Engorgement is a result of insufficient emptying of the alveoli because of poor sucking, or infrequent or inadequate nursing. With milk backup clogging of ducts can occur and cause a predisposition to mastitis or breast abscess. If the baby cannot suck sufficiently to empty the breast then milk needs to be expressed from the breast either by hand or with a pump. Sore nipples are caused by poor latching on as a result of incorrect positioning, poor tongue placement, or traction on the nipple, sore nipples are directly related to the pressure on the nipple incorrectly placed in the baby's mouth. To prevent problems the following directions are helpful to the new mother:

- Express a few drops of milk before putting the baby to the breast
- Make sure the baby is properly fixed on the breast and is sucking on the areola
- Remember, the reflex takes several minutes to operate in the new nursing mother
- Nurse in differing positions so the pressure of suction affects a different portion of the nipple.
- Avoid pulling the baby off the breast; break the suction first.
- Expose the nipples and let them air dry for at least 10 minutes after feeding; the longer the better. Apply a few drops of breast milk before drying to aid in the healing process
- Keep nursing pads and bras dry at all times. Remove any plastic linings
- Avoid using soap on the nipples, instead apply pure lanolin or vitamin E oil
- Apply cold compresses or ice to the nipples if the pain is severe.

Plugged ducts: If undue pressure is applied to the breast, as from a poorly fitting brassiere or pressure of the baby's chin during nursing, stasis can occur in a duct. The water content of the milk there is absorbed by the tissue, leaving a thick viscous substance that irritates the tissue, inflammation occurs as a response (noninfective mastitis).

Mastitis: Mastitis is a bacterial infection of the connective tissue surrounding the breast glandular tissue and is not an infection of the glands or ducts themselves. The means by which bacteria gain entrance and colonize the tissue around the mammary gland are unknown. Sore, inflamed, or crackod nipples are thought to precipitate mastitis. Most likely, bacteria shared between the infant's oropharynx and the maternal areola gain entrance through small cracks or fissures within the areola and cause infection. *Staphylococcus aureus*, group A and B streptococci, or other skin or mouth flora generally are believed to cause mastitis.

Infective mastitis occur infrequently in 0.8% to 2.5% of lactating women. Symptoms usually occur within the first 2 weeks after birth, with another peak 5 to 6 weeks later. Delay of more than 24 hours in initiating antibiotic treatment may contribute to abscess formation.

Signs: Women with mastitis usually note breast tenderness or pain localized to one specific area. In addition, general malaise, fever often higher than 101°F, increased pulse rate, and local erythema and warmth may be present. Complaints of flu-like symptoms in the postpartum or breastfeeding woman should always initiate evaluation for some type of postpartum infection. Catecholamines released in response to pain may inhibit the let down reflex and disturb breast-feeding. Symptoms usually improve within 36 to 48 hours of antibiotic treatment.

Clinical management: Care includes antibiotic therapy, analgesia, education, and support for continued breastfeeding. Antibiotic choices include oral dicloxacillin, a cephalosporin, or erythromycin if the woman is allergic to penicillin. Continuation of breastfeeding is strongly encouraged by use of both the affected and unaffected breasts. There appears to be no additional risks to the newborn in as much as the bacteria causing the infection probably are part of the newborn's normal oropharyngeal flora.

Although mastitis is not a contraindication to breastfeeding, an abscess is. The baby should not nurse on the affected side but may continue on the unaffected side. The abscessed breast can then be emptied by pumping until the infection is resolved. The mother should be instructed that the full course of antibiotic therapy must be completed, usually 10 to 14 days.

The best way to treat these conditions is to be sure the breasts are empty after each feeding. The woman can assist this process by taking a warm shower or applying warm compresses before feeding and gently massaging the breast. Severe discomfort may be relieved by lying in a hot bath on the affected side and allowing the breast to float. Milk may then be expressed into the hot water. Because of oedema associated with mastitis and abscess, milk flow will be impaired and increased sodium content in the milk may taste unpleasant to the infant. Even though the affected breast is offered to the infant, it may be refused; a breast pump is then used to empty the breast.

Maternal illness: In the past the mother was not allowed to breastfeed if her temperature had become elevated over 100.4° F in the previous 24 hours. Today, on the basis of the understanding that dehydration, fatigue and early healing processes may elevate temperatures in the first 24 hours, most infants are at the breast as soon as is feasible. Colostrum contains helpful antibodies, and the infant may have already been exposed in utero to the mother's early signs of an infection. Only in the presence of active tuberculosis, hepatitis B, human immuno-deficiency virus (HIV), chickenpox, or high fever of unknown origin is breastfeeding interrupted. Urinary tract, respiratory tract or local infections are not indications to stop, especially if treatment with antibiotics has begun. Nursery staff personnel, however, need to know the current temperature and condition of the mother and take precautions to avoid the spread of infection to other babies in the nursery. Other conditions interfere if the mother is unable to care for herself or the baby because of recent anaesthesia, pain or weakness.

Breast infections: Infections of the breast are not as common today as formerly, but occasionally they still occur. Most infections are introduced at the nipple area, which may be fissured or cracked because of poor nursing techniques or exceptionally fragile breast tissue. Because of early discharge practices, such a complication is usually not found while the patient is in the postpartum area. It becomes the subject of an office call and rarely an admission to another part of the hospital for excision and drainage of an abscess. Fortunately, most cases of mastitis do not progress as far as abscess formation. The nurse should always observe the patient's breast or inquire about their condition. Signs of inflammation or cracked and bleeding nipples should always be reported. Breast infections are most often caused by the organism *Staphylococcus aureus*. The application of cold or heat to the breast may be ordered. The treatment prescribed depends on the stage of the infection and any organism cultured. Systemic antibiotics are commonly given. Nursing the infant is usually continued, although opinions differ regarding the advisability of continuing breastfeeding until the infection subsides. An antibiotic is chosen that is not harmful to the infant.

Elimination: Constipation, caused by diminished intestinal and abdominal muscle tone, may be a problem to the postpartum patient. Physicians often order a mild laxative the evening of the first or second postpartum day. If this medication does not produce results, a suppository or a gentle enema is often scheduled. Since many of these patients have haemorrhoids or adjacent episiotomy or laceration repairs, one must be careful when inserting the suppository or well lubricated enema tip. Early ambulation, increased fluids, and a diet containing roughage and cereal food fibre may prevent constipation. If stools are difficult to pass, a stool softener may be prescribed. During the secondary the patient may experience diuresis with a urinary output as high as 3,000 ml.

Supportive Care and Educational Opportunities

Aims of Postpartal Hospitalization

The Postpartal hospital stay should ideally provide safety, rest, constructive encouragement, and instruction for the recent parturient, as well as opportunities to initiate parent-infant attachment. However, in some areas the actual hospitalization period is so brief that it is difficult to realize the ideal. Discharge on or before the second postpartum day is almost routine in many parts of the United States, and short stays of 24 hours or less are frequent. The pendulum has swing a long way from 40 years ago, when 5 to 10 days passed before the new mother stirred from her ged.

The need for a swing in the pendulum of postpartum management is not debated. Certainly early ambulation and self-care techniques have reduced the incidence of many complications associated with prolonged bed rest, such as thrombophlebitis, pneumonia, and subinvolution of the uterus. However, the shortened postpartal stay necessitates a prenatal reevaluation of the needs of the new mother and her provisions for help in the home setting. The average primipara has had less opportunity than her counterpart of past generations to learn the art of child care in her own family circle while growing up. Often her first responsible contact with a newborn infant arrives the day she takes her own baby home from the hospital unless she has had the benefit of rooming in with her baby. Many times she has adequate and loving help at home. Too many times she does not.

Education Resources

There do not seem to be enough hours in the hospital day to teach a new mother what she needs to know about herself and her baby and to give her sufficient time to regain her strength and composure. Of course, for multiparas, perhaps education needs are not as great, but in these days of early discharge most primiparas cannot gain the desired assurance even if hospital classes and practice sessions could be held all day long and they could attend them all.

At present one answer seems to lie in the introduction of parentcraft courses into the regular school curriculum. Also, greater use of the prenatal and postnatal courses offered by such community agencies as adult school programme, childbirth education associations, YWCA, Red Cross, and public health departments and greater involvement by the visiting nurse should be encouraged. More single room care facilities in hospitals, an increased awareness by all postpartum staff members of their teaching roles, and the possibility of family telephone contacts and home visitations with postpartum and nursery representatives following discharge are needed.

Parent Education Needs or Teaching Topics

1. Recognition of postpartum complications and what is normal.
2. Perineal and breast care.
3. Fluid needs, nutrition, and weight loss.
4. Rest and exercise.
5. Birth control concerns (if wished).
6. Anticipating and dealing with "postpartum blues."
7. Physician's appointment.
8. Prevention of infection.
9. Infant care and feeding.
10. Prevention no accidents.
11. Coping mechanism-support groups.

The nurse may not find herself involved in any formalized classroom teaching, but the quality of nursing care given, the importance she place on personal hygiene (her own and her patient's), and the skill she develops in observing, listening to, and responding to her patient's needs will make her an important teacher nonetheless, with the use of primary nursing and care of the mother and infant together, opportunities for teaching a mother to care for her own infant are increased.

Of course, in places where postpartum stays are longer and facilities and staff are available, actual classes in baby care, bathing formula preparation and nursing techniques may be offered to mothers. Some maternity departments have started closed circuit television classes. If the prerequisites are present, the maternity department should not neglect its opportunity.

At her arrival on the postpartum unit, the mother's needs should begin to be assessed. It is important to focus on the individual mother's needs. Since the time available is often short. After teaching, it is important to gain feedback from the mother to evaluate what she has learned. Listening to the mother describe lessons in her own words or observing her as she performs the skill are two ways to evaluate her learning.

Family centred postpartum care makes it possible for both parents to get to know their baby and to begin functioning as a family unit under the guidance of skilled maternity nursing personnel. This is also an especially adaptable method for providing learning opportunities for the mother and whatever extended family is present. Because the baby is cared for at the mother's bedside, she has an opportunity to observe and ask questions of the nurse. Both the father and the mother (when she feels strong enough) may choose to participate in the care of their child. Visiting regulations vary in different hospital settings; however, siblings and other family members are often encouraged to visit and hold the new family member. Careful attention must be paid that good handwashing is done by anyone touching the baby. Cover gowns may or may not be used, as dictated by hospital policy. Multiple studies have shown no increased infection rate when gowns are not used.

Family centered care, unlike the rooming in concept is a flexible concept of individualized care, which permits the parents to share the childbearing experience and to have access to their baby during the postpartum period to the extent they desire. This does not preclude the baby from being taken to a nursery when the parents so wish.

Continued Care and Support

The new mother usually has many questions, some of which the nurse will be able to answer immediately. Others she must refer to the physician.

One of the first things the mother wishes to investigate after she has seen her baby and recovered some of her strength is her own weight loss. She is usually dissatisfied with her initial loss the first time she steps on the scale. She needs to be reassured that under normal conditions she will approximate her pre-pregnant weight in about 1 month. However, to regain a good figure, she must regulate her caloric intake to her metabolic needs. The weight gained during pregnancy in normal conditions is caused by the size of the infant, the weight of the placenta (about 1 pound), the amniotic fluid (about 2 pounds) the increased size of the uterus (about 2 pounds), breast enlargement (about 3 pounds), and increased circulating and tissue fluids and reserves.

Sometimes students are taken a back when they see postpartum patients ambulating for the first time. They confide to one another that Mrs. Lalitha does not look as though she has delivered yet. Multiparas, because of the repeated stretching of the abdominal muscles, particularly need time and effort to regain a nonpregnant shape. Occasionally a hernia develops because of the separation of the rectus abdominis muscles, which are supposed to support the abdominal contents. The condition adds to the "pregnant look." A number of years ago the use of straight or many tailed scultetus abdominal binders for support were common. Now they are seldom binder is ordered in the postpartum period, it should be applied upside down with the wrapping starting at the top to avoid forcing the uterus up and out of place.

Now a days it is thought better to rely on the abdominal muscles for support and to build up their strength instead of advocating indiscriminate use of abdominal binders. Various postpartum exercises are recommended to restore muscle tone as well as improve circulation, promote involution and regain general strength. These exercises are graded according to difficulty, ranging from deep breathing and gentle range of motion to pelvic tilts, leg lifts, and modified sit-ups. The progression of exercise should be directed by the attending physician because some may be too strenuous or even dangerous if done too early. (The knee-chest position done in early puerperium has been associated with a few cases of air embolism).

Mothers often ask what they may do when they return home. They should be advised to increase their activities gradually and to avoid fatigue, lifting heavy objects and older children, and climbing stairs. They should be encouraged to have midmorning and midafternoon rest periods and arrange to have extra help at home. Newly delivered mothers have a tendency to try to do too much and then to regress it. Even while mothers are in the hospital the provision for rest is sometimes limited. Nurses should make every effort to provide their patients with a restful environment and periods of relaxation. Showers and shampoos at home are allowed as soon as desired. Many physicians allow tub bathing equally as early. Douching should be deferred until after the routine postpartum examination by the physician in 3 to 6 weeks. If it is resumed at all. The physician's advice should be sought regarding resumption of sexual intercourse. Couples are usually asked to wait until lochial discharge has stopped and discomfort has been minimized. Methods of contraception may need to be discussed.

In the interim women should be encouraged to contact their health care providers if any problems arise. Accessible and knowledgeable nursing staff members, a good physician-patient chat, and the distribution before discharge of printed instructions and hints for a smooth adjustment to life with the baby solve some of the predictable difficulties. Problems that should be reported when the patient notes them include pain or localized tenderness in the legs, increased vaginal flow, painful breasts or cracked nipples, painful urinatioin, backache, and fever.

In nonnursing mothers, menses usually return in 5 to 8 weeks. The nursing mother may not experience menstruation until several weeks after the weaning of her infant. This does not mean, however, that she cannot become pregnant during this period. Success in nursing the infant may be enhanced by support groups and sponsored food supplementation programme for women, Infants and children.

Discharge of the Mother and Child

The discharge of the mothers and child from the maternity service is an exciting time for the family. A calm and, literally, collected patient the morning of discharge is the exception despite all efforts to smooth the departure. Before the patient leaves, any instructions that are to be carried out after discharge concerning the mother or baby must be clarified. Great care should be taken that all her belongings leave with her.

The baby is identified again and dressed for the short trip outdoors to the car. The mother is usually discharged in a wheelchair. For maximum safety, the baby should ride home in an approved infant seat, not in his mother's arms.

Special Considerations

Postpartum haemorrhage, the most common serious problems in the postpartum period, has been previously discussed. Preeclampsia-eclampsia has been discussed.

Caesarean birth patient: If a cesarean birth is anticipated, the mother may be admitted initially to the postpartum unit and prepared for surgery by its staff. For a review of what this preparation entails and other related information.

Nursing care postsurgery: The physical care of the post-caesarean-birth patient is similar to that of any patient who has had abdominal surgery. However, in addition, this patient has become a mother. She requires special attention to her postpartal needs.

Immediate observation: Blood pressure, pulse, and respiration rate should be taken at least every 15 minutes for a minimum of 2 hours and until stable. A falling blood pressure and a rising pulse are among the first signs of difficulty. Other signs of shock include pallor, cold, clammy skin, apprehension, disorientation or unresponsive behaviour, and dilated pupils. But do not wait to observe all the classic signs of shock before seeking help. The dressing should be observed for drainage and any staining reported. The lochia must be observed and any staining reported. The lochia must be observed and evaluated. As a rule caesarean with patients have less lochial flow. After the placenta is extracted during surgery, the uterus is inspected and gently sponged, emptying the cavity of some of the drainage that would otherwise sponged, emptying the cavity of some of the drainage that would otherwise be expelled vaginally. The fundus may be gently palpated after surgery to determine its position, but it should not be massaged routinely.

The patient usually receives intravenous fluids during the first 24 to 48 hours. The first ordered fluids may contain an oxytocic to cause the uterus to contract. The intravenous infusion should be frequently observed for rate of flow and signs of infiltration. An indwelling Foley catheter is usually maintained for 12 to 24 hours or until the IV fluids are discontinued. The catheter should be checked for the rate of flow and the type of urine being expelled. The tubing must be stabilized, without dependent loops. Routine temperature checks are resumed.

Pain control and psychologic postpartal support: Timely analgesia makes the recent caesarean birth patient much more comfortable. The nurse must be attentive to the patient's needs. A variety of medications and methods of administrations may be used. Intermittent intramuscular injections have been traditional. However, today patient controlled analgesia (PCA) by intravenous route or epidural narcotic administration just before the removal of the indwelling epidural catheter following surgery may be alternatives.

Although the initial physical care of the new caesarean birth mother is perhaps the primary priority, the emotional and maternal needs of the patient must not be forgotten. According to her strength and desires, she should be given opportunity to see, handle, and nurse her infant. Communication with the nursery should be frequent. If the infant can be brought to the bedside for care, perhaps this should be recommended. Often this patient feels very isolated and fearful regarding her offspring.

Dietary Considerations

Although orders may vary considerably, at first the new caesarean birth patient is usually given nothing by mouth, and then she is gradually given a progressive surgical diet based on her toleration of oral feeding. This means progressing from sips of water to clear liquid, to a soft diet, and then to a regular diet, over a period of approximately 2 to 3 days. Because of their reputations as gas-formers, milk, ice water, and citrus juices are often omitted from the diet along with other notorious food stuffs such as green peppers, cauliflower and brussels sprouts. Some observers believe that drinking through straws may also increase flatus. A new surgical patient or one with an IV infusion or an indwelling catheter should have intake and output determination taken and recorded.

Ambulation

Although orders to ambulate the patient may not be written until the day after caesarean birth, planned movement in bed should be carried out.

The patient is periodically encouraged to breathe deeply and cough as soon as she is put to bed from surgery. She is turned at least every 2 hours. How long she remains flat depends on the anaesthetic used, her general condition, and her physician's orders. When she is first allowed out of bed, she should briefly dangle her feet and then stand and mark in place only, during the second attempt, she should walk with the nurse's support. Walking the patient to a chair two steps away for a 15 minute period of sitting is not considered the best interpretation of "ambulate the patient". The sitting position does not aid the circulation in the lower extremities. It is important to follow orders for progressive ambulation should not be carried out. The nurse does not need to reiterate all the complications the physician seeks to avoid by early ambulation. Usually if the nurse simply states that it will help the patient feel stronger faster and prevent or relieve flatus, this provides the needed motivation.

Some physicians are allowing some caesarean section patients to shower relatively soon after delivery, with a plastic protector over their abdominal dressings.

Abdominal Distention

Abdominal distention caused by trapped flatus can be distressing to any patient who has undergone abdominal surgery. Frequently, it is the chief complaint of the caesarean birth patient. Although medications such as morphine or meperidine hydrochloride (Demerol) may be used for postoperative pain, it is still better to prevent or eliminate the distention. As part of her care, the nurse evaluates the condition of the abdomen. Is the area just above the dressing hard, bloated, and tender, or is it soft and relatively flat? Ambulating the patient may relieve distention, so may intermittent, small enemas, the Harris flush technique, or insertion of a rectal tube. Also helpful are suppositories, laxatives, or the use of neostigmine. Occasionally, strange to say, the use of carbonated drinks allow the patient to "bring up air" more easily and gain relief. In severe cases a nasal gastric tube connected to suction may be inserted.

Sutures

The caesarean patient receives perineal irrigations for cleanliness and comfort, but no sprays or head lamps are used, since no suturing or trauma occurred in the perineum. Abdominal sutures clips or adhesive "butterflies" are usually removed about the fifth or sixth postoperative day.

Complications

Caesarean births result in a relatively low maternal mortality. Neonatal mortality however is higher. The results depend on the condition of the mother and the foetus, the equipment available, and the skill of the operator and nursing staff. Related maternal problems reported include sepsis, haemorrhage, thrombus formation, embolism, and complications of anaesthesia, occasionally abibrinogenaemia, causing bleeding problems, complication the recovery.

The Sorrowing Mother

Not all mothers admitted to the postpartum area leave with healthy babies. Some leave without a child because the infant did not survive birth or died in the early hours of life. Some leave alone because their infant is premature or has some abnormality. It is especially and when a new mother who has waited for her child with anticipation finds that for all are waiting and care, she has either no child or a child with gross deformities. Parents need each other at this time. For the nurse to give parents the support they need in this crisis, she must acknowledge her own feelings. Only then can she really begin to understand the parents reactions. Nurses are in a position to give a great deal of help and support to parents during infant sickness or death. Most parents have an overwhelming need to talk about the experience and should be allowed to do so with whomever they choose. Some of the things a nurse can do to facilitate the parent's acceptance of the deformity or death are showing concern, allowing the parents to cry, relaxing visiting hour regulations, supporting the parents in their need to see and touch the infant, providing adequate and appropriate information, and allowing expressions of anger (recognizing these to be part of the grief process). Listening is probably the most important part of emotional support; platitudes are not helpful. Groups of bereaved parents are being organized in some settings to allow parents to share feelings and benefit from group counsel. Supportive nurses who are available, who listen, who recognize the stages of mourning, and who respond to the patient's cues, by touch or voice, will be much appreciated.

Some mothers leave the maternity area without babies because they are not keeping their infants. If a mother is planning to give up her baby for adoption, the nursing staff should be alerted regarding her wishes for infant care and comfort. An emotionally healthy mother with support of friends and family may work through the crisis better when give an opportunity to perform care taking activities for her baby.

Nurses on the postpartum unit should be in contact with the nursery when a baby is not "doing well". Team members need sharing of information by everyone working with the family. Early parental contact with the infant usually should be encouraged. Referral to helping agencies may be needed.

Maternal Postpartal Challenges and Tasks

It has been said that all postpartum patients, regardless of their different individual backgrounds and specific strengths and problems, must respond successfully to certain challenges related to changes in body image, roles, and responsibilities before they can develop a satisfactory sense of progress, wellness, and fulfillment "The nurse and maternal tasks of early postpartum, "speaks of the mother's need to review and integrate her childbirth experience into her total self-concept and to put a side the fantasies that she may have entertained regarding her unseen baby by identifying, claiming, and learning to care for her real infant. It indicates that as the mother adapts to the reality of her changing body and her new role as both mother and mate, she is performing a type of necessary "grief work", the nurse can be an important force helping the mother cope with these changing perceptions and developing "duties" in a realistic and successful manner.

Postpartum Blues

As the body hormonal levels change and the responsibilities of an enlarging family and infant care suddenly make themselves felt, many new mothers experience some degree of transitory depression commonly called "post-partum blues", The nurse may enter a patient's room for a routine check and find the previously exuberant mother wiping away tears. While providing tissues and gently asking what she may do to help, the nurse is often told that the patient does not really know why she is crying. "The tears just come." The knowledge that many mothers sometimes are bit depressed during the week after childbirth is usually reassuring to the patients.

Postpartum Depression and Psychosis

Labour and birth often comprise a physically and emotionally exhausting period even for the normal healthy woman. For a small but seemingly growing minority of women, the weeks following delivery represent a special period of unresolved stress that can result in progressive symptoms of mental disorder. For some the intensity of their distress may eventually bear the label of "postpartum psychosis." These mothers become withdrawn and uninterested or belligerent and suspicious. They are often victims of unreasonable fears. In severe cases they may become dangerous to themselves and others.

Because of increasingly early discharge practices, the nurse in the hospital setting rarely sees the anxiety and developing delusions described. The causes of these disturbances are probably long-standing and multiple, including physiologic and psychosocial factors. The crises of parenthood may serve as only the triggering mechanism for the maladaptive patterns of behaviour observed. Often these patients have had histories of previous emotional instability or illness. The fourth postpartum week is a common time for the onset of signs and symptoms. Much more needs to be learned about this condition and its origins.

Identifying and Caring for Women with Postpartum Psychological Complications (Table 6.7)

Purpose

All women should be assessed for postpartum psychological complications. Early detection and intervention might prevent an escalation of psychological problems. Educating the patient and her family about the emotional responses possible during the postpartum period prepares them to recognize and report changes that may be associated with postpartum psychological complications.

Table 6.7: Nursing care for woman with postpartum psycological complications

Nursing action	*Rationale*
1. Assess mother's interaction with her infant, including attachment, emotional responses, and caretaking behaviours	Psychological complications may interfere with the maternal-infant attachment process as well as with a mother's ability to provide appropriate newborn care
2. Facilitate positive mother-infant interaction and provide the new mother with positive reinforcement: • Show the mother how the baby responds to her voice • Point out familial characteristics of the baby • Educate the mother on the sleep-wake cycles of the baby and on the best times to interact with the baby • Encourage eye-to-eye contact between mother and baby • Encourage maternal touch and stroking of infant	Facilitating positive mother-infant interaction and providing positive reinforcement will promote the desired behaviours
3. Evaluate mother's perceptions of the maternal role and how that role fits with her other roles. Discuss with the mother and her partner what they expect the next few weeks to be like at home	The new mother and her family need support and educational guidance with role transition to new parent as well as with integration of the new role into other roles, including spouse and career
4. Assess the mother's individual coping skills and the adequacy of her family support system by having her identify those persons who are available to provide support	Lack of adequate emotional support or dys-functional family relationships could interfere with maternal adjustmentduring the postpartum period
5. Observe the mother for signs and symptoms of psychological complications, including: • Alterations in sleeping and eating • Extreme fatigue • Tearfulness, irritability, mood swings, anxiety behaviours, agitation • Detachment from reality, thought disturbances, hallucinations • Feelings of helplessness, inability to cope with activities of daily living	Individual manifestations of depression or psychosis vary
6. Initiate appropriate referrals on the basis of individual needs: • *Psychiatric consultation*: To diagnose the disorder and make recommendations for further care • *Professional counseling*: To provide ongoing support and measures To cope with depression • *Social services*: To coordinate referrals at discharge and assist with the mother's immediate financial needs • *Public health nurse*: To asses the home environment and provide nursing care after discharge • *Community support groups*: To provide opportunities to share experiences with families in similar situations so that the mother does not feel isolated and alone • *Mental health clinics*: To provide ongoing psychological follow-up	A multidisciplinary approach is needed to ensure appropriate therapy for the mother and her family
7. Document in nurse's notes the woman's affect (e.g., flat, elated, withdrawn) and whether appropriate maternal-infant interactions are observed. Document that education was provided to the patient regarding signs psychological complications. Healthy lifestyle and symptoms of postpartum blues; signs and symptoms of postpartum depression; when to call her doctor; and the importance of exercise, communication with family, getting sleep, and eating a balanced diet	Education about signs and symptoms of postpartum blues and depression prepares the patient and her family to recognize and report changes that may be associated with postpartum behaviours promote a state of positive wellbeing

Puerperal Infection (Table 6.8)

The term "puerperal infection" may be used to describe any infection of the reproductive tract during the puerperium. In the past, a patient has been considered to have a puerperal infection if she has a temperature of 100.4°F (38°C) or more on 2 successive days during the first 10 days postpartum, excluding the first 24 hours unless another source of the temperature is determined. Now with early discharge and frequent use of antibiotics, some authorities define a puerperal infection differently using various criteria (such as temperature elevations of more than 101° F after the second day, signs and symptoms of infection, or a positive culture).

The appearance of a puerperal infection is always a serious development. It may involve the perineum proper, the uterine lining (endometritis), or the pelvic area outside the uterus (parametritis). It may extend by means of blood vessels and lymphatics to areas relatively far removed, as in the case of septic thrombophlebitis of the leg. It is most often localized, but it can become a generalized peritonia or septicaemia.

Although the classic causative organisms implicated are the streptococi and *Staphylococcus aureus*, puerperal infections may be caused by multiple organisms. Many times the bacteria that invade the uterine wound at the former site of the placenta and produce infection are those also commonly found in the intestines or colonized on the cervix, vagina, and perineum of the patient without causing any local tissue invesion or damage.

The incidence of puerperal infection is thought to be infuenced by numerous factors, including the length of time the bag of waters has been ruptured before delivery, the number of cervical examinations performed, the types and number of incisions and lacerations, and the general health of the mother. Delivery by caesarean section has been associated with higher rates of infection than vaginal birth. The use of prophylactic antibiotics before and/or after surgery has decreased infection rates markedly.

If puerperal sepsis is diagnosed in the caesarean birth patient, all efforts should be made to determine the original source of the infection. This would involve a knowledge of the patient, the personal health of attending personnel and visitors, and nursing and modified techniques used careful handwashing and aseptic techniques continue to be an important priority.

Accompanying Signs and Symptoms

Along with the appearance of fever, pelvic infection is often accompanied by abdominal tenderness or pain, foul-smelling lochial drainage, an abnormally large uterus, and the presence of chills. The patient may complain of general malaise and lack of appetite and display a rise in pulse rate. Such signs and symptoms should be reported immediately. Detection of a puerperal infection should initiate isolation procedure and perhaps even the removal of the patient from the maternity service proper. Such a diagnosis may also affect the nursing procedures in the care of the infant.

Identifying and Caring for Women with Postpartum Infection (Table 6.8)

Purpose

All women should be assessed for postpartum infection. The presence of certain risk factors, however, makes some women more likely to experience this complication. Early detection and intervention can help prevent worsening of the condition.

Treatment of a case of puerperal infection depends on the extent of involvement. Antibiotics to which the causative organisms are sensitive are ordered. In case of pelvic infection the patient most often is placed in owler's position to encourage drainage of the affected area.

Extension of Infection

Observation for signs of the extension of the infection or generalized peritonitis should be constant. Such indications are increased abdominal tenderness and distension, and nausea and vomiting, as well as those previously listed.

Thrombophlebitis (Table 6.9)

Not all cases of thrombophlebitis involve the presence of infection, but many do. Clots may form anywhere in the body where a slowdown in circulation, a repair of damaged tissue, or plugging of bleeding vessels occurs. During the postpartum period, clots or thrombi may form in the pelvis or the lower extremities. They may localize and

Table 6.8: Nursing caring for women with postpartum infection	
Nursing action	*Rationale*
1. Identify factors that predispose the woman to the development of a postpartum infection	Numerous risk factors predispose a woman to postpartum infection, including prolonged rupture of membranes, traumatic or operative delivery, labour longer than 24 hours, anaemia, postpartum haemorrhage, and diabetes
2. Obtain and record the woman's temperature in the first hour after delivery. Recheck temperature according to hospital policy. Notify the physician of temperature above 100.4º F (38ºC). Administer antipyretics as ordered	Temperature elevations in the postpartum period may be due to dehydration or infection. Antipyretics, whether pharmacologic or nonpharmacologic (e.g., cool cloths), reduce fever
3. Observe the woman for signs and symptoms of a postpartum infection, including: • Elevated temperature • Increase in pulse rate • Foul-smelling lochia • Complaints of pain or tenderness at site of infection • Infection site that is red and warm to touch • Drainage of pus or blood, or separation of incision site • Malaise, chills, backache, headache	Signs and symptoms of postpartum infection vary with its location and the infective organisms
4. Obtain laboratory tests as ordered by the physician. Laboratory tests may include culture and sensitivity, complete blood count, and chest radiograph. Review all laboratory findings and report abnormalities to the physician	Cultures are done to identify the infective organism so that appropriate antibiotic therapy can be initiated. The white blood cell count normally increases in the postpartum period. To identify an abnormality, look for upward trends or for an increase of more than 30 percent in the white blood cell count during a 6 hour period. (Normal values may be as high as 25,000/mm^3 to 30,000/mm^3 on the first postpartum day. On the second postpartum day, nomal values decrease, ranging from 6,000 to 10,000/mm^3. Values return to normal 4 to 7 days postpartum. A chest radiograph is obtained to rule out pneumonia or pulmonary tuberculosis
5. Start antibiotic therapy according to the physician's orders	Antibiotic therapy based on culture and sensitivity reports is the recommended treatment of postpartum infections
6. Ensure adequate fluid and nutrient intake. Monitor intake and output	Adequate fluids, nutrition, and rest are therapeutic measures that contribute to the return to a healthy state. Continuous monitoring of intake and output gives the nurse information needed for determining whether the patient is dehydrated, well hydrated, or overhydrated (fluid overload)
7. Encourage ambulation balanced with adequate bed rest.Administer analgesics as needed	Ambulation to promote circulation, respiratory clearing, and a feeling of well-being, should be balanced with bed rest so that the woman does not get fatigued. Analgesics reduce fever and provide some relief for muscle aches
8. Instruct the woman in proper pericare techniques, wound care, disposal of contaminated items, and importance of hand washing	Infection control measures are essential to prevent the spread of infection
9. Assess the need for a breastfeeding mother to pump her breasts and discard milk to maintain lactation until she can resume breastfeeding	Maternal condition or the specific type of antibiotic ordered might prevent breastfeeding or feeding the baby mother's breast milk in a bottle. Pumping must be done early and on a regular basis to initiate and maintain lactation

Table 6.9: Nursing care for woman with thrombophlebitis

Nursing action	*Rationale*
1. Identify women at risk for thrombophlebitis. Encourage early ambulation after delivery to prevent thrombophlebitis	Factors that place a woman at increased risk for development of thrombophlebitis in the postpartum period include advanced maternal age, multiparity, obesity, immobility related to anaesthesia, and varicosities. For these women, preventive measures such as early ambulation and the wearing of support hose might be warranted. Early ambulation after delivery decreases the occurrence of thrombophlebitis.
2. Obtain and record vital signs. Check for the presence of Homans' sign by extending the woman's leg, supporting it under the knee, and dorsiflexing the woman's foot. Pain in the calf or behind the knee is the Homans' sign	Women with thrombophlebitis might demonstrate a slight increase in pulse rate. In more severe cases, a fever is usually presence of Homans' sign may indicate a deep vein thrombosis. It is important to differentiate what might be Homans' sign from the muscle tenderness often felt by women after a long labour. Further testing is needed to diagnose thrombophlebitis when the Homan's sign is present
3. Inspect lower extremities from the groin to the foot, noting color, presence of oedema, and warmth or coolness. Evaluate the woman's complaints of tenderness and pain in the affected extremity or groin	Redness, heat, tenderness, and localized oedema are indicative of superficial involvement. Pallor and coolness of the extremity suggest femoral thrombophlebitis
4. Place the woman on bed rest and elevate the affected extremity. Apply heat to the affected area according to the physician's orders	Elevating the legs above heart level empties the superficial veins and increases venous return. Heat application relieves pain and promotes circulation.
5. Administer analgesic agents to relieve the pain associated with thrombophlebitis as needed. Nonpharmacologic pain measures include elevating the legs and changing position at least every 2 hours	Inflammation and arterial spasm contribute to the pain
6. Start anticoagulant therapy according to the physician's orders. Review laboratory results including clotting times	Therapeutic anticoagulation is achieved when the activated partial thromboplastin time is 1.5 to 2.5 times normal
7. Administer antibiotics as ordered	A fever is usually indicative of deep vein thrombosis; antibiotics are used to control infection
8. Apply support hose and gradually increase the woman's ambulation	Support hose and ambulation improve venous blood flow in the lower extremities
9. Provide education as follows: • Instruct the patient to avoid rubbing or crossing her legs and to avoid constrictive clothing in the acute phase of the disease • Instruct the patient to avoid activities that might contribute to venous stasis, such as prolonged standing or sitting and crossing of the legs • Review the importance of taking anticoagulant therapy as ordered and keeping appointments with the physician on a regular basis to monitor therapy • Inform the patient that both nonfarin and heparin are compatible with breastfeeding	Document all education provided to the patient. Education of the patient is critical, because the woman with thrombophlebitis must demonstrate responsibility for porforming self-care. If she is unable to assume responsibility, she may need the services of a visiting nurse after discharge from the hospital

interfere with local circulation, set up areas of inflammation, or actually become foci of infection. Rarely, they may break away from the original site of formation and travel about in the circulation. Then they are called emboli. These clots are particularly dangerous because they may enter some small but vital vessel and cause grave damage or sudden death. This most often occurs in the case of an embolus or emboli to the long field or brain.

Fairly common sites of deep vein thrombophlebitis are the calf and thigh. The patient may experience calf pain when her foot is firmly dorsiflexed, while her leg is supported in an extended position (positive Homan's sign). Sometimes circulation is so impeded that the leg swells considerably, is extremely painful, and may demonstrate red streaks or locally inflammed areas. The skin may be so tense that it appears lighter in colour. Signs and symptoms may vary considerably.

Treatment of thrombophlebitis usually involves bed rest with elevation of the affected leg, analgesics, and the possible application of heat with a heat cardle. Antibiotics may be indicated. Some physicians may prescribe anticoagulants to cut down on the formation of further thrombi. The nurse must recognize that use of anti-coagulants for a postpartum haemorrhage. Observations of any abnormal bleeding must be quickly reported. Blood pressure should be taken periodically. Prothrombin determinations by the laboratory are expected.

After the acute phase when ambulation is approved, an order for support stockings is common. Applied correctly, they help speed the venous circulation back to the heart and discourage the formation of clots. No massage of the legs is permitted for fear of dislodging previously formed clots. Ambulation is ordered only after assessment of the day by day progress of the patient, revealed by the presence of absence of fever and her general condition. Thrombophlebitis may occur in all degrees of severity. As a preventive measure, some physicians automatically order that elastic stockings be applied to the legs of their patients, who have had difficulties with varicosities.

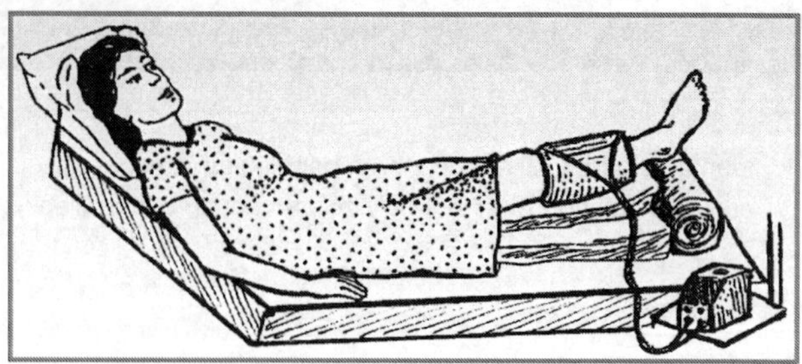

Fig. 6.9: Caring thrombophlebitis patient

The postpartum hospital stay is brief in many parts of the United State. However, the nurse can do much, even in this short interval, to help the patient face her increased responsibilities with added knowledge, skill. Identifying and Caring for Women with Thrombophlebitis (Fig. 6.9)

Purpose

All women should be assessed for thrombophlebitis every shift during the postpartum period. The presence of certain risk factors, however, places some women at higher risk for development of this condition. When postpartum thrombophlebitis is diagnosed early, prompt intervention may help prevent complications and a worsening of the condition. Education of the patient is a large component of the nursing role.

CHAPTER 7

Assessment and Management of Normal Neonate

INTRODUCTION

Neonate is a newborn infant. The neonatal period include the time from birth through the twenty eighth day of life. Newborn infants usually are considered to be tiny and powerless, completely dependent on others for life. Although this is true as far as obtaining food and water, it is not so regarding basic life process. Within one month of birth, the normal new born adapts from a dependent foetal existence to an independent one, capable of oxygen and carrying on life processes. Now there is trend, the care of the newborn is towards specialization. The branch of medicine specializing in the care of the newborn is called "neonatology".

The nurse frequently is the first health care provider who has contact with the neonate. In some birth settings it can be as long as 24 hours before a physician is required to examine a new baby. These first hours are crucial because multiple organ systems are making the transition from intrauterine to extrauterine functions. Understanding and appreciating this transition are vital to the assessment of the newborn. The nurse requires the skill to identify the baby who is having difficulty so that proper therapy can be instituted. The use of universal precautions with barriers such as gloves until the newborn has first bath is important to protect both and client from communicable diseases.

The numerous biologic changes the neonate makes during the transition to extrauterine life. The first 24 hours of life are critical because respiratory distress and circulating failure can occur rapidly and with little warning. Although most infants make the necessary biopsychosocial adjustment to extrauterine existence without undue difficulty, their wellbeing depends on the care received from others. The assessment and care of the newborn from immediately after birth until discharge are follows.

NEONATAL ASSESSMENT

Apgar Score (Table 7.1)

- A–Appearance
- P–Pulse
- G–Grimace
- A–Attitude (form)
- R–Respiration

The first assessment of the newborn is done immediately after birth by using Apgar score.

The Apgar score permits a rapid assessment of need for resuscitation based on five signs that indicate the physiologic state of the newborn.

1. Heart rate based on auscultation with a stethoscope.
2. Respiratory rate based on observed movement of the chestwall.
3. Muscle tone based on the degree of flexion and movement of the extremities.
4. Reflex irritability based on response to gentle slaps on the soles and feet.
5. Colour described as pallid, cyanotic, or pink. Evaluations are made at 1 and 5 minutes after birth and can be done by the nurse or birth

Table 7.1: Apgar score

		Score	
Sign	*0*	*1*	*2*
Heart rate	Absent	Slow (<100)	Over 100
Resp. rate	Absent	Slow week cry	Good cry
Muscle tone	Flaccid	Some flexion and extremities	Well flexed
Reflex irritabillty	No response	Grimace	Cry
Colour	Blue,pale	Body pink, extremities blue	Completely pink

attendant. Scores of 0 to 3 indicates severe distress, scores of 4 to 6 indicate moderate difficulty and scores of 7 to 10 indicate that the infant should have no difficulty adjusting to extra uterine life.

Neonatal physical assessment is similar to adult assessment that is the same methods of data collection used. A major focus will be on assessment of growth and development. The object of the assessment is to identify any alteration in health status that would make adjustment difficult. Usually physical assessment is begun with the head and proceeds downward, (based on the principle of growth and development i.e. caphalocaudal direction). Infants are stimulated by physical assessment and may lose heat quickly when undressed. Therefore, the order of the examination has been changed to minimize heat loss and to enlist the infants co-operation. Attention is given to prenatal development, developmentally related body systems are reviewed at the same time. In addition, the examiner notes differences in behaviours and vital signs during the early periods of reactivity.

General Examination

The nurse begins with a through, but quick scan of the infant, looking for overt signs of difficulty for which immediate intervention is necessary. These manifest as abnormalities is vital signs, colour, tone, movement and size. The following questions, provide a focus for the procedure.

Vital Signs

Vital signs: Temperature, heart rate, respiratory rate and B.P. within normal limits.

Assessing Vital Signs in the Newborn (Table 7.2)

Purpose To determine the newborn's respirations, heart rate, and temperature so that abnormalities can be detected and appropriate interventions

Table 7.2: Assessment of vital signs in newborn

Nursing action	*Rationale*
Respirations	
1. While the infant is quiet or sleeping, observe and count the respirations for a full minute. Observe the newborn's abdomen rising and falling; palpate the abdomen lightly to determine its rise and fall with each inspiration and expiration	1. Counting respirations for 1 minute ensures an accurate assessment because the newborn is a periodic breather (periods of apnoea lasting less than 15 seconds are normal). Observing and palpating respirations while the infant is quiet promotes accurate assessment. Palpation aids observation in determining the respiratory rate. Normal respiratory rate varies from 30 to 60 breaths per minute when the infant is not crying
2. Observe for normal characteristics of respirations as well as for signs of respiratory abnormalities	2. Breath sound should be clear. Respirations should be shallow and irregular in rate, rhythm, and depth. Respirations should come from the abdomen rather than the chest. Signs of abnormal respirations, including expiratory grunting, nasal flaring, retractions, cyanosis, and seesawing, should be absent
3. Record your findings in the newborns chart	3. Respiratory rate and characteristics should be recorded in the chart to facilitate detection of abnormalities and initiation of appropriate interventions
Heart Rate and Blood Pressure (Figs 7.1A and B)	
1. Auscultate and count, with an infant stethoscope, the newborn's heart rate for 60 seconds at the apex of the heart, which is located to the left of the midclavicular line at the third or fourth intercostal space. Listen, observe, and count the heart rate (apical pulse rate) when the newborn is quiet or sleeping. If necessary, use a pacifier to soothe a crying infant before assessing heart rate.	1. The small infant stethoscope allows better contact and more accurate determination of the heart rate and sound than the larger stethoscope does. Heart sound are more audible when the newborn is quiet
2. Note heart rate and record it in the newborn's chart	2. Recording the heart facilitates detection of abnormalities and initiation of appropriate interventions. The normal heart rate is 120 to 160 beats per minute
3. Listen for heart murmurs or other abnormalities, such as alterations in rhythm	3. If a gallop rhythm is heard, heart failure is suspected. Heart murmurs are not unusual in the first days after birth and are usually related to incomplete closure of foetal heart structures
4. Palpate brachial and femoral pulses	4. Pulses should be strong, regular, and equal bilaterally.
5. Blood pressure is not routinely assessed in healthy term newborns. If assessment of blood pressure is necessary, use a correctly sized neonatal cuff (no wider than two thirds of the infant's upper arm). Usually an electronic monitor is used because it is more accurate.	5. Blood pressure is usually assessed only if an abnormality or problem is suspected or if the infant is ill. The normal range for blood pressure in term infants 60 to 90 mm Hg for systolic pressure and 40 to 50 mm Hg for diastolic pressure

Contd...

Contd...

Nursing action	*Rationale*
Axillary temperature (Fig. 7.2)	
1. *Prepare the thermometer.* A glass or an electronic thermometer may be used. If an electronic thermometer is used, place a cover on the probe and turn it on. Wear gloves if the neonate has not been bathed.	1. Gathering and preparing the appropriate equipment facilitates completing the procedure effectively. Placing a cover on the prevents cross-contamination. Wearing gloves before the first neonatal bath is consistent with Standard Precautions
2. Expose the baby's axilla; if it is moist, pat it dry	2. Moisture can interfere with an accurate temperature reading. Friction can raise the temperature
3. Place the thermometer in the axilla; fold the infant's arm over the chest and hold	3. Keeps thermometer in place
4. Leave glass thermometer in place for 5 minutes. Leave electronic thermometer in place until digital reading appears	4. Leaving the thermometer in place for the prescribed amount of time helps ensure an accurate reading
5. Remove thermometer and read temperature. Normal axillary temperature is 36.0 to 36.5°C (97.1 to 97.8° F). Discard probe cover of electronic thermometer.	5. A separate probe cover is used for each infant to prevent the spread of microorganisms
6. Record findings in newborn's chart. Record immediately for accuracy	6. If temperature is not within the normal range, interventions must be initiated to maintain temperature within the normal range
Rectal temperature	
1. *Prepare thermometer.* If a rectal glass thermometer is used, wipe the cleaning solution off if necessary (use a circular motion, proceeding from the end opposite the bulb to the bulb). Shake down the thermometer. If an electronic thermometer is used, place a cover on the probe and turn the unit on	1. Gathering and preparing the appropriate equipment facilitates completing the procedure effectively. Wiping a glass thermometer ensures removal of faecal material and allows better visualization of temperature. Shaking down the thermometer helps ensure an accurate reading. Placing a cover on the probe prevents cross-contamination
2. Lubricate the thermometer or probe cover 1.5 to 2.5 cm (0.5 to 1.0 inch)	2. Lubricating the thermometer or probe cover facilitates insertion by reducing friction
3. Place the baby either on the back (while holding legs up) or on the abdomen. The baby must be held securely so that he or she cannot move	3. These positions facilitate insertion of the thermometer. Holding the legs firmly ensures that the baby does not sustain injury from the thermometer
4. Insert the thermometer into the baby's rectum no more than 0.5 inch. Do not force	4. Gentle technique minimizes trauma; the newborn may not have a patent anus
5. Hold glass thermometer in place for 5 minutes, holding legs. Hold electronic thermometer in place for 10 to 20 seconds until digital reading appears. (Note: Neonates will often have a stool)	5. Leave the thermometer in place for the prescribed amount of time to ensure an accurate reading. Peristalsis or passing a stool may force the thermometer out of the rectum
6. Remove thermometer and read temperature. Normal rectal temperature is 36.5 to 37.0° C(97.6 to 98.6° F). Discard probe cover of electronic thermometer.	6. A separate probe cover is used for each infant to prevent cross-contamination
7. Record findings in newborn's chart	7. Record route used; temperature varies by route. Recording findings facilitates detection of abnormalities and initiation of appropriate interventions
Tympanic temperature	
The tympanic membrane temperature device may be used if the infant's ear canals are free of vernix and moisture (usually after 24 hours)	
1. Attach the probe cover according to manufacturer's directions	1. Attaching a probe cover prevents cross-contamination.
2. Insert the probe into the external auditory canal gently; the probe must occlude the canal	2. Gentle insertion prevents injury. The external auditory canal must be occluded to obtain an accurate temperature
3. Leave the thermometer in place for 1 second or for the amount of time indicated by the manufacture	3. Leaving the thermometer in place for the prescribed amount of time helps ensure an accurate reading.
4. Remove the thermometer and read the temperature. Normal tympanic temperature is 36.5 to 37.0° C (97.6 to 98.6°F). Discard probe cover	4. A separate probe cover is used for each infant to prevent cross-contamination
5. Record findings in newborn's chart	5. Note that tympanic route was used; temperature varies by route

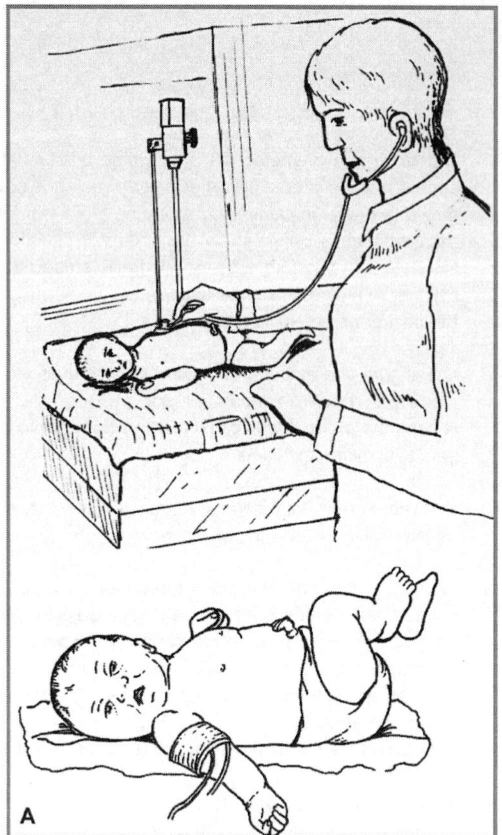

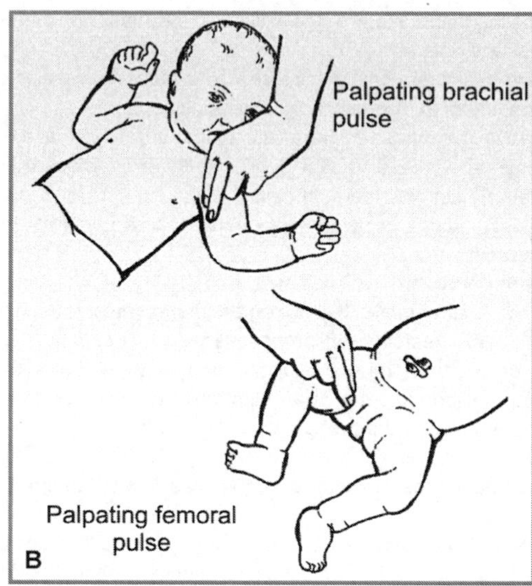

Figs 7.1A and B: Steps for measuring of heart rate and BP

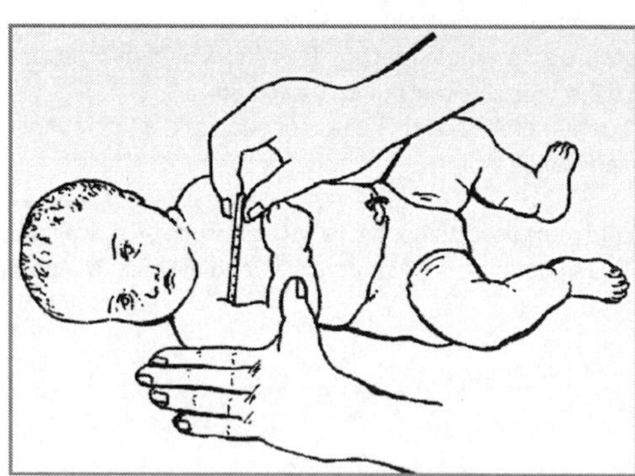

Fig. 7.2: Taking axillary temperature

initiated. Respirations and heart rate are usually measured every hour for the first 4 hours of life and then every shift. Temperature is usually assessed every hour for the first 4 hours of life, every 4 hours for the remainder of the first 24 hours, and then every shift.

Equipment

- Infant stethoscope
- Doppler device
- Glass thermometer or electronic thermometer
- Probe cover
- Tympanic temperature device

Temperature

An axillary temperature can be taken within minimal distrubance by gently slipping the thermometer into the axillary space. Rectal temperatures are not routinely taken because the vagus nerve is stimulated and there is risk of rectal perforation. Normal ranges of axillary temperatures are 36.1° to 36.5°C (97.0° to 97.7°F).

Heart Rate

An apical heart rate of 110 to 160 beats /min. should be heard on the left side of the chest near the nipple and the examiner may listen for less than 1 minute and multiply appropriately.

Respiration

The irregularity of respirations requires counting for a full minute. A range of 30 to 60 breaths/min is normal. The rate is irregulea and abdominal, with a possibility of brief (less than 3 to 5 seconds) periods of pause or apnoea. Some otherwise healthy infants may show tachypnoea during the first hour as excess lung fluid is absorbed. The examiner listens for the quality of breath sounds at each midaxillary line.

Blood Pressure

Initial readings are taken with the Doppler device (Diomap) on an arm and a leg and compared. In the first 3 days the range is from 75/45 to 50/30, with an average of 65/41. If there is a reading above or below these levels, further evaluation of blood volume is done.

Colour

The infant's colour should be pink, with the exception of hands and feet.

Acrocyanosis (peripheral cyanosis) is normal in the first 12 hours of birth. Later it may be a sign of difficulty controlling temperature or glucose. The rest of the body and mucous membranes should be pink. The examiner looks especially during feedings to see, if the infant's mouth becomes bluish.

Measurements

The weight and length, as well as head and chest circumstances, should be consistent with the estimated gestational age.

The examiner needs an infant scale and paper barrier, a paper tape measure, and a growth chart. The head circumference is measured from occiput to forehead and the chest circumference is measured at the level of the infant's nipples. Length is measured by stretching the paper tape measure under the infant from tip of head to sole of foot. A very active infant can be positioned with the head touching the top of the crib and one leg gently extended. This distance can then be marked and measured.

Compare the infant's birth weight, length and head circumference with the criteria in Table 7.3. These values can be plotted on a growth and development chart after gestational age assessment is completed. The range in weight if from 2,500 to 4,000 gm. Measurements of length range from 44 to 55 cm. Head circumference averages from 33 to 35 cm, with chest circumferance always 1 to 2 cm less. If the chest is larger than the head, they should be closely observed for microcephaly. A head circumference less than the 10th percentile indicates microcephaly associated with congenital malformations and infections. A head circumferance greater than the 90th percentile indicates macrocephaly, caused perhaps by hydrocephaly. Some infants whose parents are constitutionally large or small may exceed or fall short of these limits, but the measurements should not fall in widely divergent percentiles. For example, an infant whose weight and height fall within the 75th percentile should not have a head circumference in the 25th percentile. If the infant's head is greatly molded, the head and chest circumstances may be equal until the molding resolves. Remeasurement within 3 days is advised (Table 7.4).

Weighing and Measuring the Newborn (Table 7.3)

Purpose The newborn is weighed to determine whether weight loss after birth is normal and to determine whether nutritional intake is adequate for growth. The newborn is weighed at birth to provide a basis for evaluating further growth and daily thereafter (daily weights are compared with birth weight).

Equipment

- Scale
- Cover sheets
- Paper tape measure.

Movement and Tone

After assessing measurement, consider the following questions:

- Does the infant move all four extremeties and return to a symmetric position of flexion?
- Does any motion seem limited or hypotonic in comparison with the other body parts?

Table 7.3: Nursing action in weighing and measuring newborn

Nursing action	*Rationale*
Weighing	
1. Place cover sheet (Chux pad or other disposable paper pad) on scale. Wear gloves if newborn has not been bathed	1. The cover sheet prevents cross-contamination and lessens heat loss by conduction. Wearing gloves is consistent with standard precautions
2. Adjust the scale balances to 0, or push the appropriate pads on the digital scales, using a protective barrier on your hand	2. Adjusting the scale appropriately ensures an accurate reading. Using a paper towel or other protective barrier prevents cross-contamination
3. Place naked newborn supine on scale, holding your hand above the newborn compare weight with birth weight (Fig. 7.3)	3. Newborns should not lose more than 10 percent of birth weight. Newborns regain their birth weight by 7 to 10 days of life and then gain about 1 ounce per day in the first 6 months of life. Holding your hand above the newborn is a protective measure (Fig. 7.3)
4. Record weight on baby's chart. Weight baby at the same time each day	4. Findings need to be recorded on the chart to determine whether weight loss is normal and to determine whether nutritional intake is adequate for growth. Weighing each day allows comparison of daily weight with birth weight to note whether weight loss is normal or excessive
Measuring	
1. To measure length, place the newborn in the supine position on the crib mattress, with the head against the top of the crib. Place the paper tape measure beside the infant, with the 0 end of the tape against the top of the crib. Some scales include a built-in ruler for measuring length. Wear gloves if the newborn has not been bathed	1. An infant's length is measured from the top of the head to the heel of the extended leg, with the body kept in alignment. The tape must be placed next to the infant to measure the length
2. Hold the newborn's head straight with one hand, and extend one leg with the other hand. Watch that the tape measure remains straight (Fig. 7.4)	2. An infant's length is measured from the top of the head to the heel of the extended leg (Fig. 7.4)
3. Note the length and record it in the infant's chart. Compare your finding with the normal range; most infants are 48 to 53 cm (19 to 21 inches) in length.	3. Measurements are taken to note abnormalities and provide a baseline value
4. To measure head circumference, place the paper tape under the newborn's head. Wrap the tape around the newborn's head, measuring just above the eyebrows so that the largest area of the occiput is included. Record your finding in the infant's chart (Fig. 7.5).	4. Head circumference of a term newborn is normally 33 to 35.5 cm (13 to 14 inches). The head circumference is approximately 2 cm larger than the chest circumference. Measuring head circumference provides a baseline value for detection of abnormalities, such as hydrocephalus or microcephaly (Fig. 7.5)
5. To measure chest circumference, place the paper tape under the newborn's chest, at nipple level. Wrap the tape around the chest, at the nipple line. Note the circumference and record it in the infant's chart (Fig. 7.6)	5. Chest circumference is measured at the nipple line. Average chest circumference of a term newborn is 30.5 to 33 cm (12 to 13 inches). Recording chest circumference facilitates detection of abnormalities
6. To measure abdominal circumference, place the paper tape under the newborn's abdomen, at umbilical level. Wrap the tape around the abdomen, at umbilical level. Note abdominal circumference and record it in the infant's chart	6. Abdominal circuferences vary but are typically similar to the chest circumference. Recording abdominal circumference provides a baseline value and facilitates detection of abnormalities, such as abdominal distention (Fig. 7.7)

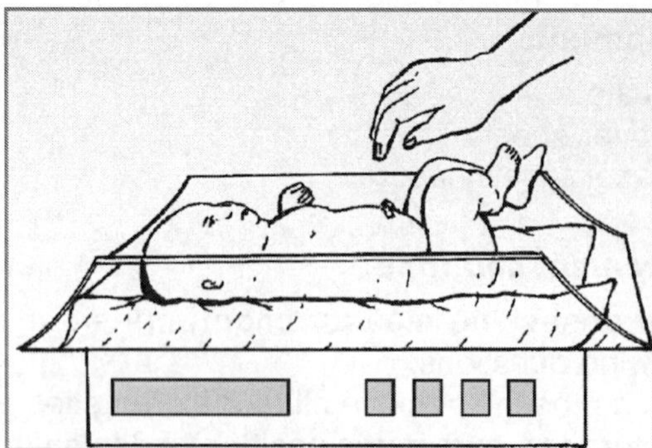

Fig. 7.3: Measuring the weight of infant

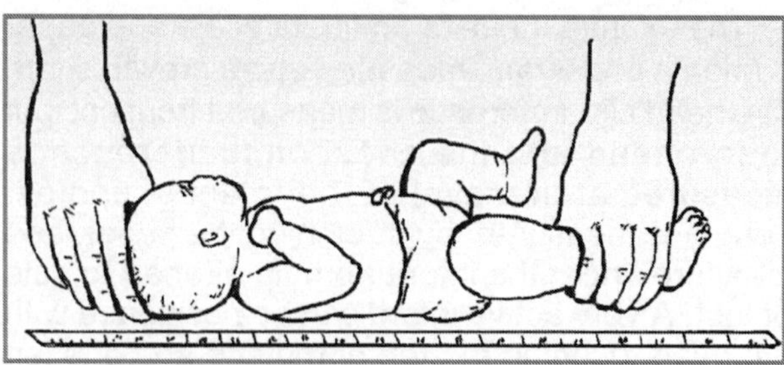

Fig. 7.4: Measuring the length of infant

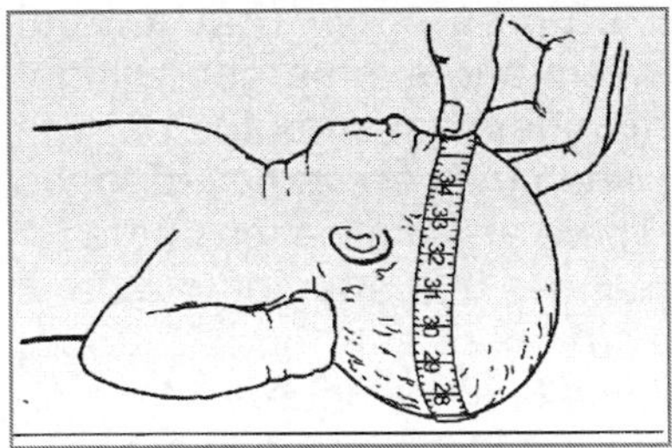

Fig. 7.5: Measuring the head circumference of infant

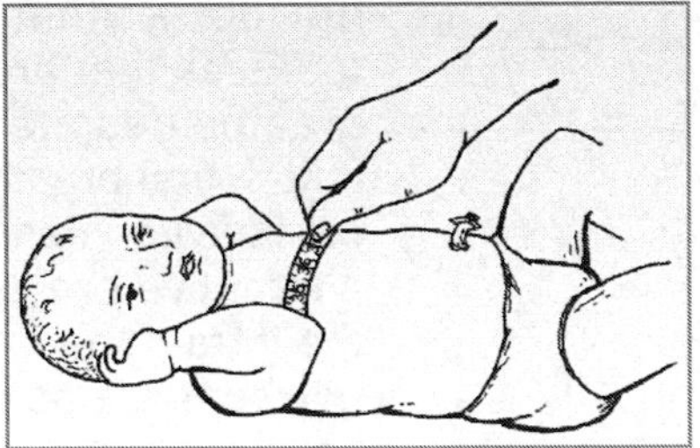

Fig. 7.6: Measuring the chest circumference of infant

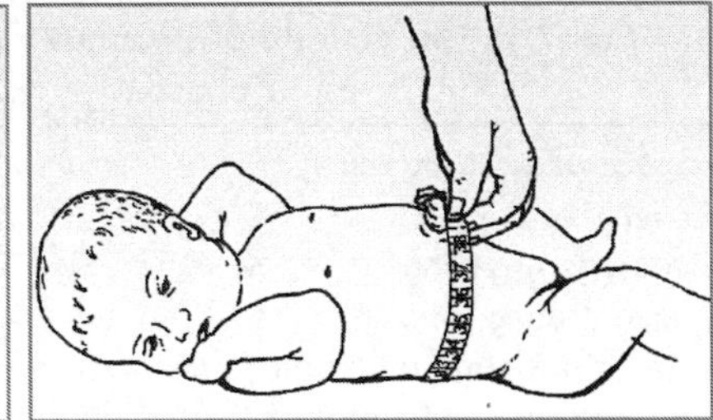

Fig. 7.7: Measuring the abdominal circumference of infant

Table 7.4: Normal term newborn measurement

Value	*Normal range*	*Variations*
Weight	2500-4000 gm	Average is 3400 gm (7 1/2 Pounds) or 2500 gm for Indian babies.
Length	44-55 cm	Average is 50 cm x 20 inches): because molding of head can influence this value, remeasure before discharge
Head circumference	32-37.5 cm, average 33-35 cm	Check/molding of head
Chest circumference	1-2 cm less than head circumference	Breast engorgement or molding of head can influence this ratio
Axillary temperature	36.1° -36.5° C (97.0° -97.7° F)	Environmental temperature extremes, sepsis and altered neurologic function can cause hypothermia or hyperthermia
Respirations rate	30-60 breaths/min	Respirations may be relatively tachypnic (rate over 60) during first hour but should not rise
Quality	Easy, abdominal without use of accessory muscles	Infant may have period of grunting, flaring and retractions during first hour
Apical pulse	110-160 beats/min	Rate of 100-120 is normal during sleep but should accelerate with stimulation, rate over 160 common with increased activity and crying.
Blood pressure (take in arm and leg)	Systolic 50-75 mm Hg Diastolic 30-45 mm Hg	Hypotension may mean low blood volume Should be equal in upper and lower extremity

Note especially birth injuries or anaesthesia effects on muscle responses. A hypotonic infant also may have acidosis, hypoglycaemia, hypothermia, or congenital problems.

Behavioural State

Assess the behavioural state in terms of the following questions (Box 7.1):

- Is the cry appropriate?
- Does the infant seem interested in the environment?
- Is the transition from sleep to wake a smooth one?

Because the behavioural state will influence assessment, it is important to relate the infant's period of reactivity to these questions (Box 7.1) to the findings.

Although a "Yes" answer to the seven questions under vital signs, colour, measurements, movement and tone, and behavioural state does not guarantee an uneventful recovery, it indicates that the infant is in no immediate distress. The following warning signs may indicate a need for intervention.

- Axillary temperature less than 36.1° or over 37.2°C (97° or over 99° F). Heart rate less than 110 or over 160 beats/min (if asleep may fall to 100 or if active may rise to 180)
- Respiratory rate less than 30 or over 60 breaths/min (may rise transiently if active)
- Cyanosis other than acrocyanosis
- Jaundice
- Periods of apnoea lasting over 15 seconds.
- Lack of movement and responsiveness.

Box 7.1: The periods of neonatal reacitivity are in phases

First phase (30-60 min)
Active, alert
Eyes open, gazing
Active rooting, sucking
Vital signs labile: Rapid, irregular heart rate and respirations, may have rales, grunting, retractions, flaringnares
Activity labile: Observe for tone, symmetric movement.
First sleep (2-4 hr)
Quiet sleep, no interest in feeding.
Stabilized vital signs
Onset of bowel sounds
Second reactivity period (4-10 hr afterbirth)
Infant awake and alert
Rooting and sucking strong
Variable vital signs with mild cyanosis
Mottling, increased mucus
Passage of meconium and urine

- Hypotonic or hypertonic position.
- Lack of interest in the environment.
- Birthweight < 5 pound or > 9 Pounds.
- Head circumference less than the 5th percentile.
- Large or small for gestational age.

Cardiorespiratory Assessment

The respiratory and cardiovascular systems are considered together because of their obviously related functions to survival, and proximity during assessment.

Respiratory

The First Breath

There are several stimuli to breathing. During vaginal delivery, the infant's thorax is first compressed and then rapidly re-expands, or recoils. This draws in a small amount of air. The comparative cold of the extrauterine environment, the bright lights, noises, pressure on the infant's body and sensation of weight from the addition of gravity all stimulate the newborn to take a deep gasping breath.

Mild asphyxia (hypercapnia, hypoxia, and acidosis) normally accompanies labour and delivery. Mild asphyxia is a chemical stimulant to respiratory control centres in both the adult and newborn. Animal studies show that animal foetuses that are warm and submerged will not breathe despite this chemical stimulus but will take a first breath, when they are exposed to the cool environment. There are implications here for alternative birth practices that attempt to extend the intrauterine environment after birth. Several newborn deaths related to home under-water birth have been documented. These infants were submerged for upto1 hour, with the parents thinking that the infant "enjoyed" the water.

Establishment of Respiration

An adequate supply of surfactant is needed if normal respirations are to continue. In its absence, alveoli collapse with each exhalation, and there is no residual volume. With each breath the preterm infant must try to inflate lungs that are collapsed. The tremendously increased respiratory effort soon leads to respiratory failure. This is the basis of respiratory distress syndrome (RDS).

Once respirations are established the range will be between 30 and 60/min and will be irregular in rate, rhythm and depth. The face and trunk will have a pink tone, although the extremities may still show a bluish colour.

As the infant breathes, the partial pressure or (pO_2) in the blood increases, whereas the partial pressure of carbon dioxide (pCO_2) decreases. As acidosis resolves, blood pH approaches adult values. The pulmonary blood vessels constricted in foetal life, dilate in response to the increased oxygen levels and allow a dramatic increase in blood flow to the new born lungs. The results of normal transition occur as follows:

1. Surfactant production is maintained.
2. Residual volume is established.
3. Physiologic acid-base balance continues.
4. Blood flow to the lungs is increased.
5. Vital signs are within normal limits.
6. A pink, oxygenated colour is evident.

Cardiovascular

Transitional Circulation

Foetal circulation should be reviewed before transitional circulation is studied.

Changes that occur during the transition from foetal newborn circulation are closely linked to changes in the respiratory system. These changes are caused by the alternations in systemic and preliminary pressures that result from the first deep breath and the establishment of respirations. Therefore, clamping the umbilical cord does not cause the reversal from foetal to adult circulation. Circulatory patterns will change from foetal to newborn even if the infant is born unattended and the cord is not clamped immediately after birth , illustrates the following description of transitional circulation:

1. The infant's first breath raises the pO_2, which causes the pulmonary arterial blood vessels to dilate and allows blood to flow freely to the lungs. Now the pulmonary blood pressure is decreased.
2. The umbilical arteries constrict in response to increased pO_2 levels and the cord is cut.
3. Circulation through the umbilical vein ends.
4. As the ductus venouses closes, the systemic blood pressure rises.
5. These changes in pressures cause blood flow through the ductus arteriosus to reverse its direction, thus changing one of the right-to-left shunt. The ductus arteriousus then constricts (also in response to increased pO_2 levels) preventing blood flow through it by the end of the first day. It will later become the ligamentum arteriosum.
6. Because of increased blood flow to the lungs, there must be increased flow from the lungs through the pulmonary veins and to the left atrium.
7. The increased pressure of this blood against the foramen ovale force it to close against the interatrial septum. The reverses the other right-to-left shunt. (The site of the old foramen ovale will later become the fossa ovalis).
8. These allow blood to flow to the newborn lungs for gas exchange and return to the heart for distribution to the body. All foetal vessels, first functionally and then anatomically, adapt to adult circulation by atrophy.

The rate of the neonatal heart will be relative to the foetal heart rate but will gradually become slower. The rate continues to be irregular in rate rhythm, but variability also decreases. The rate responds to stimuli as did the foetal heart rate. The results of normal transition are as follows:

1. Decrease in pulmonary blood pressure with resultant increase in pulmonary blood flow.
2. Closure of the foramen ovale.
3. Constriction of the ductus arteriosus.
4. End of flow through umbilical vein.

Failure of this transition is a life-threatening disorder. *Persistent Foetal Circulation (PFC) or Persistent Pulmonary Hypertension of the Newborn (PPHN).*

Assessment of PPHN

Inspection: The infant is observed at rest and during activity. The examiner looks for skin colour and symmatric expansion of the chest. The infant's colour should be pink centrally, but there still may be acrocyanosis. Bulging of the chest may indicate that air is trapped in the pleural space below (Pneumothorax). The respiratory rate is counted by watching the lower portion of chest and the abdomen rise and fall (watching the cord can be helpful) for a full minute because the neonate's normal irregular pattern of respiration will cause the total to be inaccurate if the counting is discontinued before 60 seconds have lapsed. Although respiration range from 30 to 60 breaths/min, there may be flares according to state and period of reactivity. The quality of respiration is assessed by noting retraction or nasal flaring. Retractions are caused by use of accessory muscles of respiration and are seen as inspiratory "pulling in" of the chest wall above and below the sternum (suprasternal and substernal retrac-tions) and between the below the ribs (intercostal and subcostal retractions). Recognition of retractions as mild, moderate, or severe requires practice. When nasal flaring is present, the nares seem to dilate with each inspiration, indicating that the fluid that fills the lungs during foetal life has not yet been absorbed or that more serious difficulties in extrauterine adjustment may be present.

The presence of meconium staining of the skin, nails and cord should be noted. This staining may be associated with respiratory distress if meconium aspiration has occurred during labour. While assessing respiratory status, the examiner notes the number and spacing of the nipples and the presence of gynaecomastia, or breast engorgement. A few infants may have extra nipple tissue, that is supernumerary nipples. The special impulse of paint of maximal impulse (PMI) also may be seen.

Auscultation: The best place to listen to breath sounds is the midaxillary line, but all lobes should be examined. An equal amount of air entry on each side of the chest should be heard. Scattered rales (sounds of moisture within the lungs) are considered normal during the first few hours of life, especially in the infant delivered by surgical intervention. There should be no stridor or noise during inspiration. Grunting is an abnormal expiratory sound heard as the infant forcibly exhales against a closed glottis to keep the alveoli from collapsing. It may be possible to hear this grunting without a stethoscope. It is a warning of respiratory distress.

The examiner concentrates on the heart sounds, auscultating the entire cardiac region. One pattern is to begin at the apex, found on the infant at the point of maximal impulse where the pulse is best felt. The PMI is found just the left of the midclavicular line at the fourth intercostal space. This point is higher than in the adult because the neonatal heart lies in a more horizontal position. The examiner works from the apex, up the left sternal border, towards the base of the heart and then listens along the right sternal border, turning the infant over and listening between the scapulae.

The normal neonatal heart rate ranges from 110 to 160 beats/min, but a rate of 100 may be observed when the infant is at rest, and a rate of 170 to 180 may occur during periods of activity. If a rate of less than 110 is heard, stimulating the infant to cry should make the rate rise. Although neonatal heart rates have variability similar to foetal heart rates, obvious irregularities in the cardiac rhythm should not occur. Gestational age also influences heart rates (with faster rates earliar in gestatic because of the dominance of the sympathetic nervous system).

The next focus is the quality of heart sounds and the presence of extra sounds. S1 and S2 are the first and second heart sounds. S1 is heard when the atrioventricular valves (mitral and tricuspid) close, and S2 occurs when the semilunar valves (aortic and pulmonary) close. The "Lub-dub" sounds are S1 and S2, respectively. The time between S1 and S2 respectively. The time between S1 and S2 is systole, and the time between S2 and S1 is diastole.

In evaluating heart sounds, a separate and distinct S1 and S2 should be heard, usually with no extra sounds during systole or diastole. The sound should be easy to hear (i. e, it should not seem as though the heart is far from the stethoscope). However, "Closeness" of heart sounds to the chest wall is a parameter that can be assessed accurately only with experience. A good order to use when auscultating the hear is as follows:

1. Count the rate, noting its regularity and variability with the infant's activity.
2. Locate the place where the sounds are best heard in the chest.
3. Differentiate between S1 and S2.
4. Decide if there are extra sounds.

Palpation: Brachial pulses are palpated at the antecubital space and the femoral pulses bilaterally along the inguinal ligament halfway between the iliac crest and the symphysis pubis. Their relative rates and volumes should be equal.

Percussion: Percussion of the neonatal chest generally is not undertaken because any questions concerning the size and condition of organs are investigated by radiographic or ultrasonic examination.

Cardiorespiratory warning signs: Require intervention:

- Sustained heart rate < 110 or >180 beats/min.
- Respiratory rate < 30 or > 60 breaths/min.
- Central cyanosis.
- Apnea for more than 15 seconds.
- Muffled heart sounds or heart shifted to right
- Cardiac murmur.
- Unequal breath sounds.

Metabolic Control Assessment

Heat Transfer

The newborn enters an environment at least 20° to 25° F cooler than core body temperature. Unless the infant is protected against heat loss, deep body temperature can drop 0.5° to 2° C (0.9° to 3.6° F within 5 to 10 minutes of birth. Thermal receptors are present on the body surface, with many on the face. When they are triggered, the response is peripheral vasoconstriction. The head, 20 per cent of the body surface is wet at birth and difficult to dry completely. Because most of the heat loss is through evaporation and radiation, drying is a priority, use of radiant overhead warmers has significantly reduced initial heat loss. Incubators also useful to control heat loss from convection.

The temperature gradiant is the difference between the skin and the environment (external gradient) or between the core of the body and the skin (internal gradient). Temperature control in the newborn is influenced primarily by this temperature gradient.

When ambient temperature falls in the adult, increased metabolism raises internal or core temperature by means of involuntary high intensity rhythmic shivering, and voluntary muscle activity. This muscle activity is physical thermogenesis. However, the newborn infant can use only chemical thermogenesis. A special form of fat, brown adipose tissue (BAT) is deposited during foetal life. New borns produce body heat by increasing their metabolic rate and by metabolizing this tissue. They do not shiver. A decrease in ambient temperature stimulates production of norepinephrine, which increases brown fat metabolism. This response is impaired when an infant has hypoxia or if lipid stores are already depleted. Certain drugs also block this response. During BAT metabolism oxygen is consumed and fatty acids and glycerol are produced. Newborns are vulnerable despite these mechanisms because (1) there is large skin surface to body weight ratio, which promotes a more rapid loss of heat from core to the skin surface, and (2) the presence of substantial layers of white fat as additional insulation depends on gestational age and birth weight.

Extremes of environmental temperature, therefore, will stress the infant. This may lead to overbeating, which will cause an elevated body temperature, vasodilation with flushed skin, and tachypnea as the infant tries to dissipate the extra heat. For this reason an infant should never be left unattended under a radiant warmer without a continuous Servo mechanism for temperature feedback.

More commonly the environmental temperature will be too low and initiate the adverse affects termed cold stress.

Cold Stress

The infant responds to low environmental temperatures with peripheral vasoconstriction, which leads to increased anaerobic metabolism and acidosis, Initially, peripheral vasoconstriction will make the skin temperature drop while the core temperature is maintained. Later, core temperature is maintained. Later, core temperature will fall.

One goal of nursing care is maintenance of a thermal neutral environment in which heat production (measured as oxygen consumption) is minimal, yet core temperature is within the normal range. Infants cared for in such an environment need not expend extra energy nor consume extra oxygen to maintain normal internal temperature. Althought this may not make a tremendous difference to the healthy, full-term infant, the added stress can be disastrous for the sick infant.

Glucose and Calcium

Maintenance of adequate blood glucose levels is vital because of the brain dependence on glucose to energy; lack of glucose may cause tremors, seizures, and permanent neurologic damage. Maintenance of serum calcium levels also is necessary for normal neuromuscular function; low calcium levels may tremors, tetany, and seizures. Abnormally increased calcium levels are rare in the neonate.

Assessing Blood Glucose Level Using Dextrostix or Chemstrip with Accu-Check II Device (Table 7.5)

Purpose To assess the newborn's blood glucose level for presence of hypoglycaemia when ordered or when symptoms of hypoglycaemia are present. Hypoglycaemia is diagnosed when blood glucose level is below 30 mg/dL in the first 72 hours or below 45 mg/dL after the first 3 days of life.

Equipment

- Lancet or Tenderfoot
- Alcohol swabs
- Sterile 2 x 2 gauze pads
- Small round adhesive bandage
- Cotton balls
- Container of glucose strips (Chemstrip or Dextrostix)
- Gloves
- Accu-Check II device
- Squeeze water bottle

Glucose is needed for the increased energy demands that occur after delivery. The newborn infant must breathe and maintain body temperature. The infant's movements also are more vigorous than those in uterus. At birth, glucose levels are maintained by glycolysis of hepatic glycogen and gluconeogenesis. These prenatal stores will be the primary source of energy until feedings are well established.

Table 7.5: Nursing action in assessing blood glucose

Nursing action	*Rationale*
1. To achieve free flow of blood for an adequate sample, follow steps 1 through 5 of Procedure 31-3, using the Heel Stick Method to obtain blood	1. Accurate assessment of blood glucose evel requires an adequate sample of the newborn's blood
2. Completely cover the treated area of the reagent strip with the blood sample from the newborn's heel. For Chemstrip with Accu-Check II, use the first drop of blood as the sample. For Dextrostix without the Accu-Check device, discard the first drop of blood	2. Completely covering the treated area of the reagent strip helps ensure accurate test results. For Chemstrip with Accu-Check II, test results are more accurate if the first drop of blood is used rather than subsequent drops. The first drop of blood is discarded for Dextrostix used without the Accu-Check device, since the first drop is typically diluted with tissue fluid from stick site
3. Leave the blood sample on the glucose strip for exactly 60 seconds. The treated area of the strip will change colour during this time. (Note: If the Accu-Check II device is used, press the "time" button to activate the timing mechanism)	3. Leaving the blood sample on the strip for the prescribed amount of time helps ensure accurate test results. (With Accu-Check II, three high beeps sound at seconds 57, 58, and 59; one low deep sounds at second 60)
4. At 60 seconds, clean blood from the strip. For Chemstrip, use clean cotton balls to wipe away blood completely, leaving no blood on the treated area of the strip. For Dextrostix, use a forceful stream of water from a squeeze bottle to rinse away blood completely from the strip	4. Executing the procedure carefully and according to directions is crucial for obtaining an accurate reading
5. Determine blood glucose value. With the Accu-Check II device, insert the Chemstrip into the adapter slot of Accu-Check II before the timer display reads 120 seconds. At 120 seconds, a high beep sounds, and the screen displays a blood glucose value (in mg/dL). For Dextrostix, wait for the amount of time recommended on the container and compare the colour of the Dextrostix strip with the colours on the Dextrostix container to ascertain the blood glucose value (Fig. 7.8).	5. False readings can result from inaccurate timing
6. Apply small, round adhesive bandage to heel	6. An adhesive bandage creates pressure needed to minimize bleeding, and it protects the site from contamination
7. Check the heel stick site frequently for bleeding	7. The baby's normal motions, such as kicking and rubbing, can remove the adhesive bandage and cause bleeding

Fig. 7.8: Checking blood glucose by analyzer

Large amounts of glucose infused during labour may result in foetal hyperinsulinaemia with a postnatal rebound hypoglycaemia. For this reason glucose is usually not infused during labour. There also may be transient neonatal tachypnoea, hyponatraemia, and elevated bilirubin, levels when fluid intake during labour has not been carefully regulated.

Several factors influence neonatal calcium metabolism and increase the risk for hypocalcaemia. At delivery, maternal calcium supplies end. Levels of hormones that control calcium metabolism are low at birth. In addition, the foetus that is stressed in utero also is at high risk for hypocalcaemia.

Results of a normal transition show serum glucose levels in the normal range or 50 to 100 mg/dl and calcium in the normal range of 7 to 8 mg/dl. A difficult transition may manifest in several ways. Tremors are most commonly seen, but

Lethargy, Tachypnoea, Pallor and Cyanosis also are common signs of hypoglycaemia or hypocalcaemia. It is important to anticipate metabolic imbalances in infants who are especially at risk: those who are small or large for gestational age, LGA, SGA infants of diabetic mothers (IDM), and premature and postmature infants.

Warning signs of poor metabolic control, are as follows:

1. LGA, SGA, IDM, preterm, or post-term infants.
2. Temperature less than or above normal range.
3. Tremors, tachypnoea, pallor, cyanosis
4. Glucose < 50 mg/dl
5. Calcium < 7 mg/dl.

Integumentary System

The integumentary system is the next system to be evaluated as the nurse continues to undress the infant. The information obtained from assessing this system often is related to the integrity of other systems (e.g. skin colour provides information as to the health of the cardiovascular and haematologic systems).

At birth the skin and its structures are exposed to the dry. colder extrauterine environment. Any vernix that remains is absorbed. Therefore skin commonly becomes dry and may crack at the ankles and wrists. The term infant's skin normally will peel within two days of birth; peeling before that time is not normal. Desquamation (peeling) over the entire body is a classic sign seen in the premature infant.

If the infant is chilled, Cutis Marmorata, which is mottled or marbled appearance over thin body, may be observed. It is caused by dilation of the small blood vessels, not an expected reaction to chilling. It usually is seen only during early infancy but may persist longer in infants with certain congenital problems. The Barlequi sign is a phenomenon seen only in the newborn infant, more often in low birth weight. The infant who is lying on one slde will becomo bright red over the dependent half of the body and very pale over the half that is superior. There is a definits line of demarcation between the two colour, which will reverse sides if the infant's position is reversed. This sign is benign and lasts a short while.

Pigmentation is genetically determined and influenced by the extra-uterine environment. After birth, when the infant is exposed to light, the skin of black infants will continue to darken. Above 90 per cent of all infants of black, Asian, or Latin origin will have mongolian spots which result from the deep dermal infiltration of melanonocytes. These flat, irregularly shaped, pigmented lesions are seen most commonly over the lumbosacral region, They vary in size (some may be quite large) and colour from grey-blue to blue-black. With age these lesions appear to fade but actually become less obvious as the overlying skin loses its transparency. After age 4, these mongolian spots may seem to have disappeared.

The most common skin variation seen during the transition period is Erythema Toxicum. The cause of this is not known, but its appearance has alarmed the mothers of many full-term infants. These pale-yellow to white pustules and papules with reddened bases usually erupt first on the trunk but then may spread to the entire body, with the exception of soles and palms. The lesions disappear spontaneously within hours to days after their appearance.

Many full-term infants are born with Milia, or epidermal inclusion cysts. These small white or yellow papules are commonly found on the nose, chin, and forehead, when they appear on the palate or gums, they are called Epstein's Pearls. Both types disappear early in infancy. Sweat may be retained in small, noninflammatory vesicles called miliaria. These also are seen over the forehead, as well as the neck and diaper area. Because this condition usually occurs in infants who live in a hot, humid environment, cooling and drying the infant will cause the vesicles to resolve.

Inspection of the integumentary system takes place during the examination of other systems. It is presented here to provide guidance for the balance of the examination.

The skin colour is observed in natural light. If this is not possible the examiner should recognize that fluorescent light tends to alter true colour. Skin thickens as gestational age increases; therefore the less mature infant's skin is more transparent.

The pigmentation, which ranges from pale to dark brown, is assessed. Mucous membranes should have underlying pink tones, and no cyanotic changes should be seen with crying or activity. Acrocyanosis and mottling occur early but may be abnormal if they persist. The examiner notes whether the infant is *pink* or has *pallor* (pale pink or white underlying tone) or *plethore* (ruddy, purplish colour). The skin of the forehead or abdomen is blanched by applying finger pressure momentarily and observing the return of colour (capiliary filling), which should be prompt. This is an indication of perfusion. The presence of jaundice also is noted.

It is important to examine the entire skin surface including the neck and inguinal and axillary folds. At term, vernix caseosa is found only in these deep skin folds. Skin turgor, an indication of adequate intrauterine growth, is examined by gently pinching a fold of skin on the abdomen or thigh, any oedema or extra folds of skin also are noted.

The quality and distribution of hair are important parts of both gestational age assessment and evaluation of the infant at risk for genetic disease. Unusual patterns and distributions of hair growth are associated with some genetic syndromes (e.g, Cornelia de Lange syndrome). In addition certain racial groups have heavier hair distribution at birth. Lanugo is fine, downy hair that covers the back, shoulders, and forehead of a preterm infant and is present on the shoulders at term. Nail growth increases with gestation; nails will have grown to the end of the fingers at term and past the finger tips after term. The skin thickens and begins to peel (Desquamation) if the infant is postmature.

The examiner looks for birth marks, skin injuries, and meconium staining and gently palpates masses for consistency, tenderness, and return of colour noting whether a reddened lesion blanches with pressure, which indicates a vascular connection. Tiny red spots that do not blanch with pressure may be petechiae or microhaemorrhages within the skin, possibly caused by pressure during birth. Another cause, thrombocytopenia can be life threatening but is also a sign of congenital infection. Oval reddened areas (forceps marks) may be observed on the cheeks of infants whose delivery has been assisted with forceps. Most of these marks gradually disappear.

Some integumentary structures are subject to prenatal stimulation by maternal hormones. One manifestation is secretion of a colostrum-like fluid ("witch's milk") by the breasts during the neonatal period, which is seen in both male and female infants.

Other structures also may appear to mature early. Occasionally a tooth may erupt during foetal life and be seen at birth (natal teeth). It is almost always a prematurely erupted deciduous tooth rather than an extra or super-numerary, one. An attempt is made to save the tooth, if possible. Before the infant is discharged, however, a loose tooth is removed to prevent possible aspiration.

Nevi are genetic changes in the skin. There are many types of nevi, some spontaneously disappear and others do not. Within each of these groups are two other subdivision: telangiectatic or flat and haemangiomatous or raised. Salmon patch or strawberry haemangiomata are flat, pale pink, irregularly shaped lesions called "stork's bites" when found at the nape of the neck. About 50 per cent of all white newborns have a simple haemangioma either on the sacrum, the back of the neck, the face, or eyelids. These are small at birth, then grow, and eventually disappear. Although they fade with age, parents may express concern when they are first noticed. Nevus flammeus, or port-wina stain, is seriously disfiguring and most often found on the face; unfortunately, this does not disappear. Giant haemangiomata are larger and raised; these can be dangerous if they trap platelets and thereby lower the amount of circulating platelets.

Most skin lesions are harmless, although they usually are a source of concern to parents who naturally hope for the perfect infant. Parents need to know which of these will disappear spontaneously and which need treatment. Common skin lesions described in the following list are warning signs of of integumentary system problems:

- Long nails and desquamation indicating postmaturity.
- Thin translucent skin with abundant vernix and lanugo, indicating prematurity.
- Pallor, possibly caused by hypothermia, anaemia, sepsis or shock.
- Cyanosis, possibly caused by cardiorespiratory disease, hypoglycaemia, polycythaemia, sepsis, or hypothermia.
- Petechiae, possibly caused by thrombocytopaenia, sepsis, congenital infection, or pressure sustained during delivery.
- Plethora, possibly caused by polycythaemia.
- Meconium staining, possibly caused by intrauterine asphyxia.
- Abnormal hair distribution (unrelated to gestational age) or extra skin folds, possibly associated with genetic syndromes.
- Poor skin turgor associated with intrauterine growth retardation and hypoglycaemia.
- Large (cavernous) haemangiomas, which may trap platelets within their borders and cause thrombocytopenia.

- Bullae or pustules, possibly caused by staphylococcal infection.

Common neonatal skin lesions will include the following:

- Naevi
- Haemangiomata (Developmental vascular abnormalities)
  - Flat (telangiectatic) haemangiomata: salmon-pink colour and easy to blanch; found at nape of neck, eyelids, and forehead; fade within 1 year.
  - Naevus flammeus (port-wine stain): Red to black in colour; if found on face along trigeminal nerve tract, may be associated with cerebral vascular mal-formation.
  - Raised and giant (cavernous) haemangiomata: Bright red to reddish blue in colour; tend to increase in size after birth; cavernous type may trap platelets, causing thrombocytopenia.
- Pigmental lesions:
  - Mongolian spots: Grey to blue; found on lumbo-sacral area in black, fade in first few years of life.
  - Cafe-au-lait sports; small, brown patches; if more than six are present or any are larger than 4 x 6 cm, infant may have neurofibromatosis: with aging these may undergo precancerous changes.
- Erythema toxicum:
  - Maculopapular rash that may include small pustule-like lesions containing sterile fluid and eosinophils (white cells indicative of an allergic response rather than infection); found on the trunk and face; fades within a few days.
- Milia neonatorum:
  - Epidermal cysts containing keratogenous material; look like whiteheads found over the nose and chin; fades within a few days.
- Miliaria:
  - Retention of sweat in unopened exocrine glands causing clear vesicles on the face, scalp, and perineum; resolve in a few days if environmental heat and humidity are not extreme.
- Bullae:
  - Blister over 1 cm in diameter.
- Pustules:
  - Small lesion containing pus; may be signs of Staphylococcal infection; needs to be differentiated from erythema toxicum.

Gastrointestinal System

For the first 15 minutes to half hour after birth (first period of reactivity), the healthy, full-term infants will be alert and eager to suck-this is the ideal time to initiate breastfeeding. Newborn gastric capacity at term is about 10 to 20 ml. Although the stomach will not empty completely during the first few hours of life this is not a concern because the breastfeeding infant will consume only a small amount of colostrum.

The suck-swallow mechanism that has been functioning prenatally further matures after birth to prevent aspiration. The result of this maturation is the rapid opening of the epiglottis during swallowing and closing during respiration. The cardiac sphincter between the oesophagus and stomach in the newborn infant frequently is less than fully functional; therefore reflux of gastric contents into the oesophagus and upward into the pharynx may occur during the second period of reactivity from about the second to sixth hour after delivery when the infant demonstrates variability in several areas of adjustment to extrauterine life. It is also during this time that the infant may become 'mucousy', or have difficulty with mucus secretions. The infant may gag or choke and it may be necessary to clear the airway by changing the position or by suctioning any secreations.

Bowel sounds can be heard as the first period of reactivity ends. Meconium usually is passed during the second period of reactivety, although it may occur *in utero* or at delivery.

There are several congenital defects that affect the gastrointestinal system. Early general assessment may detect if there is an Imperforate Anus, with feeding, lack of an intact oesophagus would immediately cause an infant to choke.

Inspection

The abdominal wall should be free of defects. The cord is observed for colour and amount of Wharton's jelly Umbilical cord changes should be consistent with the age in days; it will blacken and become dry within 2 to 3 days. An umbilical hernia may be present. This mass protrudes more when the infant cries and is seen more commonly in black infants. The abdominal girth is measured just above the umbilicus. The rectum should be patent, and meconium should be passed within 24 hours. Some meconium filled loops of bowel may bulge through the abdominal wall until this occurs.

Auscultation

The examiner always auscultates for bowel sounds before palpating the abdomen because bowel motility can be affected by palpation. Bowel sounds should be present several hours after birth.

Palpation

Palpation of the newborn abdomen requires gentle firmness. It should be done at least 2 hours after a feeding. The entire abdomen is palpated in a systematic manner, noting masses. The liver should be evaluated for size by palpation from the right iliac crest upto the right costal margin until the lower liver edge is felt to slip against the fingers to 1 to 3 cm below the right costal margin. The spleen tip may be felt at the left costal margin.

There should be no masses, but the examiner may feel some loops of bowel. There may be diastasis or separation of the rectus muscles, which feels like softness in the midline between the two hands of rectus muscles.

Observation of any of the following warning signs for the GI system requires intervention:

- Obvious defects in the abdominal wall, possibly gastroschisis or omphalocele.
- Single umbilical artery associated with congenital, especially renal anomalies.
- Meconium stained or shriveled umbilical cord associated with intra-uterine growth retardation or perinatal asphyxia.
- Imperforate anus, which may be associated with a tracheoesophageal fistula or oesophageal atresis.
- Hepatosplenomegaly (enlarged liver and spleen) associated with congenital infections and haemolysis.
- Flat or scaphoid abdomen, which may be associated with a diaphragmatic hernia (congenital defect in which abdominal contents are in the thorax).
- Failure to pass meconium stool within 24 hours.
- History of polyhydramnios during pragnancy.
- Masses anywhere in abdomen.

Genitourinary System

Renal

The removal of the placenta at birth ends the neonate's dependence on the maternal kidneys for renal function. The quality of renal function in the term infant generally is adequate for the infant's needs. However, the ability of the newborn kidney to adapt to stress is limited. This deficiency improves during the first week of life and continue. During the neonatal period, urine composition changes from dilute (specific gravity 1,004 to 1,010) to more concentrated as renal function matures. By 2 months of age, the infant's urine has a strong odour and the specific gravity of adult urine.

Adrenal

The normal foetus responds to the stress of labour and delivery with secretion of catecholamines, which cause foetal heart rate accelerations and help to mobilize hepatic glycogen for energy in the immediate neonatal period.

Assessment

Kidneys and bladder The quantity of amniotic fluid is the first clue that the kidneys are functioning . After birth the infant should void within the first 24 hours. The first voiding is easy to miss, because newborn urine is quite dilute and may not be noticed in the excitement immediately after birth. Newborns then void frequently, wetting six to eight diapers a day. If measured, the normal infant's output of urine is 1 to 3 ml/kg of body weight per hour. The kidney are palpated bimanually (using both hands). The examiner, supporting the infant's lumbar region from below, palpates the flank deeply in the spine just under the costal margin.

Female genitalia The examiner assesses the configuration of the labia and hymen and notes the placement of the urinary meatus and rectum and the length of the perineum, as well as the size of the clitoris and labia, which vary with gestational age.

In the full-term female, the labia almost completely cover the clitoris. There should be no fusion of the labia; hymenal tags (small tags of mucous membrane extending from the vaginal are not significant. A white mucous discharge, sometimes streaked with light pink blood (Pseudomenstruation), often is present and is the result of withdrawal of maternal hormones for a few days after birth. The labia may be edmatous and darker than usual in response to birth pressure and maternal hormones.

Fused labia, clitoral hypertrophy, and placement of the urinary meatus anterior to the clitoris are signs of sexual ambiguity. With prematurity, there are widely spaced labia majora and a large clitoris. Bulging of the hymen may be caused by the pressure of fluid behind an imperforate hymen.

Male genitalia: The examiner inspects the penis for correct placement of the urinary meatus which should always be at the tip of the penis. The scrotum is observed for colour, size and rugae (deep wrinkles), which vary with gestational age. The scrotum is larger and covered with rugae close to term. The colour is dark because of the passive transfer of maternal hormones. After a breech delivery, the infant may have bruises and oedema of the genitalia, which resolves after several days, but gross abnormalities should not occur.

The examiner palpates the testes by blocking the inguinal canal with one finger while gently palpating the scrotum with a thumb and forefinger. The fullness of the scrotal sac is noted. By 36 weeks each testis should have descended into the scrotum and is palpated separataly. Each should be smooth, about 1 cm in diameter, and freely movable. The testes may retract into inguinal canal if the infant is cold.

Male infants frequently have erections, which also may surprise new parents. Infants have been observed engaged in pelvic rocking. The possibility of infantile sexual reactions is disturbing to some. Cutaneous sensation, however, is the first sensory capability to develop and remains a major source of sensory input during the neonatal period.

The following conditions are warning signs of genitourinary system problems:

Female and male
- Oligohydramnios
- Mass palpated in abdomen
- Defects of the abdominal wall
- Failure to void within 24 hours.

Female genitalia
- Clitoris hypertrophy
- Fused labia
- Abnormal placement of the urinary meatus.

Male genitalia
- Hypospadias (urinary meatus opening on ventral surface of penis)
- Epispadias (urinary meatus opening on dorsal surface of penis)
- Micropenis
- Bifid or split scrotum (not fused in midline)
- Scrotal masses
- Hydrocele fluid within scrotal sac).

Haematologic Systems (Table 7.6)

At birth, the haematologic system is infused with oxygen. The relatively low oxygen tension of umbilical venous blood is replaced with the higher oxygen tension now supplied by the lungs via the pulmonary artery. Adjustment from a foetal to adult state of function occurs gradually. Observations focus on the ability of this system to carry oxygen, rid itself of its foetal haemoglobin load, and maintain normal coagulation.

Using the Heel Stick Method to Obtain Blood

Purpose

To obtain the newborn's blood for assessment of blood glucose levels, haematocrit, phenylketonuria, or bilirubin level as ordered or when symptoms of hypoglycaemia occur.

Equipment

- Alcohol swab
- Lancet or Tenderfoot capillary tubes
- Dextrostix
- Gloves
- Small round adhesive bandage
- Sterile 2 x 2 gauze pads.

Haemoglobin vs Haematocrit

The normal term infant has a blood volume of about 80 ml/kg of body weight. Haematocrit values will range from 45 to 65% if drawn from a vein or artery; because of the normally sluggish peripheral circulation, it will be higher if a capillary sample is examined. Haemoglobin levels are about one-third of total haematocrit; that is, an infant whose haematocrit value is 60% will have a haemoglobin level around 20 g/dl. Within the first few days, the red cell mass decreases from a prenatal 5 to 6 million/mm^3 to a more adult level of 4 to 5 million/mm^3. This extra red cell destruction contributes to the bilirubin load to be metabolized.

Blood volume is affected by birth technique. If the neonate is held above the level of the placenta before the cord is clamped, enough blood can flow back into the placenta from the infant to produce

Table 7.6: Nursing action and rationale for heel stick method

Nursing action	*Rationale*
1. Wash hands and apply gloves	1. Standard precautions require gloves for contact with blood and body fluids.Washing hands helps prevent cross-contamination
2. Warm the baby's heel for 15 to 30 seconds by wrapping the foot in a warm pack(warm a diaper by running it under warm water; do not cover with plastic or use a disposable diaper with plastic)	2. Wrapping the foot in a warm pack is somtimes helpful to increase circulation to the site (heat causes local vasodilation and increased blood flow). Application of hot pack can cause thermal burns. Plastic covers prevent heat dissipation and can result in thermal burns
3. Choose either side of the heel (either the lateral or medial aspect of the heel) as the puncture site. The lateral aspect of the heel is the preferred heel stick site	3. Puncturing the side rather than the middle of the heel prevents damaging the posterior tibial nerve and artery and the longitudinal fat pad, which could interfere with walking (Fig. 7.10).
4. Cleanse the site with an alcohol swab. Dry the site with a sterile 2 × 2 gauze pad	4. Cleansing the site alcohol minimizes contamination. Drying the site is important because alcohol can be irritating and can cause haemolysis
5. Puncture the heel with the lancet or Tender-foot to achieve free flow of blood. (Tenderfoot is a small plastic case that houses a needle. When the case is placed on the baby's foot, the needle can be automatically ejected) (Fig. 7.9)	5. Free flow of blood ensure an adequate sample. Use of Tenderfoot ensures controlled depth of entry and makes optmal penetration possible (i.e; penetration is deep enough to obtain an adequate specimen yet superficial enough to prevent damage to tissues, nerves, and bones and to prevent fibrosis and scarring caused by repeated sampling)
6. Collect blood into capillary tubes, onto Dextrostix, or onto Chemstrip. If necessary, gently apply slight pressure to the foot or ankle above the puncture site to obtain enough blood	6. The collection device needed depends on the test being done. Application of slight pressure is sometimes necessary to obtain enough blood
7. Cover heel stick site with small circular bandage	7. Applying on adhesive bandage creates pressure needed to minimize bleeding, and it protects the site from contamination
8. Check the heel site frequently for bleeding	The baby's normal motions, such as klicking can remove the adhesive bandage and cause bleeding

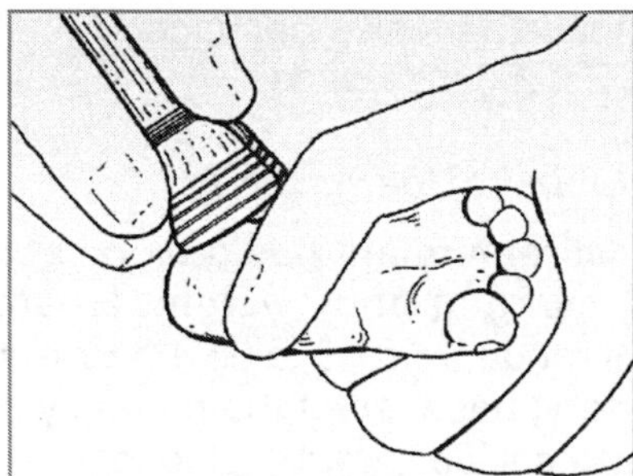

Fig. 7.9: Application of lancet to achieve free flow of blood

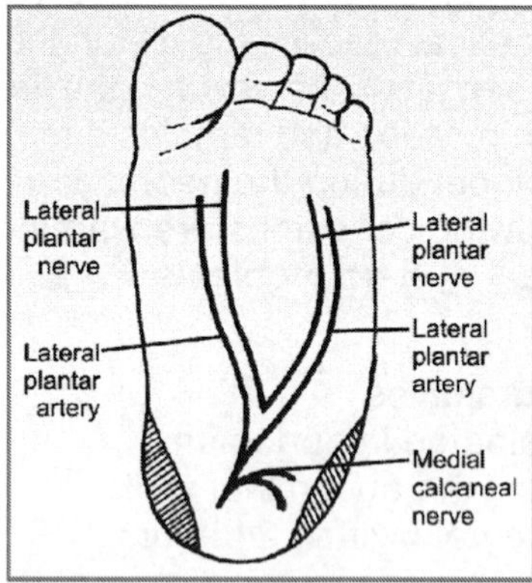

Fig. 7.10: Position of arteries and nerves in the sole

anaemia. If the baby is held below the level of the placenta, or if the cord is squeezed along its length towards the infant ("milked") there will be enough extra blood transfused to cause Polycythaemia. Because each condition is dangerous, if is recommended that the infant be held in level with the placenta until cord clamping is accomplished.

The function of haemoglobin is the same in foetal and adult life. Adequate growth and metabolism cannot proceed without a constant supply of oxygen. The infant's ability to provide this depends on the concentration of oxygen in the air, the level of pulmonary maturity, adequate cardiac output, adequate volumes of blood and haemoglobin, and ability of the blood to carry and deliver oxygen to the tissues. The concentration of oxygen in the blood (pO_2) and the ability of the blood to carry oxygen (determined chiefly by the amount and type of haemoglobin) contribute to oxygen saturation. Normally between 96% and 98% of haemoglobin is saturated with oxygen. During foetal life, oxygen is supplied via umbilical venous blood flow in a concentration far lower (pO_2 is 30 mm Hg) than that which is normal during extrauterine life. Thus foetal oxygen saturation must still be kept in the normal range, although less oxygen is available. The following adaptations have evolved in the human foetus to allow for this:

1. Total haemoglobin concentration is increased (1.5 to 20 g/dl vs 11 to 13 g/dl in the adult
2. Red cell mass is increased in the foetus to 5 to 6 million/mm3
3. Foetal haemoglobin has a high haemoglobin-oxygen affinity (haemoglobin-oxygen binding)

The increased affinity of foetal haemoglobin of oxygen makes it harder to detect hypoxia by observing cyanosis in the neonate, because a greater amount of haemoglobin is associated with oxygen at any pO_2.

Bilirubin

Bilirubin is produced when the haeme portion of the hemoglobin molecule is catabolized. The destruction of 1 g of haemoglobin yields 35 mg of bilirubin. Bilirubin is produced in the reticuloendothelial system and is bound to albumin, a plasma protein for transport to the liver. In the liver, two acceptor proteins remove the bilirubin from the circulation. The bilirubin at the point is indirect, also called unconjugated, it is available for diffusion across cell membranes. Conjugation, the most important step in bilirubin metabolism, occurs in the liver. Conjugation is a process by which fat-soluble, indirect bilirubin is converted to a water-soluble substance called conjugated or direct bilirubin, Bilirubin must be metabolized in this way to be excreted. If the metabolic process is delayed, high levels of bilirubin for hyperbilirubinaemia will produce jaundice or yellow discolouration of the skin and sclerae. More important, high levels of indirect bilirubin are toxic to the brain and will produce kernicterus.

Jaundice

At birth most infants, even those severely affected with intrauterine haemolytic disease, will not have jaundice. The situation quickly changes, however, when the maternal system is no longer available for metabolism of bilirubin. Jaundice is not apparent until the serum bilirubin level rises above 5 mg/dl of blood and should not develop until the infant is more than 24 hours old. The timing of its appearance is influenced by the factors that produced it. The large haemoglobin load is one factor contributing to the frequency of physiologic jaundice because unconjugated bilirubin produced prenatally is easily carried across the lipid-rich cell membrane of the placental endothelium and transported to the maternal liver for metabolism and secretion into bile. It is then excreted via the mother's small and large intestine.

Coagulation

The newborn infant's bowel is sterile at birth and thus does not support the normal production of vitamin K until adequate food and bacteria are in the intestine. Because vitamin K will not be produced before adequate food intake has occurred, parenteral administration of vitamin K soon after delivery is an established way of correcting this lag in production. Most term neonates are deficient in factors II, VII, IX, and X. These deficiencies are even more prevalent in the premature infant. It may take weeks to several months for the neonate to develop adult levels of clotting factors. The normal newborn, however, has adequate platelets for haemostasis.

The examiner integrates assessment of the haematologic system with that of the skin, eyes, gastrointestinal, and cardiorespiratory systems. In natural light, the infant's skin tone is observed for pallor, plethora (ruddy colour caused by a high haematocrit level), and jaundice. Firmly pressing the skin over the forehead, sternum, or calf, the examiner looks quickly for the first colour in the pressed spot; If it is yellow, it indicates jaundice. In infants with brown skin it may be necessary to look at the mucous membranes and sclera of the eye. Jaundice proceeds from head to foot in a cephalocaudal direction as bilirubin levels rise although the sclera become yellow last. Thus this examination provides some idea of the severity of the hyperbilirubinaemia, but a serum level always should be established for confirmation. The neonatal laboratory values are as follows:

- Haemoglobin: 13.5-21 g/dl
- Haematocrit: 45%-65% (central)

- Red blood cells: 4-6 million/mm^3
- White blood cells. 10,000-30,000/mm^3
- Platelets > 100,000/mm^3

Total serum Bilirubin

- First 24 hrs < 5 mg/dl
- Second 24 hrs < 10 mg/dl
- Third 24 hrs < 12 mg /dl
- Decreases thereafter.
- No jaundice after the first week.

Palpation of the liver add spleen aids the assessment because enlargement of these organs often accompanies newborn haemolytic disease. The examiner also checks the maternal and neonatal blood types and indirect and direct Coomb's test results.

Small red spots that do not blanch with pressure are *Petechiae* (microhaemorrhages within the skin). Large bruises (areas of ecchymosis) called Purpura also may be present on the face of an infant whose cord was around the neck or on areas of pressure during the birth process (vertex or breech). These bruises may indicate thrombocytopenia, which must be investigated.

Warning signs of haematologic system problems are as follows:

- Pallor
- Plethora, hypoglycaemia (associated with polycythaemia)
- Jaundice
- Hepatosplenomegaly
- Petechiae or purpura not over pressure area
- Thrombocytopenia.

Immunologic System

Although developed prenatally, the immune system begins to function sluggishly at birth. The normal full-term newborn will experience exposure and colonization with an endless number of organisms. Infection should not develop. Whether infection occurs is a function of the infant's own immunity, the presence of IgA and other immune factors found in breast milk, and the handwashing diligence of the neonatal staff. Sepsis has been called the "great pretender" because its signs and symptoms are so varied in the neonate.

The examiner observes the infant or pallor, cyanosis, jaundice, lethargy or irritability and poor or shrill cry, with special attention to an infant with the following risk factors:

1. Low birth weight
2. Prematurity regardless of birth weight
3. Birth more than 24 hours after rupture of membranes
4. Mother a known hepatitis B carrier, drug user, or lacking in prenatal care.

A complete blood cell count, culture of blood, cerebrosoinal fluid, and urine may be ordered for infants at risk for sepsis.

The following warning signs pertain to immunologic system problems:

- "Doesn't look right"
- Foul-smelling amniotic fluid.
- Maternal fever during labour
- Pallor/cyanosis/lethargy/petechiae.
- Respiratory distress
- Hypoglycaemia
- Hypothermia.

Head and Neck

Examination of the head, ears, eyes, nose, and throat, as well as special senses, will precede neurologic assessment because the condition of these structures is a sign of the integrity of the neurologic system. Many anomalies of the head and neck are associated with neurologic dysfunction.

Head

The head is inspected from all sides for size, shape and evidence of trauma, Molding may be present with vaginal or caesarean delivery, if the foetus has been in the breech position, the vertex may be flattened and the occiput prominent.

The condition of the scalp and cranial bones is considered. If internal foetal heart rate monitoring or foetal blood sampling was performed during labour, lacerations of the scalp may be present. Occasionally an infant delivered by caesarean birth sustains a scalp laceration during incision of the uterus. The quality of the hair also is noted, premature infants have woolly hair, whereas the hair of full-term infants is soft and silky.

The examiner palpates the head from the frontal bone, following the suture line to the diamond-shaped anterior fontanelle, then along the coronal suture, and next along the sagittal suture to the triangle-shaped posterior fontanelle. The occiput is palpated, and the assessment continues laterally to the parietal bones until the entire skull has been examined. If there is molding, the suture lines may be overriding, or there may be only a small space between the cranial bones. Premature closure of one or more sutures (Craniosynostosis) retards brain growth and causes the skull to develop an odd shape.

Fontanelles should feel soft and flat. The normal anterior fontanelle measures 2 x 3 cm and closes about 18 months after birth. The posterior fontanelle is much smaller and closes by the fourth month. Abnormally large fontanelles may be a sign of hydrocephaly, osteogenesis imperfacta, or congenital hypothyroidism. Unusually small fontanelles also may be normal or associated with microcephaly.

During birth the head is subjected to pressure from the forces of labour. The sutures and fontanelles provide space for movement of these bones during labour and delivery, causing temporary molding of the foetal head however the transitional stage of labour is excessively long, the pressure of the ischial spines on the foetal parietal bones may cause subperiosteal bleeding, or cephalohaematoma Pressure on the presenting part may cause it to become edematous. In a vertex presentation this is seen as caput succedaneum or oedema of the scalp.

Examination of the head may reveal the following warning signs:

- Widely spaced suture lines or abnormally large fontanelles
- Abnormally small fontanelles or suture lines that do not override or that have spaces
- Bulging fontanelles, a sign of increased intracranial pressure
- Depressed fontanelles, possibly associates with dehydration
- Large cephallohaematoma, possible associated with skull fracture, extreme molding, or intracranial bleeding
- Lacerations of the scalp with widely separated wound edges, which may need suturing
- Malformations of the head, face or spine
- Abnormal head circumference.

Eyes

The examiner observes for symmetry and size of the eyes, colour of the sclera and iris, and the presence of exudate of any other deviations from normal. The eyes should be equal to size and symmetrically placed. The angle of slant from inner to outer canthus is noted. A mongolian slant is upward from inner to outer canthus, the opposite is an anti-mongolian slant. The sclera may be white to blue-white; subconjunctival haemorrhage can result from the pressure on the infant's face and head during delivery. The iris varies with heredity from darker or lighter slate blue to brown. Speckling of the iris (Brushfield's spots), Epican that Folds (a vertical fold of skin covering the inner canthus), and a slant up or down from the inner canthus to the outer are associated with trisomy 21. Chemical conjunctivitis from eye prophylaxis may produce whitish exudate within the first 24 hours. Pressure during the birth may cause the eyelids to become edematous. The sun-setting signs appears as a crescent of sclera over the iris and is caused by retraction of the upper lid; it is seen with hydrocephalus, when open, the lids should cover only the top part of the iris; drooping or ptosis is a sign of neuromuscular weakness. The examiner turns the infant's head from side-to-side and observes for doll's eyes movement, a lag in eye movement is normal in the newborn.

The examiner places the infant in the supine position and inspects the pupillary reflex by shining a light first into one eye and then the other. Pupillary reflexes appear at 30 weeks' gestational age and should be equal. The red reflex, a circular red area of light at the pupil is noted. The red reflex indicates congenital cataract (opacity of the lens). The observation is commonly documented when checking Perrl (Pupils equal round, reactive to light).

Ocular movements are observed when the infant is alert. The examiner holds a light or red object 10 to 12 inches from the eyes and tries to get the infant to follow. The full-term infant should be able to follow a bright object or a face for 180 degress horizontally and for 30 degress vertically; however the eyes may not move smoothly and in unison because of immature muscular control. This is seen as crossing of the eyes or strabismus. The infant should blink in response to bright light (optical blink reflex) but will show habituation to this response.

Newborn infants are relatively nearsighted and focus best on an object held at a distance of 10 to 12 inches.

The normal newborn shows interest in highly contrasting, brightly coloured patterns. This is why the human face, with its sharply contrast in features hold the neonate's attention.

The bright lights and hasty administration of eye prophylaxis in conventional delivery room settings are deterrents to neonatal vision. In spite of their normally decreased visual acuity, infants delivered in an environment where the lighting is dimmed will open their eyes and scan the area. When eye prophylaxis is delayed, the neonate will make eye-to-eye contact, an important part of early parent-infant interaction and bonding.

Ears

The placement of the ears is noted by using a straight edge and visualizing a line between the pinna and the inner canthus of the eye. The configuration, firmness, and degree of incurving of the pinna are observed. (This is an important part of gestational age assessment). Examination of the canal and tympanic membrane (eardrum) soon after birth usually is not possible because vernix fills the canal. After vernix is absorbed, the membrane is visualized by pulling the ear lobe down and back. The membrane should appear light, pearly gray, and translucent. Often this examination is not included in the initial neonatal inspection.

Skin tags and preauricular sinuses may be innocuous or associated with renal malformations, and low-set or otherwise malformed ears are associated with chromosomal aberrations.

Hearing

Hearing may be impaired in the normal neonate if the external auditory canal is filled with amniotic fluid or vernix. This usually resolves within days.

The examiner observes the infant's startle reflex in response to loud noise and preference for high-pitched voices. The normal newborn will turn to the sound of the human voice and shows preference to the mother's voice. Refer to the Brazelton's neonatal behavioural assessment (P-383) for a description of the infant's ability to habituate to repetitive, noisy stimuli.

Warning signs for eye and ear problems follows:

- Exudate that is copious, greenish yellow, or persists or appears after 24 hours of age, possibly caused by an infectious process.
- Jaundice of the sclera caused by hyperbilirubinemia.
- Ptosis
- Sun-setting sign
- Brushfield's spots, epicanthal folds, and mongolian slant associated with Down's syndrome.
- Antimongolian slant associated with chromosomal abnormalities.
- Cataract associated with congenital rubella.
- Lack of optical blink reflex or failure to follow objects associated with blindness.
- Short palpabal fissures associated with foetal alcohol syndrome.
- Failure to respond to loud noise or human voice, or both.
- Low-set or malformed ears.

Nose

The examiner observes for gross abnormalities of the nose and face for nasal patency by closing the infant's mouth and noting slight nasal flaring as the baby breathes. A soft catheter can be passed through both nares, but the previous method is less traumatic. Air should easily enter through the nose. A small amount of clear or white nasal discharge may stimulate the sneeze reflex, which is not a sign of illness. Copious nasal discharge may be a sign of congenital syphilis, and difficulty with nasal breathing may be associated with choanal atresia (blocked posterior nasal passages). Neonates are obligate nasal breathers—they will not breathe through the mouth if nasal passages are blocked. Therefore assessment of nasal patency is vital.

Mouth

While the infant is quiet, the lips and mouth are inspected for external defects and symmetry. There should be no obvious defects. Mucous membranes should be moist and pink. All movements of the mouth should be symmetric; facial movement may be caused by facial nerve palsy (commonly associated with forceps delivery). The examiner places a gloved-finger near the mouth to note rooting, then places a gloved finger near the mouth to note rooting, then places the finger in the infant's mouth to test sucking, and runs the finger over the hard and soft palates or uses a tongue blade to stimulate the gag reflex, which should be easily elicited. Sucking and rooting reflexes should be strong and coordinated with swallowing. Weak or absent root, suck, or swallow reflexes may be associated with neonatal depression caused by maternal medication or perinatal asphyxia.

When the infant cries, the examiner notes the size of the tongue and its coordination with the soft palate and uvula during movement and oberves for the presence of natal teeth.

Neck

To properly visualize the anterior aspect of the normally short neonatal neck, the examiner extends it by placing one hand behind the neck and allowing the head to fall back slightly. The neck is inspected for skin tags, masses and pits and the posterior portion is abserved for skin folds, the hairline, and the contour of the neck. The head should rotate freely during this process.

The examiner pulls the infant to a sitting position and looks for head lag, noting how well the infant can use the neck extensors and flexors to control the head in the upright position. This is the only time that the examiner does not support the infant's head.

The clavicles are palpated. Fractures may be sustained if a large baby has shoulder dystocia delivery. The examiner may note a "crunchy" feeling (crepitus) or actually feel the two ends of the broken bone. The eternocleidomastoid muscle is palpated and any masses noted.

The following warning signs require further investigation for nose, mouth and neck problems:

Nose

- Occluded nares
- Copious nasal discharge.

Mouth

- Cleft lip or palate, or both
- Large or small mouth
- Thin upper lip and smooth philtrum (bow of lip)
- Weak or absent root, suck, swallow or gag reflexes.
- Poorly coordinated suck and swallow
- Asymmetric facial movement or appearance
- Large tongue
- Natal teeth or other masses.

Neck

- Masses, pits, or skin tags
- Abnormal hair line
- Head lag
- Crepitus, poor arm movement.

Neuromuscular System

During intrauterine life the normally developing foetus exhibits voluntary and involuntary activities that increase in complexity and frequency with maturity. These prepare the infant for many behaviours vital for healthy extrauterine life. Chest wall movements encourage pulmonary development; rooting, sucking, and swallowing reflexes prepare or feeding, arm and leg movements keep limbs supple and promote symmetric muscular growth. Increasing muscle tone produces a posture of increasing flexion as pregnancy advances. This will help the newborn conserve body heat by exposing less body surface to the colder environment as well as keeping the handle positioned close to the mouth, encouraging rooting and sucking. Although reflexes such as the Moro and grasp must have had a positive survival value for our evolutionary ancestors, they now have no critical use.

The normal intrauterine environment provides only minimal variations in temparature, tactile sansation, light, and louder sound of the extrauterine world. These are functional because they provide the neonatal nervous system with necessary stimuli, as do rising carbon dioxide levels during the second stage of labour. Efforts can be made, however, for a gentler transition during the immediate neonatal period by shielding the newborn's eyes from harsh, direct, lighting and by handling and speaking gently to the infant. A gentle delivery is especially important, a time when pressure from maternal structures and assisting hands or instruments can injure delicate nerves, bones and connective tissue.

The close relationship of the neurologic and musculoskeletal systems, other functionally and anatomically, allows simultaneous assessment. Normal structure and behaviours both voluntary and indicators of normal foetal development and future neonatal function.

Assessment of foetal neuromuscular status begins during the observation of heart rate variability and accelerations with movement. These initial observations of the neonate's neurologic status are included in the Apgar score. The rest of the neurologic examination may be delayed for 24 hours to allow for recovery from birth and partial metabolism of any medications given to the mother. The examination is devided into three parts; general assessment; evaluation of motor function, development reflexes, and cranial nerve function; and behavioural assessment. This assessment is time consuming the tiring for the infant. It may not be completed in the setting; the demands in a busy unit may requirs an abbreviated examination.

General Assessment

Overall assessment should take place when the infant is quiet and neither too sleepy nor too hungry. The examiner should always remember to maintain warmth and especially to note the following:

1. Weight, height and head and chest sizes (abnormal growth and development are associated with neurologic dysfunctions).
2. Presence of any obvious congenital anomalies.
3. Resting posture; position other than flexion (in a fullterm infant) may be due to the effect of maternal medications, sepsis, or congenital neuromuscular disease.
4. Tremors (repetitive vibratory motions); may be due to metabolic imbalance, neonatal drug withdrawal, or neurologic disorders.
5. Abnormal eye movements or repetitive leg movements such as bicycling (leg movements in a cycling motion), tonic posturing, lip smacking, or rapid flexion extension (clonic movements).
6. Level of responsiveness (see behavioural assessment).

Changes in neurologic status often are early markers for abnormalities of other systems; for example, lethargy is an important sign of sepsis and quality of cry a sign of some congenital syndromes.

Back

The back is inspected for anomalies by placing the infant in a prone position and observing; observe for birthmarks, hair distribution dimples, or hair tufts anywhere along the spine (associated with spina bifida occulta). There should be no obvious defects. Mongolian spots and naevi may be seen.

The extremities are observed for symmetry of movement and size, posture and rest, fractures, lacerations, bruising or deficiencies in function. No evidence of trauma should be noted. The full term in infant should lie in a position of flexion (normal intrauterine posture) at rest.

Extremities

An infant who has assumed the frank breech position in utero will lie with the hips flexed, with knees fully extended. These infants are high risk for congenital dislocation of the hip. The following characteristics indicate dislocation:

1. There is limited abduction of the affected hip.
2. The femur will appear shortened on the affected side.
3. The placement of thigh creases (gluteal folds) is deeper on the affected side.

The examiner inspects for number of digits, normal formation of the hands and feet, and condition of the nails. There should be no deformities. Fingernails should not be stained with meconium and should reach the ends of the fingertips at term. The degree and pattern of sole and palmar creases are noted. At term, creases are found over the entire sole. A single crease in the palm, the simian line, is associated with Down's syndrome, More reflex is elicited to evaluate whether there is any damage to the structure of the extremities and the function of the peripheral and central nervous systems. The Moro reflex should be brisk and complete bilaterally. The extremities should move symmetrically and return to the flexed position when movement ceases. Warning signs are listed at the end of this discussion.

The back is palpated by holding the infant under the chest and lifting horizontally, allowing the spine to flex. The examiner stimulates the trunk incurvation reflex by firmly running a fingertrip along the back from shoulder to hip just lateral to the spine and then running the fingers over the entire spine from neck to sacrum. The examiner palpates for masses and absent vertebrae, Flexion and extension of the spine should be smooth and regular. Flexion should be elicited with the incurvation reflex.

Obvious defects may be a meningocele or meningomyelocele associated with hydrocephalus and deformities of the feet. Ortolani's test is performed during examination for the presence of congenital hip dislocation, with the infant placed in the supine position. The examiner places the middle fingers on the outside of the femur (at the greater trochanter) and the thumb on the inside (at the lesser trochanter), flexing the infant's legs until the hips and knees are at right angles. The kness are abducted by pressing them towards the examining table. A click is heard and felt during this motion if the hip is dislocated.

If the feet seem to be abnormally positioned, an attempt is made to manipulate them gently into a neutral or midline position. This- should be easy to do if the malposition has resulted from pressure *in utero* rather than structural deformity.

The following are *warning signs for back and extremity problems:*

- Absence of limbs or digits, usually isolated deformities.
- Deformities of digits, including fusion (syndactyly) and an extra digit (polydactyly), also usually isolated deformities.
- Simian line associated with Down's syndrome.
- Lack of movement of limb, possibly from brachial nerve palsy caused by excessive traction and flexion of the neck during delivery (arm held adducted and internally rotated) or fracture.
- Limited abduction and unequal femur length.
- Asymmetric thigh creases or positive orrolani's manoeuvre (clicks indicating congenital hip dislocation)

Motor Function

The infant's posture is observed for tone and movement on the basis of the head, back and extremity examination results.

Developmental Reflexes

Assessment of neonatal reflexes should be performed with expectations appropriate for the infant's gestational age. Table 7.7 reviews assessment of developmental reflexes.

Cranial Nerves

Observation of cranial nerve function is more detailed than other parts of the neurologic assessments however, many parameters are assessed during other parts of the physical examination. For instance, as the examiner looks for forcep marks, the mouth can be observed for symmetric movement because the same excessive pressure that damaged the skin can cause facial nerve palsy. Pupillary response and eye movements indicate functioning of optic and oculomotor nerves. Rooting and sucking reflexes test the trigeminal and facial nerves. Startle response to a loud noise indicates the health of the eighth nerve.

These *Neuromuscular Warning Signs* must be assessed with consideration of gestational age:

- Low birth weight, short height, and/or small head size.
- Hypertonia or hypotonia.
- Lethargy, irritability, abnormal cry.
- Tremors.
- Repetitives movements of the eyes or limbs.
- Asymmetric development, movement, and/or strength.
- Deformities of back or limbs.
- Limited abduction and unaqual femur length.
- Asymmetric thigh creases or positive ortalani's manoeuvre.
- Poor or weak Moro reflex and grasp.
- Absent or uncoordinated root, suck and swallow.
- Lack of self-quieting behaviours.
- Failure to change behavioural states smoothly (see Brazelton's assessment).

Brazelton's Neonatal Behavioural Assessment Scale

Brazelton's research during the past two decades has changed the way health care personnel think about a newborn infant's capabilities. Previously, neonates were thought to be passive receivers of environment stimuli. It is now known that the normal full-term infant can influence the amount of stimuli intake and the care giver's responses (Brazelton 1984). Neonates can attend to their surroundings or sleep or can remain agitated and distressed or use self-quieting activities for consolation. Normal infants differ in these abilitis, but the normal full-term infant should make the transition between states smoothly. Use of the Brazelton Neonatal Behavioural Assessment Scale (BNBAS) as a research tool is limited to those who have completed an examiner's workshop training programme. Nurses, however, can use items from this tool to assess the responses of infants and increase parental understanding of infant temperament and behaviour patterns.

The Brazelton scale consists of 28 items in 7 categories

The Brazelton's neonatal behvioural assessment scale is as follows:

1. *Habituation:* Infant's ability to decrease response to external stimuli (bright light, rattle, bell, and tactile stimulation to the foot).
2. *Orientation:* Infant's ability to attend to, focus on, and interact with animate and inanimate stimuli (auditory and visual).
3. *Motor Performance:* Infant's ability to organize and control motor activity.
4. *Range of State:* State of consciousness during the entire examination period.
5. *Regulation of State:* Infant's self-quieting abilities.

Table 7.7: Developmental reflexes (Figs 7.11A to I)

Technique	Normal response	Abnormal response
1. *Moro reflex* (Fig. 7.11A) Use your hand and forearm to support infant's head and back as you lift upper body off the surface and drop supporting hand to simulate falling. (This allows you to test response to sensation of falling. Using loud noise to elicit startle reflex tests response to sound)	Abduction and extension of arms and at least fingers three to five occurs followed by adduction and flexion of upper extremities. Infant may startle and cry. Disappears: 4 months	Asymmetry means hemiparesis, fractured humerus or clavicle, or brachial plexus injury. Sluggish responses are seen in premature and ill infants
2. *Tonic neck reflex* (TNR) (Fig. 7.11B) position infant on back and turn head to side	Same sided arm and leg show extension and increased tone, whereas arm and leg on opposite side flex and show extension and increased tone, whereas arm and leg on opposite side flex and show decreased tone ("fencing position"). Infant's response may vary. Disappears: around 4 months	Infant who is unable to break this it is elicited exhibits abnormal obligatory response
3. *Stepping reflex* (Fig. 7.11C) Hold infant upright and place one foot in contact with firm surface	Leg in contact with surface extends while other flexes. Infant then appears to take steps	Hypertonic means both legs will be in extension. Hypotonic means infant will not extend legs
4. *Babinski's reflex* (Fig. 7.11D) Stroke lateral aspect of infant's sole from heel to toe	Dorsiflexion of great toe with extension of other toes occurs. Disappears; by 2 years	Response may indicate neurologic dysfunction
5. *Plantar grasp* (Fig. 7.11E) Press your finger to infant's sole just below toes	Toes flex around your finger Disappears: 10 months	Absence of reflex is seen in infants with hypotonia or spinal cord or lumbosacral plexus injuries
6. *Palmar grasp* (Fig. 7.11F) Place object in palm of infant's hand	Flexion of fingers with grasping of object occurs (see photo). This grasp is strong enough to allow infant to be lifted from bed (see traction response)	Lack of grasp seen in infants with hypotonia perinata asphyxia
7. *Traction response* (Fig. 7.11G) Place infant on back and firmly place one finger in each palm. After infant grasps your fingers, pull up	Infant grasps your fingers and can be pulled to sitting position	Lack of response indicates hypotonia
8. *Rooting reflex* (Fig. 7.11H) When infant is awake, touch cheek	Infant turns head and mouth toward stimulus. Disappears; 6 months	Response may not be elicited in normal infants who have just beefed; it is weak infants with fade nerve palsy or central nervous system depresssion
9. *Sucking reflex* (Fig. 7.11I) When infant is awake, place clean finger or nipple in mouth	Infant beging to suck	Weak or absent suck
10. *Swallow and gag reflex* (Fig. 7.11I) Observe infant swallowing during feeding	Infant sucks and swallows fluid without distress. Coughs or gags appropriately	Drooling, lack of swallow, and lack of coordination between suck and swallow

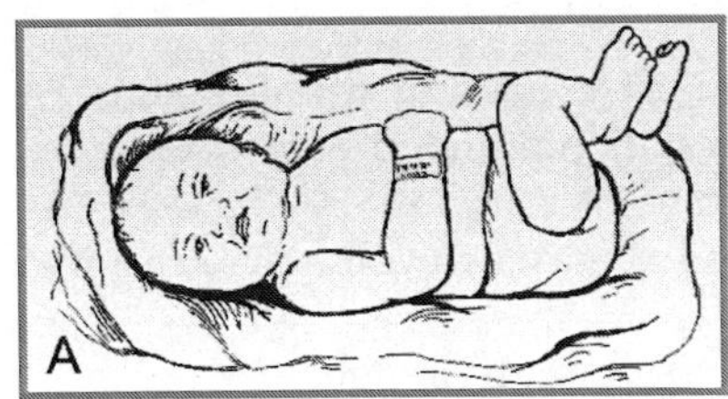

Moro Reflex

- Elicited by a variety of stimuliloud noise, sudden movement of the surface the infant is lying on, or the sudden drop of the infant's head backward about 30 degrees into the examiner's hand
- Portions of the Moro reflex are present at 25 to 27 weeks of gestation
- Complete Moro reflex is present at 34 weeks of gestation
- Disappears at approximately 6 months of age.

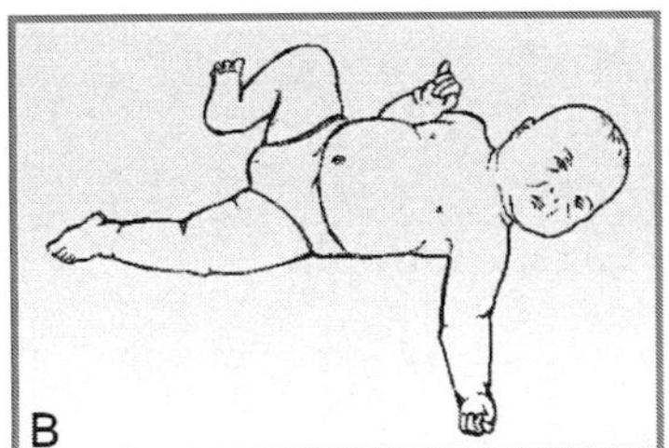

Tonic Neck Reflex

- Elicited by rotation of the head to one side
- Present as early as 35 weeks of gestation
- Most prominent at 1 month after term
- Disappears by approximately 7 months of age.

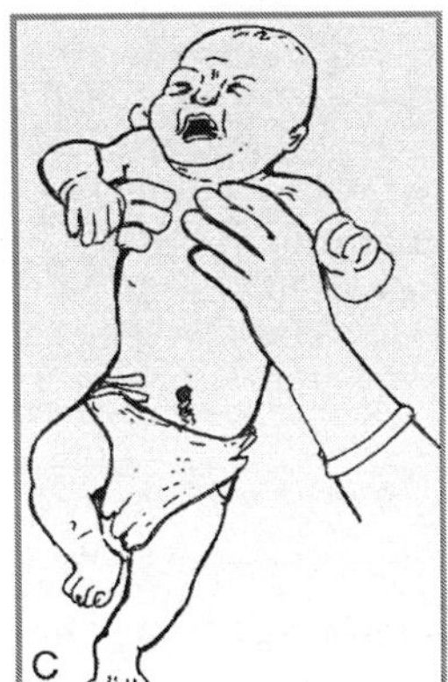

Stepping Reflex

- Elicited by holding the infant upright so that the sole of a foot is in firm contact
  with a flat surface
- Appears at 34 weeks of gestation, immature toe-heel stepping
- Mature, heel-toe stepping, at 38 weeks of gestation.
- Disappears at approximately 1 to 2 months of age.

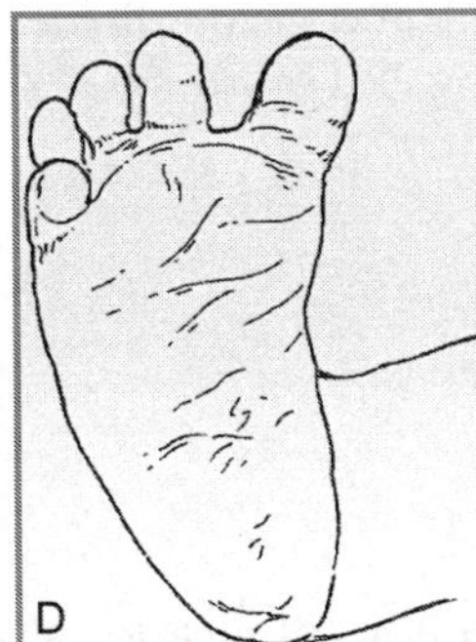

Babinski Reflex

- Elicited by stroking the lateral aspects of the sole of the foot from the heel upward and across the ball of the foot with the fingernail
- Disappears at approximately 12 months of age.

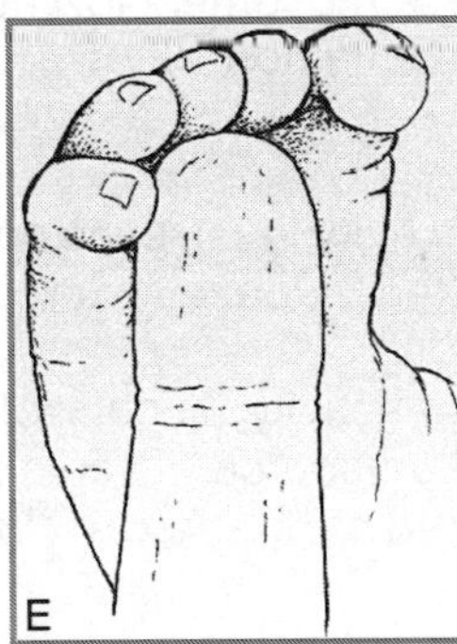

Plantar Grasp Reflex

- Elicited by stimulating the ball of the foot by firm pressure
- Appears at 26 to 27 weeks of gestation, immature.
- Mature at 34 weeks of gestation
- Disappears at approximately 6 to 9 months of age.

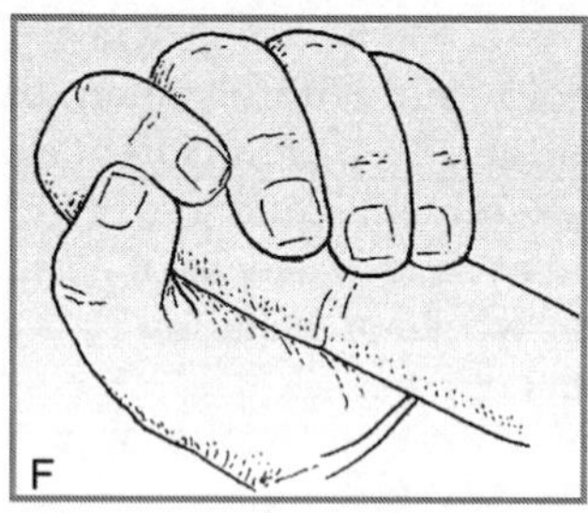

Palmar Grasp Reflex
- Elicited by stimulating the palm of the hand by firm pressure
- Appears at 26 to 27 weeks of gestation, immature.
- Mature at 34 weeks of gestation
- Becomes inconsistent at 2 months of age when voluntary grasping begins
- Disappears at approximately 6 to 9 months of age.

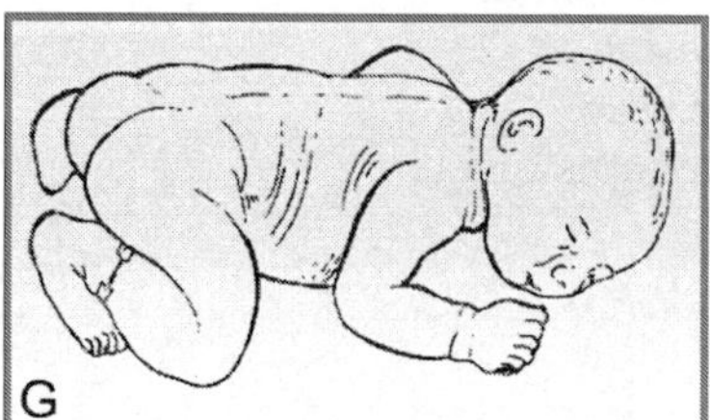

Trunk Incurvation
(Galant Reflex)
- Elicited by gentle stroking of the fingers down the paravertebral area with infant in prone position
- Appears as early as 24 weeks of gestation
- Disappears by 12 months of age.

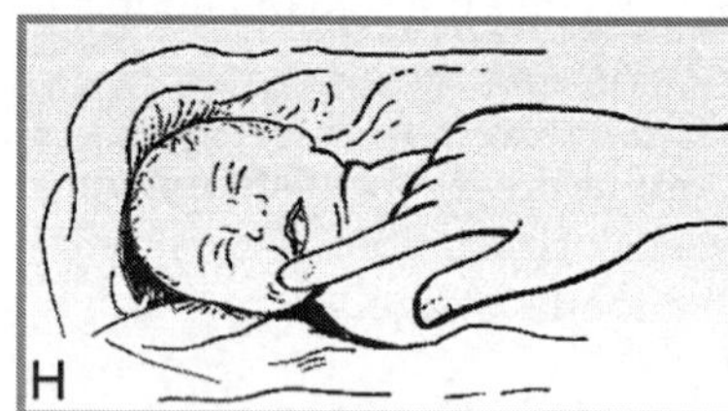

Rooting Reflex
- Elicited by stimulating the perioral area with the finger
- Appears at 28 weeks of gestation, immature
- Disappears at approximately 4 months of age.

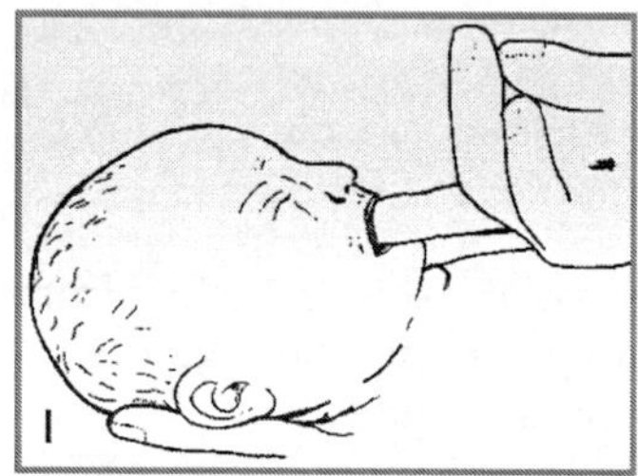

Sucking Reflex
- Elicited by stimulating the mucous membranes of the mouth with gloved finger
- Appears at 28 weeks of gestation, weak and uncoordinated suck
- Mature at 34 weeks of gestation, strong and coordinated suck
- Disappears at approximately 4 months of age.

Figs 7.11A to I: Showing different developmental reflexes in newborn baby

6. *Autonomic requlation:* Skin colour.
7. *Reflexes:* Primary neonatal reflexes.

   Before the assessment is begun, the infant's state of consciousness is determined as given below:

Neonatal States of Consciousness

1. *Sleep States*

   State I
   - *Deep Sleep:* Regular breathing, eyes closed with no movements, no spontaneous activity except startles.

   State II
   - *Light Sleep:* Irregular respirations, eyes closed with rapid eye movement low activity level with sucking behaviours.
2. *Awake States*

   State III
   - *Drowsy:* Variable activity level, eyes open or closed with lids fluttering, dazed expression.

   State IV
   - *Alert:* Minimal motor activity, bright look with attention focussed on source of stimulation, may appear dazed but easy to "break through" to infant.

State V

- *Eyes Open:* Much motor activity, thrusting movements of extremities, reacting to stimuli with increasing activity and/or startles.

State VI

- *Crying:* High motor activity and intense crying difficult to "break through" to infant.

Recognition of their infant's state is especially improtant to parents because it can cue them to the appropriateness of their parenting behaviours. For example, it is not appropriate to attempt to play with an infant who is sleeping, to do so only encourages a sense of failure. However, the parent who recognizes the alert state and initiates play will more likely be rewarded by responese. Parents also can be made aware that their infant's hand-to-mouth activity is a self-quieting behaviour not a bad habit to be eliminated. Fostering this king of awareness may help new parents to understand their newborn.

Gestational Age Assessment

The gestational age of the newborn infant is calculated in weeks from the last menstrual period (LMP). Prenatally, foetal age can be assessed by various indirect means (e.g. ultrasonic determination of biparietal diameter and crown rump length. After birth physical examination leads to a more accurate assessment of maturity. It is important to determine the maturity of each infant because complications of the neonatal period vary greatly with maturity; premature and postmature infants have the most difficulty adapting to extrauterine life.

Method: Several attempts have been made to develop a system of gestational age assessment that is easy to perform, is replicable by many examiners, and has a high correlation with actual gestational age. Physical characteristics may be assessed soon after birth, some of which may have been noted during an early assessment.

The examiner assesses the skin first by noting colour, peeling and/or cracking, and visible blood vessels. The skin thickens with maturity, causing peeling and making the blood vessels less visible. The amount and distribution Lanugo, which appears early in gestation and disappears as pregnancy progresses, are observed, Next the sole creases are inspected; these increase in number and depth with gestational age. The breast areolae are palpated and their diameter measured. The areolae will be barely visible in the very immature infant and grow to 5 to 10 mm in diameter close to term. The pinnae to the infant's ear curve in with increasing gestational age. Cartilage formation also causes the pinnae to become stiffer and recoil after being folded in the more mature infant. Last, the genitalia are examined. In the male infant the testes descend through the inguinal canal as gestational age increases. As this occurs, the scrotum becomes larger with rugae. In the female infant the labia majora grow to cover the clitoris and labia minora. At the conclusion of physical assessment, the examiner totals the sum of the physical characteristics and records the number in the space provided.

Neuromuscular assessment should be postponed for 24 hours to allow the infant to recover from the stress of birth. First the infant's resting posture is observed. The preterm infant lies in a position of extension, which becomes gradually more flexed with maturity. Next the angle of the square window is determined by flexing the hand on to the forearm and noting the angle at which resistance is felt. The angle decreases with increasing gestational age. The degree of arm recoil is assessed by first flexing and then extending the infant's arms for 5 seconds and then releasing them. The angle formed as the arms recoil also decreases with increasing gestational age. The popliteal angle is assessed by placing the infant on his or her back. The examiner extends one leg, taking care not to allow the buttocks to lift off the bed and noting the point at which resistance is met. The angle becomes more acute as gestation progresses. While the infant is on his or her back, the scarf sign is assessed by wrapping one arm across the baby's chest until resistance is met and noting where the elbow lies in relation to the infant's midline. Finally, heel-to-ear flexibility is assessed by grasping the foot loosely, extending it toward the ear and letting up (allowing the back to rise up off the bed if necessary) and noting the point at which the foot slips out of grasp. The score for neuromuscular assessment is totaled as for the physical characteristics.

Add the two scores and find the corresponding gestational age. After gestational age is determined, it is plotted against birth weight on the graph and the infant is diagnosed as small, appropriate, or large for Gestational age (SGA,

AGA, or LGA). Normally there is a positive relationship between gestational age and birth weight. This relationship, however, can be disturbed as a result of complications of pregnancy such as infection, diabetes and hypertension. The weight of an infant who is AGA falls between the 10th and 90th percetile. SGA or LGA infants fall below and above these limits, respectively. The Interaction of gestational age and birth weight greatly influences neonatal well-being. In addition, appropriateness of size and gestational age influences clinical decisions.

Assessment of neonatal health will not be completes for 25 hours, when all three areas of assessment history, physical examination, and gestational age are completed. Every infant should be completely assessed soon after birth and then just before discharge. Assessments for skin colour and cardiovascular and neuromuscular status are performed as necessary.

CARE OF THE NORMAL NEONATE

The nurse is responsible for the care of the newborn immediately after birth, verifies that respirations have been established, dries the infant, assesses the temperature, and places identical identification bracelets on the infant and the mother. The infant may be wrapped in a warm blanket and placed in the arm of the mother, given to the partner to hold, or kept undressed under a radiant warmer. In some setting, immediately after birth, the infant is placed on the mother's abdomen to allow skin-to-skin contact. This contribution to maintenance of infant's optimum temperature and parental bonding. The infant may be admitted to a nursery or remain with parents throughout the hospital stay.

Today one encounters recovery or transition nurseries devoted to the care of the infant less than 24 hours old or newborn surgical patients, neonatal intensive care units (NICU) designed for small premature or sick infants and intermediate progressive care units for those infants whose nursing needs are not as intensive. Such care opportunities now make possible the survival of many babies who formerly would have died or suffered severe damage. Along with the trend towards specialization, there continues to be a growing emphasis on family centered maternity care. It is now recognized that normal healthy newborns need not be separated from their mothers. In some hospitals a mother and her baby are seen as a unit and are cared for by one nurse. This is referred to as mother-baby nursing or couplet care. Many hospitals provide opportunity for the baby to "room-in" with the mother and for the father to visit and participate in infant care. Some centres permit other healthy siblings and grand-parents to see and hold the baby as well. Even when the infant is sick and must be in a NICU the parents are encouraged to spend time with their baby. But no matter what the circumstances or locate, of birth or the type of care facilities available, all newborn infants have certain need that must be met for them in thrive and take their place in society. Some of these needs take priority, some can be met simultaneously, and still others are important but need not be rushed. Following are listed nine universal needs of the newborn infant:

1. A clear airway
2. Established respiration
3. Warmth
4. Protection from haemorrhage
5. Protection from infection
6. Identification and observation
7. Nourishment and fluids
8. Love-parent-infant attachment
9. Rest.

Clear Airway

The first two needs must be met immediately or the baby will not survive, and no amount of oxygen, mouth-to-mouth resuscitation, or intermittent positive pressure will stimulate a newborn infant to breathe, if its airway is not open. Conversely, if the airway is not clear but filled with amniotic fluid, meconium particles, or blood and the infant does try to take breath and inhale, the respiratory tract may become plugged, irritated, or contaminated. The airway may be cleared by using these methods:

1. Wiping off the child's nose and mouth at the time of the birth of the head.
2. Gently suctioning first the mouth and then the nose with a small, soft, short bulb aspirator or a soft catheter attached to a trap and low wall suction before birth is complete.
3. Holding the child's head down to drain immediately after birth while gently compressing the throat toward the mouth-to-milk out secretions.
4. Visualizing the larynx with a laryngoscope and suctioning the trachea by trained personnel for unresponsive infants.

Suctioning the Newborn with Bulb Syringe or Catheter

Purpose: To use a bulb syringe or catheter to remove secretions or fluids when they obstruct the newborn's respiratory passages. A catheter rather than a bulb syringe must be used to remove fluids that are lower in the respiratory tract.

Equipment

- For bulb syringe suctioning
  - — Bulb syringe (each baby has a separate, initially sterile bulb syringe).
- For catheter suctioning
  - — French rubber catheters (sizes 10, 12, 14), whistletip or two-hole tip sterile for each baby.
  - — French plastic disposable catheters (sizes 8, 10, 12), finger control, two-hole tip, sterile for each baby.
  - — External suction source (as on radiant warmer)
  - — Container of sterile water (typically a sterile water feeding bottle).

Established Respiration

With the introduction of closed chest cardiac massage techniques and appliances to stimulate the heartbeat electrically, perhaps, "established respiration" should read "Established respiration and heartbeat. If respiration does not occur spontaneously after the airway is clear, the child should be stimulated to cry. Many infants respond to gentle rubbing of the back or gentle suctioning of the nose with a soft catheter. More vigorous stimulation consists of slapping the heels or rubbing the sternum. If breathing is not initiated soon after stimulation, methods of breathing for the infant must be employed. Sometimes this means the use of intermittent positive pressure by means of orotracheal tube or mask and bag. Sometimes the operator will blow directly through a patent endotracheal tube. No matter what method is used, it should be emphasized that an airway must be maintained through proper head positioning and /or use of a small oropharyngeal airway to keep the infant's tongue from falling back and obstructing the pharynx.

When a child is being resuscitated, is breathing poorly on his own, has generalized cyanosis, or has a heart rate under 100 beats per minute, supplimentary oxygen should be administered.

Warmth

Newborns may suffer from depressed body temperature or hypothermia not because they produce heat poorly but because they are so vulnerable to heat loss. They lose heat easily because the body surface area is so great in relation to weight, and they have relatively little subcutaneous fat to provide insulation. Heat is provided for the infant in most delivery room settings through the use of unenclosed infant warmers, which provide easy accessibility for care by utilizing overhead radiant at panel. The baby should be dried immediately after birth with a warm towel or blanket to decrease heat loss. An interesting study, comparing heat loss in heated cribs with heat loss in the mother's arms, confirmed that the mother is a reliable source of heat for the normal, dry, wrapped infant placed on the mother's chest. This has implications for early maternal-infant attachment processes.

The importance of maintaining the infant's body heat immediately after birth and in the extended neonatal period has been emphasized because the temperature of the infant affects the number of calories the baby must burn to keep warm, as well as his oxygen consumption, the incidence of apnoea, and the acid base balance of his blood. When the infant is sick, the provision of appropriate heat is critical.

The way in which the baby is dressed depends on the temperature of the nursery or rooming-in area. Current recommendations are the nursery air temperature be maintained at 24°C (75°F) with a relative humidity in the range of 34 to 60% for personnel comfort. Some babies are perfectly warm in only a cotton shirt and diaper, covered by a light cotton blanket. Except for an initial rectal temperature reading when a check is made for imperforate anus, 3-minute axillary temperature determinations are now advocated. An electronic thermometer may be employed. Axillary temperatures for the normal newborn should range from 36.5° to 37.0°C (97.7° to 98.6°F).

Protection from Haemorrhage

Today most babies born in hospitals have their cords clamped with some type of compressive band. These commercial clamps have proved to be satisfactory, and althought the cord must still be frequently observed for bleeding, incidents of difficulty are extreme rare. When a ligature of any kind is being used, it is usually tied twice approximately 1 inch from the abdominal wall in a depression in the cord made by a previously placed haemostat, if one is available. The tie is secured by a square knot for stability and checked frequently during the first few hours to detect any loosening or bleeding.

Protection from haemorrhage in the newborn infant also becomes important when caring for the male infant after circumcision.

In an effort to decrease the possibility of abnormal cerebral pressure and subsequent intracranial bleeding, newborns are not placed in a prolonged head-down position.

Vitamin K to decrease coagulation time is routinely administered in most hospitals (Table 7.8).

Administration of Vitamin K (Fig. 7.12)

Purpose To administer vitamin K one time within 6 hours as prophylaxis for bleeding.

Equipment
- 1-mL syringe
- 25-gauge 5/8 inch needle
- Ampule of Aquamephyton or Konakion
- Alcohol sponges.

Protection from Infection

Protecting the newborn infant from infection is a constant challenge to delivery room and nursery nurses. It involves the entire environment of babies and the techniques used in handling and nourishing them. It can be said to reach back to the prenatal period when efforts are made to prevent any contamination of the foetus by organisms that are able pass over the placental barrier (viruses, spirochetes). The baby, while in the hand of the delivering physician or nurse midwife is considered and maintained sterile. The cord is clamped and cut aseptically. Then the baby is usually handed to a circulating nurse who, having carefully washed her hand and put on clean

Table 7.8: Nursing action and rationale vitamin K therapy

Nursing action	*Rationale*
1. Check vitamin K order	A physician's order is required for administration of vitamin K
2. Wear gloves. Shake medication to bottom of ampule. Protect fingers and break top off ampule	Wearing gloves is consistent with standard precautions. Shaking medication to bottom of ampule allows medication to flow to large and of ampule where it can be drawn up
3. Remove needle cover; maintain sterility. Draw up dosage ordered	Sterility must be maintained to avoid infection
4. Steady the injection leg with one hand	Restraint ensures placement of needle in appropriate location
5. Follow these steps to find the preferred injection site, which is the lateral aspect of the middle-third of the vastus lateralis muscle in the baby's thigh: • Use the baby's greater trochanter and knee as landmarks • Visually divide the distance between the landmarks into three equal sections • Identify the area that is the middle-third of the distance between the landmarks	The vastus lateralis muscle is the preferred injection site because it is free of major blood vessels and nerves and is big enough to absorb the medication
6. Cleanse the injection site with alcohol, holding the thigh between the thumb and forefinger. Insert the needle at a 90-degree angle, aspirate (as you would with any medication), and then slowly inject the medication. Give the injection within 6 hours of birth	Positioning the needle at a 90-degree angle ensure injection into the muscle rather than the subcutaneous tissue. Injection within 6 hours of birth is recommended so that the newborn receives the prophylactic effect of the medication
7. Withdraw the needle, massage the area, apply pressure, and record administration of medication	Massage hastens absorption. Application of pressure helps prevent bleeding at the site of injection. Recording documents administration
8. Observe injection site for bleeding	Until vitamin K prophylaxis has take effect, bleeding may occur.
9. Notify physician if bleeding from any site (i.e. umbilical cord, nose, gastrointestinal tract) occurs after sufficient time for absorption of vitamin K has elapsed	If the prophylactic dose of vitamin K proves insufficient to prevent neonatal bleeding, additional vitamin K will be administered

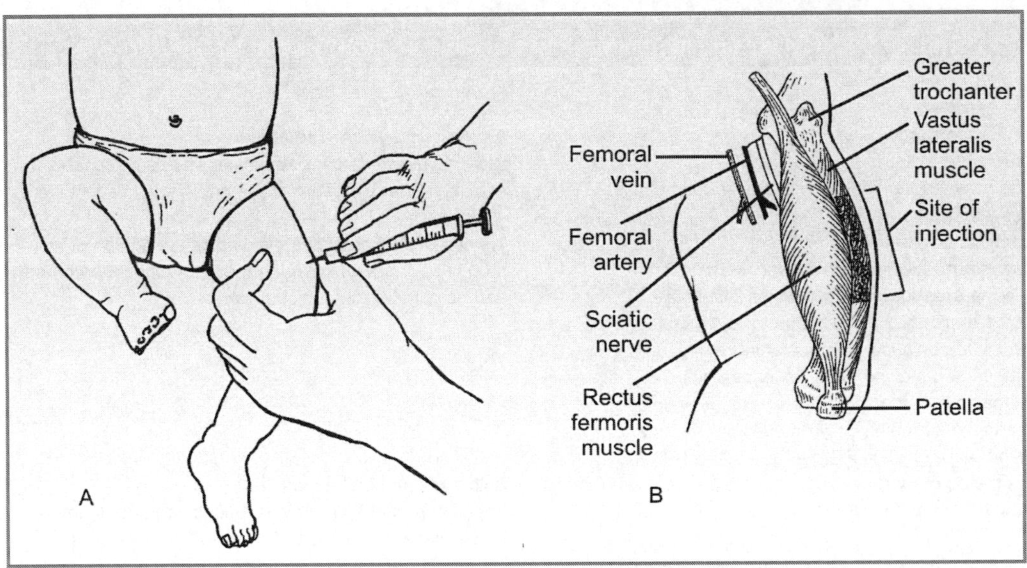

Fig. 7.12: Vitamin K therapy

gloves and overgown, receives him for further care (see umbilical cord care).

Umbilical Cord Care

Purpose: To minimize contamination by microorganisms and prevent infection of the umbilical cord and to foster drying and "falling off" of the cord by applying prescribed preparations two-to-three times per day.

Equipment

- Prescribed preparation: Triple dye, silver sulfadiazine cream, bacitracin ointment, or isopropyl alcohol.
- Cotton-tripped applicator, cotton ball, or alcohol swab.
- Gloves

In most countries protection of the infant from infection involve the use of some prophylacting against ophthalmia neonatorum caused to the gonorrhoeal organism. The prophylactic agent may be drops of silver nitrate 1% or (see procedure below) an ophthalmic ointment containing tetracycline 1% or most commonly erythromycin 0.5%. Although the agent should be installed shortly after birth, a delay of upto 1 hour is acceptable. This delay may facilitate the intial maternal-infant attachment by allowing the newborn unimpaired eye with the mother. Care must be taken in administering the drops or ointment; no pressure should be put on the eyeball itself. Occasionally, if the eye area has not been previously touched, shading the baby's eyes from the light will cause them to open spontaneously, making instillation comparatively easy. If this helpful reaction does not occur, the nurse pulls down on the lower lid to instill the agent into the conjunctival sac. All the while the nurse guards the child from cold and continues to observe skin colour and respiration patterns. Parents should be told that the eyedrops may cause some swelling and drainage within the next 24 hours.

Instillation of Erythromycin, Tetracycline, or Silver Nitrate Eye Treatment (Table 7.9)

Purpose: To administer prophylactic eye treatment one time soon after birth to prevent ophthalmic infections of the newborn.

Equipment

- Tube of erythromycin eye ointment (0.5%) or tetra-cycline eye ointment (1%).
- Silver nitrate ampules (1%).

Thermoregulation of Newborns

Purpose: To use the overhead radiant warmer or the servomechanism controlled incubator to help the newborn achieve and maintain a stable body temperature that is within normal limits.

Table 7.9: Showing nursing action and rationale of prophylactic agents for eye

Nursing action	*Rationale*
1. Check physician's order	A physician's order is required
2. Wear gloves	Wearing gloves is consistent with standard precautions
3. If necessary, clean the eyelids with sterile cotton balls moistened with sterile water	Allows greater exposure to the prophylactic agent
4. If erythromycin or tetracycline ointment is ordered, retract the infant's lower eyelid outward with forefinger to expose the area for instillation of the ointment. Instill a strip (typically 1 inch or 2.5 cm) of ointment along the lower conjunctival sac, starting at the inner canthus and moving to the outer canthus. Carefully manipulate the lid to spread the ointment. Only one dose per eye and one tube per baby	Method of administration maximizes absorption of the prophylactic agent, ensuring that it reaches the cornea and all parts of the conjunctiva
5. Repeat in the other eye	Both eyes need treatment
6. Do not irrigate or rinse the eyes	Irrigation probably minimizes efficacy and does not seem to decrease occurrence of chemical conjunctivitis
7. Check for side effects such as oedema, inflammation, and drainage. Also observe for hypersensitivity	oedema, inflammation, and drainage may interfere with the newborn's ability to focus. Drainage can be cleansed from the eye. The newborn may be allergic to the medication
8. If silver nitrate (1%) is ordered, use a needle to puncture the ampule the ampule, which is made of wax, and squeeze the ampule to release the drops. Instill 2 drops in each conjunctival sac, carefully manipulate the lids. After 1 minute, wipe any excess solution from the eyelids with sterile water	Lid manipulation spreads the silver nitrate solution. One minute is needed for silver nitrate to be effective. Wiping excess silver nitrate drops from the eyelids removes excess and minimizes irritation
9. Chart administration of prophylactic agent	Charting provides a written record of administration of prophylactic agent as ordered and document fulfillment of legal requirement to help prevent ophthalmia neonatorum
Silver Nitrate (1%) *Action:* Causes disruption of the microbial cell membrane and death of the organism. Prevents gonococcal eye infection; not effective against chlamydial infection *Dose:* 1% silver nitrate in wax ampule (to prevent evaporation and precipitation of the silver caused by glass). Two drops in each eye. Must be administered within 1 hour of birth. *Side Effects:* Chemical conjunctivitis **Erythromycin (Ilotycin) Ointment (0.5%)** *Action:* Bactericidal (destroys the bacteria) or bacteriostatic (inhibits growth of the bacteria), depending on the organism. Effective against both *Neisseria gonorrhoeae and Chlamydia trachomatis*. No effect on viruses, yeasts, or fungi. Inhibits protein synthesis and bacterial cell multiplication	*Dose:* At least 0.5-inch (1- to 2-cm) or 1 inch (2.5-cm) ribbon of ointment to conjunctiva of lower eyelids *Side Effects:* None **Tetracycline (Achromycin or Aureomycin)** *Ointment (1%)* *Action:* Bacteriostatic for gram-positive and gram-negative organisms, including gonococcus and chlamydia. Inhibits protein synthesis *Dose:* At least 0.5 inch (1-to 2-cm) or 1-inch (2.5-cm) ribbon of ointment to conjunctive of lower eyelids *Side Effects:* None

Equipment

- Thermometer
- Overhead radiant warmer
- Servomechanism controlled incubator.

A central nursery for normal newborn infants and a separate postpartum area for mothers have been the principal pattern of hospital infant care for over 50 years, and recognizes that many hospitals are still organized in this way. However, a growing number of hospitals are offering mother-baby care units of have initiated single room maternity care. In these settings one nurse for the needs of both mother and baby. One of the benefits of these newer types of hospital maternity care is the reduction of the risks of infection. No matter how patient care is organized, all hospital personnel must be aware of the potential hazard of sepsis.

After birth the infant has his own individual bassinet and should also have his own bath equipment, supply of linen, and layette. Infants should be bathed in their own beds and not on a common bathing table. The scale used for determining weight should be protected and balanced and handled in such a way that no cross-infection could take place. Any instruments or appliances that must be used for more than one infant because of lack of supply must be carefully disinfected or sterilised after use. This would apply to stethoscopes, circumcision and instruments, resuscitators, and other equipment.

Staff members should wear simple, hospital-supplied and laundered clothing on duty, keep their fingernails short, restrict jewelry, and evaluate their own health. No personnel should assume responsibility of caring for newborns while suffering from a contagious respiratory condition, skin infection or diarrhoea.

Personnel entering the nursery usually wash their hand and arms above the elbow with an antibacterial product much as povidone-iodine (Betadine) before starting patient care. Hand-washing is mandatory after the care of each baby or individual unit and in the care of the same baby after changing a soiled diaper and proceeding with further needs. The hands should always be washed before treating the cord, since it can become the site of serious infection, It should be observed for signs of inflammation and drainage. A nurse who leaves the maternity area should wear a cover gown to protect her clean nursery gown. If her gown should become soiled in the nursery with urine emesis, or stool at any time, it should be changed. unless wrapped in a protective blanket or on a protective cover, the infant should be held away from the nurse's gown during care and feedings to protect the nurse's dress from becoming a source of cross contamination to other infants. Precautions not necessary at home are essential, when many infants from many backgrounds and families are being cared for in a small area, such as the hospital nursery.

Parents and ancillary staff (e.g. X-ray personnel) should also be taught the importance and technique of good handwashing when visiting the nursery or caring for infants in the mother's hospital room or in the home.

Professional organizations take an active part in making recommendations and requirements governing the construction, maintenance and operation of the nursery as well as other parts of the hospital. They are concerned about floor space available, distance between bassinets, type of ventilation, control of temperature and humidity, privision for adequate lighting, safety of electrical appliances, elimination of possible fire hazards appropriate dressing and hand washing facilities, and safe formula preparation as well as optimum techniques.

Identification and Observation

Identification of the infant may be accomplished in various ways, but it should always be done beyond doubt before the baby leaves the delivery room. In multiple births, the infants should be identified immediately after birth to avoid confusion. Identification that can be easily counter-checked—the use of double or triple bands—is recommended.

Admission Bath

Most infants have their admission bath in the nursery after being checked in, identified, weighed and measured. Many infants are not bathed completely until several hours after birth when the baby temperature is higher. Newborn infants are covered with varying amount of vernix and blood. They may also be soiled with meconium. During the admission bath the nurse reaffirms identification, inspects the infant more carefully than was possible in the delivery room, takes his temperature, dresses him appropriately, and places him in a warm incubator or bed depending on his body temperature and observational needs. An admission bath usually employs a mild soap solution or an antibacterial product. The following description outlines procedures for the admission bath, although details may differ from hospital to hospital. The nurse's hands are carefully washed before starting. Depending on the circumstances of the birth and the condition of the baby the nurse may wear gloves.

Admission Bath

Materials

1. Basin of warm water.
2. Mild soap or antibacterial product.
3. Paper mesh squares.
4. Sterile cotton balls

5. Triple dye, bacitracin, or alcohol, 70% for cord care.
6. Applicators for cord care.
7. Two towels or soft diapers for covering and drying.
8. Individual thermometer.
9. Small plastic comb.
10. Laundry hamper.
11. Appropriate clothing, diaper, shirt and receiving blanket.

Procedure

1. The temperature is taken:
   a. Axillary temperature is taken by placing a thermometer deep in the axilla while holding the arm gently but firmly against the chest.
   b. Usual time is 3 minutes or until the mercury stops rising.
   c If the infant is cold, the bath is delayed unitl the temperature reaches the normal range.
2. The newborn infant is usually partially-wrapped with a towel or blanket to prevent chilling.
3. The eyes may be wiped with cotton balls moistened with water. Irrigation or wiping starts at the nose and proceeds outward to prevent unwanted drainage from the inner canthus of the eye from entering the lacrimal duct leading to the nose. (One cotton ball is used for each wipe.)
4. The face is cleaned with a paper mesh square or cotton balls dipped in clear water. No soap is used since be drying to the skin.
   a. If necessary, the opening of the nose is cleared with water moistened cotton balls, but the canal is never probed.
   b. The external ears may be gently wiped with water moistened cotton balls, but the canal is never probed.
5. The head is gently but efficiently handled and rinsed over the wash basin:
   a. A football hold on the baby is best.
   b. A small comb, gently used, helps to lift out particles of vernix that are difficult to dislodge.
6. The bath is continued by washing, rinsing, and drying the neck, chest, arms hands, abdomen and back.
   a. The recently clamped cord and its base are usually avoided until later when an antiseptic is applied. Nurseries today put no gauze dressing on the cord and have found that it dries much faster and has no greater incidence of infection for having been left exposed.
   b. Vernix caseosa may be thick and difficult to remove, particularly from the creases. To avoid skin irritation only what wipes off easily should be removed. Special attention should be paid to the neck creases.
   c. After turning the baby on his side to wash, rinse, and dry, a partially folded towel may be placed under the washed portion of the infant to be completely unfolded when the "bottom half" is clean.
   d. A small undershirt may be put on at this time, rolled up away from the cord to conserve warmth until the bath is completed.
7. The bath is continued, washing the legs, feet, and then the buttocks and perianal region.
8. The nurse's hands are again washed, and any ordered antiseptic is applied with an applicator to the cord end and the inner rim of the skin cuff surrounding the base of the cord. The vessels in the cord may be counted at this time.
9. The genitalia are inspected and cleansed with cotton balls previously moistened with clear water.
   a. For a baby girl the cotton balls may be wiped gently from front to back between the labia, never using a ball more than once.
   b. For an uncircumcised baby boy paediatric urologists do not recommend attempting to retract the foreskin of the newborn until about 5 months of age-since most are adherent. The glans that is visible should be gently cleansed with a moistened cotton ball.
10. The diaper is put on, and the infant tucked into bed. The crib identification card is checked against the infant's personal identification.
    a. Newborn infants are frequently propped on their right sides with a rolled blanket. For the older infant a right-side position is better because of the aid that gravity

gives to the flow of food from the stomach and because any air or bubble remaining will rest near the entrance of the stomach and be more easily expelled.

b. No newborn infant should be left unattended on his back because of the danger of aspiration.
c. In some hospitals the new-born infant is not dressed until shown to the parents and waiting relatives.

11. Notations regarding voidings, stool, or any pertinent observations should be appropriately recorded.

Bathe the Newborn

It is not advisable to bathe a baby after a feeding because handling may cause regurgitation. Since bathing is thought to be relaxing to the infant, before feeding may be the best time.

Sponge bathing is necessary until the cord has fallen off and circumcision, if applicable, has healed (approximately 2 weeks).

All supplies should be gathered before the bath is started so that supplies are accessible. Suggest that your client keep supplies together in the place so that they can be easily assembled each time the baby is bathed. Typical supplies include washcloth, towels, mild soap with out perfume (examples are Neutrogena and Dove; perfumes can irritate the skin), baby shampoo, cord care items (70% rubbing alcohol, cotton balls or cotton-tipped applicators), clean clothing, diaper, and infant washbasin or sink.

The baby should never be left alone during the bath.

The environment should be prepared so that it is warm and disruptions are minimal. Room temperature should be maintained (about 75°) to help the baby maintain body temperature. Suggest that your client minimize disruptions by taking the phone off the hook or ignoring it if it rings.

A clean basin or sink should be filled with 2 to 3 inches of warm water; your client can check the temperature with her wrist. The water is used to wet the washcloth and to rinse the baby.

When the baby graduates to a tub bath, again only 2 to 3 inches of water should be used in the clean infant tub or sink. A washcloth or towel should be placed in the bottom of the tub or sink to prevent slipping.

Be mind your client that it is important to maintain the baby's temperature because infant lose heat easily. Bathing quickly, exposing only the part of the body being bathed at that time, and drying thoroughly help to keep the infant warm.

Bathing should start at the eyes and face, generally the cleanest area. Wrapping the washcloth over the index finger and wetting with water (no soap is necessary for the eyes, ears, and face since it could be drying and irritating), gently wipe from the inner to outer corner of one eye. Explain that this will help prevent irritation and infection of the lacrimal duct. The process is repeated on the other eye.

Next, the external ear and behind the ear are cleansed, again with the washcloth over the index finger. A cotton tipped applicator should not be used because it could be inserted too far and damage the eardrum, or it might push discharge farther into the ear canal. Another part of the cloth should be used for the other ear. Now the baby's face may be cleansed.

Explain to your client that it is important to wash the infant's hair regularly to avoid cradle cap (or scaling of the scalp). The process is the same for both the sponge and tub bath.

Pick the baby up in a football hold, holding the head over the washbasin and tilted slightly downward. The infant's hair should be rinsed with clean water with a washcloth or cupped hand, allowing the excess to drip into the basin. A small amount of shampoo in the free hand is lathered into the scalp. Teach your client to cleanse and rub the scalp including the soft spots. Then rinse over the basin with washcloth or cupped hand and dry well. A soft brush may be used every day. Should seborrheic dermatitis develop, baby oil may be applied to the scalp a half-hour before the bath.

Emphasize to your client that the baby must be held at all times when in the tub. Have your client cradle one arm at the back and under the baby's shoulders, and grasp the baby's arm or thigh with that hand. This will leave the other hand free to wash and rinse the baby.

For a sponge bath, the blanket is unwrapped and the T-shirt removed; the blanket is then used to loosely cover as much of the infant as possible to prevent heat loss. Each area is soaped, rinsed, and gently patted dry. Explain to your client that the baby's skin is fragile and easily irritated.

The infant's neck should be exposed by placing a hand under the baby's back at the shoulders and lifting slightly, allowing the head to fall back slightly. Formula, breast milk, or lint will often accumulate in the folds of the neck.

Hands and arms are washed by soaping with a washcloth or hand, making sure to gently cleanse the vernix where secretions may collect. The chest should be cleansed and rinsed while being careful to keep the cord dry. Patting dry and putting on a clean T-shirt or wrapping the upper body with a blanket will decrease heat loss.

Soaping and rinsing the baby's neck, chest, and arms with washcloth or hand is done in the same manner for a tub bath. To wash the baby's back, teach your client to place the non-cradling arm across the baby's chest and grasp the baby's arm. Then the baby may be gently tipped forward into a supporting arm, leaving the other hand free to wash the back.

Expose the baby's legs and cleanse with soap and water. Then rinse and pat dry.

For a sponge bath, the diaper should be removed now. Clean from the urethral area back to the rectal area for girls, using a different part of the washcloth each time. For boys, teach your client to cleanse the urethral area of the penis, then down the penis, next washing the scrotum, and finally the rectal area. Using these steps will help avoid faecal contamination of the urethral area. Dry and apply a diaper.

After cleansing the diaper area during a tub bath, the baby may be removed from the tub, patted dry thoroughly, and dressed.

Cord care may aid drying of the cord and decreases microorganisms.

When the bath is completed, additional clothing may be needed. The infant may then be wrapped in a blanket if necessary.

Throughout the bath procedure the nurse is inspecting and evaluating the infant. As cleans the eyes, she watches for discharge, conjunctival haemorrhage, or areas of opacity. As she feels the head, she checks the contour, the relative size of the fontanelles, and the presence of areas of swelling, pushing down on the chin, she peers into the mouth, continuing the bath procedure, the nurse evaluates respirations, counts and separates fingers, and judges skin turgor and muscle tone. As she washes each part, she inspects the infant. She wants to be able to report significant findings so that the paediatrician or family practitioner may be called if necessary. Every new baby should be completely examined by a physician or nurse practitioner within 24 hours of birth, and the condition of some may necessitate a much earlier examination.

Inspection bath On the following days the bath of the newborn infant serves two main purpose- inspection and stimulation. An example of this procedure follows. Details of possible eye care and genital cleaning are similar to those observed during the admission, both described previously.

Daily Inspection Bath

1. Each infant should have its own individual unit including:
   a. Thermometer
   b. Diapers, shirts
   c. Linen supply
   d. Blankets.
2. Papermesh squares or two wash cloths.
3. Mild soap or tap water alone.
4. Alcohol 70%, triple dye, or other cord antiseptic.
5. Applicators for cord care.
6. Scales and scale paper if baby has not been weighed earlier.
7. Scratch paper and pencil.
8. Laundry hamper.
9. Disinfectant for equipment clean up.

Procedure

1. Wash hands; check crib for needed materials.
2. Identify the baby
3. Undress the baby as necessary to take temperature and drop clothing into hamper.
4. Take the temperature (axillary or rectal) following appropriate technique.
5. Weigh if necessary, placing the baby on a clean paper on the scale.
6. Replace the baby in the crib on the scale paper.
7. Apply alcohol or other ordered antiseptic to the cord at the base by the skin margin and at the tip.
8. Wash the face with a paper mesh square and clear water. Wash the rest of the baby with mild soap and water solution or plain tap water in the following order; external ears, head, neck, arms, front of baby (avoiding the cord), back, legs and feet, lower back, and anus, pat dry. (Genitalia are cleansed as necessary with newly washed hands and a separate paper mesh square or cotton ball.)
9. Dress the baby and change the bed as necessary.

10. Place the baby on his abdomen, head to one side. Tuck one or more blankets over the infant.
11. Record weight, temperature, general condition, stool, and urine on work paper as appropriate. Loose, watery stools should be reported.
12. Hands should be washed before and after each baby's care and after caring for the anal genital area before proceading with additional with the same child. Hands should also be washed before removing a cord clamp when the cord is dry. Students should not remove cord clamps without appropriate supervision.
13. Avoid chilling the baby during the procedure.
14. All equipment that becomes contaminated while weighing should be washed with disinfectant before it is reused. Scales, cart and all equipment are washed with disinfectant at the end of daily care.
15. As the infant is bathed, inspect for the following:
    a. Colour-jaundice, cyanosis, pallor
    b. Rash
    c. Petechiae
    d. Braise marks
    e. Edematous area on the head.
    f. Condition of the mouth-excess salivation.
    g. Condition of the eyes (cleaned onl if a discharge is present)
    h. Condition of genitalia
    i. Condition of the cord (signs of inflammation, discharge, bleeding)
    j. Signs of possible paralysis of spasticity
    k. General level of alertness and actidity
    l. Indications of respiratory distress.
    m. Possible congenital malformations.

Lifting and holding The positioning, handling, and transporting of young babies can sometimes be alarming to new or beginning student nurses. Both need to bo reassured of their ability, to learn to care for their charges and to learn comfortable and safe methods of handling a baby. A baby does not break, and knowledge of certain principles will help to give the infant greater support and confidence.

The newborn infant usually tries to maintain a foetal position. With a little coaxing, the child usually readily assumes his unborn posture. This is sometimes useful to the paediatrician or family practitioner who is trying to evaluate the placement of a foot or the line of a mandible.

The newborn infant has one continuous antero-posterior spinal curve and no real control of head movements, although in the prone position the baby may raise its head slightly and briefly. Whenever the baby is lifted or transported, the head, being so large and heavy in relation to the rest of the body, must be supported for comfort and to prevent muscle strain. For safety all lifts must have at least two contact points so that is one fails, another is still available. Babies, even small ones, can be wriggly and sometims slippery. Following is one of the most common methods of lifting an infant on his back from a bed:

1. Facing the soles of the feet, lift the legs and buttocks slightly by grasping the feet, ankle separated by a finger.
2. Slide the opposite hand, palm up, under the full length of the baby until finally the entire back and head are supported.

A second method follows:

1. Facing the baby's side, slide one hand from the side under the hand and neck to grasp the outside arm. The head is supported by the forearm or the head and neck may be supported by the grasping hand.
2. With the other hand reach under the legs to grasp the farther thigh, or grasp the feet holding one finger between the ankles. This is a good lift for weighing the baby or putting him into a tub.

A baby should not be lifted by the arms. When head stability if attained at about 3 months of age, the child may be lifted by grasping the trunk with both hands below the arms. A newborn infant should not be left alone flat on his back. The baby may be propped with a rolled blanket along his back to maintain a side position or may be placed on its abdomen with the head turned to one side. Some newborn infants when placed in this position for protracted periods, seem to object and rub their knees up and down on the linen, causing reddened shins. Baby beds should have firm mattresses regardless of the style. No pillow should be used. A child should not always be placed in the same position, since this can distort the shape of his head or chest or cause localized baldness.

Babies have been carried in many ways; some methods are more comfortable for the one who carries and others give the baby a greater sense of safety and support. Three ways are common and are recommended:

1. *The traditional crade hold:* The child's head is cradled in the bend of the elbow; the forearm reaches around the outside of the body to grasp the outer leg with the fingers. The nurse's opposite hand and forearm helps support the back and buttocks. This additional support may be momentarily withdrawn if the hand is needed for a task.
2. *The football hold*: About half the length of the baby's body is supported by the nurse's forearm with the head and neck resting in her palm. The rest of the body, legs and buttocks are firmly wedged between the nurse's elbow and hip. This is a fine hold, and it was definitely designed to provide the parent or nurse with a free hand. However, one should not carry the baby in this position, since the head is some what unprotected.
3. *The shoulder hold*: The baby is held up against the chest and shoulder. The palm of one hand supports the baby's buttocks. The other hand keeps the head and back from sagging. Two hands are needed to support the baby's back correctly. This is the hold used often for burping the baby.

Most newborn infants love to be cuddled, and the way they are handled, touched and fed is how nurses and caregivers can show love and respect for them as individuals and as important members of humanity.

Nourishment

Nourishment, though not the most pressing of a newborn infant's needs, eventually becomes paramount. In modern society there are two ways of meeting this need; breastfeeding and formula feeding.

Breastfeeding

Breastfeeding, of course has an ancient biologic basis and is still the most universally recommended way of providing an infant with nourishment. A mother should carefully consider the advantage of breastfeeding when deciding how she will feed her infant. A father who is supporting of breastfeeding will influence the mother's success. Therefore, he should also be given information regarding the advantages of breastfeeding.

Teaching the Mother Breastfeeding Procedure

Purposes

1. To provide psychological and emotional satisfaction for the infant and the mother.
2. To feed the infant in natural and ideal food that will supply him with adequate nutrition.
3. To have milk always available at the right temperature.
4. To prevent chance of gastrointestinal disturbances and development of allergies.
5. To provide physical closeness of baby to mother during feeding (Fig. 7.13).
6. To provide comfort.

Procedure (Table 7.10)

Breastfeeding for the Ill or Hospitalized Infant (Table 7.11)

Equipment

1. Clear water
2. Cotton balls
3. Procedure (Table 7.11):

Advantages

Putting the baby to breast contributes to the mother's wellbeing in that the stimulation of the infant's nursing causes the recently emptied uterus to contract and helps in the return of the organ to its proper size and position, a process called involution. A further benefit is the relaxing effect that prolactin, the milk producing hormone has on the mother. Many investigators believe that the baby receives certain immune factors through the breast milk that help protect the baby against disease to which the mother may have been previously exposed. It is agreed that as a general

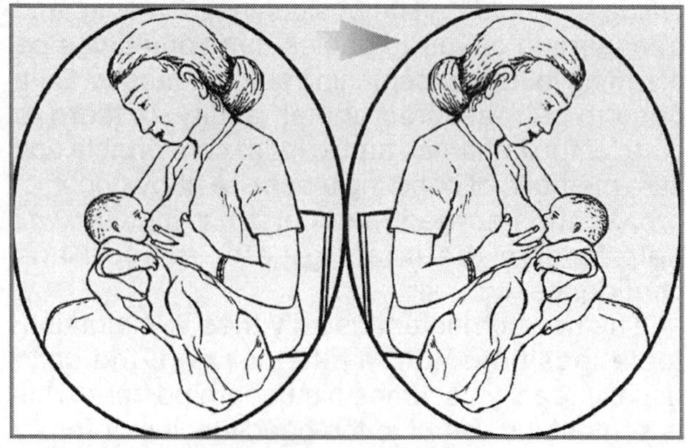

Fig. 7.13: Breastfeeding

Table 7.10: Teaching point, nursing action and rationale of breastfeeding

Teaching points	*Rationale*
1. Wash hand before breastfeeding	Protects infant and breast from infection
2. On demand feeding the advantages for mother and infant	a. Frequent suckling stimulates the mother's secretion of prolactin which, in turn, contributes to an increased milk supply b. Breast engorgement very rarely occurs
3. Once lactation is established, feeding intervals will vary between one and a half and six hours	Nursing pattern will fit into family life
4. Milk production continues by night, and day and night feeds for the baby are important in providing satisfaction	Will minimize or prevent engorgement and provide the baby with a substantial proportion of his twenty four hour intake
Position of Mother	
1. Lie on side with pillow under head. A pillow in the small of her back and one between her knees may provide added comfort and support. Position left arm above head; or	The mother should be relaxed and comfortable
2. If sitting, use a chair with back support. Place pillow on lap to hold infant	The infant's head should be higher than his abdomen to prevent regurgitation
Nursing action	*Rationale*
1. Allow time for mother and baby to interact. The mother may speak to and stroke her baby	The baby's rooting reflex may be stimulated by the tactile and oil factory sensations he receives
2. The baby should be guided gently to the breast. With the right hand, press darkened area around nipple into infant's mouth	
a. Make sure that the infant has both the areola and nipple in his mouth	Sucking on only the nipple causes pain and trauma for the mother, whilst the baby will receive inadequate milk supply, Indications for sound attachment i. The baby's mouth will be wide open ii. The baby's bottom lip will be curled back and some way from the base of the nipple, and further away from the base of the nipple than the top lip iii. If the baby's cheeks are sucked inwards, the baby is not properly attached
b. If breast is full and firm, use one finger to press breast way from infant's nose	Prevents obstruction of airway, infant breathes mainly through his nose
3. Use both breasts at each feeding	Empties each breast and maintains milk supply
4. At each feeding, alternate the breast that is used first. Pin a safety pin to the bra so a reminder of which breast to start with at the next feeding	The infant will empty the first breast, nursing at the second breast will increase milk production
5. Allow infant to have breast naturally alternately, break the suction by putting a finger into the corner of the infant's mouth	Pulling the nipple abruptly away from the infant will result in sore nipples
6. Have the mother 'burp' infant midway through the feeding. Pat gently on the back or hold in upright position	Releasing air in the infant's stomach will make him more satisfied and less fretful
7. Alert the mother that uterine cramping may occur, especially in multiparous women	Nursing stimulates release of oxygen hormone, causing uterine contractions, which can be worse in women with lessened uterine tone
8. Teach the mother to provide for adequate rest and to avoid tension, fatigue and a stressful environment	maternal fatigue stress and tension inhibit the letdown reflex and make breast milk less available to the infant at feeding
9. Avoid taking medications and drugs	Many substances pass into breast milk and can reduce milk production or have a deletarious effect on the infant

Table 7.11: Nursing action and rationale of breastfeeding of hospitalized infant

Nursing action	*Rationale/amplification*
1. When an infant who is breastfeeding is hospitalized, it is the nurse's respensibility to encourage the mother to continue breastfeeding if the infant's condition does not contraindicate it. Explain to the mother that a. Supplementary infant formula can be given to the infant if she is not available; or b. She can express her breasts by hand or by using a pump and bring in her milk to be given to the infant via bottle when she is not available	Some mothers have very strong feelings about wanting to breastfeed their baby, it gives them an emotional satisfaction that is vitally important to the mother-child relationship since it is an integral part of the total mothering process. The nurse must help to foster this relationship as much as she can
2. When nursing is to be done in the hospital paediatric setting, the physical surroundings may need to be altered somewhat. Provide the mother and infant with a relatively quiet area that is as private as possible and free from interruption	This will provide the mother and infant with an opportunity to continue to develop their relationship during the crisis of illness and hospitalization
3. Provide the mother with a comfortable armchair or pillow so that she can assume a comfortable position during the feeding. A footstool should also be available so that she can support her feet and the infant	Proper and comfortable position of the mother will enable her to hold the baby correctly and support him while he is at the breast
4. The infant should be awake and dry before the feeding is started	If the infant is awake and comfortable he will settle down and feed better.
5. Dress the infant appropriately so that he is not too warm or too cool, during the feeding. The infant should also be hungry	If he is too warm, he may fall asleep after the first few sucks of milk. A sleepy baby will not nurse well. If he is too cool, he may be fussy and restless
6. Have mother washed her hands. Then mother should wash her nipples with clear water and cotton balls	Washing the nipples will remove any old milk that may have leake and dried on them, providing a good medium for growth of bacteria
7. Position the baby at breast. Put him in a semi-sitting position with his face close to the breast and supported by one arm and hand. A pillow may be used under the baby to support him	Proper positioning will provide the infant with comfort and security and make it easier for him to suck and swallow
8. The breast may need to be supported by mother's hand	This makes the nipple more easily accessible to the baby's mouth and prevents obstruction of nasal breathing
Performance phase	
1. When the feeding is to start, let the breast touch the infant's cheek. Do not hold his cheek and try to help him find the nipple	The rooting reflex will over and the infant will turn his head towards the breast with his mouth open. If his cheek is touched with a hand, he will become confused, perhaps turning towards the hand.
2. The infant's lips should be out over the areaola and not just around the nipple before he begins to suck	Since the nipple is so small, suction cannot be achieved merely by grasping it. The areola must be in the infant's mouth in order to establish suction and make the suck effective
3. Note the presence or absence of the 'let down' reflex during the nursing period	Milk flowing from the other breast during nursing is quite normal. It is not usually present when the mother is worried
4. The length of feeding time may vary from five to twenty minutes. Let the infant feed until he is satisfied	When the infant is satisfied, and has nursed well, he is relaxed and usually falls asleep. He will stop sucking
5. Instruct the mother to burp the baby during and at the end of the feeding	When the infant is sucking he swallows some air. Burping will help abdominal distension and discomfort as well as regurgitation
6. One or both breasts may be used at each feeding. It makes no difference as long as (a) baby is satistified at the end of the feeding and (b) one breast is completely emptied at the feeding	Regular and complete emptying of the breast is the only stimulation for the production to milk.
Follow-up Phase	
1. When the infant has finished feeding, change his happy if it is wet or soiled	To provide comfort for a restful sleep and to prevent happy rash
2. Position infant on his right side or on his abdomen on his bed	This facilitates emptying of the stomach and decreases the possibility of regurgitation
3. Note if baby appears satisfied or still seems to be hungry	
4. Record descriptively and accurately: a. How baby fed. b. How baby went to breast. c. Satiety or hunger after feeding d. Breast or breasts used; which breast was nursed from thereafter	If both breasts were used, the second breast is not usually emptied and should be used first at the next feeding.

Contd...

Contd...

Nursing action	*Rationale/amplification*
5. For the new mother-infant nursing team: a. Provide the mother with anticipatory guidance for possible problems (i.e, breast engorgement)	To help establish and maintain successful breastfeeding that will be continued following discharge. Encourage mother to continue to get adequate rest and nutrition during and following infant's discharge
b. Promote maternal confidence in handling and nursing her infant c. Increase mother's knowledge about the mechanics of breastfeeding d. Provide mother with literature and resources	

rule breastfed babies have fewer respiratory tract infections and alimentary tract disturbances. Certainly when environmental hygiene is poor, breastfeeding is preferred over the great possibility of contaminated artificially prepared feeding because breast milk is normally sterile.

The observation that cow's milk was first designed for calves, whereas mother's milk is specifically designed for babies, is indisputable. The curd of human milk is softer than that of cow's milk and is easier for a baby to digest, Breastfed babies have fewer allergy problems. At first, breastfed babies have more frequent stools than formulafed infants. The stools are yellow-orange and aromatic but not offensive. Later on they may have fewer stools than their formulafed counterparts. No prolonged preparation time is necessary, and in the long run, successful nursing is less expensive. Obesity is seen less often in children who have been breastfed. If the mother nurses her baby, the return of menstruation may be delayed until several weeks after weaning, but nursing is no guarantee that pregnancy will not occur. However, the nursing may experience such a sense of closeness to her baby, fulfillment, and motherliness that this becomes the primary reason she continues to nurse.

Contraindications

Even thought some mothers may want to nurse, occasionally thc condition of the mother or baby make it in advisable. Maternal illness that is particularly protracted, severe, or contagious in nature may preclude breastfeeding. A mother who is in a high-risk group for acquired immune deficiency syndrome (AIDS) (for example, has used intravenous drugs should receive a HIV blood test before nursing. Mothers who have newly diagnosed active tuberculosis should be separated from their newborn infants until they have received appropriate medications and are judged noncontagious (usually 2 or more weeks). The mother then will be individually evaluated regarding her own health, and the condition of her infant. A woman with cardiac disease or established renal disease may be discouraged from nursing because of the demands on her own body resources that nursing may make. Mentally disturbed mothers may not be allowed the close contact needed for feeding their infants wither artificially or by breast unless closely supervised.

Other Considerations

The nursing mother must have a good diet to maintain her resources and provide sufficient nourishment for her infant. She produces about 25 ounces of milk when lactation is fully established in the second half of the first year, production typically drops about 20%. She needs more calories-approximately 500 to 1000 more calories per day than when she is not pregnant nor breastfeeding. Some of these calories can come from the stores of maternal fat built up during pregnancy. Therefore, an additional 500 calories per day is adequate unless the mother is under weight.

She also needs increased fluid inake to maintain her milk production. Her diet should include at least 1¼ quarts (4 to 5 glasses) of skimmed or low fat milk in liquid form or cooking mixtures a day to protect her personal calcium supply and to avoid possible osteoporosis, or weakening of the bony skeletion. Calcium supply and to avoid possible osteoporosis, or weakening of the bony skeletion. Calcium in the form of medication can be supplied if necessary, but a balanced diet containing calcium-rich foods would give her other healthful nutrients, benefit the whole family, and eliminate the need for pills.

The new Recommended Dietary Allowances (RDAs) indicate two different levels of nutritional requirements reflecting the higher needs of the first 6 months of lactation compared with the normal moderate decrease in milk production typical of the second 6 months. If is suggested that the nursing mother maintain a daily protein intake of about 65 g in the first period and about 62 g in the second. The recommended intake during pregnancy is 60 g.

During the first 6 months the RDAs of vitamins A, most B complex, C, and E in addition to the minerals zinc, iodine, and magnesium are expanded above those advised during pregnancy. In the second 6 months, requirements for these same nutrients remain above or at the level recommended during pregnancy. Only the recommendations for folate, iron, and vitamin B6 are lower during lactation than during pregnancy.

Some foods eaten by the mother have been said to cause the nursing baby abdominal distress, such as cramping or diarrhoea, and in the past women have been given lists of foods to avoid while nursing. There is no scientific basis for limiting "gassy" foods to prevent gas in a breastfed baby. Many babies do not seem aware of any deviation in the mother's diet. However, while some babies do not seem to tolerate certain foods, no one food affects every baby. Examples of foods that have caused problems are " strong" vegetables, such as cabbage, brussels sprouts, asparagus, and onions, and certain fruits such as prunes. By omitting the suspected food from her diet for a day or two and observing the baby's response, a mother can usually determine whether the baby is reacting to that food. Fussiness also has been reported in babies whose mothers drink large amounts of coffee or cola drinks.

Most, if not all, drugs taken by the mother may pass through the milk to the baby. The drug thiouracil used in treating hyperthyroidism actually becomes more concentrated in the maternal milk and may affect the infant severely. Certain laxatives are as effective on the baby as the mother and should be avoided or used only judiciously. Common medications to be avoided include cascara, Epsom salts, and Ex-Lax, but not inert mineral oil. It is wise to counsel mothers to remind their physicians that they are nursing when receiveing new prescriptions. Concern has been expressed regarding the amount of DDT and other environmental contaminants found in some human milk samples. However, discontinuation of breastfeeding is not recommended by authorities unless the level of DDT is judged to be high.

Some cultures teach that an intake of low-percentage beer or, for those more affluent, the addition of champagne to the diet increases milk production. The benefits from these are probably caused by increased fluid intake and a feeling of relaxation. It is true that a tense, worried mother may have difficulty in maintaining an adquate milk supply. However, alcohol does pass into breast milk and it consumption should be discouraged while breast feeding.

More and more mothers who must or who prefer to work outside the home are successfully continuing to breastfeed. This requires extra effort because to maintain a milk supply the breasts must be stimulated and emptied at fairly frequent intervals. A nursing mother may manually empty her breasts when unable to feed her infant because of separation, but this procedure may not always be convenient. Electric or manual breast pumps may be preferable.

The nursing mother needs good breast support. The typical nursing bra, with the liftdown cup, is efficient and easily used. Many mothers use freshly laundered or paper handkerchiefs or soft cellulose pads strategically placed to absorb leakage.

A mother with severely cracked nipples, mastitis, or breast abscess is no longer required to terminate nursing. Many authorities recommend continuation of breast feeding while antibiotics and other remedies are used with proper initial management and frequent nursing such conditions are avoidable.

The condition of the baby may influence the decision of whether to nurse. Small premature infants usually do not have the strength to suckle at breast, but they may benefit from the expressed maternal milk. For this reason, mothers of premature infants may wish to maintain their milk supply for the immediate use of the baby in the hospital (to be given by means of gavage) and for later use when the baby goes home. Other babies, unable to suckle may benefit from maternal milk, a child with a cleft lip or palate may be able to breastfeed, depending on the extent of the defect. If household freezing techniques are used, maternal milk may be stores for 1 to 2 weeks, Longer storage necessitates quick freezing and deep freezer storage.

To be completely successful, most nursing must really want to nurse have supportive family members, be convinced of its advantages, and receive prenatal instruction regarding the care and normal function of their breasts, as well as encouragement and assistance in the postpartum period. If a woman has flattened or inverted nipples, they may be treated during this preparation period by prescribed nipple stretching exercises, use of special breast cups, or suction. In some localities groups of mothers particularly interested in promoting breastfeeding have formed organization to help the new mother or mother to be.

Some babies nurse well from the start; others take a little while to get the idea of what they are supposed to do. However, with breastfeeding the nurse and mother have some powerful allies-inborn reflexes and hunger. By using his own natural behaviours and reflexes the baby can be assisted to begin nursing at the breast. In preparation for breastfeeding the mother first washes her hands. Then she and her baby should be comfortable positioned. The mother needs to be in good body alignment and well-supported in the position of her choice. If sitting up in bed or in a chair, she usually finds it more comfortable to place the baby on a pillow in her lap. This brings the infant closer to the breast with less strain. She may lie on her side with her lower arm cradling the baby if the baby has no history of ear infections.

To empty the breast effectively and to preserve the nipple in good condition the baby must nurse with the areola in his mouth and not just the nipple. This is important because, if the baby is allowed to chew on the end of the nipple, painful, cracked or fissured nipples may result. The following will help the baby to get a good grasp. While in a comfortable sitting position the mother holds the infant using the cradle hold. The infant should then be turned onto his side so that his entire body faces his mother and his lower arm can be tucked underneath him or around his mother's waist. In his position does not have to turn his head or strain to reach the breast, and he is close enough to fit his open mouth well back onto the areola. Now the mother can support her breast, using her free hand, by placing her fingers under the breast, and her thumb above in preparation for the infant's mouth. By lightly tickling the baby's lips with her nipple the mother can stimulate the baby to open his mouth. After a few moments of tickling the baby will open his mouth wide. While the mouth is open wide, the mother quickly pulls the baby toward her as closely as she can. The tip of the baby's nose should touch her breast. If he needs more room to breathe, her thumb is conveniently there to press the breast gently away from his nose.

The same steps apply to a mother who is nursing lying down, except that the infant is placed on the bed so that he is lying on his side facing the mother. It is possible to nurse infant's using various modifications as necessary.

Sometimes if the baby has difficulty getting started or is new at the breast, gently expressing a drop of milk on the tip of the nipple will serve as an appetizer and help give the baby the basic idea. If the breasts are engorged, expressing some milk before begining to nurse will relieve tension of the breast and make it easier for the baby to grasp the areola. Nipples should be allowed to air day after feeding. Soaps and antiseptics should not be used. Washing the breasts and nipples once a day with clear water is sufficient. Repeated washing of the nipple even with clear water removes the protective oils and predisposes it to cracking. Therefore the use or creams or ointments that need to be washed off before nursing should be avoided.

When removing the baby from the breast, the nurse should remember that babies are capable of considerable tenacity. To convince an infant that is best to let go, the nurse can gently pull down on the chin or insert a finger into the corner of the infant's mouth between the jaws to release them and break the suction.

The first few days the baby obtains an "introductory milk, "called colostrum, which has a laxative effect and contains protective antibodie maternal milk becomes "complete"—that is, possesses its characteristic content-serveral weeks later.

It must be emphasized that the greatest aid to milk production is frequent stimulation and emptying of the breast. If the breasts are not emptied, milk production may dwindle.Probably the ideal maternity accommodations for a nursing mother, particularly if the child involved is her first, is the rooming in plan or a modification of rooming-in. In this setting the baby may be but to the breast as desired and is not limited to the 4 hour feeding schedules followed by many hospitals without family centered postpartum care programmes. Babies seem to do the best when allowed to feed on demand without limitations as to frequency or length of feeding. Nursing infants are often fed every 2 to 3 hours when breastfeeding is initiated. The length of the feeding varies considerably from baby to baby and is usually somewhere between 10 to 30 minutes.

Limiting the time the baby nurses at the breast is no longer considered effective in preventing sore nipples. It is generally recommended that a mother nurse from both breasts at each feeding. Perhaps the most important consideration is that the breast be emptied. If it is not emptied by the baby, the mother should empty it manually or with the aid of a pump to maintain milk production.

Breasfed babies, like formula-fed babies, must be purped to remove swallowed air. Sitting the infant up or holding him over a protected shoulder while gently rubbing his back, in addition to patience, produces results for both breast and bottle babies.

Artificial Feeding

Today, with present knowledge of nutrition and increased understanding of food processing and preservation, the bottle-fed baby need not be threatened with malnutrition or disease. Although mothers should be told the advantages of breastfeeding, they should not be considered or made to feel like maternal failures if they cannot or choose not to nurse. To assume such a position is unrealistic and unkind. To force a mother to nurse against her will may cause an unhappy cyele of rebellion, failure, and regret and may make those few mothers who cannot or should not nurse feel lacking in maternal virtue. Some have schedules that are difficult to combine with nursing; some are concerned that their youngsters are not getting enough to eat; and some have felt like failures in past nursing experiences. For others, the process of nursing is physically unattractive and may lack approval from their mates. Many healthy children have been formula fed. A loving mother cuddling her baby while tilting a milk-filled bottle need not consider her self a "poor mother".

The primary health care provider should guide the selection of formula. It has been recommended that nonbreastfed infants receive iron fortified formula during the first year of life. Numerous commercially prepared proprietory formulas that contain the necessary iron and vitamins are available. These may come in liquid or powder form. Directions must be carefully followed since some are ready to use and others must be diluted or mixed. Their use saves preparation time and bother. The cost involved differs with the type, form and vendor. The less modification needed before use, the more expensive the product. A number of companies are manufacturing disposable prefilled nursing units.

Gavage's Feeding (Table 7.12) (Figs 7.14 and 7.15)

Purpose To provide either breast milk or formula to those infants unable to feed orally.

Equipment
- Paediatric stethoscope
- Gastric tube (6 to 8 French for oral feedings, 3.5 to 5 French for nasogastric feedings)
- Breast milk or formula
- Tape
- Blanket roll
- Syringe
- Suction equipment
- Infusion pump.

Preparation of Formula

If the more costly ready-to-feed bottle formula is not purchased, the most frequently recommended method of formula preparation today is the so-called tap water method, using prepared formula in the form of liquid concentrate, or powder.

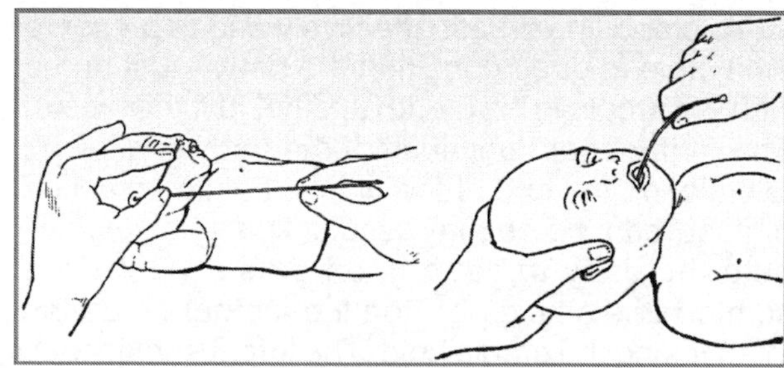

Fig. 7.14: Gavage's feeding: Use of catheter

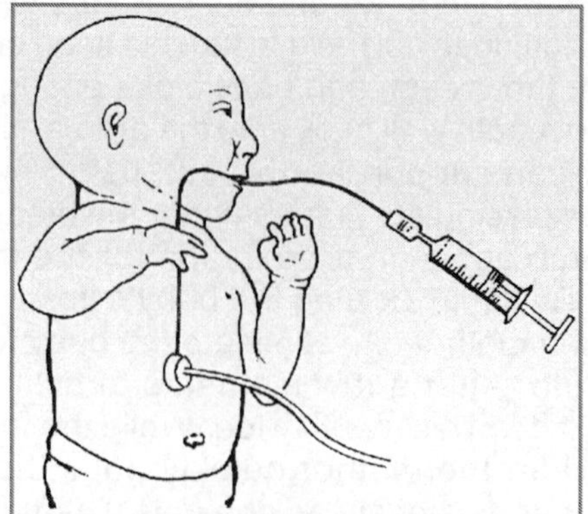

Fig. 7.15: Gavage's feeding

Table 7.12: Nursing action and rationale of Gavage's feeding

Nursing action	*Ratonale*
1. Select the appropriate size tube. For nasogastric tubes, measure (with the tube itself) from the tip of the infant's nose to the ear-lobe and either to the distal end of the xiphoid process or to a point midway between the distal end of the xiphoid process and the umbilicus. Mark the tube at the measured point with tape. For orogastric tubes, follow the same steps but use the mouth as the initial landmark	The smallest bare tubling that will deliver the feeding but not occlude the naris should be selected for nasagastric feedings. Using these steps to measure the tube before it s insertion helps ensure that the tube will be long enough to reach the infants stomach
2. Place the infant in a supine position and gently insert the catheter through the nose or mouth, with the head in a slightly extended position, until the tape market is positioned at the orifice. If the infant should being to cough, gag, or turn cyanotic, remove the tube immediately. If regurgitation occurs, suction the airway until it is clear and then resume tube placement	Slight extension promotes entry of the tube into the oesophagus. Hyperextension or under extension may decrease air entry
3. Secure the orogastric or nasogastric tube in place by taping it to the infant's cheek. Limit the amount of tape to the minimum required to ensure security. A pectin barrier may be placed under the tape if there are concerns about skin integrity	Removing adhesives can result in epidermal stripping. This loss of skin integrity may lead to increased risk for infection, increased water loss, and thermal instability
4. Before each feeding, check tube placement by using a syringe to inject 0.5 to 1.0 mL of air into the tubing while listening with a stethoscope over the epigastric area for a "swoosh"	Correct tube placement is critical to avoid delivery of the feeding into the lungs
5. If indicated by hospital protocol aspirate for gastric contents by pulling gently with the syringe; replace secretions	Aspiration of gastric contents is an indication of correct tube placement; however, the absence of gastric contents does not mean that the tube is positioned improperly. Routine aspiration of gastric contents can cause irritation of the stomach lining
6. The infant may be held by a parent or nurse during the feeding or placed in the prone or right lateral position with the head of the bed slightly elevated.	Elevation of the bed reduces the risk for gastroesophageal reflux. Oxygenation can be affected by the infant's position; therfore, the position that best supports adequate oxygenation should be considered. The infant may be supported or nested into position with blanket rolls. Having parents hold the infant during the feeding promotes parental attachment.
7. Deliver the prescribed amount of breast milk or formula by the method designated by the physician. Feedings can be delivered on either a continuous or an intermittent schedule by either gravity flow or an infusion pump	There are no reparts that convincingly support one method over another. Clinician preference and the infant's ability to tolerate the feeding without physiologic compromise (such as apnoea, bradycardia, or gastroesophageal reflux) most often determine the method of choice
8. Offer the infant non-nutritive sucking during Gavage's feeding	Research indicates that nonnutritive sucking may improve the sucking reflex and promote weight gain
9. Document the date and time the feeding and how the infant tolerated the procedure	Some feeding tubes are made of tube was placed polyvinyl chloride, a plastic that hardens over time. The rigidity of the tube increases the risk for gastric perforation. If this type of tube is left in place for subsequent feedings, it should be changed every few days
10. Carefully remove the tube by pulling on it in one continuous motion. Cotton balls moistened with water can be used to assist with removal of any unwanted tape from the infant's skin	Removing the tube in one continuous motion helps minimize potential agitation

Tap Water Method—Formula Preparation

This method of formula preparation has become popular because of its simplicity. Used conscientiously, it is safe. Abused by lack of cleanliness or improper technique, it may be associated with infant illness.

Materials

- Capped formula bottle
- Nipple
- Bottle brush
- Soap or detergent
- Sauce pan
- Can opener
- Spoon

Formula as prescribed: ready to use, liquid concentrate, powder.

Procedure

1. Use a clean formula bottle that has been *Meticulously washed* in warm sudsy water, rinsed in hot water, and air dried.
2. Use a nipple that has been carefully washed and rinsed. Make sure that the nipple holesare open. (Some references also recommend boiling the clean nipple 3 to 5 minutes).
3. Measure the ingredients needed for one feeding into the bottle. Besure that you understand what dilution (if any) is to be made because formula is sold in many different forms and concentrations. Read the directions: Babies have become ill and even died because caretakers have not realized this. Add warm water from the tap to the bottle in the amount the formula directions indicate. (Boil tap water that is unapproved). Mix with clean spoon. Feed Immediately; do not save formula from one feeding to the next or for more than an hour.

Special handling of infant formula is necessary because milk is such an ideal medium for the nourishment and growth of other living things in addition to human babies. Microorganisms that are not at all compatible with the baby's digestive system may multiply rapidly in milk if it is improperly bottled or is left open to air and warmed for an extended period. Typhoid organisms were fairly common contaminants of milk and milk products before pasteurization became widespread. Because of the baby's succeptibility, certain methods of disinfection or "sterilization of the formula (aseptic or terminal) were considered necessary until the last decade. Now it is believed that in most instances a conscientious clean technique is sufficient unless formula must be prepared in advance and stored. However, hospitals usually use sterile precautions until an infant has reached 3 months of age. Plastic bottles employed for older infants who hold their own, if reused, should be sterilized between patients.

Feeding an infant is formula can be an enjoyable experience. The hands should be clean; the milk usually should be tepid (no sensation of hot or cold) falling on the inside of the parent's or nurse's wrist.

Experiments using cold formula for feeding the new born have demonstrated no undesirable effects, even on premature babies. However, it is psychologically difficult to give a young infant a COLD meal. Many nurses have discarded formula warmers because of problems with elevated bacterial count on the equipment. Feedings are offered at room temperature. The rate of nipple flow should be almost one drop per second when the bottle is inverted. Nipple holes may by enlarged by a hot needle mounted on a cork.Vigorously sucking babies should be given a resistant nipple. Babies who tire easily and premature babies do better with a soft, pliable nipple.

Be sure the nipple is on top of the tongue, and do not push it too far back; it may stimulate the Gag reflex. Babies seem to drink best when held closely on a definite incline. Studies indicate that such positioning minimizes the possibility of retrograde infection through the eustachian tubes to the middle ear and helps prevent aspiration. The neck of the bottle should always be tipped so that it is full of milk. Air in the baby's stomach may cause pain, decrease appetite or promote regurgitation. Bubbles may be expelled by rubbing the baby's back in an upright position. This may be done after each ounce with newborn babies, particularly finger suckers and those who have been crying, before feedings as well. Newborns should be carefully observed before and during feedings for indications of any abnormality in the digestive or respiratory tracts. Prefeeding coughing, cyanosis, and excessive mucus may be associated with anatomic abnormalities. Regurgitation of a feeding through the nose and mouth should be reported at once. Many babies are offered water before they are put to the breast or fed formula to evaluate their ability to drink without difficulty.

After feeding, the infant may need to have his diaper changed. He sould be placed on his right side or abdomen to sleep. The amount taken should be recorded in nursery records. The newborn infant may take only 1 ounce the first day and 2 or 3 ounces per feeding on the second and third days. Newborns usually are fed every 3 or 4 hours.

Evaluation of Nutritional Status

There are numerous ways to judging whether a newborn infant, either formulafed or breastfed, is receiving enough to eat.

1. *Observing his behaviour*—does he seem content, or is he a short sleeper and irritable? (Note that babies cry for reasons other than hunger pangs; for example, if they are wet, too tightlybundled or too warm, have gas pains, or want to be held).
2. *Watching for signs of dehydration* from poor fluid intake:
   a. Fewers than 6 to 8 wet diapers per day.
   b. Dark, concentrated urine, dry, hard stools.
   c. Dry mucous membranes.
   d. Dry skin with little "bounce" (poor turgor).
   e. Low-grade fever (note that the most common cause of low grade fever is dehydration, although the nurse shouldn't overlook the possibility of infection).
   f. Elevated specific gravity (above 1,020)
   g. In severe cases, sunken fontanelles.
3. *Measuring intake*:
   a. This is routine with bottle fed babies
   b. If measuring is ordered, breastfed babies are weighed dressed and wrapped directly before the feeding and directly after the feeding, before any diapers are changed with the same clothes and blankets (1 gm 1ml)
   c. Intake should be evaluated in terms of a 24-hour period and not individual feedings.
4. Measuring weight gain:
   a. This method is of little use currently because of the short hospital stays of most newborn infants (sometimes less than a day).
   b. All babies lose weight directly after birth, which should cause no concern unless the weight loss approaches 10% of the birthweight.
   c. After weight gain is reestablished, a gain of about 1 ounce a day is average, equaling about 6 ounces a week. At the end of 5 months most babies have doubled their birth weight.

Love-Parent-Infant Attachment

The birth of a child is a special occasion and although the child needs to be protected against infection and over-handling, the way that the child is introduced to the parents are siblings is of great importance. If possible, both the father and the mother should have an opportunity to see and handle the infant without hurry directly after birth.

The importance of this early postpartum period to the formation of positive mother-child and mother-father-child relationships is being explored attentively. The newborn has been reported to be often more alert during the first hour after birth than in the immediate subsequent hours. Many agree that birth and the immediately postpartum period when the baby is first seen, touched, and cared for are sensitive periods in the development of attachment. If the mother is also alert and willing and the circumstances of the labour and birth are conductive, early parent-child interaction followed by frequent visits appear to her young parents develop gratifying maternal-paternal identities.

The nurse is an excellent position to assess and facilitate attachment. Numerous investigators have described the typical initial exploratory behaviour of human mothers and fathers. Gentle fingertip touching of the hands and feet progresses to massage like motions of the palm on the baby's trunk. Eye-to-eye contact is remarkable, and a characteristic "enface" positionis often demonstrate (the mother's face poised directly in front of and in line with that of her infant). This eye-to-eye observation helps establish the new born's identity as a person and provided rewarding feedback to the mother. However, many parents establish strong attachments to their infants without having experienced early "hands on" contact. If for some reason such early interaction is not provided, it should be remembered that human beings are very adaptable. Future relationships can still be rewarding and meaningful.

Nurses must recognize that many expectant fathers want to be involve not only in the preparation for parenthood but in the actual birth and care of the infant. Mothers must be helped in understanding that just as they have many adjustments to make, so do new fathers. A father often has a need to handle and touch his newborn. Typically he has experienced various concerns including the health of his wife, the outcome of the pregnancy, changes in sexual practices, and increased financial responsibility.

If the newborn's siblings, grandparents and other family members visit, they should be able to see the baby and visit with the new mother according to her wishes. Newborn infants may receive all other things, but if they do not receive true love, they will not thrive.

Although it is important for newborns to receive stimulation, they also need times of relatively little input to "organize" their world and grow. Overstimulated babies are likely to be more nervous, with shorter attention spans.

Special Needs

Parent education: The new parent will have a lower level of anxiety if she is equipped with a comprehensive knowledge of her child. Although she is in the hospital for a brief time in the postpartum period, it is the nurse's responsibility to build on teaching in the following areas:

- Importance of stimulation
- Developmental milestones
- Possible sibling rivalry
- Infant care
- Bathing
- Skin care
- Cord care
- Circumcision care
- Nutrition
  - Breastfeeding
  - Formula preparation
  - Introduction to solids
- Sleep patterns
- Elimination patterns
- Safety
- Car seats
- Never leaving child unattended
- Cool vs hot mist vaporizer
- Pacifiers
- Cribe
- Available community resources
- Additional teaching can be begun or continued in high school family education classes, Prenatal and postnatal parent education programs, clinic and office waiting rooms, and well-child visits.

Circumcision

Circumcision involves the slitting or surgical removal of all or part of the foreskin, or prepuce of the penis. Advocates of the procedure believe that it makes hygiene easier, decreases irritation of the area from an accumulation of cellular debris (smegma) under the foreskin, and may help to avoid urinary tract infaction and cancer. Other practitioners declare that circumcision is unnecassary and a possible source of infection, hemorrhage, and meatal stenosis. The outcome of this surgery appears to depend a great deal on the skill and teachinque of the operator. It has been stated that there are no valid medical indications for circumcision in the newborn period. Routine circumcision of all male infants appears to be decreasing.

Physicians usually have individual preferences regarding the techniques used, but the following set up list and procedure may be helpful.

Circumcision Procedure

Materials

1. Sterile set up including:
   a. One circumcision drape
   b. Two 4 x 4 squares (flats or gauze compresses)
   c. Two cotton balls
   d. Three small haemostats (mosquito clamps)
   e. One Yellen (Gomco) clamp, 1.3 t 1.1 cm in diameter.
   f. One scalpel handle and added blade.
   g. Possible, needle holder, needle and suture materials (chromic 3-0)
   h. One grooved director and probe.
   i. One thumb forceps.
2. Sterile groves, appropriately sized
3. Ordered antiseptic for skin preparation such as povidone iodine (Betadine)
4. Dressing materials
   a. Petroleum-impregnated gauze
   b. Tincture of benzoin application
5. A circumcision board, diapers, pins, or special restraining halter that ties over the board.
6. Lidocaine HCl 1% (Xylocaine), 1 ml without epinephrine if anaesthesia is used.
7. Syringe, 1 ml. with 27-gauge, 0.5 inch (1.2 cm) needle if anaesthesia is used.

Procedure

1. *Preliminary*
   a. Obtain a signed informed consent from parent before procedure.
   b. Properly identify the baby. Check for possible reasons for not proceeding with the

operation (presence of inflammation, tendency to bleed). Clean diaper area.
c. Restrain the baby gently but firmly on a padded or plastic circumcision board.
d. Ensure good light. A stool or chair may be appreciated by the operator.
e. Use of a pacifier may comfort the baby during the procedure.

2. *Technique*
a. The technique of circumcision differes considerably from surgeon-to-Surgeon. Local anaesthetic is being used more frequently as the entire question of pain perception in infants and small children is being re-examined.
b. The Yellen (Gomco) clamp may be used to cut off circulation, and the foreskin excised. Sutures may or may not be used.
c. The foreskin may be feed from the glans with probe, cut away, and bleeders controlled and sutured.
d. A nonconstrictive dressing is applied. Petrolatum-impregnated gauze is often used.

3 *Aftercare*
a. Notice of the recent circumcision should be attached to the crib.
b. Frequent checks should be made to determine possible swelling and bleeding.
c. Voidings, especially the first after the procedure, should be carafully charted. There is a danger of urinary retention.
d. The area should be kept clean, soiled of displaced dressings should be replaced with clean mate-rials.
e. The infant is positioned on his side.

Table 7.13: Nursing action of newborn's circumcision and rationale

Nursing action	*Rationale*
1. Assess level of pain (facial expression, body movements, crying)	Assessing for pain allows initiation of interventions to minimize or lessen pain.
2. Dress, wrap, cuddle, and talk to the baby	These measures provide comfort after a painful procedure.
3. Attach diaper more loosely	A loose diaper decreases pressure and pain at the circumcision site.
4. Position the baby on his side	This position minimizes pressure and pain at the circumcision site.
5. Take the baby to the mother for feeding and comfort right after the circumcision	The baby will not have been fed for serveral hours before the procedure, so he will be hun-gry. The mother will want reassurance that the baby is okay.
6. If bleeding occurs, apply gentle pressure to the site intermittently with a folded sterile 4 x 4 gaize pad. Wear gloves. If the bleeding is not controlled, notify the physician, who may inject epinephrine or put in a suture	Pressure decreases bleeding. Wearing gloves is consistent with standard precautions.
7. Assess voiding for amount and adequacy. Instruct the mother to call the physician or midwife if the baby has not urinated within 24 hours	Swelling or damage may obstruct urine output
8. Change diaper. Reapply vaseline gauze or A and D ointment per physician's order. Wear gloves. If the diaper adheres, squeeze water over the penis to loosen it from the diaper. Use only water to cleanse the area, and squeeze it over the glans	Frequent changing prevents contamination of the site. Reapplying vaseline gauze or A and D ointment helps keep the diaper from sticking to the site. Squeezing water over the penis helps remove the diaper without causing more bleeding because soap may irritate the area and cause discomfort. Wearing gloves is consistent with standard precautions
9. Observe the site for infection	Contact with microorganisms may cause infection. A whitish-yellow exudate appears around the in 24 hours or so. This is granulation tissue and is part of the healing process. If persists for 2 to 3 days. Symptoms of infection include pus, foul odour, fever, increased redness/swelling/ tenderness after healing has started, or no healing within 72 hours
10. Show parents how to care for circumcision	The baby and mother are usually discharged the same day the circumcision is done. Careful observation and care of the circumcision site must continue until healing has occurred (usually about 2 days)

Table 7.14: Nursing action and rationale for neonatal transport

Nursing action	*Rationale*
1. Assess the neonate to ensure that he or she is stable for transport. A thorough risk assessment includes review of maternal history and delivery; the neonate's vital signs, neurologic status, colour, and muscle tone; blood glucose evaluation; weight and measurement; anomalies; and gestational age assessment.	A neonate in stable condition will handle the stress of a transport better and be less likely to require emergency intervention enroute.
2. Communicate with family and physicians. It is the responsibility of the referring physician to ascertain that room is available at the receiving hospital, to communicate with the receiving physician regarding the baby's history and status , and to discuss transport with the parents. The nurse may witness informed consent for transfer and give parents information on the receiving hospital including unit phone numbers and local motels.	Open, frequent communication between nurse, physician, and parents helps to decrease uncertainty and confusion, thereby improving the efficiency of the transport. Witnessing informed consent is necessary because the form is a legal document.
3. Plan for the transport. Estimate times of transport arrival at referring hospital, departure, and arrival at receiving hospital. Discuss equipment and personnel need.	Planning needs ahead of time prevents delays during which the condition of the baby could change.
4. Provide the receiving hospital with a photocopy of the maternal record and of the neonate's complete chart, X-ray films, and a tube of the mother's blood.	The receiving hospital needs all information regarding the neonate's stay to develop an appropriate plan of care and provide continuity of care.
5. When the transport team arrives, give an up-to-date report on the baby's status. Document in the chart that a verbal report was given and the time of arrival and departure of the team.	Up-to-date information on the status of the newborn helps the transport team anticipate problems that might occur enroute. The transport records become part of the baby's permanent record, so accurate documentation regarding all aspects of the transport is important
6. Allow parents contact with their baby and provide parental support	Parents will be grieving the loss of an ideal birth outcome and be fearful about their baby's condition. For some parents, it may be their last opportunity to see their baby alive.
7. Call the receiving hospital when the transport team leaves	This provides the receiving hospital with an estimated time of arrival.

Nursing Care after Circumcision (Table 7.13)

Purpose To care for the newborn's circumcision, to observe for bleeding, and to prevent infection.

Equipment

- Sterile 4 × 4 gauze pads
- A and D ointment or vaseline gauze

Sometimes circumcisions are performed not long before the baby's discharge home. In this event the parents should be carefully instructed regarding observation and care of the area.

Neonatal Transport

Purpose: Neonatal transport to a tertiary care centre is indicated when the condition of a neonate warrants more intensive evaluation or intervention than can be provided where the infant is currently hospitalized. Adequate communication and information are imperative for effective neonatal transport (Table 7.14).

Equipment

- Consent form
- Copy of maternal chart
- Copy of baby's chart including X-ray films
- Transfer form
- Tube of mother's blood
- Information, about the receiving hospital for parents.

Discharge Procedure

Discharge is an exciting, somewhat trying time for most parents. Before the actual time of departure, the physician's order for discharge is checked and home orders are reviewed. The mother's belongings are packed, and clothes are put out for the infant. Mothers should have ready at least 2 diapers, pins (or 2 disposable diapers), a baby shirt, kimono and receiving blanket or comparable wardrobe. Identification should be established, and the baby viewed and dressed in his own clothes. The discharge record should be signed and witnessed. If the mother has chosen to bottle-feed, a supply of formula may be available to take home.(Some people believe that sending formula home with breastfeeding mothers, sets them up for failure.) Before saying goodbye to the family, the nurse should make sure discharge instructions are understood and preferable written out, with any questions answered. Ideally, the baby's first car ride home from the hospital should be in an approved automobile safety restraint. Many hospitals and insurance plans are making this item available to new parents.

Before leaving the infant, the nurse should take one last peek at his face to assure herself of his condition and wish him well.

Nursing Management of Normal Newborn (Please See Nursing Care Plan Table 7.15)

Table 7.15: Nursing care plan of normal neonate/newborn

Problem (1)	*Reason (2)*	*Objective (3)*	*Nursing Intervention (4)*	*Evaluation (5)*
1. Risk for ineffective breathing pattern Related to • Prenatal or intra-partum stressors (such as pain medication, cord compression • Excess mucus (increased oxygen needs, which contribute to acidosis) • Respiratory acidosis • Ineffective airway clearance	*Subjective Data* Absence of crying. *Objective Data* • Acrocyanosis • Central cyanosis • Gagging or choking • Persistent alterations in respiration (< 30/min > 60/min) • Abdomen immobile with respirations • Pronounced thoracic/ chest movement with respirations • Sternal/intercostal retractions • Grunting • Nasal flaring	Client will demonstrate effective breathing patterns	• Assess gestational age (surfactant develop in the third trimester) • Differentiate period breathing pattern from apnoea • Assess and observe raspiratory rate as frequently as needed. Typical frequency is every 15 minutes for four times, then every hour until stable then every shift. • Observe characteristics indicating normal respirations, charactaristics of normal respiration are shallow, irregular in rate, rhythm, and depth; nose breathing; abdomen move with inspiration and expiration, thoracic area remains relatively immobile with respiration periodic breathing.; colour indication oxygenation • Observe for symptoms indicating that respirations are normal-persistently abnormal rate, retractions, grunting, nasal flaring, or central cyanosis. • Auscultats breath sounds, Breath sound be symmetric with it rales and/or bonchi. • Position on side with blanket roll behind back • Clear airways as needed. Suction as needed with bulb syringe or wall suction/catheter, keep bulb syringe in ingant's crib at all times • Assess colour for cyanosis • Maintains newborn temperaturs. • Have emergency respiratory resuscitation aquipment available • Provide tactile stimulation if necessary.	Client will evidence a patent airway, normal respiratory rate absence of aerocyanosis normal characteristics of newborn respiration absence of retractions. absence of grunting and nasal flaring
2. Risk for altered tissue perfusion related to • Persistent foetal circulation; shunts not closing • Respiratory distress • Haemoloysis of RBCs	*Subjective data* *Objective data* • Tachycardia • Rales • Tachypnoea • Absence of bowel sounds • Absence of bowel elimination	Client will demonstrate adequate tissue perfusion	• Assess apical rate as frequantly as needed. Typical frequency in every 15 minutes for four times, then every hour until stable, then every shift. • Observe colour for cyanosis. Blanch skin on trunk and extremities periodically to assess capillary fill time. • Assess for brachial, radial, femoral,	Client will evidence absence of central cyanosis; heart rate of 120 to 160 beats/mm normal respiratory bowel sounds bowel elimination

Contd...

Contd...

Problem (1)	Reason (2)	Objective (3)	Nursing Intervention (4)	Evaluation (5)
associated with Rh factor and blood incompatibility • Excessive amount of RBCs	• Absence of urine elimination • Decreased capillary filling • Poor feeding • Vomiting • Symptoms of respiratory distress		popliteal and dorsalis pedia pulses. • Ausculate heart sounds and report murmurs for evaluation. • Auscultate breath sounds. • Note intensity of cry. • Obtain heel stick sample of blood for haematocrit. Assess haemoglobin level and haematocrit. • Note blood group and Rh factor of mother and newborn. Note results of coombs' test. • Assess bowel sounds and bowel elimination • Assess urinary output. • Assess feeding behaviours and note if vomiting occurs	urine elimination absence of vomiting feeding well normal peripheral pulses
3. Risk for hypothermia or hyperthermia related to *Hyperthermia* • Large body surface in relation to body mass • Minimal insulating fat and limited brown fat • Thin epidermis with proximity of blood vessels to skin • Exposure to colder environment from a warm intra-uterine environment • Inability to shiver • Decreased metabolic rate • Inadequate clothing	*Subjective Data* Both conditions *Objective Data* Hypothermia • Auxillary temp below 97.7° F • Increased activity (restless, agitated hyperactive) • Poor appetite Poor feeder • Decreased heart rate • Cold stress syndrome • Drop in skin temperature, increased activity. pallor, or rottling cool skin, hands and feet Symptoms of respiratory distress Hyperthermia • Axillary temparature 99.5° F • Perspiration on face, hand • Apnoea, seizures • Tachypnoea • Flushed skin	Client will demonstrate normal body temperature	Hyperthermia • Dry newborn place stockinette cap on infant's head. Dress and wrap inwarm blankets • Place newborn on prowarmed matters on in Parent's arms. Warm colder objects coming in contact with the newborn (stethoscope, scale, hands) • Maintain environmental and room temperature. Maintain controlled heat source at 98.6°F • Position crib away from cold airconditioner. Cold walls, or cold window, Maintain radiator, Warmer 98.6°F. Position crib away from heater and sunlight • Adjust clothing in relation to room temperature • Cover newborn as much as possible when diaper, providing bathing/cleansing postpone first bath until baby temperature is stable • Assess axillary temperature. Typical frequency in everyhour in the first 4 hours, then every 4 hours, in the first 24 hours of life and than every shift • Observe for symptoms of cold stress • Assess for symptoms of respiratory distress-apnoea, central cyanosis, grunting, retractions nasal flaring bradycardia and abnormal respiratory rate	Client will evidence axillary temp 97.7 to 96.6° F absence of increased activity; absence of apnoea, seizures Cold stress symptoms resp. distress normal skin. temperature normal heart rate; adequate intake

Contd...

Contd...

Problem (1)	Reason (2)	Objective (3)	Nursing Intervention (4)	Evaluation (5)
Hyperthermia • Excessive clothing • Overwarming • Inability to sweat • Dehydration • Inadequate intake of fluids	becoming dry • Tachycardia		• Feed regular schedule • Assess heart rate Hyperthermia • Assess for symptoms of hyperthermia and dehydration • Note infant's clothing and covering. • Assess feeding behaviour • Treat accordingly	
4. Altered nutrition: Less than body requirement related to • High-metabolic rate and calorie requirement. • Poor sucking feeding. • Inadequate or depleted glocose store	*Subjective data* Cries at intervals. *Objective data* • Regurgitation (Relaxation of sphincters • Infrequent stools • Distention of stomach • Crying at frequent intervals • Poor suck: dribbles or gags • Sleepy at feeding times • Weight loss. • Does not settle or sleep for 2-3 hours after feeding • Dehydration symptoms • Less than 6 weet diapers a day • Inadequate intake • Jitteriness with hypoglycemia	Client will have nutrition adequate for body requirements	• Initiate sterile water feeding of approximately 10 ml. sterile water. Then feed glucose water, breast milk or formula depending on protocol • Assess readiness for feeding signs of readiness include rooting, sucking, hand-to-mouth activities, alert state, nose breathing, stable heart rate, and respirations, and presence of bowel sounds. • Weigh shortly after birth and daily thereafter compare daily weight with initial baseline weight and determine percentage of weight loss. Weigh at check-up and compare with growth chart • Correctly position nipple in newborns mouth • Note and record amount and frequency of infant feeding • Feed on demand within appropriate parameters. • Note and record feeding behaviours. • Assess and record frequency, amount and colour of urine. • Observe and record frequency, colour and characteristics of stools. Assess for constipation or diarrhoea. • Observe for symptoms of gastrointestinal abnormalities – Intestinal distraction, cystic fibrosis or tracheo-esophageal fistula • Observe for signs of hypoglycaemia • Feed iron-supplemented formula if ordered. • Assess for dehydration—sunken fontanelle temp, poor skin turgor, delayed or decreased voiding	Client will evidence regaining birth weight by 10 days of life and then gaining 1 to 2 ounce per day in the first six month absence of dehydration symptoms setting after feedings at least 6 wet diapers a day and absence of hypoglycaemia

Contd...

Contd...

Problem (1)	Reason (2)	Objective (3)	Nursing Intervention (4)	Evaluation (5)
			• Assess parent's knowledge about feeding • Assess mother's knowledge about preparation of formula and mother's diet – teach accordingly	
5. Altered nutrition more than body requirement related to • Overfeeding • Addition of solid foods too early	*Subjective data* Cries frequently *Objective data* • Gains more than 1 oz/day or 4 ounces/week	Client will have nutrition adequate for body requirement.	• Weight newborn—Compare growth chart • Assess amount and frequency of feedings • Include assessment of solid food intake • Assess parents feeding behaviours • Education about proper time to introduce solid foods	Client will evidence gaining 1 ounce a day or 7 ounces a week
6. Risk for bleeding injury. related to • Minimal Vit K. • GI tract without bacterial flora which inhibits absorption of Vitamin K	*Objective data* • Bleeding from circumcision • Oozing cord; bleeding from cord • Ecchymosis • Haematuria • Blood in stools • Bleeding from injection site • Bleeding or bruising with handling	Client will remain free from injury	• Administer vitamin K injection intramuscularly • Assess newborn for signs of bleeding Assess stools, urine, injection site, circumcision site for bleeding • Handle newborn gently, reducing trauma	Client will evidence absence of bleeding
7. Risk for injury hypoglycaemia related to • Minimal intake after birth • Sleepiness • In ability to suck well or vigorously • High demand for glucose right after birth (to initiate breathing to maintain temperature)	*Subjective data* Sleepy, lethargic, weak, high pitched cry *Objective data* • Poor suck • Jitteriness • Tremors (sponteneous or with stimulation) • Hypotonia • Weak, high pitched cry • Poor feeding • seizures • Listlessness	Client will demonstrate absence of hypoglycaemia	• Check blood level by Dextrostix or by Chemstrip with Accu-check II Device. • Assess for symptoms of hypoglycaemia. • Feed at intervals	Client will evidence normal blood glucose level; demonstrate absence of jitteriness tremors, hypotonia weakness, high-pitched cry seizures
8. Risk for injury Physiologic	*Subjective data* Lethargy	Client will demonstrate	• Assess colour for jaundice. Blanch skin over bone prominence at sternum, fore-	Client will evidence bilirubin levels

Contd...

Contd...

Problem (1)	Reason (2)	Objective (3)	Nursing Intervention (4)	Evaluation (5)
jaundice, related to • Immature liver, (inability to produce enzyme needed for conjugation)	*Objective Data* • Jaundice after the first 24 hours of life, typically the second or third day of life • Serum bilirubin level not higher than 12 mg/dL • Hypotonia • Diminished • Rooting and sucking	absence of injury from elevated bilirubin level	head and knees • Check oral palate, and conjunctival sac for dark skinned babies in day light. • Assess for conditions associated with greater risk for pathological jaundice • Assess bilirubin level in blood. Obtain blood specimen by heelstick • Feed at regular intervals	within physiological range, absence of hypotonia without diminished rooting and sucking
9. Risk for infection related to • Deficiency of neutorophils deficiency of specific immu-noglobulins • Deficiency of IgA in bottlefed newborn (IgA protects surface of respiratory urinary and GI tracts) • Exposure to microorganisms from a rela-tively large number of portals of entry • Lack of normal intestinal flore until feeding are established	*Subjective data* • Crying • Listless, Lethargic *Objective data* • Skin rash • Diaper rash • Cracking skin • Umbilical cord moist with discharge and odour • White curdy patches on oral mucosa • Low temperature • Respiratory infection symptoms • Poor feeding • Purulent discharge from eyes	Client will demonstrate absence of infection	• Assess gestational age (IgG antibodies can be transferred *in utero* in the last trimester protects against bacteria and some virus) • Assess mother's history for factors predisposing newborn to infection • Do arm and hand-scrub with appropriate prepa-rations before working in nursery. Wash hands before handling each newborn (nurses, parents and others) • Maintain separate equipment and supplies for each neonate • Screening visitors for illnesses and ask them to wash hands before handling newborn. Advise client to stay away from crowds until infant is 1 month of age • Assess newborn symproms of infection • Administer prophylactic eye treatment • Expose umbilical cord to air by folding diaper below and T-shirt above the cord stump. Apply alcohol to cord stump according to protocol • Monitor laboratory values. Lab-test may evidence WBC count, serum levels for IgG, IgM, and IgA blood cultures, culture of lesions • Administer appropriate topical, oral or parenteral antibiotics • Wash newborn clothes separately, using hot water, mild detergents, and double rinsess • Instruct client in treatment of URTS. Symptoms include poor feeding, breathing difficulty, nasal congestion, and cough • Administer hepatitis B immune globulin-HBIg, HBr and others according to protocol	Client will evidence norm-al temperature absence of dia-rhoea, absence of skin irri-tations, and rashes, absence of resp. infections, absence of eye infections

Contd...

Contd...

Problem (1)	*Reason (2)*	*Objective (3)*	*Nursing Intervention (4)*	*Evaluation (5)*
			• Administer zero polio, BCG according to protocol	
10. Risk for constipation or diarrhoea, related to Constipation: • Allergies • Inadequate fluid/milk intake • Inactive bowel at birth • Diet and drugs of laxating mother Diarrhoea • GI infection • Overfeeding	*Subjective data* Constipation: • Straining with stools • Perspiration with passing stools • Cries *Objective data* Constipation • Absence of meconium stools • Absence of transitional stools (yellowish colour) • Abdominal distension • Stools change to firm, hard, infrequent stools Diarrhoea • Watery ring on diaper • Anal irritations • Stool change is frequent, watery, forcefully expelled stools	Client will demonstrate normal bowel elimination.	Constipation: • Check records for passage of meconium *in utero* or at delivery • Auscultate bowel sounds • Monitor and record passage of meconium. • Perouss abdomen for distention. Note if vomiting occurs • Assess for symptoms of necrotizing enterocolitis (NEC) or Hirschsprung's disease. • Assess frequency, amount, character and odour of stools • Assess feeding behaviour-teach or advise accordingly Diarrhoea • Assess for diarrhoea • If diarrhoea present , assess for dehydration, • Assess skin turgor; fontanelles • Assess feeding behaviour-advise and treat accordingly	Client will evidence anal patency, soft undistended abdomen, meconium to transitional to breastfeed or bottle-fed stools absence of diarrhoea, absence of constipation
11. Risk for altered urinary elimination related to • Immature kidneys at time of birth • Low glomerular filtration rate at birth • Limited tubuar reabsorption, which can contribute to acidosis or electrolyte imbalance • Limited or minimal oral intake	*Objective Data* • Absence of urine output dry diapers • Minimal saturation of diapers, infrequent voiding/less than 6 wet diapers in 24 hours. • Sunken fontanelles • Poor skin turgor	Client will demonstrate normal pattern of urinary elimination	• Monitor and record initial voiding and then frequency of voiding • Monitor intake • Note degree of saturation of diapers • Note colour of urine • Assess for dehydration assess skin turgor and fontanelles • Palpate bladder distention	Client will evidence voiding at least six times a day. each diaper saturated with urine; normal fontanelles normal skin turgor

Contd...

Contd...

Problem (1)	*Reason (2)*	*Objective (3)*	*Nursing Intervention (4)*	*Evaluation (5)*
• Excessive re-gurgitation • Increased insensible water losses • Renal anomaly				
12. Risk for impaired skin integrity related to • Skin contact with ammonia in urine • Skin contact with stools • Most diaper area in contact with skin	*Subjective data* • Cries at intervals and is not hungry • Cries when diaper area is cleared *Objective data* • Rash/lesions in diaper area • Inflammation/erythema in diaper area	Client will demonstrate normal skin integrity	• Assess diaper area for erythema, inflammation, and rash • Teach parents how to prevent or minimize diaper rash (changing frequently with gentle cleansing, with nonirritating nonperfused soap or water) • If using cloth diapers, use nonirritating detergent. Follow interventions to minimize • Diaper rash (some) prefer protective quoting of petroleum jelly or A and D ointment • Instruct parents to contact health care providers if diaper rash worsens or persists • Reinforce teaching concerning prescribed medicated topical ointments or creams	Client will evidence normal skin or diaper areas
13. Risk for injury related to • Lack of safety measures	*Objective Data* • Choking on small objects toys • Strangling from over-crib toys, from drapery cards, or between slats of crib • Suffocation from stuffed animal, pillow soft mattress • Aspiration from fluids • Injury from falls • Drawning in bath water	Client will remain free from injury	• Maintain newborn in side-lying position • Keep one hand on infant at alltimes to prevent rolling and falling from changing table or bed • Maintain safely during bath, test water temperature. Do not leave infant in bath water until the baby is able to sit alone, hold on to baby's arm • Use a safe crib and mattresses, pillow, no slat-narrow, painted or stained without lead. no stuffed animals • Place crib away from window • Do not place over crib toys with sprints • Do not place small objects, toys, or rattles in crib • Use appropriate care seat. Don't use infant carrier in car • Advise parents to take infant CPR classes	Client evidences absence of injury
14. Risk for altered parent-infant attachment related to • Dysfunctional family relationship	*Subjective Data* • Nonverbal behaviour does not indicate attachment (minimal gazing at newborn, few smiles, little touching , touches newborn roughly	Client will demonstrate adequate parent-infant attachment behaviours	• Inform parents about newborn care and routines in hospital • Give newborn to mother and father to hold right after delivery. Suggest they touch and examine the newborn • Point out behaviour and responses of the newborn to parental interactions	Client will evidence adequate parenting tasks and parental attachment behaviour

Contd...

Contd...

Problem (1)	*Reason (2)*	*Objective (3)*	*Nursing Intervention (4)*	*Evaluation (5)*
• Parental illness. • Lack of external resources • Unrealistic expectations of newborn or spouse • Lack or knowledge about parenting • Inability or unwillingness to assume parenting role • Poor problem-solving techniques • Daily stressors			• Explain behavioural capabilities of newborn if parents are unaware • If mother wishes to breastfeed, inquire whether she wishes to breastfeed soon after delivery and assist if she does • Assess strength, demographic factors such as age, socioeconomic status, cultural group, and support network that foster development of parenting skills and emotional attachment. Assess mothers physical status for conditions that may influence ability to interact with newborn	
	Objective data • Respond inappropriately to baby's cries • Does not place newborn. enface ensuring eye contact • Handles baby roughly • Incongruent verbal and non-verbal behaviours • Inappropriate visual, tactile or auditory stimulation of newbron • Growth and developmental lag in newborn • Frequent accidents or illnesses of newborn • Minimal parental attachment behaviours • Inattention to newborns cries and needs		• Act as a role for parenting behaviours and identify other role models within the parents' social network. Assist client in learning care-taking skills • Assess infant's condition and interactional responses • Provide for rooming-in and privacy, but be available to support as needed • Provide experiences in which parents can demonstrate caretaking skills and ask for information as needed, giving reinforcement as appropriate. Provide phone number for client to take home • Refer client to appropriate support groups • Assess and record behavioural indications of attachment	

8 CHAPTER

Assessment and Management of High-Risk Pregnancy

INTRODUCTION

Pregnancy is a physiological state (*i.e.,* biological situation) considered as "at risk group". The central purpose of prenatal nursing is to identify "high-risk cases (as early as possible) from a large group of antenatal mothers and arrange them for skilled care while continuing to provide appropriate care to all mothers. Early recognition and management of complication during this period is very essential.

EARLY COMPLICATIONS

Hyperemesis Gravidarum

Hyperemesis gravidarum is excessive vomiting in pregnancy occurring in the first trimester. The patient may vomit throughout the day till she empties both the stomach and duodenal contents. In such circumstances the vomitus contains bile. On the other hand, she may feel continuously nauseated and can scarcely eat. In both cases, the patient's general health is usually affected as the vomiting, nausea and anorexia can produce a state of malnutrition and metabolic disturbance which may be fatal.

Aetiology

The cause of vomiting in 50 per cent of pregnant women is not known, nor it, known why the mild state of vomiting or nausea in the morning results in hyperemesis gravidarum in some women. It has been suggested that the vomiting could be of a pyschological origin as in the case of an unwanted pregnancy. It may also occur if the pregnant woman seeks sympathy and attention from her husband and relatives. Hyperemesis gravidarum is more common amongst educated and nervous women. It is also known to be associated with multiple pregnancy, hydatidiform mole, acute hydramnios, infective hepatitis, and pyelonephritis. Histamines and histamine-related substances are said to have an aetiological role in hyperemesis. This is the reason why hyperemesis gravidarum is treated with antihistamines.

Signs and Symptoms

The patient usually cannot eat or retain her food. This, coupled with the effort of retching and vomiting, makes her weak, emaciated, dehydrated and miserable. The eyes are sunken and the skin is dry and inelastic. The tongue is coated or red and raw with sordes on the teeth. The urinary output is scanty, the urine is concentrated and contains acetone. The patient is often constipated. In very severe cases there is gross acidosis with consequent electrolyte disturbance. In such cases the patient's breath smells of acetone. Hypotension and proteinuria may occur. The patient may eventually become jaundiced, delirious and comatose. Death may supervene.

Management

From the above, the seriousness of the condition and the necessity for prompt and adequate treatment can be appreciated. The patient is admitted into a hospital and nursed in a side room or at the end of the ward where she will have maximum rest. A thorough examination of the patient by the physician is necessary to exclude other causes of vomiting such as infective hepatitis, pyelonephritis, strangulated hernia, intestinal obstruction and cerebral tumour.

The management of hyperemesis gravidarum is based on the replacement of lost fluid and electrolytes. Intravenous infusion of glucose and normal saline is given to provide hydration, energy and correct acidosis. Vitamin B complex is usually added to the infusion.

Serum electrolytes are estimated daily and corrected as necessary. Antiemetic drugs (some of which also have a sedative effect) such as Largactil (25-50 mg) or Phenergan (25-50 mg) are given intramuscularly twice daily. Oral fluids are withheld till the vomiting abates. Further vomiting may be prevented by the administration of oral Avomin (25 mg) or Ancoloxin (25 mg) once or twice a day. Multivitamins, iron and Daraprim are also given.

Nursing Interventions

The patient is usually miserable and feels sorry for herself. The nurse midwife must, therefore, be tactful, understanding, kind but firm in her approach and management of the patient.

Complete bed rest is necessary because the patient is weak and is usually on intravenous infusion. Daily bed baths are given and the pressure areas treated at least twice daily. Mouth toilet is done daily using glycerine to keep the lips moist and free from cracks. The patient should be made to gargle or rinse her mouth with diluted lemon juice to keep the mouth fresh and to prevent excessive salivation. To assess the amount of fluid given and to detect oliguria (a possible complication of this condition), an accurate intake and output chart is kept. The urine should be tested daily for proteins, acetone, bile and chlorides. Any abnormality is reported to the physician.

If the patient is constipated, a mild aperient such as magnesium hydroxide (30 ml-1 fluid ounce) is given. Suppositories are used when the patient cannot retain anything taken orally. The temperature, pulse, blood pressure, and respiration are checked and recorded four-hourly. Low blood pressure and weak, rapid pulse should bc reported to the physician. Other unfavourable signs and symptoms which must be reported to a physician are:

1. The presence of jaundice.
2. Undue excitement or excessive drowsiness.
3. Presence of lower abdominal pain which may denote onset of abortion.

With good medical and nursing care, a majority of the patients improve and carry their pregnancies to term. Very rarely, therapeutic abortion may be necessary to save the patient's life.

EARLY HAEMORRHAGIC COMPLICATIONS

Vaginal Bleeding

Vaginal bleeding in pregnancy, however slight, is abnormal. It is a cause of concern to mothers, particularly those who have had previous experience of foetal loss. Any reports of bleeding should be viewed seriously by the nurse or midwife. Because bleeding, the pregnancy may jeopardize both maternal and foetal well-being. Maternal blood loss decreases oxygen carrying capacity, which predisposes the woman to increased risk for hypovolaemia, anaemia, infection, preterm labour, and preterm birth and adversely affects oxygen delivery to the foetus. Foetal risks from maternal haemorrhage include blood loss, or anaemia hypoxaemia, hypoxia, anoxia and preterm birth. Antepartal haemorrhage is a leading cause of maternal death, with ectopic pregnancy, rupture and abruptio placentae being responsible for most maternal deaths.

If the woman presents with a history of bleeding in the current pregnancy, it is important to establish when it occurred, how much blood was lost, the colour of the loss and whether it was associated with any pain, should be noted. If the symptoms have subsided, it is important to advise the mother to report any recurrence. Bleeding during early pregnancy is alarming to the woman and of concern to the health care provider, midwife and/or the nurse. Clients must be taught to report without delay the slightest vaginal bleeding. The midwife must never attempt to examine a patient vaginally, in order not to aggravate the condition.

Aetiology of Early Pregnancy Bleeding

There were two types of causes for early pregnancy bleeding, which includes extra gestational or incidental causes and gestational causes.

In early pregnancy, an extra gestational or incidental causes refer to those conditions which could have caused vaginal bleeding in any woman. The incidence is high in pregnancy because of increased vascularity of the genital organs. These incidental causes are as follows:

i. Cervical erosion which produces slight blood stained discharge often mixed with mucus. This seldom requires treatment during pregnancy.
ii. Cervical polypus—a small mucoid growth often pedunculated. If its surface becomes

ulcertated, it bleed freely on touch or after intercourse.

iii. Carcinoma of the cervix— This is a serious condition but luckily very rare in pregnancy. It is more common amongst multigravious patients. The history of haematrorrhagia prior to pregnancy should arise the nurse-midwife suspicion. Prompt medical care is necessary because pregnancy accelerates growth of malignant cells.

iv. Any trauma or laceration in the genital tract will cause bleeding.

v. In the areas where schistosomiasis is common, a patient may confuse haematuria with vaginal bleeding.

Gestational causes for early pregnancy bleeding includes the following:

i. Abortion or miscarriage
ii. Incompetent cervix
iii. Ectopic pregnancy.
iv. Hydatidiform pregnancy (molar pregnancy).

In this chapter the gestational causes for early pregnancy bleeding are discussed.

Abortion or Miscarriage

Abortion may be defined as the interruption of pregnancy before the 28th week. The placenta is usually separated and this may result in the death of the foetus and its subsequent expulsion. The term "miscarriage is commonly used in preference to the term "abortion". But in this text, the term "abortion" is also used. Abortion may be spontaneous or induced. The classification of abortion is shown below in flow chart:

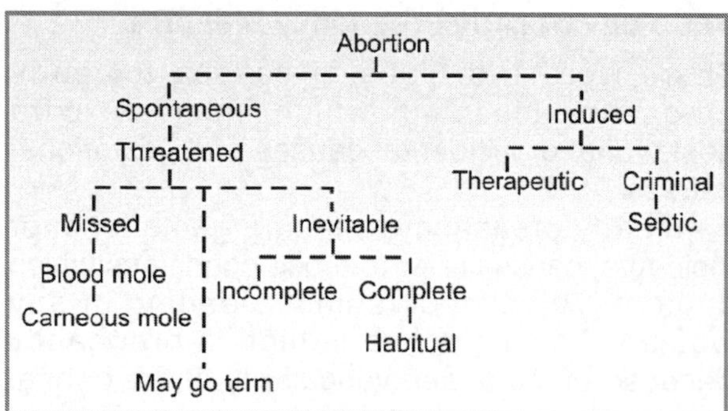

Spontaneous Miscarriage

Obstreticians generally define miscarriage as the natural termination of pregnancy during the first 20 weeks of gestation (Delivery between the 21st and 38th weeks is considered as premature birth), even if the foetus does not survive).

At least 20 per cent of all pregnancies end in a miscarriage between sixth and tenth weeks. Recent studies indicate, however, that the figure may be as high as 50 per cent, but that many go unnoticed, because women do not realize that they are pregnant.

Typically, a miscarriage begins with vaginal bleeding or a brownish discharge, which may be accompanied by cramps and lower back pain. If the woman is unaware of being pregnant, she may simply assume them she is having a heavy menstrual period.

The definition of spontaneous miscarriage is the termination of pregnancy before 24th week of pregnancy. This definition is modified to termination of pregnancy before foetal viability or less than 50 percent.

Aetiology

The Maternal causes of spontaneous miscarriages include general ill health and disability, especially associated with hyperpyrexia in either malaria, anaemia, diarrhoea and dysentry, tuberculosis, pyelonephritis and chronic nephritis, hypertention, untreated syphilis and diabetes. Other maternal causes include hormonal imbalance (hCG), extreme emotional stress, e.g. grief or freight, accidents, violent exercises, and certain drugs and also some local conditions in the birth canal such as submucus fibroid infantile uterus and incompetent internal os of the cervix because miscarriage.

The possible causes of early miscarriages include endocrine imbalance, (insulin dependent diabetes) immunologic factors (such as antiphospholipid antibodies), infections (such as bacteriuria, rubella and *chlamydia trichomatis*), systematic disorders (SLE) and genetic disorders.

A late miscarriage is one that occurs between 12 and 20 weeks of gestation. Late miscarriages usually result from maternal causes, such as advancing maternal age and parity, chronic infections, premature dilation of the cervix and other anomalies of the reproductive tract, chronic debilitating diseases, nutrition, and recreational drug use, and excessive use of alcohol and coffee along with cigarette smoking.

Types of Miscarriages and their Management

The type of miscarriage include threatened, inevitable, incomplete, complete and missed.

Threatened Miscarriage

As any vaginal bleeding in pregnancy is abnormal, to any vaginal blood loss in early pregnancy should be thought of as a threatened miscarriage until shown otherwise. In them, the disturbance to the pregnancy is so slight that the pregnancy may continue to term with good management. On the other hand, the damage may be progressive, resulting in massive separation of the placenta and dilatation of the cervix.

Clinical manifestation: The first sign of an impending miscarriage in the development of vaginal bleeding in early pregnancy (Fig. 8.1). The uterus is found to be enlarged and the cervical os is closed. A period of amenorrhea often proceeds the onset of slight vaginal bleeding. The patient may complain of backache, and intermittent low abdominal pain. Backache and pain are less commonly encountered than vaginal bleeding in cases of threatened miscarriage. A speculum examination done by the physician will reveal a closed cervical os. The membranes are intact.

In a threatened miscarriage, blood loss may be scanty with or without low backache and cramps like pains. The pain may resemble dysmenorrhea or period pains. The cervix remains closed and the uterus soft, with no tenderness when palpated. The presence of a foetal heart in conjunction with a closed cervical os is often reassuring. About 50 per cent of women presenting with a threatened abortion will continue with the pregnancy irrespective of the method of management.

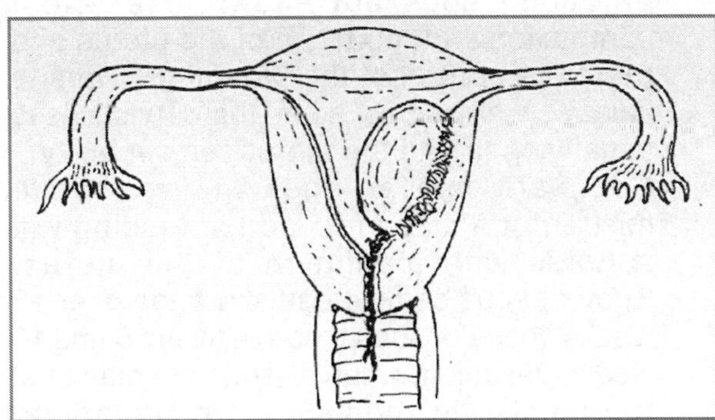

Fig. 8.1: Threatened abortion: Blood loss in early pregnancy

Management: Traditionally, mothers have been advised to rest. Threatened miscarriages should be treated by rest in bed until the bleeding subsides. Bed rest is essential. The patient is reassured, made to wear a vulval pad and remain in bed while the nurse informs the physician. In rural health centre, some sedation such as chloralhydrate (2 grams) may be given to the patient before her transfer in the best available transport to the nearest hospital. Articles stained with blood should be taken along with the patient. In the hospital the patient continues to rest in bed. Phenobarbitone 30-60 mg may be given twice or thrice daily (as per standing orders to ensure both mental and physical calmness. If there is increasing lower abdominal pain or uterine contractions, heavy sedations with sodium amytal 200 mg, six hourly may be given for 24 to 48 hours according to the physician instructions.

Nursing interventions include complete bed rest is maintained till all vaginal bleeding ceases. Daily washes and bed bath are given and the patient is encouraged to clean her teeth. Vulval toilet is done twice daily with aseptic precautions using antiseptic lotions, e.g. hibitane 1:2000. The vulval pads are inspected, noting the colour, odour and contents of the discharge. If bleeding continues, report it to the doctor concerned.

Examination of the patient should include gentle vaginal or speculum examination to ascertain cervical dilatation. Some women may prefer not to be examined, because of apprehension that the examination may promote miscarriage and their wishes should be respected.

Nurses should ensure that the patient passes urine well and if she is constipated, mild aperients such as two Dulcolix suppositories or magnesium hydroxide (30 ml) should be given. Enemas and strong purgatives stimulate uterine contractions and must never be given.

Temperature, pulse and respirations are taken and recorded twice daily, except where the patient is febrile, When a four hourly record is kept. The blood pressure is checked daily, except where the patient is febrile when a four hourly record is kept. The blood pressure is checked daily and urine is examined daily for albumin, sugar, and acetone. If there is pyrexia, high vaginal swab should be taken for bacteriological culture. If miscarriage may be complicated by haemorrhage and severe pain and may necessitate blood transfusion and relief of pain with opiates.

If there is evidence that products of conception have been passed, the uterus must be evaluated by direct curettage or suction curettage as early as possible products of conception should be submited for histological examination.

If there is evidence of infection, antibiotic therapy should be started immediately and adjusted subsequently if the organism identified is culture is not sensitive to the prescribed antibiotic. Septic abortion complicated by endotoxic shock is treated by massive antibiotic therapy, large doses of corticosteroids and adequate carefully controlled fluid replacement.

Complications of treatment include perforation of the uterus and continuing bleeding associated with incomplete evacuation of the uterus. Intrauterine infection may result in tubal infection and tubal obstruction. With subsequent infertility. If uterine perforation is suspected and there is evidence of intraperitoneal haemmorrhage or damage to the bowel, then laparatomy should be performed. Accordingly, nursing care will be provided.

Good feeding is encouraged and supplements such as ferrous sulphate (200 mg b.i.d.), folic acid (5 mg/day) and vitamin C (50 mg t.i.d.) are given and prescribed drugs are administered to prevent malaria and anaemia. On discharge, the patient is advised to have adequate rest and at home; avoid lifting heavy objects, strenuous exercises and intercourse for at least one month. The importance of regular clinic attendance and making an immediate bleeding reoccurrence is emphasized.

Inevitable Miscarriage

When the blood loss persists, the pain may become rhythmical and the uterus contracts to expel its contents as the miscarriage becomes inevitable. In the case of the pregnancy cannot be saved, because of a good portion of the placenta has been detached and the cervical os is dilating. The vaginal bleeding is severe and some clots may even be passed. The accompanying backache and intermittent lower abdominal pain are intense. Where the uterus is palpable, strong uterine contractions may be felt abdominally. The membranes may rupture and part of the products of conception may protrude through the dilating cervical os.

Inevitable miscarriage may end up as one or other of the following:

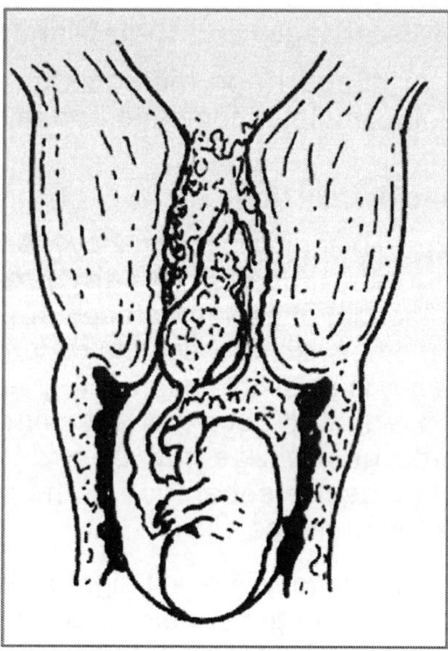

Fig. 8.2: Incomplete abortion: Progression to expulsion of part of the conceptus is accompanied by pain and bleeding

i. *Incomplete miscarriage*: Threatened miscarriage may either settle and the pregnancy continue or proceed to about. The patient develops abdominal pain, and bleeding becomes worse. The cervix opens, and (Fig. 8.2) eventually, products of conception are passed into the vagina. However, if some of the products of conception are retained, then the abortion remains incomplete. In this variety of miscarriage, part of the product of conception, usually the foetus is passed and the placenta and membranes are retained. The patient is often more than 12 weeks pregnant, so the placenta firmly embedded and the slender cord breaks. The bleeding continues and may become profuse, because of the presence of retained products, does not allow for efficient contraction and retraction of the uterus and therefore control of the bleeding. There is pain, as well as backache, the cervical os is usually open and the uterus remain bulky.

ii. *Complete miscarriage:* An incomplete miscarriage may proceed to bleeding will subside with involution of the uterus. Spontaneous complete miscarriage over 16 weeks gestation than those between 8 and 16 weeks gestation, when retention of placental fragments is common. In complete miscarriage, the whole product of conception is expelled. After expulsion of the conceptus, pain and vaginal bleeding decrease. The cervix if inspected, is found to be closed or reforming and the uterus becomes smaller in size. It is more common before the 8th week of pregnancy. In this, the uterus is firmly contracted on palpation, and an empty cavity is seen on ultrasound examination. No further medical intervention is required although support through the aftermath of pregnancy loss should be available. Mother should be advised to seek advice of bleeding recurs or a pyrexia develops.

Management: Management of inevitable miscarriage may require hospital admissions. The diagnosis should be made by physician. The nurse could however, suspect the condition if the patient bleeds profusely and may in the absence of a physician she/he can follow standing orders– i.e. can give an ergometrine 0.5 mg or any prescribed medication to the patient. A good analgesics (Pethidine 100 mg) may be given to relieve pain. If the patient is in a shocked or collapsed state, she should be kept warm and the foot of the bed raised to keep the vital centres supplied with blood. Intravenous infusion may be given to correct hypovolaemia. In desperate cases, when bleeding endangers life and the patient is in a remote place, a second dose of ergometrine may be given. The nurse scrubs her hand, cleans the patient's vulva and makes attempts to remove the retained products. Arrangements made for the immediate transfer of the patient to the nearest hospital. The nurse should ideally accompany the patient to report on any treatment given and take along some relatives to donate blood. Soiled articles also are taken along for the assessment of blood loss.

As stated earlier, inevitable miscarriages may require hospital admissions. In the hospital, the factor is notified of the patient's arrival. Initial medical assessment ought to bo carried out within locally agreed time limits, ideally within an hour. The use of transvaginal ultrasound is specific in detecting retained products and its use can prevent mothers having undergo repeated vaginal examinations to confirm diagnosis.

The nurse assesses the patient's general condition. The general condition of the patient depends on the amount of the blood loss. Excessive blood loss leaves the patient shocked and anaemic. The blood pressure falls, the pulse is weak and rapid. The patient feels cold and clammy. Other signs of shock such as air hunger may follow. The nurse keeps a quarter hourly record of all vital signs. Morphine (15 mg) may be ordered. A urine sample is taken for a pregnancy test and baseline observations of pulse and blood pressure and general well being are noted. Blood should be taken to confirm Rhesus factor, if not already known. Blood is taken for grouping and cross matching and also estimation of haemoglobin or packed cell volume, after which, intravenous infusion of 5 per cent glucose is set up to combat circulatory failure. Ergometrine (0.5 mg) given intravenously if the bleeding is not controlled and five units of Pitocin (Oxytocin) may be added to the infusion. Evacuation to remove retained tissue should be under general anaesthesia.

Evacuation of the uterus under general anaesthesia is undertaken when the patient's condition improves, and blood is available. The nurse obtain consent for operation and prepares the patient for dilation and currettage. Patient's pubic hair is shaved and the pubic area washed. The bladder is emptied and the patient's stomach aspirated. Premedication usually atrophine (0.6 mg) is given intramuscularly to dry up bronchial secretions.

Nursing interventions of the patient after the dilatation and curettage entails observing her to exclude shock and vaginal bleeding. Half hourly B.P. and 4th hourly T.P.R. to be recorded. the lochia are examined to ensure that vaginal bleeding has ceased. The urinary output should be carefully watched, especially where there has been severe haemorrhage, to detect early oliguria, which may be due to acute tubular necrosis of the kidneys. A wellfitted brassiere or breast binder should be worn. Stilboestrol tablets (0.5 mg) may be given t.i.d. for 5 days to suppress lactation in late miscarriages.

Recurrent or Habitual Miscarriage

The recurrent or habitual miscarriage is used when a patient has had three or more consecutive spontaneous miscarriages. Recurrent miscarriage is defined as the loss of three or more consecutive pregnancies. Most women who have had two or more consecutive miscarriages are anxious to be investigated and reassured that there is no underlying cause for the miscarriage (Figs 8.3A and B).

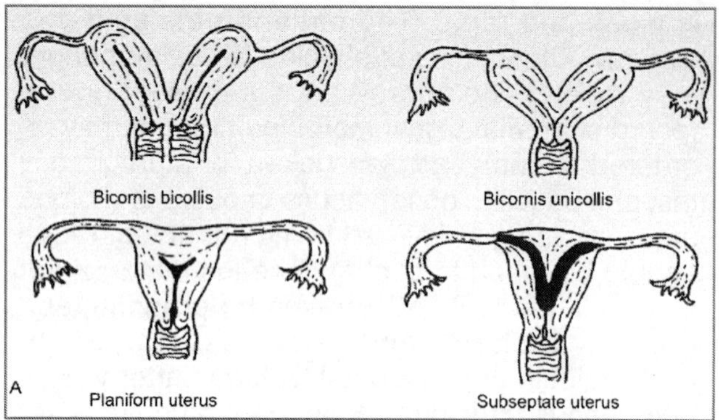

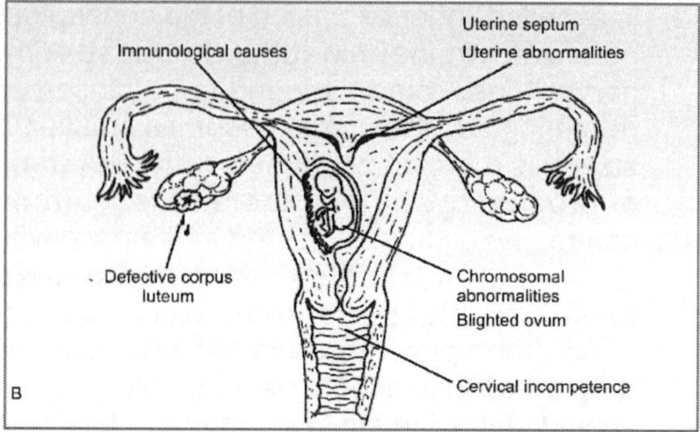

Figs 8.3A and B: A. Anomalies of the genital tract are sometimes a cause of recurrent abortion; **B.** Causes of recurrent abortion

The factors associated with recurrent miscarriage include:

i. *Genetic factors:* In any form of spontaneous abortion, there is a 50 per cent of chromosomal imbalance. The most chromosomal defects are autosomal trisomies, which account for half of the abnormalities. While polyploids and monosomy × (20 percent each) Parental chromosomal abnormalities are mainly translocations or mosaicisms. There are molecular mutations which which may operate in the foetus which has a normal karyotype and these include mutations in genes which code for products critical to development and mutations which lead to foetal metabolic diseases.
ii. *Structural anomalies*:Impact of the abnormality depends on the nature of the anomaly congenital uterine malformations may lead to recurrent miscarriages. And *intrauterine adhesions*. Following damage to the endometrium and inner uterine walls, the surfaces may become adherent, thus partly obliterating the uterine cavity. The presence of these Synechiae may lead to recurrent loss. And Cervical incompetence clinically results in midtrimester spontaneous abortion or early preterm delivery. The abortion tends to be rapid, painless and bloodless. The causes will be cone biopsy of congenital weakness of the cervix. The diagnosis is established by the passage of a Hegar-8 dilator without difficulty in the nonpregnant woman or by ultrasound examination or by premenstrual hysterogram. Cervical incompetence may be congenital but most commonly result from physical damage caused by mechanical dilatation of the cervix or by damage inflicted during childbirth.
iii. *Immunological*: Woman with recurrent miscarriage have been found the possibility of a failure to most of the normal protective immune response or if expression of relatively non-immunogenic antigens of the cytotrophoblast may result of the foetal allograft. Women with history of recurrent loss have also been found to lack an IgG blocking agent. In normal pregnancy. IgG coats prevent the foetal antigens and prevents rejection of the foetus. There is evidence that unexplained spontaneous loss as associated with couples who share abnormal number of HLA antigens of the A,B,C or loci.
iv. *Hormonal abnormalities*: Hypersecretion of LH may act on the oocyte causing it to age, or on the endometrium resulting in errors in implantation. Mother with polycystic ovaries have reduced fertility and an increased risk of early pregnancy loss. Corpusluteum deficiency may result in pregnancy loss.
v. *Infection:* Individual pregnancies may be affected by infections particularly with organisms such as *Listeria monocytogenes* and Mycoplasma. *Toxoplasma gondii* and cytomegalovirus are infective agents associated with pregnancy loss. But the role of infection in recurrent loss is unclear since their action in pregnancy failure remains uncertain.

Clinical features of miscarriage due to incompetence of the internal os of the cervix are:

- The abortions occur late in the second trimester, usually between the 22nd and 24th week of pregnancy
- There may be no previous warning such as vaginal bleeding; the membranes may rupture suddenly followed by expulsion of the products of conception
- The abortus looks fresh.

Diagnosis: Recurrent loss should be investigated. Thorough investigation is carried out between pregnancies to exclude diseases such as diabetes, nephritis, and tuberculosis. Local lesions such as cervical erosion, abnormalities and displacements of the uterus and fibroids are excluded on pelvic examination.

Vaginal bleeding may prompt a woman to think, she has had a miscarriage when, in fact, the foetus is still in the uterus. This type of threatened abortions can sometimes be stopped. If miscarriage has taken place, a woman should undergo a careful physical examination which may include viewing of the uterus by ultrasound. The uterus may also be examined by hysteroscopy using a lighted magnifying instrument inserted through the cervix. If possible, the foetus and other material expelled from the uterus should also be examined for abnormalities that might explain what went wrong.

Repeated miscarriages call for other test to seek a possible cause; these might include:

- Genetic chromosomal studies
- Hormonal evaluations to check for thyroid disease and diabetes, or, more importantly, the presence of hormones needed for normal ovulation
- Blood tests to identify possible immunologic abnormalities, such as production of antibodies that can cause miscarriage
- Hysterography or hysteroscopy to assess the anatomy of the uterus.

Management: If minor bleeding signals that a miscarriage is imminent, is likely to recommend bed rest to save the pregnancy. If bleeding stops, and the foetus appears to be normal, the pregnancy may still continue to term. When miscarriages truly begin, however, it usually cannot be prevented. If it is incomplete, then the remaining foetal and placental material must be removed from the uterus. In first trimester miscarriage, this can be accomplished by suctioning the uterus or performing a D and C in which the cervix is widened (dilated) and the uterus is scraped with curette.

An incomplete miscarriage during the second trimester may be treated by giving the woman an intravenous infusion of oxytocin, a hormone that causes uterine contractions to expel all the remaining tissue in a process similar to that of normal labour. In some cases antibiotics are prescribed to treat or prevent infection.

The couple are advised to improve their general health by taking food rich in proteins, minerals and vitamins; and to start another pregnancy, as soon as possible. The patient should report as soon as she thinks she is pregnant. She is then given some advice as a patient who has had threatened miscarriage. It must be stressed that coitus should not take place during the rest of pregnancy. In case where patient is unlikely to have adequate rest at home, hospital admission is recommended during the first half of the pregnancy. The treatment of incompetent cervix is the Shirodkar operation. A purse-string stitch of mersilene tape or any non-absorbable suture material is tied round the cervix at the level of the internal os at the 14th to 16th week of pregnancy. The operation is boldly and conspicuously recorded in the patient's notes. The suture must be removed at about the 38th week or as soon as the patient goes into labour. The patient should be made aware of the implication and the possible danger of ruptured uterus on failing to remove the suture on time.

If there is a risk of future miscarriages, these preventive steps may be taken, depending on the cause:

- When certain antibodies have been found in the blood, anticoagulant drugs are given, generally to doses of heparin or aspirin
- When uterine abnormalities, such as polyp or fibroids have been found, corrective surgery may be undertaken before attempting another pregnancy
- When the cervix has been opened prematurely, the incompetent cervix may be stitched, closed during the next pregnancy.

Although no alternative therapies can prevent miscarriage, psychotherapy may be beneficial as part aftercare. It is normal to feel sad after miscarriage and psychological counselling or participation in a support group can help ease unwarranted feelings of guilt as well as anxiety about future pregnancies.

Many women have some vaginal bleeding during early months of pregnancy. This does not necessarily signal a miscarriage but it should be reported to the physician. Complete bed rest for a week or longer may stop a threatened miscarriage but it should be reported to the physician. Complete bed rest for a week or longer may stop a threatened miscarriage from progressing. Also sexual intercourse and strenuous physical activity should be avoided until the crisis is past.

Missed Miscarriage

Sometimes the foetus dies *in utero* but is not immediately expelled. There is usually some pain and bleeding and the uterus does not increase in size. The term is used when the foetus dies and is retained *in utero*. Subsequently, the signs of threatened miscarriages subside except for some brownish discharge which is associated with pain. The uterus fails to grow, the breast become soft and the other signs of pregnancy disappear. The dead foetus may be retained for varying periods of time 3 to 4 weeks. Its prolonged retention may occasionally lead to profuse vaginal bleeding as a result of hypofibrinogenaemia.

On account of this, the obstetrician usually takes steps to encourage the expulsion of the foetus as soon as the diagnosis of missed miscarriage is confirmed. Usually medical induction in the form of a castor oil enema and bath, followed by 2.5 units of IM pitocin injection or half hourly intervals for six doses is given. On the other hand a continuous infusion of pitocin (oxytocin) or synthocinon in 5 per cent glucose solution is given intravenously until the products of conception are expelled. There is no place for surgical induction in late cases of missed miscarriages. When the conceptus has been expelled and there is no haemorrhage, the obstetrician may arrest the haemorrhage by curettage of the uterus and the administration of oxytocic drugs. There may be bleeding into the choroidecidual space which forms a mass of clot. This becomes organized and laminated and forms what is termed a *carneous mole*. Blood mole may arise in cases of missed abortion in which the decidual capsularis remains intact and permits the zygote to be surrounded by layers of blood. When fluid is extracted from the blood, the fleshy, firm, hard mass is known as carneous mole. The management is the same as for missed abortion.

Therapeutic Miscarriage/Induced Abortion

Therapeutic abortion is evacuation of the uterus done by qualified medical practitioners in the interest of the mother's life or her total well being. It is the termination of pregnancy before 24 weeks gestation, legally on following grounds certified by the two medical practitioners:

- Continuation of pregnancy would involve risk greater than if the pregnancy were terminated, of injury to the physical and mental health of the pregnant woman or any existing children of her family.
- Termination necessary to prevent grave permanent injury to the physical or mental health of the woman
- The continuation of the pregnancy would involve risk to the life of the pregnant woman, greater than if the pregnancy were terminated
- There is a substantial risk that if the child were born it would suffer such physical or mental abnormalities as to be seriously handicapped
- In addition certain reasons mentioned in MTP Act 1971.

The indication for therapeutic abortion are usually medical condition threatening the mother's life or likely to cause gross foetal abnormalities. These conditions include cardiac diseases, chronic nephritis and German measles contracted in the first 12 weeks of pregnancy. Both the husband and wife must give written consent for the termination of the pregnancy. The uterus is usually evacuated vaginally following dilatation of the cervix under a general anaesthetic. Abdominal hysterectomy is performed when the pregnancy is over 16 weeks.

Therapeutic abortions should be performed as early as possible in pregnancy to avoid complications. Suction evacuation is advised before 12th week of pregnancy. Mid trimester termination should be avoided. When mid trimester termination has to be done it can be accomplished surgical by abdominal hysterectomy or by nonsurgical methods using intrauterine abortifacients, e.g. intraamniotic prostaglandines, hypertonic saline, urea and high glucose concentrations. These methods are not always free from risks (Fig. 8.4).

Medical methods of termination of pregnancy, include Mifepristone (antiprogesterone compound) and prostaglandin are licensed for use upto 63rd day from the first day of woman's LMP (used on prescriptions). It is taken orally, in the presence

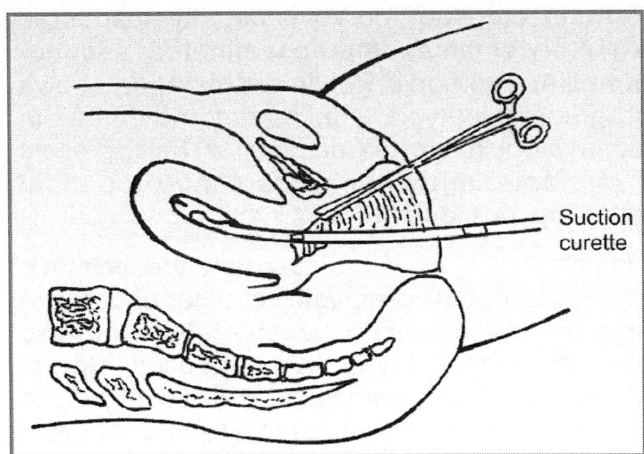

Fig. 8.4: Evacuation of retained products of conception

of physician or nurse. By blocking progesteron the sensitivity of the uterus to prostraglandin rises. A low dose vaginal prostaglandin Pessary is inserted to effect the termination. In second trimester, Extrauterine prostaglandin, accompanied by large doses of oxytocin, produces uterine contractions. The mother experiences labour and process may be protracted. Prophylactic antibiotics may be given following termination.

The mother needs to be cared for in a single room, her privacy being protected at all times. She should be offered information about the process so she is aware of what is happening. Adequate analgesia should be available and supportive staff identified to care for the mother and her family throughout the procedure.

Criminal Abortions

Criminal abortion is abortion illegally procured. Abortion induced by a variety of techniques make suprasubstantial percentage of abortion in some countries including India. Where the indications for legal abortions are liberal, criminal abortions is infrequent, but in many countries, it contributes to a high percentage of apparently spontaneous miscarriages. Such abortions are often done by the unqualified persons having little regard for the consequences. Risks of sepsis, uterine perforation, conical lacerations and haemorrhage are associated with criminal abortion. Other dangers are sudden death and acute renal failure. Criminal abortions are largely responsible for a high percentage of infertility and maternal morbidity. A nurse must under no circumstances give advice or information which could lead to an illegal abortion, nor should participate in such practice.

Septic Abortion

During the process of abortion either spontaneous or induced infection may be introduced into the uterine cavity. The condition is most commonly a complication of induced abortion and incomplete miscarriage, and is due to ascending infection. Septic abortion is usually a sequel of incomplete abortion. Often criminally induced. In this, in addition to the signs of miscarriages, the mother complains of feeling of unwell and may have a headache, nausea and pyrexia. It may present as either a localized infection in the uterine tubes and the uterine cavity, or as generalized septicaemia with peritonitis (Fig. 8.5).

The patient is usually anaemic, ill with a high temperature, rapid pulse, vomiting, lower abdominal pain (especially if there is pelvic peritonitis). The lochia are profuse and offensive. The patient becomes jaundiced and looks toxic, especially if the condition is complicated by septicaemia.

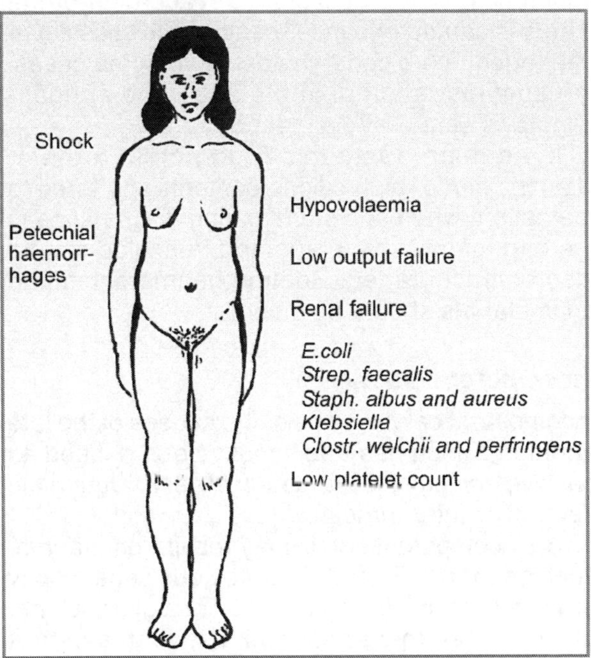

Fig. 8.5: Manifestation of endotoxic shock complicating septic abortion

Management: Blood culture and vaginal swabs should be taken to identify the cause of the infection and intravenous antibiotics administered commencing with both broad spectrum antibiotics and one effective against anaerobic infection.

The patient should be admitted into a single room in an isolation unit or barrier-nursed at the end of the ward. She is confined to bed and her pain is relieved with injections of pethidine (100 mg 6 to 8th hourly) or any latest analgesia as prescribed. A four hourly record of her temperature pulse and respirations is kept. If the temperature is about 39°C, the patient is tepid sponged or exposed and fanned. Her personal toilet in the form of bed bath or washes and month toilet must be taken care of. Vulval toilet is done twice daily and pads changed whenever they are soiled. During the initial stages when the patient is very ill, intravenous infusion of glucose saline is setup to correct dehydration and electrolyte imbalance.

A careful fluid chart is kept because renal failure may complicate the situation. Mild apperient could be used to relieve constipation if present.

The patient's blood loss would be replaced by massive blood transfusion and any infection should be treated with appropriate broad spectrum antibiotics. When necessary, evacuation of the uterus is carried out under heavy antibiotics cover after adequate blood transfusion. In some cases, the administration of antitetanus and antigas-gangrene sera may be mandatory.

In addition, tasteable food rich in protein, vitamins and of high caloric contents is offered to the patient when she starts eating. Extra fluids in the form of milk, beverage and fruit juice should also be encouraged. Routine haemotonics and antimalarials should be given.

Incompetent Cervix

Incompetent cervix is one of the causes of the late abortion, which has traditionally been defined as passive and painless dilatation of cervix during the second or third trimester.

An incompetent cervix may result from trauma, such as forceful D and C, a previous cone biopsy procedure, cervical cauterization or a difficult birth, or from anatomic abnormalities, such as short cervix, abnormal uterus or decreased collagen in the cervix. It may also be caused by drug DES taken by the woman's own mother during pregnancy.

An incompetent cervix is usually suspected when a woman experiences habitual second-trimester abortions. Pelvic examination shows progressive cervical effacement and dilatation along with bulging of the membranes, which present a characteristic hour glass shape (cervical funneling) or effacement of the internal cervical os.

Management: The nurse assesses the woman's feelings about her pregnancy and her understanding of reduced cervical competence and also evaluate with the woman's support systems. Management of incompetent cervix usually begin with bed rest (some times in Trendelenberg's position), fluid replacement, no sexual activity (vaginal rest) and tocolysis (inhibition), of uterine contractions. If these measures not successful, a cervical cerclage procedure may be performed. This procedure uses either a McDonald's cerclage, nonabsorbable ribbon (Merseline) or a band of homologus fascia to constrict the internal os and prevent dilatation. These cerclages are left in place until term and then removed, to allow labour to begin. If removed cerclage, placement must repeated with each successive pregnancy.

If a cerclage is performed, the nurse monitors the woman postoperatively for contractions, ROM, and signs of infection. Discharge teaching focuses on continued monitoring of these aspects at home. The woman must understand the importance of the activity restriction at home and need for close observation and supervision. Instructions include rationale for bed rest or activity restrictions and warning signs of preterm labour, ROM, and infection to report.

The woman must be instructed on the importance of taking a oral tocolytic medication if prescribed; the expected response and possible side effects. Tocolytics may be given prophylactically to prevent uterine contractions and further dilatation of cervix. If home uterine monitoring is implemented the woman is taught to how to apply the uterine contraction monitor and transmit information to hospital. The woman should know the signs that warrant immediate transfer to the hospital, including strong contractions less than 5 minutes apart, rupture of membrane, severe perineal pressure, and urge to push.

If the management is unsuccessful and the foetus is born before viability, appropriate grief support should be provided. If the foetus is born prematurely, appropriate anticipatory guidance and support will be needed.

Ectopic Pregnancy

The term 'Ectopic Pregnancy' refers to any pregnancy occurring outside the uterine cavity. An ectopic pregnancy is one in which the blastocyst does not implant within the uterine cavity. The most common site of implantation is the fallopian tube; the other site will include ovary, cervix, and the abdomen. Ectopic pregnancy is a significant cause of maternal death. The risk factors for ectopic pregnancy will include any one of the following alterations; the normal functioning of the uterine tube in transporting the gametes:

- Previous ectopic pregnancy
- Previous surgery on the uterine tube
- Exposure to diethylstilboestrol (DES) *in utero*.
- Congenital abnormalities of the tube
- Previous infections including chlamydia, gonorrhoea, and PID
- Use of intrauterine contraceptive devices
- Assisted reproductive technique.

In uterine pregnancy the blastocyst embeds in the decidua and the trophoblast erodes the maternal tissue anchoring the developing embryo. In tubal cyesis, the blastocyst rapidly erodes the epithelium and becomes attached to the muscle layer. It grows and expands within the wall, distending the tube. Maternal vessels are exposed and pressure caused by the resultant blood flow can destroy the embryo. The uterus increases in size and changes associated with early pregnancy occur in the body. Degrees of change take place within the endometrium, under the influence of hormones. Vaginal bleeding associated with ectopic pregnancy. The outcomes of tubal pregnancy will be tubal abortion, tubal mole, tubal rupture, abdominal pregnancy and maternal death.

Tubal Pregnancy is the most common type of ectopic pregnancy. It is very common in the tropics, because of the high incidence of blocked tubes resulting from gonorrhoea, puerperal postabortal sepsis.

The ovum is fertilized in the fallopian tube but the zygote is unable to reach the uterine cavity because of loss of tubal motility and ciliary action. The ovum, therefore, develops where it is arrested in the parts of the tube listed below:

- The fimbriated end of the tube is an uncommon site
- The ampulla is the most common site
- The isthmus is the most dangerous site because of the frequency of tubal rupture
- The interstitial part of the tube is uncommon site.

Clinical Features of Ectopic Pregnancy (Figs 8.6 and 8.7)

There is usually a history of amenorrhoea of about six to eight weeks duration. A missed period, adnexal fullness, and tenderness may suggest an unruptured tubal pregnancy. The tenderness can progress from a dull pain to a colicky pain when the tube stretches. Pain may be unilateral, bilateral or diffuse over abdomen.

The patient may experience a transient feeling of faintness and dizziness when rupture takes place. Abnormal vaginal bleeding that is dark red or brown occur in 50 to 80 per cent or women. If the rupture is a small one and there is not a great deal of haemorrhage, the patient may feel better and set about her daily work at home. There will however be a slow but steady trickle of blood into the pouch of Douglas as a result of rupture. The patient later presents with a mass in the pouch of Douglas, anaemia, abdominal pain. Vaginal examination confirms the mass and there is pain when the cervix is moved.

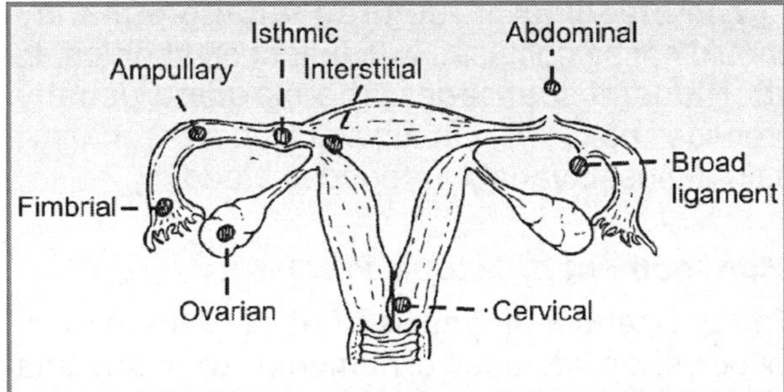

Fig. 8.6: Sites of implantation of ectopic pregnancies

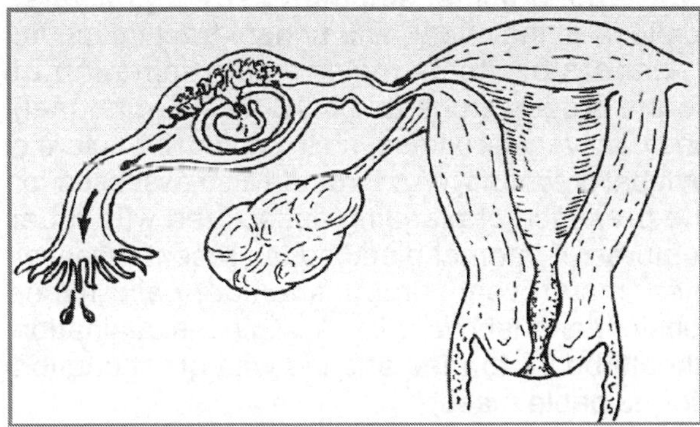

Fig. 8.7: Penetration of the tubal wall by trophoblastic tissue

If the ectopic pregnancy ruptures, pain increases. Usually tubal rupture results in massive bleeding into the peritoneal cavity. The patient feels faint, and all the signs and symptoms of shock soon appear. There is a marked increase in pulse rate, severe hypotension and beads of cold sweat can be seen on the patient's forehead. The skin is cold and clammy.

The patient complains of great pain which may be felt in the iliac fossa or hypogastrum and radiates to the shoulder tip if she lies down. The pain may be generalized, unilateral, or acute deep lower quadrant pain caused blood irritating the peritoneum. Referred shoulder pain can occur as a result of diaphragmatic irritation caused by blood in the peritoneal cavity. There may be slight vaginal bleeding because of the decidual reaction in the uterus. The woman may exhibit signs of shock related to the amount of bleeding in the abdominal cavity and not necessarily related to the amount of bleeding in the abdominal cavity and not necessarily related to obvious vaginal bleeding. An ecchymotic blueness around the umbilicus indicating hemaperitoneum, may develop in a neglected ruptured intra-abdominal ectopic pregnancy.

The bleeding of ruptured tubal pregnancy should not be confused with that of an abortion. In abortions/miscarriages, the bleeding usually precedes pain, while in ruptured tubal pregnancy, pain almost invariably precedes bleeding.

Management of Ectopic Pregnancy

The differential diagnosis of ectopic pregnancy involves consideration of numerous disorders that shares many signs and symptoms, which includes miscarriages, ruptured corpus luteum cyst, appendicitis, salpingitis, ovarian cysts, torsione of the ovary, and urinary tract infection.

Laboratory tests include determination of serum progesterone and hCG levels (< normal) and transvaginal ultrasound to confirm intrauterine or tubal pregnancy. And woman also assessed for the presence of bleeding associated with tubal ruptures. If internal bleeding is present, assessment may reveal vertigo, shoulder pain, hypotension, and tachycardia. A vaginal examination should be performed at once with great caution (for palpable mass).

Once the diagnosis has been established, the ectopic pregnancy must be removed by one of the following techniques:

- Salpingectomy
- Laparoscopic surgery
- Salpingostomy
- Methotrexate
- Tubal compress.

Treatment involves the removal of the ectopic pregnancy by salpingostomy is possible before rupture. Residual tissue is dissolved with a dose of methotrexate postoperatively. Methotrexate is a folic acid analog that destroys the rapidly dividing cells. It may also be used in a single dose of IM injection to treat unruptured tubal pregnancies.

All cases of suspected or diagnosed ectopic pregnancy should be referred to the hospital. In the hospital, physician must be summoned at once. Preparation should be made for intravenous (IV) infusions and blood collection for the estimation of haemoglobin and packed cell volume as well as grouping and cross matching. The physician usually prescribes morphine (15 mg) by intra muscular (IM) injection. An IV infusion of dextrose or dextrose saline will be set up pending the arrival of properly cross-matched blood. A blood transfusion is setup while arrangements and preparations are made to transfer the patient to the operation theatre, where salpingectomy is carried out on the affected side (Fig. 8.8).

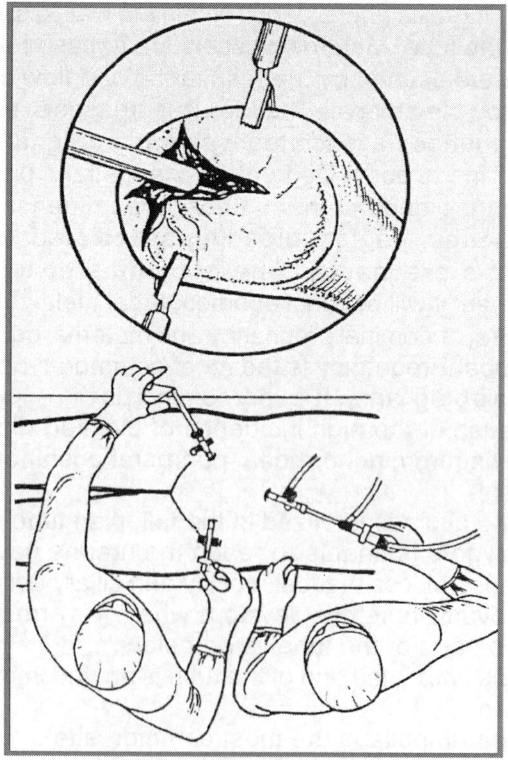

Fig. 8.8: Laparoscopic surgery for tubal disease and tubal pregnancy

The postoperative medical and nursing care of the patient is important and is the same as after any major obstetric or gynaecological operation/ surgery.

Abdominal pregnancy is rare. If happens foetal development may take place in the abdominal cavity and follows early rupture or abortion of a tubal pregnancy, but expands and attaches to neighbouring organs. The foetus develops within the peritoneal cavity but rarely survives. Infection develops causing peritonitis and septicaemia. In very rare cases, baby survives pregnancy proceeds to term, and baby may be found to have compression, deformities due to oligohydramnios.

Cervical pregnancy also extremely rare, but poten-tially foetal owing to massive haemorrhage.

Hydatidiform Mole (Molar Pregnancy)

Hydatidiform mole is a gestational trophoblastic disease. Abnormality of early trophoblast may arise as a developmental anamoly of placental tissue, and results in the formation of a mass oedematous and avascular villi. There is usually no foetus but the condition can be found in the presence of a foetus. The placenta is replaced by a mass of grape like vesicle known as hydatidiform mole.

Aetiology

The actual cause is unknown, although there may be an ovular defect or a nutritional deficiency. Women at higher risk for hydatidiform mole formation are those who have undergone ovulation stimulation with clomiphene and those who are in their early teens or older than 40 years of age.

There are two distinct types of hydatidiform moles. Complete (or classic) mole and partial mole. *The complete mole* results from fertilization of an egg whose nucleus has been lost or inactivated. The mole resembles a bunch of white grapes. The fluid filled vesicles grow rapidly, causing the utorus to be larger than expected for the duration of the pregnancy. Usually the complete mole contains the foetus, placenta, amniotic membrane, or fluid. Maternal blood has no placenta to receive it; haemorrhage into the uterine cavity and vaginal bleeding therefore occur. There may be progression towards choriocarcinoma. *A partial mole* often has embryonic or foetal parts and an amniotic sac present. Congenital anomalies usually present. There is potential for malignant transformation.

Pathophysiology

Hydatidiform mole is an abnormal development of the primitive chorion resulting in cystic proliferation of the chorionic villi and hydropic degeneration of the centre of the villi. The extended villiform vesicles of variable sizes and the whole mass looks like a bunch of grapes or the arrangements of papaya seeds. Usually the embryo is absorbed in the process and no foetus nor placenta can be identified. At times the cystic generation may be part of an otherwise normal placenta and occasionally it coexists with normal healthy twin. The exuberant proliferation of the trophoblast gives rise to a tremendous increase in the level of the human chorionic gonadotropin (hCG) and large amounts are excreted in the urine. This causes the pregnancy test to be very strongly positive. In addition, these hormones stimulate the ovaries resulting in formation of large lutein cysts which may grow to gigantic dimensions.

Clinical Manifestations

The signs and symptoms of a complete mole in the early stages cannot be distinguished from that of normal pregnancy. There is usually a period of amenorrhoea varying from 3 to 4 months. The usual symptoms of early pregnancy such as morning sickness, ptyalism, etc. May be exaggerated. Later vaginal discharge may be dark brown (resembling prune juice or bright red and either scant or profuse). The diagnosis is confirmed by the passage of small vesicles that look like small grapes. In some cases, the vesicles may not be seen until the entire mole is expelled. Bleeding may continue for only a few days or intermittently for weeks. Early in pregnancy, the uterus in approximately half of affected women is significantly larger than expected from menstrual dates. Anaemia from blood loss, excessive nausea and vomiting (hyperemesis gravidarum) and abdominal cramps caused by uterine distension are relatively common findings.

Abdominal examination reveals a uterus which is larger than the period of amenorrhoea suggests. A patient who gives a history of three months, may have a uterus the size of 24 to 26 weeks pregnancy. The abdomen is quite soft and usually no foetal parts are felt. No foetal heart sounds are heard and no feotal movements are seen, felt or heard. There may be signs of pre-eclamptic toxaemia, i.e. hypertension, oedema and albuminuria.

Vaginal examination will confirm soft bulky uterus and if the cervix is open, the vesicles may be felt or they may be discharged on the examining fingers. The bilateral thecalutien cysts of the ovaries may be felt with careful examination.

The diagnosis of the hydatidiform mole is made on the basis of the above signs and symptoms. But confirmatory diagnosis is obtained from ultrasonography and serial hCG immuno assay.

- There is high level hCG in the early morning urine of the patient or a positive Hogben's test in dilution of 1:500
- A straight X-ray of the abdomen and pelvis reveals no foetal skeleton even though the uterus is the size of 26 weeks gestation
- Pelvic angiography—A radio-opaque dye fails to continue the patterns of the placenta in hydatidiform mole
- Ultrascanning is very useful diagnostic tool.

Management

Nursing assessment during prenatal visits should include observations for signs of molar pregnancy during the first 24 weeks of hydatidiform mole is suspected patient should be referred to physician. The patient as admitted to the hospital for investigations and treatment. If she is bleeding, IM ergometrine 0.5 mg is given to induce uterine contractions and control bleeding. If bleeding is profuse or the partientis shocked, IM morphine 15 mg is given and an intravenous infusion is set up by the physician. Blood is sent for grouping and cross-matching. The nurse-midwife should do the following:

- Shave and wash the vulva
- Obtain consent for operation
- Empty the patient's bladder and rectum and
- Prepare for evacuation of the uterus.

After evacuation, the patient's pulse rate, blood pressure, and respiration are checked half-hourly. The nurse should look for evidence of vaginal bleeding. If the patient bleeds, ergometrine (0.5 mg) is given intramuscularly and a report is made to the physician. Hysterectomy is performed if the patient is over 40 years of age. This ensures a complete removal of the mole, minimises the risk of bleeding and uterine perforation, and the subsequent development of chorioepithelioma.

Patients with confirmed diagnosis of hydatidiform mole who are not bleeding much, are treated medically. The vulva is shaved and swabbing is done twice daily. The pads are carefully inspected. Usually castor oil (60 ml), an enema and bath are given. These are followed by pitocin or syntocinon infusion using 5 per cent glucose in water. During the intravenous infusion the nurse should observe the patient carefully noting her pulse rate, blood pressure, and respiratory rate which are checked at half-hourly intervals. The time of onset, duration of which contraction and its effects on the patient should be recorded. When the mole is expelled, it should be kept for examination by the physician. Anything passed for vaginum by the patient must be sent for histological examination.

The complication of hydatidiform mole will include:

- *Shock* from excessive haemorrhage
- *Uterine perforation* during curettage: In hydatidiform mole, the uterus is very soft and friable and can be likened to wet blotting. So it is easily perforated
- *Sepsis:* This may occur if a septic and antiseptic techniques are faulty or if profuse haemorrhage lowers the resistance of the patient to infection
- *Malignant changes:* Choriocarcinoma is a serious complications of hydatidiform mole. It may develop several months after the expulsion of the mole.

A patient who has been treated for hydatidiform mole should be followed up for a long time. hCG estimation or pregnancy tests to be carried out at three months interval. The nurse provides the woman and her family with information about disease process, the necessity for a long course of follow-up, and the possible consequences of the disease, frequent physical and pelvic exam and b-hCG estimations.

Choriocarcinoma (Chorioepithelioma)

Choriocarcinoma is a malignant neoplasm which can develop as a consequence of the molar pregnancy. It is sometimes referred to as malignant trophoblastic disease. It may follow a hydatidiform mole, a normal full term pregnancy, an abortion or an ectopic pregnancy and it is characterized by irregular vaginal bleeding which may sometimes be profuse.

In choriocarcinoma the growth invades not only the lining of the uterus, but also the muscle wall, and sometimes it perforates the uterus and appears in the peritoneal cavity. The growth actively invades the myometrium, putting the mother at risk of severe haemorrhage in the first instance. The mother also is at risk for developing lung, hepatic, and cerebral metastasis if the neoplasm goes undetected. The secondary deposits may be found in the lungs give the appearance of miliary tuberculosis giving rise to a generalized mottlings of lungs (snow storm appearance) secondaries also sometimes are found in the vagina. In very bad cases, secondary deposits are found in the ovarain at postmortem examination.

Choriocarcinomas can also occur after a normal term gestation, ectopic pregnancy or a termination of pregnancy. The diagnosis of choriocarcinoma includes the following:

- The human chorionic gonadotrophin level is usually very high
- Pelvic angiography shows a typical pattern diagnostic of choriocarcinoma, such as dilatation of the blood vessels supplying the uterus and the adnexa and the prominence of the spiral myometrial vessels, as well as the opacified irregular vascular spaces
- Chest X-ray may reveal the typical "Cannon ball" or 'snow storm secondaries'.

Management

When the nurse see a woman with the history of pregnancy, abortion, ectopic pregnancy, should suspect choriocarcinoma and refer the patient to the doctor. All cases of choriocarcinoma are treated in major hospitals with facilities for frequent hCG estimations and routine blood tests and blood transfusions.

The drug used in the treatment of choriocarcinoma are called cytotoxic drugs, because of their ability to destroy rapidly growing cells. They are folic acid anagonists and, therefore, they are referred to as antifolates. Examples of these drugs are:

- Methotrexate (dose 0.4 mg/kg body weight per day)
- 6-mercaptoprurine (dose 6-10 mg/kg body weight per day).

  The side effects of cytotoxic drugs are anaemia, low white blood cell count (Leucopenia) and low platelet count (thrombocytopenia). In addition, they cause alopecia (falling off of scalp hair), buccal ulcerations, glossitis, angular stomatitis, and gastrointestinal upsets. Other drugs used in the treatment of choriocarcinoma include actinomycin D and vincristine.

Patients with choriocarcinoma are usually followed up for life if possible. The hCG estimation is carried out at frequent intervals. The routine nursing care should be given accordingly as in other such cases.

Antepartum Haemorrhage (APH)

Antepartum haemorrhage is defined as bleeding from the genital tract after the 28th week of pregnancy and before the birth of a baby. In other words, some places, bleeding from the genital tract in later pregnancy after 24 week of gestation and before the onset of labour is referred to as an APH. Severe APH may cause still birth and neonatal death, and also if bleeding is severe, it may be accompanied by shock and DIC (disseminated intravascular coagulation), the mother may die or will be left with permanent ill health.

Aetiology

The bleeding is often due to premature separation of the placenta. Lesions of the cervix or trauma along the genital tract may also cause bleeding and there is no means of telling where the bleeding is coming from on merely looking at the patient. The factors which cause APH may be present before 24th week but the original distinction between a threatened abortion and an APH was based on the potential viability of the foetus. Vaginal bleeding may be due to (Fig. 8.9):

- Haemorrhage from the placental site and uterine cavity
- Lesions of the vagina or cervix

  The major causes of the uterine bleeding are:
- Placenta praevia
- Abrupto placentae or accidental haemorrhage.
- Uterine rupture
- Unknown aetiology

  Based on these causes, APH is classified.

Classification of APH

APH is classified according to the site of the placenta.

i. Accidental APH or abrupto placentae is bleeding from premature separation of the placenta situated in the upper uterine segment.
ii. APH due to placenta praevia or unavoidable APH is bleeding from a placenta situated

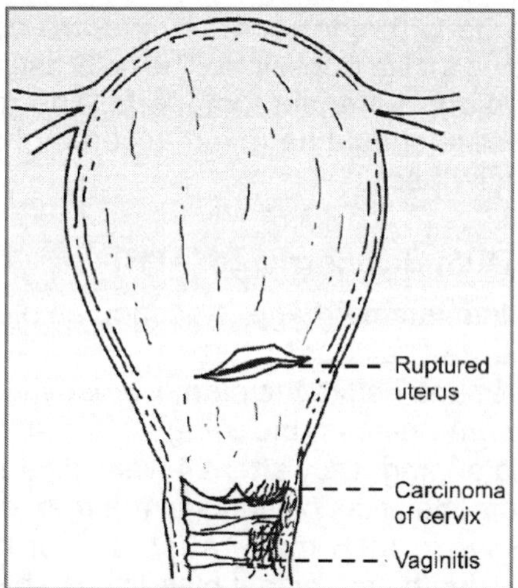

Fig. 8.9: Non-placental causes of antepartum haemorrhage

partially or wholly in the lower uterine segment. The term "unavoidable" explains the fact that placenta is bound to separate prematurely following the contraction of the lower uterine segment and subsequent dilatation of the cervix.

iii. Unclassified APH in which group of patients, there is neither evidence of placenta praevia nor of accidental haemorrhage. The cause of the bleeding may not be determined even after delivery. Usually such bleeding may be due to incidental findings such as cervical erosion, vascular ulcerated polypus, and rarely carcinoma of the cervix.

Placenta Praevia (PP)

The placenta is said to be praevia when all or part of the placenta implants in the lower uterine segment and, therefore, lies in front of the presenting part. Actually, the placenta is implanted in the lower uterine segment near or over the internal cervical os.

Aetiology

Placenta praevia is due to delay in implantation of the blastocyst so that this occurs in the lower part of the uterus. It is common in high parity and in conditions where the placental area is large, such as multiple pregnancy or placenta membranacea. The most important risk factors are previous placenta praevia, previous caesarean births, and induced abortion and also with multiple gestation.

Classification of PP

From the point of view of management, following types of placenta praevia have been described (Fig. 8.10).

i. *Lateral or type I or I degree:* In this type the placenta is situated mainly in the upper uterine segment with only a tip of its encroaching on the lower uterine segment. The placenta is not easily reached through the undilated cervical os by the examining finger.
ii. *Marginal* or type II placenta praevia (PP).
iii. *Complete or type III PP:* In this type the placenta completely covers the undilated internal os, but its lower margin is still within reach of the examining finger. As such it covers the os when it is only 6 cm dilated but not when it is fully dilated.
iv. *Central or type IV PP:* In this case, the placenta completely covers the undilated internal cervical os and the margin cannot be reached by the examining finger. It completely covers the entire os, even at full dilatation. An anterior or posterior variety is described for each of the four types of placenta praevia. This was previously described as fourth degree PP

The classification is important in relation to management because spontaneous delivery is extremely rare where there is a central placenta

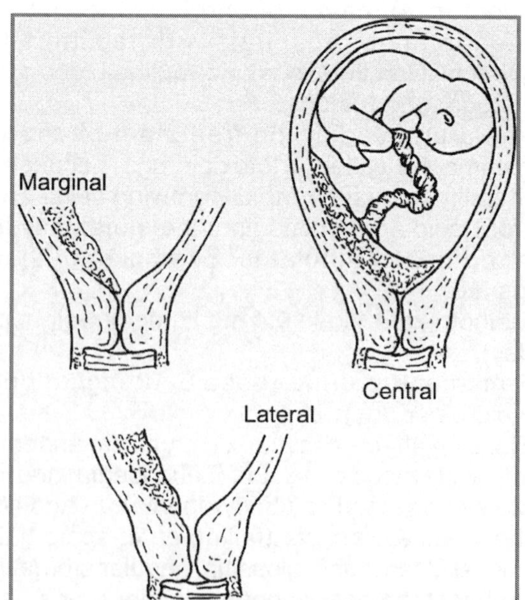

Fig. 8.10: Classification of placenta praevia

praevia, but normal labour and delivery may occur with lateral or marginal implantation.

Bleeding results from separation of this placenta the formation of the lower segment occurs and the cervix effaces. This blood loss occurs from the venous sinuses in the lower segment. Occasionally foetal blood loss may occur, particularly where one of the placental vessels lies across the cervical os—a condition known as 'vasa-praevia'.

Pathophysiology of PP

In this condition the placenta is situated wholly or partially in the lower uterine segment. The stretching and dilatation of the lower uterine segments during the later weeks of pregnancy causes premature separation of the placenta and subsequent bleeding. The bleeding is not associated with any pain or exertion. Development of lower uterine segment begins at 28 weeks gestation and thus bleeding is likely to occur during the second trimester. Bleeding is unpredictable and may vary from minor shows to massive and life endangering bleeding.

Clinical Manifestation of PP

The main symptoms of placenta praevia is painless vaginal bleeding. There may sometimes be lower abdominal discomfort, where there are minor degrees of associated placental abruption. The signs of placenta praevia are, *vaginal bleeding, malpresentation of foetus and uterine hypotonus*. The first few episodes of bleeding are usually slight but subsequent episodes may be profuse and may endanger the patient's life. The small painless haemorrhages are often called warning haemorrhages and the patient usually ignores the first two or three episodes of bleeding. It is the profuse bleeding that brings many of our illiterate patients to the hospital.

The presence of the placenta in the lower segments tends to displace the presenting part and when the placenta is posterior, the head is pushed forward over the pelvic brim and is easily palpable. When the placenta is anterior, the presenting part is difficult to feel. Lateral placement of the placenta results in contralateral displacement of the presenting fact. Where there is central placenta praevia, the foetal head is held away from the pelvic brim and the lie may be transferse, or oblique. If the head does not approach the pelvic brim when the erect posture is adopted, it is strongly suggestive of placenta praevia.

Diagnosis of PP

Diagnosis of the placenta praevia will be made on the basis of:

i. *Clinical findings:* Painless bleeding occurs suddenly and tends to be recurrent. When labour starts and cervix dilates, profuse haemorrhage may occur. Although sometimes in a later placenta praevia the presenting part compresses the placental site and bleeding is controlled.
ii. *Abdominal examination*
    - Displacement of the presenting part—the lie may be oblique or transverse. If the placenta lies on the posterior uterine wall, the presenting part will be easily palpable. If placenta is anterior the presenting part is difficult to palpate
    - Flaccidity of the uterus—uterine muscle tone is usually low and the foetal parts are easy to palpate.
iii. *Diagnostic procedures:* Ultra scanning, MRI, Placentography, angiograph. Placenta praevia can be diagnosed using transabdominal ultrasound. Transvaginal ultrasound examination may also be used.

Management of PP (Table 8.1)

A woman with third-trimester vaginal bleeding requires immediate evaluation. Necessary history data include gravidity, parity, and description of bleeding (how long, precipitatory event, estimation of amount). Other assessment data to be collected are the woman's general status, estimated gestational age, current amount of bleeding vital signs and foetal status. Laboratory studies include CBC, determinates of blood type and Rh status, a coagulation profile and possible type and cross match.

The management of placenta praevia when the diagnosis is established depends on the amount of blood loss, the maturity of the foetus and the degree of the placenta praevia. The aim is to control haemorrhage and save the mother and her foetus from excessive blood loss.

Immediate termination of pregnancy is referred to as acute treatment. This is instituted when the bleeding is severe or the patient fails to respond

Table 8.1: Nursing care plan of placenta praevia (PP)

Problem	*Reason*	*Objective*	*Nursing intervention*	*Evaluation*
Decreased cardiac output related to bleeding secondary to PP	S* O*	Patient will exhibit signs of increased blood volume and restoration or cardiac output	• Palpate uterus for tenderness and tone • Assess bleeding rate, amount, colour, degree of bleeding, CBC value and coagulation profile to determine severity of situation • Do not perform vaginal examination because it may stimulate further bleeding • Establish baseline data for cardiac output (vital signs, heart and breath sounds; skin colour, tone turger; capillary refill; level consciousness; urinary output, pulse oximetry) to use as a basis for evaluating effectiveness of treatment • Initiate intravenous therapy or blood transfusions and medications per physian's order to restore blood volume and prevent organ compromise to mother and foetus • Place woman on bedrest to decrease oxygen demand • Monitor vital signs, intake and output haemodynamic status and laboratory values to evaluate treatment response Provide emotional support to woman and her family (i.e, explain procedures and their rationale; explain what is happening and what to expect, keep support person present) to allay fears and provide to the family with some sense of control • After stabilization, teach the woman home management including bed rest, watching for spotting/bleeding, close follow-up with her health care provider and preparation for immediate return to hospital if needed to prevent or stem further complication	
Risk for injury related to decreased uterine/placental perfusion secondary to bleeding		Patient will exhibit ongoing signs of foetal well being (adequate foetal movement, normal FHR, reactive NST, normal BPP	• Monitor foetus daily of tachycardia, decreased movement, loss of reactivity on NST to identify and treat changes in foetal status • Obtain BPP per physician's order to assess for signs of chronic asphyxia • Maintain maternal side-lying position to prevent compression of aorta and vena cava	
Risk for infection related to anaemia and bleeding secondary to placenta praevia		Patient will show no signs of intrauterine infection	• Monitor vital signs for elevated temperature, pulse and blood pressure • Monitor laboratory results for elevated WBC count, differential shift • Check the uterine tenderness and malodour vaginal discharge to detect early signs of infection resulting from exposure of placental tissue • Provide perineal hygiene to decrease the risk for ascending infection.	

*S = Subjective data, O = Objective data

to conservative treatment; that is, there is an onset of further brisk loss or intrauterine death of the foetus. For the active treatment, the patient is managed as described under APH.

An urgent vaginal examination under anaesthesia is made of the foetal heart sound is present, a Lower Uterine Segment - Caesarean Section (LSCS) is carried out. If the baby is dead, the membranes are rupture and a leg is brought down and a 450 grams weight is attached to the baby foot to compress the placenta and control bleeding. If types II posterior II or IV placenta praevia are diagnosed, caesarean section is performed to avoid massive haemorrhage and consequent foetal exsanguination and death.

The reason for doing caesarean section in type II posterior placenta praevia is that bleeding is difficult to control and the descending head could compress the placenta against the sacral promontory, thus causing foetal hypoxia and intrauterine death. In the absence of profuse bleeding and cephalo-pelvic disproportion, amniotomy or artificial rupture of membrane is done for type I and II anterior placenta praevia whether foetus is dead or alive. The patient usually goes into labour and delivers spontaneously.

Conservative treatment is given to a patient whose bleeding is slight and the gestational age is less than 36 weeks. Expectant treatment is an attempt to prolong the pregnancy, prevent prematurity and give the baby a reasonable change of survival. In addition management for slight bleeding, the patient is kept under careful supervision. Ultrasonographic examination may be done every two to three weeks. At about the 38th week, of gestation and examination under anaesthesia is carried out in the operating theatre which is set for caesarean section. The patient should be having blood at the time of examination and another one or two litres of blood are kept in handy in an icebox or Refrigerator, in the theatre. Equipment for resuscitation of a collapsed patient and *as phyxiated* baby should also be ready.

The woman with placenta praevia should always be considered a potential emergency because massive blood loss with resulting hypovolaemic shock can occur quickly if bleeding resumes. The possibility that she may require an emergency caesarean for birth always exists. Emotional support for the woman and her family is extremely important. The main danger of placenta praevia is PPH and increased risk of placenta accreta, air embolism and maternal death, foetal hypoxia, foetal death.

Abruptio Placentae/Accidental Haemorrhage (Figs 8.11A and B)

Accidental haemorrhage is bleeding from premature separation of a placenta situated in the upper uterine segment. The term "abruptio of placentae "means to tear apart and it describes the situation better than accidental haemorrhage. The term 'accidental' implies separation as the result of trauma, but most cases do not involve and occur spontaneously.

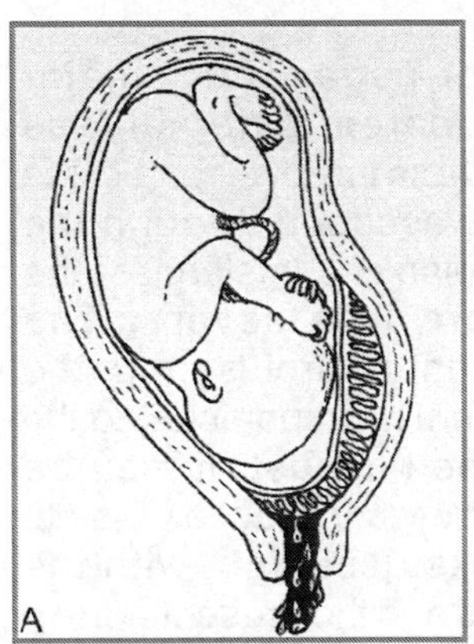

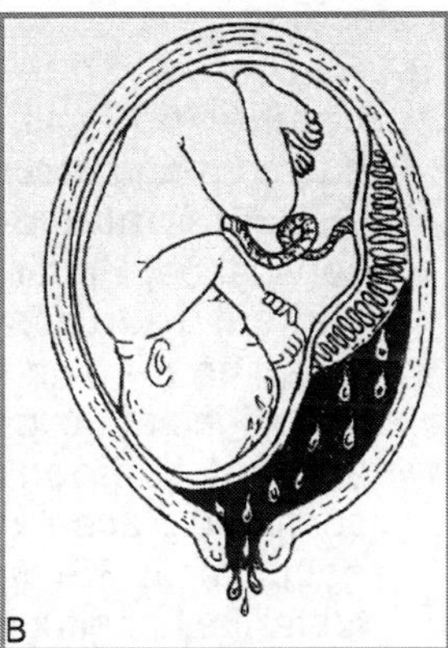

Figs 8.11A and B: A. A type of total placenta praevia, **B.** Abruptio placentae, or separation of normally inserted placenta

Aetiology

Premature separation of the placenta is a serious event that accounts for significant maternal and foetal morbidity and mortality rates. Abruptio placentae may be associated with severe hypertension, pre-eclampsia and eclampsia. A strenuous physical effort on acute emotional stress may precipitate the occurrence of accidental haemorrhage. Abruptio placentae has been known to occur following external cephalic version and artificial rupture of membranes. The bleeding of abruptio placentae is associated with pain due to uterine contractions. The bleeding may escape through cervix and vagina, it may be retained in the uterus with very little vaginal bleeding, and there may be a combination of both types. Placental abruptio tends to occur more frequently under conditions of social deprivation in association with dietary deficiencies, folic acid deficiency in particular.

Whatever factor predisposes to placental abruptio, they are well established before the abruptio occurs. The foetus is more likely to be male and the birth weight is often low, indicating pre-existing growth retardation. Trauma is relatively uncommon cause of abruptio and in the majority of cases, no specific factor can be identified.

Classification (Fig. 8.12)

The most common classification of placentae abruptio is according to type and severity. The terms revealed, 'concealed' and 'mixed' respectively are used to describe these varieties of bleeding.

i. *Revealed haemorrhage:* The major haemorrhage is apparent externally as haemorrhage occurs from the lower part of the placenta and blood escapes through the cervical os. Under these circumstances, the clinical features are less severe. The bleeding may be slight or profuse, but the conditions of the patient is proportional to the amount of blood she has lost. It may be confused placenta praevia. Abruptio tends to occur after 36 weeks gestation, with the foetal lie. Longitudinal and the presenting part sitting well into the pelvic brim. In this, uterine activity may be increased, but this finding is not constant.
ii. *Concealed haemorrhage:* It is the most severe variety of accidental haemorrhage, which occurs between the placenta and the uterine wall. The uterine content increases in volume and the fundal size appears larger than would be consistent with the estimated date of confinement. Uterine tonus increased and pain and shock are common features. The uterus may become broad, rigid and tender.

The bleeding is concealed and there is wide area of placental separation with the formation of a large retroplacental blood clot. The clinical picture is typical. The patient is usually in a state of shock, because of the massive concealed bleeding and her condition is far out of proportion to the amount of external bleeding if any. The pulse rate is rapid and the volume is small. The blood pressure is low. The patient looks ill and anxious.

It is important to realize that initially blood pressure may be raised and the pulse rate slowed but eventually, the patient becomes shocked with the development of tachycardia, hypotension, anuria and oliguria. The peripheral circulation becomes vasoconstricted and there may be physical signs of this condition even before hypotension develops.

Extensive myometrial bleeding damages the uterine muscle. If blood accumulates between separated placenta and the uterine wall, it may produce "Couvelaire uterus". The uterus appears reddish or purplish; it is ecchymotic and contractility lost. Shock may occur and is out of proportion to blood lost.

There may be signs of pre-eclampsia. There is constant excruciating abdominal pain. The abdomen is woody hard and tender to touch. Foetal parts are very difficult to palpate and foetal heart sounds are absent, because of separation of greater part of the placenta might have resulted in intra-uterine death of the foetus. The blood coming from the vagina may fail to clot due to hypofibrinogenaemia.

iii. *Mixed haemorrhage:* In most cases of concealed accidental haemorrhage present as mixed haemorrhage for there is usually some revealed bleeding even in the so called concealed bleeding. Haemorrhage occurs close to the placental edge and after no interval when the haemorrhage is concealed, blood loss soon appears vaginally. The patient may be shocked, depending on the amount of blood lost, and the degree of shock is usually out of proportion to the amount of external bleeding (Fig. 8.13).

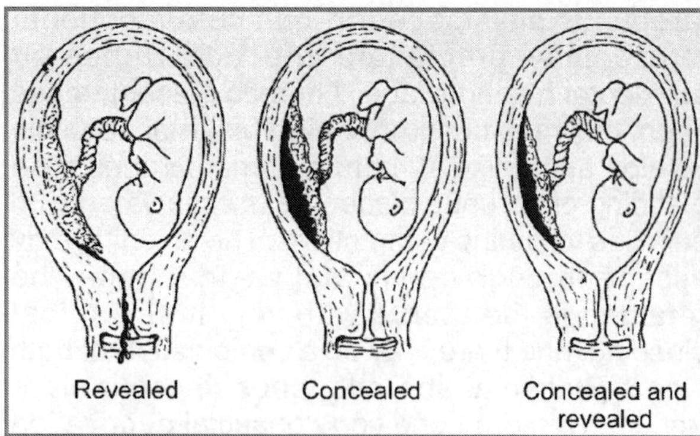

Fig. 8.12: Sites of placental abruptio

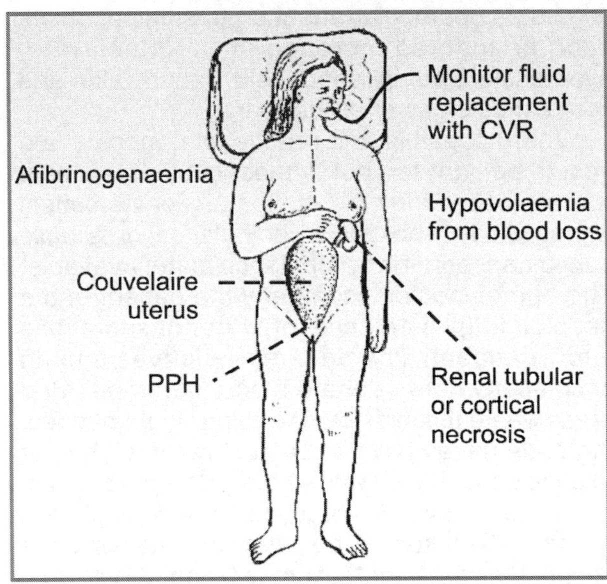

Fig. 8.13: Complications of placental abruptio

Management

Abruptio placentae should be highly suspected in the woman with a sudden onset of intense, usually localized, uterine pain, with or without vaginal bleeding. Nursing diagnosis are similar to that of placenta preavia.

Treatment depends on the severity of blood loss and foetal maturity and status. The patient must be admitted to the hospital, and the diagnosis established on the basis of the history and examination findings. Mild cases may be treated conservatively and the placental site localized to conform the diagnosis. If the haemorrhage is severe, resuscitation is the first pre-requisite. First aid treatment may be given before the transfer of the patient to hospital. The nurse or midwife should accompany the patient to the hospital, taking some of the patient's relatives to donate blood. Records kept, including that of total blood loss, are taken to the hospital.

In the hospital, the patient is admitted and a good history of the patient's previous health, onset of the bleeding and any resuscitative measures already given are obtained. The patients general condition is assessed including abdominal examination, but vaginal examination avoided. Pethidine (100-150 mg) is given intramuscularly and oxygen administration if necessary. Blood is taken for haemoglobin estimation or packed cell volume (PCV), grouping and cross-matching. Clotting time and fibrinogen index are estimated. Intravenous infusion of 5 per cent glucose may be given pending arrival of blood transfusion. Fresh blood which is rich in fibronogen, should be given after cross matching. About 3 liters of fresh blood may be needed; so that patient's relatives should be asked to donate blood. The first liter of blood is run in rapidly (depending on the degree of shock). The blood coming from the vagina is examined for evidence of clotting. In small hospitals some blood is withdrawn in a glass capillary tube and held in the palm for the clotting time to be determined. Transfusion of triple strength plasma is given if there is evidence of hypo-fibrinogenaemia. Fresh blood and figrinogen are also given if available.

The nurse should keep accurate records of blood loss, the pulse rate, respiratory rate, and blood pressure of the patient. A fluid chart is kept, and urinary output is carefully observed. This ought to be 30 ml per hour. Specimens of urine should be tested for albumin.

The patient is prepared for operation and asked to sign a consent form. She is then taken to the operating theatre where an examination under anaesthesia is done to exclude placenta praevia. In the absence of placenta previa, the membranes are ruptured and an intravenous Pitocin infusion is set up. Caesarean section is not done because the foetus often dies *in utero* and the risk of bleeding from hypofibrinogenaemia is increased.

Postpartum haemorrhage is common after concealed antepartum haemorrhage. Further blood loss should therefore, be prevented by the prophylactic use of intravenous ergometrine given with the delivery of the anterior shoulder of the presentation of the foetus is cephalic or, with the crowning of the head if the presentation is breech. If no doctor is available at the time of delivery, the nurse or midwife should give intra-muscular syntometrine with the delivery of the anterior shoulder or crowning of the head. After delivery the placenta must be examined for evidence of retro-placental blood clots which are found on the material surface of placenta. These blood clots must be weighed and the weight recorded.

A patient with concealed accidental haemorrhage is usually not out of danger until several hours after delivery. So she must be watched for evidence of further vaginal bleeding. The pulse rate and blood pressure should be checked at halfhourly and two hourly intervals respectively and this is done during the first 24 hours after delivery. It is very important to record the urinary output and keep an accurate fluid chart because oliguria or anuria due to acute renal failure is not uncommonly seen in cases of severe concealed bleeding. Once good urinary output has been maintained and the pulse rate and blood pressure have remained normal for 48 hours, the patient does not need more than the usually routine observations.

Nursing care of patients experiencing moderate to severe abruption is demanding because it requires close monitoring of the maternal and foetal condition. All procedures should be explained to the woman and her family.

Emotional support is also extremely important because the woman and her family may be experiencing grief over foetal loss in addition to the mother's critical illness.

In unclassified APH, there is usually no evidence of placentae praevia or accidental haemorrhage. The management is the same as described under placenta previa or abruptio placentae.

Management of Patient with Unclassified Bleeding

The midwife may not be faced with the responsibility of diagnosing this type of antepartum haemorrhage but she has a duty to see that the patient does not lose her life and that of her baby. As such, she gives the best first aid treatment she can, before transferring the patient to a good modern hospital with facilities to cope with massive antepartum haemorrhage. The patient is kept warm and calm in bed. The foot of which may be raised to prevent shock. Intramuscular injection of pethidine (100 mg) or any other simlar drug is given if available, otherwise choralhydrate (2 g) is given to allay anxiety. The patient's general condition is quickly assessed by noting her pulse, presence of pallor, blood pressure and oedema. A gentle abdominal examination is carried out to determine the lie of the foetus and the engagement of the presentation. Presence of pain, tenderness, uterine consistency and malpresentation are also noted. On no account should a vaginal examination be done. Vaginal examination may provoke further haemorrhage which could endanger the patient's life. A rough examination of blood loss is made by the midwife and all clothes and pads removed from the patient should be kept for the doctor to see. A quarter-hourly record of the blood pressure pulse and respiratory rates should be kept. The midwife should pay particular attention to signs of shock such as marked increase in the pulse rate, hypotension, perspiration, cold clammy skin and sometimes signs of air hunger.

Where possible and practicable, medical aid should be sent for, but in most circumstances it is much better and practical to transfer the patient without delay to hospital by ambulance, or suitable public transport if an ambulance is not available. The nurse should accompany the patient to the hospital to give an account of her observations and treatment. The patient's relatives should accompany her to donate blood. In remote rural areas where the midwife is working single-handed, the patient may have to be accompanied by her relative while the midwife writes a detailed account of her examination findings and treatment given in a letter to be taken by the patient's relatives to the hospital to which the patient is being transferred.

Medical Aid

If the patient is first seen in the hospital, the midwife should inform the physician immediately of the patient's arrival. She may still have to give the prescribed first aid management where the physician arrival is delayed. In some rural maternity centres there are no physician to send for, or it may not be easy to get in touch with a physician. In such a situation, the midwife should do her utmost to get the patient into a fit state to travel to the nearest hospital.

Management in the Hospital

The management of antepartum haemorrhage in the hospital depends on the severity of the bleeding and the duration of pregnancy. On the patient's arrival the midwife puts her to bed, informs the physician and carries out the first aid treatment if necessary and also prepare for the investigation and treatment of the patient by the physician.

Equipment is got ready for:

a. Taking blood for A, B, O and Rhesus blood grouping and cross matching of the blood.
b. Haemglobin or packed cell volume estimation.
c. Haemoglobin genotype determination.
d. Clotting time and fibrin index.
e. Intravenous therapy with dextrose, blood and Pitocin.
f. Injection of pethidine, atrophlne, etc or any such drug prescribed.
g. Oxygen.

The midwife then shaves the patient's pubic and vulval hair, tests her urine for sugar, albumin, acetone and sets up Esbach's quantitative test if there is albuminuria. Abdominal examination as previously described is carried out. Permission for operation and anaesthesia should be obtained from the patient or her next of kin. Blood banks are few and blood is not readily available in most hospitals in developing countries. The midwife should, therefore, persuade and explain to the patient's relatives to come forward and donate blood. In some cases arrangement could be made to bleed them before they are allowed to go home.

Severe Antepartum Haemorrhage

Active treatment or termination of pregnancy is indicated when the bleeding is severe and there is great danger of maternal collapse and foetal death. In such circumstances, the following should be done;

a. Steps are taken to resuscitate the patient immediately by giving intravenous infusion while blood is being procured, but intravenous dextrans should not be given before the blood specimen for grouping and cross-match obtained from the patient.
b. Maternal pulse, blood pressure and foetal heart rate are recorded at quarter hourly intervals.
c. Oxygen is administered by mask.
d. Blood is taken for grouping and cross-matching and haemoglobin estimation.
e. The theatre is prepared for caesarean section.
f. The anaesthetist to be called.
g. The patient is prepared for examination under anaesthesia.

Slight Antepartum Haemorrhage

When bleeding is light and the patient in good condition, conservative treatment is given. This entails resting the patient, observing her closely and making some investigations with a view to prolonging the pregnancy until the baby Is mature and preventing further bleeding. The patient is confined to bed and not allowed up for any purpose. Her vulva is shaved and washed and sterile perineal pads are worn. To ensure complete rest and relaxation, phenobarbitone (30 to 60 mg) is given twice daily and sodium amytal (200 mg) at night. Blood investigations, described under 'Management in the hospital' are carried out and one to two litres of blood are cross-matched and kept ready incase the patient bleeds profusely. The perineal pad should be inspected at least four times daily noting evidence of fresh bleeding. If such is present, the pads are kept for inspection by the physician. Vulve toilet is done twice daily since the patient is confined to bed and cannot clean herself. A gentle abdominal examination noting pain, tenderness, foetal heart sounds, and the size of the baby is done twice daily. The blood pressure, pulse, temperature and respiration are also recorded twice daily. Routine urine testing is done daily to exclude albuminuria. Magnesium hydroxide (30 ml) may be given daily to avoid constipation and straining at defaecation. Drugs such as daraprim (25 mg weekly), folic acid (5 mg daily) and ferrous sulphate (200 mg) are given to prevent anaemia and promote good health.

Diet

The patient's food should be rich in protein and vitamins. In non-catering hospitals, the relatives must be instructed on what kinds of food to bring. Such food must be inspected by the midwife before delivery to the patient.

In addition to the alone, following to be carried out:

1. The doctor often does a speculum examination 48 to 72 hours after all bleeding has stopped. This is to exclude cervical lesions such as carcinoma of the cervix and other incidental causes of antepartum haemorrhage.
2. Pre-eclampsia and hypertension are excluded by the routine recording of blood pressure, urine testing and examination of the patient for oedema.
3. Packed cell volume is estimated at least twice weekly.
4. An attempt at placental localization is done by way of placentography or angiography. Chest X-ray may be done in unbooked patients to exclude pulmonary tuberculosis.
5. Ultrasound scanning is a helpful diagnostic tool where facilities are available.

The patient is allowed up five days after cessation of bleeding, but she must be kept under close observation. The decision to keep the patient in hospital or discharge her is the physician. Usually, it is wise to keep the patient in hospital until examination under anaesthesia, even if placentography or ultrasound scanning fails to reveal placenta praevia.

ANAEMIA IN PREGNANCY

Anaemia is the most common medical disorders of pregnancy. Anaemia results in reduction of the oxygen-carrying capacity of the blood. When it occurs, the heart tries to compensate by increasing the cardiac output. This effect increases the workload of the heart and stresses ventricular function. Therefore anaemia that occurs (e.g. preeclampsia may result in congestive heart failure.

Anaemia can be defined as a reduction below normal in the number of red blood corpuscles per cubic millimeter, the quantity of haemoglobin and the volume of packed red cells per 100 ml of blood. The average female patient in health has a haemoglobin of 14.5 grams per 100 ml of blood (cent per cent Hb) 450,000 R.B.C. per cubic millimetre of blood and packed cell volume of 45 per cent. Sometime these values are considerably reduced during pregnancy and the condition of anaemia in pregnancy results. Folic acid deficiency is the most important cause of non-hemorrhagic anaemia in pregnancy. Approximately 90 per cent of cases of anaemia in pregnancy are of the iron deficiency type. The remaining 10 per cent of cases embrace a considerable variety of acquired and hereditary anaemias, including folic acid deficiency, sickle cell anaemia and thalassemia.

Clinical Manifestation of Anaemia

Pallor is the constraint feature of anaemia. The areas to be examined for pallor are the conjunctiva, the tongue, the lips, the palms of the hands, the nail beds and the soles of the feet. In the severe cases of anaemia there is breathlessness, ankle oedema and a low grade fever. The spleen and liver may not be enlarged. Usually anaemia secondary to malaria give rise to enlargement of spleen and liver.

When anaemia is very severe, the patient may go into heart failure when she will have Pallor and very marked dyspnoea, cough, oedema of ankles. The liver is enlarged, soft and tender. There are signs of congestion in the bases of lungs.

Diagnosis

Anemia can be diagnosed from the symptoms and signs mentioned above. The objective diagnosis is, however, made by taking a specimen of blood for the determination of haemaglobin and packed cell volume. The laboratory methods of determining these values are not relevant. The nurse should be conversant with the use of Salhi's Haemoglobinometer. The Talquist's paper method is grossly inaccurate and should be employed only in the absence of other better and more accurate methods. In a few selected case of severe anaemia in pregnancy, it becomes necessary to do the bone marrow biopsy which is obtained from the sternum or the iliac crest with great precautions. Other investigations that may be carried out in anemic patients include examination of the stool for hookworm ova, examination of urine to exclude urinary infections and liver function tests. Chest X-ray examination is done to exclude pulmonary tuberculosis.

Effects of Anaemia on Pregnancy

Anaemia increases the incidence of abortion, premature labour and intrauterine death of the foetus with the delivery of a macerated foetus. The more severe anaemia, the greater is the perinatal loss (stillbirths and deaths occur first week of life). The foetal loss rate in severe anemia in pregnancy may be related to intrauterine hypoxia (reduced O_2 supply to foetus *in utero*).

The resistance to infection is lowered and thus the incidence of puerperal sepsis may be increased. Severe anaemia may lead to heart failure. Untreated anaemia leads to chronic ill health. Women with sickle cell trait usually do well in pregnancy although they are at increased risk for urinary tract infections and may be deficient in iron.

If the woman has sickle cell anaemia, the anaemia that occurs in normal pregnancy may aggravate the condition and bring on more crises. Foetal complications include being small for gestational age, IUGR and skeletal changes. Pregnant women with sickle cell anaemia are prone to pyelonephritis, leg ulcers, bone abnormalities, strokes, cardiomyopathy, congestive heart failure, and pre-eclampsia, UTIs and haematuria are common.

Thalassaemia major complicates pregnancy. Pre-eclampsia is more common and there may be an increase in low-birth weight infants and foetal death.

Management

Anaemia pregnancy is preventable. Prevention is achieved by referring all cases at risk, such as those giving previous history of anaemia, PPH, APH, and all short primigravidae, to a major hospital or by observing following regimen.

- A loading dose of 800 mg chloroquine sulfate or 750 mg of chloroquine phosphate is given to eradicate malarial parasite from the bloodstream in areas where malaria is endemic.
- A prophylactic dose of 25 mg of pyrimethamine (Daraprim) is given weekly throughout pregnancy and puerperium. In lieu of this Paludrine 100 mg daily given
- Folic acid 5 mg daily given throughout pregnancy and puerperium
- Iron in the form of ferrous gluconate 32.5 mg or ferrous sulfate 200 mg is given twice to thrice daily.

In addition, patient should be advised on what food to eat. Food rich in iron and Folic acid should be encouraged throughout pregnancy. The richer source of folic acid are fresh green vegetables, yams, liver and kidney. Meat is the other source of folic acid. Iron is found in liver, beef, muscle, eggs and dry fruits. In giving dietary advice, the patient the nurse must remember that the majority of clients may not be able to afford expensive food items usually suggested to them in the hospital. The important thing to study the patients dietary habit and work out pattern for her that will ensure adequate supply of the essential nutrition in pregnancy.

From the point of view of treatment it will be convenient to classify all cases as mild, moderate and severe. The mild cases with a PCV of between 28 per cent and 33 per cent (Hb. 60-70%) can be treated as out patients and reviewed weekly at the clinic. At each visit the PCV and Hb% should be checked and the weekly dose of pyrimethamine as well as oral iron (t.i.d) should be given.

The moderate cases with PCV of 22 to 27 per cent should be admitted to the hospital for rest. They should have daraprim, iron and folic acid as stated above, but the PCV and Hb should be checked at least twice weekly and if possible once daily. The need for blood transfusion will be dictated by the period of gestation at which the anaemia is diagnosed. If the diagnosis is made before the 28th week of pregnancy, blood transfusion may not be necessary unless the patient condition worsens or the patient fails to show improvements.

The severe cases with PCV of 5 to 21 per cent must, of course be sent to hospital without delay. Usually the ones with PCV of 5 to 13 per cent are at very great risk of not going into heart failure but also losing their babies if adequate and prompt treatment is not instituted. This class of patients if given direct blood transfusion, runs the risk of going into premature labour and heart failure. Such patients are usually treated with exchange of blood transfusion. Exchange blood transfusion, however, a big undertaking far beyond the scope of small hospital which are usually understaffed. In such a situation direct transfusion with packed cells are given slowly, into the pint of packed cells are transfused. Ethacrynic acid in a very quick acting diuretic. By causing her to pass copious amounts of urine simultaneously with or shortly after transfusion of the patient is relieved of the load of the extra fluid which might lead to right heart failure. This method of treatment is also good for patient, who are already in heart failure irrespective of the level of the PCV. All patients whether transfused or not given, oral treatment with prescribed drugs can be continued.

Sickle cell crisis is due to rapid haemolysis and destruction of the red blood cells. The patient is severely anaemic, often jaundiced and very ill with severe pain including other signs and symptoms. The nursing care is as for that of severely anaemic patient. A bed cradle should be used to take the weight of the bed linen off the painful legs of the patient. Analgesics must be given as prescribed. Tepid sponging or fanning of the patient may be necessary to lower the temperature if it is too high. Urine is tested daily for protein, acetone and bile. The nurse should observe for degree of jaundice. If puerperal patient, observe for lochia and any possibility of haemorrhage.

PULMONARY DISORDERS IN PREGNANCY

As pregnancy advances and the uterus impinges on the thoracic cavity any pregnant woman may experience increased respiratory difficulty. This difficulty will be compounded by pulmonary diseases. The common pulmonary disorders affecting pregnancy are asthma, cystic fibrosis and pulmonary tuberculosis.

Asthma

Bronchial asthma is an acute respiratory illness characterized by periods of exacerbations and remissions. Exacerbations are triggered by allergens, marked change in ambient temperature, or emotional tension. In many cases, the actual cause may be unknown although a family history of allergies is common. In response to stimuli, there is a wide spread but reversible narrowing of the hyperactive airways, making it difficult for the woman to breathe. The clinical manifestations are expiratory wheezing, productive cough, thick sputum and dyspnoea.

Asthma is a common pulmonary disorder in the general population; it may also affect the pregnancy. Pregnancy does not make the woman more prone to asthmatic attack. Women often experience few symptoms of asthma in the first trimester and in the last weeks of pregnancy. The severity symptoms usually peak between 29 and 36 weeks of gestation. Women with severe disease and those who have poor control of asthma seem to have an increased incidence of adverse maternal and neonatal outcomes including preterm labour and birth, hypertensive disorders in pregnancy, babies of small gestational age, abruptio placentae, chorioamnionitis and caesarean birth.

Management of asthma has three objectives:

- Relief of the acute attack
- Prevention and limitation of later attacks
- Adequate maternal and foetal oxygenation.

These goals can be achieved in pregnancy by eliminating environmental triggers (e.g. dust, mites, animal) and patient education. Respiratory infections should be treated and mist or steam inhalation employed to air expectoration of mucus. Acute episodes may require albutrol, steroids, aminophylline, beta adrenergic agents and oxygen. Almost all asthma medications are considered safe in pregnancy.

Asthma attacks can occur in labour, thus medications for asthma are continued in labour and postpartum. An increase in Cortisone and adrenaline from the adrenal glands during labour is thought to prevent asthma attacks during labour. If an asthma attack does occur, it should be treated with the same rapidity and medication as an attack outside of pregnancy. Pulse oximetry should be instituted during labour. Epidurals are recommended for pain relief. Morphine and meperidine are histamine releasing narcotics and should be avoided. Any woman who has received corticosteroids in pregnancy should have increased dose for the stress of labour, as prescribed. During postpartum, woman who have asthma are at increased risk for hemorrhage. If excessive bleeding occurs, oxytocin is the recommended drug. The woman usually returns to her prepregnancy status within 3 months after giving birth. Breastfeeding should be encouraged, particularly as it may protect infants from developing certain allergic conditions.

Cystic Fibrosis (CF)

Cystic fibrosis is a common autosomal recessive genetic disorder in which the exocrine gland produces excessive viscous secretions causing problems with both respiratory and digestive functions. Respiratory failure and early death may occur. An incidence in 1:2000 live births.

In women with good nutrition, mild obstructive lung disease and good chest X-rays, pregnancy tolerated well. In those with severe disease the pregnancy, the pregnancy is often complicated by chronic hypoxia, and frequent pulmonary infections. Women with cystic fibrosis show a decrease in their residual volume during pregnancy, as do normal pregnant women and are unable to maintain vital capacity. Presumably, the pulmonary vasculature cannot accommodate the increased cardiac output of pregnancy. The results are decreased to the myocardium, decreased cardiac output, and increased hypoxaemia. A pregnant woman with less than 50 per cent of expected vital capacity usually has a difficult pregnancy. Increased risk of maternal and parental mortality is related to severe pulmonary infection.

Once pregnancy is confirmed a multidisciplinary approach is essential. Specific diagnostic measures will include pulmonary function tests, arterial blood gases, sputum, culture, liver function tests, glucose tolerance tests, chest radiogram, electrocardiogram, echocardiogram and monitoring of weight gain. An essential component of CF care is the use of postural drainage techniques in order to keep lungs clear of mucoid secretions. An early recognition of CF and pulmonary infection are also vital. In addition, pay attention to nutrition and CF-related diabetes because poor nutrition and deterioration in lung function will affect the supply of nutrients and oxygen to the foetus resulting in IUGR and preterm labour and birth.

During labour, monitoring for fluid and electrolyte balance is required. The amount of sodium lost through sweat can be significant, and hypovolaemia can occur. Conversely, if any degree of corpulmonale is present, fluid overload is a concern. Oxygen is administered by face mask during labour, and monitoring by pulse oximetry is recommended. Epidural or local analgesia is preferred analgesic for birth. Breastfeeding appears to be safe as long as the sodium content of the milk is not abnormal. Pumping and discarding the milk is done until the sodium content has been determined. However, in order for breastfeeding to be successful, when need to be well nourished and maintain an adequate caloric intake.

Pulmonary Tuberculosis

Tuberculosis is caused by an acid fast bacillus, known as *Mycobacterium tuberculosis*. It is infection and can be transmitted through the sputum of an open case (i.e. a case with tuberculous cavities in the lungs). It is a disease which rapidly spreads in congested, unhygienic surroundings. The lungs are the organs most commonly affected, although it may involve any organ.

As stated earlier, it is transmitted through inhalation of infected airborne droplets from a person with active tuberculosis or it may also be contracted from infected cattle through the consumption of milk and dairy products that have not been pasteurised.

Clinical Manifestation

The onset of primary tuberculosis is often insidious and the symptoms are non-specific fatigue, malaise, loss of appetite, loss of weight, alteration in bowel habit and low grade fever. These can be interpreted as usual symptoms occurring in pregnancy. The classic symptoms of chronic cough, night sweats, haemoptysis, dyspnea and chest pain occur quite late in the disease process and are often absent, when TB is extrapulmonary.

Pulmonary tuberculosis causes fever which may be very high, cough with expectoration and, in severe cases, haemoptysis (coughing out of blood). Night sweates are experienced by the patient and loss of weight is not unusual.

Pulmonary tuberculosis is very important because it is common in the tropics where It can run a rapid course. It may adversely affect the course of pregnancy if there is inadequate medical and antenatal care. The nurse should therefore refer all suspicious cases to hospital for assessment and diagnosis.

Diagnosis

The diagnosis of pulmonary tuberculosis is made on a family history of tuberculosis, and the symptoms and signs, and on X-ray examination of the chest. In the presence of cavities in the lungs, the sputum may be positive for acid fast bacilli. In order to detect pulmonary tuberculosis in a population of antenatal patients, routine X-ray examination of the chest is advocated in some quarters. This has, however, been found to be impracticable in developing countries where there may be shortage of personnel and material to cope with the large and expanding antenatal clinics. All cases attending the antenatal clinic are thoroughly examined by the physician and suspicious cases are subjected to radiological examination of the chest. By the same token emergency antenatal and puerperal admissions are routinely examined radiologically.

The Effect of Pulmonary Tuberculosis on Pregnancy

In the past, patients with pulmonary tuberculosis seldom got married and the outlook for conception was poor for those who did get married. Those who were lucky to have live babies might not be able to breastfeed their infants.

The outlook for tuberculosis has improved since the advent of antituberculous drugs. Untreated or inadequately supervised cases of pulmonary tuberculosis in pregnancy usually about or have intrauterine death of the foetus leading to the delivery of a macerated foetus. Anaemia may develop. The condition may worsen and the patient may die of fulminating tuberculosis.

In the management of a patient with a history of pulmonary tuberculosis, four categories are recognized.

1. Those in whom, the disease has been adequately treated and is quiescent. These cases usually require the usual antenatal and intranatal care. The prognosis is usually good for the mother and baby although the possibility of a relapse cannot be ruled out if supervision is inadequate. The baby can be breastfed. Ordinary BCG vacclnation is all that is required to protect the baby against pulmonary tuberculosis.
2. Those in whom the disease is still active who have been receiving treatment to which they are responding satisfactorily before the onset of pregnancy. The outlook in these cases is usually good provided supervision is adequate. Treatment is usually continued with streptomycin (1 gram daily for 3 months), PARA-

aminosalicylic acid (PAS) (12 grams daily in three divided doses), iso-nicotinic acid hydrazide (isoniazide; INH)(100 mg three time daily). The latter two drugs are continued for at least 18 months, or until the disease becomes inactive as evidenced by negative sputum and X-ray of the chest. The babies of these women are protected against tuberculosis by giving them 10 mg INH per kg of body weight daily for 2 weeks and later giving INH-resistant BCG vaccination to all such babies. On this regimen, the mother can safely breastfeed her infant if she is fit enough to do so.

3. Those in whom the disease is first diagnosed in pregnancy or in the puerperium. The prognosis here is very poor. Such patients should be treated as an acute emergency requiring immediate admission to hospital and immediate therapy. They may not be fit to breastfeed their infants, but in those who can breastfeed their infants, the regimen of giving INH and INH-resistant BCG to the infant is observed as stated above.
4. Those who have had the disease for a very long time and have been adequately treated but without a satisfactory response to treatment. Such cases are referred to as resistant cases and are usually give 600 mg of isoniazid daily. They may or may not be fit to breast their infants. If they should breastfeed their infants, the above stated regimen on INH and INH-resistant BCG should be observed for the baby.

Management of TB in Pregnancy

The TB is treated in two phases. The first involves taking rifampicin, isoniazid and pyrizinamide daily for the first two months. In the second phase, rifampicin and isoniazid are taken for a further 4 months. These drugs are considered to be safe and are not associated with human foetal malformations. Congenital deafness has been reported in infants with exposure to streptomycin *in utero* and's therefore, this drug is best avoided in pregnancy. Nowadays, bacillus becoming resistant to drugs. So care is planned individually, so that those women at risk of non-adherence have thrice weekly directly observed therapy (DOTs) whereby health workers directly observe the woman taking her medication and evaluate her progress. Attention should also be placed on rest, good nutrition and education with regard to preventing the spread of disease.

The management of pulmonary tuberculosis entails very good antenatal care in which anaemia is prevented or energetically treated when present, pre-eclampsia is looked for and routine X-ray examinations at three monthly intervals are carried out. The sputum is periodically examined and cultured for acid-fast bacilli.

Management in Labour

In labour, exhaustion should be avoided by the liberal use of analgesics. The midwife should not give inhalation analgesics to tuberculous patients. The second stage of labour should be shortened by a timely vacuum extraction or forceps delivery. The physician must therefore be informed as soon as the patients cervix is fully dilated and the foetal head is visible in the vagina. Where there is cephalo-pelvic disproportion or foetal distress before full dilatation of the cervix, caesarean section is usually done.

In the puerperium, the nurse must watch for signs of relapse such as a troublesome cough, dyspnoea and haemoptysis. All these signs must be reported to the physician. Breastfeeding and BCG vaccination have been discussed above. The babies of tuberculous mothers should be followed up in the infant welfare clinic and should have a Mantoux test at 6 to 8 weeks after BCG vaccination. If the test is negative, another BCG vaccination should be done. The patient herself should continue to attend the chest clinic until she is discharged fit.

METABOLIC DISORDERS IN PREGNANCY

Diabetes Mellitus

Diabetes mellitus is the most common medical condition to affect pregnancy. Pregnancy complicated by diabetes is still considered high risk. It is most successfully managed, i.e. collaborative health care team.

Pathophysiology

The term "Diabetes Mellitus" describes a metabolic disorder of multiple aetiology that affects the normal metabolism of carbohydrates fats and protein. It is a group of metabolic disease characterized by hyperglycaemia resulting from defects in insulin secretion, insulin action or both. Insulin, is produced by the beta cells in islets of Langerhans in the pancreae, regulate blood glucose levels by enabling glucose to enter adipose and muscle cells, where it is used for energy. When insulin is insufficient or ineffective in promoting glucose uptake by the muscle and adipose cells, glucose accumulates in the bloodstream and hyperglycemia results. Hyperglycaemia causes hyperosmolarity of the blood, which attracts intracellular fluid into the vascular system, resulting cellular dehydration and expanded blood volume. Consequently the kidneys function to excrete large volume of urine (polyuria) in an attempt to regulate excess vascular volume and to excrete the unusable glucose (glycosuria), polyuria, along with cellular dehydration causes excessive thirst (polydipsia).

Clinical Manifestation

The classic signs and symptoms of DM are polydipsia, polyuria and unexplained weight loss. The body compensates for its inability to convert carbohydrate (glucose) into energy by burning proteins (muscle) and fats. However, the end products of this metabolism are ketones and fatty acids, which in excess quantities produce ketoacidosis and acetonuria. Weight loss occurs as a result of the breakdown of fat and muscle tissue. This tissue breakdown causes a state of starvation that compels the individual to eat excessive amounts of food (polyphagia). The long-term effects of DM are reflected in the development of macrovascular and microvascular disease producing coronary heart disease, peripheral arterial disease, diabetic retinopathy (loss of vision), diabetic neuropathy (nerve damage), premature, atherosclerosis.

Classification of DM

Classification of DM includes four groups as follows:

i. *Type 1 DM*: It occurs when beta cells in the islets of Langerhans in the pancreas are destroyed, stopping insulin production. Insulin therapy is required in order to prevent the development of keto acidosis or can occur at any age and thought to be caused by autoimmune process.
ii. *Type 2 DM:* It is the most prevalent form of the disease and include individuals who have insulin resistance and usually relative (rather than absolute) insulin deficiency. The risk of this type increases with age, obesity, and lack of physical activity. It occurs more frequently in women with pregestational DM and individual with hypertension.

    Pregestational diabetes mellitus is the label sometimes given to type 1 or type 2 diabetes that existed before pregnancy.
iii. *Gestational DM:* It is defined as carbohydrate intolerance resulting in hyperglycaemia of variable severity, with its onset or first recognition during pregnancy. This definition is appropriate whether or not insulin is used for treatment or the diabetes persists after pregnancy.
iv. *Other specific DM* types: They are caused by infection or drug induced.

Effects of Diabetes on Pregnancy

Pregnancy has some adverse effects on diabetes is that increases the insulin requirements of the patient and also lowers the renal threshold for sugar. This lowering of renal threshold leads to a great loss of carbohydrates in the urine and makes the control of diabetes difficult. Diabetes exerts its effects on pregnancy by increasing the incidence of foetal loss as a result of intrauterine death of the foetus, still birth, and early neonatal deaths. The incidences of pre-eclampsia, hydramnios, and congenital foetal abnormalities is known to be very high in diabetic pregnancies.

Management of Diabetes in Pregnancy

WHO (1999) recommended following criteria for diagnosis of diabetes mellitus:

- Diabetes symptoms of increased thirst, increased urine volume, unexplain weight loss plus
- A random venous plasma glucose concentration of > 11.1 mmol/L or a fasting plasma concentration >11.1 mmol/L 2 hours after 75 g any drop glucose in an Oral Glucose Tolerance Test (OGTT).
- Without symptoms, diagnosis should not be based on a single glucose determination but requires confirmatory plasma venous determination on another day.
- The OGTT should always be used to diagnose gestational DM and impaired glucose regulations.

Treatment

Almost all women with pregestational diabetes are insulin dependant during pregnancy. Patients should be given instruction regarding dietary management, self administration of insulin, self-testing of blood glucose level, treatment of hypoglycaemia and what to do when illness occurs.

i. *Dietary management of diabetes in pregnancy:*
   - Follow the prescribed diet plan
   - Eat a well-balanced diet, including daily food requirements in normal pregnancy
   - Divide daily food intake between three meals and two to four snacks, depending on individual needs
   - Eat a substantial bedtime snack to prevent a severe drop in blood glucose level during the night
   - Limit the intake of fats if weight gain occurs too rapidly
   - Take daily vitamins and iron as prescribed by the health care provider
   - Avoid foods high in refined sugar
   - Eat consistently each day; never slip meals or snacks
   - Reduce the intake of saturated fat and cholesterol
   - Eat foods high in dietary fibre
   - Avoid alcohol and caffeine.

ii. *Self-administration of insulin:* Procedure for mixing NPH intermediate acting and regular short acting insulin will be as follows:
   - Wash hands thoroughly and gather supplies. Be sure the insulin syringe corresponds to the concentration of insulin that you are using
   - Check insulin bottle to be certain, it is the appropriate type and check the expiration date
   - Gently rotate (do not shake) the insulin vial to mix the insulin
   - Wipe of rubber stopper of each vial with alcohol
   - Draw into syringe the amount of air equal to total dose
   - Inject air equal to regular insulin dose into regular insulin vial. Remove syringe from vial
   - Invert 'regular' insulin bottle and withdraw regular insulin dose without adding more air to NPH vial, carefully withdraw NPH dose
   - Without adding more air to NPH vial, carefully withdraw NPH dose. The procedure for self injection of insulin is followed
   - Select proper injection site (Remember to rotate sites)
   - Injection site should be clean. No need to use alcohol. If alcohol is used, let it dry before injecting
   - Pinch the skin upto form a subcutaneous pocket, and holding the syringe like a pencil, puncture the skin at a 45 to 90 degree angle If these is great deal of fatty tissue at the site spread the skin taut and inject the syringe at a 90-degree angle
   - Slowly inject the insulin
   - As you withdraw the needle, cover the injection site with sterile gauze and apply gentle pressure to prevent bleeding
   - Record insulin dosage and time of injection.

Self-testing of Blood Glucose Level

- Gather supplies, check expiration date, and read instructions on testing materials. Prepare glucose reflectance meter for use according to manufacturers directions
- Wash hands in warm water (warmth increases circulation)
- Select site on side of any finger (all fingers should be used in rotation)
- Pierce site with lancet (may use automatic, spring loaded, puncturing device). Cleaning the site with alcohol is not necessary
- Drop hand down to side, with other hand gently squeeze finger from hand to finger tip
- Allow blood to drop on to testing strip. Be sure to cover entire reagent area
- Determine blood glucose value using the glucose reflectance meter following manufacturer's instruction
- Record results
- Repeat as instructed by health care provider and as needed for signs of hypoglycaemia or hyperglycaemia.

Treatment of Hypoglycaemia

- Be familiar with signs and symptoms of hypoglycaemia (nervousness, headache, shaking, irritability, personality change, hunger, blurred vision, sweaty skin, tingling of mouth or extremity

- Check blood glucose level immediately, when hypoglycaemia symptoms occur
- If blood glucose is < 60 mg/dl, immediately eat or drink something that contains 10 to 15 g of simple carbohydrate. Example
  - ½ cup (4 Oz) unsweetened fruit juice.
  - ½ cup (4 Oz) regular (not thick) soda.
  - 5 to 6 life savers candies.
  - 1 table spoon honey or corn (Karo) syrup.
  - 1 cup (8 ounces) milk.
  - 2 to 3 glucose tablets.
- Rest for 15 minutes, then recheck blood glucose
- If glucose level is still < 60 mg/dl, eat or drink another serving of one of the glucose booster listed above
- Wait 15 minutes, then recheck blood glucose. If it is still< 60 mg/dl, notify health care provider immediately.

And also nurse has to instruct the patient "what to do when illness occurs; which include:

- Be sure to take insulin even though appetite and good intake may be less than normal (Insulin needs are increased with illness or infections).
- Call the health care provider and relay of the following information:
  - Symptoms of illness (e.g., nausea, vomiting, diarrhoea)
  - Fever
  - Most recent blood glucose level
  - Urine ketone
  - Time and amount of last insulin dose.
- Increase oral intake of fluids to prevent dehydration
- Rest as much as possible
- If unable to reach health care provider, and blood glucose exceeds 200 mg/dl with urine ketone present, seek emergency treatment at the nearest health care facility. Do not attempt to self treat for this.

Nursing Intervention

The nurse should refer all patients to physician. Routine testing of urine for glucose is important. It is equally important to test the urine for acetone. Because of the difficulty to control of diabetes in pregnancy, the patient should be admitted at about the 16th to the 20th week of gestation for stabilisation (i.e. finding out the insulin requirement which will present glycosuria, hyperglycaemia and hypoglycaemia). This is done by series of tests on the blood and urine. After stabilisation, if the patient is discharged from the hospital and seen weekly at the antenatal clinic. At each visit, the urine is tested for sugar and acetone and the presence of these are reported to the concerned physician. In addition, signs of toxaemia, infection and anaemia are looked for and appearance of any of these warrants admission of the patient to hospital.

Diabetic patients are usually admitted to the hospital in about the 32nd week of gestation and kept there until induction of labour is carried out at about 37th week. Sometimes this ideal of admitting patients to hospital 5 weeks before delivery may not be easy to achieve especially the tropics where the demand for hospital bed far exceeds the number of available beds. It is better in such cases to see the patient weekly at the antenatal clinic and admit her whenever there is a bed, but certainly before the 37th week of pregnancy.

The urine should be tested 4-hourly for sugar, acetone and albumin. During labour patient is not given any food by mouth. Glucose infusion is given to ensure adequate hydration and calories and to prevent hypoglycemia. A close and accurate observation of the foetal heart sound is made in order to detect hypoxia early. The physician must be informed if the patient is not delivered within 18 hours of labour. In a small number of patients, elective caesarean section is performed either because it is felt that induction of labour may fail or because of suspected cephalopelvic disproportion.

Some basic principles of preoperative care are employed here. Usually, the patients blood sugar is estimated 2-4 hours prior to operation and soluble insulin is given as indicated by the result of the blood test. A glucose infusion is also set up. It should be noted that the insulin requirements of the patient increases in pregnancy but decreases in the puerperium. The daily insulin requirement of the patient should therefore be reassured. Urinalysis is also carried out six hourly or before meals. Infection must be avoided. The patient should be encouraged to breastfeed her baby.

Care of the Diabetic Baby (Fig. 8.14)

The diabetic baby is usually fat, flabby and edematous, weighing 4 to 4.5 kg or over. Despite its enormous size, it is a premature or immature baby that needs the same special care and attention as a full term baby weighing about 1.5 kg.

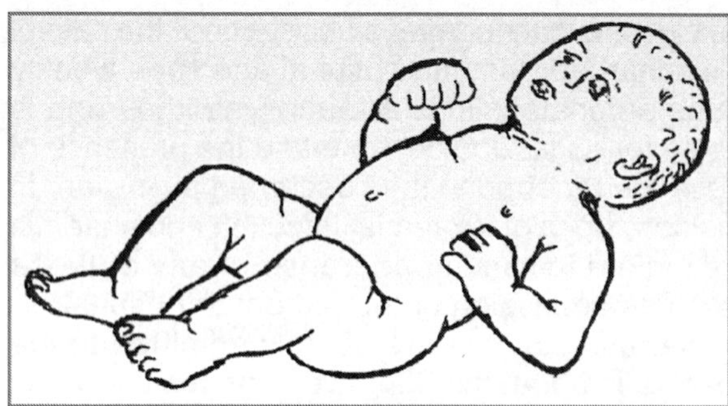

Fig. 8.14: The infant born to the diabetic mother may exhibit macrosomia and abnormal birth weight

The first 48 hours of the life of a diabetic baby are fraught with hazards and the baby runs the risk of respiratory complications often caused by poor expansion of the lungs, inhalation of stomach contents and hyaline membrane disease. As the oedema subsides, the baby loses weight very rapidly and tends to chill very easily.

At birth, the airways must be adequately cleared and a stomach tube passed to empty the stomach and prevent regurgitations and subsequent aspiration of stomach contents. If the baby has a lot of mucus it should be put on side with a slight head down fist to allow for the drainage of mucus. The airways should be aspirated at regular intervals and the baby closely observed. Oxygen by mask or nasal catheter is administered as often as necessary.

The neonate is watched for signs of cyanosis and respiratory embarrassment, Feeding is managed as that of a premature baby. Where the baby is ill, or disinclined to suck, spoon feeding may be employed. Over feeding is avoided so as to prevent regurgitation and subsequent aspiration of the stomach contents. Precautions are also taken to prevent infection.

CARDIAC DISEASES IN PREGNANCY

Pregnancy is associated with increase in cardiac output and, therefore, creates considerable hazards for the mother if there is underlying cardiac disease. The maternal risk varies according to the nature of the cardiac lesion. Cardiac diseases take a variety of forms, those more likely to be seen in pregnancy are described below.

Rheumatic Heart Disease (RHD)

RHD causes inflammation and scarring of the heart valves and results in valve stenosis, mostly mitral valve stenosis. The condition classically remains asymptomatic, when diagnosed most women with valvular heart diseases can be managed with the use of drugs such as diuretics, beta blockers or digoxin. If severe, surgical procedure such as ballon valvoplasty or valve replacement.

Congenital Heart Diseases

The most common congenital heart defects include ASD, VSD, PDA. Pulmonary stenosis, aortic stenosis and tetrology of Fallot. These lesions may be corrected surgically in childhood. Uncorrected lesions give rise to pulmonary hypertension cyanosis and LVF. Congenital heart conditions, include—Eisenmenger's syndrome, Marfan's syndrome, ischemic heart disease, endocarditis and peripartum cardiomyopathy. Septal defects, PDA, pulmonary and tricuspid lesions may have low risk in pregnancy. Mitral stenosis, aortic stenosis. Marfan's syndrome, previous MI, coarctation are associated with significantly greater risk and the condition with maximum high risk includes Eisenmenger's syndrome, pulmonary hypertension, Marfan's syndrome involving the aorta and cardiomyopathy.

The risks generally are those of cardiac failure and acute pulmonary oedema. Adequate rest and the avoidance of infection are important. The use of antibiotic cover should be routine during labour. Anticoagulant therapy may also be necessary where there has been a valve replacement. It must be remembered that the risk of cardiac decompensation is maximal disorder "please read author's text on Medical Surgical Nursing."

In normal pregnancy the hemodynamic progress alters in order to meet the increasing demands of the growing fetoplacental unit. Although this increases the work load of the heart, quite normal healthy pregnant women are able to adjust these physiological changes quite easily. In that certain changes taken place which increase the work of the heart. Some of these changes include an increase in blood volume and cardiac output. This haemodynamic changes start early in pregnancy at about the 10th or 12th week of pregnancy and gradually reach their maximum effect between 38 and 32 weeks of pregnancy. During labour there is significant increase in cardiac outputs as a result of uterine contractions. There are periods of cardiovascular stress leads to critical and fatal to women with heart lesion.

Clinical Manifestation

Heart disease is difficult to diagnose in pregnancy because some of the signs and symptoms of heart diseases resembling to those if normal pregnancy such as breathlessness on exertion, oedema, and heart murmurs. The fatigue, shortness of breath (dyspnea) difficulty in breathing unless upright (orthopnoea), palpitations, bounding, collapsing pulse, chest pain development of peripheral oedema, distended jugular veins and progressive limitation of physical activity. The majority of pregnancies complicated by maternal heart disease can be expected to have a favourable outcome for both mother and foetus. The risk factors of mother will include:

- The nature of the cardiac lesion
- Its effect on the functional capacity of the heart and
- The development of pregnancy-related complication such as hypertension, infection, thrombosis and haemorrhage.

Management (Table 8.2)

All patients who have undue breathlessness on exertion should be suspected of having heart disease and referred to hospital. In addition, oedema, irregular pulse, unexplained tachycardia, palpitations, cough, anaemia and loss of energy should bring about the suspicion of heart disease and the patient must undergo proper investigation. Along with signs and symptoms, laboratory tests can assist with diagnosis of cardiac disease and determine the types of lesions together with an assessment of current functional capacity of the heart. The tests include:

- Complete blood count
- Electrocardiography
- Chest radiograph to assess cardiac size and outline, pulmonary vasculature and lung fields. (X-ray are considered safe in pregnancy)
- Clotting studies
- Echocardiography.

The types of lesions that are encountered in a patient with cardiac disease are mitral stenosis, mitral incompetence, aortic stenosis, aortic incompetence, Congenital heart disease and puereperal heart disease. In the management of cardiac diseases in pregnancy four grades of patients are recognized.

Grade 1

Patients who have the signs of cardiac lesions such as cardiac murmurs and radiological and electrocardiographic evidence of cardiac evidence of cardiac disease but no symptoms. These patients can be seen at fortnightly intervals at the antenatal clinic until the 32nd week, after which, they should be seen weekly. Such patients should be admitted between the 29th and 32nd week a time when the cardiac output is maximal. In this, no limitation of physical activity, ordinary activity does not cause undue fatigue, palpitation, dyspnoea or angina.

Grade II

The patients in this grade have sign of cardiac disease and are breathless on ordinary exertion. They are *symptomless* at rest. These patients can be seen weekly at the antenatal clinic. They should be advised to rest for at least 2 hours in the day and 10 hours during night. No heavy work should be advised, and effort should be made to provide the patients with home help and transport to the antenatal clinic. Where possible, they should be admitted between the 28th and 32nd weeks of pregnancy. In this slight limitation of physical activity, comfortable at rest, ordinary physical activity results in fatigue, palpitations, dyspnoea or angina.

Grade III

This grade refers to patients, who have signs of cardiac disease and are very breathless after very little exertion. They are unable to do their daily work at home and are breathless after a short argument. Such patients are admitted to the hospital from the time they are first seen in the antenatal clinic and kept in hospital until about three weeks after delivery. Here marked limitation of physical activity, comfortable at rest, less than ordinary physical activity results in fatigue, palpitation, dyspnoea or angina.

Grade IV

The patients, in this grade who have signs of cardiac disease as well as signs of cardiac failure. They are breathless even at rest and are orthopnoeic (breathless, when they are lying flat on their back) and usually have to be cropped up. These patients are admitted to the hospital and

Table 8.2: Nursing care plan of the pregnant woman with heart diseases

Problem	*Reason*	*Objective*	*Nursing intervention*	*Evaluation*
Activity intolerance related to effects of pregnancy on the patient with RHD and mitral valve stenosis.		Woman will verbalize a plan to avoid risk of cardiac decompensation.	• Assist the patient to identify factors that decrease activity tolerance and expose extent of limitation. to establish a base for evaluation • Help women to develop an individualized program of activity and rest, taking into account, the living and working environment as well as support to family and friends to maintain sufficient cardiac output • Teach woman to monitor physiologic response to activity (i.e. pulse and resp. rate) and reduce activity that causes fatigue or pain to maintain sufficient cardiac output and prevent potential injury to foetus. • Enlist family and friends to assist woman in pacing activities and to provide support in performing role functions and self-care activities that are too strenuous to increase chances to compliance with activity restrictions • Suggest that woman maintain an activity log that records activities, time, duration, intensity and physiologic responses to evaluate effectiveness of and adherence to activity programe • Discuss various quick diversional activities which could be done by the woman to decrease the potential boredom during the rest period.	
Risk for ineffective therapeutic regimen management related to woman's first pregnancy and perceived sense of wellness.		Woman will participate in an effective therapeutic regimen for pregnancy complicated heart disease.	• Ideology factors, such as insufficient knowledge about the effect of cardiac disease on pregnancy which could inhibit the woman from participating in therapeutic regimen to promote early intervention such as teaching about importance of rest. • Teach woman and family about factors such as lack of rest, or not taking prescribed medications that could adversely affect the pregnancy to provide information and promote empowerment over the situation.	

Contd...

Contd...

Problem	*Reason*	*Objective*	*Nursing intervention*	*Evaluation*
			• Encourage expression of feelings about the disease and its potential effect on the pregnancy to promote a sense of trust • Identify resources in the community to provide shared sense of common experiences • Encourage woman to verbalize her plan for carrying out the regimens of care to evaluate the effects of teaching	
Decreased cardiac output related to increased circulatory volume secondary to pregnancy and cardiac diseases.		Women will exhibit signs of adequate cardiac output (normal pulse, blood pressure, normal heart and breath, sound, normal skin colour, tone and turger normal capillary refill normal urine output and no evidence of oedema.	• Reinforce the importance of activity/rest cycles, to prevent cardiac complications • Plan with woman a frequent visit schedule to caregiver to provide adequate surveillance of high-risk pregnancy. • Teach woman to lie in lateral position to increase utero-placental blood flow and to elevate legs while sitting to promote venous return. • Monitor intake and output and check for oedema to assess for reveal complications or venous return problems. • Measure FHR and foetal activity, perform NST as indicated to assess foetal status and detect utero-placental insufficiency.	

treated for heart failure. They are kept in hospital until at least three weeks after delivery. In this grade, patients have inability to carry any physical anxiety without discomfort. Symptoms of cardiac insufficiency or angina may be present even at rest, and are intensified by activity.

Nursing Intervention

The antenatal supervision of patients with cardiac disease is of great importance. Anaemia and signs of pre-eclampsia should be looked for. Signs of infection should be watched for on infection may bring about cardiac failure. Subacute bacterial endocarditis is a frequent complication of valvular heart disease. It may occur during pregnancy or lead to the suspicion of their serious condition and a report must at once be made to the physician. Subacute bacterial endocarditis is treated with massive doses of penicillin or any recent antibiotics can be prescribed for it.

All pregnant women with heart diseases should be managed in obstetric units with multidisciplinary approach involving nurses, midwives, obstetricians, cardiologists and anaesthetists. During the antenatal period, women with heart diseases are often monitored more frequently than heavy pregnant women and monitor the foetal well being with:

- Ultrasound examination to confirm gestational age and congenital abnormality
- Assessment of foetal growth and amniotic fluids volume both clinically and by ultrasound
- Monitoring foetal heart rate by CTG
- Measurement of foetal and placental blood flow indices by Doppler ultrasonography.

The nurse can give advice with regard to modifying and adjusting physical activity during pregnancy. Consideration must also be given to the emotional stress and other psychological support. And also prompt dietary advice, and the aspects of prevention of infusion also emphasized.

In the management of labour, the following points must be borne in mind:

- The first stage of labour should not be allowed to exhaust the patient. Liberal doses, if but not indiscriminate use of analgesics should be encouraged in the first stage of labour. The patients in Grade II and IV should be propped up to prevent orthopnea. Inhalation analgesia such as trilene, or gas and air mixutes should be avoided by the nurses or midwives. A forceps trolley should be prepared. Maintaining fluid balance, pain relief, positioning are very important. Proper method of induction of labour can be used accordingly.
- The second stage of labour should not be long. Thus when the cervix is fully dilated and the head is visible in the vagina, the doctor must be informed. Labour is, as a rule, quick in the cardiac patients but nurse should report any delay in the first or second stage of labour. A prophylactic forceps delivery early in the second stage of labour minimizes the exhaustion of the patient.
- The routine use of ergometrine should be avoided in cardiac cases as this may lead to heart failure. Ergometrine should only be used if there is postpartum haemorrhage.
- After delivery, patient may collapse as a result of heart failure and the need for adequate supervision cannot be over stressed. The pulse and blood pressure should be checked at regular intervals. Breathlessness cough, etc. should be looked for any abnormality should at once be reported to the concerned physician. Breast feeding should be encouraged where possible, because the strain of artificial feeds may be too much for the cardiac patient without home help. In addition patient may not be able to afford the artificial milk. In developing countries with a high degree of illiteracy, the standard of preparation of artificial feeds may fall short of the minimum accepted hygienic requirement and the infant may develop diarrhoeal diseases because of contamination of its feeds. Signs of infection should be looked for in the puerperium. These should be reported to the physician.

When discharging cardiac patient from the wards/hospital, adequate arrangement for home health care should be made and they are given appointment for postnatal clinic. Patients with severe cardiac disease should be advised against future pregnancies. Contraceptive advice should be given. In the not so severe cases, it may be necessary to advise spacing of the children so as to avoid frequent repeated pregnancies. Two or three years between pregnancies should be advised. The woman and her husband will need to discuss the implications of future pregnancy with the cardiologist and obstetrician. Following this, the nurse can provide advice in the woman and her husband/partner about contraception.

HYPERTENSION IN PREGNANCY

Hypertension is most common medical complications of pregnancy. In its most severe form, the condition is associated with convulsions, proteinuria and edema and may lead to maternal death. In its mildest form, hypertension alone in later pregnancy. It appears to be of minimal risk.

Hypertension is defined as a systolic pressure of at least 140 mmHg or a diastolic pressure of at least 90 mmHg on two or more occasions after 20 weeks of pregnancy. The hypertensive disorders of pregnancy encompass a variety of conditions featuring an elevation of maternal blood pressure with a corresponding risk to maternal and foetal well being.

Classification

Working group on high blood pressure in pregnancy describes five categories of hypertension during pregnancy.

Chronic Hypertension

Chronic hypertension is known hypertension before pregnancy or a rise in blood pressure more than 140/90 mm Hg before 20 weeks gestation and persisting 6 weeks after delivery.

Gestational Hypertension

Gestational hypertension is the development of hypertension without other signs of pre-eclampsia. It is diagnosed, when after resting the woman's blood pressure rises above 140/90 mmHg on at least two occasions, no more than 1 week apart after the 20th week of pregnancy in a woman known to be normotensive. Hypertension that is diagnosed for the first time in pregnancy and that does not resolve postpartum is also classified as gestational hypertension.

Pre-eclampsia

Pre-eclampsia is diagnosed on the basis of hypertension with proteinuria, when proteinuria measured as above 1 on dipstick or above 0.3 g/L of protein in a random clean catch specimen or an excretion of 0.3 g protein per 24 hours.

In the absence of proteinuria, pre-eclampsia is suspected when hypertension is accompanied by symptoms including headache, blurred vision, abdominal/epigastric pain, or altered biochemistry, specifically low platelet count and abnormal liver enzyme levels (ALT, AGT, GGT).

Eclampsia

Eclampsia is defined as the new onset of convulsions during pregnancy or post-partum, unrelated to other cerebral pathological conditions in woman with pre-eclampsia.

Pre-eclampsia Superimposed on Chronic Hypertension

Pre-eclampsia superimposed on chronic hypertension may occur in woman with pre-existing hypertension (< 20 weeks gestation) who develop:

- New proteinuria (> 0.3 g/24 hours)
- Sudden increase in pre-existing hypertension and proteinuria
- Thrombocytopenia (Platelet count< 100 < 105—L)
- Abnormal liver enzyme.

Clinically, there are two basic types of hypertension during pregnancy—chronic hypertension and pregnancy- induced hypertension (PIH) with the distinction based on the onset of hypertension in relation to pregnancy, chronic hypertension is hypertension that predates the pregnancy or hypertension continuing beyond 42 day postpartum. Pregnancy induced hypertension is the onset of hypertension generally after the 20th week of pregnancy, appearing as marker of a pregnancy specific vasospastic condition. Both may occur independently or simultaneously.

Pregnancy induced hypertension (PIH) further classified according to the maternal organ system affected.

Pre-eclampsia

Mild: Pre-eclampsia is a pregnancy specific condition in which, hypertension develops after 20 weeks of gestation in a previously normaly tension women, is a multisystem, vasospastic disease process characterized by haemoconcentration, hypertension and proteinuria. Proteinuria: a concentration of 0.1 g/L (1+ to 2+) on dipstick measurement or more at least two random urine specimen collected at least 6 hour apart.

Pathologic oedema is clinically evident, generalized accumulation of fluid of the face, hands or abdomen that is not responsive to few hours bed rest. It may also be manifested as rapid we eight gain of more than 2 kg in 1 week. The presence of oedema is no longer considered for the diagnosis of pre-eclampsia.

In *severe pre-eclampsia* the presence of any one of the following in the woman diagnoses pre-eclampsia:

- Systolic blood pressure of at least 160 mmHg or a diastolic blood pressure of at least 110 mmHg.
- Proteinuria of greater than 0.5g protein excreted in 24 hours specimen or greater than 3+ to 4+ on dipstick measurement
- Oliguria, less than 400 to 500 ml of urine output over 24 hours
- Cerebral or visual disturbances such as altered level of consciousness, headache, scotomata, or blurred vision
- Hepatic involvement
- Thrombocytopenia with a platelet count less than 1,50,000/ mm^3
- Pulmonary cardiac involvement, or
- Epigastric pain, nausea, vomiting.

HELLP syndrome is laboratory diagnosis for a variant of severe pre-eclampsia characterized by haemolysis (H) elevated liver enzyme (EL) and low platelet (LP).

Eclampsia

Eclampsia is the occurrence of seizures or coma in a patient with pre-eclampsia that cannot be attributed to other causes. Approximately, half of all cases of eclampsia occurs before labour begins with the other half equally divided between the intrapartum and postpartum period.

Chronic Hypertension

Chronic hypertension is the hypertension present before the pregnancy or diagnosed before the 20th week of gestation. Hypertension that persists longer than 6 weeks postpartum is also classified as chronic hypertension.

Chronic Hypertension with Superimposed Pre-eclampsia

Woman with chronic hypertension may acquire pre-eclampsia or eclampsia. Superimposed pre-eclampsia is the development of proteinuria (0.5 g. Protein or more in 24 hr. specimen) and an increase in blood pressure (30 mmHg systole or 15 mmHg diastolic) in woman with chronic hypertension.

Gestational Hypertension

Gestational hypertension is the development of hypertension during pregnancy (often 37 weeks of gestation) without other signs of pre-eclampsia or pre-existing hypertension. It is the most common cause of hypertension in pregnancy. The incidence is higher in multipara and in twin gestation.

Effects of Hypertension on Pregnancy

Pre-eclampsia progresses along a continuum from mild disease to severe pre-eclampsia, HELLP syndrome, or eclampsia. The pathophysiology of pre-eclampsia reflects alterations in the normal adaptations of pregnancy. Normal adaptations include increased blood plasma, volume, vasodilation, decreased systemic vascular resistance, elevated cardiac output and decreased colloid osmotic pressure. Pathologic changes in the endothelial cells of glomeruli (glomerulo-endotheheliosis) seen in pre-eclampsia. Particularly in multipara. There will be poor perfusion as a result of vasospasm. Arteriolar vasospasm diminished the diameter of blood vessels, which impedes blood flow to all organs and rises blood pressure. Functions in organs such as the placenta. Kidneys, liver and brain is depressed leads to many problems.

Essential hypertension can cause an increase in maternal morbidity. The higher the level of blood pressure at the commencement of pregnancy, the worse the prognosis. The younger the patient, the worse is the outlook. When the blood pressure is very high, e.g. 160/100 mmHg or more, the patient may develop albuminuria and frank pre-eclampsia may set in. In some cases a very high level of blood pressure causes cerebral haemorrhage which may be fatal. In addition, occasionally, a very high blood pressure may later in pregnancy cause concealed accidental haemorrhage (abruptio placentae) and this may lead to renal complications, particularly acute renal failure.

The effect on the foetus may be serious. The worse the hypertension, the higher the incidence of abortion, intra-uterine death of the foetus and premature onset of labour. In cases complicated by pre-eclampsia, eclampsia or abruptio placentae, more than half of the pregnant women thus afflicated lose their babies. Thus it can be seen that this is a serious condition which the midwife should never undertake to manage on her own.

Management

The essential point in the management of hypertension in pregnancy is bed rest. This is nearly as important as, if not more important than, the use of hypotensive drugs. Adequate rest during the day and a good sleep at night must be ensured. These can be accomplished by the use of sedatives such as sodium amytal (200 mg 6 or 8 hourly). The nurse should realize that sedatives have little or no effect on hypertension. Their usefulness lies in removing fears and anxieties and, thereby, ensuring adequate sleep. During the day, the patient should remain for most of the time in bed, but occasionally she should be allowed to sit in a comfortable chair to relax. The medical management of hypertension in pregnancy depends on the severity of the case. In mild and moderate cases, the patient may, in addition to the sedatives, be given hypotensive drugs. The hypotensive drugs usually prescribed are reserpine (0.5 mg to 0.75 mg daily), guanethidine (10-25 mg initially, rising to a maximum dose of 150 mg daily) and methyl-dopa (250 mg thrice daily) or any recent drugs prescribed for the same.

The blood pressure is checked at least twice daily, and in severe cases it is checked at 4 hourly or 2 hourly intervals.

When the blood pressure is unusually high (e.g. 200/120 mm Hg the patient should be heavily sedated and should be nursed in a cool quiet, slightly darkened room in order to prevent the occurrence of a fit.

Obstetric Management

Patients with essential hypertension are not allowed to carry their pregnancies beyond term. In the mild to moderate cases, labour is induced by artificial rupture of membranes at about 38-48 weeks. In severe cases labour is induced at about 36 weeks and if progress is slow, labour is terminated by caesarean section to avoid eclampsia.

Investigations

These include routine testing of the urine for albumin. A midstream specimen of urine is examined microscopically for evidence of pus cells and sent to the bacteriological laboratory for culture of organisms and sensitivity. When there is albuminuria, a twenty four hour collection of urine is made for the purpose of estimating the total amount of protenuria, of Esbach's albuminometer is used to estimate the quantity of albumin in the urine. Renal function tests are carried out to determine the degree of kidney involvement. The blood urea is checked oedema is looked for and the patient is weighed twice weekly.

Pre-eclamptic Toxaemia (Pre-eclampsia)

This is a condition occurring after the 28th week of gestation, characterized by the presence of any two of the following signs.

1. Oedema or excessive gain in weight
2. Hypertension
3. Albuminuria.

Of these signs, albuminuria is usually the last to occur and its occurence may mean a worsening of the condition because of impaired renal function.

Causes of Pre-eclampsia

Many theories have been advanced for the aetiology of pre-eclampsia but without adequate support. One thing that it may be certain about is that pre-eclamptic toxaemia is not caused by toxins.

From the nurse's point of view, it should suffice to know that pre-eclampsia is more commonly seen in the following types of patients:

a. Primigravida, usually the short obese woman with short study finger very young primigravidae (e.g. 14 years of age); elderly primigravida (35 years and over).
b. Any patient with overdistension of the abdomen, as in a multiple pregnancy and hydramnios.
c. A patient with severe hypertension in pregnancy.
d. A diabetic patient.
e. A patient suffering from chronic nephritis.
f. A patient with hydatidiform mole.

Diagnosis of Pre-eclampsia

The diagnosis is made when a patient who has previously been known to have any of the signs (i.e. excessive weight gain or oedema, hypertension and albuminuria) suddenly develops any two of them.

Weight gain and oedema: After the 28th week of pregnancy, a weight gain of 0.45 kg per week is usually accepted as normal. Anything much in excess of this constitutes excessive weight gain and must be taken seriously by the nurse midwife, even in the absence of pitting oedema.

Pitting oedema is best felt over the ankles (the medial maleolus, the lower end of the tibia) and the dorsum of the foot, the abdomen (e.g. the indentation made by a foetal stethoscope), the fingers (for example, a very light or non-fitting wedding ring), the face and, in patients who have been lying down for a long time, the sacral region. The greatest the depression made by the pressure of the finger the worse the oedema. Even in the absence of hypertension and albuminuria, gross pitting oedema or excessive weight gain (e.g. 1 to 1.5 kg in one week) should be taken as a serious indication for admission of the patient to hospital.

Hypertension A blood pressure of 140/90 mmHg or above is regarded as hypertension. If, however, there is a big rise in blood pressure, though the level of 140/90 mmHg has not been reached. Rising blood pressure is also significant. A patient with a blood pressure reading of 90/50 at one attendance, then 100/60, 110/70, 120/70 mmHg in subsequent visits should be closely watched and advised on rest and restricted salt intake.

Nurses should be aware that a blood pressure of 130/80 mmHg is significant between the 16th and 30th week when the usual fall in blood pressure occurs.

Albuminuria: This is usually the last sign to appear and it usually implies renal involvement. All patient in whom albuminuria is present along with one other sign should be admitted to hospital.

Management of Pre-eclampsia (Table 8.3)

Every patient with signs of pre-eclampsia must be referred by the midwife/nurse to the physician, preferably one working in a big hospital with facilities for adequate and proper management of the case. A midwife/working in a rural community may have difficulty in convincing a patient to travel to a hospital in an urban district where she probably known nobody. The patients with pre-eclampsia often feel well and, therefore, see very little need for hospitalization.

However, a majority of the patients are admitted to the hospital for bed rest which is of paramount importance in the management of pre-eclampsia. The patients generally find it difficult to rest well at home because of their domestic commitments. Moreover, rest at home is not advisable because a close observation of the patient is not possible.

To ensure adequate rest, the midwife has the responsibility of seeing that the patient spends most of her time in bed. She may be allowed up to the toilet if her case is mild. Fear, anxiety and worry do not make for proper rest. Thus the midwife/nurse should eliminate orally these in her patient through careful counselling and advice. The help of a medical social worker may be sought if there are problems beyond the midwife/nurse's scope. Sedatives such as phenobarbitone (30-60 mg given thrice daily) keep the patient calm during the day. Sodium amytal (200 mg) is given at night to ensure adequate sleep. Severe cases of pre-eclampsia may be given sodium amytal (200 mg) at six to eight hourly intervals. The usefulness of hypotensive drugs in the management of pre-eclampsia is uncertain. However, it is believed that these drugs lower the blood pressure with subsequent improvement of placental circulation and foetal prognosis. Diuretics such as hydroflumethiazide may be used to reduce massive oedema, but they improve neither the pre-eclampsia not the prognosis for the foetus.

Observation

Observation in order to assess the patient's response to treatment, the following records are kept:

a. The blood pressure is measured at least twice daily but a four-hourly record is kept in severe cases of pre-eclampsia (Fig. 8.15)
b. The urine is tested daily for albumin. Esbach's quantitative test for albumin is done if the patient has albuminuria.
c. A fluid chart is kept to exclude oliguria (a possible complication of pre-eclampsia). Illiterate ambulant patients should be advised to pass the urine into a graduated jug or into a bed pan and show this to the nurse for measuring and recording.
d. The patient is examined daily for the presence of oedema. She is also weighed twice weekly to exclude occult oedema.

Table 8.3: Nursing care plan of mild pre-eclampsia (at home)

Problem	*Reason*	*Objective*	*Nursing intervention*	*Evaluation*
Risk for injury related to signs of pre-eclampsia	(SOAP)	Patient will demonstrate ability to assess self and foetus for signs of worsening pre-eclampsia; no adverse sequale will occur as a as a result of pre-eclamptic conditions	• Review warning signs and symptoms of pre-eclampsia to ensure adequate knowledge base exists for decision making • Assess home environment, including woman's ability to assume self-care responsibilities, support systems, language, age culture, beliefs and effects of illness to determine home care in viable option • Teach woman how to do a self-assessment of clinical signs of pre-eclampsia (take and record blood pressure, measure, urine protein, maintain daily weight lag, assess edema formation, assess foetal activity) to provide immediate evidence of worsening condition • Teach woman to report any increase in blood pressure, +2 proteinuria, weight gain, greater than 1 lb per week, presence of oedema, and decreased foetal activity to her health care provider to prevent worsening of pre-eclamptic condition. • Teach woman about use of rest and relaxation as palliative treatment options to decrease blood pressure and promote diuresis.	
Fear/Anxiety related to Pre-eclampsia and its effect in the fetus	S* O*	Patient's feelings and symptoms of fear/anxiety will decrease	• Provide a calm, soothing atmosphere and teach family to provide emotional support to facilitate coping. • Encourage verbalization of fears to decrease intensity of emotional response • Involve woman and family in the management of her pre-eclamptic condition to promote greater sense of control. • Help woman identify and use appropriate coping strategies and support systems to reduce fear/anxiety. • Explore use of densitization strategies, such as progressive muscle relaxation, visual imagery, or thought stopping, to reduce fear related emotions and related physical symptoms.	
Deficient diversional activity related to imposed bed rest	S* O*	Patient will verbalize diminished feelings of boredom.	• Assist woman to explore creatively personally meaningful activities that can be pursued from the bed to ensure that have meaning, purpose and value to the individual. • Maintain emphasis on personal choices of woman to promote control and minimize imposition of routines by others. • Evaluate what support and system resources are available in the environment to assest in providing diversional activities. • Explore ways for women to remain an active participant in home management and decision to promote control. • Engage support of family and friends in carrying out chosen activities and making necessary environmental alterations to ensure success • Teach woman about stress management and relaxation techniques to help manage tension of confinement.	

** S = Subjective data, O = Objective data A = Assessment, P = Plan*

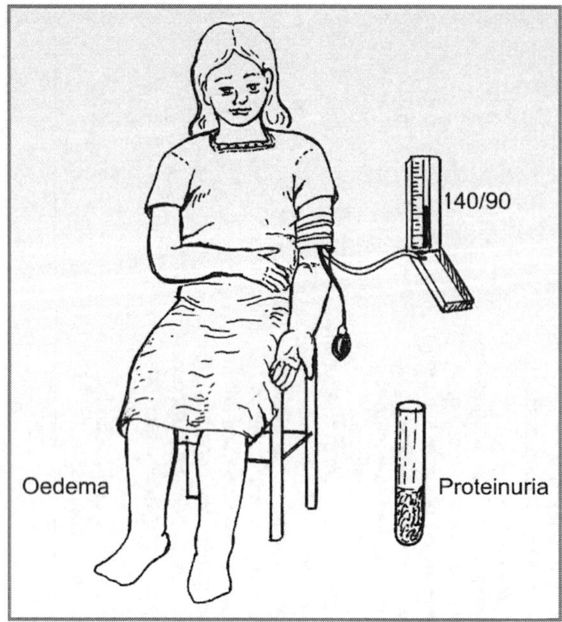

Fig. 8.15: The signs of pre-eclampsia include hypertension, proteinuria and oedema

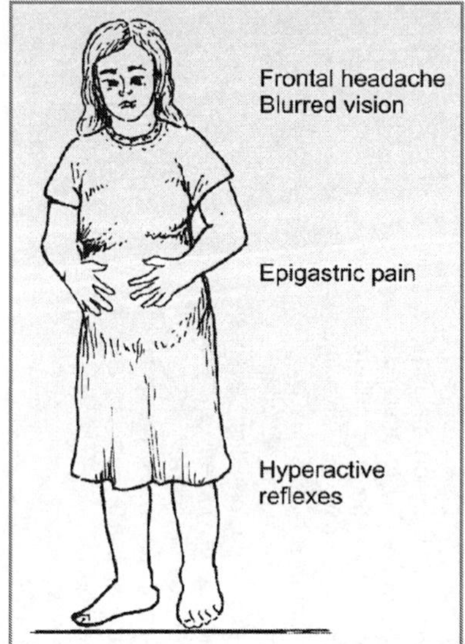

Fig. 8.16: Presenting signs of eclampsia

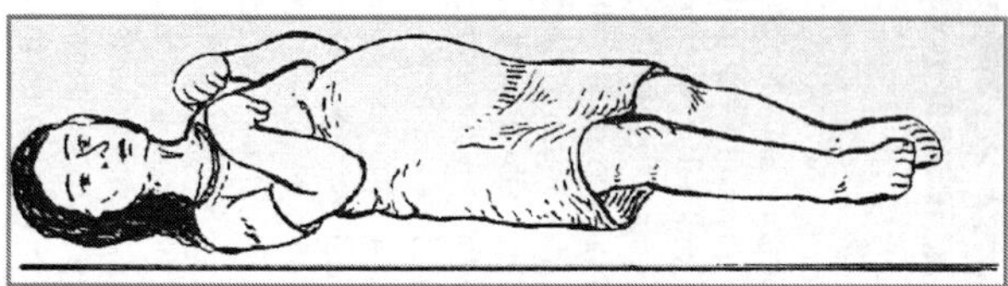

Fig. 8.17: The differentiating feature of eclampsia is the development of convulsions

e. Abdominal examination is done twice daily. The foetal heart sounds are auscultated. Placental insufficiency should be suspected if the foetus feels very small in comparison to its gestational age. Presence of abdominal pain in a pre-eclamptic patient could donate:
   i. Massive abruptio placentae, in which case the pain is constant and excruciating, the uterus is tender and board-like.
   ii. Onset of labour, in this case the pain is intermittent and other signs of labour will be present.
   iii. Deterioration of the condition leads to pain in the epigastric region and is described by the patient as acute indigestion pain. This is a sign of imminent eclampsia and must not be ignored.

Serious Signs and Symptoms (Figs 8.16 to 8.18)

The nurse midwife must be constantly on the alert for the development of serious signs and symptoms which often herald eclampsia. These signs and symptoms are:

1. Sudden sharp rise in the blood pressure.
2. Increasing oedema and albuminuria.
3. Diminished urinary output.
4. Severe headache, usually frontal.

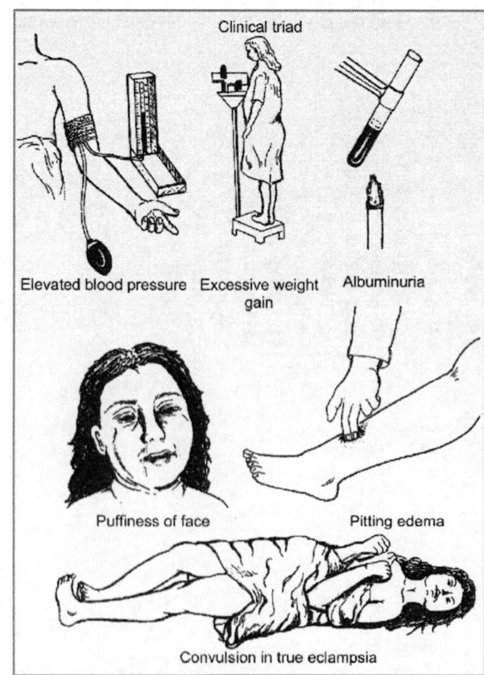

Fig. 8.18: Symptomatology of pre-eclampsia and eclampsia

5. Visual disturbance, e.g. dimness or blurring of vision, flashes of light, coloured spangles.
6. Epigastric pain.
7. Vomiting.
8. Drowsiness.

The physician must be informed immediately and a heavy sedative must be given at once. The patient should from thence be nursed as an eclamptic patient in a quiet corner of the ward, in a separate side room or in a special eclamptic room.

Routine Nursing Care

Routine care of the patient includes the four-hourly recordings of temperature, pulse and respiration, care of the bowels and prevention of constipation. Bed washes or baths if the patient is confined to bed are also carried out. It is debatable if reduction of salt in the patient's diet has any therapeutic value in pre-eclampsia. Where reduced salt intake is advocated, the patient is instructed not to add extra salt to her food at table. In non-catering hospitals, the midwife/nurse should instruct the relatives to use salt sparingly in cooking. Food such as tinned and smoked fish, sausage meat, cheese and Bovril contain high amounts of salt and should be avoided. A high protein diet is recommended for patients with low haemoglobin. It is also advisable to give oral iron and folic acid. Daraprim (25 mg) is given weekly to prevent malaria.

Investigations

Patients with pre-eclampsia admitted to big hospitals usually have the following investigations carried out:

a. Blood urea.
b. Total albuminuria in 24 hours.
c. Serum cholesterol.
d. Renal function tests.
e. Liver function tests.
f. The packed cell volume is checked at regular intervals.

Unbooked cases have these additional investigations done:

a. Chest X-ray to exclude tuberculosis.
b. Blood group and Rhesus factor.
c. Haemoglobin genotype.

Termination of Pregnancy

It is important that no patient with pre-eclampsia should be allowed to carry her pregnancy beyond term, because of placental insufficiency. As a rule, labour is induced at about 38-40 weeks. When serious signs manifest and there is no apparent response to treatment after 48 hours, pregnancy is terminated. Surgical induction of labour is often carried out. Intravenous Pitocin drip may be preferred in elderly primigravidae or for cases of failed induction of labour.

Care of Pre-eclamptic Patient in Labour

The risk of pre-eclamptic patient having eclamptic fits is higher during labour. As such, adequate sedation of the patient is necessary. A vigilant observation is made on the blood pressure and foetal heart sounds which are taken and recorded at least hourly. Every urine specimen is tested for albumin. Enemas may not be given to patients with severe pre-eclampsia. The use of nitrous oxide and air is contraindicated for fear of foetal hypoxia. Gas and oxygen or trilene is safe. An episiotomy may be made or a low forceps delivery carried out in the second stage of labour to avoid fits occurring from the effort and strain of pushing. At the completion of labour the blood pressure is taken. An hourly recording of blood pressure is imperative. Heavy sedation in the form of sodium amytal (200-500 mg) is given intramuscularly to prevent postpartum eclampsia. Sedation is repeated at 6 to 9 or 8 hourly intervals until the patient is out of danger. When there is a marked reduction in the level of the blood pressure the patient is transferred to a lying in ward. She is nursed in a single room or a quiet corner in the ward. Phenobarbitone (60 mg) may be given thrice daily and sodium amytal (200 mg) is given at night. The blood pressure is recorded four-hourly for 24 hours then twice a day and finally daily.

Outcome of a Pregnancy Complicated by Pre-eclampsia

The outcome of pregnancy depends on the severity of the condition. Mild cases usually end well for the mother and baby if very good antenatal and intranatal care is ensured. The following material complications may occur in severe cases:

1. Eclamptic fits.
2. Abruptio placentae.
3. Cerebral haemorrhage.
4. Oliguria or anuria resulting from acute renal failure.

The foetal complications are:

1. Intrauterine death may result from placental insufficiency. This will lead to the delivery of a macerated still born baby. Still birth may also result from severe abruptio placentae but in this case the foetus may not necessarily be macerated.
2. Neonatal death associated with prematurity or severe intrauterine hypoxia may occur.

Eclampsia (Fig. 8.18)

Eclampsia means fits. It is a condition characterized by repeated fits which may endanger the patient's life if nothing is done in good time. It may result from a severe pre-eclampsia, or it may arise suddenly without any previous evidence of pre-eclampsia. In the latter case, the patient's blood pressure may show a sudden sharp rise followed by the aura and later the fits characteristic of eclampsia.

An eclamptic fit may be preceded by what is usually referred to as warning signs. These are:

1. Failure of pre-eclampsia to improve, i.e. increasing hypertension, oedema and albuminuria as well as diminished urinary output (oliguria)
2. Visual disturbances, i.e Double vision, flashes of light in the eyes rolling of the eyes
3. Severe frontal headache
4. Epigastric pain
5. Vomiting.

There are four stages to an eclamptic fit. These are listed below:

1. *Premonitory stage:* In this stage, the patient may fall unconscious. She rolls her eyes and the head is drawn to one side. She may have twitching in the muscles of the face and hands. This stage lasts about 20-30 seconds.
2. *Tonic stage:* The patient becomes rigid because, there is generalized contraction of the muscles of the body. The teeth and fists are cleanched, eyes staring, the feet are inverted with the toes flexed. There is respiratory arrest with cyanosis. This state lasts about 30 seconds and is followed by the next stage.
3. *Clonic stage:* This is a stage during which the muscles relax and contract alternately. There is a great deal of jerky body movement and the patient can easily be thrown out of bed if not supervised. The alternate opening and closing of the jaw may cause the patient to injure her tongue by biting it. A great deal of blood-stained frothy saliva is produced in unconscious state. The respiration is laboured and noisy. The patient's face is usually congested and distorted. This stage lasts about one or two minutes. During the eclamptic fit, a great deal of energy is generated, the temperature may rise to as high as 40°C and the blood pressure may be very high. The pulse is full and bounding.
4. *Coma:* The patient soon goes into coma after the tonic stage. She becomes deeply unconscious and her breathing is stertorous. The coma may be punctuated by one or two fits before the patient recovers.

Varieties of Eclampsia

Eclampsia can occur in pregnancy (antepartum eclampsia), in labour (intrapartum eclampsia) and after delivery (postpartum eclampsia). Ante and postpartum eclampsia may be very severe. A majority of cases of postpartum eclampsia occurring four weeks or more after delivery may not be true cases of eclampsia but may be due to severe brain damage as a result of hypertension.

Management of Eclampsia

An eclamptic fit constitutes an obstetrical emergency demanding urgent and effective treatment to prevent death. The management is aimed at the prevention of further fits and expediting delivery. The pregnancy is almost invariably terminated, for the patient may go into labour during the fit, or labour may be induced to prevent recurrence of fits which may cause cerebral damage to the mother, foetal hypoxia and intrauterine death of the foetus.

First Aid Management

During a fit, the patient must not be held down but her head should be turned to one side and objects which are likely to cause injury should be removed. If possible a padded spatula or spoon is placed between the teeth to prevent injury to the patient's tongue. At the end of the fit, the foam or froth from the patient's mouth is wiped off and the nasopharynx is aspirated. Oxygen, if available, should be given and a rubber airway may be used to keep the tongue in position and thus maintain a clear airway. The patient must be sedated to prevent further fits. A midwife on her own may give any sedation at her disposal. This could be chloral hydrate (3 grams given rectally), or paraldehyde

(8-10 ml intramuscularly). Pethidine may be the best sedative available to midwives practising in some rural districts. In such cases, the midwife may give pethidine (100 mg) and, if possible, Largactil (50 mg intramuscularly). When the patient has been sedated, the midwife must hourly intervals. The foetal heart sounds are auscultated. It is worth ascertaining if the patient is in labour. Restlessness in spite of heavy sedation is indicative of uterine contractions: so the midwife must feel for the contractions.

Arrangements are then made to transfer the patient to a hospital if the fit occurred on the district. The midwife must accompany the patient to the hospital and take with her, on the journey the following:

1. Delivery bag.
2. Sterile gauze swabs.
3. Sponge-holding forceps.
4. Mouth gag.
5. Tongue forceps and tongue depressor.
6. Mucous extractor.

These may not be available in some rural maternity centres. In such cases, the midwife takes her delivery bag, a padded spoon or spatula, towel and a bowl in case the patient vomits. In addition sedative drugs are taken because the nearest hospital may be 80 km away. In some situations, the midwife may work single-handed and may be faced with the difficult decision of accompanying the patient and leaving her station, or remaining in her station and sending the patient with a relative no medical knowledge.

If possible the hospital should be informed to expect the patient. In places where the services of an ambulance are not available, suitable public transport is hired and the driver is ordered to drive slowly. It may be useful if the patient's ears are plugged with cotton wool so that the noise of the traffic does not precipitate more fits.

Preparation for the Reception of the Patient

Ideally, a quiet, slightly darkened room, kept very cool in the corner of labour wards in each hospital should be reserved for the nursing of eclamptic patients. Where this is not available, a bed should be got ready in a quiet corner of the ward. The sides of the bed should be padded and the head end should be padded with two pillows in a drawsheet.

Other things to get ready in the room or at the bed sides are: suction apparatus; oxygen and face mask; anaesthetic tray with spatula, airway swab-holder and gauze swabs; oral hygiene tray; things for intravenous injection and infusion; rectal tray with fine catheter for rectal administration of Avertin; catheterization tray and Aldon bag's or Winchester's bottle for draining the bladder; sphygmomanometer, binaural stethoscope. Pinard's foetal heart stethoscope; thermometer and pulsometer; blocks for raising the foot of the bed when necessary; tray for vaginal examination. It is advisable to get ready in the room a delivery trolley with Wrigley's forceps, cot and equipment for the resuscitation of the baby because the patient is often delivered in the room in which she is nursed.

Reception of the Patient at the Hospital

The nurse midwife should inform the physician as soon as the patient arrives at the hospital. If the fit occurred in the patient's home and she is brought into the hospital by her relatives, the midwife must obtain a history of the number of fits the patient has had, the resuscitative measures employed and any drug which might have been administered to the patient.

Medical Management

For the initial control of the fit in hospital, intravenous thiopentone (250 mg) is given slowly after making sure of a clear airway and good oxygenation of the patient. Tribromoethanol (Avertin) is used to maintain sedation. Avertin is given by rectal infusion and the dose is calculated according to the patient's weight. Usually 0.1 ml is given per kg body weight, an average dose of 5 ml diluted with water at 40°C to a strength of 1-40 will make the patient sleep quietly for 3-4 hours. Further sedation may be maintained by repetition of the dose of Avertin or by the use of lytic cocktail in the form of chloropromazine (largactil) (50 mg) promethazine (Phenergan) (50 mg) and pethidine (100 mg) intramuscularly at six-hourly intervals.

Sodium amytal (500 mg) intramuscularly may also be given 4 to 6 hourly. However, the prescribing of drugs is the physician responsibility, but the midwife must report to the physician when the patient shows any sign of restlessness. Effects of drugs often wear off in 3 to 4 hours so another dose is usually given after this period. Magnesium sulphate is at times used in the management of eclampsia. It has a diuretic action thereby relieving cerebral oedema and controll in convulsions; 20 ml of a 20 percent solution of magnesium sulphate could be given intravenously or intramuscularly every 6 hours.

Other drugs: Antibiotics, e.g. procaine penicillin (600000 units) are administered intramuscularly daily to combat chest infection. Sometimes the use of broad spectrum antibiotics such as tetracycline, given intramuscularly because the patient is unconscious, is preferable to penicillin.

Hydration intravenous infusion of 5 per cent glucose is given for the period the patient is unconscious and does not take oral fluids. The total fluid given in 24 hours should not exceed 2,000 ml. The amount should be reduced in the presence of pulmonary oedema and in oliguric patients. Now tribromethanol (*Avertin*) has been withdrawn from the market and also its rectal infusion.

Nursing Intervention

Good nursing care is a necessary factor in saving the patient's life. The patient should never be left unattended for she might have a fit of roll out of bed while still unconscious.

The midwife should go about her duties quietly. The treatment of the patient should be planned to commence about half an hour after the administration of a sedative.

Clear airway: Because the patient is unconscious, secretions from the bronchi and saliva must be sucked out frequently to maintain a clear airway. The patient is nursed in a semi-prone position, obliquely across the bed with her head to one side towards the edge of the mattress. In this position, there is less risk of inhalation of mucus and saliva. The patient is turned at 2 hourly intervals to avoid hypostatic congestion of the lungs.

Oral hygiene: The mouth and nostrils should be cleansed after fit or at 4 hourly intervals to avoid hypostatic congestion of the lung care of the bladder. A self retaining catheter is used to drain the bladder into an Aldon's bag or Winchester's bottle. The bag or bottle is emptied hourly and the amount of urine is measured. A specimen of the urine is collected via the catheter into a receiver and urinalysis is done twice daily. An Esbach's albuminometer is set up twice daily or as ordered by the physician to assess the amount of albumin in the urine.

Care of the bowels: An enema should not be given to an eclamptic patient even if she is in labour. The patient usually takes nothing by mouth Dulcolax or glycerine suppositories may be used to evacuate the rectus.

Bed bathing: This should be done at least once daily when the patient has been well sedated. Pressure areas are treated 4 hourly and the patient face, hands and groins are sponged at the same time.

Diet: No oral fluid is given to the patient when she is unconscious, for the swallowing reflex may be absent and the fluid may run into the trachea. Any necessary fluid is given intravenously. However, as the patient recovers and regains consciousness, nourishing fluid (about 200 ml) may be offered 3 hourly. The patient is gradually weaned onto an easily digestible diet.

The midwife sitting with the patient should observe and note the following:

1. *Fits* The premonitory signs of eclampsia call for further sedation of the patient. The time of occurrence, length, severity and number of fits must be recorded.
2. *Signs of labour* These are restlessness or moaning accompanying uterine contractions; slight vaginal bleeding and rupture of membrane dilatation of the cervical os as revealed by vaginal examination.
3. The patient's general condition. This is assessed by the following:
   a. The pulse, respiration and blood pressure are usually taken and recorded half hourly; the arm band of the sphygmomanometer could be left on the patient's arm to avoid undue distrubance of the patient; the temperature is taken and recorded 4 hourly.
   b. The colour of the patient is also noted to exclude cyanosis and jaundice.
   c. The degree of oedema on the face, hands, feet, legs and sacrum should be assessed and recorded by a series of signs such as oedema of the feet.
   d. A fluid chart is kept for the record of the urinary output and fluid intake.
   e. The foetal heart sound is auscultated every half hour; any abnormal sign should be immediately reported to the physician.

The following signs are considered unfavourable and when they occur the doctor must be informed immediately:

1. A rise in the pulse rate, temperature and respiratory rate. These signs may indicate the onset of infection or cerebral haemorrhage.
2. Slow respiration may also be due to cerebral haemorrhage. Moist respiration often indicates pulmonary oedema.
3. A sharp rise or fall in the blood pressure. The fall in the blood pressure may be due to the drugs given or the death of the foetus and subsequent improvement in the women's condition.
4. Oliguria or anuria—These are highly suggestive of acute renal failure.
5. Presence of jaundice.
6. Frequent fits.

Most obstetricians think that after the control of fits, it is essential to deliver the patient by the quickest and safest method. A vaginal examination should be done to determine the state of the cervix and the adequacy of the pelvis. An amniotomy (rupture of the membranes) is performed if the cervix is ripse and the pelvis adequate. Intravenous Pitocin drip should also be given as an adjunct to amniotomy. In cases in which rupture of the membranes is unlikely to be fruitful, consideration is given to delivering the patient by caesarean section. Patients who progress satisfactorily in labour after surgical and/or medical induction, are usually delivered by forceps when the cervix is fully dilated.

Care after Delivery

The patient must continue to be supervised until the acute stage of the conditon is past and all unfavourable signs have disappeared. Sedatives are reduced as the blood pressure falls and the patient regains consciousness. Breastfeeding is not possible when the patient is still unconscious or drowsy. The breasts should be manually and impairment of vision may exist for a few days. The period of convalescence should be extended until the blood pressure is near normal and albuminuria clears.

Complications of Eclampsia

The patient is liable to injuries as a result of the violence of her fits. Blockage of the airways by blood stained saliva and mucus can cause severe asphyxia which may lead to death. The major causes of death are cardiac failure, cerebral haemorrhage, liver damage, and renal failure secondary to acute tubular necrosis or bilateral renal cortical necrosis.

The foetal prognosis is bad in eclampsia. The majority of babies are lost. The prognosis is further worsened in the presence of massive placental separation resulting in abruptio placentae.

INFECTIONS IN PREGNANCY

Diarrhoeal Diseases in Pregnancy

Diarrhoea may be caused by a variety of conditions. Patients usually refer to diarrhoea as dysentery, irrespective of the cause of the diarrhoea. All patients complaining of diarrhoea should be referred by the nurse to the physician. Although it is true that in some cases examination of the patient's stools to determine the cause of the diarrhoea is of vital importance.

Bacilliary Dysentery

In tropical countries bacillary dysentery may occur at any time of the year but it is most commonly encountered during the rainy season. House flies play an important role in the transmission of the infection. Poor sanitation and inadequate purification of drinking water contribute in no small measure to the spread of the disease.

The patient with bacillary dysentery is usually ill and toxic looking. There may be fever and the patient may pass blood stained mucous stools. In severe cases, there may be rapid destruction of the lining of the large bowels leading to death of the patient. When the disease is mild there may be only a simple diarrhoea with no blood or mucus.

Amoebic Dysentery

Amoebiasis is caused by *Entamoeba histolytica*. There are various types of amoebiasis, e.g. intestinal amoebiasis and hepatic amoebiasis. Pregnancy seems to influence the course of amoebiasis adversely. Consequently, the morbidity and mortality from amoebiasis are greater in the pregnant than in the nonpregnant women.

The symptoms of amoebic dysentery are almost similar to those of bacillary dysentery. In amoebic dysentery, however, there is much less abdominal tenderness than there is in bacillary dysentery. The diagnosis of both conditions can be made by examination of the stools.

The diarrhoeal diseases are important in pregnancy because they can cause abortion and premature labour, presumably by causing uterine contract one. Amoebic or bacillary dysentery may worsen the condition of patients who already have anaemia or malnutrition. Puerperal cases must be carefully look for and isolated. The danger of cross infection is a real one and newborn babies may be infected, with fatal outcome.

Treatment

Since dehydration may result from excessive diarrhoea, adequate fluid replacement should be ensured. Blood transfusion may be necessary in anaemic patients. Bacillary dysentery usually responds to sulphathiazole (2 grams initially and 1 gram six hourly for 5 days or more). Mist, Kaolin ET Morphine is given to diminish excessive bowel action.

Amoebic dysentery is treated by injections of emetine hydrochloride (60 mg daily for 10 days administered deep into the subcutaneous tissues or by intramuscular injection). This is followed by a course of EBI (emetine bismuth iodide, 200 mg daily for 10 days). Attention is paid to fluid replacement and treatment of anaemia. Metronidazole, (Flagyl) has been introduced in the treatment of amoebiasis (400 mg is given three times daily for 7 days).

Nursing Care of a Patient with Diarrhoeal Condition

As already dicussed, most of these conditions are infectious. The patient has to be nursed in an isolated ward or unit. Where this is not possible, she must be barrier nursed in a side room or at the end of the ward.

Pyrexia, dehydration, weakness and often prostration are the common features of these conditions. As such, the patient must be confined to bed and nursed as an ill patient. Temperature pulse rate and respiratory rate are recorded four-hourly. If the temperature is very high, the patient should be tepid sponged or fanned. Particular attention must be paid to the pulse of the patient on emetine. This drug causes weakness of the heart muscle thus making the pulse weak and thready. Often electrocardiography may be indicated in such cases and the physician will usually order one.

Where there is severe dehydration, the patient is given an intravenous infusion. Oral fluids should be encouraged in cases with less severe dehydration. Nourishing fluid rich in glucose and protein, as well as fruit juice should be offered. A fluid chart should be kept to assess the daily intake and output of the patient. Food, if tolerated, should be light and easily digestible. The serving of a large quantity at a time must be avoided and the meal should be attractive. Vitamins and iron are given to augment the diet.

Stools are disinfected with lysol (1-80) or carbolic lotion. The patient must be taught and encouraged to wash her hands after defaecation. The midwife too must wash her hands thoroughly. The bedpan must be sterilized and kept separate for the exclusive use of the patient. Faecal odour often gives the room an unpleasant smell. Windows should be left open to allow in fresh air and Airwick or air freshener may be used to counteract the bad odour.

Ambulation is encouraged as the patient's condition improves. When the stool specimen is negative (contains no organisms) the patient may mix freely with the other patients.

VIRAL DISEASES IN PREGNANCY

The important diseases in pregnancy caused by viruses are:

1. Rubella or German measles.
2. Measles or morbilli.
3. Smallpox (variola).
4. Chickenpox (varicella).
5. Viral hepatitis.
6. Common cold and influenza.

Rubella

Rubella is of importance because its occurrence before the 12th week of gestation may result in the birth of an abnormal baby. The abnormalities include mental deficiency, hare-lip, cleft palate, congenital cataract, deafness, mongolism, spina bifida and congenital heart disease and osteitis.

The nurse can recognize rubella by the help of the following:

1. A long incubation period lasting about 18 days.
2. The rash appears on the first day.
3. There are catarrhal symptoms such as redness of the conjunctiva, coughing and sneezing but these are not as serious as in measles (morbilli).

4. There is slight enlargement of the glands at the back of the neck and in the region of the occiput. Sometimes the glands in the axillary and inguinal regions are enlarged.

The diagnosis of rubella during pregnancy can be made on the clinical manifestation of the infection which includes a fine macular rash lymphadenopathy, in cervical region and mild pyrexia and confirmed by throat wash or from blood culture. Injection of g Globulin where contact with rubella has occurred may help to prevent infections.

Measles (Morbilli)

Infection a paramyxovirus with droplet transmission placental transmission, does occur, and may result in neonatal death and abortion.

Measles is important because of the possibility of the development of congenital foetal abnormalities, as listed under rubella, if the mother comes in contact with it, in the early weeks of pregnancy. The following points will help the nurses to recognize measles:

- The incubation period of 14 days
- The prodromal phase which is characterized by catarrh of the eyelids and the upper respiratory tract. This is evidenced by lacrimation, a running nose, coughing and sneezing
- The three or four days of high fever preceding the appearance of the rash
- The appearance of the rash on the fourth day The distribution of the rash behind the ears, along the hair margin of the forehead, temples and neck. The face is soon covered with the rash and later the whole body. The rash is usually more marked on the face and trunk than on the more distant parts of the body. It is macular type of rash
- The bluish-white Koplik's spots at the level of the upper molars further confirm the diagnosis. The glands at the back of the neck are not enlarged
- The typical circumoral pallor.

Smallpox (Variola)

Smallpox is a very serious complication of pregnancy. In an epidemic of smallpox, pregnant women are much worse than non-pregnant women of the same age group. Smallpox can lead to a very high incidence of maternal morbidity and mortality. The foetal loss rate is very high from abortions, prematurity, intrauterine death and early neonatal death due to congenital smallpox.

The nurse should recognize smallpox by the following points:

- The incubation period of 12-14 days
- The prodromal phase characterized by sudden occurrence of shivering and high fever (39-40°C), with severe headache and pain in the back. Vomiting, cough and bronchitis are common.

The patient is very ill, the tongue is furred and the conjunctiva is red. After two to three days, these symptoms disappear and the patient feels slightly better. Later the rash appears. The earliest lesions are often seen in the mouth. Sore throat results from the involvement of the larynx and pharynx.

At first the rash is macular, and later papular. The papular rash is hard and surrounded by a reddish area (or areola). The distribution of the rash is on the forehead, the front of the wrists and on the feet. Later, it reaches other parts of the body. Smallpox is an ostentatious disease. When it appears on the face, the rash is concentrated on the bony prominences such as the forehead, the malar eminence, the sides of the nose and the chin. In the upper limbs the rash is orominent on the ulnar and radial eminences of the wrists, the knuckles, the thenar and hypothenar eminences. On the lower limbs, the rash crowds round the prominences of the ankle joint the malleoli, the ball of the foot and the heel. On the trunk the rash is high up in the back over the shoulder blades. It is rare on the abdomen. The rash is always in the same stage of development, i.e. macules first appear, later papules appear and are followed by vesicles and pustules. Two different types of rash do not appear together.

Smallpox is a serious disease which must be referred to the medical help. It is preventable and the nurse in her health education talks must stress the importance of vaccination against smallpox.

Due to the efforts of the World Health Organization small pox has been eradicated. The occasional case of smallpox is, however, still being encountered in developing countries.

Chickenpox (Varicella)

Chickenpox (varicella) is caused by a herpes virus.

Chickenpox is not usually characterized by the constitutional upsets found in smallpox. Its distribution is different from the distribution of small pox in that it affects the trunk more than the face, although occasionally the rash of chicken-pox may spread to the face. In such cases, however, the density (the number of rashes per unit area) of the rash is not as great on the face as is that of smallpox.

The rash of chickenpox appears on the first day. In adults the appearance of the rash may be preceded by fever (38.3-39°C), malaise, headache and backache. These may occur 12 to 24 hours before the appearance of the vesicular rash of chickenpox. Chickenpox is a much milder disease than smallpox and the course of pregnancy is not usually altered by chickenpox. Infection occurs between 8 and 20 weeks, there is a risk of congenital malformations, including muscular atrophy, microcephaly, cerebellar or cortical atrophye, cataracts and chorionotinitis.

Jaundice in Pregnancy

Jaundice is a yellow discoloration of the skin and mucus membranes due to excessive bile pigments in the blood. It is serious condition in pregnancy because the liver is usually affected. There are three types of jaundice in pregnancy which include:

i. Haemolytic jaundice due to excessive destruction of the RBCs as occur in malaria, sickle cell disease, septicaemia, and incompatible blood transfusion.
ii. Viral or infective hepatitis due to poor liver functions. This is the most serious form of jaundice for it may result in acute necrosis of the liver, hepatic coma and death.
iii. Obstructive jaundice is rare in pregnancy. It may be due to obstruction of the bile duct by a gall stone or carcinoma of the head of the pancreas.

Infective Hepatitis

This is caused by a virus carried in the blood or in the faeces of an infected person. There are two types of viral hepatitis—infective hepatitis (virus A) and serum hepatitis (virus B). Virus A is associated with a short incubation period and virus B with a long incubation period. Hepatitis B surface antigen is known as Australian antigen.

Acute infection affects approximately 1:1000 pregnancy, has an incubation period of 3 to 5 weeks and it is during this period that the patient is infectious. Viral hepatitis B mainly spread by blood, blood products and sexual activity. The virus can also be transmitted across the placenta. Hepatitis B is more common in tropical and developing countries especially where nutrition is poor.

Clinical Manifestation

The signs and symptoms of hepatitis include nausea, vomiting, anorexia, loss of appetite, pain over the liver, mild diarrhea, jaundice, lasting several weeks and malaise. Fever rare and for many, the disease is asymptomatic. As soon as jaundice develops, the patient is no longer infectious. In the advanced stage, of the disease, the liver function is disturbed, blood urea rises, the serum bilirubin is raised. There may be necrosis of the liver and acute yellow atrophy. Coma and death supervene. Often the jaundice clears up after some weeks and the patient recovers completely. Another type of viral hepatitis is that caused by the virus of homologus serum resulting from plasma or blood transfusion. The incubation period is 90 to 120 days. Clinically it is not distinguishable from infective hepatitis.

The effects of viral hepatitis on pregnancy include abortion, premature labour, stillbirth, PPH and maternal death. The risk to the foetus of the maternal infection appears to be minimal. The infant may become infected by swallowing maternal blood or amniotic fluid during labour and infant may develop hepatitis. Few mothers will develop hepatic failure, which can result in death unless liver transplantation is available. If hepatitis B is transmitted from mother to foetus, and immunization does not prevent infection in the baby, the child will be at increased risk of liver cancer in later life.

Diagnosis and Management

A jaundiced patient must be sent to hospital immediately for physician to decide the cause of her jaundice by doing the liver function test as well as other relevant tests. Diagnosis is made from the woman's history of her symptoms and lifestyle.

Admission of the patient into a hospital for close observation is essential. The patient should be examined daily and the abdomen palpated. An accurate fluid chart is kept. The urine is tested daily for proteins, bile and acetone. Blood pressure, temperature, pulse and respirations are recorded twice daily or more often if necessary. The degree of jaundice, the mental state of the patient, delirium or excessive drowsiness should be reported. Flapping tremors (fine tremors of the un-stretched fingers) should be watched for; these and a poor mental state of the patient often herald hepatic coma. It is advisable to keep the patient in bed till the jaundice clears. A low protein and high carbohydrate diet should be given regularly.

Treatment is of the symptoms they arise. Infection control measure should be instituted where the woman is considered to be infectious, and information not only of the disease, but also nutrition and sexual advice should be offered. Drugs excreted by the liver, e.g., barbiturates, paraldehyde and chloropromocaine should never be given to the patient. Sometimes the physician uses steroids and neomycin in the course of treatment. Despite energetic treatment the patient may fail to improve. The bad signs are:

- Deepening of the jaundice
- Poor mental state, e.g. delirium or drowsiness
- Epigastric pain often associated with vomiting
- Highly concentrated and very dark urine
- Increasing proteinuria
- Acetenuria
- Bleeding from the alimentary tract; from the nose, etc
- Coma.

In hepatic coma, the patients are unconscious and very ill. Good nursing and medical care is necessary to keep her alive. Nothing is given by mouth. Intracaval infusion of 40-50 per cent glucose is given. Vitamin B complex is given through the drip. Neomycin 2g at six hourly intervals, and magnesium sulphate enema are given to clear the gut of bacterial organisms. Injection of vitamin K may be given to prevent bleeding. Cortisone or hydrocortisone may be used in the course of treatment. Drugs and sedatives normally excreted by the liver must never be given.

In coma patients, a clear airway should be maintained by lying the patient on her side and the nasopharynx should be sucked as often as may be necessary to clear it of mucus. Daily bed baths should be given and mouth toilet should be done. The patient should be turned two hourly to avoid pressure sources and hypostatic pneumonia. An accurate fluid intake and output chart should be kept. The level of consciousness should be assessed from time to time.

Prevention

Australia antigen positive women are managed with particular precautions as cross infections may occur from maternal faces, urine, maternal blood amniotic fluid. These patients should be managed with barrier nursing, taking precautions with the disposal of excreta. The risk of vertical transmission is substantially reduced by the concurrent administration of immunoglobulin and vaccination after delivery. Liver function will be monitored and foetal condition assessed.

House hold contacts should be offered immunization once their HBsAg seronagatively is established. Sexual partners be traced and offered testing and vaccination. Postnatally, the mother will be encouraged to accept vaccination for the baby.

Herpes Hominis

Herpes infections are due to two antigenic types, 1 and 2. Type 2 is responsible for 95% of genital tract infections, whereas type 1 occurs in non-genital sites such as the mouth, eyes and central nervous system. Type 2 infections are sexually transmitted.

Genital herpes is associated with a five fold increase in the incidence of abortion during the first 20 weeks. Genital infection at term results in a 40 percent incidence of infection in the foetus and this may be manifested in skin vesicles and in infections involving the brain, liver and adrenals.

At the present time, it is generally considered advisable to deliver the infant by caesarean section to minimize the risk of infection acquired during vaginal delivery, if the culture from the vagina remains positive.

Other Infections

Cytomegalovirus

It has been estimated that 4% of women acquire the infection during pregnancy. Both the placenta and foetus may be affected by the viraemia which may result in the development of microcephaly and be the cause of mental retardation of infants in the first 6 years of life. The diagnosis can be established by the presence of a rising antibody titre. Newborn screening is based on raised cord blood IgM levels (>20 mg).

Pregnancy Bacteriuria

Bacteriuria in the mother is associated with an increase in low birth weight infants. Urine specimens yielding more than 105 colonies/ml are considered bacteriuria and should be treated with appropriate antibiotic therapy.

Toxoplasmosis

Toxoplasmosis gondii is a protozoal infection which is found throughout the world. The mode of infection involves the domestic cat. Congenital toxoplasmosis may occur if the mother acquires the infection during pregnancy, and its incidence has been estimated in England at 1 in 20,000 births. In France it may be as high as 1 in 2,000 births. Maternal infection may be a cause of recurrent abortion.

Chlamydiosis

The intracellular bacterium *Chlamydia trachomatis* is a cause of neonatal conjunctivitis and trachoma. The infection can be diagnosed by immunoassay, and treated with 7 to 14 days of erythromycin.

Herpes Zoster

First-trimester infection is associated with an increased risk of abortion and rarely, embryopathy with intrauterine growth retardation and limb scarring. The major risk to the foetus comes from neonatal chickenpox, which is most likely to occur when delivery is within 4 days of the onset of symptoms in the mother. This develops 2 to 3 weeks after delivery and has a 20 percent mortality. Infants born within this time and mothers who are known not be immune should be given immunoglobulin.

Listeriosis

Listeria monocytogenes if found in soil, unwashed vegetables, birds, insects and constaceans. The organism can be transmitted transplacentally or by inhalation of amniotic fluid at delivery. It affects 1/20,000 births. There is an increased risk of intrauterine death and abortion, and untreated neonatal infection has a 90 percent mortality rate in the infant. The diagnosis can be established by blood and urine cultures, and should be suspected in any women presenting with a flulike illness with conjunctivitis, pharyngitis, loin pain and diarrhoea. The organism is sensitive to ampicillin or gentamicin.

HIV Infection

Women are the fastest-growing population of individuals with HIV infection and AIDS. An estimated 16.4 million women are infected worldwide (CDC 2001). Human immunodeficiency virus (HIV) is a retrovirus which affects human lymphocytes and other cells in the central nervous system. There are three levels of manifestation of HIV infection:

1. *Asymptomatic* a positive test for HIV but no clinical symptoms.
2. *Acquired immunodeficiency syndrome (AIDS)* related complex (ARC) persistent generalized lymphadenopathy, weight loss, lethargy
3. *AIDS* includes the clinical symptoms plus opportunistic infections such as *Pneumocystics carinii* and the presence of kaposi's sarcoma.

Infection is usually asymptomatic and incubation takes 15-58 months. Transmission is sexual or blood borne and transplacental. There is no evidence to suggest that airborne infection occurs.

Incidence: AIDS is largely confined to homosexual or bisexual individuals (27%). However, 50% of cases occur in intravenous drug abusers and 10% after blood transfusion. Obviously, these clinical incidence figures will continue changing.

In pregnancy, there is no evidence that HIV infection is clinically accelerated. AIDS and ARC depress the T-helper cell population. It does not affect fertility.

There is a higher incidence of pre-term labour and low birth weight infants in affected mothers, but there are complicating social factors. There are three routes of infections of the child:

1. Transplacental.
2. At birth.
3. Breast milk.

Incidental perinatal transmission occurs in 30 to 50% of cases.

Foetal AIDS

This syndrome is manifested by intrauterine growth retardation, microcephaly, prominent forehead and blue sclerae.

Prognosis: The outlook for survival is infected children is very poor, with a high mortality rate. There is some evidence that the extent of maternal illness may determine the risk of infection in the baby.

All HIV positive pregnant women should be managed jointly with a physician who specializes in HIV. It is not considered essential to nurse these mothers in isolation unless there is abnormal haemorrhage or infective complications. Early signs and symptoms include malaise, fevers, night sweats, and weight loss. There are numerous gastrointestinal and dermatological symptoms, including Kaposi's sarcoma. There is some evidence to suggest that delivery by elective caesarean section may reduce the incidence of vertical transmission but, as yet, there are insufficient data to justify routine operative delivery.

During the second stage of delivery, staff should wear full protective clothing with face protection and overshoes, with double gloves for suturing.

Foetal blood sampling should be avoided whenever possible.

The placenta should be double-bagged and incinerated. The newborn infant should undergo the following investigations:

1. Full blood count and differential white cell count.
2. Urine culture for cytomegalovirus.
3. Hepatitis B and C serology.
4. HIV serology.
5. Virology.
6. Immunology including T lymphocyte and immunoglobulin levels.

The breastfeeding appears to double the risk of transmission of HIV and, therefore, these women should generally be advised against breastfeeding.

Nursing Management of HIV in Pregnancy

Transmission of the human immunodeficiency virus, a retrovirus, occurs primarily through exchange of body fluids (Seven, blood, vaginal secretions) Severe depression of the cellular immune system associated with HIV infection characterized AIDS. Although behaviours that place women at risk have been well documented all women should be assessed for the possibility of HIV exposure.

Once HIV enters the body, seroconversion to HIV positivity usually occurs within 6 to 12 weeks. Although HIV seroconversion may be totally asymptomatic, it usually is accompanied by a viremic, influenza like response. Symptoms include fever, headache, night sweats, malaise, generalized lympadenopathy, myalgia, nausea, diarrhoea, weight loss, sore throat and rash. Laboratory studies may reveal leukopenia, thrombocytopenia, anaemia and an elevated ESR. HIV has a strong affinity for surface maker proteins of T-lymphocytes. This affinity lends to significant T-cell distribution HIV infection is usually diagnosed by using HIV-1 antibody tests-ELISA and Western blot test:

On entry to the health care system, a woman can be hand written information about the risk factors for the AIDS virus and asked to inform the nurse if she believes she is at risk. She should be told that she does not have to say why she may be at risk, only that she thinks she might be. Counselling before and after HIV testing is standard Nursing Practice. It is a nursing responsibility to assess a woman's understanding of the information such a test would provide and to be sure the woman thoroughly understands the emotional, legal and medical implications of a positive or negative test before she is ready to take an HIV test, when providing or negative test before she is ready to take an HIV test, when providing post test counselling to an HIV positive woman privacy with no interruptions is essential. Referral for appropriate medical evaluation is essential.

During the initial contact with an HIV infected woman, the nurse should establish what the woman knows about HIV infection. The nurse should ensure that the woman is being cared for by a physician or at a facility with expertise in caring for persons with HIV infection, including AIDS. Psychologic referral also may be indicated. Resources such as counselling for financial assistance, legal advocacy, suicide prevention and death and dying may be appropriate. All women who are drug users should be referred to a substance abuse programme. A major focus of counselling is prevention of transmission of HIV to partners.

Nurse counselling seropositive women who wish contraceptive information may recommend oral contraceptives and latex condoms. Norplant implant latex condoms, spermicides, female condoms or abstinence can be offered to women, whose partner refuse to use condoms. No cure is available for HIV infections at this time. Rare and unusual diseases are characteristics of HIV infections. Opportunistic infections and concurrent diseases should be managed vigorously with treatment specific to the infection or disease. Routine gyaenecologic care of HIV positive women should include a pelvic examination every six months. Careful pap screening is essential because of the greatly increased incidence of abnormal findings on examination. In addition, HIV-positive woman should be screened for syphilis, gonorrhoea, chlamydia and other vaginal infections and treated if infections are present.

Common Cold and Influenza

These conditions are caused by viruses. For common colds, simols measures such as bed rest and analgesics may suffice. Influenza on the other hand should not be treated lightly because of the complications such as sinusitis, ottis media, bronchitis and bronchopneumonia. All cases must be referred to the physician.

Pyelonephritis

Pyelonephritis is common in the pregnant woman because of certain physiological changes in the urinary tract during pregnancy.

Under the influence of progesterone, there is marked dilatation of the ureters. Pyelonephritis may be acute or chronic. Acute pyelonephritis is characterized by fever, tachycardia, rigors and loin pain. The patient is ill and the tongue is dry and furred. There is usually vomiting and there may be dysuria and frequency of miturition. The pain and vomiting may lead to erroneous diagnosis of appendicitis.

The urine may be cloudy and offensive. A microscopic examination of the urine reveals the presence of numerous pus cells. Culture of the *urine may* reveal organisms such as *Escherichia coli (Esch. coli), Proteus vulgaris* and *Streptococcus faecalis.*

Treatment: Patients with acute pyelonephritis should be admitted to hospital and made to rest in bed. It is advisable to have the patient lying on the non-affected side. Liberal fluid intake is encouraged and an intake and output chart is kept. Application of heat on the affected areas may relieve pain but often analgesics such as two Panadol tablets, Buscopan (20 mg) are given. Fanning to reduce the high temperature often alternates with provision of blankets when the patient has rigors. Bed baths, washes and changing if the bed linen are comforting when the patient sweats profusely.

The nutritional needs of a patient must not be forgotten and her general condition should be built up as soon as possible. Supplementary vitamins, iron, calcium and antimalarial drugs are given. Usually a course of sulphonamide, e.g. sulphadimidine, is given unless the organisms are known to be sulphonamide resistant. The dose is 2 grams immediately followed by one gram at six hourly intervals for seven days.* MIST, Potassicitrate in the dosage of 30 grains (1.8 g) at six hourly intervals for five to seven days is often given along with the antibiotics to make the urine alkaline and less scalding when passed.

Complications: The high fever of acute pyelonephritis may cause abortion or the premature onset of labour. Acute pyelonephritis may become chronic.

Chronic Pyelonephritis

This is the chronic phase of acute pyelonephritis in which case there are fewer constitutional disturbances. Apart from occasional dull pain in the loins, dysuria and general feeling of ill health, numerous pus cells are usually found in a midstream specimen of the urine. There may be a moderate iron deficiency anaemia. Occasionally there may be acute exacerbation of chronic pyelonephritis resulting in fever, prostration and loin pain.

Complications of chronic pyelonephritis are hypertension area retention and renal failure. The incidence of abortion, premature labour and intrauterine death of the foetus is also increased.

Chronic pyelonephritis is difficult to treat as the organisms are deepseated in the kidneys and are difficult to eradicate.

Treatment with sulphadimidine as previously stated or Furadantin (50 to 100 mg six-hourly for seven days) may suffice. Recurrent cases are treated with long acting sulpha drugs (500 mg) daily throughout pregnancy.

---

*Nowaday's Mist or mixtures are not in use but their use give good results

Other Urinary Complications in Pregnancy

Haematuria

Haematuria is not an infrequent complication in pregnancy in the tropics. The causes include the following:

1. Infection with *Schistosoma haematobium* (schistosomiasis): In this case the haematuria is usually terminal and is not painful. Its diagnosis is made by looking for the ova of Schistosoma in the urine of the patient. Treatment is with Ambilhar (500 mg daily), or any recent substitute but the nurse must report all cases of haematuria to the physician and should not attempt treatment unless ordered to do so.
2. Haemoglobinopathies: Patients with haemoglobin SS or SC may have haematuria. Occasionally haemoglobin as is associated with haematuria. All such cases should be referred to the physician.
3. Ureteric stones (calculi): In this condition the patient has spasmodic pain in the loin before passing urine. The urine may be blood stained.

Vesical Calculi

Stones in the urinary bladder can cause painful haematuria.

Thyroid Dysfunction in Pregnancy

The effect of pregnancy on the normal thyroid gland : There is slight enlargement of the thyroid gland during pregnancy. There is also an increased blood flow. A bruit (murmur) may be heard over the thyroid during pregnancy. In addition, certain biochemical changes take place in the thyroid. Thyrotoxicosis, Grave's disease and hypothyroidism (myxoedema) are not common complications in pregnancy. This is because both conditions cause impaired fertility. Pregnancy has, however, been reported in women suffering from thyroid dysfunction.

The main abnormal conditions of the thyroid which are sometimes associated with pregnancy are:

1. Thyrotoxicosis (hyperthyroidism)
2. Myxoedema (hypothyroidism)
3. Endemic goitre: This is due to dietary deficiency in iodine. It occurs in areas of iodine deficiency.

Although thyrotoxicosis, myxoedema and even endemic goitre have been associated with intrauterine growth retardation and increased perineal mortality rate, adequate treatment of these conditions prevents any adverse effect they may have on the course of pregnancy. This is because of the transplacental transfer of the foetal thyroid hormones to the mother. On the other hand, inadequately treated thyrotoxicosis may result in a poor foetal outcome, e.g. increased abortion and still birth rates. Inadequate treatment of maternal thyrotoxicosis may result in hyperplasia of the thyroid gland of the neonate and lead to the development of a goitre.

Thyrotoxicosis

Thyrotoxicosis is sometimes difficult to diagnose in pregnancy because of the altered thyroid function brought about the pregnancy.

The symptoms usually complained of by a patient with hyperthyroidism may also be complained of by a euthyroid (normal thyroid) pregnant patient. These symptoms are:

- Fatigue
- Breathlessness
- Palpitation
- Tachycardia
- Intolerance to heat
- Enlargement of the thyroid gland
- Increased appetite but without any weight gain
- Sweating, which is part of the heat intolerance
- In addition there may be exophthalmos.

The above symptoms are typical of hyperthyroidism or thyrotoxicosis. Added to these symptoms is the tremor of the fingers of the outstretched hands of a woman who has thyrotoxicosis. Certain biochemical tests are done to confirm the diagnosis of thyrotoxicosis. A simple diagnostic test is the measurement of the basal metabolic nurse rate (BMR), which is high in thyrotoxicosis. The nurse midwife must, however, realize that other conditions much as fever, anaemia, cardiopulmonary insufficiency etc, can cause an increase in the BMR.

Myxoedema (Hypothyroidism)

In myxoedema, thyroid function is inadequate. In a number of women amenorrhoea is the rule. There is usually infertility, but, as indicated above, pregnancy may occur in the myxoedematous patient and myxoedema is improved by pregnancy.

Management

Thyroid disease in pregnancy should be reported to the physician. The treatment is medical or surgical, or both. As far as possible medical treatment is to be preferred, Drugs include:
1. Methyl thiouracil
2. Carbimaezole

Carbimazole is the drug of choice. It is usually given at a dose of 15 mg four times daily for one month. Thereafter, 5 mg of carbimazole is given twice daily for six weeks. At the end of this period the patient's symptoms will have subsided. Sometimes it may be necessary to give a maintenance dose of carbimazole for three to six months. Instead of carbimazole, any drug choice discovered recently may be used with proper instructions.

Endemic Goitre

Endemic goitre is treated with iodine rich diet. In addition, if the goitre causes pressure symptoms, the patient is referred for surgical treatment.

ACUTE RENAL FAILURE

Acute renal failure is said to occur when the daily urinary output of a patient is greatly diminished or when there is a total suppression of urine. The terms oliguria and anuria are used to describe these conditions. In oliguria, the urine is usually dark in colour with a very low specific gravity. The quantity passed per day is about 400 ml or less. Anuria is a rare condition but oliguria is more commonly seen in obstetric patients.

Causes of Acute Renal Failure in Obstetrics

1. Severe haemorrhage leading to shock as usually occurs in concealed accidental antepartum haemorrhage, incomplete abortion, ruptured ectopic gestation and postpartum haemorrhage.
2. Excessive loss of fluids and electrolytes as in hyperemesis gravidarum or in any of the diarrhoeal diseases.
3. Septicaemia is in septic abortion, *E. coli* septicaemia and *Clostridium welchii* infections.
4. Incompatible blood transfusion.
5. Shock from any other cause.
6. Eclampsia.
7. Pre-existing renal disease, e.g. chronic nephritis and chronic pyelonephritis.

Acute renal failure may be due to acute tubular necrosis (lower nephron necrosis) or bilateral renal cortical necrosis. Acute tubular necrosis is a reversible condition from which the patient usually recovers if she is well treated. Bilateral renal cortical necrosis is an irreversible and fatal condition. Since one of the two conditions is reversible, all cases of acute renal failure are energetically treatment in the hope that the patient is suffering from the reversible condition.

Clinical Features of Acute Renal Failure

Four phases are recognized in acute renal failure. These are listed below:
1. *Warning phase:* During this phase the patient passes a diminished quantity of urine which is highly concentrated. This phase usually lasts about 24 hours.
2. *Phase of oliguria or anuria:* In this phase the patient passes very little or no urine. The blood urea begins to rise and there is a great deal of electrolyte disturbance. The serum potassium level usually rises to well above 5 milli-equivalents per litre and the patient may be acidotic. She is usually very ill even though she may be mentally alert.
3. *Phase of early diuresis:* In this phase the kidneys have begun to recover. The patient begins to pass urine but the daily urinary output is still well below the daily output of a normal patient. The blood urea and the serum potassium may begin to fall. In this phase the tubular function has not yet caught up with the glomerular function and so there may be loss or electrolytes resulting from failure of reabsorption by the tubules.
4. *Phase of late diuresis and recovery:* In this phase, the kidneys have almost fully recovered and the patient passes copious amounts of urine daily. The patient is, however, in danger of gross electrolytic depletion, and dehydration if she is not adequately hydrated. The blood urea and the serum potassium fall but it may take weeks before the normal levels are reached.

Management of Acute Renal Failure

Acute renal failure can be prevented in any of the following ways:
1. Prevention or adequate treatment of haemorrhage.

2. Prompt and adequate replacement of fluid and electrolyte loss.
3. Prevention of infection through strict aseptic and antiseptic precautions and energetic treatment of existing infection.

During the oliguric or anuric phase, fluid restriction is imperative because a liberal fluid intake will result in pulmonary oedema and heart failure and subsequent death. The patient is usually allowed 500 ml of fluid plus and equivalent volume to the vomitus and urine passed in 24 hours. Thus if a patient passed 300 ml of urine and vomited 800 ml of gastric contents in a day, her fluid requirement for that day is 500 ml + 300 ml + 800 ml = 1600 ml.

Glucose is given liberally to ensure adequate caloric intake of 2000 to 2400 calories daily. Since the end products of protein metabolism result in the accumulation of nitrogenous compounds and potassium in the blood, protein is either restricted or completely removed from the patient's diet in the oliguric or anuric phase.

The majority of patients in the oliguric or anuric phase vomit a great deal and cannot keep food in the stomach. To ensure adequate caloric intake, intragastric feeding with a special mixture consisting of 400 grams of glucose and 100 grams of peanut oil and gum acacia to emulsify is added to one litre of fluid and given to the patient through a stomach tube (Now mixtures are not in use). The patient must not be given fruit juices or other food rich in potassium. Experience with obstetric cases is that nausea and vomiting may be troublesome and the patient usually requires an intravenous infusion of a high concentration of glucose. This is usually given through a large vein like the inferior vena cava to prevent thrombosis, 500 ml of 50 per cent glucose, to which 1000 units of heparin and vitamin B complex and ascorbic acid (vitamin C) have been added, is infused in 24 hours. As previously stated, the daily volume of infusion is determined by the amount of vomitus and urinary output of the patient.

The serum electrolytes and urea are checked twice or thrice daily during the oliguric phase. When diuresis begins, any electrolyte depletion must be corrected. The patient is not out of danger until diuresis is well established, the serum potassium is normal and there is a diminution in the level of blood urea. When all these conditions have been fulfilled the intragastric tube feeding or intravenous infusion may be discontinued. The patient may be allowed to return to normal diet gradually.

In some severe cases of acute renal failure when oliguria or anuria persists and the blood urea and serum potassium are rising steeply, the patient may have to be given peritoneal or haemodialysis. The physician usually decides when the patient requires dialysis.

Renal Disease in Pregnancy

Pregnancies complicated by renal disease should be regarded as high risk pregnancies. Pregnant women who have renal disease should be referred to the physician and managed in a hospital with facilities for dealing with high risk cases.

Among renal conditions that may complicate pregnancy, pyelonephritis is about the most common. This conditions has already been described. Acute renal failure, a very serious condition complicating massive ante and postpartum haemorrhage, excessive loss of body fluids as in hypereme is gravidarum, etc. The other renal conditions encountered in pregnancy are:

1. Acute glomerulonephritis.
2. Subacute glomerulonephritis.
3. Chronic glomerulonephritis.

The above classification of renal disease (Bright's disease) has given way to another classification by Ellis. Bright's disease has been divided by Ellis into separate groups, viz.

1. Ellis type I nephritis.
2. Ellis type II nephritis.

Before going any further, it is necessary to distinguish between the clinical features of Ellis type 1 and those of Ellis type II nephritis (Table 8.4).

Ellis Type I Nephritis: Acute Nephritis

As a rule, acute nephritis (Ellis type I) is very rarely complicated by pregnancy. In many cases in which pregnancy complicates acute glomerulonephritis the women usually abort. Only a few cases of Ellis type I nephritis (acute glomerulonephritis) associated with pregnancy have been reported.

Ellis Type II Nephritis: Chronic Nephritis

A number of women with chronic nephritis remain infertile. Those who become pregnant have gross albuminuria and oedema very early in pregnancy. Hypertension is a late occurrence in chronic nephritis. The phase of nephritis characterized predomi-

Table 8.4: Differences between Ellis type 1 and Ellis type II nephritis

Events	*Ellis type I*	*Ellis type II*
Onset	Sudden manifested by fever, vomiting, headache and pain in the loins	Insidious (slow in showing itself)
Previous history of infection	There is, in the great majority of cases, a history of streptococcal infection	There is usually no previous history of streptococcal infections
Age incidence	The great majority of patients are under the age of 20 years	Occurs at any age
Urine	There is usually gross haematuria but only slight albuminuria	There is gross albuminuria. There is no obvious haematuria any haematuria present can only be detected microscopically
Oedema	Very little or no oedema. When oedema is present it does not last long	Progressively increasing oedema
Blood pressure	Usually raised	Elevation of blood pressure occurs only in very late cases
Course	About 80 per cent recover completely. Foetal and rapid onset occurs in about 10 per cent. Slow progressive hypertension. resulting finally in renal failure in the remaining 10 per cent	90 to 95 per cent of the patients die within ten years as a result of progressive hypertension and uraemia

nantly by gross albuminuria and oedema is what is usually diagnosed as nephrotic syndrome. Women with nephrotic syndrome have albuminuria and oedema early in pregnancy. The serum cholesterol is high and there is hypoalbuminaemia (reduced plasma albumen) and lipiduria. Nephrotic syndrome in the child is sometimes associated with infection with *Plasmodium malariae*. Other causes of nephrotic syndrome include diabetes, syphilis, disseminated lupus erythematosus and secondary amyloidosis.

Management of Nephritis

All cases with albuminuria or haematuria should be referred to the physician. Patients with nephritis are high risk patients. They should be managed in specially equipped hospital centres.

The investigations done are listed below:

1. Urinalysis including microscopic examination.
2. Blood tests such as:
   a. Packed cell volume
   b. haemoglobin genotype
   c. Serum electrolytes and urea
   d. Liver function tests
   e. Serum cholesterol.
3. Renal function tests, which include;
   a. Tests for glomerular function
   b. Tests for tubular function.

A description of renal function tests is beyond the scope of this book.

Prognosis in Renal Disease

The prognosis for the mother and the baby in cases of renal disease manifested only by gross oedema and albuminuria is usually good, provided the woman receives good antenatal and intranatal care. When hypertension complicates oedema and albuninuria the prognosis is not so good for the mother and her baby. In such cases the perinatal mortality rate is high. It may be as high as 35 per cent. The worst prognosis is found in cases in which oedema and albuminuria are associated with hypertension and azotaemia (very high blood urea level 200 mg per 100 ml or more). In such cases, maternal morbidity and mortality are high. Perinatal mortality rate is very high. Sometimes it may be necessary to terminate pregnancy to prevent deterioration in the maternal condition. The above account further underlines the need for the nurse midwife to refer all pregnant women with signs and symptoms of renal disease to a physician with the minimum of delay.

MALARIA IN PREGNANCY

Malaria is the commonest cause of pyrexia in many parts of the tropics. It is a serious disease but it is preventable.

Malaria is caused by *Plasmodium* parasites of which there are four species, viz.—*Plasmodium malariae, P. ovale, P. vivax and P. falciparum*. The predominance of the species varies from one country to another. Thus in India *P. falciparum* is the chief cause of malaria in adults. The vector of the malarial parasite is the female Anopheles mosquito of which there are many species.

Malaria causes fever which may be very high. The patient may be very ill and rigors and sweating are common. Headache may be severe and generalized aches are quite common. Sometimes there may be gastrointestinal symptoms such as vomiting and diarrhoea. Occasionally, when there is excessive haemolysis resulting from destruction of the red blood cells, the patient may be jaundiced and there may be anaemia.

Effect of Pregnancy on Malaria

Pregnancy is said to lower the acquired immunity to malaria. This is particularly so in first pregnancies. Subsequent pregnancies do not seem to have a great deal of influence on the patient's acquired immunity to malaria.

Effects of Malaria on Pregnancy

Because of the hyperpyrexia caused by malaria, abortion or premature labour may occur. The hyperpyrexia may also cause intrauterine death of the foetus with the birth of a macerated foetus.

The rapid destruction of the red blood cells by malarial parasites causes haemolysis of the red cells and leads to the development of anaemia of the folic acid deficiency type.

When the malarial parasites have invaded the placenta they cause a condition known as parasitization of the placenta. This causes placental insufficiency which leads to the delivery of low birth weight babies even at term. This fact is not universally accepted throughout the tropics. Studies confirms that malarial parasitization causes the delivery of low birth weight babies. Some workers have confirmed the findings, although some workers have not confirmed these findings.

To summarize, malaria has the following effects:

1. On the mother:
   a. Hyperpyrexia and ill health;
   b. Haemolytic anaemia with deficiency in folic acid.
2. On the foetus: abortion, increases perinatal loss, prematures LBW.

Prevention of Malaria

In the prevention of malaria it is essential to avoid stagnant pools and bush surroundings which encourage the breeding of mosquitoes. In areas in which malaria is endemic, the patients should be advised to sleep under mosquito nets or in houses with mosquito proofing. In early pregnancy a loading dose of chloroquine (800 mg) is given to each patient. This is followed by pyrimethamine (Daraprim) (25 mg weekly) throughout pregnancy and puerperium. One tablet of chloroquine or Resochin taken twice weekly is also said to suppress malaria. Paludrine, one tablet (100 mg) daily, is also a good suppressant.

Treatment of Malaria

A patient with an attack of malaria should be referred to a doctor for treatment. In the absence of the doctor the midwife should 800 mg (4 tablets) of chloroquine sulphate or 750 mg of chloroquine phosphate (3 tablets), or three tablets of camoquine or 4 of Resochin to the patient. Codeine phosphate (2 tablets) may be given with the initial dose of antimalarial to relieve headache and generalized aches. The patient should be confined to bed. Treatment is continued with 200 mg of chloroquine sulphate or 250 mg of chloroquine phosphate twice daily for 5 days if chloroquine was initially given.

Nursing Interventions

A severe attack of malaria leaves the patient ill, weak and often anaemic. Hospitalization is sometimes necessary. Bed rest is recommended during the acute phase of the illness. The high temperature which characterizes the disease should be reduced by tepid sponging, fanning or the use of antipyretic drugs such as 600 mg of aspirin at 6 hourly intervals.

Rigors are also a common feature. The patient must be kept warm during attacks. An extra blanket should be given or a hot water bottle used to provide warmth.

Frequent washes and changes of bed linen are necessary because the patient sweats a lot.

There is usually a loss of appetite but the patient should be encouraged or persuaded to take plenty of nourishing fluid diet. Light diet such as pap or gruel and milk, boiled egg and bread should be served. Vitamins and iron should also be given.

Temperature, pulse and respiration are recorded four hourly until the patient's condition improves. Jaundice may be present as a result of the blood destruction and the urine is concentrated and scanty. These signs should subside with treatment.

A period of convalescence is recommended before the patient rent home.

9 CHAPTER

Abnormal Labour: Assessment and Management

INTRODUCTION

All pregnant women are at risk of complications. The complications of pregnancy that cause high risk for women and infant are presented in previous chapters. When complications arise, during labour and birth, risk of perinatal morbidity and mortality increases. Nurses should be alert to identify all high risk pregnancies as early as possible. In some women, there may be one or more high risk factors as follows.

RISK FACTORS ASSOCIATED WITH LABOUR

Obstetric Factors

- *Gravidity*: If primigravida is the only risk factor, one has to consider if she can be handled at peripheral health centre. Grandmultipara (more than 4 pregnancies) should be referred to higher health facilities.
- *Age*: Elderly at and above 35 years, below 10 years.
- *Height*: All gravidas less than 145 cm (4 ft.10 inches).
- *Weight*: Under weight (a prepregnancy weight of less) or overweight (20 per cent or over) as per height-weight standard.
- *Multipara*: With bad obstetric history like difficult labour and loss of previous baby, caesarean section, hypertension in previous pregnancy, recurrent premature labour and abortion, intrauterine foetal death, previous third stage abnormalities, congential malformations and neonatal death.
- Cases of disproportion (evident or suspect) due to pelvic contraction, pelvic tumour, or primigravida with nonengaged head at or near term.
- Malpresentations and multiple pregnancy.
- *Obstetric complications*: Pregnancy haemorrhage (threatened abortion, APH, PIH (pre-eclampsia and eclampsia).
- *High-risk foetus*: Premature labour, IUGR foetus, Rh incompatibility foetus and post-maturity.
- *Infertility*: Conceived after treatment of infertility.

Medical Factors

Anaemia, undernutrition, cardiac diseases, hypertension, diabetes mellitus, STDs, pulmonary tuberculosis and chest diseases, hepatitis, psychiatric disorders, thyroid disorders, obesity and other medical problems.

Some complications are anticipated, especially if mother is identified as high risk during the antepartum period, others are unexpected of unforeseen. The woman, her family and the obstetric team can feel devastated when things of worn. Nurses must recognize these feelings if they are provided effective support. It is crucial for nurses to understand the normal birth process to prevent and detect deviations from normal labour and birth and to implement nursing measures when complications arise. Optimal care of the labouring women, foetus, and family experiencing complications is possible only when the nurse and other members of the obstetric team use their knowledge and skills in a concerted effort to provide care.

THE ELDERLY PRIMIGRAVIDA

An elderly primigravida is a patient going through her first pregnancy at or over the age of 35 years. This definition may be adopted in the developing countries but it must be remembered that the reproductive activity of the women in developing countries starts at a much earlier age than that of the women in devloped countries. Although the agelimit is being raised from 35 to 40 years in Britain and other European countries, it may be wise to regard as an elderly primigravida, any woman who is pregnant for the first time at the age of 30 years or more in developing countries.

The elderly primigravida is likely to develop the following complications in pregnancy and labour.

1. Tendency to abort.
2. Increased incidence of hypertension, pre-eclampsia and eclampsia. This is understandable because the older the woman gets the more likely to develop hypertension.
3. The long period of infertility may induce the development of uterine fibroids which may complicate pregnancy.

Labour tends to be longer in the elderly primigravida than in the multipara. Posterior positions of the occiput are also common. Abnormal uterine action may complicate labour. There is increased need for obstetric intervention because of the rigid perineum and prolonged labour

The neonatal morbidity and mortality are increased because of prematurity, prolonged labour and the need to intervene, as well as the increased evidence of congenital foetal abnormalities (e.g. mongolism, hydrocephaly, anencephaly, etc.) with increasing maternal age.

Maternal morbidity and mortality are higher in elderly primigravidae than in young primigravida is faced the nurse midwife must refer all elderly primigravidae to a big hospital for delivery.

THE GRAND MULTIPARA

A patient who has had five or more previous viable babies is said to be a grande multipara. Some obstetricians put the lower limit at seven, but it is better to regard five or more as the criterion.

The following are the hazards of grande multiparity.

1. The increased tendency to hypertension and other cardiovascular complications because of advancing age.
2. Anaemia—This may be the result of successive pregnancies with little or no rest in between. The patient may not have recovered from the anaemia of a previous pregnancy before she is again pregnant. Usually women who have large families are poor and their diets are grossly deficient in iron, folic acid and vitamins, all of which they greatly need.
3. Poor health due to anaemia, under nutrition, poor living conditions and family worries. The patient is far too busy attending to the health.of her children and has very little time to attend to herself. Whilst she is caring for a child with measles another one is developing pneumonia. As one child is just recovering from an attack of diarrhoea, the other is developing malaria. Soon the woman becomes a nervous wreck. Sleep eludes her and she becomes more and more irritable.
4. There may be increasing weight resulting from too frequent deliveries. The overstretching of the abdomen may lead to laxity of the abdominal muscles and a pendulous abdomen results. This leads to malpresentation and abnormal lie of the foetus.
5. Multiple pregnancy is more common in grand multiparae than in women of low parity.
6. Antepartum haemorrhage: There is a higher frequency of placenta praevia and concealed accidental haemorrhage in the grande multipara than in women of lower parity.

The complications in labour are:

1. Precipitate labour
2. Prolapse of the umbillical cord due to malpresentation, abnormal lie (transverse) and premature rupture of the membranes.
3. Rupture of the uterus due to excessive thinning of the uterine muscular wall, replacement of muscle by elastic and fibrous tissue, malpresentation (e.g.brow, face, occipito-posterior position and shoulder) causing obstructed labour.
4. Postpartum haemorrhage resulting from poor retraction of the uterus, retainad placenta or rupture of the uterus.

In view of all the serious complications listed above all grande multiparae should be referred to hospitals with facilities for dealing with complicated deliveries.

HIGH-RISK WOMEN

A high-risk pregnancy can be defined as a pregnancy in which the outcome is bound to be poor for the mother and the foetus. Examples of high risk pregnancies are those complicated by antepartum haemorrhage, severe hypertension, severe pre-eclampsia, diabetes mellitus, cardiac disease and active pulmonary tuberculosis to mentions a few. To the above list can be added short maternal stature with the likelihood of foeto-pelvic dispropotion and consequent obstructed labour, previous caesarean section with the possibility of uterine rupture during pregnancy or labour and premature rupture of membranes with the attendent risk of intrauterine infection, amnionitis and eventual intrauterine foetal death. First pregnancy, a high parity, pregnancies at frequent intervals, pregnancies at a tender (teenagers under 17 years) or advancing age all carry a high risk, In addition, conditions like maternal malnutrition, poor sanitary conditions, in the house, overcrowding, large families and ignorance further increase risk for the neonate-especially the risk of gastroenteritis, neonatal tetanus, etc.

A highrisk pregnancy requires special care. The most important thing is identification of women at risk and referral of such women in well equipped and adequately staffed hospitals.

The nurse midwife, during her training, should be encouraged to develop the risk approach to maternal and child care. She should be taught to develop the risk strategy. By a careful history taking and a thorough clinical assessment, the nurse midwife should be able to identify the women at risk, and refer them to the appropriate clinics or hospitals. The ability to detect risk factors will depend not only on the level of training of the health personnel but also on the available facilities. History taking allows the nurse midwife to measure risks related to maternal age and parity. The availability of a weighing scale and facility for measuring the women's height will make it easy for the midwife to identify risk related to excessive weight gain and short stature. The possession of a sphygmomanometer facilitates the identification of women at the risk of developing hypertensive disorders, pre-eclampsia. In the big urban centres, with excellent facilities for monitoring foetal growth, etc. the ability to detect risks is further enhanced.

There should, however, be a standardized method of measuring risk. Risks are not necessarily confined to the prenatal period. In the assessment of women at risk, the risks in pragnancy, labour and puerperium should be considered. Even if the pregnancy is normal, labour may be difficult. Thus a short woman with a contracted pelvis may have an uneventful pregnancy but labour may be prolonaged and subsequently obstructed due to fosto-pelvic disproportion. A grande multipara whose prenatal period was uncomplicated and who had a spontaneous live birth might have post partum haemorrhage in the third stage of labour.

In the assessment of risk a scoring system which will lead to a better management of the patient should be adopted.

A method of screening is necessary in the antenatal clinic to identify high and low risk women.

The following conditions should place any pregnent woman in the category of high risk:

1. Cardiac disease.
2. Hypertension.
3. Renal disease.
4. Diabetes mellitus.
5. Pulmonary tuberculosis.
6. Anaemia.
7. Abnormal haemoglobins e.g., Hb, SS and Hb SC.
8. Pre-eclampsia.
9. Eclampsia.
10. Pyelonephritis.
11. Short stature contracted pelvis.
12. Multiple pregnancy.
13. Abnormal lie of the foetus in late pregnancy.
14. Antepartum haemorrhage.
15. Advancing maternal age, e.g. a woman of 30 or more years.
16. First pregnancy (irrespective of maternal age).
17. Teenage pregnancy, especially with maternal age below 17 years.
18. A previous history of:
    a. High pregnancy wastage, e.g. recurrent abortions, still births and neonatal deaths.
    b. Caesarean section.
    c. Postpartum haemorrhage with or without blood coagulation problems.
    d. Retained placenta.
    e. Rupture of the uterus.
    f. Prolonged labour/obstructed labour.
    g. Five or more deliveries.

Other include:

i. Premature rupture of membranes.
ii. Premature onset of labour.
iii. Postmaturity.
iv. intrauterine growth retardation (IUGR).

All women with any of the above conditions should be regarded as being at risk and referred to a physician for thorough assessment. The management of high risk cases should be in a well equipped and adequately staffed hospital.

THE MANAGEMENT OF LABOUR IN HIGH-RISK CASES

All high-risk pregnancies must be transferred to a well equipped hospital staffed by experienced nurse midwives and physicians. As soon as the patient is admitted in labour the midwife/nurse should use all available resources to ensure a successful outcome. Effective foetal heart monitoring is important. Only very few hospitals have the sonic aid for monitoring the characteristics of uterine contractions and the foetal heart rate but also the strength and frequency of uterine contractions. The patient's pulse should be recorded at quarter hourly intervals and the blood pressure at the same time as the pulse rate. An intake and output chart must be scrupulously kept. All specimens of urine should be tested for sugar, albumin and acetone. Any untoward development should be reported to the physician. Preparation for intravenous infusions, blood transfusion, forceps delivery, vacuum extraction or caesarean section should be made in all high risk cases in labour.

Even in hospitals where it is not possible to use sophisticated equipment to monitor the progress in labour a partography can be used. This is a graphical recording of all the events taking place from the onset of labour to the time intervention is deemed necessary. One quick glance at the chart will give all the information necessary to take a decision for positive action.

Use of a Partograph (Flow chart 9.1A and B)

By noting the rate at which the cervix dilates, it is possible to identify women whose labour is abnormally slow and who require special attention. The foetal and maternal conditions are also monitored on the partograph. Partograph should be started after checking that there are no complications of pregnancy which require immediate action. If history of maternal complications or signs of obstetric emergencies are present, the patient should be immediately referred to a hospital.

In the centre of the partograph dilatations of the cervix are plotted. Along the left side are figures 0-10 against squares. Each square represents 1 cm dilatation. Along the bottom of the graph are numbers 0-24. Each square represents one hour. The dilatation of the cervix is recorded with an 'X' in the appropriate square. When labour goes from latent to active phase, plotting of the dilatation is transferred to the active phase by a broken line. If progress is satisfactory the plotting of cervical dilation will remain on or to the left of the ALERT line.

Descent of head is plotted on the same part of the graph which is used for plotting cervical dilatation. On the left side of the graph is the word 'descent' with lines going from 5 to 0. Descent is plotted with an 'O' on the graph.

Below the time line there are 5 blank squares going across the length of the graph. Each square represents one contraction. If there are 2 contractions in 10 minutes two squares are filled. If the contractions last for 20 seconds or less fill the squares with dots; if between 20 to 40 seconds by diagonal lines and if more than 40 seconds fill the square completely.

The foetal heart rate is recorded at the top of the partograph. It is recorded half hourly and each square represents one half hour. The lines 120 and 160 are darker as these are the limits of a normal foetal heart rate.

The maternal condition is plotted on the partograph by recording pulse rate (half hourly), blood pressure (4 hourly, or more frequently if indicated), temperature (4 hourly, or more frequently if indicated), urine volume (encourage woman to pass urine 2 to 4 hourly), albumin or sugar in the urine and drugs (IV fluids, oxytocin, etc.) if used.

Illustration of Plotting of a Partograph

In this example a normal partograph has been shown. The purpose is to make you understand the plotting of different parameters on the graph. A complete partograph is provided and you are required to refer to the recordings as you read through the example.

The graph has five sections for recording:

1. Foetal heart rate;
2. Cervical dilatations;
3. Descent of head;
4. Uterine contractions and;
5. Maternal condition.

Foetal Heart Rate

This is recorded every half hour and is plotted as a line graph.

Flow chart 9.1A: Partograph

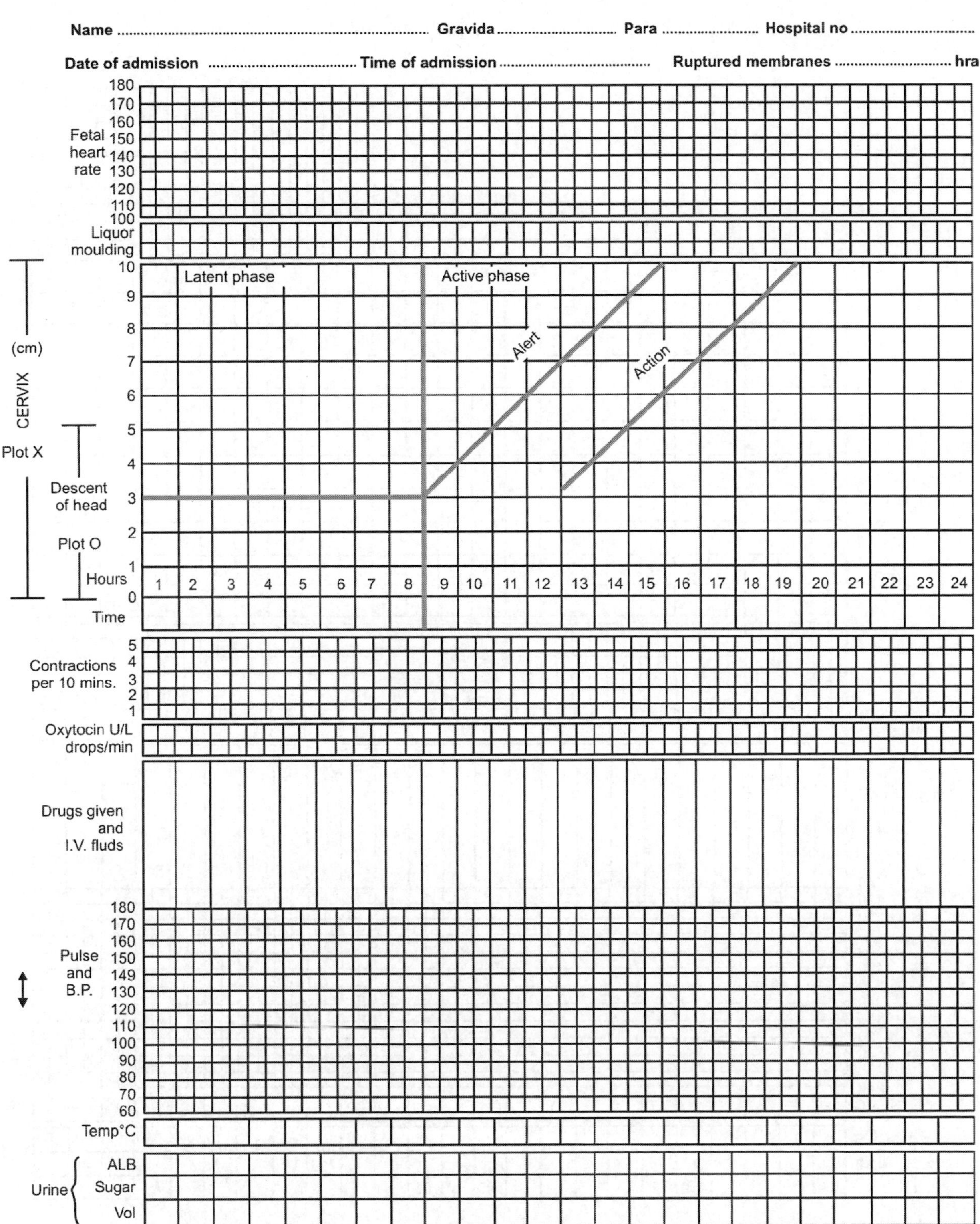

Flow chart 9.1B: Partograph

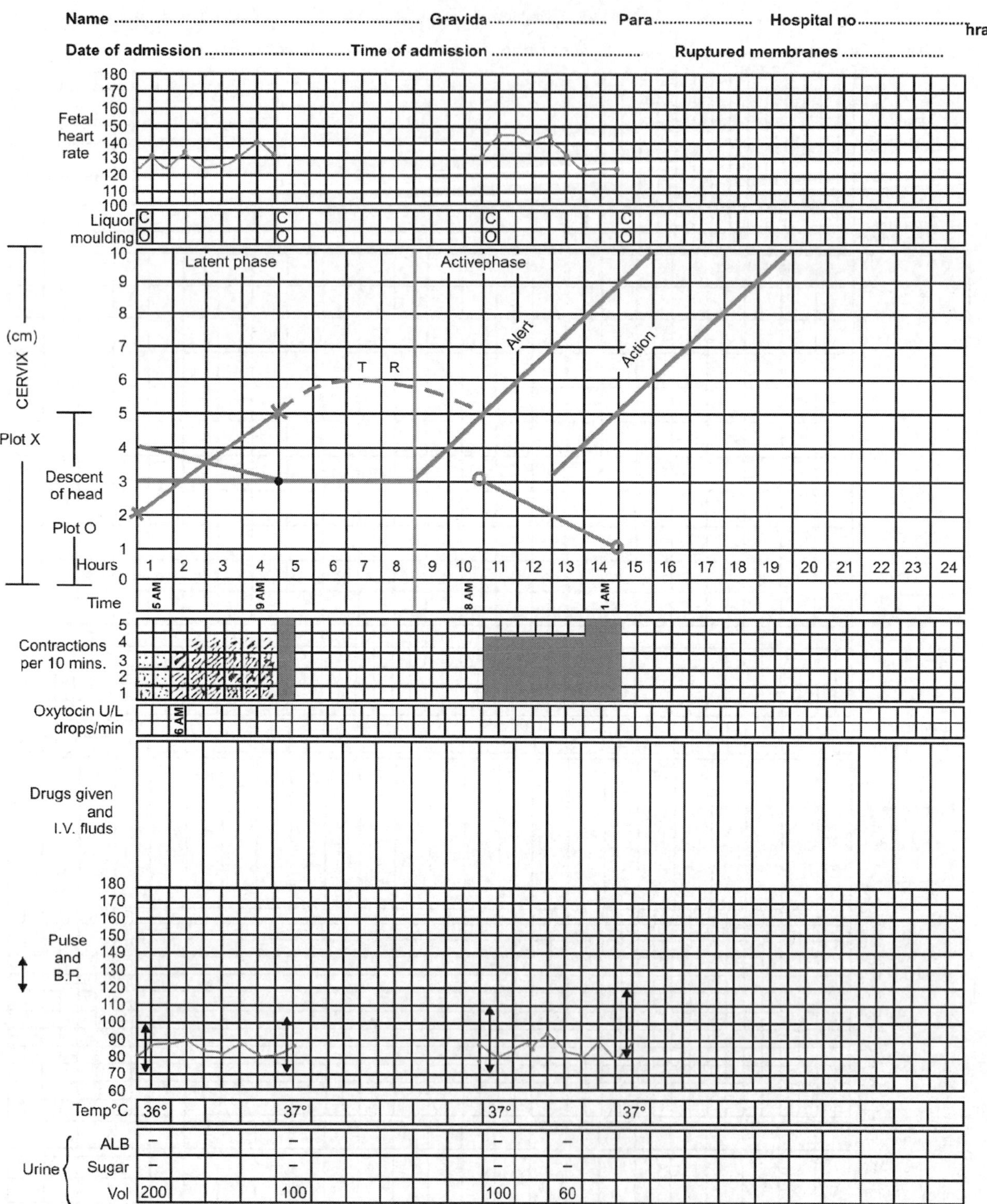

Cervical Dilatation

- The patient was admitted at 5 am with 2 cm dilatation. It is marked as 'X' at 2 on the left line. In place of the time '0' on the bottom line the actual time of 5 am is recorded.
- Second observation (PV examination) was done after 4 hours at 9 am. Cervical dilation was found to be 5 cm. It is marked as 'X' against 5 on the left line.
  Five cm dilatation means that cervical dilatation is in the 'Active Phase'. The plotting, i.e. 'X' at 5 is, therefore, transferred to the active phase on the graph with a dotted line.
- Third observation was made again after 4 hours at 1 pm. Cervical dilatation was found to be 10 cm and is marked as 'X' against 10 on the graph.

The cervix at this stage is fully dilated and the line joining 5 (the earlier reading) to 10 (the present reading) is to the left of the 'Alert Line'.

Inference

- Progress of cervical dilatation is normal.
- Length of the first stage in the hospital was 8 hours.
- Delivery of the baby could be expected any time before 3 pm. In the present case a live female infant was born at 1.10 pm.

Descent of Head

- When patient was admitted at 5 am, the head accommodated 4 fingers (four-fifths) and is marked as '0' at 4 on the left line.
- At 9 am, the head accommodates 3 fingers (three fifths). This is marked as '0' against 3 on the left line.
  As cervical dilatation at 9 am is in the active phase, the descent of head is also transferred to the active phase as was done for cervical dilatation ['0' at 3 in the active phase].
- At 1 pm, the head accommodates only one figure (one fifths) above the pelvic brim. This is marked as '0' against 1 on the left line.

Uterine Contractions

These are recorded every one hour in the latent phase and every half hour in the active phase.

- On admission at 5 AM the patient had 3 contractions in 10 minutes. Duration of each was less than 20 seconds. To depict this three squares are marked with dots.
- Second observation on this was made after 1 hour at 6 AM. Patient had 3 contractions in 10 minutes. The duration of each contraction had, however, increased to 26 seconds. This is marked on the graph by filling three squares with lines.
- At 7 AM the frequency of contractions increased to 4 in 10 minutes. Duration remained same as at 6 am. This is depicted on the graph by filling four squares with lines.
- At 9 AM, though the frequency remained same (4 in 10 minutes), the duration of each contraction had increased to above 40 seconds. This is marked by filling four squares completely.
  Since at 9 AM, labour is in active phase, observations are to be repeated every half hour.
- At 12 noon, the frequency of contractions increased to 5 in 10 minutes. Duration remained above 40 seconds for each contraction. This has been recorded by completely filling five squares.

Maternal Condition

At the bottom of the graph space has been provided for recording maternal condition (drugs and IV given, pulse, BP, temperature and urine output). Recording of medication is made in the space provided.

Special Tests for Assessing High Risk Preganancies

The management of high risk cases should be carried out in well equipped, adequately staffed hospitals with facilities for antenatal monitoring of foetal and maternal well being. All high risk women should be referred by the midwife to the physician.

In many teaching hospital facilities are available for carrying out special tests which will give necessary information on the foeto-placental unit. In addition, facilities are available for determining the maturity of the foetus and ascertaining whether it is safe to terminate a high risk pregnancy.

Some of these tests will be briefly described to enable the nurses-midwife to appreciate their significance.

Oestriol Estimation

Oestriol is an end product of the metabolism of oestrogen. In the presence of placental insufficiency the level of oestriol excretion in the urine is low-less than 5 mg/litre. On the other hand, if placental function is good, urinary oestriol is of the order of about 10-12 mg/litre. Measurement of urinary oestriol is, therefore, an indirect method of assessing placental function.

Lecithin/Sphingomyelin Ratio (L/S Ratio)

Lecithin and sphingomyelin are phospholipids. They are found in the amniotic fluid. They are known as pulmonary surfactants. When they are in a particular ratio to one another, they indicate maturity or non-maturity of the lungs of the foetus. The normal L/S ratio is 2 of lecithin to 1 of sphingomyelin. Anything above this indicates foetal lung maturity. An L/S ratio of less than 2 indicates immaturity of the foetal lungs. The L/S ratio is measured by withdrawing a little quantity of amniotic fluid and sending it to the laboratory. In the laboratory, by special techniques, the levels of the amniotic lecithin and sphingomyelin are measured and the L/S ratio is determined. A low L/S ratio is usually found in preterm babies and premature babies in general. A low amniotic L/S ratio is the rule in cases of infants dying of respiratory distress syndrome of the newborn.

There are other methods of determining foetal lung maturity. These include the measurment of amniotic lecithin-palmitic acid, or amniotic cortisol-cortisone ratio, etc.

Oxytocin Challenge Test (OCT)

The oxytocin challenge test is used to assess foetal well being as reflected by the foeto-placental unit. In the adult, cardiac function and the amount of cardiac reserve can be roughly estimated by observing the tolerance of the individual to exercise or stress. The same principle is involved in the oxytocin challenge test, in which the reaction of the foeto-placental unit is observed in relation to stress. The oxytocin challenge test attempts to duplicate the stresses of labour by induced uterine contractions and observance of the foetal heart response. By this, the placental reserve or foetal well being can be assessed.

The oxytocin challenge test is carried out at weekly intervals in all high risk pregnancies. It is done in a specialized unit with specially trained physicians and nurses in attendance.

To perform the test the patient is placed in a semi-fowler position. The blood pressure the pulse rate are checked at ten-minute intervals. The transducer of an external monitor (Sonic aid capable of measuring and recording uterine contractions and foetal heart beats) is placed on the patient's abdomen. Baseline recordings of the uterine contractions and foetal heart rate are made in the first ten minutes. Oxytocin infusions, regulated by an infusion pump, is then administered to excite uterine contraction every three to four minutes with each contraction lasting about thirty to eighty seconds. The test is continued for thirty minutes.

The test may be positive, negative, suspicious or unsatisfactory.

A positive test In this case there is a uniform slowing of the foetal heart at the height of a uterine contraction or just beyond the height of a contraction. This slowing of the foetal heart is repeated with every induced uterine contraction.

Negative test This is found in women who show no late deceleration (slowing of foetal heart rate) with the oxytocin-induced uterine contractions.

Suspicious test A test is said to be suspicious when foetal heart slowing is not associated with every induced contraction.

Unsatisfactory test A test may be unsatisfactory because of technical difficulties in carrying it out.

Interpretation of the OCT A positive test implies that all is not well for the foetus. The foeto-placental unit is not functioning normally. The foetus is, therefore, at risk and serious considerations should be given terminating the pregnancy.

A negative test augurs well for the baby. It means that the placental reserve is good and there is no urgent need to terminate pregnancy because the foetus as at that time is not at risk.

Reliance is not always placed on any one test. A number of tests are done and it is only when the result is consistant that a decision is taken. The decision to act is based on other measurements such as the urinary oestriols, the L/S ratio and other tests. A positive OCT in the presence of normal oestriol level and normal L/S ratio may indicate induction of labour and termination of the pregnancy. A negative OCT indicates that there is no urgency in terminating the pregnancy. Eventually when the infant is delivered, cases in which the OCT is persistently negative show infants with a high Apgar scores at birth. The perinatal mortality is usually very low.

Contraindications to OCT: The OCT should not be done in:

1. Cases of previous classical casearean section.
2. Cases of placenta praevia
3. Women who run the risk of going into premature labour, i.e. women with incompetent internal os of the cervix or those with premature rupture of membranes.

It is important that the nurse midwife should know that there may be false negative and false positive OCT. This is why it is important not to place reliance on only one test. It is also important to consider the result of the OCT with results of other tests before the obstetrician takes a final decision on the case.

Non-stress Test

In the non-stress test, the reaction of the foetal heart in response to foetal movements is observed. If, in response to foetal movements, the foetal heart rate increases, it is presumed to be a sign of foetal-well-being and good placental function.

Measurement of the pH of the Foetal Scalp Blood

Foetal acidosis is a cause of hypoxia and depression of respiration in the immediate neonatal period. In a high-risk pregnancy the determination of foetal blood pH may be very important in deciding on the next line of action to be taken to save the foetus. A pH less than 7.22 may imply that the foetus will suffer acidosis and severe intrauterine hypoxia. A pH of 7.3 or above is of good prognostic importance provided other tests are normal.

The application of all the above tests to high-risk pregnancies has led to a drastic reduction in antepartum stillbirth rate, a decrease in morbidity and increased foetal survival rate as well as improved prognosis for the survivors.

It should be noted, however, that the tests described in this chapter are not suitable under all circumstances. They can only be performed in the large urban hospitals with facilities for doing them.

TRIAL OF LABOUR (TOL)

A trial of labour may be initiated if the mother's pelvis is of questionable size or shape, if the foetus is in an abnormal presentation or if she wishes to have a vaginal birth after a previous caesarean birth. It is a form of care likely to be beneficial when implemented after a previous low segment caesarean birth. Foetal sonography or maternal pelvimetry may be done before a trail of labour to rule out CPD (Cephale pelvic disproportion). The cervix must be soft and dilatable. During trial of labour, the woman is evaluated for the occurrence of active labour, including adequate contractions engagement and dilatation of cervix. Nurses must recognize that the woman and her partners are often anxious about her health and well-being and that of their baby. Supporting and encouraging the woman and her partner and providing information regarding progress can reduce stress, enhance the labour process and facilitate successful outcome.

Trial of labour is conducted in the presence of a minor or moderate degree of cephalo-pelvic disproportion in an attempt to achieve a vaginal delivery. The factors aiding the achievement of vaginal delivery in trial of labour are:

1. Effective uterine contractions.
2. Moulding of the foetal head.
3. The give of the pelvis.
4. The fortitude of the patient.

Since there is a possibility of obstruction during trial of labour, it should only be conducted in a hospital with facilities for emergency caesarean section. The nurse should on no account undertake the conduct of trial of labour on her own responsibility.

The Nurse's Responsibilities during a Trial of Labour

Duties to the patient: It is advisable to explain the situation to the patient and forewarn her of possible operative interference. The patient should be carefully assessed on admission to ascertain the following:

i. The establishment of labour.
ii. Thc presentation of the foetus, its position and relation to the pelvic brim.
iii. The flexion of the head.
iv. The foetal heart rate.
v. The general condition of the mother.

The physical and the emotional states of the patient are very important factors in trial of labour so the nurse should endeavour to improve the morale of the patient. The patient is confined to bed to prevent early rupture of membranes. Sedation is given liberally to promote rest and avoid exhaustion and undue anxiety. Adequate hydration of the patient is ensure by giving intravenous infusion of 5 per cent glucose. Nothing is allowed by mouth since operative interference may be necessary at short notice. The danger of inhalation of vomitus during anaesthesia is thus averted.

The bladder and rectum should be emptied to facilitate descent of the foetal head. Encouragement of the patient and a friendly attitude on the part of the nurse will be a long way to boost the patient's morale.

Assessment of progress of labour The progress of labour is determined by vigilant observations made by the nurse in constant attendance of the patient. The observations are made on:

i *The uterine contractions* The type of utering contractions (that is their frequency, strength and duration) are noted and recorded hourly and half-hourly towards the end of labour; the effect of these contractions on the patient and the foetus is also noted.

ii *The descent of the presentations* The uterine contractions should aid flexion and descent of the head into the pelvis, the descent of the head is determined abdominally hourly.

iii *The foetal condition* An half hourly observation and record are made of the maternal pulse, blood pressure and respiration; the temperature is recorded hourly, every specimen of urine, the patient passes is tested to exclude albuminuria and acetonuria; a fluid chart is also kept; the nurse midwife should inform the physician at once if the patient can no longer endure the ordeal.

Conditions to report to the physician. The physician should be contacted for the following conditions:

1. Abnormal uterine actions-especially hypertonic or incoordinate uterine action.
2. Abnormal presentation-that is, a change from vertex to brow or face presentation.
3. Rupture of membrances-the time of its occurrence and number of hours the patient has been in labour, this is done so that the physician may do a vaginal examination to exclude cord prolapse and no determine the progress of labour; it is not advisable for the patient to have many vaginal examinations as these predispose to infection.
4. Failure of descent of the presenting part in the presence of good uterine action-that is, a high head after six to eight hours of strong uterine contractions.
5. Signs of foetal and maternal distress.

Advantages of Trial of Labour

Trial of labour prevents unnecessary elective caesarean section in case of minor degree of disproportion. This is particularly important in developing countries like India where facilities for maternity services are poor and the patients may not return for antenatal supervision after delivery by caesarean section. These patients run the great risk of uterine rupture in subsequent confinements.

The second advantage is the avoidance of premature induction of labour with its attendent risk, which used to be widely practised in cases of suspected disproportion. Premature induction of labour is believed to forestall the delivery of a baby which may be too big for the maternal pelvis if delivered at them. It is, however, not without risks. The patient may fail to go into labour and intrauterine infection may supervene. If the patient goes into labour a grossly premature baby may be delivered.

Wherever possible, a vaginal delivery is to be preferred to an abdominal delivery. If, therfore, trial of labour ensures a safe vaginal delivery, so much the better for all concerned.

Disadvantages of Trial of Labour

Trial of labour may fail, and when it fails the patient is naturally disappointed. She may have gone through a great deal of psychological trauma. Her failure to deliver per vias naturales (by the natural route may affect her adversely). She may consider herself of her baby abnormal and she will think of several reasons why she is unable to do what other women seem to do without much mental or physical trauma.

Apart from the mental agony the patient and her attendants go through if trial of labour has gone on too long, the risk of intrauterine infection with its consequences on the mother and baby cannot be dismissed lightly.

Factors which Influence the Prognosis in Trial of Labour

1. *The membranes:* In trial of labour, early rupture of the membranes prejudices the outlook for mother and baby. Early rupture of the membranes may be complicated by prolapse of the cord, malpresentation, abnormal lie and intra-uterine infection.
2. *The foetal head:* Moulding of the foetal head is of great importance poor moulding means that the head will not be able to go through a borderline pelvis. If malpresentation occurs during the course of labour, the prognosis for the trial of labour is poor.
3. *Maternal distress:* The onset of maternal distress may put an end to trial of labour.
4. *Foetal distress:* Foetal distress from prolapse of the cord or any other cause may make it necessary to terminate a trial of labour.

Contraindications of Trial of Labour

Trial of labour should not be attempted in the following conditions:

1. Gross pelvic contraction
2. Elderly primigravida
3. In the presence of pre-eclampsia, diabetes mellitus, severe hypertension, cardiac disease, etc.
4. In cases in whom a previous trial of labour has been unsuccessful.
5. In the presence of malpresentation.
6. In cases of previous caesarean section.

Outcome of Trial of Labour

Trial of labour is said to be successful if the delivery of the infant is accomplished per vaginum spontaneously or by forceps or vacuum extractor. It is only when unfavourable conditions, such as foetal or maternal distress make the delivery of the baby by caesarean section necessary that trial of labour can be said to have failed.

Induction of Labour (IOL)

Induction of labour is an attempt to bring about regular uterine contractions artificially. There must always be a good reason for induction. If must only be done in the interest of the life or health of the mother or foetus. Induction of labour is the chemical or mechanical initiation of uterine contractions before their spontaneous onset or the purposes of bringing about the birth. Induction may be indicated for variety of medical and obstetric reasons. These include:

- Pregnancy-induced hypertension (Pre-eclampsia and Eclampsia).
- Chronic hypertension/Severe hypertension.
- Diabetes mellitus.
- Chronic nephritis.
- Post-term gestation.
- Suspected foetal life jeopardy for, e.g. IUGR, IUDF-death of foetus.
- Prolonged pregnancy.
- Antepartum haemorrhage (etc, abruptio placentae or minor placenta praevia).
- Congenital foetal abnormality.
- Hydatidiform mole.
- Previous history of repeated intrauterine death of foetus.
- Cross hydramnios causing a great deal of discomfort to the mother.
- Rhesus isoimmunization.
- Fulminating hepatitis as in acute yellow atrophy.
- Logistics factors such as history of previous rapid birth or distance of the women's house from the hospital.

Induction may be medical or surgical.

MEDICAL INDUCTION OF LABOUR

In this, less commonly used methods, include nipple stimulation (manual or with a breastpump), the ingestion of castor oil or herbal preparations, a soap-such enema, stripping of the membranes and acupuncture. Prostaglandins are also used for inducing labour but their use for this purpose continues to be investigated.

Prostaglandin

A prostaglandin E2 gel has been used as a cervical ripening agent. Curently preparations of prostaglandin E1 and prostaglandin E2 can be used before induction to 'ripen' (soften and thin) the cervix, This treatment usually results in a higher success rate for induction of labour, the need for lower doses of oxytocin during inductions, and shorter induction times. In some cases, women will go into labour after the administration of prostaglandin, thereby eliminating the need and administer oxytocin to induce labour.

Prostaglandin E1 (PGE1PM isoprostol-cytotex)

PGE1 ripens the cervix, making it softer and causing it to begin to dilate and efface, stimulates uterine contractions. It is used for preinduction-cervical ripening (ripen cervix before oxytocin induction of labour when the Bishop's score is 4 or less) and to induce labour or abortion.

Administration

Insert 25 to 50 µg (¼ to ½ of 100 µg tablet) intravaginally into the posterior fornix using the tips of index and middle fingers without the use of a lubricant. Repeat every 4 to 6 hours as needed to a maximum of 30 µg in a 24 hour period or until an effective contraction in 10 minutes, cervix ripens (Bishop's score of 8 or greater) or significant adverse reaction occur.

Higher dosages are more likely to result in adverse reactions such as nausea and vomiting, diarrhoea, fever, tachysystole (12 or more uterine contractions in 20 minutes without alteration of FHR pattern) hyper stimulation of the uterus (tachysystole with non-reasuring FHR pattern) or foetal passage of meconium.

Nursing Intervention

- Explain procedure to woman and her family. Ensure that an informed consent has been obtained as per hospital policy.
- Assess maternal-foetal unit, before each insertion and during treatment following hospital protocol for frequancy. Assess maternal vital signs and health status, FHR pattern and status of pregnancy, including indications for cervical ripening of induction of labour, signs of labour or impending labour, and Bishop's score. Recognize that a non-reassuring FHR pattern; maternal fever, infection, vaginal bleeding or hypersensitivity and regular progressive uterine contractions, contraindicates the use of PGE1 (misprostol).
- Use caution if the woman has history of asthma, glaucoma, or renal, hepatic, or cardiovascular diseases.
- Assist woman to maintain a supine position with lateral tilt or sidelying position for 30 to 40 minutes after insertion.
- Prepare to swab vagina to remove unabsorbed medication using a saline soaked gauze wrapped around figuers and to administer terbutaline 0.25 mg subcutaneously or intravenously if significant adverse reactions occur.
- Initiate oxytocin for induction of labour 2 to 4 hours after last dose of misoprostol was administered, following hospital protocol, if ripening has occurred and labour has not begun.
- Document all assessment findings and administrate procedure.

Note: oxytotic is not yet approved. Use cautiously.

PGE_2 Dinoprostone (Cervidi) Insert

PGE_2 ripens the cervix, making it softer and causing it to begin to dilate and efface; stimulates uterioecontractions.

PGE_2 is used for preinduction cervical ripening and to induce labour or abortion.

Administration of PGE_2

Place cervidil (10 mg dinoprostone gradually released over 12 hours) intravaginally into the posterior fornix. Insert syringe containing 0.5 mg of dinoprostone) into cervical canal just below internal cervical os. Repeat gel insertion in 6 hours as needed to maximum of 1.5 mg in a 24-hours period. Continue treatment until an effective contraction pattern is established (3 or more uterine contractions in 10 minutes). Cervix ripens (Bishop's score of 8 or more) or significant adverse reactions occur. Adverse reactions are as in PGE1.

Nursing Intervention

Explain procedure to woman and her family. Ensure that an informed consent has been obtained as per hospital policy. Assess maternal-foetal unit, before each insertion and during treatment following hospital protocol for frequency. Assess maternal vital signs and health status, FHR pattern and status of pregnancy, including indication for cervical ripening or induction of labour, signs of labour and impending labour and Bishop's score. Recognize that non-reassuring FHR pattern, maternal fever infection, vaginal bleeding or hypersensitivity and regular progressive uterine contraction contraindicates the use of dinoprostone.

- Use caution if the woman has a history of asthma, glaucoma, or renal, hepatic or cardiovascular disorders.

- Bring gel to room termperature before administration. Don't force warming process by using warm water bath or other sources of external heat (microwave).
- Have woman to void before insertion.
- Assist woman to maintain a supine position with lateral tilt or a side lying position for 30 to 60 minutes after insertion of gel or for 2 hours after placement of insert.
- Prepare to swab vagina to remove remaining gel using a saline soaked gauze wrapper around fingers or pull string to remove insert and to administer terbutaline 0.25 mg subcutaneously or intravenously if significant adverse reaction occurs.
- Initiate oxytocin for induction of labour within 6 to 12 hours often last insertion of gel or within 30 minutes after removal of insert.
- Follow hospital protocol for induction if ripening.

Dystocia, premature rupture of membranes, post-term pregnancy, choxio amniotis, maternal medica problems, PIH, foetal demise, multiparous women with history of precipitations labour or who live far the hospital. The management of stimulation of labour is the same regardless of indications. Contraindications to oxytocin stimulation of labour include, but are not limited to the following:

- Non-reassuring FHR
- Placenta praevia or vasa praevia.
- Prior classic Uterine incision or uterine surgery.
- Active genital herpes infection.
- Invasive cancer of the cervix.

Certain maternal and foetal conditions, although not contraindications to the use of oxytocin to stimulate labour, do require special precautions puting administration. These conditions include—multifoetal presentation, breech presentation, presenting part above the pelvic inlet, abnomal FHR pattern, not requiring emergency birth, polyhydramnios, grandmultiparity, maternal cardiac disease and hypertension.

Pitocin Administration

Pitocin is secreted by the posterior pituitary and its action on the uterus is well known. It produces intermittent uterine contractions and may initiate the onset of labour. In the synthetic form it may be used intramuscularly or intravenously. Intramuscular pitocin should not be used to induce labour when the baby is alive and viable. This is because it may cause uterine spasm, which may prejudice placental circulation and cause asphyxia of the foetus in utero. Intramuscular pitocin is, therefore, used to induce labour only in cases of intra-uterine death of the foetus or missed abortion. In such cases it is given in doses of 2¼ units half hourly upto a maximum of six doses. An enema is given to the patient after the second dose of pitocin. The midwife is advised never to undertake this procedure on her own responsibility in rural practice.

Buccal Pitocin

Buccal pitocin is so called because it is absorbed in tablet form from the buccal mucous membranes. Its action is unpredictable. It may also cause uterine spasm and its action cannot be easily controlled. Pitocin or Syntocinon may also be given by nasal spray.

Intravenous Pitocin

Intravenous pitocin is commonly used to induce labour because it is easily controlled and is more reliable in effect than that given by the intramuscular route. It is usual to start with a small dose, gradually increasing it until the desired effect is obtained. Two units of pitocin in 500 ml of 5 per cent glucose is the usual starting point. A Y-shaped giving set is used. In one limb of the set 5 per cent glucose in water containing pitocin is infused. In the other lab 5 per cent glucose in water without pitocin is set up. The drip is usually started at the rate of 20 drops per minute, increasing by 5 drops every fifteen minutes until contractions are adequate or a rate of 40 drops per minute is reached. If no progress is made the amount of pitocin may be increased from 2 to 5 units and the number of drops reduced to 20 per minute. This may also be increased by 5 drops every quarter hour until contractions are adequate or a rate of 40 drops per minute is reached. The drip is continued throughout labour unless tonic contractions occur and until one hour after the completion of the third stage to prevent postpartum haemorrhage.

Care of the Patient

Before the drip is started the presentation of the foetus must be ascertained and cephalo-pelvic disproportion rule out. The maternal pulse is taken at frequent intervals and recorded every hour, the blood pressure and respiration are also recorded at the same interval. The temperature is recorded every four hours. The time, duration and strength of every uterine contraction should be recorded every half hour. The foetal condition is assessed by auscultating and recording foetal heart sounds every 15 minutes. Ideally a nurse midwife should stay with the patient all the time.

The drip should be stopped and the physician informed if a contraction lasts over 60 second or if there is no relaxation between contraction. If there is foetal distress or deterioration in the patient's general condition a report must be made to the physician. Other uses of pitocin drip in obstetrics are to stimulate uterine contractions in case of hypotonic uterine inertia and for treatment of postpartum haemorrhage.

A synthetic preparations—Syntocinon (the action of which is similar to that of pitocin) may also be used. The precautions that are taken with pitocin apply also to Syntocinon. Syntocinon can be given intravenously in exactly the same way as pitocin.

Quinine Hydrochloride

Quinine hydrochloride in the dose of 300 mg half-hourly up to a total of six doses may be given. The occurrence of 8th nerve symptoms such as dizziness, buzzing in the ears, etc. warrants the discontinuation of quinine therapy even if the total dose envisaged has not been given.

Quinine therapy as a method of induction is only suitable in cases of missed abortion and intra-uterine death. it must on no account be used when the foetus is alive.

Oestrogens

Oestrogens in the form of high doses of still-boestrol are used in induce labour. If is believed that oestrogens sensitize the uterus to the action of pitocin or Syntocinon, i.e., if a patient is previously given a high dose of oestrogens responds very well to induction by pitocin or Syntocinon drip. Oestrogens are not frequently used to induce labour.

SURGICAL INDUCTION OF LABOUR

In this method foetal membranes are ruptured artificially. Prior to the rupture of membranes, the physician often does a through pelvic assessment to exclude cephalo-pelvic disproportion. He makes a vaginal examination and insinuates a finger through the cervix, sweeps round the area beyond the internal os, detaching the chorion from the dacidua. The procedure is referred to as stripping or sweeping of the membranes. Some physician also stretch the cervix manually, the idea being to stimulate the uterus before the rupture of membranes is carried out. In artificial rupture of membranes a forewater of hindwater rupture may be done. A pair of kocher's forceps or special amniotomy forceps is used by the doctor to carry out forewater rupture. A Drew Smythe catheter is used for hindwater rupture.

Other Methods of Induction

These include the use of intravenous or intra-amniotic prostaglandins, intra-amniotic injection of hypertonic saline or concentrated glucose solution. Hypertonic saline and concentrated glucose are only used in the termination of an unwanted pregnancy.

Prostaglandins are products of fatty acids related to linoleic acid. They are found in body tissues such as the uterus in the female and the prostate gland in the male. Naturally occurring or synthetic prostaglandins may be used. When given intravenously, they cause a great deal of constitutional upset, e.g. anorexia, vomiting, tachycardia, etc. They are well tolerated when given through the uterine cavity or amniotic sac.

Labour can also be induced by other mechanical means such as the introduction of bougias, catheters and hydrostatic bags. The last three methods are old fashioned and are seldom used in modern obstetrics.

Preparation of the Patient

The situation sould be explained to the patient. Her general condition is assessed and her vulva is shaved and washed. An enema saponis is often given on the morning of the day and the artificial rupture of membranes is to be performed. An anaesthetic is not usually required but apprehensive patients are often given pethidine (100 mg) or substitute 1 hour prior to the procedure. The patient is placed in the lithotomy position for the procedure. A pair of Kocher's or amniotomy forceps is used to rupture the forewaters. It rupture of the hindwater is desired a Drew Smythe's catheter is used.

The Risks of Induction

Certain grave risks are associated with induction of labour.

1. The induction may fail. The patient may be disappointed and depressed. If surgical induction fails there is the great risk of infection and uterine sepsis which may result in intranatal pneumonia or intrauterine death of the foetus. Surgical induction may also lead to a dry labour if all the liquor amnoil drains out before the patient goes into labour. In such a case, the possibility of foetal hypoxia is increased.
2. Prematurity—In women, who are not very sure, of the date of their last menstrual period a premature baby with poor chances of survival may be born.
3. Induction may be inadvertently done in the presence of cephalopelvic disproportion which was not anticipated at the time of induction. This is a serious matter. No patient should be induced in the presence of cephalopelvic disproportion, however mild.
4. In the presence of an unsuspected low lying placenta, surgical induction may produce bleeding usally described as a 'bloody tap'. The bleeding may be of foetal or maternal origin and can be dangerous to both.
5. Sudden release of pressure following induction of labour from gross hydramnios may cause premature separations of the placenta and lead to antepartum haemorrhage.
6. Cord prolapse—Prolapse of the cord may follow artificial forewater rupture of membranes.
7. Amniotic fluid embolism—This is a very rare but serious complication of surgical induction.
8. Rupture of the uterus—The uterus may be perforated by the Drew Smythe's catheter during hindwater rupture of membrane. Intravenous or intramuscular oxytocin may cause uterine rupture in a grand-multipara or in patients with a previous history of caesarean section. Oxytocin given when there is cephalo-pelvic disproportion can cause uterine rupture in a multigravida.

The physician or nurse-midwife writes the order for the induction of augmentation of labour with oxytocin. The nurse implements the order by initiating the primary intravenous infusion and administering the oxytocin solution through a secondary line. The nurse's actions related to assessment and care of women whose labour is being induced are guided by *hospital protocol* and professional standard.

Patient/Family Teaching

Explain technique, rationale, and reaction to expect:

- Route and rate for administration of medication.
- What "Piggyback" is for.
- Reasons for use: Induce labour, or Improve labour.
- Reactions to expect concerning the nature of contractions; the intensity of contraction increases more rapidly, holds the peak longer, and ends more quickly; contractions will come regularly and more often.
- Monitoring to anticipate: Maternal blood pressure, pulse, uterine contractions, uterine tone, foetal-heart rate, activity.
- Success to 'expect' a favourable outcome well depends on inducibility of the cervix (e.g., Bishop's score).

Administration

- Position woman in side lying or upright position.
- Assess status of maternal foetal unit.
- Prepare solutions and administer with pump delivery system according to prescribed orders.
  - Infusion pump and solutions are set up (e.g., 10 IU/1000 ml isotonic electrolyte solutions).
  - Piggyback solution is connected to IV Line at proximal port (portnearest point of venous insertion).
  - Solution with oxytocin is flagged with medication label.
  - Begin induction at 0.5 to 2 mU/min.
  - Increase dose 1 to 2 mU/min at intervals of 15 to 60 minutes until a dose of upto 20 to 40 mU/min. is reached.

Maintain Dose

- Intensity of contractions results in intrauterine pressure of 40 to 90 mmHg (shown by internal monitor).
- Duration of contractions is 40 to 90 seconds.
- Frequency contractions is 2 to 3 minutes intervals.
- Cervical dilatations of 1 cm/hour in the active phase.

Maternal Foetal Assessment

- Monitor blood pressure, pulse and respirations every 30 to 60 minutes and with every increment in dose.
- Monitor contraction pattern and uterine resting tone every 15 minutes and with every increment in dose.
- Assess intake and output; limit IV intake to 1000 ml/8 hours; output should be 120 ml or more every 4 hours.
- Perform vaginal examination as indicated.
- Monitor nausea, vomiting, headache, hypotension.
- Assess foetal status using electronic foetal monitoring, evaluate tracing every 15 minutes and with every increment in dose.
- Observe emotonal response of women and her partner.

Reportable Condition

- Uterine hyperstimulation.
- Non-reassuring FHR pattern.
- Suspected uterine rupture
- Inadequate uterine responses at 20 mU/min.

Emergency Measures

Discontinue use of oxytocin per hospital protocol.

- Turn woman on her side.
- Increase primary IV rate upto 200 ml/hr unless patient by water intoxication, in which case, the rate is decreased to one that keeps the vein open.
- Give woman oxygen by face mask at 8 to 10 L/min or per protocol or physician or nurse-midwife's order.

Documentation

- Medication; kind, amount, time of beginning, increasing dose, maintaining dose, and discontinuing medication in patient's record and on monitor strip
- Reactions of mother and foetus.
  - Pattern of labour
  - Progress of labour
  - FHR and pattern
  - Nursing intervention and woman's response.
- Notification of physician or nurse midwife.

OBSTRUCTED LABOUR

Labour is obstructed when there is no advance of the presenting part despite strong uterine contractions. The obstruction usually occurs at the pelvic brim; but may occur at the outlet—For example, deep transverse arrest in an abdroid pelvis.

Obstructed labour refers to a situation in which the descent of the presentation is arrested, despite good and efficient uterine contractions. Obstruction usually occurs at the brim but it can takes place at the mid-cavity or outlet of the pelvis.

The incidence of obstructed labour is quite high in developing countries because the women are relatively short in stature. There is inadequate antenatal and intranatal care, Partly because patients do not make good use of the available antenatal clinics. Marriage at an early age when the development of the pelvis has not attained its full capacity is also common in these countries.

Obstructed labour accounts for a high percentage of maternal mortality and morbidity.

Effects of Obstructed Labour

Most cases of obstructed labour have had no antenatal care. They often labour at home for hours or days thus arriving at the hospital exhausted, septic and dehydrated. At times the uterus may rupture and the women die of haemorrhage or a combination of the above complications. Other ill effects if obstructed labour are recto-vaginal and vesico-vaginal fistulae which occur as a result of bruising of the rectum and the bladder or injury sustained during a difficult instrumental delivery. Foot drop is another complication due to pressure on the sciatic nerve. The foetal prognosis in obstructed labour is usually poor. The foetus often does in utero, therefore, the stillbirth rate is high. Neonatal death is common as a result of severe asphyxia or intracranial injury at birth.

Causes of Obstructed Labour

The usual causes of obstructed labour are:

1. Contracted pelvis.
2. Cephalopelvic disproportion.
3. Persistent occipito-posterior position.
4. Abnormal presentation such as shoulder presentation, brow presentation and face presentation with the chin in the posterior position.

5. Pelvic tumours such as a large ovarian cyst, a large cervical fibroid, etc.
6. Stenosis of the cervix from a previous operation such as Manchester repair, previous curettage, or from carcinoma of the cervix.
7. Foetal abnormalities, particularly hydrocephaly, or tumours in the baby's neck or head. These may cause obstructed labour.

Clinical Features of Obstructed Labour

The labour is usually prolonged. A good nurse should be able to detect early signs of obstruction and report to the physician. The contractions are usually strong and hypertonic with little relaxation between contractions. Labour is prolonged because the os dilates slowly and is usually not well applied to the presenting part. The presentation is high and does not descend with good uterine contractions. Signs of obstruction are the uterus becomes tonic and moulds round the foetus, especially as the membranes usually rupture early; an excessive retraction ring known as Bondl's ring can be palpated at a depression across the abdomen in the region of the umbilicus; the lower uterine segment which is stretched and thinned out into the form of a balloon distends the lower part of the abdomen; the abdominal distension is further increased by the presence of a full bladder and gas in the colon and intestines and there is difficulty in catheterizing the bladder and the urine obtained is usually concentrated and often bloodstained.

If a vaginal examination is made, the presenting part is found wedged or impacted in the pelvis; a large caput succedaneum is felt and there is overlapping of the skull bones (excessive moulding) in a cephalic presentation. The cervix is usually thick and oedematous if it is not fully dilated. If hangs lossely over the presenting part. The vagina feels warm because the patient is hot and dehydrated. The vulva may be oedematous especially if the patient has been bearing down for a long time. Vaginal bleeding may be a warning sign that the uterus has ruptured. Evidence of foetal and maternal distress is usually manifest.

Management of Obstructed Labour

Since obstructed labour rarely occurs in patients whose pregnancies have been properly supervised, the majority of these cases are admitted in a poor state as emergencies. However, if labour becomes obstructed in a patient, supervised a nurse, medical aid must be sought immediately or the patient transferred to a hospital. If the nurse cannot accompany the patient, she must write a full account of all the events preceding the obstruction. Details of drugs administered, the time of onset of labour and rupture of membranes must be included in the letter which a relative takes with the patient to a hospital.

In the hospital The physician is informed of the patient's arrival. A history of the labour as well as social, medical and obstetrical history is obtained from the patient. Inquiry is also made about drugs, especially native herbs and their extracts taken at home. The patient's general condition is assessed by recording her pulse, blood pressure, temperature and these are continued quarter-hourly till the patient delivers.

A specimen of urine is obtained by catheterization and tested for albumin, sugar and acetone. The foetal heart is auscultated to ascertain whether the baby is alive or dead. Blood is collected for grouping and cross matching followed by intravenous infusion of 5 per cent glucose given to correct dehydration and ketosis. Pethidine (100-150 mg) is given intramuscularly to relieve pain and sedate the patient. Vulval toilet is done and preparations for operation including emptying the stomach with a wide bore stomach tube are carried out, though no operative delivery will be undertaken unless dehydration and ketosis are effectively controlled. A consent for anaesthesia and operation is obtained from the patient or her relative. A premedication of atronopine 0.6 mg is usually given prior to the administration of anaeathesia. Labour is usually terminated in one of the following ways.

1. Caesarean section is done if the baby is alive and there is gross disproportion or malpresentation if the cervix is not completely dilated.
2. Forceps delivery or vacuum extraction is done if the cervix is fully dilated and foetal head is arrested in the midcavity of the maternal pelvis.
3. Destructive operation such as craniotomy and decapitation is done if the baby is dead.

Management after Delivery

After delivery, the general condition of the patient is closely watched. The quarter hourly record of pulse and respiration and the hourly blood pressure recording are maintained till the patient's general condition improves. The temperature is recorded four-hourly. A course of antibiotics is usually given. The bladder is drained continuously with an indwelling catheter for ten days. This will rest the bladder, and prevent in formation of a fistula or bring about spontaneous closure of a very small existing fistula. Gastric aspiration is done hourly and oral fluids are withheld till the abdomen is less distended and bowel sound are present and normal. Fluids are given intravenously and a fluid chart is kept. Before unbooked patients are discharged, the following investigations are made:

1. X-ray pelvimetry is done to exclude contracted pelvis. Patients found to have contracted pelvis are instructed to have their subsequent confinement in hospitals.
2. Chest X-ray is done to exclude tuberculosis.
3. The haemoglobin genotype is determined.
4. Any other relevant investigation to be done.

RUPTURE OF THE UTERUS

Rupture of the uterue is a serious obstetric accident seen commonly in developing countries because of the high incidence of contracted pelvis as well as poor antenatal and intranatal supervision.

Rupture of the uterus is usually encountered in women of high parity. It is very rare in primigravid patients unless there has been a previous trauma to the uterus; such as previous myomectomy or perforation at dilatation and curettage for infertility. Ruptured uterus may be complete or incomplete and it may occur in the anterior or posterior aspects of the uterus. Incomplete uterine rupture does not involve the peritoneal covering of the uterus but in complete ruputure, uterus as well as its peritoneal covering is usually torn.

Causes of Rupture of the Uterus

1. Obstructed labour resulting from cephalopelvic disproportion, impacted shoulder presentation, or any malpresentation is very likely to cause rupture of the uterus in women who have had one or more children if the obstruction is not relieved.
2. *High parity* One of the most important predisposing factors is high parity. The uterus of a grand multiparous patient is most likely to rupture even in an apparently normal labour because nearly all its smooth muscle fibres have been replaced by fibrous tissue and the babies are usually big.
3. *Previous trauma to the uterus* The most important cause under this heading is a previous caesarean section, particularly a classical caesarean section. Other causes include a previous vigorous uterine curettage, previous perforation of the uterus at D and C operation, previous myomectomy and previous manual removal of a morbidly adherent placenta. In respect of caesarean section, the classical section scar is far more likely to rupture than the lower segment scar. In this regard the scar of a previous classical caesarean section may rupture during the pregnancy. The scar of a previous lower uterine segment caesarean section is not likely to rupture before the onset of labour.
4. *Difficult obstetric manipulations* These include external or internal version, especially in the presence of a previous uterine scar or if a great deal of force is used. Instrumental deliveries such as forceps delivery, destructive operations such as craniotomy, decapitation, etc. may result in rupture of the uterus.
5. *Abuse of oxyocin drugs* Oxytocic drugs should never be given to induce labour if there is a history of previous caesarean section. The inadvertent use intravenous pitocin may lead to uterine rupture, especially in cases of diaproportion and grande multiparity.

Intramuscular and buccal administration of pitocin have also been associated with uterine rupture.

Clinical Features of Ruptured Uterus

The clinical features of ruptured uterus depend to a certain extent on the causative factor and on the extent of the rupture. Uterine rupture associated with a previous lower segment caesarean section usually occurs during the last four weeks of pregnancy or at the beginning of labour, and as the signs may not be dramatic as in obstructed labour, the term's silent rupture is used. The usual symptom is low abdominal pain which may be accompanied by vaginal bleeding. Shock, comas on slowly in some cases and abruptly in others. Some cases of rupture of a previous scar may only be discovered on routine exploration of the uterus of a delivered mother or at repeat caesaran section operation.

In cases where the uterine rupture follows obstructed labour, there is usually a great deal of constitutional disturbance. The patient may feel faint at first. Later she goes into a state of severe shock, because of the large collection of blood in the peritoneal cavity. She is cold, and clammy and beads of perspiration may be observed on her forehead. The blood pressure is low and the pulse is rapid and thready. If she has not yet been delivered, and the rupture is incomplete the abdominal pain persists uterine contractions. As soon as the foetus is extruded into the peritoneal cavity, the pain of uterine contractions ceases.

On abdominal palpation, there is usually an area of tenderness. The foetal parts are very easily palpable in cases of large rupture as the foetus has been led into the peritoneal cavity. Foetal movements cease and the foetal heartsound is not heard. There may be some vaginal bleeding.

Management of Ruptured Uterus

If the rupture is dagnosed in the hospital, the nurse midwife must inform the physician in charge without any delay. The patient should be kept cool and comfortable. Usually the physician prescribes an intramuscular injection of morphine (15 mg). The nurse midwife should check the patient's pulse and blood pressure at quarter hourly intervals. Preparation for an immediate intravenous infusion should be made. When setting up a intravenous infusion, blood should be collected for grouping and cross matching. The patient and her husband should be informed of the possibility of hysterectomy or sterilization and their consent should be obtained. The patient should be prepared for laparotomy.

In the operating theatre, the surgeon may, after removing the foetus placenta and blood clots, do one of the following, depending on the finding at operation.

1. Repair of the uterus only.
2. Repair of the uterus and sterilization (bilateral tubal ligation).
3. Removal of the uterus-total or subtotal hysterectomy.

If, at operation, the surgeon finds a clan and linear tear of the uterus and if the patient has only one or two children, he will repair the uterus but without sterilizing the woman. If, however, the tear is a very big one or if there are several points of rupture, the surgeon may either repair the uterus and sterilize the woman or do a total or subtotal hysterectomy. A grand multiparous patient who ruptures her uterus will invariable be sterilized.

If the rupture occurs outside a hospital not equipped for dealing with such an emergency, the nurse midwife must at once make arrangements to transfer the patient to a big hospital. She should keep the patient cool and administer any pain relieving drug (such as pethidine, 100 mg) at her disposal, shock is treated by raising the foot of the bed and giving an intravenous infusion of saline or glucose-saline, or a rectal infusion of tap water if sterile solutions of glucose, saline or glucose saline are not available.

As soon as possible, the patient should be transferred to a big hospital in an ambulance and a midwife or nurse should accompany her to the hospital. The patient' s husband and some relatives should be asked to go along to the hospital and donate blood. An account of the treatment given to the pattent and the records kept by the nurse should be taken to the hospital. In the hospital, the patient is resuscitated and treated as stated above.

Silent ruputures are usually small and, if discovered after delivery at routine uterine exploration, no treatment is necessary. The patient's pulse rate, blood pressure and general condition must be watched carefull for 48 to 72 hours after delivery.

Nursing Interventions

If a patient with rupture of the uterus is not sterilized, she should be advised to avoid pregnancy for at least 9 to 12 months. In addition she should be told to report to the nearest hospital whenever she is pregnant. She should carry a note indicating what operation she has had. All such patients must be delivered by elective caesarean section at about 38 weeks gestation patients who have had bilateral tubal ligation or hysterectomy need no obstetric follow-up, but the nature of the operation and its consequences must be thoroughly explained to them.

Prevention is the best treatment. Woman who have had a previous classic caesarean birth are advised not be attempt vaginal birth in subsequent pregnancies. Women at risk for uterine rupture are assessed closely during labour. Women whose labour induced with oxytocin or prostaglandin are monitored for signs of uterine hyperstimulation, because this can precipitate uterine rupture. If hyperstimulation occurs, the oxytocin infusion is discontinued or decreased and tocolytic medications may be given to decrease the intensity of the uterine contractions. After giving birth, women are assessed for excessive bleeding, especially if the fundus is firm and there are signs of haemorrhagic shock.

If the rupture occurs, the type of medical management depends on the severity. A small rupture may be managed with laparatomy and birth of the infant, repair of the laceration, and blood transfusion if needed. For a complete rupture, hysterectomy and blood replacement is the usual treatment.

The nurse's role may include starting intravenous fluids, transfusing blood products, administering oxygen, and assisting with the preparation for immediate surgery. Supposing the women's family and providing information about the treatment, are important, during the emergency, providing information about spiritual support services or suggesting that the family contact their own support system may be warranted.

PROLAPSE OF THE UMBILICAL CORD

Umbilical cord prolapse may be occult (hidden, not visible) at any time during labour whether or not the membranes are ruptured. It is most common to see frank (visible) prolapse directly after rupture of membrane when gravity washes the cord in front of the presenting part. Contributing factors include a long cord (longer than 100 cm), malpresentations (breech transverse lie or unengaged presenting part).

The cord (funis) is said to prolapse when if lies below the presenting part of the aby after the membranes have ruptured. When the cord lies in front of the presenting part with the membranes intact, cord presentation (funic presentation is diagnosed).

Prolapse of the cord occurs about once in 400 deliveries if both normal and abnormal presentations are considered. The incidence is lower in vertex than in other presentations.

Causes of Cord Prolapse

1. Abnormal presentation and position of the head. Prolapse of the cord is possible in any presentation in which the presenting part is not well applied to the cervix. Examples of these abnormal presentations are (Figs. 9.1 to 9.4):
   a. Breech presentation-cord prolapse is common in breech presentation especially the footling and full breech. It is uncommon in breech with extended legs.
   b. Face and brow presentations.
   c. Shoulder presentation resulting from transverse lie, about one-fifth of cases of cord prolapse occur in this presentation.
   d. Occipito-posterior position.
2. Contracted pelvis—This is one of the most important causes of cord prolapse because all the malpresentations mentioned above are sometime the direct result of contracted pelvis.

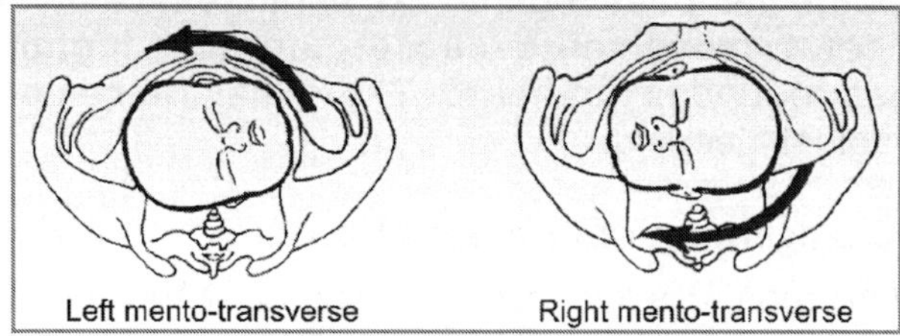

Fig. 9.1: Position of the face presentation; the denomination is the chin

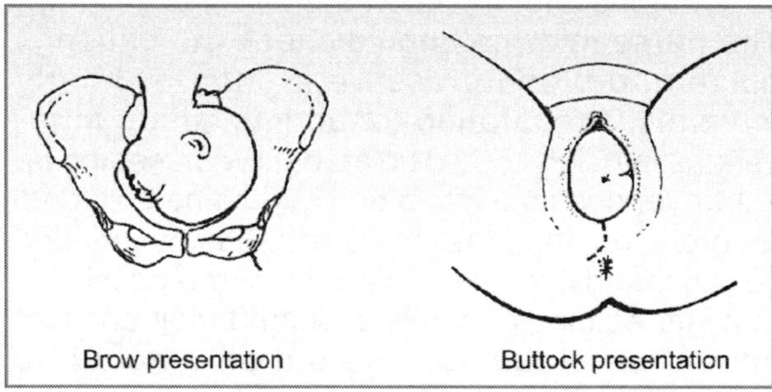

Fig. 9.2: Brow and breech presentation at delivery

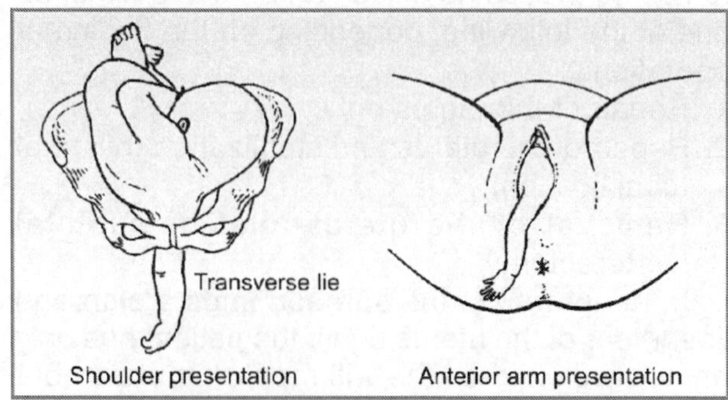

Fig. 9.3: Prolapse of the arm into the vagina sometimes results in a shoulder presentation

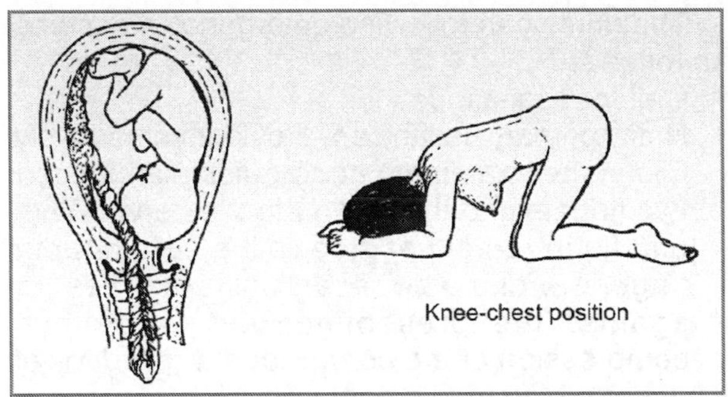

Fig. 9.4: Cord prolapse (left); pressure on the cord can be minimized by placing the mother in the knee-chest position (right)

3. Certain placental and cord conditions predispose to prolapse of the cord. These include low implantation of the placenta, marginal insertion of the cord and unusually long cord.
4. Premature rupture of the membranes especially when the head is high and the patient is walking about.
5. Grande multiparity is a contributory factor because the foetal head may not be engaged when the membranes rupture.
6. Prematurity predisposes to prolapsed cord because the foetus is small and is presenting part is high and poorly applied to the cervix.
7. Hydramnios—The cord is liable to be swept down in the rush of fluid when the membranes rupture.
8. Multiple pregnancy—Hydramnios, malpresentation and prematurity occur in twins and they cause cord prolapse.
9. High head—In this case the head is not well applied to the cervix, so the cord is liable to prolapse.

Diagnosis of Cord Presentation and Prolapse

It is not usually possible to diagnose cord presentation or prolapse until the patient is in labour and the cervix is dilated sufficiently to admit one or two fingers.

In cord presentation a soft pulsating mass may be felt in front of the presenting part with the membranes intact.

A prolapsed cord may be felt in the vagina or seen lying outside the vulva as a soft mass which may or may not be pulsating. The nurse must determine whether the cord is pulsating or not because a favourable prognosis for the baby depends on good and strong pulsation of the cord. In order not to mistake pulsations in her own fingers or maternal pulsations for cord pulsations, the nurse midwife should hold the cord between here two fingers and test for pulsation. If only one finger can be inserted into the cervix, the cord may be tested for pulsation by pressing it between the examining finger and the foetal presenting part.

Auscultation of the foetal heart sounds also helps to confirm the diagnosis of cord prolapse, especially if there is associated compression of the cord or spasm of the umbilical vessels. In such cases, the foetal heart may be rapid, slow or irregular.

Treatment

Cord Presentation

The treatment for cord presentation is to prevent rupture of the membranes, compression of the cord and to arrange for the immediate delivery of the baby, preferably by caesarean section. The nurse should seek medical aid. The foot of the bed should be raised high or the patient put in the genu pectoral (knee chest) position pending the arrival of the physician. The genu-pectoral position is efficient in preventing cord compression but is very uncomfortable for the mother. A third and perhaps the most comfortable position for the patient is the Sim's lateral position. In this position, the patient's pelvis is raised on pillows. She is less uncomfortable and immediate preparations should be made for the performance of a caesarean section if the cord is still pulsating and the foetal heart is audible.

Cord Prolapse

If the prolapsed cord is pulsating, the nurse should prevent pressure on the cord by putting the patient in any of the three positions previously mentioned under cord presentation. If the presenting part is high, any attempt to replace the cord may fail. It is better to prevent spasm of the umbilical vessels (caused by prolonged exposure) by wrapping the cord in sterile gauze dipped in warm saline solution. The physician must be informed at once.

If cord prolapse occurs during the first stage of labour, the nurse should prepare the theatre and the patient for caesarean section after giving the emergency treatment discussed above.

If the patient is in the second stage of labour and the physician is not immediately available, an episiotomy should be done and delivery has tend by fundal pressure, Forceps delivery may be done if a physician is present.

For the ANM in the rural areas cord prolapse is a trying complication. The emergency treatment is as for the hospital, but after this, an attempt should be made to transfer the patient to hospital by the quickest and safest method of transportation. As long as the cord is pulsating and cord compression is prevented, the ANM should not despair. It is amazing how determined to live some babies are.

Prognosis

Cord presentation and prolapse are serious complications, which, unfortunately, are not easy to prevent. About 50 per cent of foetal mortality occurs with cord prolapse through and rest for susceptible cases may be considered prophylactic. The prognosis is better in footling or full breeches than in cephalic presentations. The babies usually die of anoxia secondary to compression or spasm of the umbilical vessels.

Nursing Management

Prompt recognition of a prolapsed umbilical cord is important, because foetal hypoxia resulting from prolonged cord compression, i.e. occlusion of blood flow to and from the foetus for more than 5 minutes usually results in CNS damage or death of the foetus. Pressure on the cord may be relieved by the examiner putting a sterile gloved hand into the vagina and holding the presenting part off the umbilical cord. The woman is assisted into a position such as modified Sims. Trendelenburg or knee-chest position in which gravity keeps the pressure of the presenting part off the cord. If the cervix is fully dilated, a forceps or vacuum assisted birth can be performed for the foetus in a cephalic presentation. Otherwise, a caesarean birth is likely to be performed non-reassuring foetal status, inadequate uterine relaxation and bleeding can also occur as a result of prolapsed umbilical cord.

In cases of emergency, where woman shows signs of:

- Foetal bradycardia, with variable deceleration during uterine contraction
- Woman reports feeling the cord after membranes rupture.
- Cord is seen or felt in or protruding from the vagina.

The nurse can following emergency measures as follows:

- Call for assistance
- Notify primary health care provider immediately
- Glove the examining hand quickly and insert two fingers into the vagina to the cervix. With one finger on either side of the cord or both fingers to one side, exert upward pressure against the presenting part to relieve compression of the cord. Place a rolled towel under the woman's right or left hip.
- Place woman into the extreme Trendelenburg or a modified Sim's position or a knee-chest position
- If the cord is protruding from vagina, wrap loosely in a sterile towel saturated with warm sterile normal saline solution.
- Administer oxygen to the woman by mask at 8 to 10 L/min. until birth is accomplished.
- Start IV fluids or increase existing drip rate
- Continue to monitor FHR by internal foetal scalp electrode if possible.
- Explain to woman and support person what is happening and the way it is being managed
- Prepare for immediate vaginal delivery if cervix is fully dilated or Caesarean birth if it is not.

DYSTOCIA/PROLONGED LABOUR

Prolonged labour is most common in primigravidae and may be caused by ineffective uterine contractions, Cephalopelvic disproportions and occipito posterior positions. Dystocia literally means "difficult labour" and is associated with slow progress and failure to progress in labour. This can be caused by problems with contractions, which include—not being effective in dilating and effacing the cervix; being uncoordinated, where the two segments of the uterus fail to work in harmony; giving inadequate involuntary expulsion.

Dystocia is long, difficult or abnormal labour; it is caused by various conditions associated with the five factors affecting labour.

- Dysfunctional labour, resulting in ineffective uterine contractions or maternal bearing down efforts (the powers).
- Alterations in the pelvic structure (the passage) Pelvic dystocia, Soft tissue dystocia.
- Foetal causes including abnormal presentations or position, anomalies, excessive size, and the number of foetuses (the passengers).
- Maternal position during labour and birth.

- Psychologic responses of the mother to labour related to past experience, preparation, culture and heritage and support system.

These factors are interdependent. In assessing the woman, for an abnormal labour pattern, the nurse must consider the way in which these factors interact and influence labour progress. Dystocia is suspected when there is an alteration as the characteristics of uterine contractions, a lack of progress is the rate of cervical dilation, or a lack of progress in foetal descent and expulsion.

ABNORMAL UTERINE ACTION/ DYSFUNCTIONAL LABOUR

Abnormal uterine action refers to dysfunction of the uterine muscles caused by neuromuscular disharmony which manifests itself as follows:

1. Hypotonia (uterine inertia).
2. Incoordinate uterine action comprising:
   a. Hypertonic lower uterine segment.
   b. Colicky uterus.
   c. Constriction ring dystocia.
   d. Spurious labour.
3. Cervical dystocia.

Hypotonia (Uterine Inertia)

Hypotonia refers to low or poor tone in the uterine muscle fibres. This results in weak uterine contractions which are infrequent and do not give rise to much pain. The uterus can be indented even at the height of a contraction. The contractions are ineffective. Therefore cervical dilatation is slow and labour is usually prolonged.

Uterine inertia may be primary or secondary. When it occurs from the onset of labour it is primary. Occasionally it occurs in an established labour especially if the uterus is exhausted. In such cases it is secondary. It may be the cause of a retained second twin.

Effects of Hypotonic Uterine Action

Labour is prolonged and may go on for several days. The mother could be distressed, dehydrated and demoralized and the risk of foetal distress and infection is increased unless the membranes are intact and the nursing care is efficient. Postpartum haemorrhage is likely in the third stage of a labour.

Management of Hypotonia

Management usually consists of performing an ultrasound examination to rule out CPD, and assessing FHR and pattern, characteristics of amniotic fluid if membranes are ruptured, and maternal wellbeing, if findings are normal, measures such as ambulation, hydrotherapy, on enema stripping or rupture of membrane, nipple stimulation and oxytocin can be used to augment the progress of labour.

The patient should be admitted to hospital if labour is over 18 hours. She is reassured and sedated to keep her calm, and induce a good sleep. Abdominal and pelvic examinations are done to exclude cephalopelvic disproportion and possibly determine the cause of the inertia. In the absence of gross cephalopelvic disproportion good uterine contractions are stimulated by:

a. Repeat enema after 18 hours.
b. Emptying of the bladder as may be necessary.
c. Oxytocin drip of 2 to 5 units of pitocin in 500 ml of 5 per cent glucose water.

Ketosis should be prevented by fluid and electrolyte replacement. Vigilant observation is kept on maternal and foetal conditions. Nursing care is the same as for prolonged labour. Labour is often terminated by operative measures. Caesarean section is performed for maternal and foetal condition. Nursing care is the same as for prolonged labour. Labour is often terminated by operative measures. Caesarean section is performed for maternal and foetal distress, occurring before the os is 6 cm dilated. The vacuum extractor may be used when the os is half dilated and the head is below the midcavity.

Forceps delivery is often necessary because the patient is too tired to push in the second stage of labour. The possibility of postpartum haemorrhage ought to be kept in mind and ergometrine (0.5 mg) or syntometrine (1 ml) given with the delivery of the anterior shoulder of the baby.

INCOORDINATE UTERINE ACTION

There are four varieties of incoordinate uterine action, viz.

i. Hypertonic lower uterine segment.
ii. Colicky uterus.
iii. Constriction ring dystocia.
iv. Spurious labour.

General Description

In incoordinate uterine action the uterus is very irritable. More placing of the hand on the uterus causes it to contract. The contractions are usually strong, painful and erratic. They may be frequent but the cervix dilates slowly. Clinically, the condition is recognized by the fact that the patient experiences a great deal of pain long before and after a palpable uterine contraction. Severe back pain, which may be referred to the rectum, causes the patient to bear down prematurely and this effort makes the cervix oedematous. The patient is usually exhausted with diminished morale. There may be distension of the bowels and urinary retention. Foetal hypoxia ensues because the hypertonic state of the uterus interferes with placental circulation.

A brief description of the varieties of incoordinate uterine action is given below:

a. *Hypertonic lower uterine segment* In this condition, the lower uterine segment is hypertonic, so there is loss of polarity. Clinically it is recognized by the very severe backache and intermittent abdominal pain which come before and persist long after a palpable uterine contraction.
b. *Colicky uterus* In this condition, the upper uterine segment contracts strongly and spasmodically. There is intense cramp-like pain and the uterus is tender. Sometimes the whole of the uterus contracts spasmodically and painfully but there is no severe backache.
c. *Constriction ring dystocia* This is a form of Colicky uterus in which there is a localized spasm of a group of circular muscle fibres. The spasm of these fibres forms a constriction ring between the upper and the lower uterine segment and it may encircle the foetus. The spasm is likely to arise following intrauterine manipulation such as internal version or when membranes rupture early and the uterus becomes irritable and moulds round the foetus. Constriction ring may be palpated on the inner aspect of the uterus at vaginal examination. Inhalation of an amould of amylnitrite or administration of general anaesthesia may be necessary to effect immediate relaxation of the constriction ring.
d. *Spurious labour* This is a form of incoordinate uterine action in which uterine contractions occurring before the onset of labour are painful and accompanied by backache. It can be abolished by an intramuscular injection of morphine or pethidine. This enables one to differentiate between spurious labour and true labour.

Management of Incoordinate Uterine Action (Fig. 9.5)

Cephalopelvic disproportion is usually the underlying cause of this type of abnormal uterine action and should therefore be excluded. If a major degree of disproportion is diagnosed arrangements are made to deliver the patient by lower uterine segment caesarean section. Cases where, after thorough pelvic and radiological assessment, the physician is satisfied that there is absence of disproportion, are allowed to continue in labour. The nurse midwife should keep a careful record of the patient's blood pressure, pulse, respiratory rates, fluid intake and output. The urine should be tested for albumin and acetone. The foetal heart should be auscultated at quarter-hourly intervals. Adequate fluid should be given by the intravenous route to prevent dehydration and ketosis. The signs of maternal and foetal distress should be reported without delay. Progress in labour is determined by the progressive dilatation of the cervix and progressive descent of the presenting part of the foetus. Strict aseptic and antiseptic precautions should be observed when making vaginal examinations. The number of vaginal examinations should be reduced to the essential minimum.

In a small proportion of cases, spontaneous delivery takes place usually with the aid of an episiotomy. In the majority of cases, labour is terminated by vacuum extraction, forceps delivery or caesarean section. The nurse must, therefore, anticipate and make adequate preparation for any of these procedures.

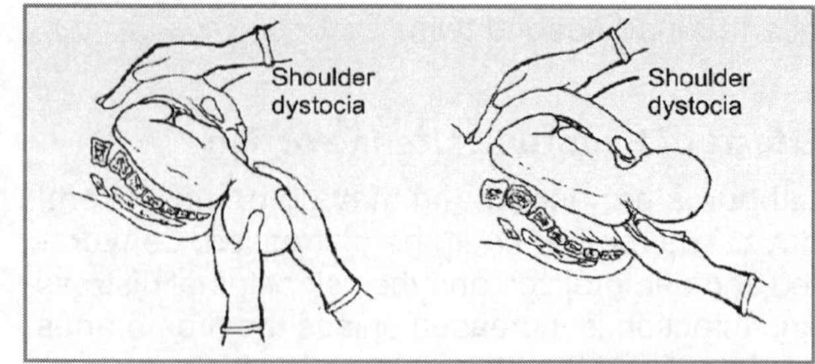

Fig. 9.5: Disimpaction of the anterior shoulder, impacted shoulders: It is sometimes necessary to rotate the foetus to disimpact the posterior shoulder

Cervical Dystocia

Cervical dystocia may be primary or secondary. In primary cervical dystocia, the uterine contractions are normal; the presenting part is low down in the pelvis but the cervix fails to dilate. The delay is often due to the cartilagenous ring round the cervix, and incision of the cervix by the physician usually hastens delivery of the baby.

Secondary cervical dystocia is caused by previous trauma to the cervix, such as previous Manchester repair operation or previous forcible dilatation and curettage. Carcinoma of the cervix is another cause of secondary cervical dystocia. The cervix fails to dilate in spite of very good uterine contraction. The labour is usually terminated by caesarean section.

Factors which Predispose to Abnormal Uterine Action

The factors which predispose to abnormal uterine action are listed below:

1. *Age* The older the patient, especially if she is to have abnormal uterine action.
2. *Parity* Abnormal uterine action is more frequently seen in primigravidae, particularly elderly primigravidae.
3. *Disproportion or malpresentation* Cephalopelvic disproportion and occipito-posterior position of the foetal head may cause hypotonic uterine action or incoordinate uterine action.
4. *Postmaturity* A pregnancy prolonged beyond the expected date of confinement may be associated with abnormal uterine action.
5. Other factors associated with abnormal uterine action are overdistension of the uterus as in multiple pregnancy and hydramnios, premature rupture of the membranes and emotional tension in the patient.

Labour is said to be prolonged when it exceeds 24 hours. Since labour is usually quick amongst women and medical aid is not easy to get, nurses practising in developing countries are advised to regard a labour as prolonged if it exceeds 16 hours, especially in multiparous patients. This is because by the time the patient is transferred to a hospital and medical aid is available, the said 24 hours would have been reached and exceeded. Moreover, prolonged labour is often associated with cephalopelvic disproportion in most developing countries; therefore, it is wise to look for help early before maternal and foetal conditions deteriorate and labour becomes obstructed.

The common causes of prolonged labour are:

1. Cephalopelvic disproportion.
2. Contracted pelvic.
3. Abnormal uterine action, the hypotonic and the inordinate types are more common.
4. Occipito-posterior position of the foetal head.
5. Deep transverse arrest, rigid perineum and big baby usually cause delay in the second stage of labour.
6. Malpresentation such as shoulder, brow and face presentations.
7. Pelvic tumour preventing descent of the presenting part.

The Course of Prolonged Labour

As previously mentioned, prolonged labour is often associated with some degree of disproportion between the pelvis and the foetal presentation. As such, application of the cervix to the presentng part is poor, thus making dilatation of the cervical os slow and painful. Early rupture of the membranes and prolapse of the umbilical cord may occur as a result of the ill fitting presenting part. Risk of infection of the genital tract and at times of the foetus is increased by the need to repeat vaginal examinations to assess the progress of labour. This risk is great when the membranes rupture early in labour. When labour is prolonged, the mother becomes exhausted. Dehydration, ketosis and other signs of maternal distress become apparent. Abdominal distension, a full bladder, and blood stained urine are common features of prolonged labour associated with obstruction. Signs of foetal distress may be present, caput succedaneum and excessive moulding may be found on the foetal head in cephalic presentations.

Patients have been known to develop fulminant pre-eclampsia and eclampsia as a result of prolonged labour.

Management of Prolonged Labour

All cases of labour exceeding 16 hours must be referred to hospital. A good history is obtained with particular attention to the time of onset of labour, time of rupture of the membranes, frequency and strength of uterine contractions and the amount of pain the patient experiences. The patient's general condition, with particular reference to her mental outlook and state of hydration, is assessed. Her temperature, pulse, blood pressure and respiration are taken and recorded. A specimen of urine is obtained and tested for albumin, sugar and acetone. Anaemia is excluded by estimation of the packed cell volume.

An abdominal examination to determine the foetal lie, the presentation and its engagement is done. The type of uterine contractions are noted and foetal heart sounds auscultated. A vaginal examination is necessary to ascertain the degree of cervical dilatation, the state of the membranes and the position of the presentation.

If the membranes are intact, maternal and foetal conditions are satisfactory and there is evidence of progress, the labour is allowed to take its course even if it is prolonged. A sedative or analgesic such as pethidin or fortuin is given to calm the patient and relieve pain. Intravenous infusion of 5 per cent glucose solution is setup to prevent or correct ketosis.

The patient is not allowed anything by mouth because labour may be terminated by operative delivery. It is, therefore, advisable to obtain operation consent from the patient or her relative. Blood should be grouped and cross-matched in readiness. If the membranes have ruptured for longer than 18 hours, a cervical swab should be cultured and prophylactic antibiotic therapy instituted while awaiting the laboratory results. Oxygen may be given to the mother if the foetus is distressed.

Nursing Interventions

Patience, tact, good companionship, and supervision are required to manage a patient who is almost exhausted because of her long and difficult labour. The patient and her relations should be reassured by the nurse midwife. Rest and sleep are encouraged to conserve the patient's energy. The patient may feel reassured if a nurse midwife sits with her to check her pulse rate, blood pressure, respiratory and foetal heart sounds which should be monitored quarter-hourly. The type of the contractions and the descent of the presentation are noted hourly. A fluid chart is kept and the patient is encouraged to pass urine hourly. The urine specimens are tested for acetone and albumin. The general comfort of the patient as regards her personal toilet should be kept in mind.

Complications of Prolonged Labour

Maternal

1. Maternal conditions may deteriorate due to dehydration, electrolyte imbalance and exhaustion.
2. Pre-eclamptic toxaemia and even eclampsia have been known to complicate prolonged labour.
3. Risk of infection is increased because of early rupture of membranes, repeated vaginal examinations and operative delivery.
4. Postpartum haemorrhage is likely to occur due to uterine atonia.
5. The uterus may rupture if labour is obstructed.
6. The pelvic floor may be unduly stretched especially in the second stage of labour. Utero-vaginal prolapse, cystocoele and stress incontinence are rare complications.
7. Perineal lacerations are common.
8. Drop foot, vesico and rectovaginal fistulae are other maternal complications associated with prolonged labour, particularly when obstructed labour complicates the picture.
9. Poor mental outlook to future child bearing is a serious psychological complication.

Foetal

1. Foetal hypoxia may occur because of prolonged compression of the placenta, especially if the amniotic fluid has drained away.
2. Intracranial injury and hypoxia could arise as a result of excessive moulding and compression of the head as it is being forced through the birth canal.
3. Infection of the foetus is also likely if the membranes have ruptured early.
4. Perinatal mortality rate is generally increased.

In view of the above complications nurses, midwives, especially those working in rural areas, must never let the sun set twice on a labouring woman in their case.

FOETAL DISTRESS

Foetal distress refers to foetal hypoxia in utero. This occurs when conditions which interfere with the supply of oxygen to the foetus are present.

Conditions which Predispose to Foetal Distress

1. Maternal conditions such as pre-eclampsia and eclampsia, severe hypertension, chronic nephritis, chronic pyelonephritis and diabetes. These conditions may lead to placental insufficiency.
2. Severe anaemia in pregnancy, severe cardiac disease and pulmonary tuberculosis result in deficient oxygen supply to the mother.
3. Abnormal uterine action, especially of the hypertonic type.
4. Prolonged labour, especially if the membranes have been long ruptured, interferes with placental circulation.
5. Antepartum haemorrhage due to premature separation of the placenta.
6. Presentation or prolapse of the umbilical cord and its compression by the presenting part.
7. True knots in the umbilical cord.
8. Prematurity.
9. Postmaturity is associated with degeneration of the placenta.
10. Congenital foetal abnormality. Experience has shown that abnormal foetuses do not with stand labour well.

The diagnosis of foetal distress is based on the following findings:

1. *Tachycardia:* Increase in the foetal heart rate is the earliest sign of foetal distress. An increase of 20 beats per minute on the normal of 120-140 beats is a sign of mild hypoxia. A rate of 160 or more per minute should give cause for concern.
2. *Bradycardia* Or slow foetal heart rate usually follows the tachycardia and is a sign of severe hypoxia. A decrease of 20 beats in the normal rate is significant. The heart rate may become progressively slower until a rate of 100 or less is reached. Heart rates of 80 per minute or below may result in foetal death.
3. *Irregular heart rate:* Later, irregular foetal heart beats (arrhythmia) follow the slow heart rate.
4. *Passage of meconium:* The passage of meconium in a cephalic presentation suggests severe intra-uterine anoxia causing relaxation of the anal sphincter and passage of meconium. Slight green staining of the liquor may be due to previous distress from which the foetus has recovered. The presence of fresh meconium in the liquor denotes foetal distress which needs urgent attention. Passage of meconium in breech presentation does not necessarily constitute foetal distress.
5. *Convulsive movements of the foetus* Sometimes precede intrauterine death. Treatment of foetal distress at this stage is usually fruitless.

Other methods of detecting foetal hypoxia, such as the determination of blood Rh, pH as in foetal scalp sampling in utero, and the uses of the Sonic aid are not readily available in many hospitals in developing countries.

Management of Foetal Distress

Prophylaxis Prevention of foetal distress is not very easy. All patients pregnancy complications mentioned above should be referred for hospital delivery and should not be allowed to have prolonged labour. If the membranes have ruptured and the presenting part is high, the patient should be confined to bed to prevent prolapse of the umbilical cord.

Some of the severe clinical signs of foetal distress might be prevented if it were possible to detect very early signs of foetal distress. In this regard, the Sonic aid and foetal blood sampling would have been of immense help. In the present stage of development in many countries of, reliance will have to be placed on the conventional method of detecting foetal distress, that is, auscultating the foetal heart at quarter hourly intervals in susceptible cases.

Treatment: As soon as the first sign of foetal distress is detected preparations should be made for immediate delivery of the baby and the physician must be informed at once. If oxygen is available, it should be given by mask to the mother, especially to those mothers with cardiac failure, eclampsia, severe anaemia, etc., who are likely to be deficient in oxygen. Administration of nikethamide or Coramine (2 ml) and 10-40 ml of 10 per cent glucose in conjunction with the oxygen has yielded good results. Whenever possible, the cause of the distress should be determined. Since this is not always possible a vaginal examination may be carried out to determine the degree of cervical dilatation and exclude cord prolapse. If the patient is in the second stage of labour and the head is being held up by a right perineum, a nurse midwife could expedite the delivery with episiotomy. Forceps delivery under pudendal block may be necessary in cases of established foetal distress in the second stage of labour. Caesarean section should be anticipated and the necessary preparations made if foetal distress occurs in the first stage of labour.

MATERNAL DISTRESS

Maternal distress means maternal exhaustion, i.e. the strain and stress of labour have proved too much for the mother. The exhaustion is not necessarily related to the duration of labour, for maternal distress can occur at any stage of labour, though it is unusual in early labour. Maternal distress of exhaustion is an indication that the labour should be terminated.

Signs of Maternal Distress

a. Increase in the pulse rate is one of the earliest signs of distress and it may be 90 to 120 or more per minute.
b. Rise in temperature of 37.2°C and over in an otherwise uncomplicated labour.
c. Increase in respiratory rate of 24 per minute and above.
d. Signs of dehydration, such as dry furred tongue, dry skin, presence of acetone in the breath and in the urine.
e. Distension of the bowel with gas.
f. Vomiting occurring at times.
g. Restlessness, weakness and sweating.
h. The patient looks ill, anxious and worried.

The above signs are indications that things have gone wrong and the mother's life is threatened. No midwife should allow all these signs to be present in a woman before summoning the physician. For early diagnosis, maternal distress should be anticipated in certain labours, e.g. trial of labour, induction of labour with Pitocin drip and when there is malpresentation and abnormal position of the foetus. Other groups of patients likely to get easily exhausted during labour are elderly primigravidae, and those with cardiac disease, pulmonary tuberculosis, diabetes, severe hypertension, pre-eclampsia and eclampsia and severe anaemia. These patient's condition may deteriorate quickly if they are exhausted during labour. They must, therefore, be closely watched, well managed during labour and delivered in a hospital.

Management

Adequate rest, sedation, hydration and avoidance of prolonged labour are preventive measures against maternal distress.

Labour is usually terminated if the patient is exhausted and the method employed depends on the degree of cervical dilatation. The nurse midwife should therefore, determine the state of labour and send for medical aid where possible. Nurses working in rural areas are advised to try in addition to determine the cause of the distress, sedate the patient and hasten delivery with episiotomy in the second stage.

An intravenous infusion of 5 to 10 per cent glucose solution should be given to correct dehydration and ketosis.

Termination of Labour

If the cervical os is less than 6 cm dilated, caesarean section is usually performed. Forceps delivery or episiotomy is performed to shorten the second stage of labour in cases in which full dilatation of the cervix has been achieved.

MULTIPLE PREGNANCY (FIGS 9.6 AND 9.7)

The term "multiple pregnancy" issued to describe the development of more than one foetus in utero at the same time. Multiple or plural pregnancy refers to the presence of more than one foetus in the uterus. The number of foetuses may be two as twins, three as triplets, four or quadruplets, five or quintruplets, etc. Multiple pregnancy results either from the fertilization of two ova during the same intermenstrual period or by the division of one fertilized ovum into two three or four embryos in the early stage of pregnancy.

Families expecting a multiple birth have different health needs requiring extrapractical support and understanding throughout pregnancy, the postnatal period and the early years. Information and support from well informed health care professionals from the time to time that multiple pregnancy is diagnosed will help to prepare the parents and avoid potential problems.

Twins are the common form of multiple or multifoetal pregnancy and they can be formed in two ways. The first is by the division of one fertilized ovum to form two embryos which later becomes identitical twins or uniovular twins. The second is the fertilization of two ova to form two embryos.

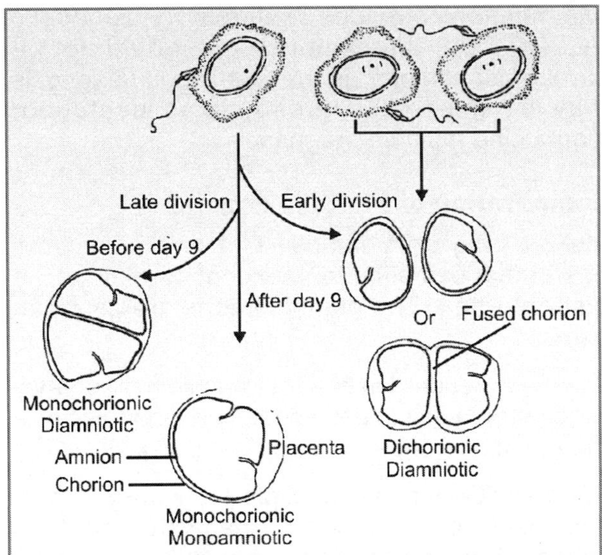

Fig. 9.6: Types of twinning indicating the structure of the membranes and placenta. Note that twins of different sexes are always dizygous and those with a single chorion always monozygous. Dichorionic twins of the same sex can be either monozygous or dizygous

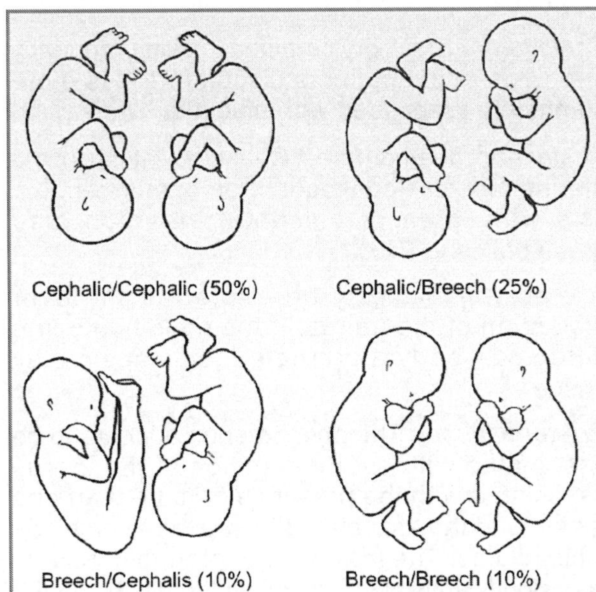

Fig. 9.7: The four major presentations of twin pregnancy. The 5% of other variations are not listed in these major groups

These develop into unidentical or binovular twins. In utero, uniovular (or monozygotic or monochorionic twins share the same placenta and chorion but separated from each other by their respective amnions. They are of the same sex and bear a very close resemblance of each other. Developmental abnormalities, such as fusion of the two foetuses usually known as conjoined twins or Siamese twins are usually encountered in uniovular twins. At times one of the foetuses develops at the expense of the other. The deprived foetus dies, becomes compressed and is called foetus papyraceous or compressus. Hydramnios is a common complication of uniovular twins and the perinatal mortality is high in these cases. Binovular (or dizygotic, bichorionic) twins have two separate placentae but in some cases, the placentae do fuse. There are two chorions and amnions. The foetuses may or may not be of the same sex. At birth, unidentical twins bear no more resemblance to one another than any two brothers or sisters.

Causes of Multiple Pregnancy

A familial tendency to monozygotic twining is rare but transmission can occur through both maternal and paternal lines. Twining rates increase—with parity but this increase seems only to apply to dizygotic twinning. Multiple pregnancy is common following the use of drugs to induce ovulation (e.g., use of gonadotrophin therapy results in twin or triplet) and also use of fertility drugs accounts of multiple pregnancy. In vitro fertilization, (IVF) and embryo transfer, where the ovaries are hyperstimulated to enable collection of multiple oocytes may lead to multiple pregnancy.

Clinical Manifestation

A multiple pregnancy places the mother and foetuses at risk. The maternal blood volume is increased, resulting in an increased strain on the maternal cardiovascular system:

- Anaemia often develops because of great demand for iron by the foetuses.
- Marked uterine distension and the increased pressure in the adjacent viscera and pelvic vasculature and diastasis of the two recti abdominis muscle (in the midline) may occur.
- Placenta praevia develops because of the large size or placement of placenta.
- Premature sepration of placenta may occur before the second and any subsequent foetuses are born.
- Multiple pregnancy often end in preterm birth
- Spontaneous rupture of membranes before term is common.

- Congenital malformation are twice as common in monozygotic as in single tons, though there is no increase in the incidence of congenital anomalies indizygotic twins.

In addition two vessel cords—that is cords with a single umbilical artery—occur more often in twins than in singletons, but it is more common in monozygotic twins. The most serious problem for the foetus is the local shunting of blood between placentas (twin to twin transfusion) causing reciprocal twin to be larger and the donor twin to be small, pallid, dehydrated, malnuourished, and hypovolaemic. In addition congenital heart failure may develop in the larger twin during the first 24 hour after birth.

Diagnosis

The diagnosis is seldom missed where there is high index of suspicion, such as a family history of twins, especially on the wife's side, and if the patient has previously given birth to twins or triplets. The clinical diagnosis of multiple pregnancy is increased if any one or a combination of the following factors is revealed during a careful assessment.

- History of dizygot twins in the female lineage
- Use of fertility drugs
- More rapid uterine growth for time in pregnancy
- Hydramnios
- The palpation of an excessive number of small or largeparts.
- Asynchronous foetal heart beat or more than one foetal electrocardiographic tracing
- Ultrasonographic evidence of more than one foetus.

The usual symptoms may be exaggerated. The early morning sickness may be severe, and may go on to hyperemesis, gravidrum. Varicose veins become more prominent and painful. Later in pregnancy, the patient becomes easily breathless. She may find walking difficult and feel generally heavy.

On abdominal examination, there is an apparent discrepancy between the especially the presence of three foetal poles, such as two heads and a breech or two breeches and a head are obvious signs of multiple pregnancy. At times, there may be difficulty in abdominal palpations and hydramnios may be present. On auscultation two foetal heart sounds are heard at two separate points and at different rates. Radiological examinations provides confirmatory diagnostic evidence but the examination should not be carried out earlier than the 26th week (diagnosis may be missed). Ultrasound is useful for diagnosing multiple pregnancy.

Complication of Multiple Pregnancy

Multiple pregnancy carries a high risk of almost all obstetrical complications except cephalopelvic disproportion. The complications are as given below:

Abortion: Resorption of a foetus in twin pregnancy is common event in early gestation, and this basis the incidence of partial abortion is high.

Anaemia: Common in multiple pregnancy with its extra demands on the already inadequate maternal stores of iron and folic acid, worsens a pre-existing anaemia.

Antipartum haemorrhage: May be result of a wide area of placental insertion with a portion of the placenta being complanted in the lower uterine segment.

Polyhydramnios: Very common in twin pregnancy and adds to the patients discomfort. It is more commonly associated with uniovular twins.

Postpartum haemorrhage: Caused by atonia of the uterine muscles consequent on overdistention. The wide area of placental insertion also predisposes to PPH.

Pre-eclampsia: May be related to the over distention of the uterus. If the condition is not detected—early and treated, eclampsia may ensue.

Pre-term labour: The phenomenon appears to be associated with over distension of the uterus associated with the presence of more than one foetus and the associated increases in amniotic fluid volume. The incidence of preterm labour is also significantly higher in uniovular than binovular twins.

Prolonged labour: In multiple pregnancy is more likely to be associated with malpresentation than overdistention of the uterus. It has been seen, that labour progresses normally in multiple pregnancy.

Malpresentation: Such as shoulder may complicate multiple pregnancy. The risk of prolonged labour and ruptured uterus is a real one which must be guarded against by careful antenatal and intranatal assessment.

Zygosity: Monozygotic twins have a higher perinatal mortality than dizygotic twins and a higher incidence of congenital abnormalities, IUGR and preterm delivery.

Management of Multiple Pregnancy

A nurse should never undertake solely the management of multiple pregnancy because of the associated complications. In rural areas of developing countries where help is not easily available in case of an emergency, the nurse should refer all cases of multiple pregnancy to a big hospital, where facilities are available to treat and manage this type of cases.

Management in the Antenatal Period

The patient should be seen fortnightly at the antenatal clinic till about 30 to 32 weeks and thereafter, she should be seen weekly until she delivers. Complications such as anaemia, pre-eclampsia, hydramnios are watched out for and the patient is admitted into the hospital if any of these complications arises.

The nurse midwife should advise the patient on nutrition with emphasis on food rich in protein, iron and vitamin B. Regular daily intake of iron, folic acid and weekly intake of Daraprim (or any substitute) are ensured. The patient requires a lot of rest and should avoid strenuous manual work, carrying of heavy loads on her head and travelling, especially after the 28th week of pregnancy for these predispose to premature onset labour which commonly occurs between the 30th and 34th week. If premature labour occurs, the babies are usually too small to survive, especially out of a hospital. As such, some authorities recommend rest in hospital from 30th to 36th week, but this policy cannot be successfully adopted in areas where the incidence of twinning is high and there is a great demand for the few available obstetric beds. More compelling reasons such as occurrence of serious pregnancy complications are required for the admission of women expecting twins. However, the situation is different with triplets, quadruplets, etc. because the incidence of premature labour is higher. Patients expecting triplets and quadruplets, etc. should be admitted as soon as the diagnosis is made. They are kept in hospital thoroughout the antenatal period.

Management in Labour

Ideally all twin deliveries should be conducted in hospital and a high standard of anaesthesia must be available. During the first stage of labour the usual routine observations are carried out. Heavy sedation and analgesics are avoided especially where the babies are possibly premature. It is necessary to ascertain the lie and presentation of the first foetus. When the membranes rupture, a vaginal examination is done to assess the progress of labour and exclude prolapsed cord.

Preparations for the Delivery

1. Additional swabs, cord clamps and scissors, ligatures, mucus extractor episiotomy scissors, and the obstetric forceps should added to the delivery trolley. Extra cots should be got ready.
2. Equipment for resuscitation of the babies should be handy to combat asphyxia neonatorum if it should occur.
3. Ergometrine (0.5 mg) or syntometrine (1 ml) should be drawn up in readiness to be given at the delivery of the anterior shoulder of the last baby or as soon as the placentae are born.

Delivery of the First Twin

The patient may be delivered in a dorsal or lithotomy position. The delivery of the first twin seldom presents difficulty where vigilant and careful intranatal care is given. When the first twin is delivered, the time of delivery is noted and the baby's airway is aspirated. The placement end of the cord should be ligatured in two places to avoid haemorrhage. The baby is identified as twin one and put in a warm cot.

Delivery of the Second Twin

Active and immediate intervention is advocated in the delivery of the second twin. The longer the delay in delivering the second twin, the greater the foetal mortality due to anoxia resulting from separation of the placenta, excessive retraction of the placental site and prolapse of the cord. The delivery of the second twin is hazardous and causes a high foetal mortality rate, twice that of the first twin. The abdomen is palpated without delay to ensure that the lie of the second twin is longitudinal.

After swabbing the vulva a vaginal examination is done and the membranes are ruptured provided the lie is longitudinal. If the lie is abnormal, the nurse should inform the physician but she may try a gentle external cephalic version between contractions. If this is successful, the membranes are ruptured at the weight of a uterine contraction. The nurse should exclude prolapsed cord and then proceed with the delivery of the baby. If spontaneous delivery does not occur within a 3 to 5 minutes for ten minutes from birth of the first twin, the physician is informed. Usually delivery is accomplished by forceps, vacuum extraction or breech extraction.

In the case of twins, intramuscular syntometrine or ergometrine with hylase is given with the delivery of the anterior shoulder or crowning of the head. Intravenous ergometrine is given if a physician is present at the delivery. The woman's immediate postpartum condition is assessed by recording her blood pressure, pulse and respiration. These should be recorded half hourly and bleeding watched for at least 6 hours. The placentae are examined to determine the zygosity of the twins.

Complications of Twin Delivery

1. Prolapse of the cord, particularly of the second foetus, may occur resulting in hypoxia. The nurse midwife should ensure a longitudinal lie, make a large episiotomy and deliver the baby. Application of fundal pressure may aid the descent of the baby.
2. Transverse lie of the second twin (see delivery of the second twin).
3. Retained second twin: Retention of the second twin is very common and is usually due to uterine inertia after delivery of the first twin. Often a full bladder predisposes to uterine inertia. Other possible causes of retention of the second twin are abnormal presentation or position causing obstructed labour. Uterine rupture may complicate the picture. Another cause of retained second twin is the shutting down of the cervix after delivery of the first twin. If the first twin is small it may be delivered through an incompletely dilated cervix. The bigger second twin is, therefore, retained. The second twin may be retained in the horn of a double uterus. The doctor should be emptied as a routine. The management of retained second twin necessitates the checking of the lie and presentation of the twin, amniotomy if the lie is longitudinal and the administration of an infusion of pitocin if there is no disproportion and the foetal lie is longitudinal. Patients who have delivered at home and are admitted into hospital with retained second twin and ruptured membranes should have antitetanus serum and broad spectrum antibiotic. The haemoglobin or packed cell volume is estimated to exclude anaemia. The risk of intrauterine death is high with retained second twin.
4. Intrapartum haemorrhage or bleeding before the delivery of the second twin indicates separation of the placentae and possible anoxia of the second twin. In such a case the nurse midwife should massage the uterus, perform an episiotomy and deliver the baby with the aid of fundal pressure.
5. *Locked twins* Occasionally the after coming head of the first twin (presenting the breech) may be arrested by the descending head of the second foetus (presenting by the vertex). The heads become impacted and decapitation of the head of the first baby is usually necessary. Fortunately this complication is rare.

Management of the Puerperium

The mother needs help and advice with regard to the feeding of the babies. The babies should be kept in the hospital till they are gaining weight, satisfactorily. In the first few weeks of the puerperium it may be helpful to give the babies alternate breast and bottle feeds to allow the patient some rest. This practice is only suitable in hospital, particularly for educated wealthy patients who can afford artificial feeding when they are discharged. In other circumstances, it is necessary to improve the patient's general health and lactation, so that she can breastfeed the babies. Solids such as corn flour porridge and eggs could be introduced as early as the age of 3 months. The nurse could get milk producing firms or companies to sponsor the feeding of the babies of mothers from a very poor socio-economic background. Often these babies die through poor care and feeding.

HYDRAMNIOS (POLYHYDRAMNIOS)

By hydramnios is meant liquor amnii in excess of 1.5 litres (1500 ml). The average quantity of liquor amnii in the latter half of pregnancy is about 500 to 800 ml. The lower limite of normal is 300 ml of liquor amnii. The appear limit of normal is 1500 ml.

Cause of Hydramnios

The mechanism of production of liquor amnii is not quite understood. Consequently the pathophysiology of hydramnios is obscure. Certain maternal and foetal conditions are, however, known to be associated with hydramnios.

Maternal Conditions

Hydramnios is frequently associated with the following maternal diseases:
1. Diabetes mellitus.
2. Severe pre-eclampsia.
3. Congestive cardiac failure.

Foetal Conditions

The foetal conditions associated with hydramnios are listed below:
1. Twin pregnancy, particularly uniovular twins.
2. Congenital foetal abnormalities particularly of the central nervous system. Examples of these are anencephaly and spina bifida. It is believed that the normal foetus swallows liquor amnii. The anencephalic foetus is, however, incapable of swallowing liquor amnii hence hydramnios.
3. Oesophageal atresia—again in this condition, the foetus is unable to swallow liquor amnii.
4. Severe erythroblastosis fetalis.
5. Vascular abnormality of the chorion—e.g. chorioangioma. This is a small tumour growing from a chorionic villus, consisting of enlargement of the blood vessels and connective tissue.
6. Hydrocephalus, club-foot and harelip are infrcquontly associated with hydramnios.

Clinical Features of Hydramnios

Clinically there are two types of hydramnios—Acute and Chronic.

Acute Hydramnios

This is a very rare condition which usually develops very rapidly around the fourth month of pregnancy. It brings about a rapid enlargement of the abdomen. The abdominal birth is usually in excess of 100 cm. Acute hydramnios is usually associated with gross congenital foetal abnormalities or occasionally with uniovular twins.

There is severe abdominal discomfort and breathlessness (dyspnoea). There may be oedema of the ankles and legs and if varicose veins are present they become very troublesome. There may be digestive discomfort and vomiting. The abdomen is very tense and difficult to palpate. It is usually difficult to feel the foetal parts. The abdomen may be woody hard. This finding coupled with severe abdominal pain may lead the nurse midwife to suspect concealed abruptio placentae.

Chronic Hydramnios

This condition develops gradually during the second half of pregnancy. It increases the abdominal birth but, because the increase is gradual, there are no acute symptoms of dyspnoea, pain and digestive discomforts. In severe cases there may be dyspnoea, abdominal discomfort and oedema of the legs. Varicose veins, if present, may be painful. It may be difficult to palpate the foetus or hear the foetal heart sounds. The abdominal birth is in excess of 100 cm. A fluid thrill can be elicited.

Conditions that may be confused with hydramnios are:
1. Pregnancy co-existing with an ovarian cyst.
2. Hydatidiform mole.
3. A full bladder.

Management (Figs 9.8 and 9.9)

The nurse must refer all cases of hydramnios to the physician for investigation and treatment.

In all cases, radiological examination of the abdomen is important to exclude twin pregnancy and congenital foetal abnormalities. In centres where the facilities are available ultrasonography may be done.

In acute hydramnlos the patient is admittod to hospital. Invariably the pregnancy is terminated. The membranes are ruptured and the patient is allowed to go into labour. In many cases the foetus is abnormal.

Mild cases of chronic hydramnios are observed in the clinic at frequent intervals. The severe cases are admitted. Abdominal paracentesis is carefully performed as frequently as the occasion

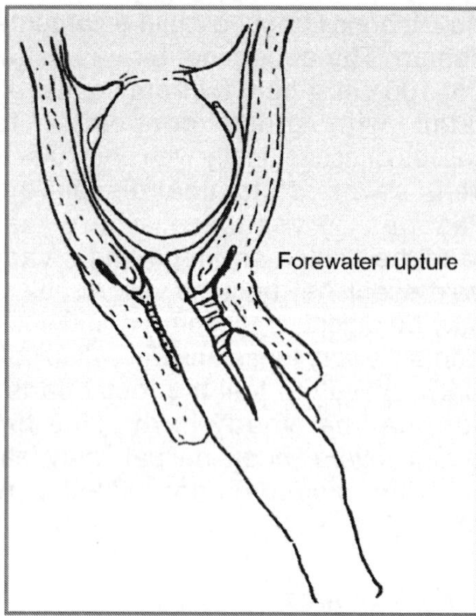

Fig. 9.8: Induction of labour by forewater rupture

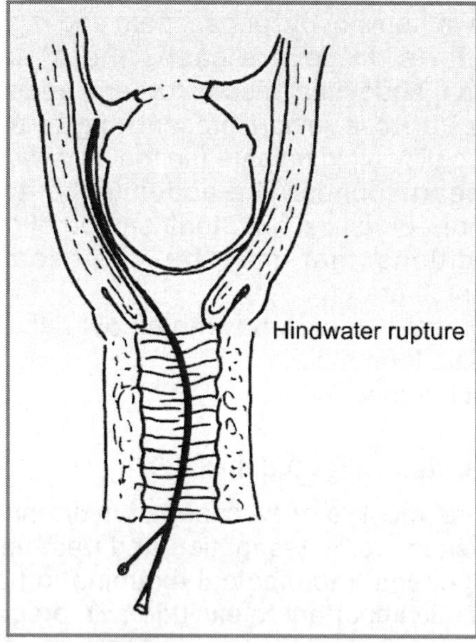

Fig. 9.9: Induction of labour by hindwater rupture

demands. If the foetus is mature, labour is induced by a slow controlled forewater or hindwater rupture of membranes. The dangers of sudden rupture of membranes in cases of hydramnios are (Figs. 9.8 and 9.9):

1. Prolapse of the cord.
2. Placental separation leading to antepartum haemorrhage.

After delivery the patient may have postpartum haemorrhage. This is because of the attendant uterine inertia due to the overdistension of the uterus.

OLIGOHYDRAMNIOS

In this very rare condition the quantity of liquor amnii is markedly diminished. It is usually less than 300 ml. It may be thick and viscid. The causes of oligohydramnios are not known. It is sometimes believed to be due to developmental abnormality of the Foetal kidney. It is therefore, associated with renal agenesis (non-development of the kidney) in the foetus. Because of the scanty liquor amnii the foetus is usually compressed by the uterus. Consequently there may be deformities of the limbs and trunk. Sometimes the amnion is adherent to the foetus. The foetal skull is sometimes compressed.

The diagnosis of oligohydramnios is made by observing that the height of the uterine fundus is much less than expected for the gestation age. Labour is usually prolonged. The foetus shows signs of compression of the trunk and limbs.

MALPOSITIONS OF THE FOETUS (FIG. 9.10)

The most common foetal malpositions is persistent occipito-posterior position, i.e. right-occipito position or left occipito position. Labour, especially the second stage is prolonged; the woman typically complains of severe back pain from the pressure of the foetal head (occiput) pressing against her sacrum.

Occipito-posterior Position (Fig. 9.11)

The head is said to be in the posterior position within the occipito either of the sacro-iliac joints. The incidence of occipito-posterior positions not known because, unless the diagnosis is made late in the pregnancy or in early labour, about 10 per cent of all vertex presentation end up with the occiput in the posterior position.

Causes of Occipito-posterior Position

The direct cause is often unknown

1. *Pelvic shape:* The most likely type of pelvis to favour the posterior position of the occiput is the anthropoid pelvis because of the large antero-posterior diameter and the small transferse diameter of its brim. The foetal head engages

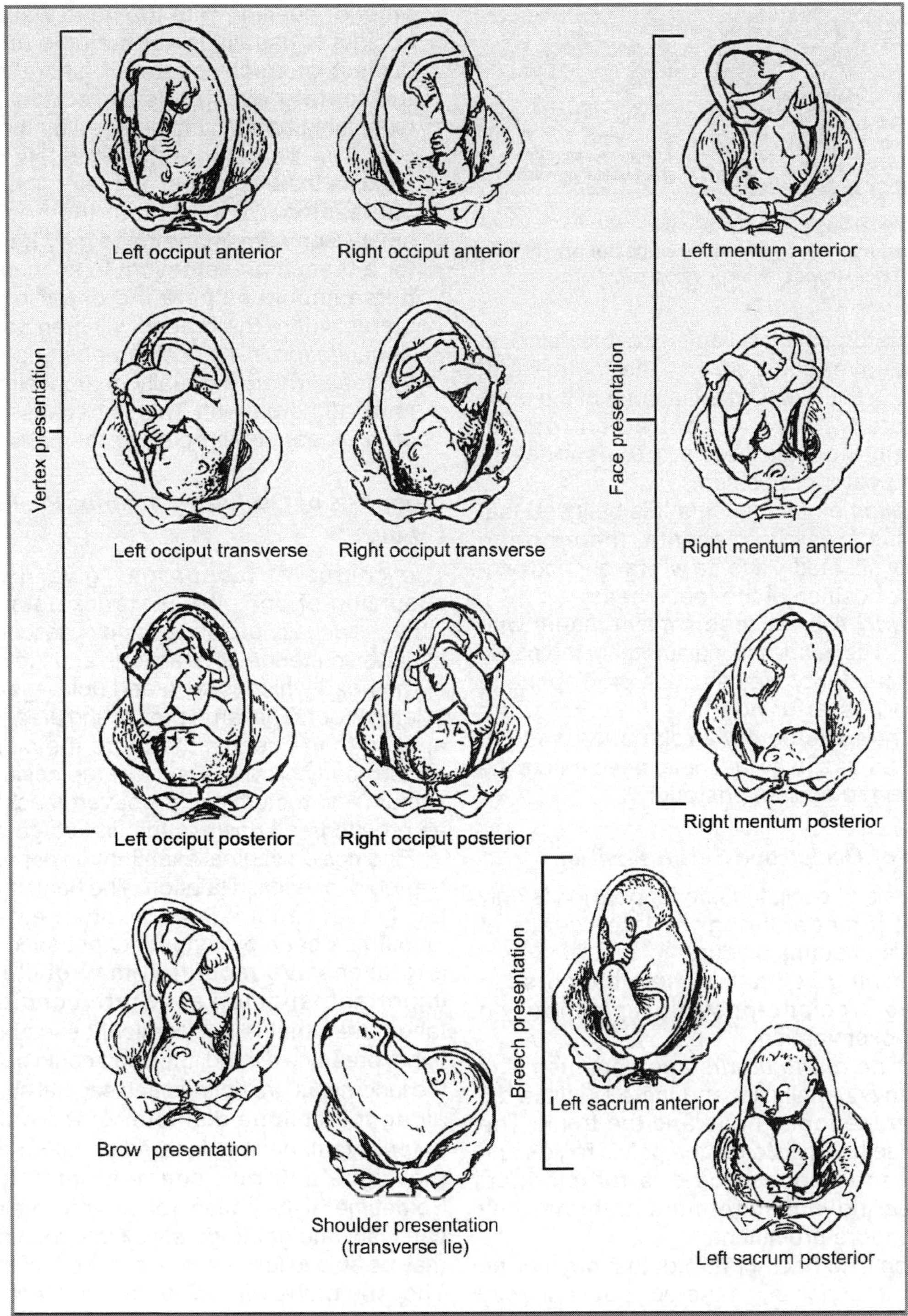

Fig. 9.10: Foetal presentations and positions. The left and right occiput anterior positions are most common

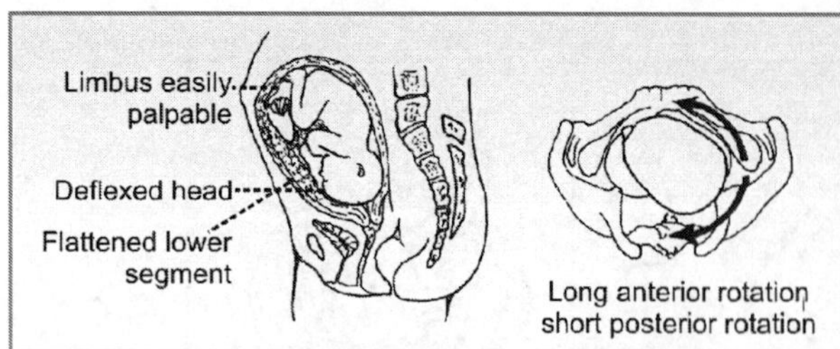

Fig. 9.11: Clinical findings in the occipito-posterior position (left); the head may rotate anteriorly or posteriorly or may arrest in the occipito-posterior position (right)

in the antero-posterior diameter of the pelvis. In a normal gynaecoid pelvis, the foetal head engages in the transverse diameter of the brim.

2. *Contracted pelvis* A contracted pelvis, especially android pelvis, predisposes to occipito-posterior position.
3. *The position of the placenta* It is believed that the foetus faces its placenta, therefore an anteriorly situated placenta will favour occipito-posterior position of the foetal head.
4. *Prematurity* A small foetus may present with any part of its head in any diameter of the pelvic brim. Prematurity may as such predispose to occipito-posterior position. In spite of the above, no satisfactory explanation has yet been given as to why the foetal head enters the brim with the occiput posteriorly.

Diagnosis of Occipitoposterior Position

The diagnosis of occipitoposterior position is only significant if made during the later weeks of pregnancy and during labour.

The following points may help the nurse in diagnosing occipito-posterior position on abdominal examination:

1. *The outline of the uterus and abdomen* The abdomen is usually flat and there is a little dip between the foetal head and the trunk. The high, large head distends the pelvic region and gives it the appearance of a full bladder. Because the limbs are more anterior, they become more prominent.
2. *Palpation* The back of the foetus may not be easily felt, especially if the occiput is directly posterior (sacral position of the occiput). In such a case, the edge of the shoulder girdle may be felt. The limbs are easily felt because of their anterior position. Palpation of the head reveals that the sinciput is prominent, is almost at the same level as the occiput. In an occipito-anterior position with the head well fixed the occiput is usually lower then the brow. If the occiput is directly posterior (sacral position), the foetal head tends to recede from the examining hand if it is grasped by the Pawlik's grip. The diameter of the head felt, in such a case, is the bitemporal diameter, therefore, an impression is formed that the head is very small. Sometimes, the head may be mistaken for a breech presentation. In such cases, the nurse should palpate the upper pole of the uterus where the breech will then be felt.
3. *Auscultation* In an occipito-posterior position, the foetal heart is usually heard well out in the flank of the patient. This is because the back of the foetus is directed to the flank.

Diagnosis of Occipito-posterior Position in Labour

The course of labour may give rise to the suspicion of occipito-posterior position. The labour is usually prolonged and is associated with hypertonic uterine contractions and slow descent of the head which is high and not engaged even in late labour. The large presenting area is not well applied to the cervix, therefore the membranes rupture early. The pressure of the occiput on the sacrum and rectum causes severe backache and an urge to bead down in the first stage of labour.

Findings on vaginal examination depend on the degree of cervical dilatation. The head may not be easily reached if it is deflexed or extended. If labour has been prolonged, caput succedaneum and excessive moulding may obliterate the important landmarks. Where conditions are favourable, that is the cervical os is about three finger breadths dilated, the head could be reached, the landmarks are defined and sagittal suture is felt along the oblique diameter of the pelvis. The anterior fontanelle is located on either the left or the right anterior segment of the pelvis. Sometimes if the patient relaxes and the examiner can insinuate her fingers well into the vagina she may be able to feel the lobe of the ear of the foetus. The lobe of the ear points in the direction of the occiput. Difficult cases may be resolved by radiographic examination. Usually, an erect lateral X-ray view of the pelvis is taken. This reveals the position of the occiput, the degree of descent and deflexion of the head.

Management of Malpositions of the Foetus (Figs 9.12 and 9.13)

There is no definite treatment of this condition antenatally. If the diagnosis is made late in pregnancy or early in labour, the patient must be referred to a physician in a well equipped maternity hospital. This measure is necessary because of the complications in labour associated with the persistent occipito-posterior position of the foetal head. The right occipito-posterior position is more common than the left, because the presence of the pelvic colon on the left prevents the occiput from occupying the left position. Also, the pregnant uterus rotates to the right that is, there is right obliquity of the uterus.

The possible outcome of labour is influenced by the flexion of the head which will be determined by the type of the pelvis and the uterine contractions. In most cases, the head flexes and the occiput becomes the leading part as it descends into the pelvis. On reaching the pelvic floor, the occiput

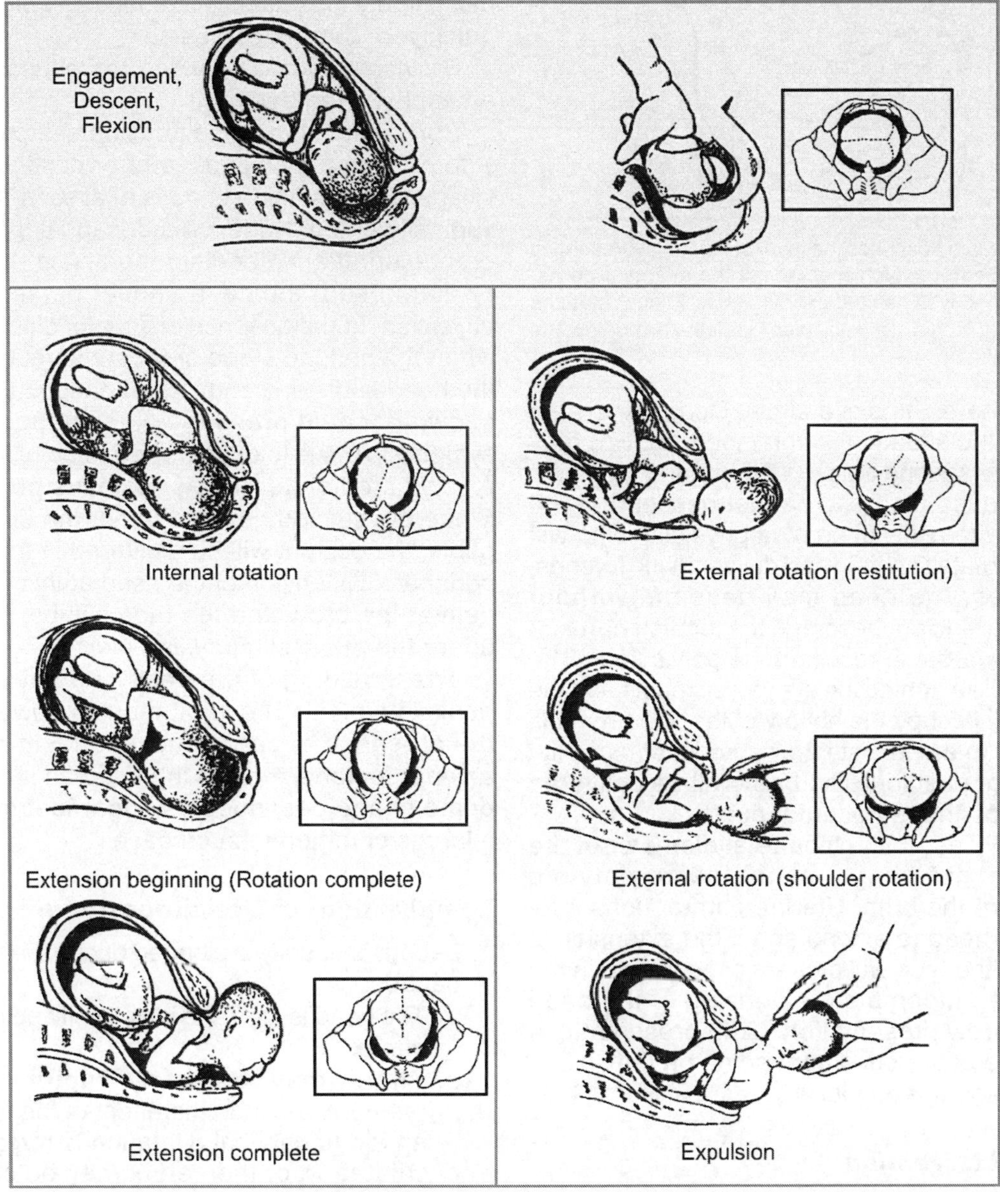

Fig. 9.12: The mechanisms of labour, also called cardinal movements. The positional changes allow the foetus to fit through the pelvis with the least resistance

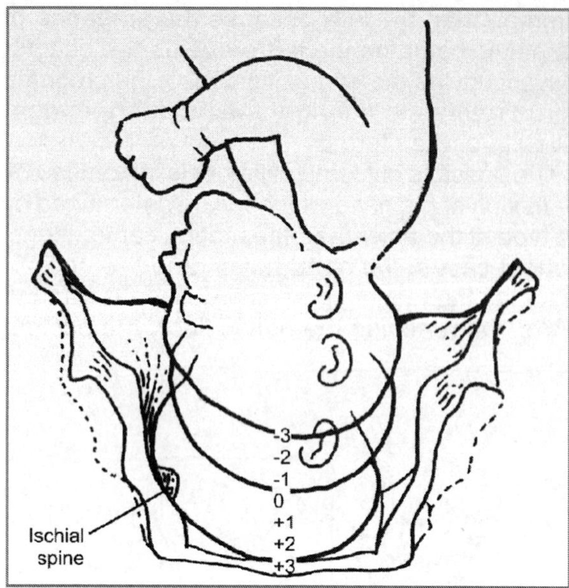

Fig. 9.13: Station describes the level of the foetal presenting part in relation to the ischial spines of the mother's pelvis. It is determined with vaginal examination. "Minus" stations are above the ischial spines; "plus" stations are below the ischial spines

rotates three-eighths of a circle. Deep transverse arrest (as the situation is commonly known) may occur in the second stage of labour and causes a delay because the head cannot descend. Such cases require assistance by a physician who will manually rotate the head and deliver it with forceps.

At times, the head may descend without flexing, the sinciput becomes the leading part and rotates forwards on reaching the pelvic floor. The sinciput will lie behind the symphysis pubis and the occiput will occupy the hollow of the sacrum. This is referred to as persistent or unreduced occipital to posterior position. The baby will be delivered with its face to the maternal pubis.

In a few cases, the biparietal diameter of the head may get caught at the sacro-cotyloid diameter of the brim. Uterine contractions may cause the head to extend and if the extension is complete, the face will present or lie lowest in the birth canal. Incomplete extension of the head result in brow presentation. Both presentations may cause obstruction depending on the size of the baby and the pelvis.

Nursing Intervention

The nursing care of the patient during labour is the same as for prolonged labour.

Equipment for performing an episiotomy should be got ready. An episiotomy is necessary because large diameters after distend the vulva in an occipitoposterior position and this predisposes to severe prineal laceration.

Neville-Barnes' or Kielland's forceps should be available on the delivery trolley in cases of occipitoposterior position because of the possible malrotation and deep transverse arrest of the foetal head. The forceps delivery may be done under general anaesthesia in which case the nurse must empty the patient's stomach and prepare her quickly for the anaesthesia.

Provision should be made for resuscitation of an asphyxiated baby.

Sometimes, the nurse finds herself confronted with persistent occipitoposterior position on the village. The first thing to do is to assess the pelvis vaginally and exclude a major caphalopelvic disproportion. If a major disproportion is suspected or diagnosed, the case should be sent to the physician. In the absence of a major disproportion when the second stage of labour is reached and the head is distending the peritoneum, the nurse midwife should press the sinciput against the symphysis pubis to encourage flexion of the head. A wide mediolateral episiotomy is performed. Since the sinciput is fixed under the symphysis pubis, the occiput will be delivered in front of the perineum. Extension of the head at this stage will deliver the brow and the face will be delivered under the pubic symphysis.

The moulding of the head of a baby face to pubis is typical. The vault moulds upwards and the presence of caput succedaneum near the anterior fontanelle gives the head an intracranial dome shape described as sugar loaf moulding injury is common in such cases.

Complications of Occipitoposterior Position

1. Labour is usually prolonged due to the following causes:
   a. The head is high and is not well applied to the cervix.
   b. There may be early rupture of the membranes, thus the effect of the forewater an aid to cervical dilatation is removed.
   c. Dilatation of the cervix may be slow and painful because of the poor application of the presenting part to the cervix.

   d. Deep transverse arrest or persistent occipito-posterior position causes delay in the descent of the head and thus labour is prolonged.
2. Risk of infection is high, because of frequent vaginal examination necessitated by the prolonged labour.
3. Instrumental delivery is also very common, especially when there is deep transverse arrest or persistent occipito-posterior position.
4. The frequency of cervical, vaginal and perineal lacerations is increased.
5. The maternal morbidity is increased and in unsupervised cases maternal mortality is increased.
6. There is increased perinatal mortality rate because the prolonged labour and abnormal moulding of the head predispose to intracranial injuries and intrapartum asphyxia.

The suggested measures to relieve back pain and facilitate rotation of the foetal occiput to an anterior position, which will facilitate birth are as follows:

1. Measures to reduce back pain during contraction:
   - Counter pressure: Apply fist or heel of hand to sacral area.
   - Heat and cold application: Apply to sacral area.
   - Double hip squeeze.
     - Woman assumes a position with hip joint flexed such as knee-chest
     - Partners, nurse, or doula place hands over gluteal muscles and presses with palms of hands up and inward towards the centre of the pelvis.
     - Woman assumes a sitting position with knees a few inches apart and feet flat on the floor or on a stool.
     - Partner, nurse or dowa cups a knee in each hand with heels of hands on top of tibia then presses the knees straight back toward the woman's hips while leaning forward toward the woman.
2. Measures to facilitate the rotation of the foetal head and may also relieve back pain:
   - Lateral abdominal stroking of stroke the abdomen in direction that the foetal head should rotate.
   - Hands and knees position (all-fours): can also be accomplished by kneeling while leaning forward over a birth ball, padded chair seat, bed or over the bad table.
   - Squatting
   - Pelvic rocking.
   - Lateral position: Lie on side toward which the foetus should turn.
   - Lunges: Widens pelvis on side towards which woman lunges:
     - Woman stands, facing forward, next to/ along side a chair so that she can lunge towards the side the foetal back is on or in the direction of the foetal occiput.
     - Places foot on seat of chair with toes pointed toward the back of the chair, then lunges.
     - Alternative position for lunges: kneeling.

MALPRESENTATIONS OF THE FOETUS

Face Presentation

When the attitude of the head is one of complete extension, the occiput of the foetus will be in contact with the spine and the face will present. In other words, when the head is fully extended, so that the occiput of the foetus is in contact with the spine, the face will present at the pelvic brim. In face presentation, the engaging diameter in subments bregmatic of 9.5 cm. In spite of this small diameter, descent of the head may be difficult and progress of labour retarded, because the bulk of the presentation is increased by the extreme extension of the head and the bone of the face do not mould.

Face presentation may be primary or secondary. A primary face presentation is present before the onset of labour; a secondary face presentation develops after the onset of labour.

Positions

The denominator of the position in a face presentation is the chin. The four positions of the presentation are:

1. Right mento-posterior (RMP)
2. Left mento-posterior (LMP)
3. Left mento-anterior (LMA)
4. Right mento-anterior (RMA)

In the first position, the chin points towards the right sacroiliac joint; in the second position it points towards the left sacroiliac joint; and in the third and fourth positions, the chin points towards the left and right pectineal eminences respectively.

Causes

The foetus normally adopts an attitude of flexion in utero, but occasionally spasm in the muscles of the spine will cause the head to become extended and face presentation will occur. An anencephalic foetus often presents with the face. At times, the head is deflexed and is caught in a small diameter at the brim. The force of uterine contractions may cause the head to extend and descend into the pelvis in that attitude. This is likely to occur in the flat type of contracted pelvis, occipito-posterior position and pendulous abdomen.

Diagnosis

It is unusual to diagnose face presentation during pregnancy and in early labour. Abdominal palpation may not be very easy because the bulky presenting part stretches the lower uterine segment making it tender, irritable and difficult to palpate.

When it is possible to palpate the abdomen satisfactorily, the nurse may be able to appreciate the following points which may help in the diagnosis.

A sulcus may be felt between the extended head and the back of the foetus especially in mento-posterior position when the back of the foetus is to the front. In mento-anterior position, this sign may not be elicited. In this case, the foetal heart is readily auscultated because of the nearness of the chest of the foetus to the maternal anterior abdominal wall. If the abdominal and uterine walls are thin, the impulse of the foetal heart may be felt by the examining hand. In mento-lateral or mento-transverse positions, the foetal heart is heard well to the side and on the same side as the limbs are palpated.

Vaginal Examination

Vaginal examinations may be misleading, especially early in labour when the cervix is only partly dilated and the presenting part is high. The face may be mistaken for a breech presentation. If the cervix is sufficiently dilated, feeling the chin and the following landmarks may help in arriving at the diagnosis of face presentation. These landmarks are:

a. The orbital ridges.
b. The prominence of the malar bones.
c. The ridge of the nose.
d. The nostrils (anterior nares).
e. The alveolar processes.

At times, some of these landmarks may be misleading. For example, the molar bones may mistaken for the ischial tuberosities. The most reliable of the landmarks are the nostrils and alveolar processes.

Radiographic Examination

Doubtful cases are usually diagnosed by X-ray examination.

Management of Face Presentation

There is very little to be said about the antenatal management of face presentation. This is because face presentation is seldom diagnosed before the onset of labour. If, however, face presentation is suspected late in pregnancy the midwife should refer the patient to the doctor for a thorough pelvic assessment and the exclusion of major cephalo-pelvic disproportion.

A thorough vaginal examination should be made to confirm the diagnosis and to determine the position of the chin. As a rule, mento-anterior positions have a good prognosis.

Whenever a nurse diagnosis face presentation with the chin in the posterior position she should, without delay, inform the doctor or, if on the district, transfer the patient to a hospital. The majority of patients with face presentation and thin posterior are delivered by lower uterine segment caesarean section unless the foetus is dead or abnormal. Sometimes, if the chin is posterior, it may rotate forwards, especially if it is lower than the sinciput.

Mechanisms of labour in face presentation mento-anterior are the same as in a vertex presentation. The course of labour may only be slightly affected provided there is no disproportion. Early rupture of membranes, prolapsed cord or prolonged labour may occur as in any other malpresentation. Caput succedaneum often forms over the face and the lips are usually swollen.

The nurse should make a vaginal examination when the membranes rupture to exclude prolapsed cord. Care should be taken during the examination not to infect of injure the eyes. In fact, some authorities are against the use of obstetric cream at such vaginal examinations. If labour is prolonged, nursing care of the patient described under prolonged labour should be given. The foetal heart is carefully monitored. If the head remains high in spite of good uterine contractions, caesarean section or forceps delivery should be anticipated.

An episiotomy may be necessary to prevent perineal laceration. Extension should be maintained by holding back the sinciput to permit the chin to escape under the symphysis pubis before the head is flexed and the occiput allowed to swap the perineum.

Prognosis and Complications of Face Presentation

For the foetus there is the great danger of anoxia secondary to prolonged labour and intracranial damage, or prolapse of the cord due to ill-fitting presenting part. There is, therefore, increased perinatal morbidity and mortality in face presentations.

In the mother, especially in mento-posterior positions, labour is prolonged because the face is a poor dilator of the cervix, and in mento-posterior positions the chin may fail to rotate forward. Prolonged labour may lead to maternal exhaustion and dehydration. The need to intervene increases the chances of infection (from repeated vaginal examinations) and extensive lacerations of the vagina and perineum. Unattended cases are likely to go into obstructed labour which, unrelieved, may lead to rupture of the uterus in multiparous women or the development of vesico vaginal fistula in primigravidae as well as multigravidae.

BROW PRESENTATION

Brow presentation is very uncommon; occurring once in about 3,000 to 4,000 deliveries. The reason for this is that the head is midway between extension and flexion and as labour progresses the head either flexes or extends further to a face presentation. If, however, a contracted pelvis is present the brow presentation may persist.

Brow presentation is rarely ever diagnosed in pregnancy. The diagnosis is usually made in labour. Abdominal examination may not be very helpful; but occasionally, as in face presentation, a sulcus or groove may be felt between the extended head and the back of the foetus. The presenting part is very high and overrides the pelvic brim. The head appears big because it is palpated across the wide mento-vertical diameter.

Vaginal examination: The determining landmarks are the two orbital ridges and the anterior fontanelle. These may be easily felt provided labour has not been prolonged and the cervical os is sufficiently dilated. They are usually obscured by a large caput succedaneum if labour is prolonged.

Progress in Labour

Spontaneous delivery is rare in brow presentation unless the baby is very small or the pelvis is very large. There is no mechanisms of labour because the presenting diameter (mento-vertical 12.8 cm is greater than the maximum diameter at the brim. Engagement of the head is, therefore, impossible. The nurse should refer all cases of brow presentation to the doctor.

Usually a caesarean section is performed to deliver the baby in brow presentation but if the baby is dead or abnormal, craniotomy is preferred. At times it may be possible to convert the brow into another presentation by vaginal manipulation under anaesthesia. The head may be further extended into a face presentation flexed into a vertex.

Since spontaneous delivery is unusual it follows that neglected cases will lead to a higher rate of foetal loss, maternal morbidity and mortality. The prognosis and complications for the mother and foetus are the same as in cases of neglected mento-posterior face presentation.

TRANSVERSE LIE AND SHOULDER PRESENTATION (FIG. 9.14)

Transverse lie is a serious complication in obstetrics. In transverse lie, the long axis of the foetus is across that of the mother and the shoulder usually presents. The foetus is across that of the mother and the shoulder usually presents. The foetus may lie with its back to the mother's front or spine. These positions are described as dorso-anterior and dorse-posterior respectively.

Causes of Transverse Lie

Transverse lie will occur:

1. When the foetus is very mobile as in case of prematurity, grande multiparity and hydramnios.
2. When the foetus is dead and has no muscle tone.

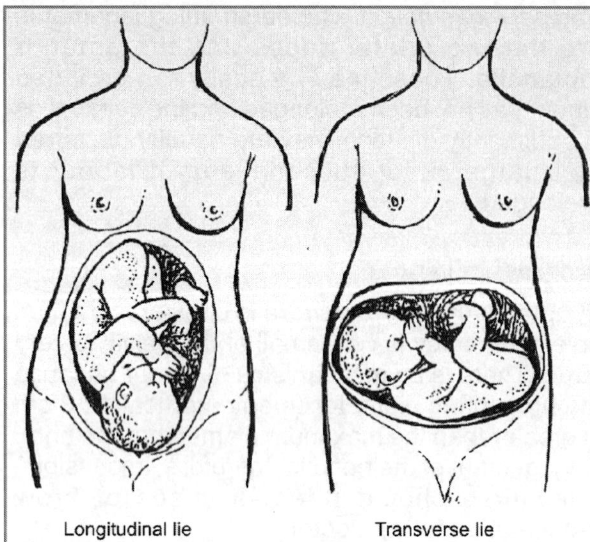

Fig. 9.14: Lie—In the longitudinal lie, the foetus is parallel to the mother's spine. In the transverse lie, or shoulder presentation, the fetus is at right angles to the mother's spine

3. When the foetus is forced into the position. Because the pelvis is contracted or there is a major degree of placenta praevia or there are large pelvic tumours.
4. When the foetus is forced into the position, because of minor degrees of uterine abnormality, as an arcuate or suseptate uterus.
5. When there are twins or triplets.

Diagnosis

Transverse lie can be suspected from the shape of the uterus. The uterus is wide and shortened in its long axis.

On palpation of the abdomen the head is felt across one side of the uterus as a round hard mass and the breech is felt to the other side as a bulky soft mass. If the back is to the front it is felt as a curved body connecting the two poles of the foetus. Palpation is easy as long as the membranes rupture or if there is oligohydramnios, palpation of the foetal parts is rendered difficult because the uterus is wrapped round the foetus. In labour, a vaginal examination is of great help. Early in labour the presenting part is high, usually beyond the nurse midwife's reach. In advanced labour the shoulder is felt as a small rounded body beyond which the nurse midwife can palpate the clavicle or the ribs. Thus the clavicles and ribs are important landmarks. The foetal heart sounds are heard low down in dorso-anterior position. It may not be tool easy to hear the heart sounds in dorso-posterior position. Finally a radiographic examination will resolve any doubt about the diagnosis.

During labour when the membranes rupture, there may be prolapse of an arm, a hand, a foot or umbilical cord. Sometimes there is a combination of a foot and an arm presenting or the elbow may appear in the vagina. In cases of prolapsed hand the nurse midwife can determine to which side the hand belongs by shaking hands with the baby. If it is possible to shake hands using one's right hand then the right hand of the baby is the hand that has prolapsed and vice versa.

Course of Labour

The shoulder is pushed into the pelvis and if the mother is not assisted, it may get impacted in the pelvis. Uterine contractions continue until the uterus is exhausted or ruptures.

In a very small number of cases and in exceptional circumstances, the baby may be delivered spontaneously. For spontaneous delivery to occur one of three things may happen.

Spontaneous version: The lie becomes longitudinal spontaneously, with either the breach or the head presenting. This usually occurs before the rupture of the membranes. Labour then progresses as for a longitudinal lie.

Spontaneous evolution: In this condition, the shoulder is driven down the pelvis and an arm may prolapse. The shoulder goes down the pelvis and is fixed under the pubic symphysis. The trunk, breech and limbs are delivered. Later the other shoulder and head escape. Spontaneous evolution is very rare. It can only occur in very small premature babies or if the pelvis is very large.

Doubling up of the foetus: The head and the chest of the foetus are pressed together and it escapes through the pelvis. This is a very rare phenomenon.

Treatment

The patient should be referred to hospital if transverse lie is discovered after the 32nd week of pregnancy. External version will be done to convert the presentation to a head and this may have to be repeated on several occasions for the foetus may revert to a transverse lie. If this occurs repeatedly and the patient is near term, admission to hospital should be advised before labour begins. In early labour an attempt should be made to convert the presentation to a head presentation by external version. If this is not possible and the os is one or two fingers dilated, the presentation is converted into a breech presentation by bipolar version. If the cervical os is fully dilated, the presentation is converted to a breech presentation. If all the liquor amnii has drained away and the uterus has closely enveloped the foetus, version is impossible without causing rupture of the uterus.

In such circumstances, the baby is delivered by caesarean section if it is alive. Caesarean section is also performed if the pelvis is contracted or the cord prolapses. If the child is dead, decapitation followed by delivery of the baby is carried out. It is important for the nurse to appreciate that there is no mechanism of labour in a shoulder presentation.

Prognosis for Mother and Baby

The mother: Unsupervised cases of transverse lie usually lead to impacted shoulder presentation, obstructed labour and subsequently rupture of the uterus in multiparous patients. Thus maternal morbidity and mortality is high. If the patient is sent to the hospital and referred to a physician late in pregnancy or very early in labour before the membranes rupture, the prognosis is improved.

The foetus cord prolapse with attendant pressure of the presenting part on it, as well as spasm of its vessels is one of the chief causes of foetal death. Intra-uterine manipulations (such as internal podalic version) of the foetus also increase the foetal morbidity and mortality.

BREECH PRESENTATION

Breech presentation is the most common form of malpresentation. In breech presentation, the foetus lies with its buttocks in the lower pole of the uterus.

Varieties of Breech (Fig. 9.15)

a. *The footling breech* This is one in which one or both of the thighs are extended to that the foot lies lowest in the birth canal.
b. *Complete breech* In complete breech the attitude of the foetus is in
c. *Frank breech* The foetus has both legs extended on the abdomen.

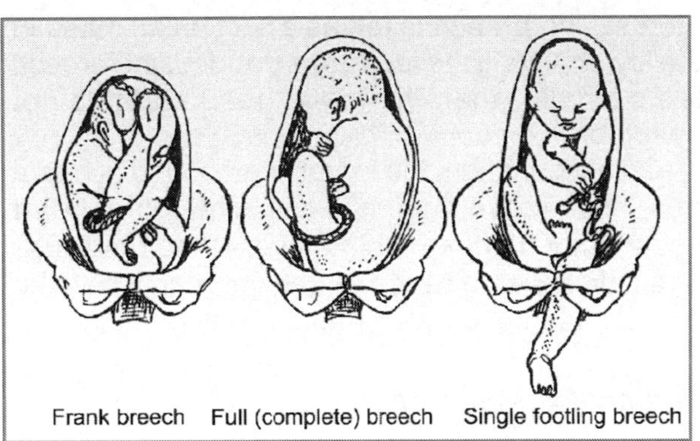

Fig. 9.15: Varieties of breech presentation

Factors Accounting for Breech Presentation

1. *Maternal factors*
   a. Contracted pelvis or any form of pelvic malformation
   b. Scanty liquor amnii or oligohydramnios; this is an important cause of breech presentation at term
   c. Hydramnios especially in association with congenital foetal abnormalities
   d. Placenta praevia
   e. Uterine abnormalities, e.g. arcuate uterus, bicornate uterus.
2. *Foetal factors*
   a. Prematurity; 50 per cent of foetuses present by the breech at about 28 weeks' gestation; the frequency of breech presentation diminishes with advancing gestation age
   b. Twin pregnancy
   c. Intrauterine death
   d. Some congenital malformation—the common ones are hydrocephaly and anencephaly

In a number of cases no explanation can be given for the occurrence of breech presentation.

Diagnosis of Breech Presentation

Antenatal Diagnosis

On inspection there is hardly any difference between the contour of the abdomen in breech presentation and cephalic presentation. Patients sometimes say that they feel a hard mass the abdomen and sometimes they complain of pain, possibly due to pressure in the area where the foetal head lies.

On abdominal palpation, the foetal head is felt as a hard ballotable object in the upper pole of the uterus. The breech is felt as a soft bulky mass in the lower pole. If the legs are extended, the breech feels smaller than the foetal head and it is not ballotable.

On auscultation, the foetal heart sound is heard at a level above the umbilicus. The foetal heart sound may be heard at the level of the umbilicus or a little lower in cases of frank breech when the breech has descended into the pelvis.

Vaginal Examination

Vaginal examination is of little or no help in the diagnosis of breech presentation before the onset of labour.

All doubtful cases should be referred to the doctor who will order radiographic (X-ray) examination to confirm the diagnosis after the 34th week of pregnancy.

Management of Breech Presentation (Figs 9.16 to 9.20)

Antenatal Period

The nurse midwife should refer cases of breech presentation to the physician as soon as possible.

The usual routine antenatal care such as regular weighing of patient checking of haemoglobin, blood pressure, giving of iron folic acid. Dataprit tablets and urine testing should be carried out.

External Cephalic Version

If the breech presents any time after the 32nd week of gestation, an attempt should be made to convert it into a cephalic presentation provided there is no contraindication. This is known as external cephalic version. The ideal time for external cephalic version is around the 34th week of gestation, because if the baby is turned earlier than this period, it may revert back to breech. Some difficulty may be encountered because of the relative decrease in the quantity of the liquor amnii if the version is done after the 34th week. General anaesthesia may be required to relax the abdominal muscles where external cephalic version fails due to tense abdominal muscles. In such case, the patient may be admitted as a day case for preparation, or instructed to report to the hospital in the morning without breakfast.

Complications of External Cephalic Version

1. Premature rupture of the membranes causing prolapse of the umbilical cord and occasionally premature onset of labour.
2. Premature separation of the placenta leading to antepartum haemorrhage.

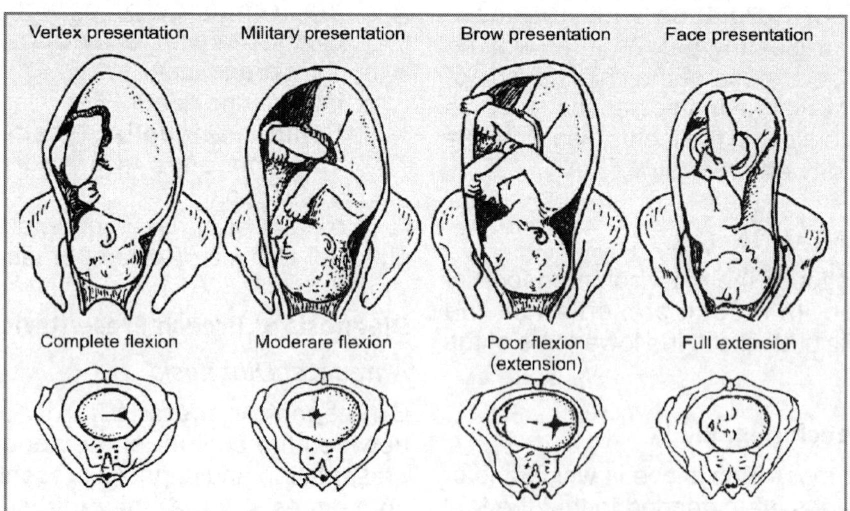

Fig. 9.16: Four types of cephalic presentation. The vertex presentation, in which the foetal chin is flexed on the chest, is the most favourable for vaginal birth because it allows the smallest diameter of the head to go through the pelvis. Note how the anterior and posterior fontanells can be used during vaginal examination to determine the foetal presentation and position in the pelvis

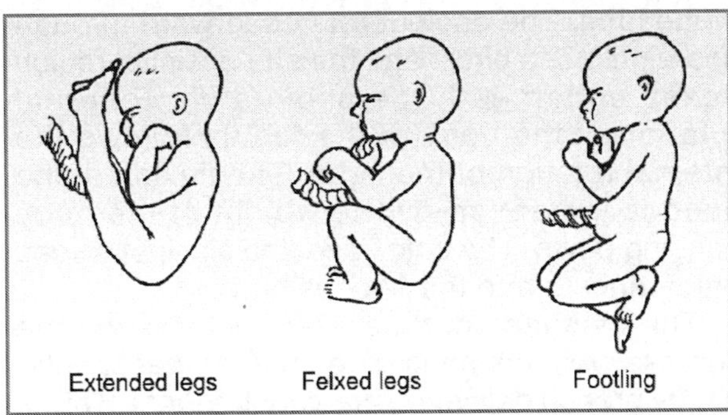

Fig. 9.17: Types of breech presentation

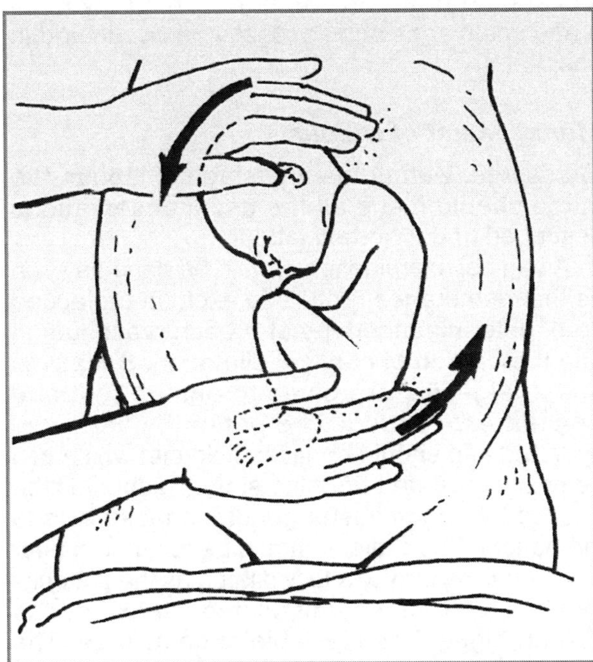

Fig. 9.18: External cephalic version: Pressure is applied in the opposite direction to the two foetal poles

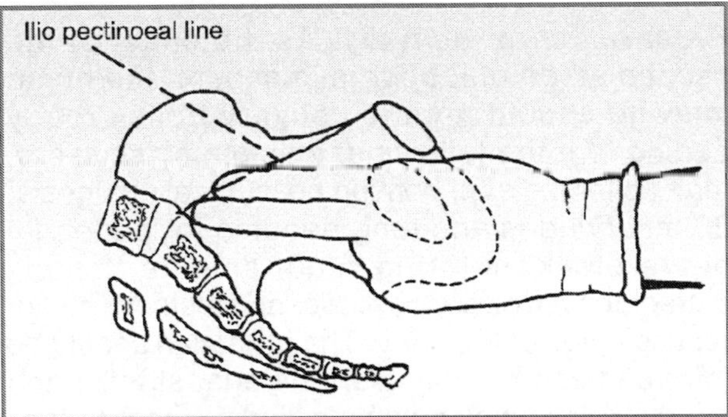

Fig. 9.19: Clinical assessment of the pelvis and breech presentation

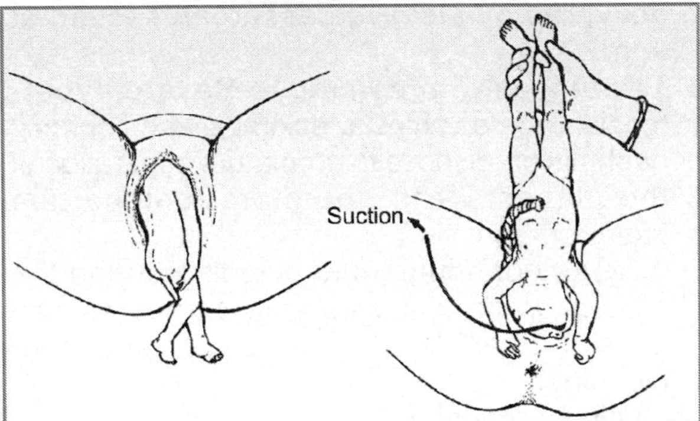

Fig. 9.20: Technique of breech delivery: initial delivery of the trunk allows descent of the head into the pelvis (left); subsequent anterior rotation of the trunk enables delivery of the foetal head with the application of forceps to safeguard the head from sudden compression and expansion (right)

Nurse's Responsibility at External Cephalic Version

Preparation for this procedure includes ensuring that the patient understands that is to be done, and also that she has emptied her bladder. X-ray, if any, should be made available at the viewing box. Equipment, e.g. foetal stethoscope, dusting powder, gloves and hibitane cream, should be handy.

If the breech has descended into the pelvis, it may be necessary to raise the foot of the bed before the version is performed. The foetal heart sound is auscultated before the procedure.

During the procedure, it is advisable to engage the woman in conversation to obtain mental and physical relaxation. At the end of external cephalic version the patient's legs and thighs are abducted so that the midwife can look for evidence of vaginal bleeding and rupture of membranes.

When practicable, the patient should be detained at the clinic for two hours and the foetal heart sound auscultated every fifteen to thirty minutes to exclude foetal distress. Painful uterine contraction should also be excluded. If the patient has to go home in less than the stated time, she must be instructed to report any vaginal bleeding or undue foetal movements.

Contraindications to External Cephalic Version

1. Contracted pelvis—No advantage is derived from external cephalic version in the presence of a major pelvic contraction. Such cases are

delivered by elective caesarean section at term.
2. Toxaemias of pregnancy—Severe hypertension, pre-eclampsia, eclampsia and chronic nephritis predispose to premature separation of the placenta and, therefore, antepartum haemorrhage.
3. A history of antepartum bleeding during the present pregnancy. Version in such cases may cause further placental separation and more bleeding.
4. Multiple pregnancy.
5. Previous caesarean section—Version should not be attempted if there is history of previous caesarean section, especially a classical section.

Diagnosis of Breech Presentation in Labour

Mechanism of labour There are four positions in breech presentation; the denominator is the sacrum. The positions are:
1. Left sacro-anterior (LSA)
2. Right sacro-anterior (RSA)
3. Right sacro-posterior (RSP)
4. Left sacro-posterior (LSP)

During labour the breech descends into the pelvis.

Left sacro-anterior position: The breech enters the pelvis with the bitrochanteric diameter 10.2 cm in the left or right oblique diameter of the pelvis. Further descent of the breech is not usually appreciable until towards the end of the first stage of labour or the beginning of the second stage.

When the cervix is fully dilated, the breech descends and the anterior buttock is the first to hit the pelvic floor. It is rotated through one eighth of a circle to the front. When the bitrochanteric diameter reaches the pelvic outlet the anterior buttock slips cut under the pubic arch and so both buttocks are born. The legs follow. Restitution of the buttocks next takes place.

With further uterine contractions the shoulders enter the pelvis with the biacromial diameter 12.1 cm in one oblique diameter or the other of the pelvis. Further descent of the shoulders takes place. The anterior shoulder reaches the pelvic floor first and is born under the symphysis pubis. The posterior shoulder sweeps the perineum and is born.

The head descends into the pelvis. It enters the pelvis with its long axis in the transverse diameter of the brim. The occiput rotates forward through one-eighth of a circle and the sub-occipital region flexes underneath the pubic arch. External rotation of the body of the foetus follows the internal rotation of the head. The flexion of the head is increased by the weight of the body hanging down. The chin, face and sinciput sweep the perineum and the head is born.

The mechanism thus described leaves the impression in the mind of the reader that spontaneous breech deliveries are very frequent. This is not always the case unless the baby is very small. The majority of breech deliveries require the assistance of an accoucheur. This is why all breech deliveries should ideally be conducted in hospital.

Management of Labour

First stage: During the first stage of labour, the nurse should make all the usual observations described under normal labour.

A vaginal examination should be done as soon as the membranes rupture to exclude prolapsed cord, determine the type of breech presentation and the degree of cervical dilatation. Sedatives and analgesics are given to ensure rest and prevent exhaustion. The patient is kept well hydrated and should be given fluid diet which can be easily aspirated from the stomach should it be necessary to administer general anaesthesia to the patient. The patient should be told not to bear down until the cervix is fully dilated as the buttocks may pass through a half dilated cervix and the harder, bigger head is liable to be help up. The patient should be instructed to breathe through her mouth if she has an urge to push. In fact, she must not be allowed to bear down until the foetal buttocks are visible at the vulva.

Preparation for delivery: As the onset of the second stage of labour is imminent, the nurse midwife should get the delivery trolley ready adding to it the following: episiotomy scissors, forceps for the after coming head, local analgesia, 20 ml sryinges and long needles for pudendal nerve block, suturing requirements, mucus extractor a full oxygen cylinder and instruments for resuscitation of the baby. The physician should be informed and he may alert the anaesthetist and paediatrician who could be called if complications occur. it is not always possible to get these specialists to be present at each breech delivery in many hospitals. Nevertheless, it is desirable to have at lease one physician present at every breech delivery.

Second stage of labour: When the breech is distending the perineum, the patient should be put in lithotomy position or be made to lie across the bed with her buttocks at the edge of the bed, knees flexed and abducted. The breech should descend with the uterine contractions and the bearing down efforts of the patient. The foetal heart is checked after every contraction.

Delivery of the buttocks and the trunk: After the usual toilet, the patient is draped with sterile bowels. Stretching of the vagina and 'ironing' of the perineum are usually done before the episiotomy to prevent pelvic resistance and make it easy for the baby to come through easily. The physician, who should by this time be present in the labour ward will carry out infiltration of the perineum with local analgesia or do a pudendal nerve block. When the breech is distending the perineum, a right mediolateral episiotomy is done by the physician. It is important that the epiosotomy should not be done too soon. If there are bleeding points from the episiotomy they should be caught with artery forceps to prevent bleeding.

Usually with good uterine contractions the buttocks are delivered by maternal effort. All that needs to be done by the nurse or physician is to assist in freeing the legs. In breech with extended legs, this freeing of the legs can be achieved by applying pressure with the fingers on the popliteal fossa of the baby. This flexes the knee which is then gently splinted between the first and second fingers and delivered by a backward and outward movement.

With further uterine contractions the trunk is born as far as the umbilicus. A loop of umbilical cord is pulled down and brought to lie between the baby's legs.

If the patient is a primigravida a general anaesthetic may be given at this stagel, arrangoment had not previously been made for general anaesthesia the patient should have had, early in the second stage of labour and before commencement of delivery, caudal or pudendal block analgesia. For a parous woman all that may be needed is the preliminary local infiltration to facilitate the making of an episiotomy.

Delivery of the shoulders: The weight of the buttocks will bring the shoulders down to the pelvic floor where they will rotate into the antero-posterior diameter of the outlet. The baby is grasped at the iliac crests and a downward traction may be used when the patient is pushing to aid the expulsion of the shoulders. The baby's back must not be turned uppermost until the shoulders have been born, to avoid extension of the head. With the next uterine contraction the elbows usually come down and the arms freed. it is usualy easier to free the posterior arm first, because there is more room posteriorly (in the hollow of the sacrum) than anteriorly (because of the pubic arch).

Delivery of the baby after coming head: This is the most critical, stage of delivery, for usually it determines the fate of the baby. If the after coming head is delivered too hastily it results in intracranial injury and subsequent death of the foetus. If it is delivered too slowly, it results in premature inspiration and severe asphyxia.

The after coming head of the breech can be delivered by the Burns-Marshall technique, by the use of obstetric forceps and by the Maurican-Smellie-Viet technique. Only the first is recommended to the nurse. The second and third methods should be done by physician.

The burns-marshall technique: The baby is allowed to hang down with the back uppermost at the vulva, for about two minutes. This encourages descent and flexion of the head and allows the head to be born as far as the nape of the neck (that is the suboccipital region of the foetal head). If the head does not descend to the pelvis in one or two minutes a genteel suprapubic pressure may facilitate its descent. When the suboccipital are appears at the pubic arch, the legs of the baby are grasped and the nurse exerts a firm outward traction and the body is lifted towards the mother's abdomen. This causes the suboccipital area to be fixed at the subpubic angle. The foetal head is delivered by a movement of flexion.

At this stage the left hand of the nurse midwife is used to guard the perineum and to prevent the head being delivered too quickly, as soon as the mouth and nose of the foetus are free an assistant sucks out all mucus from the airway. This will facilitate the breathing of the baby and prevent asphyxia.

The type of breech delivery described above is an assisted breech delivery. This is because most of the delivery is achieved by maternal effort and all the nurse midwife or physician needs to do is to free the legs and arms and deliver the after coming head. Another method of breech delivery is known as breech extraction. In this method, the patient is anaesthetized and the physician has to put his whole hand into the vagina and uterus to effect the delivery of the baby. This is seldom necessary except in complicated cases, a though some authorities recommend it for breach deliver in primigravidae.

Complicated Breech Delivery

The following are the conditions that may complicate breech delivery:

1. *Extended legs breech:* With extended legs is continuously encountered in primigravidae. It usually presents no major problem during labour provided the pelvis is adequate. In fact, a franck breech behaves like a vertex presentation in that it is well applied to the cervix and it thus aids dilatation of the cervix. The nurse could diagnose extended legs from the fact that the legs do not disengage easily when the buttocks are born and the external genitalia are more evident. The nurse should flex the baby's knees and sweep the feet over the perineum as described under "*Delivery of the Buttocks*".
2. *Extended arms:* Extended arms are diagnosed when there is no advance after the umbilicus is born. The axillae are visible and the elbows are not felt on the chest. Breech presentation with extended arms is rare and constitutes a serious complication. If this complication occurs in hospital the physician (if not present at delivery) must be summoned at once. Unfortunately this complication may occur on the district and the nurse should know what to do in an emergency if the baby is not to be sacrificed.

The midwife/nurse should attempt to deliver the posterior arm and shoulder first. If the baby's back is to the mother's right, the nurse uses her right hand to grasp the baby's legs and by pulling the baby's trunk a little to the left of the mother, she will bring down the posterior arm and shoulder. The baby's trunk may be lifted up a bit while the nurse passes her left hand up along the spine of the baby over its shoulder to spling the humerus between the middle and index fingers. The baby's arm thus bent at the elbow is pushed over its face.

After the delivery of the posterior arm the anterior arm is delivered in the same way after depressing the baby's trunk towards the sacral hollow.

Lovsett's Manoeuvre

Lovsett's manoeuvre is recommended for the delivery of breech with extended arms. it is a combination of traction and rotation. Traction is applied till the baby's axilla is visible, the nurse then graspe the baby around the pelvic girdle with her thumbs at the sacrum of the baby. With the back of the baby anterior, the trunk is rotated through half a circle (180°) to bring the posterior shoulder into an anterior position. The arm is delivered from under the pubic arch by splinting the humerus and drawing down the elbow.

At times, the arm is delivered unaided. After delivery, the shoulder with the arm and hand of one side of the baby is then rotated in the opposite direction through half a circle (180°) thus bringing the posterior shoulder to the front and delivering it as previously described.

The Extended Head

Extended head should be suspected if the hair is not visible after the baby has been handing for two minutes. The nurse midwife must ensure that the bladder is empty and a moderate suprapubic pressure is used to encourage flexion and descend of the head.

The delivery of the head can be achieved by the mauriceau-Smellie-Veit technique. The baby is placed astride the nurse's left arm with the palm supporting the chest. The middle finger on the left hand is put far back into the baby's mouth in order to flex the head. The first and third fingers are placed on the molar bones to and flexion of the head.

The first and third fingers of the right hand are placed over the baby's right shoulder. If posssible the middle finger should press on the occiput to further increase head flexion. An assistant is asked to exert suprapubic pressure whilst the nurse midwife exerts traction in an outward direction until the head is brought into the pelvis. When the nape of the neck appears under the pubic symphysis the suprapubic pressure is stopped. The nurse midwife then carries the baby's body towards the mother's abdomen. The face and forehead are carefully guided over the perineum and the airway is cleared. The occiput is born last and the delivery of the head is completed.

This is rare complication. It may be the result of mismanagement of breech delivery. Sometimes it is the result of failure of supontaneous rotation of the foetal back to the front in unassisted breech deliveries.

In cases in which the head has not already entered the pelvis, the rotation of the foetus to the dorsoanterior position may be possible and the head delivered by the Mauricau-Smellie-Veit technique.

Sometimes rotation is not possible because the head is too well fixed in the pelvis or the chin is caught above the symphysis pubis. Delivery by the nurse in such cases is difficult. If a physician is nearby, he should be called because such cases are better delivered by forceps after a wide episiotomy.

Hazards of Breech Presentation

The hazards of breech presentation can be considered under two headings:
1. Maternal
2. Foetal

Maternal Hazards

1. During external cephalic version the patient may bleed from placental separation or rupture of the uterus. These are rare complications.
2. Labour is usually prolonged, especially in a primigravida. This necessitates separation or rupture of the uterus. These are rare complications.
3. Labour is usually prolonged, especially in a primigravida. This necessitates carrying out a number of vaginal examinations which may predispose to infection in the puerperium.
4. During delivery, there is a high incidence of cervical, vaginal and perineal lacerations. These lacerations may lead to traumatic postpartum haemorrhage which may cause shock.

Foetal Hazards

1. *Intracranial haemorrhage:* This usually results from tentorial tears which occur as a result of the sudden and excessive pressure on the head during its delivery. Tentorial tears are likely to occur if the delivery of the after coming head is hurried.
2. *Asphyxia:* The intracranial injury leads to severe asphyxia neonatorum and accounts for the high perinatal loss in breech deliveries. Asphyxia may also result from premature inspiration due to too slow delivery of the head. If the delivery of the after coming head is not accomplished in about eight to ten minutes, the foetus may die from severe asphyxia.
3. Prolapse of the cord and cord compression are common in breech delivery and they cause intra-uterine anoxia or neonatal asphyxia.
4. *Birth injuries:* Tentorial tears have been mentioned already. Other birth injuries include:
   a. Fracture of the clavicle and humerus.
   b. Fracture of the femur.
   c. Rupture of the liver, spleen or other abdominal organs.
   d. Injury to peripheral nerves, especially those arising from the brachial plexus; the injury may arise from excessive traction on the neck during the delivery of the shoulders or the after coming head; Erb's or Klumpke's paralysis may result from these injuries.
   e. Bruising of the external genitalia, particularly in male babies.

OBSTETRIC OPERATIONS

The obstetric operations commonly performed in the interest of the baby or the mother are:
1. Caesarean section
2. Forceps delivery
3. Symphysiotomy
4. Vacuum extraction (ventouse)
5. Episiotomy
6. Destructive operation such as craniotomy, embryotomy, etc. are performed in the interest of the mother when the foetus dies in utero during labour.

Caesarean Section/Caesarean Birth (Figs 9.21 to 9.23)

Caesarean section entails the delivery of a baby through an incision in the uterine and abdominal walls. If such operation is the 28th week of pregnancy, the term abdominal hysterotomy is used. Table 9.1 presents nursing care plan of unplanned caesarean birth.

Table 9.1: Nursing care plan for the woman with an unplanned cesarean birth

Problem/Objective	*Nursing intervention*	*Rationale*
Nursing Diagnosis: Anxiety related to development of complications.		
• Woman and her partner will express decreased anxiety after explanations about the planned surgery	1. Reinforce all explanations given by physician, expressing them in simpler terms, if needed	1. Anxiety tends to narrow attention; although physician may have explained need for surgery, woman and her partner may not have comprehended everything they were told
	2. Encourage woman to continue using breathing and relaxation techniques she learned in prepared childbirth classes; tell her the techniques may help with pain control after birth	2. Learned pain management techniques increase woman's sense of control; control over a situation reduces feelings of helplessness and decreases anxiety
	3. Tell woman what operating room looks like and who will be present; explain basic equipment such as catheter, narrow table, monitors for her heart and blood pressure, anaesthesia machine, and large overhead lights; explain that all personnel will wear masks, gowns, gloves, hats, and shoe covers; personnel at operating table will also have eye protection, such as goggles or face shield	3. Common place equipment and attire in an operating room can be intimidating for someone who has not seen them before; unfamiliarity increases anxiety; preparation reduces anxiety and fear of the unknown
	4. Describe usual postoperative care—assessment of the vital signs, fundus, vaginal bleeding, dressing, and catheter; tell her she will be asked to take deep breaths and change position regularly	4. If woman understands common postoperative care, she is more likely to cooperate with it, even if assessments are uncomfortable
	5. Encourage her partner to be with her during surgery and do not separate family afterward, if possible	5. Companionship of familiar persons helps reduce anxiety; keeping new family together promotes bonding
Nursing Diagnosis: Pain related to effects of surgery (incisional, slowed gastric peristalsis).		
• Woman will state that pain is manageable with the pharmacologic and nonpharmacologic methods used	1. Assess nature of pain: location, quality, intensity, duration, and factors that increase or decrease it	1. Proper assessment allows nurse to choose most appropriate interventions, such as repositioning or medication
	2. Provide analgesics as ordered, usually intramuscular or patient controlled analgesia (PCA) pump for the first 24 hr and oral analgesics after this time; do not allow pain to become too intense before medicating woman	2. Analgesics inhibit brain's ability to interpret pain; early and frequent use of measures to relieve pain allows optimal control and facilitates healing
	3. Assess bowel sounds each shift or more frequently if they are diminished; ask woman to report when she begins passing flatus (gas) rectally	3. Caesarean birth may delay the return of bowel function; accumulation of intestinal gas will cause abdominal distention and cramping; passing flatus indicates return of bowel function
	4. Encourage woman to get out of bed about 24 hr after surgery, as ordered; progressively increase her ambulation	4. Activity stimulates intestinal peristalsis, which reduces accumulation of gas and limits discomfort from this source
	5. Discourage woman from drinking carbonated drinks or drinking through a straw	5. These activities tend to increase swallowed gas and can increase gastric discomfort

Contd...

Contd...

Problem/Objective	*Nursing intervention*	*Rationale*
Nursing Diagnosis: High risk for ineffective airway clearance related to reduced breathing efforts secondary to incisional pain.		
• Woman will have a normal respiratory rate of 12 to 24 breaths/min, clear lung sounds	1. Assess vital signs and lung sounds according to length of time since surgery (usually every 15 min in the recovery area, then every 4 hours after stabilized)	1. Tachypnoea or congested lung sounds suggest that woman is not moving secretions from her airways; temperature elevation over 38ºC (100.4ºF) suggests infection, which (could have several sources, including respiratory
	2. Have woman take deep breaths and cough every 2 hours; teach her to press a pillow or folded blanket over her incision area to splint it	2. Deep breathing and coughing help move secretions from airways; splinting incision reduces strain on it and reduces pain so woman can cough more effectively
	3. Encourage changing position every 2 hours before ambulating, turning side to side	3. Helps move secretions from air-ways and prevents congestion, which is a favourable environment for growth of infectious organisms
Nursing Diagnosis: High risk for altered tissue perfusion related to bleeding secondary to uterine atony		
• Woman will have adequate tissue perfusion as evidenced by saturation of no more than one pad per hour during recovery period	1. Assess vital signs every 15 during recovery area, then according to hospital policy	1. Rising pulse and falling blood pressure suggest shock, which is most often due to haemorrhage
	2. Assess uterine fundus for firmness, height, and position (midline or deviated) with vital signs; massage fundus until it is firm if necessary; explain reason for this assessment, and have woman bend her knees and breathe slowly and deeply while you assess fundus.	2. Firm fundus compresses bleeding blood vessels at placenta site; this procedure is often painful if woman had a caesarean birth, especially with a vertical skin incision; if she understands its importance and takes measures to minimize discomfort, she is more likely to accept needed assessment
	3. Assess lochia for amount, colour, and odor when uterine fundus is assessed; report over one pad per hour saturated during recovery period or persistent clots	3. Signs of excessive blood loss require prompt medical and nursing intervention to avoid altering tissue perfusion
	4. Assess catheter for patency and for amount of urine output with vital signs and fundal and lochia checks; assess voided output until woman is urinating adequate amounts (over 100 ml) regularly	4. A full bladder inhibits uterine contraction and can lead to haemorrhage; adequate urine output verifies patency of catheter and reflects and adequate circulating blood volume
	5. Check dressing and incision with each fundal check	5. Bloody drainage on dressing suggests breakdown in incision line; gapping of incision (after dressing is removed) suggests infection and can lead to haemorrhage
Nursing Diagnosis: High risk for infection related to loss of barrier (ruptured membranes)		
• Woman's temperature will remain under 38ºC (100.4ºF), and the amniotic fluid will remain clear with a mild odour	1. Take woman's temperature every 2 hr; at same time, assess the amniotic fluid drainage for colour, clarity, and odour	1. Elevated temperature is a sign of infection; cloudy, yellow, or foul-odored fluid suggests infection; meconium (green) staining suggests fetal compromise but is also seen with prolonged pregnancy

Contd...

Contd...

Problem/Objective	*Nursing intervention*	*Rationale*
	2. Monitor foetal heart rates	2. Foetal tachycardia rate>160/min) may be the first sign of infection; poor foetal oxygenation also may occur, especially with abnormal labour
	3. After birth, continue to assess woman's temperature every 4 hours until she is stable; assess the lochia (postbirth vaginal drainage) for a foul odour or brown colour	3. Woman may not show these signs of infection until after birth
	4. Observe neonate for a temperature below 36.2ºC (97ºF) or over 37.8ºC (100°F); observe for poor feeding, lethargy, irritability, or "not looking right"	4. Neonate may become infected in utero and display these signs of infection after birth; neonatal sepsis may occur with prolonged rupture of membranes and is a potentially fatal infection
Nursing Diagnosis: Ineffective individual coping related to frustration with slow labour and delayed birth		
• Woman will use breathing and relaxation techniques that she and her partner learned in prepared child-birth class	1. If there is no contraindication, such as epidural block, encourage woman to walk or to sit upright in bed or chair; walking may not be wise if membranes are ruptured and foetus is high	1. Upright positions enhance foetal descent; walking strengthens labour contractions; walking when membranes are ruptured and foetal station is high could lead to umbilical cord prolapse
	2. Help woman use natural methods to stimulate contractions, such as nipple stimulation; encourage a shower or whirpool if available and not contraindicated	2. Nipple stimulation causes woman posterior pituitary gland to secrete natural oxytocin, which strengthens contractions; water may help woman relax, which improves labour; all nondrug methods to stimulate labour enhance her sense of control
	3. Assist registered nurse with oxytocin augmentation if it is ordered; observe contractions for excessive frequency (more frequent than every 2 min), duration (over 90 sec), or inadequate rest interval (under 60 sec); observe foetal heart rate for rates outside normal 110-160 beats/min	3. Primary risks of oxytocin augmentation or induction of labour relate to overstimulating the uterus; excessive contractions can reduce foetal oxygen supply; these are signs of potential uterine overstimulation
	4. Explain to woman how each method is expected to help her labour advance; tell her any time she makes progress, either in improved contraction or increasing cervical dilation	4. If woman understands reason for any interventions, she will more likely cooperate with them and feed more in control; knowing that her efforts are having desired effect encourages her to continue with her learned coping methods
	5. Help woman relax and use breathing techniques she learned in prepared childbirth class; praise and support her when she uses them	5. Relaxation promotes normal labour woman with a long labour may feel that there is no use in continuing relaxation and breathing if she is not making progress; praise encourages her to continue

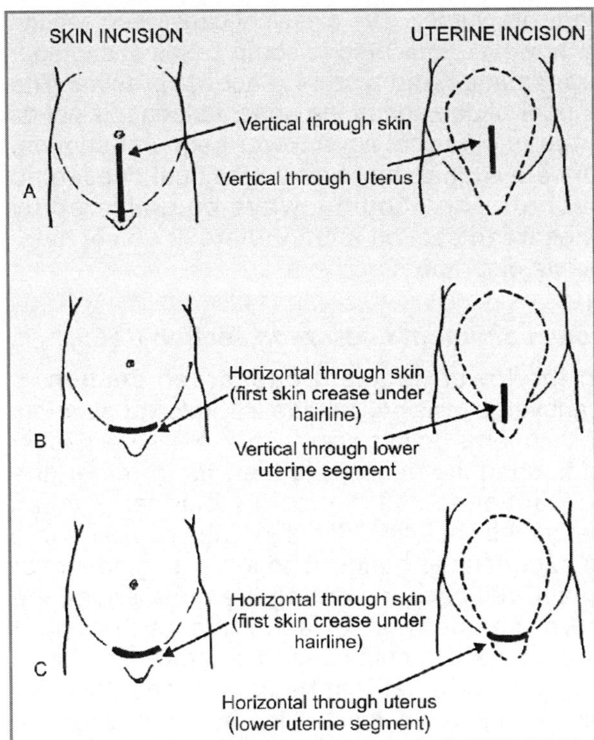

Figs 9.21A to C: Caesarean delivery: Skin and uterine incisions. **A.** Classic vertical incisions, **B.** Low cervical incision, **C.** Low cervical incision of skin and uterus

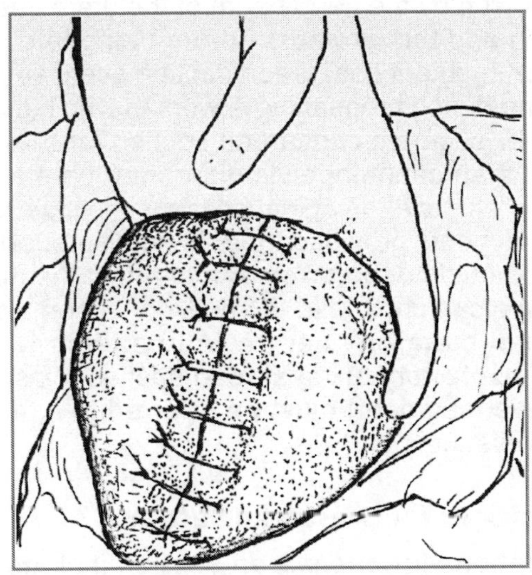

Fig. 9.22: Suture on vertical uterine incision

Types of Caesarean Section (Figs 9.24 to 9.26)

Elective Caesarean Section

An elective caesarean section is a planned operation. The obstetrician decides for some good reason to deliver the baby by caesarean section around the 38th week of gestation or at term. The patient is usually admitted two days before the operation which would have been fixed for a particular date. On the other hand, the operation may be done earlier than planned if the membranes rupture, or the patient goes into labour.

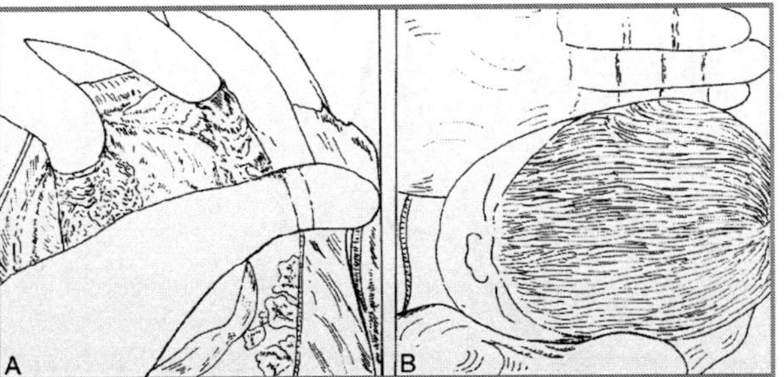

Figs 9.23A and B: Cesarean section delivery. A. The surgeon's right hand is inserted under the foetal head, which is levered out through the uterine wound. The baby's nostrils and mouth are cleared by suction as soon as the head is delivered. B, The rest of the baby is delivered by the application of traction on the baby's head. The cord is clamped and cut between two artery forceps and the baby passed to the attending paediatrician

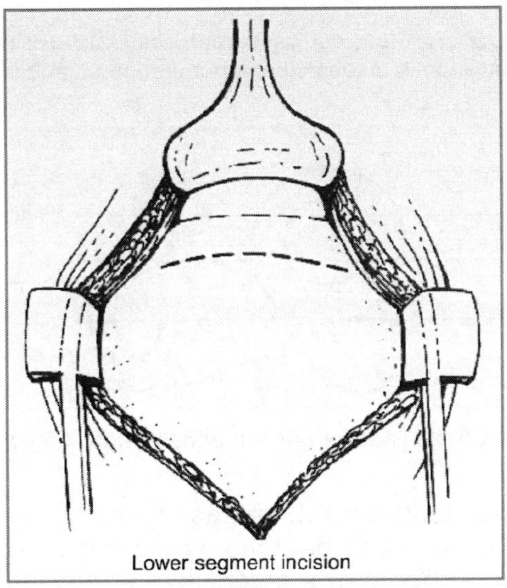

Fig. 9.24: Lower uterine segment caesarean section the bladder is reflected and a transverse incision is made in the lower segment

Emergency Caesarean Section

An emergency caesarean section is so-called, because the operation is not planned. In most cases, the patient has not been booked for a

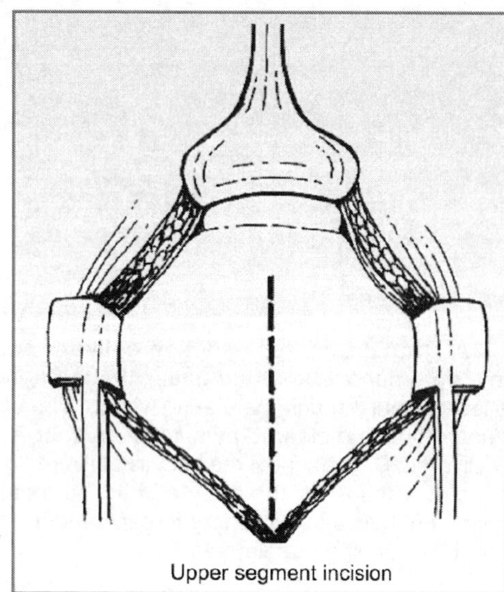

Fig. 9.25: 'Classical' caesarean section: A vertical incision is made in the upper uterine segment

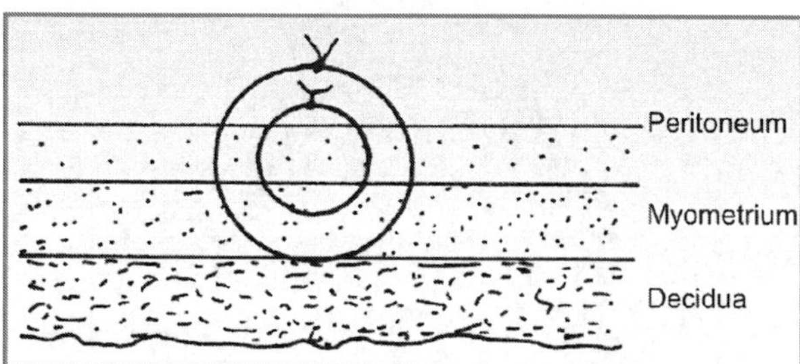

Fig. 9.26: Closure of the uterine wound in layers

hospital confinement nor has she had any antenatal care. Such patients would have been in labour at home or a maternity centre, and the operation is performed to save the baby or the mother or both.

Classical Caesarean Section

In the classical operation, a longitudinal incision is made in the middle of the anterior aspect of the upper uterine segment. Thus the classical caesarean section is an upper segment section. It is seldom performed nowadays because the wound in the uterus heals poorly and leaves a weak scar on the uterus. Because the placenta is usually situated in the upper uterine segment the classical section scar may be further weakened if the placenta is situated in the area of the previous scar. This is why classical caesarean section scars rupture during pregnancy, even in early pregnancy. The classical caesarean section is, however, indicated in some cases of shoulder presentation and type IV placenta praevia. The danger of damage to the urinary bladder is not as great in classical as in lower segment section. Once a woman has had a classical caesarean section, she should always be delivered by caesarean section even if there is no cephalopelvis disproportion.

Lower Segment Caesarean Section (LSCS)

In the lower segment caesarean section, a transverse incision is made in the lower segment of the uterus. In this operation, there is the danger of injuring the urinary bladder. If, howerver, the precaution to catheterize the bladder is taken before the operation, damage to the bladder is rare in experienced hands. The lower segment scar heals well because during the puerperium, the lower segment is not as active as the upper segment which continues to contract. The lower segment being at rest heals well and does not give rise to a weak scar like the upper segment caesarean section. The placenta is again not likely to be situated in the lower segment, except in only about 3 per cent of patients. In addition to the above, the scar of the lower uterine segment is covered by the peritoneum of the utero-vesical pouch and this protects it from being infected. Lower segment caesarean section scars seldom rupture during pregnancy. A woman who has had a lower segment caesarean section for reasons other than cephalopelvic disproportion may be allowed to have a vaginal delivery in subsequent confinements provided there is no disproportion. This should not be taken to mean that the nurse midwife can undertake the delivery at home or in a small maternity centre. All patients with a previous history of caesarean section (classical or lower segment) must be referred to a major specialist hospital.

Indications for Caesarean Section

Indications for caesarean section include the following:

1. Cephalopelvic disproportion.
2. Malpresentation and abnormal lie, e.g. transverse lie.
3. Major degrees of placenta praevia.
4. Foetal distress when the cervix is not fully dilated.

5. Maternal conditions such as eclampsia, severe pre-eclampsia, chronic nephritis, hypertensions such as eclampsia, severe pre-eclampsia, chronic nephritis, hypertension, diabetes, etc.
6. Previous caesarean section for disproportion or previous classical caesarean section.
7. Previous successfully repaired vesicovaginal fistula.
8. Previous rupture of the uterus.
9. Failed trial of labour.
10. Failed surgical induction of labour.
11. Prolapse of the umbilical cord when the cervix is not fully dilated.
12. Bad obstetric history.
13. Elderly primigravida who has for years been infertile.
14. Carcinoma of the cervix complicating pregnancy.
15. Gynaetresia—structural abnormalities of the vagina.
16. Obstructed labour due to cephalopelvic disproportion, fibroids or ovarian tumours.
17. Cervical dystocia.

Nursing Management of Caesarean Section

The nurse's responsibilities at caesarean section are:

1. Preoperative preparation and care of the patient.
2. Getting the theatre ready and preparing the required instruments and equipment.
3. Reception and resuscitation of the baby.
4. Postoperative care of the patient.

Preoperative Care

Patients for elective caesarean section are usually admitted a day or two prior to the day of operation to familiarize them with the hospital and environment and to prepare them for anaesthesia.

The nurse may have to briefly describe what the operation entails to the patient. A consent for operation is then obtained from the patient or her next of kin if she is under age. Certain specific examinations and investigations should be carried out in an attempt to reduce the risk of anaesthesia. These examinations are usually conducted by the anaesthetist. In smaller hospitals in developing countries, nurses who have acquired some experience anaesthetize the patients under the supervision of the physician. In such circumstances, the nurse should particularly ensure that these examinations and investigations are carried out and also participate in doing some of them. The examinations and investigations are listed below:

1. Blood tests done to determine:
   a. The patient's packed cell volume and exclude anaemia
   b. Blood grouping—this is usually ascertained during the first visit to the antenatal clinic and it is desirable to request two or three points of compatible blood for the patient should the need for blood transfusion arise during operation.
2. Urinalysis is done to exclude albuminuria, glycosuria and acetonuria.
3. A general examination is done to assess the patient's nutritional and general health and exclude the following hypertension, respiratory tract infection and diseases of the cardiovascular system. The teeth are examined to exclude loose teeth which could easily drop and be inhaled while the patient is being anaesthetized.

A history is obtained from the patient to find out if she has been taking any drug recently. This point is essential if the patient is admitted from home for emergency operation. It is not unusual for such a patient to have taken some traditional herbs believed to relieve labour pain. If a history of inclination to vomit easily is given by a patient, such information should be conspicuously written on the patient's notes.

Other Preoperative preparations are:

1. The patient's bowels are emptied with an enaema given the night before or on the morning of the operation. Just before the operation the bladder is emptied.
2. The vulva is shaved and the lower part of the abdomen is also shaved.
3. The patient is usually starved 8 to 10 hours before the operation. In emergency cases, the patient's gastric contents should be aspirated using a wide bore gastric tube. Some authorities recommend the giving of the magnesium trisilicate (15 ml) to these emergency cases in particular, and to all pregnant women in general. The purpose is to make the stomach contents alkaline and thus reduce the irritation of the respiratory tract caused by acidity of the inhaled gastric contents.

4. Sodium amytal (200 mg) to ensure good sleep is usually given to the patient the night before the operation.
5. An hour before the operation a theatre gown is put on the patient. A scarf and a pair of leggings are also worn by the patient. Any artificial appliances such as dentures, earrings, necklace, dressings, hair pins and make up, except the wedding ring are removed. A wristle bearing the patient's full names should be tied to the patient for the purpose of identification especially when the patient is unconscious. The patient is instructed to stay in bed.
6. The premedication, usually atropine (0.6 mg)and/or Phenargan (50 mg) is given at the specified time or 30 minutes prior to the operation.
7. The patient's notes and X-rays must accompany her to the theatre.
8. It is desirable that the nurse remain with her patient to comfort and reassure her before she is anaesthetized.
9. Just before the patient is anaesthetized, the midwife should undo the tapes at the back of the patient's operation gown. When the patient is unconscious, she should be carefully handled to avoid injury to her limbs.

Postoperative Care

After the operation, the soiled towels and the patient's gown should be changed before she leaves the operating table. The patient should be nursed on her side until she regains consciousness. During the time the patient is unconscious, her airway should be kept clear and the nasopharynx sucked out as often as necessary. Observation and recording of the patient's pulse, respiration and blood pressure are made quarter-hourly. The temperature is recorded hourly. Any abnormality must be reported without delay. The nurse should inspect the wound site and the vulva to exclude bleeding.

A midwife should not leave the operating theatre with the patient without the following:

1. A good knowledge of what has been done for the patient and any postoperative instructions which are to be carried out.
2. Clear instructions regarding the infusion or transfusion.
3. The postoperative drugs written out.

Ideally, the immediate postoperative care should be given in the labour ward or an intensive care unit of a theatre where a nurse or a midwife will be in attendance upon the patient to make necessary observation and keep records as already described. When the patient is conscious and her general condition is satisfactory, she is transferred to the ward.

In the ward: The operation notes are read carefully to familiarize the midwife with the operation performed and the instructions from the theatre. When the patient is conscious, she is gradually proppedup and analgesics are given regularly as ordered. The patient should be given her baby to hold and admire as soon as her condition permits. A record of the temperature, pulse, respiration and blood pressure is kept hourly and later two hourly or four hourly depending on the patient's condition.

General cleanliness of the patient includes: the patient is given a daily bed bath till she is ambulant. The pressure areas are treated during bath times and again before the patient is settled for the night's rest. The vulval toilet is done twice daily for as long as the patient is confined to bed. The nurse may help the patient with oral toilet on the first day of operation and wherever necessary.

Regarding diet: Usually, a physician listens for the bowel sounds 24 hours after the operation. If these are present, easily digestible diet may be given to the patient provided she is not nauseated by the food. A cup of tea or any drink may be given if the patient is hungry and thirsty before the arrival of the doctor.

Bowel action and urinary output: The patient should be able to pass urine during the first 24 hours after the operation. It is advisable to measure and record urinary output for the first 48 hours, especially if the patient is transfused. Continuous bladder drainage for 7 to 10 days is recommended in cases where caesarean section is done to relieve obstructed labour. This measure is necessary to prevent a vesicovaginal fistula. A small enema saponis is given on the second post-operative day to rid of the bowels of gas and stimulate peristalsis.

The breasts: The breasts should be well supported and breastfeeding should be encouraged as soon as the mother's condition permits. If for any reason the baby cannot suckle, the breasts should be manually expressed from the third day.

Prevention of complications: The patient is usually nursed in a sitting position and deep breathing exercises are encouraged and the patient is made to cough occasionally to rid of the respiratory tract of mucus. The services of a physiotherapist, if available should be obtained. Early ambulation is recommended to aid good respiration, drainage of lochia and to prevent thrombosis. If the patient's condition permits, she is seated out of bed for a short period on the second day after the operation. From the third day, she may be encouraged to walk to the toilet.

Care of the wound: The wound must be kept dry. Any soiled dressing should be changed. Usually the wound is left until the sixth day when the clips are removed. The sutures are removed on the eigth day. If both the doctor and midwife are satisfied that the patient has made satisfactory progress she may be discharged on the ninth or tenth day.

On discharge: It is advisable to explain to the patient why the operation was done. The need for hospital care during subsequent pregnancy and delivery must be made clear to the patient.

FORCEPS ASSISTED BIRTH/FORCEPS DELIVERY (FIGS 9.27 TO 9.33)

The obstetric forceps were invented in the 17th century by Chamberlen who kept the invention a family secret for several years. There have been several modifications to Chamberlen's forceps. Nowadays, the forceps commonly used are:

1. Neville-Barne's forceps.
2. Haig Ferguson's forceps.
3. Morris's forceps.
4. Kielland's forceps
5. Wrigley's forceps.

Each pair of these forceps consists of two blades made to accommodate the foetal head and conform with the curve of the pelvic canal. Thus the curves on the blades are referred to as the foetal and the pelvic curves respectively.

The first three forceps mentioned above are used for midcavity forceps deliveries when the occiput is in the anterior position. Kielland's forceps are specially designed to enable the obstetrician to carry out rotation occiput from the posterior to the anterior position.

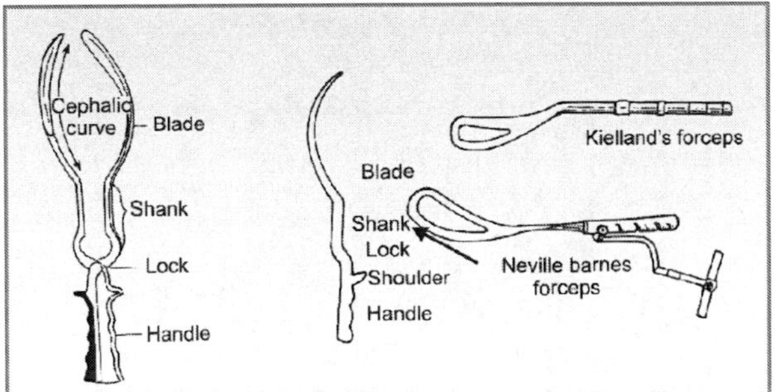

Fig. 9.27: Forceps parts (left) and commonly used forceps (right); the absence of the pelvic curve in Kielland's forceps enables rotation of the foetal head

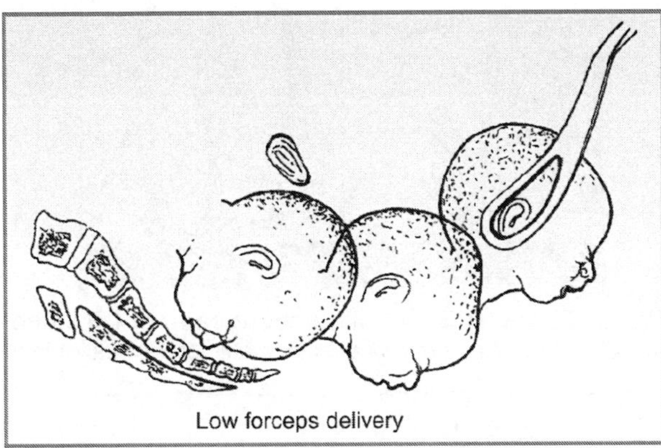

Fig. 9.28: Low forceps delivery: Traction is applied in line with the axis of the pelvis, and delivery is effected by lifting the head anteriorly once the occiput has passed beneath the subpubic arch

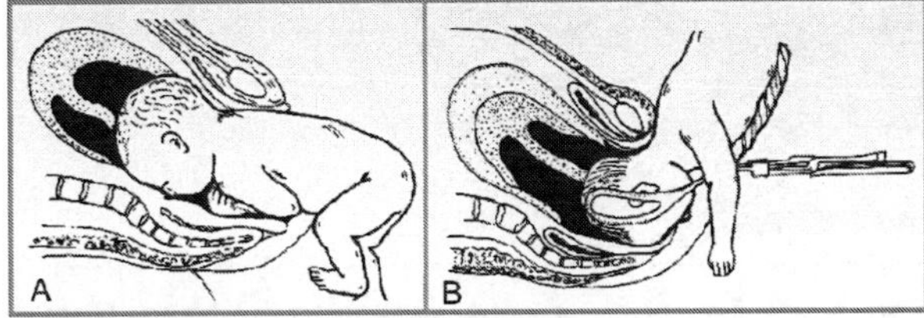

Figs 9.29A and B: Breech delivery: **A.** When infant's back is upward, a towel is wrapped around the body, **B.** Piper's forceps may be applied to the after coming head and used to initially pull downward, and then slowly and gently upward; the head is born

They are commonly used for midcavity forceps deliveries in which the head is in the occipito-lateral or occipito-posterior position. Wrigley's forceps are used for outlet forceps deliveries.

Types of Forceps Delivery

Low Forceps Delivery

Low forceps delivery is the delivery of the foetal head which has descended below the level of the

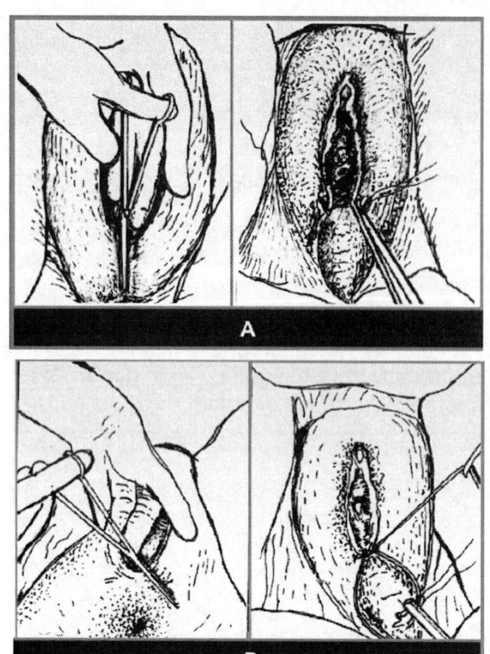

Figs 9.30A and B: A. Anatomic location of midline episiotomy, **B.** Anatomic location of mediolateral episiotomy

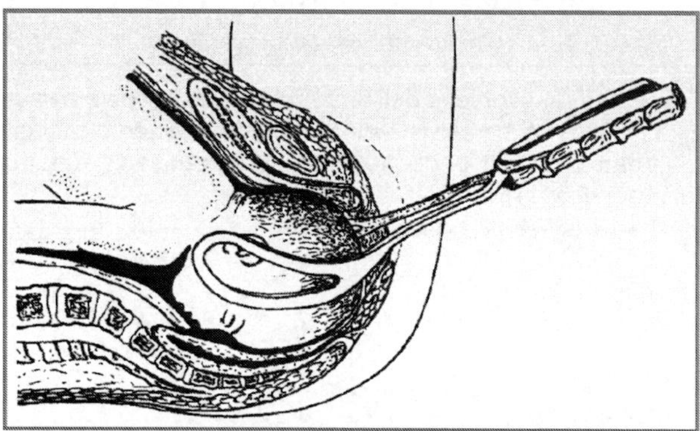

Fig. 9.31: Forceps correctly applied to the head. Note relation of curve of pelvis to curve

ischial spines. The usual indications for low forceps delivery are maternal or foetal distress in the second stage of labour. A low forceps delivery using Wrigley's forceps is carried out under pudendal block analgesia. An episiotomy is done before the delivery is carried out.

Midcavity Forceps Delivery

Midcavity forceps delivery entails the delivery of the foetal head which is engaged but its lowest part is still at the level of the ischial spines. A

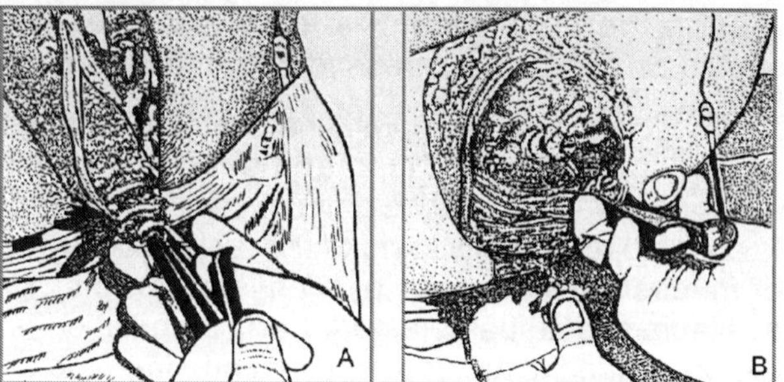

Figs 9.32A and B: The mother is encouraged to bead down with the onset of the following uterine contraction, and simultaneous traction is applied on the foetal head, **B.** During delivery of the head, the perineum is supported with a gauze pad, holding it back and preventing further distension; at the same time, traction is directed upward away from the perineum

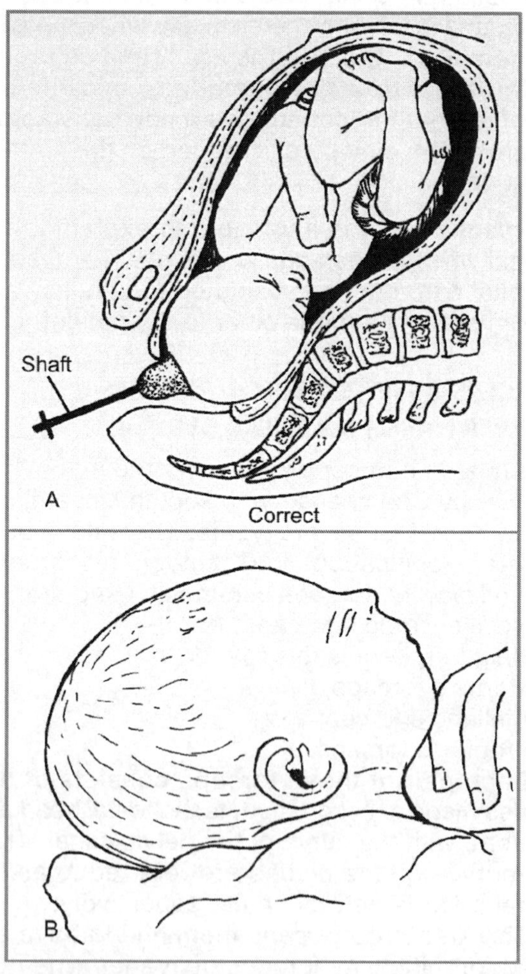

Figs 9.33A and B: Vacuum extraction. **A.** Position, **B.** The Chignon is seen in profile; it usually disappears within 24 to 48 hours

midcavity forceps delivery is carried out if there is delay in the second stage of labour. The most frequent reason for this delay is posterior position of the occiput or deep transverse arrest. The head may be manually rotated and delivered with Neville-Barnes, Haig-Ferguson, or Milne-Murray forceps or may be rotated and delivered with Kielland's forceps.

High Forceps Delivery

If the head is delivered by the forceps when it is at or above the pelvic brim a high forceps delivery is said to have been done. High forceps delivery is never done in modern obstetrics. If the delivery of the baby must be expedited when the head is not engaged, a caesarean section is usually performed. High forceps delivery is taught with complications such as rupture of the uterus, injury to the bladder at rectum and extensive perineal lacerations.

Indications for Forceps Delivery

1. Delay in second stage of labour due to minor degrees of cephalopelvis disproportion, persistent occipitoposterior position, deep transverse arrest or secondary uterine inertia.
2. Foetal distress in the second stage of labour when the foetal head is engaged.
3. Prolapse of the umbilical cord in the second stage of labour when the head is engaged.
4. In the delivery of the after coming head in breech presentation.
5. Maternal distress in the second stage of labour.
6. Prophylaxis in maternal conditions such as:
   a. Cardiac disease
   b. Hypertension
   c. Pre-eclampsia and eclampsia
   d. Diabetes
   e. Chronic nephritis
   f. Pulmonary tuberculosis.
7. Prophylaxis-in premature infants.

The nurse midwife is not expected to perform forceps delivery. She is how expected to know the indications so that she may prepare for this operation before the arrival of the physician.

Preparation for Forceps Delivery

Preparation of the patient as well as the setting of the trolley for forceps delivery is the nurse's responsibility.

The Patient

The nurse midwife should explain, what the operation entails to the patient. If forceps delivery is to be performed under general anaesthesia, a consent for operation and anaesthesia should be obtained from the patient. Preoperative preparation includes the shaving of the pubic hair, emptying of the urinary bladder, ensuring an empty stomach and general preparation of the patient for general anaesthesia.

Equipment

The equipment for performing pudendal nerve block should be got ready if the operation is to be performed under local anaesthesia. Such equipment is:

- 1-pudendal needle and guide.
- 1-20 ml syringe with long needles for local infiltration.
- Local anaesthetic agent, usually 1 per cent xylocaine.
- A pair of episiotomy scissors should be available.
- A pair of the type of obstetric forceps requested by the physician should be on the trolley.

The equipment for suturing the episiotomy wound should also be available on the trolley. This is:

- A pair of toothed dissecting forceps
- A pair of plain dissecting forceps
- 1-Mayo needle holder.
- 1-round-bodied needle.
- 1 curved cutting needle.
- No.1 chronic catgut
- No.0 mersilk.
- A pair of 12.5 cm (5 inch) scissors.
- 2 pairs of 17.5 cm (7 inch) Spencer-Wells forceps.
- 2 pairs of 12.5 cm (5 inch) Spencer-Wells forceps.

Dressing and other equipment are the same as for a normal delivery. A perineal sheet, leggings, towel clips and a urethral catheter must always be on the forceps delivery trolley. Equipment must be in readiness to treat a shocked baby, control haemorrhage and combat shock.

Other Duties of the Nurse

The nurse should put the patient in the correct position. The patient is usually delivered in the lithotomy position. Her two legs must be raised and lowered simultaneously to prevent injury to the sacro-iliac joints. Stirrup rods should be well padded to avoid trauma to the veins of the a long rubber sheet or polythene sheet is placed under the buttocks to direct fluid into the bucket. The midwife washes the punes, groin and thighs with soap and water. The doctor cleans the vulva, vagina and the whole area of the operation with swabs soaked in Hibitase. The bladder catheterized. The patient is draped in sterile sheets and leggings. And listens to the foetal heart sounds.

Certain conditions need to be fulfilled before the forceps are applied.

These are:

1. The cervix must be fully dilated.
2. The membranes must be ruptured.
3. The foetal head must be engaged.
4. The patient's bladder should be emptied.
5. An episiotomy should be made.
6. The patient should have some form of anaesthesia.

Care of the Baby

After the baby is born, the nurse has a duty to resuscitate it. Babies delivered with forceps are susceptible to intracranial injuries; they are thus observed closely and 'cot nursed' for 48 hours.

SYMPHYSIOTOMY

This operation dates back to the 17th century. It is an operation for increasing the diameters of the outlet of the pelvis. This increase in diameters of the pelvic outlet is achieved by dividing the symphysis pubis through an incision made in the skin about 3 cm (2 in) above the symphysis pubis. Separation of the symphysis pubis enables the baby's head to be delivered spontaneously or by forceps.

Symphysiotomy is only indicated in cases in which the foetal head is arrested at the pelvic outlet. Thus in a tunnal pelvis, where the transverse diameter of the outlet is small and the head is arrested at the outlet, symphysiotomy is not only indicated but beneficial. Symphysiotomy is, however, not indicated in brim and midcavity contractions. Caesarean section should be the treatment of choice in such cases. Complications of symphysiotomy such as vesicovaginal fistula and damage to blood vessels causing profuse haemorrhage are not common if the operation is performed by an experienced obstetrician.

Symphysiotomy is a useful operation in developing countries where the patients are likely to have no previous obstetric care or where they attend antenatal clinics irregularly, and live far from medical aid. These patients are particularly exposed to the risk of ruptured uterine scars in subsequent labours if a caesarean section has been previously performed.

Nursing Management of the Patient Following Symphysiotomy

The nursing care of the patient varies with the physician in charge of the case. At the end of the operation, an indwelling catheter is usually left in situ.

The patient is kept in bed for three days and she may be nursed lying on her back or sides. The indwelling catheter drains into a bottle which is emptied at least twice daily. While the patient is confined to bed her vulva is swabbed twice daily bed baths are given daily and the pressure areas are treated 6 hourly. The symphysis pubis is usually united on the second day. The patient is allowed to sit out of bed on the third day and the catheter is usually removed on the third day. Ambulation begins on the fifth day with the aid of rubber tipped walking sticks. The patient is usually walking well with minimal symptoms by the tenth day but undue muscular effort and lifting weights should be avoided for at least two months. The modern practice is to keep the patient in bed for a short time. She may be encouraged to walk round the bed from the second day of delivery provided her general condition is satisfactory.

Subsequent Pregnancy and Labour

The divided joint which heals by fibrosis usually softens during subsequent pregnancies and may lead to pelvic movements in the joint. As a result the patient may suffer from pubic pain and backache. In severe cases pain and a grating sensation may be experienced even when the patient is in bed. The patient may be greatly incapacitated by these throughout the puerperium.

Some permanent enlargement of the pelvis usually follows symphysiotomy therefore subsequent labours are often easy. However, if the foetus is much larger than in previous pregnancies and severe disproportion results delivery will have to be by caesarean section.

THE VENTOUSE OR VACUUM EXTRACTOR

An apparatus similar in principle to the ventouse was first described in 1849 by Sir James Young Simpson. The ventouse was popularized in Sweden and the present day vaccum extractor was designed by Malmstrom.

The apparatus consists of a suction cup made of metal, a rubber tubing with a chain in the centre and a vacuum pump with a manometer attached to it. The metal cup is in four sizes and the largest possible size is usually used by the obstetrician. Before the application of the cup, local infiltration of the perineum or pudendal nerve block may be necessary. The patient may be necessary. The patient may be given an injection of 100 mg of pethidine and an episiotomy may be necessary in a primigravid patient. The cup is applied to the presenting part. A pressure of 0.8 kilogram per square centimetre is gradually built up. This allows the foetal scalp to be drawn into the metal cup thus forming a circumscribed artificial caput succedaneum usually referred to as a 'chignon' (Fig. 9.33). When a pressure of 0.8 kilogram per square centimetre has been obtained, intermittent traction synchronous with the uterine contractions is carried out by pulling on the rubber tubing.

Indications for the Ventouse

These are:

1. Prolonged first stage of labour.
2. Foetal distress in first or second stage of labour.
3. Prolonged second stage of labour.
4. Uterine inertia in first stage of labour.
5. Occipitoposterior position.
6. It can be used when the cervix is not fully dilated.
7. It can be used to rotate the caput from the posterior to the anterior position.
8. Less traction force is required with the ventouse than with forceps.
9. There is less damage to maternal tissues.
10. It does not require a general anaesthetic and the patient's cooperation is easily obtained.

Hazards of Complications in the Use of the Ventouse

1. Scalp abrasions or sloughing of the scalp from frequent applications of the cup to the same area of the scalp.
2. Intracranial haemorrhage—this is not as common as thought.
3. Cephal haematoma.
4. Depressed fracture of the foetal skull.

These complications are not frequent, especially in experienced hands. The baby born by ventouse should be observed closely for signs of cerebral injury and it should be 'cot nursed' for 48 hours.

DESTRUCTIVE OPERATIONS

Destructive operations are performed in order to terminate labour which has obstructed and to reduce the bulk or size of a dead foetus. The operations are:

1. Craniotomy.
2. Decapitation.
3. Evisceration.
4. Cleidotomy.

Craniotomy

This is the perforation of the foetal skull to expel the brain matter and thereby reduce the size of the foetal head and make delivery easy. The instruments used for this operation are the Simpson's perforator and combined cranioclast and cephalotribe for crushing the head. A blunt hook and crotchet may be required to extract the after-coming head. The set up is the same as for forceps delivery. The indications for craniotomy are:

a. Hydrocephalus.
b. Contracted pelvis with cephalo-pelvic disproportion when the baby is dead as a result of prolonged obstructed labour.

Decapitation

In the operation, the head is severed from the trunk. The trunk is then delivered and later the head. It is usually performed in cases of intrauterine death of the foetus associated with impacted shoulder presentation locked twins and double headed monster. The decapitation can be performed with the Ramsbotham's decapitating hook or the Blong-Heidler thimble and decapitating wire. Other instruments which may be used during the operaion are embryotomy blunt pointed scissors, blunt hood and crochet, obstetric forceps.

Evisceration

In this operation, the abdominal and thoracic contents are removed in order to reduce the bulk of the foetus and make delivery possible. It is usually done in the case of monsters, large tumours of the abdomen or thorax in the infant, or in impacted shoulder presentation when decapitation is technically difficult. It is not an operation that should be frequently performed. Sometimes, it is better to perform a caesarean section, not withstanding than to carry out evisceration of the foetus.

Cleidotomy

In this operation, the clavicles are cut or divided in order to reduce the bulk of the shoulders.

Hazards of Destructive Operations

In craniotomy, the perforator may perforate the maternal tissues such as the urinary bladder and the uterus. In decapitation, the uterus may be ruptured or the bladder badly bruised. The rectum may also be damaged and a rectovaginal fistula results. Bone spicules may pierce and injure the cervix, bladder, rectum, vagina and perineum.

PERINEAL LACERATIONS

Perineal laceration is a tear of the preineum which occurs during the second stage of labour. The thinned and stretched out perineal body is liable to tear and this is inevitable at times. The nurse should not, therefore, consider perineal laceration a poor reflection on her skill. Modern midwives and obstetricians do not frown at perineal laceration, for it is better to repair a laceration than a uterine prolapse caused by overstretched pelvic floor. An unduly prolonged perineal phase of labour will not only cause overstretching of the pelvic floor but may also subject the foetus to intracranial injury and anoxia.

Signs that the Perineum is Liable to Tear

A midwife should anticipate perineal laceration in cases of persistent occipitoposterior position with face to pubis delivery, face presentation, a rigid and scarred perineum, or a large baby with an uncooperative mother. The warning signs of a possible perineal laceration are:

a. Cracking or tearing of the fourchette before the head is crowned.
b. Trickling of blood from the vagina.
c. Excessive thinning and stretching of the perineum.
d. Oedematous and rigid perineum.

Prevention

Most perineal lacerations occur because the nurse has no control of the patient and the head is pushed out rather rapidly.

It is important to instruct the patient on what to do before the onset of the second stage of labour. The patients are usually too distressed and distracted in the second stage of labour to take in any instructions.

It is no good saying 'do not push' to a patient whose urge to do so is over whelming. During a bearing down effort, the perineum should be allowed to stretch but the nurse/midwife should prevent the advancing head from sudden expulsion. The patient is made to pant when the head is crowned and it should be at the end of contractions. Maintenance of flexion will being a small diameter of the presenting part to passover the perineum. In a vertex presentation, extension of the head should be controlled so that the sinciput is delivered after the occipital prominence and the parietal eminences have been born. At times, perineal laceration is brought about by the delivery of the shoulders. It is, therefore, important that the nurse/midwife should await the rotation of the shoulders before she attempts to deliver them. A timely episiotomy is the best way of preventing a perineal laceration.

Types of Perineal Laceration

1. *First degree perineal laceration* Involves the skin and the fourchette only. The muscles may be exposed but are not torn. A midwife can repair a first degree perineal laceration with mersilk on a cutting needle. The sutures must be interrupted and should not be too tight.
2. *Second degree perineal laceration* The skin, fourchette, posterior vaginal wall and the pelvic floor muscles are torn. The laceration may extend to the anus but the anal sphincter is not damaged. If the laceration is very extensive medical aid must be sought for the repair.
3. *Third degree perineal laceration* This is an extensive laceration involving the fourchette and vaginal wall, pelvic floor muscles, anal sphincter and canal and in bad cases, the rectum. The repair of a third degree laceration should be carried out in hospital under general anaesthesia and by a skilled physician. Skilled nursing care is also necessary to obtain a successful result from the repair.

Repair of Perineal Laceration

The principles of repair are the same as for the repair of an episiotomy.

Management of Repaired Perineal Wound

The suture line should be kept dry and clean. Vulval toilet is therefore carried out twice daily and the suture line danned with antiseptic and drying agents such as acriflavine in spirit. Ambulant patients are encouraged to have a sitz bath with normal saline at least twice a day. The nurse midwife should inspect the perineum daily to exclude infection. Marked inflammation or oedema of the wound may be relieved with magnesium sulphate or hypertonic saline dressing. A report is also made to the physician of the state of the patient's perineum. If the patient experiences much pain mild analgesics such as Panadol (2 tablets) are given whenever necessary.

Non-absorbable sutures are removed on the sixth or seventh day. The number of sutures removed should be checked against the number inserted at the time of repair. The nurse midwife should note the union of the suture line and the healing of the wound after the suture have been removed. If the union is poor and there is no infection, sitz baths of normal saline or Hibitane solution (1:2000) are continued twice daily and the wound is dressed or danned with acriflavine (1:1000). Septic wounds are dressed with Eusol after the sitz bath. Secondary suturing may be necessary when the wound is clean.

Management of a Repaired Third Degree Perineal Laceration

The patient is allowed to rest in bed for two to three days in order to avoid strain on the suture line. She is encouraged to lie on her side while feeding the baby and rest on her knees when moving around in bed.

The care of the wound and the relief of pain are the same as in management of repaired perineal wound. There is no need to restrict the diet—ordinary diet with plenty of fruit is offered to the patient. Milk of magnesia (15 ml) may be given twice daily for the first five days to prevent constipation. If the patient defaecatex, vulval toilet must be done immediately. Antibiotics may be ordered by the physician.

On discharge, the patient is advised to avoid constipation and the strain of carrying heavy loads. It is desirable for her to attend post-natal examination to ensure that the wound is well healed and to assess the proper functioning of the anal sphincter. She is also advised to abstain from sexual intercourse for about two months to allow proper healing of the wound and avoid dyspareunia. The patient should be advised to have her subsequent deliveries in a hospital. An elective episiotomy is done in the second stage of labour in all cases of successfully repaired third degree tear.

10 CHAPTER

Assessment and Management of Abnormalities during Postnatal Period

INTRODUCTION

The puerperium is hailed as the "fourth trimester" and by definition it is the period from birth to 6 weeks postpartum, when the women is readjusting physiologically and psychosocially to motherhood. Prior to puerperium, that is, the third stage of labour is a dangerous period and until it is safely over the, nurse should not leave her patient unattended. Conditions which may complicate the third stage of labour are postpartum haemorrhage, retained placenta, inversion of the uterus and postpartum collapse or shock.

POSTPARTUM HAEMORRHAGE

Postpartum haemorrhage is bleeding from the genital tract after delivery of the baby amounting to 600 ml or more, or any amount of bleeding that can cause deterioration in the patient's condition. Therefore, a severely anaemic patient losing 300 ml of blood may be in a worse state than a woman with packed cell volume of 40 per cent who loses 750 ml of blood during delivery. A patient may bleed into the broad ligament and suffer severe shock even though the amount of visible blood may be small. Therefore it is the effect rather than the amount of the blood lost that matters.

Types of Postpartum Haemorrhage

Postpartum haemorrhage may be primary or secondary. Primary postpartum haemorrhage is the haemorrhage occurring during the third stage of labour and within 24 hours of delivery.

Secondary postpartum haemorrhage is haemorrhage occurring after 24 hours of delivery and within six weeks of delivery. It is also referred to as puerperal haemorrhage.

Causes of Primary Postpartum Haemorrhage

The main causes of primary postpartum haemorrhage are:

1. Atonic uterus.
2. Trauma.
3. Blood coagulation defects as in hypofibrino anaemia.

Atonic Uterus

Postpartum haemorrhage due to atonic uterus is the most common and is due to failure of the uterus to contract and retract efficiently. Factors which contribute to this failure are:

a. Retention of part or the whole of the placenta may prevent efficient uterine contraction and retraction and lead to massive postpartum haemorrhage.
b. Large blood clots in the uterus act in the same way as retained placenta.
c. Prolonged labour with consequent uterine exhaustion.
d. Injudicious use of analgesics in the first stage of labour or injudicious use of anaesthesia for delivery, causing relaxation of the uterine muscle fibres.
e. A full urinary bladder impairs the efficiency of the uterine action.
f. Grande multiparity causes laxity of the uterine and abdominal muscles which contract ineffectively.
g. Overd distension of the uterus resulting from hydramnios and multiple pregnancy or a large baby.
h. Meddlesome interference with the uterus during the third stage of labour causes irregular contractions and partial separation of the placenta.

i. Antepartum haemorrhage—placenta praevia predisposes to postpartum haemorrhage because the lower uterine segment on which the placenta is implanted does not contract and retract as efficiently as the upper uterine segment. In concealed accidental haemorrhage, retained large blood clots over distend the uterus and sometimes seep into the uterine muscle wall. All these factors prevent adequate contractions and retraction of the uterus.
j. Fibroids—a number of interstitial fibroids may interfere with good uterine action.

Trauma

Trauma to the genital tract varying from a bleeding episiotomy laceration of the vagina or cervix, to rupture of the uterus may cause postpartum haemorrhage.

Blood Coagulation Defect (Defibrination Syndrome)

Blood coagulation episiotomy, laceration of the vagina or cervix, to rupture of the uterus may cause postpartum haemorrhage.

Blood coagulation defect or defibrination syndrome may cause hypofibrinogenaemia and, therefore, a reduction in the fibrinogen content of the blood resulting in clotting defect. If the uterus is atonic when this condition is present, postpartum haemorrhage may be profuse.

Clinical Manifestations

In atonic haemorrhage the bleeding occurs a few minutes after the birth of the baby and tends to come in gushes. The uterus is soft, big and does not contract. It fills up easily with blood and the fundus rises above the umbilicus. In traumatic haemorrhage, the blood comes in a steady flow but the uterus is usually hard and well contracted and retracted. In cases of hypofibrino-genaemia, the blood just pours out through the vagina and does not clot. The uterus is often soft and flabby though it could sometimes be well contracted and retracted. A patient with severe postpartum haemorrhage has lost a great deal of blood and is, therefore, shocked and anaemic. The blood pressure is low, the pulse rate is rapid and the volume is small. The patient is anxious and often cold and clammy. There is pallor of the conjuctive, tongue and palms of the hands and soles of the feet.

Prevention of Postpartum Haemorrhage

It is better to prevent than treat postpartum haemorrhage. Therefore, patients at risk should be selected for hospital delivery and given an oxytocic drug at the delivery of the anterior shoulder of the baby in a cephalic presentation, or with the crowning of the head in a breech presentation. The following categories of patients are susceptible to postpartum haemorrhage:

1. Patients with a previous history of postpartum haemorrhage.
2. Grande multiparae.
3. Patients who have had antepartum haemorrhage or prolonged labour.
4. Patients with hydramnios, twins, big babies and fibroids.

These patients should be given ergometrine (10.5 mg intravenously or syntometrine (1 ml) intramuscularly with the crowning of the baby's head or delivery of the baby's anterior shoulder. A nurse midwife working on her own will need to use syntometrine because it is administered intramuscularly and midwives are not allowed to give intravenous injections. Other measures of preventing postpartum haemorrhage are:

a. Emptying the bladder at the end of the first stage of labour.
b. Sedation of patients who tend to push prematurely.
c. Avoidance of prolonged labour and traumatic instrumental deliveries.
d. Delivery of the baby slowly between contractions.
e. Allowing the placenta to separate and the uterus to contract before attempting to deliver the placenta.
f. Anticipation of hypofibrinogenaemia in cases of abruptio placentae and proloned retention of a dead foetus.

Active Treatment of Postpartum Haemorrhage

The first principle in postpartum haemorrhage is to stop the bleeding and send for the physician if there is a possibility of getting one. Immediate steps to stop the bleeding are listed below:

1. Rub up the uterus to stimulate contraction and retraction.
2. Administer ergometrine (0.5 mg) intramuscularly if possible with hylase (100 units), ergometrine may be given intravenously if a physician is present or the nurse is competent

at venepuncture. Syntometrine (1 ml) intramuscularly may be given instead of erogometrine.
3. Expel the placenta with the next uterine contraction (if it has not yet been expelled) by fundal pressure or controlled cord traction.
4. Empty the urinary bladder by catheterization.
5. A second dose of syntometrine or ergometrine may be given in ten minutes if bleeding is not controlled. The nurse midwife should stay with the patient and assess her general condition to detect or exclude shock. She should keep a quarter-hourly record of the patient's pulse, blood pressure and respiration.
6. The patient should be thoroughly examined for evidence of lacerations.

Further Treatment if the Placenta is Retained

If bleeding continues and the placenta is retained after the second dose of oxytocic, the uterus should be rubbed up until it contracts. A further attempt should be made to expel the placenta and blood clots. The patient is reassured and kept warm to prevent shock. The nurse should make preparation for manual removal of the placenta. The author does not recommend that nurses should routinely perform manual removal of the placenta outside the hospital and in rural areas, because it leads to shock if it is alone without anaesthesia and the risk of infection is high.

If a hospital is within easy reach and the patient is not shocked, the nurse should transfer her to a major hospital where manual removal can be done under any blood loss replaced, and the risk of infection reduced. On the other hand, it is dangerous to make a patient who is bleeding, travel many kilometres or miles with the placenta in situ. It is only in such circumstances that a nurse midwife may attempt a manual removal of placenta.

Method of Manual Removal of Placenta

The patient is placed in the lithotomy position or across the bed with the knees flexed and abducted. Inhalation analgesia such as trilene or gas and oxygen should be given to relax the patient and minimise pain. The vulva is swabbed with an antiseptic solution and smeared with antiseptic cream by an assistant.

The nurse scrubs with soap and water and wears sterile rubber gloves (a long gauntlet glove is desirable). Her left hand holds the umbilical cord while the right hand is shaped into a cone and is inserted into the vagina. This hand follows the cord to the placenta. The lower edge of the placenta is sought and the fingers are inserted between the placenta and the uterine wall. The left hand is now used to steady the uterus abdominally. Gradually the placenta is stripped off the uterus with a side-to-side movement. When the placenta is entirely free, it can be removed from the uterus with ease. The placenta is examined immediately. If there is doubt as to its completeness the hand should be reinserted to remove the retained placenta tissue.

A further dose of ergometrine should be given as soon as the placenta has been removed. The nurse midwife still has the duty of transferring the patient to the hospital so that the blood lost can be replaced and a prophylactic course of antibiotics can be given to prevent puerperal sepsis.

Atonic Postpartum Haemorrhage After Expulsion of the Placenta

Sometimes, even after the expulsion of the placenta, the patient bleeds profusely. The nurse midwife should, in such a case, do the following:
1. Rub the uterus to contract and expel all blood clots in the uterus
2. Give ergometrine (0.5 mg) and hyalase (100 units) or syntometrine (1 ml) intramuscularly.
3. Empty the bladder.
4. Inform the physician if one is available. If the bleeding continues in spite of the above procedures, bimanual compression of the uterus should be attempted.

Bimanual Compression of the Uterus

Bimanual compression of the uterus is an emergency method of controlling haemorrhage. It consists of the following manoeuvre.

The patient is put in the lithotomy position, the vulva and vagina with antiseptic lotion. She puts her gloved right hand, which has been adequately lubricated with hibitane cream, into the vagina and makes a fist of the right hand. The flat part of the closed fit is placed into the anterior vaginal fornix and against the anterior uterine wall. The left hand is placed on the patient's abdomen behind the uterus. The outer hand brings the body of the uterus forwards and compresses it against the clenched fist of the inner hand. This arrests or prevents any haemorrhage that take place before the oxytocic drugs already given, begin to act on the uterus. This method of bimanual compression of the uterus described is the internal method because a hand is introduced into the vagina.

In the external method of manual compression, the uterus is rubbed up until it contracts. The left hand holds the uterus up in such a way that the fingers are at the back of the uterus. The uterus is then drawn upwards and forwards over the right hand, which is clenched and applied to the abdomen in the suprapubic region so that it lies on the lower uterine segment. The uterus is compressed between the left and the right hands and this may control or stop bleeding.

It must be emphasized that bimanual compression is only a temporary method to stop bleeding in an emergency. It is not comfortable for both the contract has no place in modern obstetrics except in emergency when no oxytocics are available. Packing of the uterus with gauze swabs must be condemned because it prevents the uterus from contracting and retracting well, gives the nurse a false sence of security and predisposes to infection.

When the haemorrhage has been controlled the nurse must, from time to time check on the uterus to see if it has relaxed and filled up with blood. If such is the tendency, the uterus should be made to contract and clots expelled. A dose of ergometrine can be repeated or 2-5 units of Pitocin in 5 per cent glucose given intravenously. The total amount of blood lost should be estimated and recorded.

Traumatic Postpartum Haemorrhage

Vaginal bleeding in the presence of a firmly contracted uterus usually comes from a laceration in the genital tract or from a ruptured uterus. The bleeding is in the form of a heavy trickle and not in gushes as in atonic postpartum haemorrhage. The course of labour and the type of delivery the patient has had should arouse the suspicion of trauma to the genital tract. Forceps delivery, face to pubes delivery, breech extraction and sudden expulsion of a large baby predispose to trauma in the genital tract.

Lacerations in the perinieum and vagina are readily seen when the vagina is swabbed. Bleeding points which are easily accessible should be clamped with artery forceps and ligated. The nurse should apply firm pressure on the bleeding points with gauze swabs if no artery forceps are available. When bleeding points are not easily seen and lesions requiring stuturing are discovered, medical aid should be sought. Nurses in remote maternity centres are often capable of suturing minor lacerations.

Heavy bleeding is usually indicative of laceration in the cervix and rupture of the uterus. This poses a problem to the nurse midwife practising in rural areas. The only line of action open to the nurse if to combat shock by giving any available sedative, raise the foot of the bed, apply sponge holding forceps to bleeding points on the cervix and get the patient to the nearest hospital as soon as possible.

Vulval Haematoma

Vulval haematoma is a form of concealed traumatic haemorrhage into the connective tissue of the vulva and vagina. It is caused by rupture of subcutaneous veins. The effusion of blood may give rise to great swelling and distention of the vulva and vagina. The swelling is often discovered a few hours after delivery because the patient complains of great discomfort and pain in the vagina or vulva. Treatment entails drainage of the haematoma under general anesthesia. Antibiotics may be given as a prophylactic measure. Analgesics are given for pain.

Hypofibrinogenaemia

This is a condition in which the amount of fibrinogen in the blood is markedly reduced or absent. Hypofibrino-genaemia (reduced fibrinogen content of blood) is more common than afibrinogenaemia (total absence of fibrinogen in the blood) which is rare. Fibrinogen is required for the process of blood clotting and is converted into fibrin during this process. If the fibrinogen content of the blood is used up rapidly or if the fibrin lysed as rapidly as it is formed, the condition of hypofibrinogenaemia results. In this situation, the blood does not clot, or takes a very long time to clot.

Although hypofibrinogenaemia may be associated with postpartum haemorrhage, it is not usually the cause of postpartum haemorrhage. If the mechanism of uterine contraction and retraction is not disturbed, hypofibrinogenaemia is unlikely to cause postpartum haemorrhage. Hypofibrinogenemia is more often found in the following conditions.

1. Abruptio placentae (concealed accidental haemorrhage)
2. Prolonged retention of a dead foetus in utero, especially deaths associated with rhesus incompatibility.
3. Amniotic fluid embolism as may be found after surgical induction. This is a rare condition.
4. Septic abortion especially in the presence of anaerobic organisms, e.g. *Clostridium welchii.*

When a nurse encounters profuse and uncontrollable bleeding, she must think of blood clotting defects such as hypofibrinogenaemia or thrombocytopenia. She therefore, watches to see if the blood clots or not and how long it takes to clot. The normal clotting time is 4 to 8 minutes. All patients with conditions which predispose to hypofibrinogenaemia must be referred to the physician and should deliver in a major hospital with facilities for blood tests and transfusion.

In some places, it is not unusual for patients to admit in hospital who are severely exsanguinated after a postpartum haemorrhage which occurred at home. The placenta is usually retained for many hours or even days, and infection is probably already established. Shock is often worsened by unskilled attempts to deliver the placenta and poor transportation of the patient through rough tracts. At times, the cord breaks off and the retained placenta is discovered on exploration of the uterus.

The relatives of the patient accompanying her to hospital usually underestimate the amount of blood loss. Efficient resuscitation of the patient with blood transfusion and good antibiotic coverage are necessary before steps are taken to deliver the placenta. When a patient with retained placenta following delivery of a fresh stillbirth at home fails to respond to liberal blood transfusion, rupture of the uterus should be suspected. In such cases preparations are made for laparotomy.

Dangers of Postpartum Haemorrhage

Postpartum haemorrhage poses a serious threat to patients. The mothers are usually small and malnourished, and may start pregnancy with low levels of haemoglobin (40-60 per cent). Consequently, they can go readily into a state of shock and the shock may be irreversible.

Patients who survive the haemorrhage are susceptible to infection in the puerperium. Inadequate transfusion or failure to transfuse the patient may result in Sheehan's syndrome, a condition in which there is atrophy of the anterior pituitary gland. In its mildest form, there is failure of lactation and amenorrhoea later. In severe cases, signs and symptoms of adrenal, thyroid, pancreatic and ovarian insufficiency become manifest. There is loss of hair on the head and pubic region, as well as atrophy of the breasts.

Retained Placenta

Since the placenta is usually expelled within 10 or 15 minutes of the baby's birth in normal cases, it may be said to be retained if it has not been expelled within 30 minutes of the third stage.

Causes of Retained Placenta

1. Mismanagement of the third stage of labour, such as fiddling with the uterus or overzealous massage of the uterus, may cause an hour glass constriction of the uterus.
2. Faulty technique whereby an inexperienced midwife tries to expel the placenta before it separates or is not quite competent with expulsion by fundal pressure.
3. A full bladder may prevent adequate uterine contraction and retraction and thus impede placental expulsion.
4. Ineffective uterine contractions-secondary uterine inertia.
5. Morbid adherence of the placenta. An extreme example of this is seen in placenta acreta.

Management of Retained Placenta

The physician should be informed at once. An attempt should be made to expel the placenta by any of the methods previously described. If this fails, preparation should be made for blood transfusion and manual removal of the placenta.

If the patient is bleeding with the placenta in utero, a dose of ergometrine (0.5 mg) is given intramuscularly or intravenously. Manual removal of the placenta is usually done by the physician under general anaesthesia of using intravenous pethidine (100 mg) and chlorpromazine (Largectil) (50 mg) or intravenous morphine, 15 mg (gr. 1/4), well mixed with 10 ml of sterile water for injection and administered very slowly. If the retention is due to constriction ring, which is often diagnosed when an attempt is being made to remove the placenta manually, general anaesthesia may be administered to relax the spasm. Inhalation of one ampoule of amylnitrate may also be helpful.

Dangers of Retained Placenta

1. It may cause atonic postpartum haemorrhage, especially if it is partially separated. Its presence in the uterus impedes adequate uterine contraction and retraction. The accompanying haemorrhage may lead to shock.
2. Prolonged retention of the placenta may cause severe shock in the patient even in the absence of haemorrhage.
3. Attempts to do a manual removal of the placenta expose the patients to complications such as rupture or inversion of the uterus and puerperal sepsis.

The Hazards of Blood Transfusion

Blood transfusion is life saving in obstetrical nursing practice. Without blood transfusion many lives would have been lost as a result of massive ante- and postpartum haemorrhage. Blood transfusion is, however, not without risks, especially if incompatible blood is inadvertently given to a patient.

Certain precautions need to be taken before embarking on transfusion. Some of these are:

1. Transfusion of haemolysed blood should be avoided.
2. Blood should be stored in a refrigerator at a temperature of 4°C (four degrees centigrade).
3. Blood should not be transfused after thawing.
4. Only ABO and Rhesus compatible blood should be transfused. In cases of emergency O Rhesus negative blood may be given to the patient regardless of her blood group.

Complications of Blood Transfusion

The reactions to blood transfusion are many. They may be classified as slight, moderate and severe. In the slight reaction the symptoms are negligible. There may be rapid haemolysis of the donor blood and failure of the haemoglobin level of the transfused patient to rise.

A moderate reaction is manifested by slight pyrexia and shortlived jaundice resulting from haemolysis of the transfused blood. There is usually no rise in the haemoglobin concentration after the transfusion.

In the severe variety there is pyrexia (T = 30°C) with or without a feeling of chill but without shivering. Sometimes the temperature is raised and there is rigor.

Allergic reactions in the form of urticaria, rashes and sometimes angioneurotic oedema occur.

If the blood given is incompatible with the patient's group there is usually a haemolytic reaction. This is manifested by sudden development of fever, headache, a tightening sensation in the chest, pain in the lumbar area and breathlessness. Jaundice is the rule and haemoglobinuria develops within a few hours.

Homologus serum jaundice this is a form of transfusion reaction manifested by jaundice and symptoms indistinguishable from those of infective hepatitis. It is due to the transfusion of pooled blood from different donors. Its incubation period is about 120 days.

Other Side Effects of Blood Transfusion

Air embolism this is usually caused by an overzealous attempt to give a rapid transfusion by the use of a Higginson's syringe or when the sphygmomanometer cuff is used to 'pump' the blood in.

Right heart failure and pulmonary congestion this usually occurs if whole blood is given to a severely anaemic, pregnant woman. It may also occur as a result of the inadvertent massive transfusion of a patient with cardiac disease in imminent (impending) cardiac failure.

Transfusion reactions however mild, should be promptly reported to the physician.

The nurse-midwife must guard incompatible blood transfusion by making sure that the blood to be given is the one actually cross matched for the patient. She could check the name and hospital number on the blood bottle with those on the patient's case notes. She should also get a colleague or a physician to check the blood with her before setting up the transfusion.

Inversion of the Uterus

Inversion of the uterus is a rare but a very serious complication of the third stage of labour. Inversion often starts with a dimple in the fundus uterine and may continue till the uterus is completely turned inside out.

Causes of Inversion of the Uterus

1. *Spontaneous inversion*—Spontaneous inversion of the uterus is rare. It is usually associated with fundal insertion of the placenta.
2. *Induced inversion*—Induced inversion of the uterus is often due to pulling on the cord in the presence of an atomic uterus. Over-enthusiastic fundal pressure in the absence of good uterine contractions or Crede's method of placental expulsion with a lax uterus will cause inversion of the uterus. A well contracted and retracted uterus is not likely to be inverted.

Types of Inversion

1. *Acute inversion*—Acute inversion of the uterus occurs shortly efter delivery and is the type that the nurse is likely to encounter in her practice.
2. *Chronic inversion*—Chronic inversion of the uterus occurs several months after delivery and it is not usually associated with the particular delivery. It is usually caused by a large uterine fibroid, usually submucous.

Signs and Symptoms of Inversion of the Uterus

In minor cases of inversion, when there is just a dimple of the fundus and the rest of the uterus is not inverted, there may be no symptoms. The inversion could only be detected by very careful examination of the abdomen. In most cases it is not diagnosed.

In moderate cases, when the fundus and the body of the uterus are inverted without the uterus showing at the vaginal introitus, there may be abdominal pain, signs of shock and sometimes haemorrhage. Especially of the placenta is partially separated or has been expelled. In severe cases, where the inverted uterus is completely outside the vagina, the symptoms are usually dramatic. The patient may complain of a bearing down feeling. There is severe lower abdominal pain, shock and collapse. Acute inversion of the uterus is one of the major causes of obstetric shock. There may be profuse haemorrhage if the placenta is partially separated. On the other hand, there may be no bleeding if the placenta is morbidly adherent to the uterus.

In addition to the above, palpation of the abdomen reveals absence of the uterus.

The severe abdominal pain is usually caused by the traction on the ovaries, fallopian tubes and broad ligaments. The infundibulopelvic ligament is twisted, and dragged down by the inverted uterus.

Management

The nurse should arrange for medical help: Raising the foot of the bed will partially relieve the traction on the ovaries. Ergometrine (0.5 mg) and pethidine (100 mg) are given intramuscularly to control bleeding and alleviate pain respectively.

If the uterus is at the vulva, it should be wrapped in a warm towel soaked in hibitane lotion. The following are prepared for the replacement of the uterus by the physician:

- Equipment for blood transfusion.
- Equipment for douching with large volumes of saline.
- Anaesthesia may be used so the patient must be prepared as for a case. Receiving general anaesthesia for a major operation.
- Catheterization tray
- Hypovolaemic shock should be corrected with blood transfusion. On the other hand, shock may not improve till the uterus is replaced.

Sudden Collapse

Sudden collapse of a patient occurring during labour or shortly afterwards is usually referred to as obstetric shock. The causes are listed below:

1. *Haemorrhage* Usually from the placental site, occurring before or after delivery of the placenta. The degree of collapse or shock is usually proportional to the amount of blood lost.
2. *Inversion of the uterus* The degree of shock in this case tends to be profound and is usually not in proportion to the amount of blood lost.
3. *Rupture of the uterus* The collapse in this case is due to a combination of pain and haemorrhage especially if the foetus and placenta have been expelled into the peritoneal cavity.
4. *Embolism* Air embolism thromboembolism and amniotic fluid embolism are rare causes of the sudden collapse of an obstetric patient in the tropics. Air or some liquor amnii containing vernix caseosa could be forced into the placental blood sinuses and into the maternal circulation. This may lead to pulmonary embolism with signs of acute respiratory

distress and death. In the case of air embolism, death may be instantaneous.

5. *Exhaustion* Prolonged labour, followed by a difficult and traumatic delivery, may cause the patient to collapse especially if in addition prolonged and difficult anaesthesia had been given. Patients with serious obstetric complications such as antepartum haemorrhage or obstructed labour may collapse during transfer to hospital on rugged roads and in poor public transport.
6. *Sudden reduction in intra-abdominal pressure:* Following the delivery of twins and large babies. In cases of sudden collapse the pulse is rapid and thready; it may be imperceptible. The pressure is low with systolic pressure of 80 mmHg or less depending on the severing of the shock. When the systolic pressure is below 60 mmHg or cannot be estimated, the condition is critical. Respiration is primarily shallow becoming deep and irregular. The skin is cold and clammy. The patient is apathetic but may be restless.

Treatment

The nurse should seek medical aid urgently when the first sign of shock is noticed. In the meantime, she lies the patient down and ensures a clear airway. If cyanosis and breathlessness are present, oxygen may be given at the rate of 2 litres/ minute. Tight clothing is loosened or removed and the patient is covered with a single sheet. The foot of the bed may be raised to ensure blood supply to vital organs. The patient's pulse and blood pressure are estimated to determine the degree of shock. A thorough examination of the patient and a review of the mode of delivery should be carried out to determine the causes of shock. The blood volume should be restored by intravenous infusion if available, or tap water (600 ml) may be given rectally pending transfusion with blood. It is advisable to obtain a blood specimen for grouping and cross matching before the drip is put up. The pulse rate and blood pressure are checked at quarterhourly intervals. If there is respiratory arrest, mouth to mouth respiration should be done after the airways have been cleared. Stimulants such as coramine (2 ml) or lobelline may be given by intramuscular injection. In the presence of cardiac arrest, external cardiac massage should be done while waiting for medical aid.

Puerperal Pyrexia

Naturally more women continue to enjoy good health during the puerperium, but infection or pre-existing ill health may interfere with the patient's well being. The infection often manifests itself by elevation of the body temperature. This is referred to as puerperal pyrexia.

Puerperal pyrexia is defined as a febrile condition occurring within 14 to 21 days of delivery.

In some countries, puerperal pyrexia is a notifiable condition. With this, it is meant that a nurse must inform a doctor, who should notify the health office of that area. Notification of the condition has been recommended for the purpose of controlling the spread of infection and compiling statistics. Puerperal pyrexia is not notified in some countries because of endemic conditions like malaria which cause hyperpyrexia but are not directly related to genital tract infection in the puerperium.

The major causes of puerperal pyrexia are:

1. Genital tract infection.
2. Urinary tract infection.
3. Incidental causes such as malaria, amoebic dysentery, typhoid and pneumonia.
4. Breast engorgement, mastitis or breast abscess.
5. Thrombotic conditions such as thrombophlebitis and phlebothrombosis.
6. Pyrexia of unknown origin—In this case, no cause can be found for the rise in temperature.

Management

A patient with puerperal pyrexia should be made to rest in bed. The temperature should be reduced by fanning, exposure or tepid sponging of the patient if the temperature is over 37.9°C. The nurse midwife should inform a physician and isolate or barrier nurse the patient while investigations are being carried out. The patient should be thoroughly examined for evidence of infection respecially in the breast, chest, throat and the genital tract. The nurse should find out if thc patient has any symptoms to volunteer. The type of labour and mode of delivery of the patient are also reviewed.

Specific treatment is given when the diagnosis of the condition is known. In India and other countries where malaria is endemic, antimalarial drugs such as chloroquine (800 mg immediately and 400 mg twice daily for 3 days) are given in conjunction with the specific treatment, after a thick as well as a thin film have been sent to the laboratory for evidence of malarial parasites.

Investigations

Symptoms volunteered by the patient and the findings on general examination of the patient determine what investigations are to be done.

1. If the patient has dysuria or there is reason to suspect urinary tract infection, a midstream specimen of urine is collected for microscopic examination, culture of organisms and sensitivity of the organisms to chemotherapeutic and antibiotic agents.
2. A cervical or a high vaginal swab is cultured to exclude genital tract infection.
3. Blood film is also looked at under the microscope for malarial parasites. Blood culture may be necessary where septicaemia is suspected. Other haematological tests which may be done are white blood count, packed cell volume or Hb estimation and agglutination tests.
4. A chest X-ray and sputum examination will be done if the patient coughs or a chest infection is suspected.
5. A stool specimen is obtained if the patient has diarrhoea.
6. A swab from the wound and any other discharge may also be taken for laboratory examination.

Genital Tract Infection

Genital tract infection is otherwise called puerperal sepsis and it include infection of an episiotomy wound, perineal, vaginal and cervical laceration and the placental site. The infection may spread to the fallopian tubes, ovaries, peritoneum and the parametrium.

Urinary Tract Infection

Urinary tract infection is a common cause of puerperal pyrexia. It may be a pre-existing condition, in which case the signs and symptoms will manifest from the first day of the puerperium. At times the infection may be asymptomatic; as such, the midstream specimen of urine of patients with puerperal fever should be examined routinely for pus cells. The nurse should test the urine specimen for albumin. The nursing care and general management of patient with urinary tract infection have been described under medical complication in pregnancy.

Breast Engorgement

Breast engorgement is a venous congestion of the breasts occurring from the 3rd day of the puerperium. It is more common in primiparae and varies in degree from slight to severe. The breast are hard, tense and painful. In severe cases, the skin on the breast is stretched and shiny. Dilated veins are prominent on it. The nipples become flattened out because of the congestion. Breast engorgement may give rise to a lowgrade pyrexia.

Management

The breasts are best supported with a good brassiere or breast binder. The pain is relieved by giving Disprin (600 mg) or novalgin (2 tablets) as often as required. An initial dose of 10 mg of stilboestrol is given followed by 5 mg thrice daily for two days. The breasts are hot bathed before feeds, and gently stroked with soapy hands or warm kernel oil towards the nipples. In severe cases, the baby should not be put to the breast nor manual expression be attempted till the breasts are soft.

Breast engorgement can be prevented by educating the patient to express colostrum from the breasts in the last six weeks of pregnancy. After delivery the baby should suck at the breasts at regular intervals from six to twelve hours after birth, provided both the mother and the baby are in a satisfactory state of health.

Full breasts result from inadequate emptying of the breasts. The stagnant milk may give rise to pain, pyrexia and may even result in infection. To prevent engorgement the breasts should be manually expressed and emptied after breastfeeding.

Infection of the Breasts

Mastitis is infection of the breast tissue. The infection is confined to a lobe of the breast. The affected lobe is hard, red and painful. The patient is pyrexial and may even develop rigors. The infection is usually a sequel to cracked nipples or engorged breasts.

The treatment is to administer systemic antibiotics. The baby should not be allowed to suck on the affected breast. Masiitis may resolve or progress to abscess formation, thus resulting in a breast abscess.

Breast Abscess

When an abscess has formed in the breast, the patient is ill and the breast is more painful, and tender. It is usually enlarged and oedematous.

The treatment entails drainage of the abscess and the use of appropriate systemic antibiotics. The incision wound is dressed with magnesium sulphate and later with Eusol. The affected breast should be well supported.

Nipple Complications

Sore nipples These do not necessarily constitute a cause of puerperal pyrexia. They are described here for convenience. A nipple is sore when the mother experiences pain in the nipple during breast feeding. There may be some abrasion of the skin, thus making the nipple red and tender. Sore nipples are prevented by getting the baby to fix well on the breasts. The baby should not be allowed to suck for too long on an empty breast.

The treatment is by application of 1 per cent aqueous gentian violet to the nipples to keep them dry. If the mother experiences a lot of pain, the nipple should be rested for 24 hours, during which time the affected breast is manually expressed.

Cracked nipples: A nipple is said to be cracked when there is a fissure in it. The mother complains of pain and tenderness when suckling the baby. It is a serious condition for it predisposes to breast infection. The treatment and prevention are the same as for sore nipples. The baby is taken off the breast for 48-72 hours to rest the nipple and to promote healing. Sucking on cracked nipples causes melaena and the passage of blood in the vomitus of the new born baby. Manual expression of the breast is carried out. The nurse should never use a breast pump to empty a breast with a cracked nipple.

Thrombolytic Condition

This is a condition in which there is clot formation in the veins, usually of the legs. The clot may occur as a result of infection or trauma to the vein. When clot formation is due to infection of a vein, the term thrombophlebitis is used. Clot formation in the absence of vein infection is described as phlebothrombosis. The patient may be pyrexial if the thrombosis is associated with infection.

Thrombophlebitis

Clot formation in an inflamed vein. The clot is usually adherent to the walls of the veins and there is very little risk of embolism. A rare but a severe form of thrombophlebitis known as phlegmasia alba doolensia associated with ileo-femoral thrombosis, i.e. thrombosis of the femoral and iliac veins. It may arise as a result of spread from phlebothrombosis from the veins in the calf of the leg or a spread of the genital tract infection.

Phlebothrombosis

Clot formation is the absence of infection. The clot is attached at one end to the wall of the vein like a week in water. The risk of fragmentation and embolism is, therefore, great.

Luckily, these conditions are relatively uncommon. All the same, the nurse midwife should be on her guard, especially if the patient has varicose veins or has been in the lithotomy position for a long time. Anaemic, exhausted, generally debilitated grande multiparae of over 35 years are more susceptible to thrombotic episodes.

A patient who complains of cramps or tingling pain the calf of the leg or tenderness in the groin should be suspected of having thrombosis of the deep veins of the leg. The nurse should examine the affected leg for redness and oedema. The patient experience pain in the calf muscle if the foot is dorsiflexed. This is referred to as positive Homan's sign.

Management

The patient is hospitalized and made to rest in bed, especially if she is pyrexial and the leg is tender and oedematous. The leg is elevated with a protected pillow to aid lymphatic drainage and reduce oedema. Leg exercise is encouraged to increase the tone of the muscles.

In mild cases the use of anticoagulants is not necessary. When the area is less tender and the oedema has subsided, the patient is allowed to walk about wearing a crepe bandage on elastic stocking.

Pitting oedema, increase in the girth of the leg upto 2.5 cm and above pyrexia and tachycardia are characteristic of the sever form of thrombophlebitis or deep vein thrombosis. A bed cradle is used to take the weight of the bed clothes and allow for free movement of the leg, which is also elevated. Intravenous heparin (15,000 units) is given immediately, followed by 10,000-12,000 units 6 hourly for 24 hours. Blood clotting time is estimated before and two hours after the administration of heparin. An oral course of phenindione (dindevan) (50-100 mg daily) is usually given after treatment with heparin for 48 hours. The prothrombin time is estimated twice daily if the patient is on dindevan. Antibiotics are also sometimes prescribed.

When a delivered patient is on the above drugs, the nurse should remember the risk of haemorrhage and take measures to deal with the complication. The physician will see to it that the clotting and prothrombin times are checked regularly. The antidote for heparin is protamine sulphate solution at the dose of 1 ml to 1000 unit of heparin. The average dose 15 to 10 ml intravenously. Transfusion of fresh blood is also useful. Dindivan is not often used during pregnancy because of the risk to the foetus. Its side effect is treated with large doses of vitamin K given intravenously. Leg exercises are allowed when the acute pain subsided. The services of a physiotherapist may be used.

SECONDARY POSTPARTUM HAEMORRHAGE

The bleeding occurs any time from 24 hours after delivery upto the end of the sixth week. It is more common around the 10th to the 45th day. It may be profuse or small. The patient often seeks advice, probably because she has been warned about persistent red lochia which heralds secondary postpartum haemorrhage.

The Causes

The causes include retained products, especially a cotyledon of the placenta. The presence of this prevents adequate uterine contraction and retraction. In addition a retained cotyledon usually sloughs off between the 7th and 10th day postpartum and causes haemorrhage. Infection is also an important cause of secondary postpartum haemorrhage. Sometimes the actual cause of bleeding may not be found.

Management

The patient is made to rest in bed. The uterus is rubbed to excite uterine contractions and any clots present are expelled. Ergometrine (0.5 mg) or synometrine (1 ml) is given intramuscularly. The bladder should be emptied by catheterization. Of the bleeding is not controlled, manual compression of the uterus is done. The patient's general condition is assessed to exclude shock. A history of the onset of bleeding and the amount of blood lost should be obtained from the patient. If the haemorrhage has been profuse, anaemia is excluded or treated if present. Antitetanus serum and antigas-gangrene serum are given if the patient was delivered in an unhygienic environment. Specific treatment will depend on the cause and severity of the condition. Where the bleeding is thought to be due to retained products, the patient is admitted to hospital, given ergometrine (0.5 mg) intramuscularly and preparation is made for evacuation of the uterus after replacement of blood. In cases, complicated by infection, appropriate antibiotics are prescribed by the physician. In very mild cases of appropriate antibiotics are prescribed by the physician. In very mild cases of secondary postpartum haemorrhage, the patient is treated with a course of oral ergometrine (0.5 mg, three times a day) for two days.

The nursing care of the patient depends on her general condition. Bed rest is enforced when the patient is bleeding. The vulval pad and lochia of a patient on a course of ergometrine must be examined for retained products. A record of her temperature, pulse, respiration and blood pressure is kept four-hourly initially, then twice daily. Ferrous gluconate (300 mg, three times a day) or ferrous sulphate (200 mg, three times a day) is given orally. Folic acid (5 mg) may also be given daily.

Subinvolution

By this is meant a delay of the genital organs, especially the uterus to return to their pregravid state.

Signs and Symptoms

1. Bulky and soft uterus.
2. Lochia are profuse and reddish brown.
3. The fundal height remains stationary for a few days.

Causes

1. Anything interfering with proper contraction of the uterine, e.g. full bladder and rectum and retained products.
2. Local uterine infection.
3. Presence of uterine fibroids.
4. Grane multiparity.

Management

The nurse should palpate the uterus to exclude tenderness which may be due to infection. The suprapubic areas should be percussed to exclude a full bladder. Constipation should be excluded. Uterine drainage by early ambulation of the patient should be encouraged. The physician may order a course of ergometrine (0.5 mg × 3 days). These should be given with analgesics such as Panadol (2 tablets as required). The lochia should also be closely watched.

PUERPERAL PSYCHOSIS

Puerperal psychosis is a serious condition. Eighteen per cent start in pregnancy, 64 per cent in the first two weeks of the puerperium and 18 per cent later in the puerperium. The condition used to be referred to variously as pregnancy, puerperalor lactation insanity a most unfortunate terminology because it has a social stigma.

Causes and Manifestations of Puerperal Psychosis

1. *Infection* In many developing countries in the tropics, puerperal psychosis is due to severe puerperal infection. In such cases, the patient becomes mentally confused and there are varying degrees of clouding of consciousness.
2. *Pre-existing predisposition to mental illness:* Schizophrenia is a common psychiatric disorder found in the general population. Some women have a hereditary or personally predisposition to the development of schizophrenia. Such patients may be normal or appear normal, until pregnancy, acting as a stress factor, precipitates a breakdown in personality of the individual and psychosis develops. To some of these women (especially unmarried women or those deserted by their husbands) pregnancy and the thought of childbirth constitute a threat. There may also be an associated physical illness even though the patient looks perfectly normal.

Signs and Symptoms

In the puerperium, the disorder comes rather in an unexpected manner. At times, persistent insomnia for no apparent reason acts as a warning sign. The patient refuses her meals and loses interest in her baby. She has disorders of perception such as visual and auditory hallucinations. By this is meant that she sees people and hears voices that are nonexistent. She sometimes talks of certain members of her family wanting to harm her. She develops suicidal tendencies and may jump off the roof of the hospital or house. She exhibits a desire to destroy her infant and may show some other unusual tendencies, such as confusion, elation, talkativeness and inherent speech. In another group, the patient manifests her psychosis by extreme depression. Such a patient loses interest in her surroundings and food. She cannot concentrate and she sleeps poorly.

Management of Puerperal Psychosis

All patients showing any of the above tendencies must be referred to the physician without any delay. Patients with a previous history of mental illness should be referred for hospital confinement.

When psychosis develops, the patient is usually heavily sedated by the physician. The common drugs used are chlorpromezine (Largactil), pethidine, Librium, barbiturates, etc., in doses prescribed by the doctor. Whether there is infection or not, the patient is usually isolated and nursed single room, preferably on the ground floor of the hospital with adequate security measures to prevent her escape from the ward. Harmful instrument should not be allowed in the patient's room. Sometimes it may be necessary to get a male nurse with experience in mental nursing to stay with the patient.

In cases due to infection, massive doses of the appropriate antibiotic are given to eradicate the infection.

Nourishing and attractive diet should be presented to the patient who should be persuaded to eat her food. Attention should be paid to the parent's oral toilet and to the bladder and rectum, Bowel action may be ensured by the administration of a suppository, e.g. Dulcolax suppository daily.

The patient's infant should be taken away from her. If, however, she insists on seeing the infant, she should not be denied this pleasure, but adequate precautions should be taken to see that she does not injure the child. Lactation us usually suppressed with stilboestrol.

Some difficult patients may require electroconvulsive therapy, induction of hypoglycaemia with insulin and other types of treatment. Such patients are, of course, in a big hospital under the care of an experienced psychiatrist and an experienced team of nurses.

Prognosis

The prognosis is puerperal psychosis is usually very good. It is even better in the tropics than it appears to be in temperate countries where the prognosis is said to be good with 75 to 80 per cent of patients recovering completely.

PUERPERAL SEPSIS

Puerperal sepsis is an infection of the genital tract during the first 6 weeks of delivery or abortion. Pyrexia in the puerperium may be due to puerperal sepsis or to extragenital causes such as pyelonephritis, mastitis and pneumonia. In Britain puerperal pyrexia is notifiable if the temperature rises to 37.7 °C within 14 days (England and Wales) or 21 days (Scotland) after abortion or childbirth and remains at that or a higher level for a period of 24 hours or recurs during that period. With the discovery of antibiotics and improvement in standards of nursing practice notification of puerperal pyrexia is only of historical interest.

Even in the highly developed countries of the world puerperal sepsis was a scourge which took a high toll of maternal lives until about a century ago. Through the work of oliver Wendell Holmes, Semmelweis and Pasteur, there was a better understanding of the causes of puerperal sepsis. In the past, it was thought that a noxious constitution in the atmosphere was the cause of puerperal sepsis.

This theory was disproved by the work of Semmelweis and Pasteur who found that women who died of puerperal sepsis were those who had been attended by physician after performing postmortem examinations or by nurses after delivering an infected patient. Pasteur showed that the cause was due to the transfer of bacteria from an infected patient or from the postmortem room by the physician to the woman in labour.

There was strong opposition to the work of Holmes, Semmelweis and Pasteur. The lesson learnt from the work of Pasteur was the origin of the adoption of strict aseptic and antiseptic technique and the wearing of masks and sterile gowns by the physician and nurse when conducting a delivery.

In considering the causes of puerperal infection, the nurse should think of the following three factors:
1. The infecting organism.
2. The source of infection.
3. The predisposing factors.

The Organisms Causing Puerperal Sepsis

The organisms causing puerperal sepsis fall under four headings.

a. *Streptoccous pyogenes:* The patient may be infected with these organisms from the respiratory tract of her attendant.
b. *Eschericheia coli*: The patient may be infected with these organisms from her own perineum or gastrointestinal tract.
c. *Staphylococcus pyogenes:* The patient can be infected with these organisms from throat or skin lesions (e.g., boils and septic fingers, etc.) of her attendants or from bed clothes.
d. Anaerobic streptococci and other anaerobic organisms such as *Clostridium tetani* or *welchii*.

The anaerobic streptococci from the patient's bowels may infect the patient. Infection with *Clostridium tetani* or *welchii* may be due to delivery taking place in unhygienic situations or the use of rusty, unsterile instruments.

The Source of Infection

The source of infection may be:
a. Autogenous
b. Endogenous
c. Exogenous.

Autogenous source: The source of infection in this case is from the patient usually from her respiratory tract. Septic foci in the patient's own body may also be a source of infection.

Endogenous source: This is usually from organisms already present in the patient's vagina and bowel. These organisms are non-pathogenic in normal circumstances. They may become virulent and pathogenic if there is laceration of the birth canal.

Exogenous source: Organisms from the respiratory tracts and septic foci of the patient's attendants. The dust in the air of the ward from blankets, sheets, etc. are the main sources of infection in this variety. The majority of hospital staff (nurses and doctors) harbour staphylococci and streptococci in their respiratory tracts and will readily infect their patients if adequate precautions are not taken.

Predisposing Factors to Genital Tract Infection

a. An anaemic, malnourished and debilitated patient is more prone to develop puerperal infection than a well-nourished and healthy patient.
b. Prolonged labour, with repeated vaginal examinations during the course of the labour is potent vase of infection in the puerperium.
c. Extensive lacerations of the perineum, vagina and cervix are important predisposing factors, especially if the lacerations are not stitched in time.
d. Patients who are untreated or inadequately treated for antepartum and/or postpartum haemorrhage are in a poor state to with stand infection.

Classification of Puerperal Sepsis

Puerperal sepsis or genital tract infections may be:

1. *Localized* in which case, the infection results in local sepsis of the perineum, vagina, uterus, Fallopian tubes and ovaries.
2. *Widespread* that is, the infection extends beyond the uterus, spreading into the pelvic cellular tissues, lymphatics and pelvic veins but not entering the general circulation.
3. Infection may also spread into the peritoneum, causing peritonitis.
4. The infection may be blood born, causing septicaemia.

Localized Infection

Vagina: An unstitched or poortly stitched vaginal and perineal laceration may become infected. There is usually little or no constitutional distrubances. The temperature may be raised slightly and there may be mild tachycardia.

Cervix: Localized infection of the cervix may result from a bruised or haemolytic sreptococci may invade not only the cervix but also the pelvic cellular tissue or the blood stream. In this case, there may be marked constitutional disturbance with high fever, tachycardia, pain and tenderness in the lower abdomen and tenderness in the vaginal fornices due to parametritis.

Uterus: The placental site behaves like any large wound in the body. Depending on the type and virulence of the infecting organisms the infection may be limited to the placental site. It may cause abscess formation with severe acute endometritis and foul smelling lochia, or it may cause involvement of the muscle wall of the uterus leading to myometritis.

In such cases, there is usually marked constitutional disturbance or 4 days after delivery. The patient has pyrexia, tachycardia and sometimes rigors and there may be subinvolution of the uterus. The lochia may be scanty or may be profuse and foul smelling. The patient may complain of severe headache, vomiting and abdominal pain.

Infection Beyond the Uterus

The infection may extend from the uterus to deep cervical lacerations from where it is spread to the pelvic cellular tissues (pelvic cellulitis), to the femoral veins and rarely to the iliac veins and inferior vena cava. It may spread from the uterus to the fallopian tubes and ovaries, causing salpingo-oophoritis. The infection may cause thrombophlebitis in the veins of the oelvis and the deep veins of the legs. Pain and tenderness in the calf muscles, also pain on dorsiflexion of the foot of the affected leg are signs of deep vein thrombosis of the leg.

The patient is usually very ill, with fever, tachycardia, lower abdominal pain, tenderness on moving the cervix, tenderness in both iliac fossae and pain and tenderness in the calf muscles.

Peritonitis

Peritonitis may occur after spontaneous delivery if there is infection with haemolytic streptococcus or it may follow caesarean section for prolonged labour, especially if the membranes have ruptured for a long time before the operation. Peritonitis following ruptured uterus is quite common. The patient usually is prostrated. There is a rise in temperature the pulse is rapid, the abdomen is tender, distended and rigid an there may be a great deal of vomiting. Sometimes, paralytic ileus may result from the peritonitis and bowel sounds cannot be heard.

Septicaemia

This may occur within 18 hours of delivery or may arise from invasion of the blood stream through intestine in the placenta in which case the symptoms may be delayed until the tenth day or even later. In septicaemia, the patient is usually very ill with high fever (temperature of 39.4 to 40.5°C) tachycardia above 120/minute and, occasionally, delirium. Usually abdominal pain may be absent. The joints of the body may become painful and tender in severe infections. There may be involvement of the heart and lungs resulting in pericarditis, endocarditis, pleurisy and pneumonia. The outlook in cases like these is very poor.

Treatment

The treatment depends on the infecting organism and the extent of the lesion. Usually broad spectrum antibiotics like tetracycline are prescribed until the sensitivity of the organisms grown on culture is known. When this is known the appropriate antibiotics are given. The patient is confined to bed in an isolation ward. She is advised to take plenty of fluids if this is possible. Cases with peritonitis should have a stomach tube passed and the stomach contents aspirated. The patients are usually given intravenous infusions. If *Clostridium tetani or welchii* infection is suspected, antitetanus serum and anti-gasgangrene serum are given.

The packed cell volume should be estimated and anaemia corrected. It may be necessary to give the patients blood transfusion, but often patients respond well to chemotherapy, antibiotic therapy as well as haematinics and antimalarials.

Nursing Interventions

The nursing care of the patient is that of an ill patient. She should rest in bed and her toilet requirements should be carried out in bed. These include vulval toilet twice daily, treatment of pressure areas, mouth toilet and daily bed bath. Extra fluid in the form of fruit juice, milk, beverage is given to the patient at intervals. A chart of the fluid intake and urinary output is kept, especially if the patient is having an intravenous infusion. Attention should be paid to the bowels, which should open regularly. Four hourly observations and records are made on the patient's temperature, pulse and respiration. The nurse midwife should note the patient's mental outlook because delirium and signs of puerperal psychosis are known to be associated with puerperal sepsis. Breastfeeding may be stopped if the patient is very ill and confused.

Free and adequate drainage of the uterus should be encouraged by sitting the patient up in bed. Enema may be given to empty the rectum and also promote drainage of lochia.

Prevention of Puerperal Sepsis

1. All septic foci in the patient such as sore throat, infected teeth or tonsils should be attended to during pregnancy. The patient should be advised to abstain from sexual intercourse about 4 to 6 weeks before delivery.
2. Anaemia and other conditions that may lower the patient's resistance should be energetically treated.
3. Prolonged and debilitating labours and traumatic deliveries should be avoided.
4. Nose and throat swabs of all doctors and nurses should be examined bacteriologically and all those harbouring haemolytic streptococci or staphylococcus. Pyogenes should be treated with appropriate antibiotics and barred from attending to the patients until these organisms have been eliminated from the respiratory tract.
5. The attendant should wear masks and observe strict aseptic and antiseptic precautions (i.e., the scrubbing of the hands, the wearing of sterile gowns and gloves, the use of antiseptic lotions and lubricants during vaginal examinations or in conducting deliveries.
6. Dust in the labour and laying in wards should be avoided.
7. Isolation as well as barrier nursing of infected patients and infants is imperative.

Note: For Nursing Management of Abnormal Puerperium Please See Table 10.1.

Table 10.1: Nursing care plan of cesarean birth postnatal mother

Problem (1)	*Reason (2)*	*Objective (3)*	*Nursing intervention (4)*	*Evaluation (5)*
1. Risk for maternal injury, related to • Aspiration of gastric contents • Positioning during anaesthesic • Misplacement of surgical sponges. • Bladder injury during surgery • Injury from jewellery Contact lenses, denture • Excessive blood loss	Subjective data • Complains of incisional pain Objective data • Vomiting with aspirations of gastric contents: Resp. distress • Asymmetric breach sounds • Urine not draining into Soley drainage bag • Legs not maintained on operating table • Bloody urine drawing from catheter • Hypertension after epidural anaesthesia • Sponge or instrument count incorrect • Hypertension • Hypotension and shock • Signs of thrombophlebitis • Significant drop in Hct • Uterine atony and excessive blood loss	Client will demonstrate minimal maternal injury	• Determine time and content of last meal/intake. • Note intake and urinary output during labour. • Transport with side rails up. Assist in transfer to operating table. Position appropriately for anaesthetic administration and then for surgery • Insert Foley's catheter, maintaining asepsis • Ensure drainage floor of Foley's catheter. Do not allow kinks in tubing, place bag lower than bladder • Obtain urine specimen for culture when the Foley's catheter is inserted • Assess urinary output during surgery and in the recovery period. Note whether there is blood, in urine • Assess for untoward reactions to anaesthesia Assess BP and other symptoms. Assist with IV injections and bolus • Keep accurate instrument and sponge counts. • Assess blood pressure and pulse. Assess blood loss counting bloody sponges • Assess dressing for excessive bleeding. • Assess lower extremeties for signs of thrombophlebitis (redness, warm) • Encourage ankle and leg exercises in early recovery. Ambulate early • Hydrate the client with IV fluids • Monitor postoperative haemoglobin level haematocrit • Assess uterine fundus for firmness. Gently palpate fundus. Administer oxytocin in IV fluids	Client will evidence normal breath sounds, urine draining into Foley's draining bag, absence of blood in urine; normal blood loss
2. Risk for ineffective breathing pattern, related to: • Narcotics • Gen. Anaesthesia • Postoperative pain interfering with resp expansion of lungs.	Subjective data • Describe difficulty with deep breathing Objective data • Abnormal respiratory rate. depressed rate – Dyspnoea • Sputum	Client will demonstrate effective breathing pattern	• Assess respiratory rate and depth • Assess lung sounds • Note symptoms of respiratory distress or infection such as sputum or dyspnoea • Have client turn every 1 to 2 hours Encourage semi-up right position • Have client complete deep-breathing exercises every hours	Client will evidence normal respiration normal breath sounds, deep breathing and coughing adequate

Contd...

Contd...

Problem (1)	*Reason (2)*	*Objective (3)*	*Nursing intervention (4)*	*Evaluation (5)*
• Immobility, inactivity	• Asymmetric breath sounds • Inactive, minimal ambulation • Maintains one position in bed; little movement • Difficulty with deep breathing and cough.	•	Hydrate the patient with IV fluids and then oral fluids	ambulation
3. Pain, related to: • Bladder distention • Flatus, abd. distention • Incisional pain • Haemorrhoids • Breast engorgement • Nipple soreness. • After pains • Spinal headache. • Mastitis.	Subjective data – *Bladder distension* • Describes presence of lower abdominal dull discomfort – *Flatus abd. distension* • Describes discomfort with distended abdomen. • States not passing flatus, or only minimal flatus. • States no bowel movement *Incisional pain* • Describes incisional pain. • Describes pain that is aggravated by movement Objective data – *Bladder distention* • Lower abdominal bulging. noted with observation and palpation. • Unable to void or voids small amounts. – *Flatus, abd. distention* • Distended abdomen noted by observation and percussion • Minimal or sluggish, bowel sounds. • Absence of bowel movement – Incisional Pain • Non-verbal behaviour indicates pain with movement, sitting, walking	Client will demonstrate comfort • –	*Bladder distension* • Assess lower abdomen just above the symphysis pubis for bulging. Percuss to note dullness of abdomen and increased tympany over the rilled bladder • Encourage voiding (assist in ambulating to bathroom, runwater). Assess bladder for distension after voiding • Ambulate early and frequently • Administer pain medication 30 minutes before ambulation Obtain sputum specimen of necessary • Administer antibiotics if ordered *Incisional pain* • Assess presence, location and nature of incisional discomfort. Assess for complications. • Assess incision for healing. • Provide information about wound healing and typical regression pattern of pain. • Assess blood pressure and pulse. • Assist with measures that reduce discomfort This includes: – Repositioning to comfortable position (side, back) Demonstration and encouragement of relaxation and deep-breathing techniques, effleurage – Reduction of stimulation in the environment – Provision of backrubs • Administer pain medication, every 3 to 4 hours assess effectiveness of it, explain action of analgesics, time factors, restrictions • Encourage the client to use the football hold with pillows while feeding the baby. Administer pain medication if necessary.	Client will evidence absence of lower abdominal bulge. Voiding of adequate amounts minimal abdominal distention

Contd...

Contd...

Problem (1)	Reason (2)	Objective (3)	Nursing intervention (4)	Evaluation (5)
	• Abdominal incision. • Grimace with movement. • Nonverbal behaviour indicates pain, tenderness when incisional area is touched. • Guarding of incisions • Restricted movements		before infant feeding. • Assist with feedings and infant care as needed	
4. Risk for infection; Endometritis, Incision infection cystitis, nephritis related to • Ascension of micro-organisms into uterus • Membranes ruptured more than 6 hours before caesarean delivery Exposure to micro-organism during pregnancy Trauma to bladder • Foley's catheter Urinary retention after Foley's catheter removed	Subjective data *Endometritis* • Describes-headache, malaise, backache, • States poor appetite • Experiences pain when uterus is palpated. *Incisional infection* Describes incisional pain *Cystitis/Nephritis* Describes burning with urination Objective data *Endometritis* • Elevate temp. pulse • Uterus larger than expected on palpation. • Darkbrown, foul smelling lochia, but may be odourless. • Elevated WBC Count *Incisional infection* • Incision reddened • Incision not totally approximated • Incisional exudate *Cystitis/Nephritis* • Foley's catheter • Distended bladder • Voids small amounts • Voids frequently • Dysuria with voiding	Client will demonstrate absence of uterine, incisional urinary tract infection •	• Assess abdominal dressing or incision for tenderness, oedema, approximation, exudate. • Note whether there is an operative drain, Note moisture on the dressing and change the dressing as ordered or needed. • Assess temperature, pulse every 4 hours, until stable, then every shift. • Note WBC count. • Assess uterine fundal height and uterine tenderness every 4 hours, then every shift. • Assess lochia for amount, colour and foul odour every 4 hours then every shift • Encourage semi-Fowler position • Remove incisional dressing after 24 hours • Culture the lochia if infection is suspected • Administer expirate or Methergin if ordered Encourage a diet high in proteins, vit. C and iron • Encourage warm showers daily • Maintain medical asepsis with Foley's catheter. Provide perinea cleansing • After Foley's catheter is removed, assess output. Measure first voidings • Assess bladder distension. Assess location of fundus, firmness of uterine contractions, and amount of lochia • Assist with voiding. Assist ambulation to void • Encourage adequate oral intake • Assess for symptoms of cystitis and nephritis	Client will evidence normal temperature, pulse rate, normal sized uterus soft uterus without tenderness, normal, lochia without odour, normal WBC count, voiding adequate, amounts, absence of bladder distension, absence of symptoms of cystitis and UTI

Contd...

Contd...

Problem (1)	Reason (2)	Objective (3)	Nursing intervention (4)	Evaluation (5)
	• Costovertebral angle tenderness • Fever		• Instruct the client in Kegel's exercises • Administer appropriate antibiotics. Prophylactic antibiotics may be given	
5. Constipation, related to • Change in intro-abdominal pressure during surgery • Reduced gastro-intestinal motility • Initial bedrest • Inactivity • Altered fluid and nutritional intake • Flatus • Incisional discomfort	Subjective data • States absence of flatus • Describes discomfort with abd. distention • Describe concern to have a bowel movement Objective data • Infrequent bowel elimination • Hard stools • Straining with stools. • Absence of flatus or minimal flatus • Abd. distension. • NPO for a time. • Altered diet. • Ambulates infrequently. • Absent to minimal bowel sounds	Client will demonstrate normal bowel elimination	• Auscultate bowel sounds in all four quadrants every 4 hours • Assess abdominal distention. Palpate and percuss the abdomen • Note passing flatus • Avoid very hot or very cold oral fluids straws and carbonated beverages • Hydrate with oral fluids once bowel sounds are present • Encourage leg exercises, turning, and ambulation • Instruct the client to include fibre in the diet (fresh fruits, and vegetables, whole grains) • Administer stool softeners or cathertics as ordered • If there is abdominal dissention and minimal passage of flatus, insert rectal tube • Administer a hypertonic Fleet anaema if ordered	Client will evidence flatus, ambulating, active bowel sounds, bowel movements
6. Urinary retention, related to: • Foley's catheter for 6-24 hours • Inactivity • Handling of bladder during surgery • Diuresis postpartum • Incisional discomfort	Subjective data Describe burning with urination Objective data • Foley's catheter • Distended bladder after removal of Foley's catheter • Voids small amounts after Foley's removal • Voids frequently • Dysuria with voiding • Urgency with voiding. • Costovertebral angle tenderness • Fever	Client will demonstrate normal urinary elimination without infection	• Maintain sterile closed urinary system • Provide perineal care and instruct client in perineal care, change perineal pad frequently • Ensure that Foley drainage bag is dependant and tubing is not kink • Take measures to treat urinary track infection accordingly	Client will evidence voiding of adequate amounts, absence of bladder distension

Contd...

Contd...

Problem (1)	*Reason (2)*	*Objective (3)*	*Nursing intervention (4)*	*Evaluation (5)*
7. Altered nutritional Less than body requirement, related to • NPO after caesarean birth. • Reduced gastro-intestinal motility after surgery • Inactivity after surgery	Subjective data • Describes lack of know-ledge of four food groups, requirements for healing and breast-feeding Objective data • Absent or minimal bowel sounds • Not passing flatus, then passes flatus • Difficulty tolerating clear, full liquids • Abd. distention • Breastfeeding	Client will demonstrate nutritional intake adequate for body requirement	• Assess bowel sounds every 4 hours. • Assess abdomen for distention-palpate and percuss. • Once bowel sounds are returning and flatus is passed. Start oral gluids. Start with clear fluids, then progress to full liquids and regular diet • Administer analgesics before ambulation.	Client will evidence gastro-intestinal motility will resume normal bowel sounds, will tolerate clear liquids and regular diet
8. Knowledge deficit of caesarean birth related to • Unplanned cesarean birth. • Lack of knowledge about cesarean procedures. • Lack of retention of information. • Lack of knowledge about reason for CS • Lack of memory over previous CS.	Subjective data • States inexperience with CS procedure • Ask questions about caesarean birth • Describes concern about safety and outcome of caesarean birth Objective data First caesarean procedure symptoms anxiety	Client will demonstrate adequate knowledge of caesarean birth	• Assess learning methods • Assess level of anxiety. Intervene to reduce anxiety • Provide information in simple terms. Include rationale for action • Encourage the client to ask questions • Review procedures as they occur • Provide information about preoperative, operative and post-operative routines and procedures • Provide information regarding possible complications after caesarean birth (fever, uterine infection, urinary tract infections bleeding, abdomen distention). • Provide information related to selfcare after the caesarean birth, such as perineal care, Foley's catheter and hygiene. • Review activity and exercises after caesarean birth. • Provide information about resuming sexual intercourse and explain contraception as needed. • Plan home management with the client, assistance with housework, infant sleeping arrangements and support person availability	Client will evidence moderate anxiety, ability to attend information, minimal number of questions about procedures, compliance with instruction, verbalization of understanding of caesarean procedures

Contd...

Contd...

Problem (1)	*Reason (2)*	*Objective (3)*	*Nursing intervention (4)*	*Evaluation (5)*
9. Anxiety: moderate to severe, related to caesarean surgery and related effects	Refer to previous nursing diagram related to anxiety			
10. Risk for situational low self-esteem, related to • Caesarean birth. Loss of experience of vaginal birth • Addition of infant to family	Subjective data • Describes expectations of vaginal birth • Voices concern for safety during CS • Feelings of failure • Feelings of disappoint-ment • Un-expectations • Negative self-appraisals response to CS • Negative verbalization about CS • Expresses shame or guilt and evaluates self as inadequate Objective data • Symptoms of anxiety • Difficulty in making decisions	Client will demonstrate positive self-esteem.	• Obtain informations about the mother's conceptualization of pregnancy, labor and delivery. • Encourage verbalization of feelings. • Provide information about cesarean procedure or reinforce previous learning. Refer to caesarean delivery as a Cesarean birth • Point out similarities between vaginal and caesarean births • Encourage the significance others to be present for caesarean birth • Assist with strategies that help to restore self-esteem. Care of infant to ease transition to parenting, normalizing the caesarean birth • Assess the emotional reaction to the caesarean birth	Client will evidence expressions of expectations and feelings about caesarean birth (CB) have mild level anxiety, verbalize understanding of CB refer to caesarean delivery as a birth, relay similarities between CB and VB

C H A P T E R

Assessment and Management of High-Risk Newborn

PRETERM NEONATE

A baby with a birth weight of 2500 grams or less, regardless of the period of gestation, is premature by international standards. Assessing prematurity by weight only poses a problem in countries where babies have low birth weights. In such places, full term babies are known to weight 2,500 grams or less. Nurse midwives working in places where birth weights are low will have to determine the maturity of an infant by its general behaviour and appearance.

A premature baby is immature because its organs are not well developed at birth. Therefore, it is ill equipped for a separate existence, and the death rate amongst premature infants is high, especially in the first week of life. The shorter the period of gestation and the lower the birth weight, the less likely is the survival of the premature baby. Sixty to eighty per cent of infants with a birth weight of 1,000 grams or less die unless they are carefully and efficiently managed.

Premature Labour

Premature labour is labour that occurs before the thirty-seventh week of gestation or less than 259 days since the onset of pregnancy.

Diagnosis of Premature Labour

The diagnosis of premature labour may be difficult to make. Sometimes, it is difficult to distinguish false (spurious) labour from true premature labour. Ideally, to diagnose premature labour, there must have been some changes in cervical dilatation or effacement of the cervix should have taken place. Unfortunately, if this definition is uses as the criterion for diagnosing premature labour, it will be difficult in many cases to inhibit labour and any attempt to do so will amount to locking the stable door after the horse has escaped. It is, therefore, preferable to rely solely on uterine contractions in diagnosing premature labour if treatment is to be of any avail.

Causes of Premature Labour (Fig. 11.1)

In the great majority of cases, no cause can be found for premature labour.

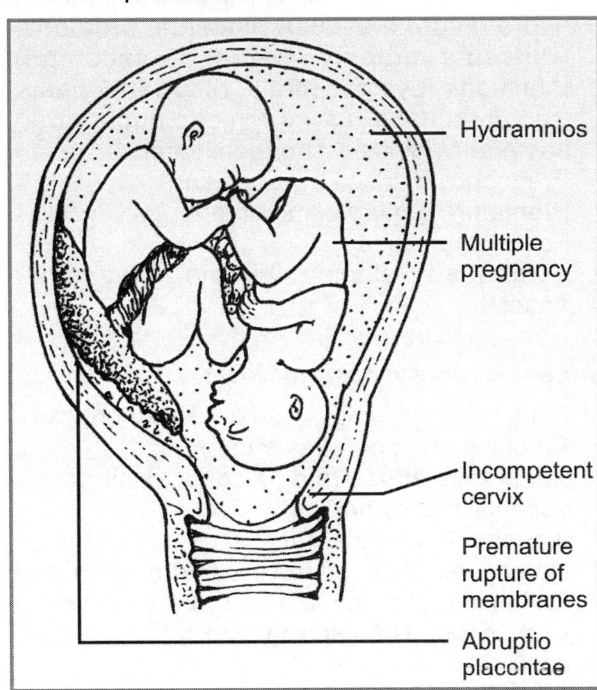

Fig. 11.1: Factors predisposing to premature labour

The known risk factors for preterm birth are as follows:

Demographic Risks

- Non-white race

- Age (below 17 above 35 years)
- Low economic status
- Unmarried
- Less than high school children.

Biophysical Risks

- Previous preterm labour and birth
- Second trimester abortion (more than two spontaneous or therapueutic) still births
- Grand multiparity: Short intervals between pregnancies (41 year since last birth), Family history of preterm labour and birth
- Progesterone deficiency
- Uterine anomalies or fibroids; uterine irritability
- Cervical incompetence, trauma shortened length
- Exposure to DES or other toxic substances
- Medical diseases (e.g. diabetes, hypertension, anaemia)
- Small stature (119 cm in height:< 45.5 kg or under weight for height)
- Current pregnancy risks: Malignant pregnancy, hydramnios, bleeding, placental problems (Placenta praevia, abruptio placentae) Infections (pyelonephritis, recurrent urinary tract infections, asymptomatic bacteriuria, bacterial vaginosis, chorioamnionitis).
- Pregnancy induced hypertension
- Premature rupture of membrane
- Foetal anomalies
- Inadequate plasma volume expansion; anaemia.

Behavioural psychosocial Risks

- Poor nutrition; weight loss or low weight gain.
- Smoking (10 cigarettes a day)
- Substance abuse (e.g., alcohol, illicit drugs, especially cocaine)
- Inadequate prenatal care
- Commutes of more than 1½ hours, each way
- Excessive physical activity (heavy physical work, prolonged standing, heavy lifting, young child care
- Excessive lifestyle stressors.

  The following conditions are usually found in association with premature labour:

Maternal Factors (Fig. 11.2)

1. Severe systemic diseases.
2. Endocrine disorders.
3. Trauma.

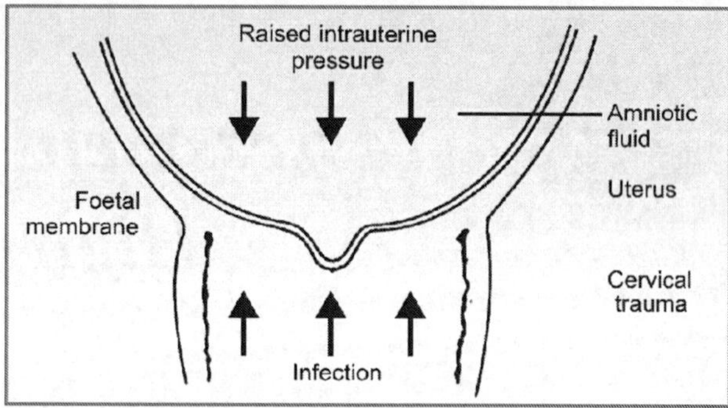

Fig. 11.2: Factors which determine the time of rupture of the foetal membranes

4. Sexual intercourse resulting in orgasm.
5. Low socioeconomic status.
6. Low maternal age.
7. Low maternal weight.
8. Heavy smoking.
9. Single marital status.
10. Previous history of recurrent premature labour.
11. Genital tract infection-genital mycoplasmas
12. Untreated hyperthyroidism and hyperparathyroidism.

Foetoplacental Factors (Fig. 11.3)

1. Genetic abnormalities.
2. Foetal death.
3. Abruptio placentae.
4. Placenta praevia.

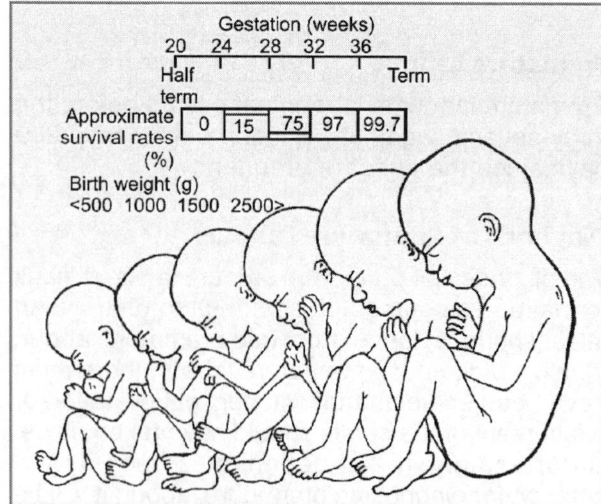

Fig. 11.3: Birth weight, gestational age and perinatal outcome

Uterine Factors

1. Overdistension of the uterus.
2. Uterine malformation.
3. Infection.
4. Foreign body—e.g., intrauterine contraceptive device.
5. Rupture of membranes.
6. Cervical trauma.

Other Factors

Iatrogenic factors—i.e., factors due to inadvertent premature induction of labour by use of drugs or artificial rupture of membranes by the physician due to an error of judgement with regard to foetal maturity.

Prevention of Premature Labour

Pregnancies complicated by premature labour or premature rupture of membranes are high risk pregnancies.

In some cases of premature labour in which it is feared that the baby is not mature enough for an extrauterine environment. In such cases, it is now possible to inhibit preterm labour by the use of certain pharmaceutical agents. Inhibition of preterm labour should not be done as a routine in all cases of suspected premature labour. There may be some cases in which it may be an advantage to terminate such pregnancies. It may not be wise to inhibit labour in cases in which the continuance of the pregnancy may aggravate maternal conditions such as fulminating pre-eclampsia or eclampsia, severe hypertension and chronic renal disease. In known cases of congenital foetal abnormalities not compatible with life it is unwise to inhibit labour. And prevention strategies that address risk factors associated with preterm labour and birth are less constantly in human and financial terms than the hightech and often lifelong care required by preterm infant and their families.

Nurses caring for those who exhibit symptoms of preterm labour should be made early recognition and diagnosis, life style modification and advise for bedrest.

Pharmaceutical Inhibition of Premature Labour

The incidence of preterm labour can be reduced by taking certain preventive measures in women who are known to be prone to premature labour. These preventive measures include prolonged bed rest, use of sedatives and the avoidance of strenuous exercise, etc. In a number of cases, these preventive measures are not enough to inhibit preterm labour. It is in such cases that the administration of pharmacological agents may prove useful in ensuring foetal maturity before delivery.

In cases in which the L/S ratio is 2 or greater, and the gestational age is above thirty two weeks, it may not be advisable to inhibit preterm labour, especially if the continuation of the pregnancy may be harmful to the mother or foetus.

Drugs Used to Inhibit Preterm Labour

These drugs fall into two main groups:

1. The drugs that act by preventing the release or synthesis of a known uterine stimulant. Examples of this group are ethanol and the prostaglandin inhibitors.
2. The second group of drugs acts by the direct effect on the myometria cells.

   Ethanol is an alcohol. It is known to inhibit uterine contractions in preterm labour. It acts by preventing the release of oxytocin. It has been known to postpone labour for 48-72 hours. It can cause signs of drunkeness in the mother. It also has harmful effects on the neonate.

Magnesium sulphate is a more potent inhibitor of uterine contractility than ethanol. When given intravenously, it causes undesirable side effects such as nausea, dryness of the mouth, perspiration, dizziness and nystagmus.

The Beta-Adrenergic Receptor Stimulants

The following are examples of these drugs:

a. Isoxsuprine.
b. Ritodrine.
c. Terbutaline.
d. Fenoterol.
e. Salbutamol.

All these are powerful inhibitors of endometrial activity. The durations of effect varies with each drug. None of the three os free side effects. Isoxsuprine is known to cause nausea, sweating, headaches drowsiness, maternal tachycardia and hypotension. Ritodrine causes maternal tachycardia and hypotension. It has, however, been widely and successfully used to prevent preterm labour. It has no known adverse effects on the foetus.

All these drugs can be given by intravenous infusion, intramuscular injection or orally. The inital dose is usually given by controlled intravenous infusion for six to twelve hours, followed by intramuscular administration for twenty four hours, and followed later by oral maintenance dose until the thirty sixth week of gestation.

It is important to emphasize that the present state of our knowledge of the actions, etc. of these drugs does not permit their routine use in all hospitals. Their use should, therefore be restricted to the hands of the experts in well-equipped hospitals.

Other prostaglandin inhibiting drugs which may be used to inhibit labour are the non-steroidal anti-inflammatory drugs such as:

1. Aspirin.
2. Indomethacin.
3. Salicylic Acid.
4. Mapoxen.
5. Mefenamic.

Contraindications to the Inhibition of Preterm Labour

The following are obstetric and medical contra-indications to the inhibition of preterm labour.

1. Eclampsia.
2. Fulminating pre-eclampsia.
3. Antepartum haemorrhage, particularly abruptio placentae.
4. Chronic renal disease.
5. Severe chronic hypertension.
6. Advanced cardiac disease.
7. Foetal distress.
8. Chorioamnionitis.
9. Foetal death.
10. Foetal growth retardation.

Tests for Foetal Maturity

Ultrasonic Cephalometry

In cases of doubt as to the maturity of the foetus, routine, antenatal ultrasonic cephalometry can be done from time to time. By measuring the biparietal diameter of the foetal head, a rough estimate of the maturity of the foetus can be made.

X-ray Cephalometry

This is not as reliable and safe as ultrasonic cephalometry. The biparietal diameter of the foetal skull increases by 0.17 cm or more per week in the last few weeks of pregnancy. A biparietal diameter of 9.9 cm indicates maturity.

X-ray for Ossification Centres

A study of the ossification centres may enable the nurse or physician to make a rough estimate of the maturity of the foetus.

1. The ossification centre of the cuboid (a bone in the foot) appears as a rule at term.
2. The ossification centre of the upper end of the tibia appears at about term, but is not as reliable as that of the cuboid.
3. The ossification centre of the lower femoral epiphysis appears between the 36th and 38th week of gestation.

Oestriol Estimation

This has already been described under 'high-risk pregnancies'. A twenty four hour collection of urine is necessary for urinary oestriol estimation oestriol levels above 5 mg/litre in 24 hours is a good sign of adequate placental function.

Lecithin/Sphingomyelin ratio (L/S-ratio): The L/S ratio has been described under 'high-risk pregnancy. An L/S ratio of 2 and above indicates maturity of the foetal lungs.

LOW BIRTH WEIGHT INFANTS

The definition of the premature infant based only on birth weight is gradually falling out of favour. Nowadays it is customary to describe infants weighing 2.5 kg or less as low birth weight infants. This is because not every baby that weighs less than 2.5 kg at birth is premature gestation age. An infant may be born at term (i.e. 40 weeks) and yet be less than 2.5 kg. Such an infant is usually referred to as being small for its gestation age-small-for-dates infants. Sometimes, such infants are said to be dysmature. A number of antenatal complications may be responsible for the delivery of a dysmature infant. These antenatal complications, (examples of which are maternal hypertension, pre-eclamps chronic nephritis, severe anaemia in pregnancy), cause placental insufficiency and stunting of the growth of the foetus in utero (intrauterine growth retardation due to intrauterine malnutrition). Sometimes, no obvious cause can be found to account for dysmaturity.

In contrast to the above, a baby may be born before term say at gestation age of about 36 weeks and weighing about 3.5 kg or more. If the original definition of prematurity based on the birth weight of the infant is the deciding parameter, such a baby would be pronounced mature. It is common knowledge that infants born to diabetic mothers tend to be large. An infant of a diabetic mother delivered at 34 weeks gestation may weigh as much as 3.5 kg. This infant, however, behaves like a premature infant weighing less than 2.5 kg. It, therefore, requires the meticulous perinatal care given to a small for date or premature infant. Low birth weight infants can be broadly classified as pre-term infants and small for dates (dysmature) infants.

It is not always that the birth weight is the determining factor in the ultimate survival of the infant. Factors such as the maturity of the foetal lungs, and the condition of the foetoplacental unit are important.

In modern well equiped hospitals facilities are available for assessing foetal well being in utero. The sonic aid can be used to monitor the pattern of uterine contractions and the foetal heart rate and rhythm. The monitoring of uterine action and foetal heart can be done before the onset of labour or during labour.

In high risk pregnancies in which it may be expedient to expedite or delay the delivery of the infant, as the occasion demands, certain tests should be carried out, the results of which reflect the status of the foetoplacental unit. Some of these tests are described in the section dealing with high risk pregnancies.

Problem of Low Birth Weight

Respiratory Difficulties

The respiratory centre of the premature infant is immature, the respiratory muscles are weak and the lung alveoli are not well developed. Initiation and maintenance of respiration in the infant are therefore, difficult. The respiration is often shallow and irregular with periods of apnoea. There is poor gaseous interchange in the lungs. Atelectasis, hyaline membrane or respiratory distress syndrome are more common in premature babies. The clinical features of these respiratory conditions are cyanosis, laboured breathing, grunting respiration with rib recession, and in drawing of the sternum. It should be noted that the cough reflex is poor in a premature infant.

Body Temperature Regulation

The premature infant is handicapped by its inability to regulate its body temperature. This inability is due partly to the immaturity of the heat regulating centre in the brain, and to the rate at which heat is lost from the large surface area of the infant's body. The absence of subcutaneous fat, the inability of the infant to shiver and the sluggish muscular activity of the premature infant result in poor heat production. A subnormal temperature is, therefore, not unusual in a premature infant.

Digestion

Sucking and swallowing reflexes are usually absent and, if they are present they are usually poor. Regurgitation of feeds is common in the premature infant, due to under development of the oesophageal and gastric sphincters. Fat is poorly tolerated by the premature infant.

Renal Function

The kidneys are immature, therefore, the urinary output is scanty. Salt excretion by the kidneys is poor. This, coupled with the inefficient circulation, predisposes to oedema of the extremities.

Circulatory Disorders

Bleeding tendency is greater due to the fragility of the blood vessels and also low prothrombin levels of the blood (hypoprothrombinaemia). Immaturity of the liver cells is responsible for the low prothrombin level as well as for the high serum bilirubin common in premature infants.

Infections

The premature infant is highly susceptible to infection. This is probably due to a low level of immune antibodies transmitted from the mother transplacentally.

Miscellaneous Hazards of the Premature Infant

These include a high incidence of congenital anomalies, cerebral haemorrhage and retrolental fibroplasia which is usually associated with faulty oxygen administration.

Clinical Features

The head of a premature infant is bigger than the rest of its body and the chest is often small in comparison to the fairly large abdomen. The cranial bones feel soft, the fontanelles are wide, sutures are widely separated and the hair on the head is very soft. The skin is usually wrinkled, delicate and soft due to reduced subcutaneous tissue. In addition, the skin is pink and almost red in colour because the blood vessels are very superficial, profuse lanugo hair and scanty vernix caseosa cover the skin at birth.

In female infants, the labia majora are smaller than the labia minora. The testes of the male may not descend. The nails are soft and short, hardly reaching the tip of the fingers. The eyes are closed most of the time.

The head of a premature infant who is a few weeks old is usually oblong in shape. The infant has a typical old man's look because of its protruding eyeballs and wrinkled forehead.

Causes

In about 50 per cent of cases, the cause of prematurity is not known. However, multiple pregnancy, severe anaemia, and acute infection during pregnancy, e.g. malaria and typhoid, are commonly associated with prematurity. Other causes of prematurity include pre-eclampsia, antepartum haemorrhage, diabetes, hydramnios and congenital foetal abnormalities. Malnutrition, hard work and illegitimacy are also known to predispose to prematurity.

Prevention

Because of the high mortality rate among premature infants, irrespective of adequate care, efforts should be directed towards the prevention of prematurity. The preventive measures are mainly concerned with good antenatal care. The nurse should advise the pregnant woman on the importance of a balanced diet and adequate rest. She should instruct the patient not to travel towards the end of her pregnancy. Obstetrical and medical conditions which predispose to prematurity should be referred to the physician for proper management. Malaria and anaemia should be prevented by regular administration of antimalarial drugs, folic acid and iron to pregnant women.

Management of Premature Infant

For good results in the management of the premature infant, labour should be conducted in such a way that the handicaps of the infant are not made worse. A woman in premature labour should be transferred to a well equipped hospital with facilities and personnel for adequate resuscitation and care of the premature infant.

Sedatives and analgesics are given to the mother cautiously, because the immature foetal respiratory centre could be severely depressed by these drugs.

When preparing for the delivery, the nurse midwife should alert the ward sister of the Special Care Baby Unit so that a warm cot or incubator can be got ready. The heated cot is transferred to the labour ward when the delivery is imminent. Where this facility is not available, a warm cot is got ready in the labour room. The nurse midwife should ensure that the resuscitation equipment, e.g. mucus extractor, oxygen, etc. is available and is in good working order. Wrigley's obstetric forceps, episiotomy scissors, local anaesthetic agents, syringes and needles should be included on the delivery trolley.

It is desirable that an experienced nurse midwife or physician delivers the infant. An episiotomy is indicated especially where the patient is a primigravida and the infant is expected to be small. This will prevent undue compression of the fragile skull. The perineal phase of the delivery is also shortened, thus reducing the risk of intracranial congestion and injury.

Immediate Care of an Infant

Efficient care of the infant at birth is equally important. The infant is received into a warm towel. The airways are cleared using a fine mucus catheter. Oxygen may be given at the rate of one litre per minute till respiration is well established and the infant's colour is satisfactory. The infant should then be put in an incubator or a covered Sorento's cot and transferred to the Special Care Baby Unit as soon as practicable. It must be allowed to recover from the stress of labour and delivery. There is no need to rush to oil or weigh it before it is transferred to the ward.

At times, patients call at maternity centres in well advanced premature labour. It is usually too late to transfer such a patient to a hospital for delivery. If the infant weighs 2 kg and over at birth, it could be nursed in the maternity centre or at home under the nurse's supervision.

Ideally, premature infants weighing under 2 kg delivered in maternity centres or rural areas should be transferred to a well equipped hospital with a premature baby unit.

Later Care of Premature Infant

Further management of the premature infant aims at:

1. Maintenance of respiration and good colour.
2. Provision of warmth.
3. Provision of fluid and adequate calories.
4. Prevention of infection.
5. Ensuring good progress and growth.
6. Education of the mother to take care of her infant.

Very few hospitals in the tropics are equipped with facilities needed for the care of premature infant. Incubators and oxygen cylinders may be lacking in some of these hospitals. The nurse midwife must, therefore, learn to improvise.

Maintenance of Respiration

The airways should be repeatedly cleared if the infant brings up mucus frequently. The infant is laid with its head to one side and the foot of the cot is slightly raised to aid drainage of mucus. The infant is closely watched for signs of respiratory distress and cyanosis. Respiratory distress is recognized by rapid and irregular respiration with periods of apnoea, in drawing of the chest walls and sternal recession, and expiratory grunt with cyanosis of the body and face. In such cases, oxygen should be given at a concentration of 30 to 40 per cent. The rates of flow to give various concentrations of oxygen are shown in Table 11.1.

In the administration of oxygen to the premature infant, high concentrations of oxygen should be avoided. The prolonged administration of high concentrations of oxygen and its subsequent sudden withdrawal may of fibrous tissue behind lance. The condition is known as retrolental fibroplasia and leads to blindness in the newborn. Where an oxygen analyser is available oxygen concentration in an incubator or cot should be measured at least thrice daily. The recommended concentration is 30 to 35 per cent. When the infant no longer requires oxygen, the rate of flow is reduced by 0.5 litre per minute every eight to twelve hours.

Table 11.1: Rates of flow of concentrations of oxygen

Concentration of oxygen (%)	*Rate of flow in mtrs/min*
20-25	¼ - 1
30-35	1½ - 2
40-45	2½ - 3

Provision of Warmth and Maintenance of Body Temperature

The nurse must do her best to prevent the baby's temperature from reaching very low levels. Very small babies of 2 kg or less should ideally be nursed in an incubator with a temperature of about 30° C and a relative humidity of 65 per cent. Unfortunately, most of our hospitals have no incubators. In such cases, premature infants are nursed in covered, Sorento's cots warmed with hot water bottles, usually three in number. A plastic bath protected with a pillow for the mattress and covered with a mosquito net could be used in the patient's home or small maternity centers to replace the Sorento's cots. Such an improvised cot is raised off the floor on a wooden box, the inside of which serves as a storage cupboard for the child's equipment. The plastic bath is easily kept clean by washing and carbolizing. A well thermometer placed in the cot will give an idea of its temperature, which should be about 29° C. Hot water bottles if used, must be well protected and placed in the pockets of the cot lining, or under the mattress, or on top of the covering blanket. These bottles could be changed in hourly rotation to ensure constant heat in the cot. An electric blanket, if available, may be placed underneath the mattress to heat the cot. The use of cotton wool and gauge tissue to keep a premature infant warm, has been condemned. The skin is deprived of air and there is danger of infection and overheating, the baby. Over clothing of the premature infant, especially with wollen material is cumbersome and may cause skin rash. Loose flannel clothing is recommended for infants nursed in cots. The infant's head may be covered with a flannel connect. The infant should not be exposed to direct rays of the sun. When the premature infant maintains its body temperature at 36°C, it is likely to do well subsequently.

Feeding

The practice of starving a premature infant for hours before feeding is considered unnecessary.

If the stomach is aspirated before the first feed, regurgitation and inhalation of the stomach contents are not likely. Feeding may be commenced after 8 to 12 hours rest. Most authorities recommend early feeding of glucose water for infants with respiratory distress because they consider that the feed counteracts acidosis, provides fluid and energy.

The first feed should be small and should be ideally given per tube. Five per cent glucose water or 10 to 15 ml of boiled water which has been cooled down may be given. If the infant tolerates this, half-strength expressed breast milk is offered next. The strength of the milk is increased gradually till full strength breast milk is taken at the end of the third day of life. The amount given depends on the size of the infant and its tolerance but 10 ml is usually offered for the first few feeds.

Breast milk is ideal for feeding small babies because it is easily digestible. Unfortunately, artificial feeding is often resorted to because the mother cannot produce adequate milk for a long period. Halfcream Cow and Gate or Lactogen diluted to half the normal strength could be used for feeding in the early days of life.

The amount of feed given depends on the infant's need and tolerance. Sixty calories, i.e. 90 ml of milk per kg of body weight per day, is recommended for the first week of life; 150 ml for the second week and 180 to 210 ml per kg body weight per day during the third week. To avoid overdistension of the stomach, subsequent vomiting and possible inhalation small feeds of greater concentration are given at 2 to 3 hourly intervals.

A nurse should always try to treat each infant individually and give the amount of milk the individual infant needs, depending also on its appetite, tolerance of feed and general condition. The method of feeding is determined by the infant's size, general health and the presence of sucking and swallowing reflexes.

Infants of 2 kg and over with good sucking and swallowing reflexes could be spoon fed or bottle fed with soft tests. Breastfeeding should be encouraged as soon as the infant's condition permits. The Belcroy's feeder may be used for infants with poor sucking reflex. The Belcroy's feeder could be given occasionally to tube-fed infants who are over 1.5 kg in weight to practise sucking.

Tube feeding, either oro-gastric or naso-gastric, could be dangerous in the hands of the inexperienced midwife. Nasogastric tube feeding is preferred because once the tube is in situ, it can be left for a week before it is changed. It carries less risk of bronchial aspiration often associated with orogastric feeding, especially if the tube is not well pinched when it is being withdrawn.

Method of nasogastric tube feeding: Small size polythene tube (Polytex) is used for feeding infants weighing 1,000 grams or less. Rubber catheter FG-10 can also be used. Though the tube comes presterilized in packets, it is advisable to boil it for five minutes before use. This makes the tube supply and easy to pass. The infant is changed, the arms are wrapped and the head of the cot raised. The nostrils are cleaned with wet cotton wool swabs. The required length of tube to be passed is determined by measuring from the bridge of the infant's nose to its sternum; the level could be marked. When the tube is passed, it should be aspirated and the contents of the syringe tested with blue litmus paper—a red discolouration indicates that the tube is in the stomach. The barrel of a syringe is used as a funnel for giving the feeds.

The amount of feed the infant has actually taken, not the amount offered, is recorded. After feeding, the infant is disturbed as little as possible and should be made to rest quietly on its back with its head turned to one side. It should also be made to lie on its right side.

Supplements: Supplements of vitamins and iron are usually given to a premature infant at a very early age. This is because it has no store of iron vitamins and mineral salts before birth. Moreover, the premature infant is subject to protracted artificial feeding because of its inability to breast feed. Artificial feeds cannot provide all the nutritional needs of the infant.

A vitamin suspension such as A,B,D,E,C is given as early as from the first week of life, starting with two drops daily and increasing till five drops are given once daily at the age of 1 month.

Iron mixtures are also given, starting with two drops twice daily from the second to third week of life. The dose is also increased gradually till a maximum of five drops are given twice daily.

Vitamin C is also given as from the age of 2 weeks. Ascorbic acid (25 mg) may be added to a feed but orange juice is preferred if it is well tolerated by the baby. One teaspoonful of half-strength fresh orange juice is given twice daily initially. The full strength could be offered as from the age of 3 weeks. It is advisable to discharge the baby on full strength orange juice.

Prevention of Infection

The need for expert nursing care and prevention of infection cannot be over emphasized. The staff of a special care baby unit should be in good health and have no foci of infection or colds. Their respiratory tracts should be free of streptococcal organisms. The nursing staff should not only be experienced but should possess the qualities of patience, devotion, observation and ability to give accurate reports. They should be meticulous in cleanliness and should be proficient at resuscitation of the baby.

Frequent hand washing is imperative in a premature baby nursery. The midwife or nurse must learn to wash her hands before touching the infant, after napkin changing, before feeding the infant and when she has finished with the infant; antiseptic hand cream such as Hibitane cream is used to provide a barrier to infection and to protect the skin of the hands.

Premature infants should be given individual attention. Each infant should possess its own equipment, e.g. thermometer, swabs, stethoscope and where possible, feeding utensils. These may be kept in a drawer under the cot or inside cup boards. The cot or incubator in which the infant sleeps should be thoroughly cleaned daily. Gowns and masks should be used in the nursery, preferably one gown for each infant handled.

Visitors are not allowed in the premature unit. If the infant is being nursed in a maternity centre or at home, only the parents should handle it. It should not be brought out to the open till it can maintain its body temperature. In hospital, parents are only allowed to view their babies through the glass windows of the incubator. The nursery must be kept clean. Damp dusting mopping or washing the floor is preferred to sweeping and dry dusting. Direct draught is avoided in the nursery to the windows are usually kept shut.

Infants nursed in the lying inwards or maternity centres must sleep under a net. Infectious babies are isolated and potentially infected ones are given prophylactic antibiotics.

Assessment of Infant's Progress

The infant's progress could be assessed through the nurse midwife's observation and records. The important observations which must be recorded include the following:

1. The respiration of the infant laboured breathing and periods of apnoea must be reported. The respiratory rate is taken and recorded four hourly, or more frequently if it is unsatisfactory.
2. Fever and hypothermia are bad signs. The infant's temperature is also recorded four-hourly. A premature infant who is progressing should be able to maintain its body temperature.
3. Auscultation of the heart and recording of the heart rate.
4. Jaundice occurring within 24 to 36 hours of birth is serious. This must be reported and the infant closely watched. Other colour changes such as cyanosis, pallor and greyness are also significant and should be reported.
5. Evidence or any suspicion of infection must be reported. Rash, discharge from the eyes or moist umbilical cord, grey colour and constantly low temperature are the usual signs of infection.
6. A part from noting the amount of feed taken by the baby, the method of feeding and the baby's eagerness to feed are also recorded. Vomiting of feeds is very significant.
7. Abdominal distension and oedema of the face, abdomen and legs, if severe, should also be reported.
8. Note if the baby is passing urine well. Absence of urine in the first 24 hours must be reported. The frequency of stools should also be noted. Loose stools may be associated with infection.
9. Premature infants may be weighed 12 to 24 hours after birth. Thereafter, weighing is usually done twice weekly because weight gain is usually slow. Weight loss in a premature infant should not alarm the nurse provided the intant's general condition is satisfactory and there is no vomiting.
10. The haemoglobin should be estimated at birth and weekly, thereafter anaemia is thus excluded.
11. The general behaviour of the infant with particular attention to its activity is also noted.

Education of the Mother

The nurse must realize that time and patience are necessary to reorientate the mother, whether she is a primipara or a multipara. The infant is often separated from the mother for several weeks, and the mother sees it as a fragile little thing and is often scared of handling it. To overcome this, it is necessary to introduce the mother gradually to the handling, feeding and general care of the infant. If possible, the mother should be readmitted and be made to manage the infant under supervision. In some hospitals the mothers stay in a mother's home and come up three hourly to the premature unit to feed and nurse their infants under supervision. There are separate cubicles in which these mothers work. They are not allowed in the nurseries.

Mothers are made to look after infants whose weights are 2 kg and over. Breastfeeding is encouraged. If for any reason the infant has to be discharged on artificial feeding, the nurse must make absolutely sure that the mother is competent to prepare the feeds. Education on how to avoid gastroenteritis and respiratory infection must be emphasized. Mothers must also be told to give vitamin and iron supplements to the infant.

It is better that a visit to the mother's home before the discharge of the infant is considered necessary and ideal. Health visitors, auxiliary nurses and domiciliary midwives would have deployed for this purpose. Where the home environment is unhealthy and the mother is illiterate, and ignorant, it is not advisable to discharge the infant till he is over 2.5 kg in weight. Other criteria for deciding when the infant goes home include its ability to feed well and maintain a constant body temperature.

Premature infants should be followed up at the Infant Welfare Clinic till they are about 2 years old. The need for this should be explained to the mother and she should be encouraged to attend regularly.

Complications of Prematurity

Cyanotic Attacks

The premature infant is prone to cyanotic attacks because of the immaturity of its lungs, the case with which *atelectasis* develops and the possibility of the developments of hyaline membrane disease. All these lead to the well known respiratory distress syndrome. Frequent cyanotic attacks usually signify a poor prognosis. Premature infants with repeated cyanotic attacks stand a very poor chance of survival.

Cerebral Haemorrhage (Figs 11.4A and B)

This is a serious complication in the premature infant because the softness of the foetal skull does not offer the much needed protection to the brain and its blood vessels. If excessive moulding occurs the fragile capillaries and small veins easily rupture. In addition, severe anoxia also leads to rupture of the veins and capillaries. Sometimes the premature infant may suffer a massive intraventricular haemorrhage if there is rupture of the vessels in the lateral ventricles of the brain. The readiness with which haemorrhage takes place in the premature infant is sometimes attributed to a low prothrombin level. This is why mothers in premature labour are given 10 mg of vitamin K or vitamin K analogue (Synkavit) as prophylaxis against intracranial damage in the unborn infant. At birth the infant is also given 1 mg of Synkavit intramuscularly.

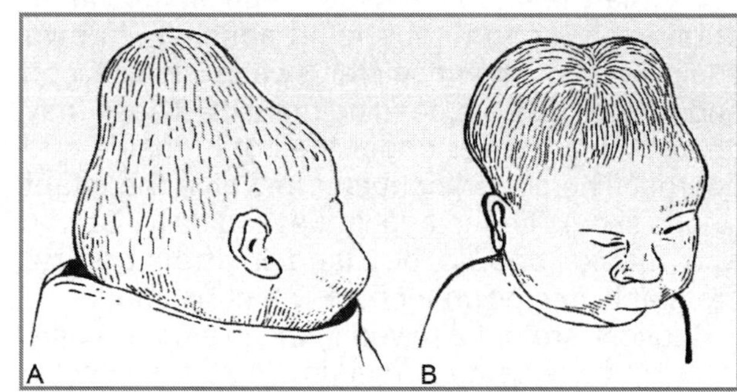

Figs 11.4A and B: A. Unilateral cephalhaematoma, **B.** Bilateral cephalhaematoma

Heart Failure and Pulmonary Oedema

The poor muscular tone of the premature infant may prevent adequate venous return causing stagnation or accumulation of the blood in the extremities. Asphyxia adds to the circulatory problems. Eventually, the infant goes into heart failure and pulmonary oedema.

The most common cause of death in prematurity is poor pulmonary ventilation resulting in severe asphyxia. The immaturity of the lungs, as well as immaturity of the respiratory centre in the brain stem, is the underlying factor. Babies dying of asphyxia show, on postmortem examination, evidence of petechial or subserosal haemorrhages in the heart, lungs and liver. Sometimes the haemorrhages affect the lining of the brain and the cerebral ventricles.

Anaemia

Anaemia is common in premature infants, especially those born before the 36th week of gestation. This is because the iron stores in the foetus are laid in the last four weeks of intra-uterine life.

Jaundice

Because of immaturity of the liver, bilirubin, cannot be conjugated. Neonatal jaundice is a common complication of prematurity. Sometimes, the level of conjugated bilirubin rises to as high as 20 mg/100 ml and causes kernicterus, even in the absence of Rhesus isoimmunization.

Infection

A common complication of prematurity, this has been mentioned above.

Poor Mental and Intellectual Development in Later Years

It is well known that prolonged asphyxia to which the premature infant is prone can lead to mental retardation and low intelligence quotient later in life. In addition, cerebral diplegia and athetosis are common in such infants if they survive the asphyxia.

Respiratory Distress Syndrome

Respiratory distress syndrome (RDS) is condition which affects a newborn premature infant, especially one delivered by caesarean section for antepartum haemorrhage. It can of course also occur in any premature baby, irrespective of the antenatal complication and the method of delivery. It is a major cause of neonatal mortality. It is not a condition found in stillborn infants.

It does not occur in still birth because, attempts at respiration by the Infant are necessary for the condition to develop. It is believed to be done to very severe anoxia in the foetus just before birth or at birth. The severe anoxia causes the foetus in utero to take a deep respiration, thus aspirating a great deal of liquor amnii.

The inspired liquor amnii contains epithelial squames which act by forming a membrane known as the hyaline membrane. The hyaline membrane lines the bronchioles and alveoli, eventually blocking them and increasing anoxia of the newborn infant. The origin of the hyaline membrane is not certain. As stated above, it is sometimes believed to arise from the squames from the swallowed liquor amnii. Another theory is that the membrane is an exudate produced by the epithelium lining the bronchioles and alveoli.

Hyaline membrane is probably due to immaturity of the lungs of the newborn. A lipoprotein referred to as pulmonary surfactant is said to be capable of preventing collapse of the lungs of the newborn infant. If the pulmonary surfactant is absent, as happens in premature infants with immature lungs, respiratory distress syndrome or hyaline membrane disease occurs. On the other hand, hyaline membrane disease may be due to inadequate pulmonary circulation. Respiratory activity is limited.

Clinically, the nurse midwife can recognize respiratory distress syndrome by the following events:

1. The infant is premature.
2. The infant is well immediately after birth and the colour is usually good.
3. Shortly after delivery, signs of respiratory distress develop. The signs are whimpering and grunting which coincide with an expiratory effort rib recession at inspiration, abnormal movement of the nose and sometimes inward drawing of the sternum. The respiratory rate is rapid about 70 or more a minute.
4. The baby's respiration is laboured and after some time the baby stops breathing and becomes intensely cyanosed.

When the nurse midwife encounters a case of respiratory distress syndrome she must at once inform the physician. The diagnosis is usually based on the clinical findings described above and radiographic appearance of the chest.

The baby should be admitted to a special care unit and given a moderate concentration of oxygen (usually not more than 35 per cent for fear of causing retrolental fibroplasia). Antibiotics are prescribed by the physician. Necessary aseptic and antiseptic precautions are taken in the handling of the infant. When feeding commences, the method of feeding is the same as for a premature infant.

The infant is of course nursed in an incubator or preferably in a respirator if one is available. Such infants are prone to decreased blood volume (hypovolaemia) and metabolic acidosis, both of which further aggravate asphyxia and worsen the prognosis for the baby. Hypovolaemia can be prevented by putting the baby below the level of the maternal abdomen and delaying severing the umbilical cord for about a minute after birth, provided Rhesus immunization has been excluded.

Trauma to Deep Structures

Sternomastoid Tumour

This condition is believed to be due to birth trauma to the sternomastoid muscle. It occurs when delivery involves excessive rotation and gross lateral extension of the neck. The tumour is hard and painless. It may be noticed soon after birth, but sometimes it manifests within the first few weeks. The first line of treatment is physiotherapy. If this fails, excision of the tumour should be considered.

Rupture of the Liver or Spleen

These injuries are rare. Rupture of either organ may occur with breech delivery if the attendant grasps the trunk forcibly below the ribs. Death is often the outcome of these injuries. Diagnosis of ruptured liver or spleen is not easy. Sudden collapse, increasing pallor, and rapid pulse are suggestive of an internal haemorrhage due to the rupture of these organs and these symptoms should prompt the nurse to seek medical aid for the baby.

Injury to Bones

Although a fracture may occur in any bone, the incidence is small. The clavicle is the most commonly fractured bone. It occurs most frequently in breech presentations. Long bones, such as the humerus and femur, may be fractured. An obvious fracture or any suspicion of one requires medical aid. The handling of the baby should be minimal. Where there is delay in obtaining medical aid and the baby is in obvious pain, the affected limb should be lightly bandaged to an improvised splint.

Skull Fracture

Skull fracture may be either depressed or complete. In depressed fracture there is either a dent or a marked depression of the skull bone. This type of fracture is usually caused by the sacreal promontory in contracted pelvis, or the blade of the forceps or in difficult delivery of the after coming head in a breech presentation. Complete fracture occurs in cases of difficult forceps delivery. The nurse's responsibility is to consult a physician once the condition is suspected or diagnosed.

Injury to Nerves

Facial nerve injury may occur in forceps delivery and cause facial nerve paralysis. In this condition, there is diminished movement of the affected side of the face. The mouth is also drawn to the uninjured side when the baby cries and the eyes on the injured side may remain always partly open. Recovery may occur within a month.

Brachial Plexus Injury

The brachial plexus may be damaged during the delivery of the after coming head of a breech presentation, or through excessive rotation, stretching or lateral flexion of the neck in a vertex presentation. There are two clinical types of injury to the plexus depending on which nerve roots are involved. The more common type is Erb's palsy in which the arm is adducted, and rotated inwards, the forearm is extended and pronated and the arm hangs down limp from the shoulders. Complete recovery occurs in mild cases but permanent paralysis may accompany a severe case. Treatment consists of splinting the arm in the correct position that is, in a position that allows for relaxation of the affected muscles.

Klumpke's Paralysis

In Klumpke's paralysis, the forearm is flexed at the elbow and supinated. The hand is flaccid.

Intracranial Injuries

The commonest intracranial injury haemorrhage which is due either to a tear of the tentorium cerebelli or falx cerebri or the small blood vessels in the brain. Premature labour prolonged labour, foetal hypoxia, caesarean section, forceps delivery and breech and face presentations predispose to cerebral haemorrhage. Those neonates whose births are associated with the above conditions should be regarded as having sustained some cerebral injury until otherwise proved. In such circumstances, the babies must be observed for signs of cerebral irritation for at least 48 hours. The term 'cot nursing' is often used to describe the minimal handling and disturbance the baby must have.

The clinical features of cerebral damage may be apparent at birth or may present themselves after a few hours or days of life. The manifestations depend on the extent and severity of the damage. Frequently a baby who has suffered severe cerebral damage is shocked and asphyxiated at birth. Respiration, if established, is of an abnormal pattern; that is difficult, irregular and rapid. The baby remains cyanosed and limp and may die within a few hours of birth. Where the general condition initially improves, the infant becomes restless and has a high pitched, shrill or a piercing cry. He is unnaturally wakeful with an alert and apprehensive look. His responses to touch, light and sound are excessive and almost violent. There may be twitching of the limbs and muscles of the face around the mouth or the eyes. In most severe cases, nystagmus and convulsions may occur. The anterior fontanelle may be tense and bulging. Neck rigidity or even retraction may also occur. The sucking and swallowing reflexes are sometimes diminished.

Signs of cerebral injury may not manifest till the second or third day of life. Vomiting, cyanosis and fretfulness are the usual warning signs in such circumstances. The temperature may be subnormal, normal or moderately raised.

Intracranial injuries can be prevented by correcting malpresentations where possible, avoiding asphyxia, delivering the premature baby with the aid of an episiotomy or forceps. The administration of vitamin K to the mother during labour and to the infant after birth may prevent the development of cerebral haemorrhage in susceptible cases.

Management

Medical aid should be sought for the baby when a nurse midwife suspects cerebral damage. The baby is usually admitted to hospital and nursed in a quiet nursery, kept warm and away from direct light and draught. The baby should be handled as little as possible, but being turned from side to side every two hours is necessary. Feeding and toileting are done in the baby's cot. Fluids should be withheld for 12 to 24 hours, especially if the baby is inclined to vomit. The method of feeding is determined by the condition of the baby. A baby who is very irritable or convulses frequently should be tube fed.

A sedative such as chloral hydrate (30-60 mg four hourly) or phenobarbitone (7.5 mg six to eight hourly) is often prescribed.

The following should be handy:

a. Oxygen to administer when the baby is cyanosed.
b. Mechanical suction or mucus extractor to remove secretions which may accumulate in the pharynx.
c. Laryngoscope and endotracheal tube.

There is great need to observe the baby for signs of improvement or otherwise. Pronounced drowsiness or extreme lethargy must be reported, this may indicate oversedation or worsening of the cerebral irritation.

Prognosis

The prognosis depends on the severity of the cerebral injury. Most babies recover with no residual brain damage, although other are subjected to mental retardation, cerebral palsy and spasticity.

Asphyxia Neonatorum

Asphyxia may be defined as a delay in the establishment of normal respiration at birth. This is associated with some degree of hypoxia. The baby is usually blue or grey in colour depending on the degree of the oxygen lack. In mild cases, the baby is blue, particularly in the extremities. He often moves his limbs and makes some attempts to breathe or gasp. The heart beat and the cord pulsations are usually good. The clinical picture given above is that of a case of mild asphyxia (asphyxia livida) of the newborn if the mild asphyxia is not treated promptly, the degree of oxygen lack is increased. This results in a state of respiratory and circulatory failure called severe asphyxia (asphyxia pallida). The baby's colour is dussy green and almost white; he is limp because of poor muscle tone. The apex beat an cord pulsations are feeble. A baby may be born in this severe state of asphyxia if he has undergone intrauterine hypoxia, the causes of which are discussed under foetal distress.

Table 11.2: Apgar score guide

Sign	Scores 0	1	2
Colour	Blue to pale	Body pink limbs blue	Completely pink
Respiratory effort	Absent	Gasping; weak cry; slow irregular respiratory movements	Lusty cry
Heart rate	Absent	Slow, less than 100	Over 100
Muscle tone	Limp	Bone flexion of limbs	Active movement
Response to stimulus	Absent	Facial grimace	Cry

Assessment of the Degree of Asphyxia

A method of assessing the degree of asphyxia neonatorum, first described by an anaesthetist—Dr Apgar—is known as the 'Apgar score'. The assessment is based on the colour, respiratory efforts, heart rate, muscle tone and the baby's response to external stimuli. Each of the above signs is awarded a maximum of two points. The grading is made at the end of the first minute of life and at five minutes after birth. The first grading is almost impracticable with a single handed midwife (Table 11.2).

A baby who scores 8-10 points is not asphyxiated. A baby who scores 5-7 points is mildly asphyxiated and will respond well to simple mucus extraction from the airways and application of external stimuli. A baby who scores 3-6 points is moderately affected, and may improve with resuscitative measures such as clearing the airways and giving oxygen, etc. On the other hand, he may deteriorate and may require endotracheal intubation. A baby who scores 0-3 points is severely asphyxiated. He requires intubation and expert management to survive.

Causes of Asphyxia

The commonest cause of asphyxia is blockage of the air passages by mucus, liquor or blood. The condition of a baby in such circumstances improves immediately the airways are cleared by simple suction. Other causes of asphyxia include:

1. Depression of the baby's respiratory centre by narcotics and anaesthetic drugs given to the mother in labour.
2. Immaturity of the respiratory centre as found in a premature baby.
3. Intracranial injury and the subsequent depression of the respiratory centre.
4. Prolonged intra-uterine hypoxia.
5. Maternal and foetal conditions, discussed under the causes of foetal distress.

Management of Asphyxia

Asphyxia of the newborn is an emergency and calls for quick, efficient management, calmness and gentle handling of the baby. The baby should be held with its head down to aid drainage of fluid and mucus from the respiratory tract. Since thick mucus cannot be removed by this method alone, the baby is laid across the mother's thigh and the air passages are cleared by suction whilst the umbilical cord is clamped and cut. A mucus extractor, an ordinary rubber catheter or a mechanical suction such as the Ambu foot sucker could be used. If the respiration is still not initiated, the baby is transferred to a warm cot with a head down tilt or taken to a resuscitating table if one is available. The baby must be covered to prevent chilling, but his chest should be exposed to enable the nurse to observe any respiratory movements. The physician should be called in urgently. Further suction of the airways is carried out till they are free of mucus. Stroking the baby's back or flicking the soles of his feet may be useful in cases of mild asphyxia.

If the baby makes efforts to breathe, oxygen is given at the rate of 1 litre per minute by a rubber funnel. Otherwise, mouth to mouth respiration should be employed to inflate the lungs. This method is very useful if oxygen is not available.

Method of Mouth to Mouth Respiration

After clearing the air passages, a direct air passage is ensured by extending the baby's head. The baby's mouth may be covered with a piece of gauze. Air from the nurse midwife's buccal cavity is gently blown down the baby's nose and mouth at the rate of 20 times per minute.

Where the nurse suspects depression of the baby's respiratory centre by narcotic drugs, such as pethidine or morphine given to the mother towards the end of labour, pethidine (0.25-0.5 mg) should be given to the baby by intramuscular injection. Respiratory stimulants are not recommended by some authorities, but nikethamide (0.5 ml intramuscularly) or vandid (3 to 6 drops sublingually) could be given in cases of mild or moderate asphyxia.

Medical aid should be summoned if the baby does not respond in one minute. Where the asphyxia is severe the medical aid is summoned immediately while the nurse prepares for intubation.

Medical Management

Medical management involves passing a laryngoscope and sucking out any mucus in the larynx and trachea. An endotracheal tube is inserted and the lungs are inflated with oxygen given under a pressure of 25-50 centimetres of water. This is repeated intermittently and the pressure is also reduced gradually. Because progressive asphyxia is sometimes associated with acidosis in the baby the physician may give an infusion of sodium bicarbonate through a scalp vein. Occasionally intravenous glucose infusion is also given to combat acidosis and protect the liver, the glycogen content of which has been depleted.

Nursing Management

During the resuscitation procedure, the nurse should keep the baby warm, note the colour, muscle tone and any respiratory attempts by the baby. The heart beat is auscultated in order to determine whether the baby is improving or deteriorating. Special nursing care is required after resuscitation. The baby is handled as little as possible, kept warm, closely observed and cot nursed for 48 hours. A 2-4 hourly record is made of the respiratory rate, apex beat and temperature. The type of respiration, including colour changes and muscle tone, is also observed. Signs of irritability, twitching and convulsions should be reported without delay. Oxygen (40 per cent) is administered if cyanosis is present. The airways are kept clear of mucus. Oral fluids are withheld till 6-8 hours after resuscitation. Antibiotics are usually given as prophylaxis against infection.

Severe asphyxia may result in permanent damage of the brain cells and the child may become spastic, mentally retarted or may develop epilepsy. It is therefore, essential for the nurse midwife to advise the mother to attend the hospital for a regular follow-up of the baby.

Congenital Abnormalities

Congenital abnormalities are malformations of the foetus, and are present at birth. Why certain foetal tissues develop abnormally is not always known but the following factors are thought to be responsible:

1. Deficient oxygen supply to the developing ovum.
2. Abnormal implantation of the ovum.
3. Abnormality of the placenta which tends to lead to abnormality of the foetus.
4. Maternal infections, e.g. rubella or German measles, in the first 12 weeks of pregnancy.
5. Maternal diseases other than infection, e.g. hypertension, cardiovascular diseases, diabetes and kidney diseases.
6. Poor maternal nutritional state, especially deficiency in protein and vitamins.
7. Physical and chemical agents such as a high dosage of X-rays in early pregnancy or drugs, e.g. thalidomide.

Other associated factors include age and parity of the mother. Malforme babies are commonly borne by elderly primigravidae or by women who are over 40 years old. High parity tends to predispose to foetal malformation.

Genetic factors also play a major role in foetal malformation, for there is a tendency for some abnormalities such as cleft palate, hare lip and mongolism to run in families (Fig. 11.6).

Foetal malformation often leads to abortion, premature birth, stillbirth and neonatal death.

Any system or organ in the baby may be malformed but those commonly affected include cardiovascular, genitourinary and central nervous systems; gastrointestinal tract; muscles; bones and skin. Some congenital abnormalities are incompatible with life. A number of the malformations can be corrected.

The discovery of a congenital abnormality in a baby indicates the need for a thorough examination of that baby for more abnormalities as these tend to be multiple. The nurse midwife is often the first to note congenital abnormalities. On her, therefore, falls the responsibility of promptly calling the attention of the medical staff to these abnormalities.

Prevention

The nurse can play an important role in the attempt to prevent congenital abnormalities. She should advise her patients to take only those drugs prescribed by the physician in early pregnancy and to report ill health, especially German measles. The patients are also advised to eat food rich in protein and vitamins in order to prevent malnutrition during pregnancy.

Abnormalities of the Central Nervous System

Hydrocephalus: Hydrocephalus is a condition in which there is an excessive and abnormal accumulation of cerebrospinal fluid in the cerebral ventricles which then become enlarged. The baby's head is abnormally big and the cranial sutures and fontanelles are widely separated. The excessive cerebrospinal fluid may be due to excessive formation, blockage to circulation or defect in the absorption of the fluid. A foetus with hydrocephalus often presents by the breech, but a cephalic presentation is not unusual. If the presentation is cephalic, the head feels big and is often high. Hydramnios may complicate the pregnancy.

Hydrocephalus may develop after birth. Widening of the sutures and fontanelles should arouse suspicion of hydrocephalus. In such circumstances, the nurse should measure the head circumference and refer the baby to the physician. Most hydrocephalic babies die during birth or within a few hours of life. Surviving hydrocephalic babies are often mentally retarded.

Spina bifidia: This is the protrusion of the meninges and sometimes the spinal cord through a gap in the vertebral arches which have failed to fuse (Fig. 11.5). Spina bifida is recognized by the presence of a reddish soft mass in the lumbo-sacral region. Paralysis of the lower limbs is usually present. The midwife should inform a doctor immediately and apply normal saline, dressing on it. Although surgical repair of the defect is possible, the prognosis is poor in severe cases. At times, spina bifida may not be easily diagnosed and is referred to as bifida occulta. It presents as a dimple on the back or a patch of hair in the lumbo-sacral region. X-ray examination of the spine will reveal the defect.

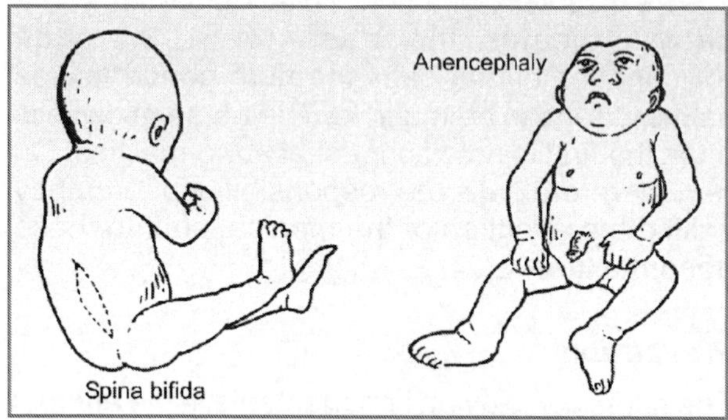

Fig. 11.5: Two common abnormalities of the central nervous system

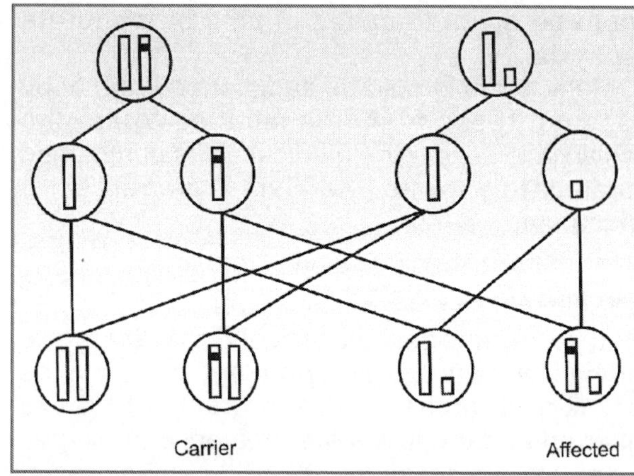

Fig. 11.6: Transmission of a recessively inherited X-linked disorder. The abnormal gene is carried on the female X chromosome

Anencephaly: (Fig. 11.5) Anencephaly is the absence of the vault of the skull and the cerebrum. It is frequently accompanied by an extensive spina bifida. Hydramnios is invariably present during pregnancy. When the diagnosis is confirmed by the aid of X-ray examination, labour is induced prematurely. Malpresentations such as face presentations, are common with the anencephalic foetus. This malformation is incompatible with life.

Microcephaly: Microcephaly is a condition in which the brain is not well developed, therefore, the head is smaller than normal. The fontanelles are either very small or closed. The condition is usually associated with mental retardation and spasticity of the limbs.

Encephalocele and meningocele: These are swellings of the baby's head caused by protrusion of part of the brain or meninges through the lambdoidal suture or a hole in the cervical region of the spinal column. An encephalocele contains some brain substance, it is usually pedunculated and it pulsates. A meningocele contains cerebrospinal fluid. It is fluctuant and becomes tense when the baby cries. Vaseline gauze or saline dressing should be applied to the lesion to avoid infection. The baby should be referred to a physician.

Gastrointestinal Tract Abnormalities

Exomphalos: Exomphalos is a defect of the abdominal wall through which the abdominal organs herniate. The organs may be enclosed in an intact peritoneal sac or lie loosely if the sac ruptures. Immediate surgery is indicated. The nurse midwife should apply a warm normal saline dressing to cover the organs and transfer the baby to a major hospital without delay.

Congenital absence of the abdominal muscles: This condition is recognized by the easy palpation of the abdominal organs which protrude readily when the baby cries. It is frequently associated with other types of congenital abnormalities. No definite treatment is available. Binders may be applied to give some support as the baby grows.

Hare lip and cleft palate: Hare lip (cleft lip) and cleft palate can occur singly or together and each may be unilateral or bilateral. They occur as a result of the failure of the frontonasal palate to unite. The malinformation may be slight or severe. Harelip and cleft palate are easily recognized, but if the defect is on the soft palate it may be missed. In order not to miss this type of defect, the infant's mouth should be inspected with a good light. Cleft palate may cause feeding problems. The mother must be reassured and taught how to spoon feed the baby, if there is a suckling problem. Herelip is usually repaired between the ages of four and six months. Repair of cleft palate is often undertaken when the child is 18 to 24 months old. Dental plates could be used to achieve alignment before operation. The dental plates also facilitate bottle feeding and reduce the risk of respiratory tract and eustachian tube infections.

Tracheo-oesophageal fistula: In this condition, there is a communication between the trachea and the oesophagus. If a pregnant woman has hydramnios, tracheo-oesophageal fistula should be suspected in the baby at birth. There is usually excessive dripping of mucus or saliva from the mouth of a baby with this condition. The baby may have respiratory distress or may be cyanotic and there may be difficulty in passing a nasogastric tube. If a neonate coughs or chokes or becomes cyanosed during the first feed, the nurse should suspect this condition and thus discontinue the feeding and inform a physician immediately. The condition can be corrected by surgery.

Obstruction of the gastrointestinal tract: Obstruction may occur at any level of the gastrointestinal tract and from various causes such as atresia, bands, meconium ileus and volvulus. Vomiting is the usual symptom. The nurse midwife should refer suspected cases to the physician for diagnosis and treatment.

Congenital hypertrophic pyloric stenosis: There is a thickening of the circular fibres or spasm of the pylorus. The symptoms usually start from about the second week of life. The baby vomits after feeds, the vomiting is projectile in character and the vomitus does not contain bile. Treatment is either medical or surgical.

Hiatus hernia: Hiatus hernia is the protrusion of the cardiac and of the stomach into the thorax. It is another cause of vomiting in the first week of life. Management consists of keeping the baby in an upright position with the aid of a firm pillow, especially after feeds.

Imperforate anus: This is easy to diagnose. Examination of the perineum reveals absence of the anal opening (the nurse may not be able to take the baby's temperature rectally). She should suspect this condition if a baby fails to pass meconium within 24 hours of birth.

Cardiovascular System Abnormalities

Some congenital abnormalities of the heart may be associated with cyanosis at birth. In some others, there is no cyanosis (acyanotic congenital heart defects). A nurse should suspect congenital heart defect in a baby who tires easily during feeding or has respiratory embarrassment. Diagnosis is often established by a physician. The baby needs good care and management especially with feeding. Infection should be avoided. Most congenital heart malformations are amenable to surgical treatment.

Genitourinary Tract Abnormalities

Difficulty in determining the sex of an infant may arise from abnormalities of the external genitalia. In females, the labia majora may be fused and the clitoris hypertrophied; in males the scrotum may be split and associated with hypospadias. The condition is known as pseudohermaphroditism.

Phimosis: Phimosis is the narrowing of the prepuce in a male child and may cause straining at micturition. Circumcision will remedy this condition.

Hypospadias: Hypospadias is the term for the condition in which the urethral orifice opens at the level of the glans penis, or at the body of the penis, or at the junction of the penis and scrotum. Plastic operations are recommended for these conditions.

Epispadias: Epispadias is a condition in which the male urethra opens on the dorsum of the penis.

Persistent urachus: Persistent urachus consists of a fistula extending from the fundus of the bladder to the umbilicus. It is a result of a failure of the foetal allantois to close. It should be suspected if urine is excreted through the umbilicus.

Ectopic bladder (ectopia vescae): This is the result of imperfect closure of the anterior abdominal wall and vesical wall. The inside of the bladder produces through a separation in the pubic bone. It is reddish in colour with urine dribbling onto the surface. The skin around the thighs and perianal region should be protected by rubbing vaseline and castor ointment on regularly bases. Cases of octopiavesicae should be reported to the physician for surgical treatment. Abnormalities of the kidneys like agenesis, horse shoe and cystic kidney are rare and clinical diagnosis is not easy.

Skeletal and Locomotor System Abnormalities

Amelia is total absence of limbs, but partial absence, ectromelia, is more common.

Polydactylism: Polydactylism means extra digits. They may be present on the hands or feet or both and they are easy to diagnose. The nurse midwife could tie off these extra digits provided no bony structure is involved. The baby should be referred to the surgeon for surgical treatment if bones are present.

Achondroplasia: Achondroplasia is a form of dwarfism in which the long bones are short but the trunk has a normal development. The babies are unusually short and often have big heads. Achondroplasia tends to run in families and there is no treatment for it. Such babies, when they reach adulthood, may end up in circuses.

Talipes or club foot: Talipes or club foot is of two forms. In talipes equinovarus, the forefoot is turned in wards (inversion) throughout its length and displaced downwards at the ankle. The condition may involve the forefoot only or the whole foot; it may be unilateral or bilateral. The other form is talipes equinovalgus in which the foot is turned outwards (eversion). The varus deformity is far more common than the valgus variety.

The treatment of talipes should commence early in life. The nurse should, therefore, seek medical opinion as soon as the baby is born. Treatment consists of manipulation and splinting or strapping the foot to an over corrected position.

Congenital dislocation of the hip This condition is not easily detected by the nurse midwife. Suspicion may be aroused by asymmetry of the lower limbs or by an abnormal position of one or both legs, or by exaggerated separation of the extended thighs. X-ray examination of the hip confirms the diagnosis. The condition is more common in girls than boys.

Birth Marks

Birth marks are usually due to abnormal collections of blood vessels in the skin and are referred to as naevi or haemangiomata. They occur in various forms at any site and may be single or multiple. Birth marks may disappear spontaneously, persist unchanged, or increase slowly in size. No treatment is necessary in the neonate.

Mental Abnormality

Mongolism is a commonly described mental abnormality. It is supposed to be associated with the presence of an extra chromosome in the genes. The diagnosis of this condition should never be made by the nurse. Moreover, she must study the features of both parents before voicing her suspicion to the physician.

The clinical features of a mongolism are as listed below:

The body has a small head with a rather flat occiput, a small mouth, short upper lip and a protruding tongue. The eyes are slanting and almost almond shaped. The hands are short and stumpy and the big toe is widely separated from the rest of the toes. There is supposed to be a peculiar skin pattern of the palm and sole of the foot. Generally, mongols have poor muscle tone and 25 per cent of them are born with congenital heart disease. They are slow feeders and weight gain is slow.

It is not the nurse's responsibility to disclose this abnormality to the mother. It often dawns on her that the baby is not normal.

Treatment with pituitary and thyroid extracts may be instituted later in life. The primary thing is to teach the mother how to get the baby to feed.

Neonatal Jaundice

Jaundice is the yellow discoloration of body tissue and fluid by bile pigments. In normal circumstances, bile pigments from haemolysed senile red blood cells are carried to the liver where they are conjugated and excreted via the urine and stools. Accumulation of the bile pigments will occur if there is:

a. Excessive destruction of the red blood cells.
b. Abnormality in the transportation of bile.
c. Abnormality in conjugation of bile pigments.

Types of Jaundice

Jaundice of immaturity: Destruction of red blood cells occurs after birth. If the liver is immature and cannot open with its normal functions, conjugation and excretion of the bile pigments are inadequate and jaundice ensues. This type of jaundice occurs in 50 per cent of full term and about 75 to 80 per cent of premature babies. It is usually not present within the first 24 hours of life, rather it is usually detected on the second or third day of life. The jaundice should begin to disappear by the end of the first week, and generally it is not noticeable within a fortnight. This type of jaundice is not accompanied by other symptoms except in severe cases, when the baby may become lethargic and sluggish with its feeds.

Management: The baby is observed closely and some glucose water is given with the baby's feeds.

Haemolytic Jaundice

Haemolytic jaundice is usually associated with destruction or haemolysis of red blood cells. Conditions which predispose to haemolysis are Rhesus and ABO blood group incompatibility. In these conditions, large numbers of red blood cells are destroyed, and there is an excessive and rapid production of bile pigments which a normal liver cannot conjugate. The bile pigment (bilirubin) accumulates in the tissues, causing clinical jaundice within 12 to 24 hours of birth. The jaundice may be associated with anaemia which can run a rapidly progressive course. In severe cases, the baby is drowsy, has rapid respiration and may develop heart failure, kernicterus and die.

Glucose-6-phosphate dehydrogenase (G-6-PD) deficiency: Glucose-6-phosphate dehydrogenase is an essential enzyme in the red blood cells. The absence of this enzyme results in easy destruction of the red cells. The haemolysis could be precipitated by drugs such as salicylates or infection. In some places approximately 20 per cent of males are deficient in this enzyme. In such places, G-6-PD deficiency is a common cause of neonatal jaundice.

Misuse of certain drugs: Neonatal jaundice of the haemolytic type may be caused by excessive administration of vitamin K and sulphonamides.

Infective Jaundice

An infection, which may be bacterial, viral or protozoal, is a common cause of neonatal jaundice, especially in babies born outside the hospital. The organism usually enters the body through the umbilical cord and may attach the liver cells. There is usually a great deal of constitutional disturbance and septicaemia may set in. The jaundice usually develops within seven days of birth and the prognosis is poor.

Obstructive Jaundice

Obstructive jaundice is usually due to congenital obliteration or absence of the bile duct. Therefore, there is an accumulation of bile in the liver and jaundice appears. In this type of jaundice, the urine is dark in colour and the stools are pale. Neonatal jaundice associated with pale stools, dark urine and persisting beyond the second week of life is suggestive of obstructive jaundice. The digestion of fat and the child's appetite are usually impaired in this type of jaundice. In a few cases, operative measures may relieve the obstruction.

Dangers of Jaundice in the Neonate

Kernicterus : This literally means a yellow staining of the brain cells in the basal ganglia. It occurs in the presence of excessive unconjugated bilirubin in the blood. Brain damage occurs and may lead to cerebral palsy or death of the baby. Clinically, a baby with kernicterus refuses feeds, is lethargic and may have convulsions. There is rigidity of the body with complete opisthotonos. Usually, babies with kernicterus die and those who survive develop permanent physical and mental handicaps. There is usually a tendency to recurrent convulsion.

Cirrhosis of the liver: Cirrhosis of the liver may occur, especially in obstructive types of jaundice, because the accumulation of bile destroys the liver cells readily.

Management

Certain types of neonatal jaundice are preventable by proper management of the mother during the 'antenatal period and delivery patients who have had previous blood transfusions or whose previous babies were jaundiced should be investigated for the presence of antibodies in their blood. Pregnant women known to be Rhesus negative should have their blood examined frequently for antibodies. All pregnant women should have Khan or Wasserman tests or the Venereal Diseases Reasearch Laboratory (VDRL) test done to exclude syphilis.

During labour and delivery, a high standard of asepsis and antisepsis must be maintained. The midwife/nurse should report yellow staining or discolouration of the liquor amnii immediately. The umbilical cord should be carefully and well treated to avoid infection.

Daily examination of the neonate is done for early detection of jaundice. The following points should be noted:

a. The colour of the skin and mucous membranes.
b. Colour of the urine and stools.
c. General behaviour and activity.
d. Any sign of infection, especially that of the umbilicus.
e. Ability to suck properly.

Any jaundiced baby should be referred to the paediatrician, especially where the jaundice develops within 24 hours of birth.

Estimation of the serum bilirubin, both total and conjugated fractions, should be done daily. The packed cell volume or haemoglobin should also be checked. Appropriate treatment of infection with antibiotics is necessary and will be prescribed by the medical staff. Exchange blood transfusion is carried out if the unconjugated fraction of the serum bilirubin rises to a critical level (usually 20 mg/100 ml) in mature babies or 18 mg/100 ml in premature babies). This method of treatment removes the excessive unconjugated bilirubin from the blood and prevents cerebral damage. The midwife's duties at exchange transfusion are discussed under "The Management of Haemolytic Disease of the Newborn".

Good nursing care of a jaundiced baby includes keeping the baby warm, giving adequate fluid and isolating the baby if there is any evidence of infection.

The baby may be tube fed if it is too lethargic to suck from the breasts or bottle. A four hourly record of the temperature, apex beat and respiration is kept. The degree of jaundice is noted daily. When the jaundice deepens, kernicterus is liable to occur. The colour of the urine and stools should also be observed. Signs of cerebral irritation and kernicterus should be promptly reported, to a physician. These are neck retraction, or rigidity of the body and limbs, muscular twitching or convulsion. Other signs include: high pitched cry, rolling of the eyes, grunting, irregular breathing cyanotic attacks.

Haemorrhagic Disease of the Neonate

Haemorrhagic disease of the newborn is a bleeding disorder commonly due to low blood prothrombin levels. Coagulation defects or reduced blood platelets may also cause the conditions. The bleeding is often in the mucous membranes of the intestinal tract, but it may also occur in the skin. Haematemesis, melaena, haematuria and bleeding from the umbilical cord are the ways in which the disease shows itself. The bleeding usually occurs within the first four days of life and may be mistaken for the 'swallowed blood' syndrome. If the bleeding is severe, death may occur unless a blood transfusion is given urgently.

Management

Presence of streaks of blood in the vomitus or stools of a neonate should put the nurse on the alert. Medical advice must be sought immediately. Where massive bleeding occurs, the nurse must act sensibly and quickly. The baby is disturbed as little as possible and is kept warm. Shock should be treated and if a physician is not easily available, the nurse should give the baby an injection of vitamin K (1 mg) intramuscularly. The blood-soiled articles are kept for the physician inspection. Blood transfusion may be necessary in severe cases of blood loss.

The baby may be fed in the absence of haematemsis, but it is advisable to withhold feeds and give the baby some subcutaneous or intravenous fluids if there is haematemesis.

A close observation is kept on the baby, noting its colour, pulse rate and the bleeding sites. The colour and any abnormal constituents of the stools and the vomitus are also noted.

Intramuscular injection of vitamin K (1 mg) is given routinely to premature and asphyxiated babies at birth as prophylaxis against this condition.

Haemolytic Disease of the Neonate

The term haemolysis refers to destruction of the red blood cells. Some causes or haemolysis have been discussed under neonatal jaundice. This is here confined to haemolysis caused by Rhesus incompatibility or isoimmunization. The condition is often referred to as "erythroblastosis foetalis."

The red blood cells are covered by different types of proteins called antigens. An antigen similar to that found in the red blood cells of the Rhesus monkey is present in 85 per cent of human beings who are known as Rhesus positive persons; the remaining 15 per cent of the population with no such antigen in their red cells form the Rhesus negative group.

If Rhesus positive red cells get into the blood of a Rhesus negative person, that person will form antibodies against the Rhesus positive cells. The mixing of Rhesus positive and negative red cells may occur through incompatible blood transfusion or when a leak in the placenta occurs during the third stage of labour. Where the latter case affects a Rhesus negative woman, she will develop antibodies which could destroy the positive cells of subsequent foetuses. This explains why erythroblastosis foetalis is not usual with the first baby unless to mother has been previously transfused with Rhesus positive blood before she becomes pregnant.

Where a Rhesus negative woman is married to a Rhesus positive man the offspring of the union are likely to be Rhesus positive individual except where the Rhesus positive antigen is of the heterogygous type. If such a case, some of the children will have Rhesus negative cells. If the positive antigen is of the homozygous type the children will always have Rhesus positive cells. This fact is illustrated below (Table 11.3).

The Rhesus antigen is represented by D, thus a Rhesus negative cell is dd, a Rhesus positive cell homozygous type is DD, and the heter zygous type Dd.

Table 11.3

Rh- mother dd homozygous	*Rh+ father DD homozygous*	*Rh– mother dd homozygous*	*Rh+ father Dd heterozygous*
Children will all be Rh positive heterozygous (Dd)		Children may be Rh negative homozygous (dd), or Rh positive heterozygous (Dd)	

The Rhesus antibodies produced in the maternal blood are capable or crossing the placental barrier, and when they do they attack and destroy the foetal red blood cells. In an attempt to make up for the destroyed cells, the foetus produces additional red blood cells, some of which are immature. These immature cells are called erythroblasts. This explains why haemolytic disease of the newborn is referred to as erythroblastosis foetalis. Bilirubin from the haemolysed cells accumulates in the tissues, and jaundice may occur at birth, or appear within twelve hours of birth. A certain degree of anaemia is always present but the accompanying pallor may not be easily detected as it is masked by the jaundice. As the antibodies derived from the mother in utero by the foetus are gradually used up, haemolysis of the infant's red cells slowly subsides and ceases completely within a few weeks.

Diagnosis

All Rhesus negative women should have their blood examined for Rhesus antibodies at booking and subsequently at the 28th, 32nd, 34th and 36th weeks of pregnancy. The presence of antibodies in the blood of a pregnant woman indicates that the baby may be affected. The level of antibodies in the blood is expressed in titre and the higher the titre the more severely would the baby be affected.

At birth, examination of both the mother's and the baby's blood will confirm the diagnosis. The maternal venous blood is examined for the presence of antibodies and the baby's cord blood is examined for the following:

a. The presence of antibodies by the Coomb's test; a positive Coomb's test confirms the presence of antibodies in the infant's blood.
b. The level of haemoglobin or packed red cell volume.

c. The serum bilirubin.
d. The blood group and Rhesus factor.
e. The presence of erythroblasts.

Clinical Features

An affected baby is jaundiced and anaemic. The jaundice may be present at birth or may become evident within 24 hours of birth. The degree of jaundice and anaemia depends on how severely affected the baby is. In a mild case, anaemia and jaundice are slight, the general condition of the baby is usually good. When the haemoglobin level of the baby is less than 100 per cent, jaundice appears very early and becomes rapidly intense and deep. The baby is lethargic and has rapid respiration. The doctor may detect enlargement of the liver and spleen in a moderately severe case. The liquor amnii in such a case may be yellow in colour and the cord is also stained yellow. Where jaundice is so intense, the term icterus gravis neonatorum is used.

The most severe form of erythroblasosis foetalis results in a still-birth or hydrops foetalis. The placenta is large and pale and the foetus shows evidence of generalized oedema. Babies who at birth are severely anaemic and jaundiced with signs of cardiac failure frequently die within 24 hours of birth, irrespective of the treatment given.

In the very severe form of icterus gravis neonatorum, unconjugated bilirubin may rise to a dangerous level and lead to kernicterus due to staining of the basal ganglia, as described earlier in neonatal jaundice.

Treatment

Increasing level of antibodies during pregnancy is an indication for premature induction of labour, or a highly specialized treatment—intrauterine blood transfusion. The later is carried out if the foetus is severely affected prior to the 32nd week of gestation. At birth, the cord is clamped immediately to avoid giving the baby more of the blood containing the offending antibodies. Examination of the core blood, as already stated, confirms the diagnosis and reveals the severity of the disease.

About 40 per cent of the affected babies do not require treatment. Others who are mildly affected with increasing anaemia are given simple blood transfusion. Exchange blood transfusion is the treatment for moderately severe and the very severe cases. However, the decision as to the method of treatment is based on the clinical condition of the infant and on the laboratory results of the cord blood.

Exchange Blood Transfusion

The aim of exchange blood transfusion is to correct anaemia, remove most of the maternal Rhesus antibodies and reduce the level of serum bilirubin. Packed cells of Rhesus negative blood of the same ABO group as that of the baby are used for the transfusion. This ensures that the maternal antibodies do not destroy the new negative red cells. Fresh, compatible, Rhesus negative blood at body temperature should be used.

Technique of exchange blood transfusion: A special polythene umbilical catheter is inserted into the umbilical vein (For this reason, the nurse midwife should not apply cord powder to the umbilicus of an affected baby). Ten to twenty millilitres of blood are withdrawn from the baby and an equivalent amount of the compatible Rhesus negative blood is put into the infant's circulation through the same catheter. The procedure of withdrawal and replacement is repeated several times until a total of 180 ml/kg of body weight of the compatible blood is used.

The responsibility of the nurse is to set and prepare the trolley with the instruments to be used for the procedure. She will also watch the baby.

Requirements

- 1 litre of normal saline for rinsing the syringe
- Complete giving set (sterilized and checked)
- Drip stand
- Polythene tubing and cannulae
- Padded cross spling
- Glass jar for discarded blood.

Instruments (sterilized and ready for use)

- 1 small Bard-Parker handle and blade
- 1 pair of plain dissecting forceps
- 1 pair of toothed dissecting forceps
- 4 pairs of mosquito artery forceps
- 1 pair of dressing scissors
- 1 pair of stitch scissors (sharp pointed)
- 3 small, curved, triangular suture needles
- 1 aneurysm needle
- 2 towel clips

- 2 20-ml syringes 1 3-way stop cocks (Luer fitting)
- Eyeless needled suture with 3/0 silk.

Other sterile items: Equipments include instrument dish, two kidney dishes, three gallipots, catgut, dressing towels, keyhole operation towel, gowns, caps, masks, gloves, cotton wool and gauze swabs and rubber tubing.

Drugs and solutions include Hibitane in spirit, heparin, 10 per cent calcium gluconate, 5 per cent sodium bicarbonate, vitamin K, digoxin, collodion and cortisone. Cardiac and respiratory stimulants and oxygen are kept handy. The room should be comfortably warm (temperature 26.6°C) with adequate lighting.

Duties to the Baby

Preparation of the baby: It is advisable to withhold feed from the baby four hours before the procedure in order to avoid overdistension of the abdomen. The baby is then bandaged to a cross splint. A stethoscope for frequent checking of the heart rate during the procedure is strapped to the left chest wall of the infant. The apex beat and respiration may be monitored by cardiorater if available. In small hospitals, a nurse sits by the head of the baby and observes it colour, respiration and heart rate every 5 to 15 minutes. A record of the blood injected and withdrawn and any drug administered is also kept by the nurse midwife. The physician is notifying the following:

- Progressive tachycardia or bradycardia
- Respiratory distress
- Tremors of twitching
- Cyanosis.

If the baby is restless, the nurse could calm it by giving a stuffed teat soaked in 5 per cent glucose for the baby to suck. After the transfusion the baby still requires special attention and observation for a few hours. He is kept warm and the quarter to half hourly record of respiration and heart beats is continued for at least six hours and the umbilical dressing is checked frequently, for any bleeding.

Neonatal Infections

Babies may acquire infections through the placenta from an amniotic fluid as they transverse the birth canal, or after birth from sources such as carers hands, contaminated objects or droplet infection. Neonatal infection is a serious problem on account of the following known facts.

a. The newborn baby has a low body resistance against infecting organisms.
b. Diagnosis of neonatal infection may not be easily made since there are usually few symptoms.
c. Infection in the newborn accounts for a high percentage of neonatal mortality.
d. In a nursery, there is the risk of spread of the infection to other infants.

The vigilance of a midwife or nurse and her prompt report of unusual signs in a baby to the physician are of great help in the early diagnosis and treatment of neonatal infections. The nurse must, therefore, be infection conscious and develop a keen sense of observation. Infants who are liable and highly susceptible to infections should be observed closely for the slightest sign of infection. Such infants are:

1. The premature baby.
2. Babies born following early rupture of membranes.
3. Babies born following prolonged and difficult labour.
4. Babies who have undergone prolonged resuscitation at birth.
5. Babies who have undergone operations for surgical correction of congenital abnormalities.
6. Infants borne by mothers who have diabetes, toxaemia of pregnancy and chronic anaemia.
7. Babies whose mothers have active tuberculosis.
8. Babies delivered in hygienic surroundings.
9. Bottle fed babies.

Diagnosis of Infection

At times, the nurse may find nothing suggestive of infection in a baby, but her suspicion should be aroused if the baby fails to thrive in spite of good feeding. The presence of one or more of the following signs is very suggestive of infection.

1. Refusal to suck.
2. Vomiting
3. Diarrhoea with or without blood or mucus in the stools.
4. Abdominal distension.
5. Irritability.
6. Weak or high pitched cry.
7. Listlessness or lethargy and loss of interest in the surroundings.

8. Twitching of limbs or generalized convulsions.
9. Diminution or absence of reflexes especially the Moro or startle reflex.
10. Full fontanelles.
11. Alteration in the rate and rhythm of respiration, especially laboured or grunting respiration.
12. Nasal discharge.
13. Small red patches on the skin due to rupture of tiny capillaries—petechiae.
14. Ecchymoses—large bleeding areas on the skin, frank bleeding from the rectum and mouth.
15. Presence of rash especially pustules, sclerema—hardening of the subcutaneous tissue.
16. Jaundice.
17. Cyanotic attacks.

The temperature may be raised, but the nurse midwife must be aware that a low temperature in the presence of infection is not uncommon in the neonates.

Investigations which may help in the diagnosis of neonatal infections include:

- Estimation of haemoglobin
- White blood cell count/complete blood cell count
- Urinalysis/testing of urine and meconium for specific organisms
- Blood culture/testing of amniotic fluid. Placental tissue, cord blood for specific organisms
- Lumbar puncture to enable examination of CSF
- MRI, CT Scans and chest X-rays.

Prevention

The role of the nurse or midwife is to be observant in order to diagnose infection early and secure good care and management for the baby. She also has a duty to prevent infection as much as possible. Good antenatal care including adequate education of the mother, goes a long way in the prevention of infection. All pregnant women should be brought into labour in good health. Conditions such as pre-eclampsia, anaemia and multiple pregnancy predispose to prematurity and should be prevented or adequately treated. Where the membranes have ruptured for more than 12 to 18 hours, prophylactic antibiotics must be given to the mother. The need for aseptic techniques during labour and delivery cannot be over emphasized. The rooming-in method, whereby babies kept in nurseries and the risk of infection. All health professionals should take universal precautions based on the routine use of techniques that reduce exposure to blood and other body fluids and tissues that may convey blood borne pathogens, every client considered as a possible source of infection.

Control of Infection in a Nursery

Nurses and midwives, especially those working in nurseries, must adopt good techniques for handling babies to prevent or control infection. This includes washing of hands before and after attending to each baby. The use of paper towels and antiseptic hand lotion is recommended where they are available. There should be a separate gown for each individual baby, kept at the side of the cot. Masks must be used always. Any attendant with a cold or any form of infection should not handle babies.

It is not hygienic to change babies in the middle of a feed. Napkins must be well disposed of in bins which should ideally have foot operated lids. These bins are best emptied by those who do not handle the babies. Since babies are likely to get infected during bath time in the nurseries, some authorities advocate the washing of the baby's face and the changing of his napkins only during the first three days of life. The use of hexachlorophane in bathing babies has recently been recommended as providing effective protection to the baby's skin.

Bathrooms must be carbolized after every use with antiseptic lotion such as cetremide (1:100) plus Hibitane (1:100). The weighing machine should also be carbolized and a separate clean towel used for each baby. Ideally, babies should be managed individually with separate equipment for each baby. The cots and lockers should be well carbolized and the equipment cleaned and sterilized weekly and after each use. It is wrong to put two babies in the same city but this practice is not infrequently seen in small hospitals due to lack of equipment. Overcrowding favours the spread of infection, so each baby should sleep in his own cost and the cot should be covered with a mosquito net. Visitors, including hospital staff other than the ward's medical and nursing staff, are not allowed in the nursery. The mothers must be made to wash their hands before feeding the babies. The milk kitchen should be fly proof. The staff of the milk kitchen should not work in the general kitchen should be fly proof. The staff of the milk kitchen should not work in the general kitchen.

Infected and/or potentially infectious babies, e.g. babies born on the farm must be isolated and may be given antitetanus serum and a course of antibiotics.

Emphasis should be placed on the importance of breast feeding because artificially fed babies are more prone to infection. The mother should not be allowed to tamper with the baby's cord. Immunization against specific infections such as tuberculosis, measles, tetanus, etc. is a positive measure for preventing infection. The traditional practice of nursing babies in a room to the exclusions of visitors also helps in the prevention of infection.

Nursing Management

A nurse should always secure good management for the baby in whom she suspects infection. But nurses working in the peripheral or rural areas may have to manage simple superficial infections such as:

1. Pustules or spettic spots.
2. Paronychia.
3. Neonatal mastitis.
4. Sticky eyes.
5. Thrush.

Septic Spots

Septic spots are often found in the flexures of skin folds. They are due to staphylococcal infections of the skin. The pustules may be punctured with a sterile needle. The infected area should be cleaned with Eusol and dabbed with 1 per cent gentian violet or Hibitaine in spirit (1:200).

Paronychia

Paronychia is an infection of the nail bed: it often occurs in babies who suck their fingers. A superficial lesion is treated as a septic spot. For the severe lesion with an abscess in the nail bed, medical aid must be sought. The abscess is incised and cleaned with Eusol. Gentian violet or acriflavine dressing is applied to the wound until it is healed. Systemic antibiotics may be prescribed by the doctor. In addition to the above, treatment, mittens made from cotton material may be worn to prevent the child from sucking his fingers.

Neonatal

Mastitis Neonatal mastitis should be left alone, but if it is secondarily infected, and there is abscess formation, the nurse should refer the baby to a physician for incision and discharge of the abscess. Systemic antibiotics may be given.

Sticky Eyes

The baby's eyes may be infected during delivery, or by the attendant. This could be prevented by treating any maternal vaginal discharge in the antenatal period. The baby's eyes should be swabbed with sterile wet wool swabs at birth.

Sticky eyes should not be confused with the severe infection of the eye called ophthalmia neonatorum. Sticky eyes are usually moist with minimal whitish discharge and there is no underlying redness or inflammation of the eyelids. Two to three hourly irrigation with normal saline and instillation of 10 per cent. Albucid eye drops constitute the treatment. If there is no improvement in 36 hours, the physician must be informed and a swab of the eye is sent for bacteriological investigation.

Thrush

oral thrush is characterized by white patches in the mouth of the baby. The patches are over and under the tongue and can be found in the cheeks. If an attempt is made to remove these patches, red raw areas will be revealed. Similar patches due to milk curds leave healthy tissue underneath when they are cleaned.

In mild cases, the baby's general health is not affected. The baby feeds and thrives well. In such circumstances, treatment could be undertaken by the nurse and this consists of painting the mouth with 1 per cent aqueous gentian violet twice daily. In severe cases, the baby go as off its feeds, becomes irritable has a greyish look, and passes loose stools. Medical aid must be sought in such cases. Treatment is with nystatin drops or syrup (200,000 units per ml given six hourly). To prevent oral thrush vaginal moniliasis in pregnant women should be treated vigorously. Other preventive measures include good nursery techniques, adequate sterilization of feeding equipment, daily inspection of babies mouths and isolation of an infected baby.

Serious Infections

Serious infections are those which interfere with the baby's well being, and constiture a threat to life. Such cases should be referred to the physician for prompt and adequate treatment.

Omphalitis

Omphalitis is an infection of the umbilical cord. It is dangerous because the infection can spread quickly and easily to the liver, resulting in hepatitis, jaundice and generalized septicaemia. It is always better to prevent this condition by the midwife handling the dressing of the chord herself. Dressing arrangements should be made for babies sent home before the cord separates.

The nurse midwife must seek medical help without delay if the area around the umbilicus is red and inflamed. Greenish discharge and an offensive small are other signs of infection of the cord.

Hot fomentations may be applied to the umbilical area where there is acute cellulitis. The nurse midwife should watch out and report haemorrhage, abdominal distension and jaundice which are serious complications of omphalitis. The treatment usually given is the appropriate systemic antibiotic after a swab specimen taken from the cord has been sent for bacteriological investigation.

Ophthalmia Neonatorum

Ophthalmia neonatorum is defined as a purulent discharge from the eyes of an infant within the first 21 days of life. The affected eye is red and oedematous with copious purulent discharge. The eyes are usually tightly shut. This serious infection of the eyes may result in blindness if not well managed. The causative organism may be a gonococcus, *Staphylococcus aureus*, a *streptococcus*, or any other bacteria. The nurse should always refer the affected baby to a physician.

The treatment consists of isolation of the baby and local instillation of antibiotic eye drops, such as penicillin or sulphacetamide (10 per cent Albucid) solutions, A swab must be taken from the ees for culture before commencing treatment. Intensive penicillin eye treatment is often instituted. A solution of crystalline penicillin (2500 units per ml) is instilled into the conjunctival sac every 5 minutes until the purulent discharge ceases. Neomycin or chloramphenicol eye ointment are also used to prevent the eyelids adhering together, thus ensuring good drainage of the conjunctival sac. Systemic antibiotics may be prescribed in addition. The eyes should be gently wiped dry with cotton wool swabs. Irrigation bathing of the eye is not recommended, especially in the acute phase. The baby should be laid on the affected side so that the pus from the affected eye will drain onto a dressing laid in the cot.

Prevention: Prevention is the main role of the nurse. To prevent ophthalmia neonatorum the nurse should do the following:

1. Examine patients regularly for vaginal discharges.
2. Ensure adequate treatment for patients with vaginal discharges during pregnancy.
3. Clean the baby's eyes with sterile wool swabs as soon as the head is born.
4. Wash the baby's face with sterile water and wool swabs at bath times to avoid infection of the eyes.
5. Instruct mothers not to tamper with baby's eyes or wipe them with their handkerchiefs.

The practice of instilling prophylactic eye drops into baby's eyes at birth no longer holds, except in epidemics.

Pemphigus Neonatorum

Pemphigus neonatorum is defined as bullous eruptions of the skin. It is characterized by watery blisters which soon become pustules. These burst leaving raw, moist areas surrounded by dead skin. A case of pemphigus neonatorum should be referred to the physician and reported to the local medical health authority, because the disease is highly contagious and tends to occur in epidemic; Pemphigus may be syphilitic in origin, in which case the palms and soles are affected. *Staphylococcus aureus* is sometimes the causative organism.

Management: A swab is taken from the affected spot and examined bacteriologically. Treatment by the administration of the appropriate antibiotics both locally and systemically, is instituted as soon as possible. The baby should be nursed naked and a bed cradle may be used to keep off the bed clothes. By so doing, the areas will be kept dry and healing is promoted. The areas are cleaned with surgical spirit or Hibitane in spirit and painted with 1 per cent gentian violet.

Good nursery technique, daily examination of babies and avoidance of skin irritation constitute the preventive measures.

Infective Gastroenteritis

Infective gastroenteritis is fairly common in the tropics and the mortality rate is high. It tends to occur in epidemic, especially where babies are bottle fed and the nursery technique is poor, or mothers have unhygienic habits. Thrush is a fairly common cause. The baby vomits an had diarrhoea. The stools are frequent and yellow. The baby loses a lot of fluid and electrolytes in this way, thus becoming rapidly dehydrated and acidotic. The eyes and fontanelle are sunken with overlapping of the skull bones. Respiration is deep and rapid. In severe cases, abdominal distension is present and the baby may collapse and become grey in colour. If untreat death ensues rapidly.

Hospitalization of the baby for immediate correction of fluid and electrolyte loss is imperative. One sixth molar lactate and Darrow's solution are the fluids which may be given intravenously or subcutaneously. Nurses practising in rural areas must transfer such babies to hospital for urgent treatment. Subcutaneous fluids may be given if the facilities are available but the baby must be transferred to hospital without delay. Sips of glucose solution (or tablespoonful to 600 ml of water to which one teaspoonful of salt and some orange juice have been added) should be offered to the baby if the journey to the hospital is likely to be long.

A course of antibiotics if often given following the stool examination and culture. Nursing care entails keeping the baby warm. Good barrier nursing or isolation and proper disposal of napkins are necessary measures to prevent spread of the infection. Zinc and castor oil ointment is rubbed into the buttocks at each napkin change to avoid sore buttocks. The baby is fed orally only when it has stopped vomiting. A small amount of clear fluid or glucose water is given first, then diluted milk may be given a little at a time. Where applicable, the mother must be educated regarding breastfeeding and hygienic methods of handling the baby's feeding equipment and preparation of feeds. Vitamin supplements are given to replace what has been lost and to aid early recovery.

Neonatal Tetanus

Neonatal tetanus is another dreadful infection with a high mortality rate. Infection usually occurs if delivery is conducted in unhygienic surroundings, or when poor methods of cutting and managing of the cord are employed. In some places bamboo barks or dirty knives and pieces of broken bottles are used to cut the cord in the erroneous belief that a baby whose cord is so cut will not steal. The cord is also treated with cow dung and herbes which are conducive to infection by *Clostridium tetani*. When the organism enters the body, it liberates some toxins which affect the nervous muscle spasm as well as spasm of the jaw muscle spasms, rigidity and opisthotonus. Generalized muscle spasm as well as spasm of the jaw muscles prevent the baby from sucking. The baby is usually irritable and cries a lot because of the frequent spasms. Its face is wrinkled and it wears an anxious look or a sardonic smile.

Treatment: To prevent neonatal tetanus, mothers should be given tetanus toxoid during pregnancy. The importance of delivery in clean surroundings under adequate supervision of a competent nurse is emphasized to the mother during the health talks. At birth, the cord should be cut under strict aseptic and antiseptic precautions. Cord dressings must be clean or, ideally sterile.

Babies born in unhygienic surroundings should be given prophylactic antitetanus serum (750 units) after an intial test dose. Immunization of all infants against tetanus is recommended and must be followed.

Established cases of neonatal tetanus must be reported to the physician without delay. Arrangements should be made for the immediate admission of the baby to a hospital.

Treatment consists of intramuscular injection of 1000 units of antitetanus serum, heavy sedation and feeding through a nasogastric tube. The usual sedatives given include Valium (1-2 mg three times a day), given usually with Largactil (chlorpromazine) (6.5 mg six hourly), or phenobarbitone (7.5 mg six hourly). Paraldehyde (2 ml) by intramuscular injection may be given at six or eight hourly intervals. Massive doses of penicillin, e.g. crystallin penicillin (200,000 units six hourly), should be given.

Effective treatment of neonatal tetanus depends on efficient nursing care. The airways must be constantly cleared of secretions and oxygen should be given as often as required. The baby should be disturbed as little as possible. All necessary procedures must be carried out when the baby has been heavily sedated.

Respiratory Infections

Babies may be easily infected by the mother or a member of staff who has a cold. Upper respiratory tract infection in a baby is recognized by snuffles and a running nose. The baby's cry may be hoarse if the larynx is also affected.

The snuffle and congestion in the nose can be relieved by the use of 5 per cent ephedrine nasal drops twice daily. Antibiotics need not be given in mild cases. The baby should be kept warm and dry.

Bronchopneumonia

The baby with bronchopneumonia is usually ill with rapid, laboured and grunting respiration. He may be cyanosed and pyrexial, but at times there may be no rise in temperature. Coughing is not a common symptom but diarrhoea and poor tolerance of feeds may feature.

Ideally, the baby should be nursed in an incubator where warmth, humidity and oxygen are provided. He is propped up and should wear light loose clothing to allow for easy breathing. A clear airway is ensured by frequent suction of mucus from the nostrils and mouth, especially if the baby is mucousy. Observation of the infant's colour, respiration and temperature is made 2 to 4 hourly to determine the baby's progress. Feeds are best given by tube to prevent respiratory distress and exhaustion. Antibiotics are given as prescribed by the physician.

Meningitis

Meningitis is infection of the meninges often caused by *Escherichia coli* or a pneumococcus or meningococcus.

The baby is fretful and cries all the time or when he is picked up. The anterior fontanelle is tense and may be bulging. The neck may be stiff, and pyrexia and twitching or convulsions may be present. The diagnosis is confirmed by lumbar puncture and culture of the cerebrospinal fluid.

Treatment: Treatment consists of the administration of a sedative to counteract convulsions and the appropriate antibiotics. Good nursing care entails keeping the baby calm, tube feeding and barrier nursing to prevent the spread of infection. A high temperature is reduced by tepid sponging or fanning. Early diagnosis and treatment are necessary if unpleasant outcomes such as hydrocephalus, mental retardation, blindness, deafness, epilepsy and paralysis, are to be avoided.

Pyelitis

Pyelitis is an infection of the pelvis of the kidney. The infection may involve the whole urinary tract. Diagnosis of this is not very easy as there is no specific sign and the baby cannot volunteer any symptoms. It is usually suspected if a baby has cyanotic attacks for no apparent reason. The baby may be limp, grey in colour and pyrexial. Reluctance to feed and vomiting are usually prevent. Vomiting is more significant in a breast fed baby. Pyelitis is supposed to be more common in female than male babies. A urine specimen should be examined in the laboratory to confirm the diagnosis.

Treatment: Treatment consists of keeping the baby warm giving extra fluid and the appropriate antibiotics.

The overall aim of management is to provide prompt and effective treatment that reduces the risk of septicaemia and life threatening septic shock in this vulnerable group. Good management includes:

- Caring for the baby in a warm thermoneutral environment and observing for temperature instability
- Good hydration and the correction of electrolyte imbalance, with demand feeding if possible and intravenous fluids as required
- Prompt systemic antibiotic or other drug therapy and local treatment of infection
- Ongoing monitoring of the baby's neurobehavioural status
- Reducing separation of mother and baby if the baby requires admission to a neonatal intensive care unit, then the nurse or midwife should encourage parents to be with their baby
- Providing evidence-based information, support and reassurance to parent
- Encouraging breastfeeding, or expressing of milk, and informing women of the important role of breast milk in fighting infections.

Nursing Management of Neonate at Risk (Please See Table 11.4)

Table 11.4: Nursing care plan of preterm newborn

Problem (1)	Reason (2)	Objection (3)	Nursing interventions (4)	Evaluation (5)
1. Risk for impaired gas exchange. related to: • Inadequate surfactant Immaturity of pulmonary vessel musculature which restricts vasoconstriction • Immaturity of CNS • Ineffective airway clearance • Anaemia • Cold stress.	*Subjective Data* • Grunting *Objective Data* • Abnormal pO_2 • Abnormal pCO_2 • Symptoms of RD (tachypnoea, nasal flaring, grunting retractions, rales) • Diminished or absent breath sounds • Central cyanosis • Cardiac arrhythmias.	Client will dominate adequate gas exchange	• Note data placing infant at high risk for impaired gas exchange or respiratory distress. These include gestational age, length of labour, type of delivery Apgar score, maternal medication during labour and need for resuscitation • Assess respiratory rate, note apnoea. • Assess symptoms of respiratory distress. • Assess for cyanosis • Suction nares and oropharynx as needed. Note transcutaneous oxygen monitor or pulse oximeter before suctioning. Limit time of airway obstruction. to 10 to 15 seconds. Administer additional O_2 needed • Assess and record oxygen levels as noted on the transcutaneous oxygen monitor or pulse oximeter • Assess skin under transcutaneous probe site at each probe change • Assess arterial blood gas values • Assess haemoglobin level and haematocrit. • Administer oxygen as needed by mask, hood ET or MV or IPPB and DEEP • Note and record oxygen in inspired air (FiO_2) every hour • Provide for and note results of chest radiographs. • Position infant on side with rolled diaper behind back or in supine position with rolled diaper beneath shoulder to produce slight hypertension • Perform postural drainage, chest physiotherapy, or or lobe vibration as ordered • Maintain baby temperature • Provide feedings by nasogastric or orogastric tubes, not by nipple until able to suck • Provide tactile stimulation • Administer medication as ordered to facilitate respiration and gas exchange.	Client will evidence minimal respiratory distress symptoms absence of broncho pulmonary dysuria, normal pO_2: pCO_2 level.
2. Altered for fluids deficit or excess related to: Fluid volume deficency • Insensible fluid	*Subjective Data* • Fluid volume excess • Fluid volume deficit *Objective Data* • Fluid Volume Deficit • Poor skin turgor.	Client will demonstrate adequate fluid volume	Fluid volume deficit. • Assess dehydration- Skin turgor, anterior fontanelle for depression, urine output (amount, frequency, colour) and specific gravity of urine. • Weight daily and record weight at some time of day with the same scale	Client will evidence adequate hydration, similar intake and output. Absence of glycosuria,

Contd...

Contd...

Problem (1)	Reason (2)	Objection (3)	Nursing interventions (4)	Evaluation (5)
losses in lungs and skin • Altered intake • Immature kidney function with inability to conserve fluids • Electrolytes instability Fluid volume excess • Excessive amounts of fluids. • Electrolyte instability Reduced glomerular filtration rate.	• Dry mucus membrane dry skin • Depressed anterior fontanella • Increased urinary output • Urine sp. gravity 1.013; diluted urine. Fluid volume excess. • Weight gain in excess 20-30 g/day • Rales, dyspnoea or tachypnoea • Oedema • Elevated BUN and creatinine levels • Elevated uric acid • Acidic pH • Oliguria.		• Monitor intake and output and compare. • Assess haemoglobin, haematocrit and electrolyte values • Do a urine specific gravity assay from urine and collections bag or aspirate urine from diaper • Assess blood pressure pulse, and mean arterial • Minimize loss of water through skin by using clothing warming, and humidifying oxygen and monitoring a neutral thermal environment • Administer IV fluids as ordered • Assess symptoms of hypocalcaemia-lethargy, high-pitched cry, abdominal distention, twitching, hypotonia, convulsions and apnoea • Assess IV site every hour. Assess oedema or swelling • Assess skin turgor. Fluid volume excess • Weigh daily. Monitor intake and output • Monitor haemodynamic status • Monitor serum electrolyte values • Monitor arterial blood gas values • Auscultate breath sounds • Assess for oedema	normal urine specific gravity, normal Hct pH, weight gain of 20-30 g/day normal BUN, pressure creatinine uric acid
3. Risk for hypothermia or hyperthermia related to Hypothermia • Decreased ratio of body mass and body surface area • Decreased subcutaneous fat; minimal fat • Limited brown fat • Exposure to a cold environment. Hyperthermia • Excessive clothing • Overwarming • Inability to seat • Inadequate fluids • Inability to shiver • Inadequate glucose Store.	*Subjective Data* Restless (for both cond) Objective Data Hypothermia. • Skin temp below 97° F • Axillary temp below 97.7 °F • Increased activity restless, hyperactive • Poor feeder • Cool, pale skin • Cool hands and feet • Symptoms of RD. Hyperthermia • Axillary temp. 99.5°F • Perspiration on face head • Apnoea, seizures • Increased resp. rate	Client will not have hypothermia or hyperthermia	• Maintain neutral thermal environment. The premature newborn may require radiant warmer, isolette, incubator, or open crib with appropriate clothing • Warm humidified oxygen to 88 to 93 °F • Monitor radiant warmer, and isoletter for temperature and humidity. Environmental temperature should be 98.6 °F, relative humidity of 50-80%. • Provide gradual warming after cold stress • Feed regularly by whatever method is appropriate nasogastric tube, prmie nipple. Monitor blood glucose levels • Weigh infant monitor weight; If there is inadequate weight gain, assess temperature of the environment • Assess ability to adopt to decreased temperature. in isolette or to room temperature. • Monitor laboratory result. If studies that may be done for hyperthermia and hypothermia. These may include serum glucose and bilirubin determination. • Administer intravenous glucose if ordered.	Client will evidence axillary temperature of 97.7 °F to 98.6 °F. Absence of perspiration, apnoea, seizures, symptoms of respiratory distress, normal heart rate

Contd..

Contd...

Problem (1)	Reason (2)	Objection (3)	Nursing interventions (4)	Evaluation (5)
• Anaerobic metabolism • Very thin epidermis with proximity of blood vessels to skin.	• Flushed skin. becoming dry.			
4. Risk for CNS injury related to • Hypoxia • Hypoglycaemia • Birth trauma • Hyperbilirubinaemia.	*Objective Data* • Respiratory distress • Hyperglycaemia (twitching jerking, eyerolling, convulsions) • Tense or bulging fontanelle • Hypotonia • Lethargy • Large head circumference • Low Hb% • Hct elevated • Elevated bilirubin level • High pitched cry • Opisthotonos • Convulsions • Anaemia.	Client will remain free from CNS injury	• Assess for symptoms of CNS damage, which includes-Lethargy; hypotonia; tense; bulging fontanelle seizures; high pitched cry; labored respirations cyanosis, apnoea; flacid guadriparesis, unresponsiveness; hypotension, tonic posturing • Assess respirations and apnoea. Support respiratory function. Provide supplemental oxygen as needed. • Assess for hypoglycaemia. Monitor blood glucose levels. Maintain glucose level by maintaining feeding or administering glucose. • Assess hypocalcaemia (twitching, eyerolling, convulsion) Administer calcium as ordered • Measure head circumference • Assess for hyperbilirubinaemia/Kernicterus. • Colour for jaundice, Lethargy, hyper-reflexion ophisthotonos-convulsions, bilirubin levels • Assist with an exchange transfusion if needed. • Administer medication to control seizures if necessary. These include phenobarbitone or phenotoin.	Client will evidence absence of hypoxia, hypoglycaemia, hyper bilirubinaemia anaemia
5. Altered nutrition: Less than body requirement, related to • Inadequate iron stores • Minimal glycogen stores • Cold stress that deplete glucose • Hypoxia that deplete glucose • Inability of kidney to	*Objective Data* • Respiratory distress unable to nurse • Gags when bottlefed. • Dribbles when bottlefed • Tires easily • Requires nipple for premature infant. • Unable to maintain adequate suction around nipple. • Loses more than 10 to 15% of birth weight. • Gains weight	Client will demonstrate adequate nutrition	• Assess to determine readiness and ability for feeding—sucking, swallowing, gag reflex. • Assess respirations and respiratory rate. • Assess energy available and degree of fatigue with feeding • Reduce situations that increase metabolism and need for calories. This includes maintaining the temperature and respirations and handling as little as possible • Weigh daily and measure head circumference and length weekly • Auscultate blood sounds • Observe tolerance of feedings-vomiting. regurgitations, diarrhoea, positive guiac test result, excessive gastric residual with tube feeding	Client will evidence appropriate weight gain (20-30 g/day)

Contd...

Contd...

Problem (1)	*Reason (2)*	*Objection (3)*	*Nursing interventions (4)*	*Evaluation (5)*
and reabsorb substances • Immature enzyme production that impairs metabolism. • Reduce Hct that hampers absorption of fat and others • Immaturity of Cardiac sphincter • Weak, absent reflexes needed for feeding.			• Administer parenteral fluids as needed for total parenteral nutrition (TPN). Assess reactions -elevated temperature, dyspnoea, vomiting, cyanosis • Administer tube feeding as needed. Insure proper placement of tube, prevention of air entry to stomach and also administration 20 mg (1 ml/minutes) • Initiate feedings when possible. Use nipple for preterm (water glucose-formula) • Initiate intermittent tube feedings as indicated. • Do not perform postural drainage for at least 1 hour after a feeding.	
6. Risk for infection related to • Immature WBCs • Reduced transfer of IgG • Lack of transfer of IgA if not breastfeed • Impaired skin integrity • Ruptured membranes • Transplacental acquired infection. • Ascending infections • Exposure to diagnostic therapeutic and monitoring procedures	*Subjective Data* • Listless • Poor feeding *Objective Data* • Active infection of parents, visitors or staff • Inadequate cord care • Injection site not wiped with alcohol • Equipment not cleaned properly • Symptoms of sepsis, eye infections, cord infection or skin infection • Sudden increase or decrease of WBC count • Low platelet count • Temp. instability • Hypoglycaemia • Hyperglycaemia • Metabolic acidosis • Culture indicating infection.	Client will demonstrate absence of infection	• Review labour and delivery records for length of time membranes were ruptured and whether resuscitation was required • Note estimated date of impairment. Assess gestational age by the new ballard score • Wash hands according to protocol. Have parents wash hands before handling the preterm infant • Ensure proper space between infants, cribs, and isolettes • Isolate infected infants in isolettes or in separate isolation rooms • Establish cohorts of infants • Follow appropriate medical aseptic practices in handling infants equipment, linens and clothing • Assess staff and visitors infections. This includes skin lesions, draining wounds, respiratory infections fever, gastroenteritis, active oral herpes simplex, and herpes zoster • Provide cord care according to hospital protocol • Wipe injection site before insertion • Use aseptic technique with suctioning according to protocol • Observe for signs of infection- hypotonia, hyper-thermia, Lethargy, resp. distress, petachiae, nasal congestion, drainage, from eyes, moist umbilical cord rash, etc.	Client will evidence cord drying, absence of phlebitis on IV Site, normal WBC counts, Platelet count normal temperature , pH, normal culture Absence of symptoms of infection

Contd...

Contd...

Problem (1)	*Reason (2)*	*Objection (3)*	*Nursing interventions (4)*	*Evaluation (5)*
			• Observe signs of late onset of infection (after the first week) • Obtain specimen assess laboratory tests done to diagnosis of infection. (urine, blood CSF, etc.)- Assist with lumbar puncture • Administer antibiotics as ordered • Assign for signs and shock or DIC (Bradycardia, low BP, temp instability listless, oedema) • Encourage breastfeeding or use breast milk	
7. Risk for bowel injury related to • Inactivity • Decreased GI motility • NEC • Altered nutritional intake.	*Objective Data* • NEC (Necrotizing Entero colitis) • Distended abdomen • Absent bowel sounds • Bloody diarrhoea • Regurgitations • Bile stained emesis • Excessive gastric residual • Reduced fluid and feeding intake • Dehydration • Diminished bowel sounds • Abnormal stools constipation or diarrhoea.	Client will demonstrate normal bowel eliminations	• Assess for stools- Frequency and characteristics. • Assess bowel sounds • Asses for abdominal distention, measuring abd. circumference and percussion of abdomen. • Assess history for risk factors predisposing to NEC • Ensure adequate fluid intake-IV fluids, intake and output and assess for dehydration. • Reduce trauma and pressure to abdomen. This includes affording use of diapers; a voiding rectal thermometer, touching and stroking extremities, head, face while talking to infant rather handling • Assess for symptoms of NEC. These include: – Abdominal distention, rigidity, tenderness – Taut abdominal skin – Visible bowel loops – Excessive regurgitation, spitting up – Bile stained emesis – All of gavage feeding not absorbed, excessive gastric residual. – Absence of bowel sounds – Assess for symptom of sepsis, shock or DIC – Assist with and monitor results of laboratory tests and radiographs-WBC count, platelet counts, PT PTT, abdominal radiographs, stool for blood APT • If NEC develops, stop oral or nasal feelings for 7 to 8 days • If NEC level ps, insert orogastric or nasogastric tube and connect to low suction • Administer antibiotics as ordered • If NEC requires surgery, prepare for surgery.	Client will evidence soft abdomen, active bowel sounds, normal consistency and frequency of stools for breastfed or formulafed neonate, absence of symptoms of NEC

Contd...

Contd...

Problem (1)	*Reason (2)*	*Objection (3)*	*Nursing interventions (4)*	*Evaluation (5)*
8. Risk for impaired skin integrity related to • Thin skin, minimal subcutaneous fat • Fragile capillaries near skin surface • Invasive procedures	*Objective Data* • Redness of areas of skin • Cracking of areas of skin • Dry skin	Client will demonstrate skin integrity	• Observe skin for redness and irritation • Change infants position routinely • Place on fleece or flotation pad. • Minimize use of tapes for equipment, such as IV Lines and nasogastric tubes, or urine collection bags • Avoid harsh agents on skin, cleanse and bathe-gently, mainly with sterile water and mild soap. • Minimize manipulation of infant's skin, handle gently • Apply petroleum jelly to lips • Apply antibiotic ointment to lips if	Client will evidence intact skin, absence of injury to skin There is irritation or cracking
9. Risk for disorganized infant behaviour related to: • Longer hospitalization than for full term infant • Immaturity of sensory perceptual systems • Restrictive environment of the hospital that limits stimulation • Reduced interactive handling • Reduced interaction with parents • Handling involved with procedures.	*Subjective Data* • Uninterpretable cues *Objective Data* • Irritability • Restlessness • Apnoea • Colour changes • Bradycardia • Inability to "alert" and "attend" • Does not quiet down does not attend to perental or staff talking • Unable to follow objects • Inadequate weight gains.	Client will demonstrate organized infant behaviour	• Assign a primary care giver for each shift. • Change position frequently. Place rolled diapers. at the back of side lying position or at sides for prone position • Talk softly to infant. Play soft music • Create uterine-like atmosphere at times. Cover isolette or cover top of radiant warmer. Reduce noise, play recordings of placental or maternal heart sounds • Place infant in the enface position when infant is held • Provide designs and pictures in the isoletts or crib • Hold the infant in the over the shoulder position for burping • If infant is receiving phototherapy, uncover eyes periodically • Assess for sensory overload or streds. This includes: – Apnoea – Colour change – Bradycardia – Changes in behaviour – Inability to alert and attend • Help parents become aware of the infant's behavioural cues. Encourage parents to interact with the infant and provide appropriate stimulation.	Client will evidence normal weight gain, appropriate responses to visual and auditory stimulations

Contd...

12

CHAPTER

Pharmacotherapeutics in Obstetrics

INTRODUCTION

Pharmacology is the study of substances (drugs) that are safe and effective to prevent, treat, and diagnose diseases. According to WHO is: "Drug is any substance or product that is used or intended to be used to modify or explore physiological system or pathological states for the benefit of the recipient." However, the term drugs should not mean the derogatory sense 'addictive substances'. Some of the important terms used in the pharmacology are given below:

Pharmacodynamics is the therapeutic effect or action (physiological and biochemical effects) of drugs and their mechanism of action at molecular, cellular and organ system levels.

- A drug can bring about physical or chemical change in the cell environment, e.g. stool softeners that act by altering surface tension, and osmotic diuretics that alter osmosis
- Cell functions and process may be altered by drug interaction with drug receptors, e.g. glucose transfer into cell is facilitated by insulin
- Drug binding to receptor that brings about pharmacological action is called an Agonist, whereas a drug, which prohibits pharmacological action is called Antagonist
- Drug effect could be Local (e.g. topical application of acyclovir for herpes simplex viral infection) that acts at the site of application, or systemic that affect more than one part of the body (example: novalgin given 1M for pain at a distant place), or Local and Systemic (e.g. xylocaine plus epinephrine given subcutaneous) an agent given for its local effect but produces a systemic effect also.

Pharmacokinetics is the study of how drugs are absorbed, distributed, metabolized, and excreted (ADME) from the body, e.g. Digoxin is absorbed orally to an extent of 80 percent, transported through the blood where 25 percent of digoxin is bound to plasma proteins, distributed widely into all tissues with its effect localized in the heart muscle, only a small fraction is metabolized to its inactive form in the liver, most of it is excreted by kidney in unchanged form, and it has plasma half time of about 40 hours.

Pharmacotherapeutics is the science of drugs used to treat various illnesses and the responses of the individual. Factors that prevent drug actions and the need to alter drug dosage will be studied latter.

- *Clinical Pharmacology* helps generate data for optimum use of drugs. It includes pharmacodynamic and pharmacokinetic in healthy volunteers and in patients to evaluate the efficacy and safety of a given drug in comparison with other forms of treatment and its adverse effects.
- *Pharmacy* is the science of compounding and dispensing drugs and preparing suitable dosage forms for administration. Which includes identification, collection, isolation, purification, synthesis, quality control and standardization of medicinal substances.
- *Pharmaceutics* is the technological science of drug manufacture in large scale.
- *Chemothcrapy* is treatment of systemic infections, and malignancy by use of specific chemical agents (chemotherapeutic agents) that have selective toxicity for the infecting organism or malignant cells with minimal adverse effect or no effect on the host cells. Drugs having only pharmacodynamic effects on the recipient are designated as pharmacodynamic agents.

Pharmacopeia is an official code containing selected list of established drugs and preparations with a description of their physical properties, purity and potency. It defines standards that these preparations must meet and their average doses for an adult.

- Toxicology is the study of adverse effects of both chemotherapeutic agents and pharmacodynamic agents, since the same agent could be a drug or poison depending on dosage used. It also includes the study of poisonous effects of drugs and other chemicals with an emphasis on prevention, detection, and treatment of poisoning.

Pharmacology in Midwifery and Obstetrical Nursing

The midwife should have thorough knowledge of the indications, actions and side effects of these drugs as well as the nursing considerations related to each of them in order to plan and implement effective nursing process.

Sedatives Analgesics—Uterine stimulants as for induction of labour—inhibit infection—destroy bacteria—Heart stimulants, coagulants and anticoagulants—Eye drops.

Childbirth is associated with much pain, fear and much danger. This being so, from the beginning of time many drugs, and remedies has been used by the old midwife and medical man. Now in this scientific age new drugs have been discovered daily with a view to reduce these hazards and easing, even to the enjoyment of the greatest moment in a woman's life—the birth of the child.

A midwife in the modern world is able to assist in this by giving certain drugs which will remove danger, but unless she has a complete understanding of these drugs with all their risks, she may do even more harm.

Pain in labour not only causes great suffering, it also exhausts the woman both mentally and physically. Every woman should have the maximum relief from pain that is constant in her own and her baby's safety. Methods employed for the relief of pain in labour.

Suggestions Childbirth is a normal physical process and acknowledging the process of labour does much to remove the anxiety and tension of the mother. Relaxation can be achieved by exercise straight in the antenatal period and by pethidine and massage of the lower back during labour.

Oxytocics

Oxytocics are the drugs that have the power to excite contractions of the uterine muscles. Among a large number of drugs belonging to this group the ones that are important and extensively used are: *oxytocin*, *ergot derivatives* and *prostaglandins.*

These are drugs that stimulate the uterus to contract. At may be administered at crowning of the baby's head, at delivery of the anterior shoulder of the baby, at the end of the second stage of labour or following the delivery of the placenta.

Ergometrine based oxytocics such as syntometrine are more likely to be associated with the risk of side effects such as maternal hypertension, nausea and vomiting.

Prophylactic Use of Oxytocics: Oxytocic is the routine administration of an oxytocic at the time of birth of the baby, given as a precautionary measure for the prevention of postpartum hemorrhage regardless of the assessed status of the woman. Prophylactic oxytocic administration is part of active management, a policy of labour management.One ml ampoule contains 5 units of syntocinon and 0.5 mg ergometrine and is administered by intramuscular injection.

The asyntocinon acts within two minutes, and the ergometrifle within 6 to 7 minutes.

The use of syntometrine or any ergometrine based drug is associated with side effects such as elevation of the blood pressure, nausea and vomiting, antidote IV fluids with 5 percent glucose saline.

Caution: No more than two doses of ergometrine 0.5 mg should be given as it can cause headache, nausea and hypertension. Great caution is required where a hypertensive state already presents and its use is usually contraindicated

Syntocinon: Syntocinon is a synthetic form of the natural oxytocin produced in the anterior pituitary is free from side effects and safe to use in a wider context than syntometrine.

It can be administered both as an intravenous and an intramuscular injection.

- *Prostaglandins.* The use of prostaglandins for third stage management has up until now been more often associated with the treatment of postpartum hemorrhage than with prophylaxis. Prostaglandin agents are also associated with side effects such as diarrhea and cardiovascular complications of increased stroke volume and heart rate.

Therapeutic Oxytocic Administration

Therapeutic oxytocic administration implies the subsequent use of an oxytocic to either stop bleeding once it has occurred or to maintain the uterus in a contracted state where there are indications that excessive bleeding is likely to occur.

Usually Emergency use indicates an event of uncontrolled hemorrhage.

Intravenous Ergometrifle 0.25 mg Prostaglandin administration is most effective when used intramurally or by intrauterine irrigation.

The procedures are time consuming and invasive and the expertise required for undertaking the procedures is unlikely to always be readily available in routine labour management.

i. Oxytocin

Oxytocin is an octapeptide synthesized in the hypothalamus and stored in the posterior pituitary.

Preparations: Synthetic oxytocin available for parenteral use includes. Syntocinon 5.4/mi in ampoules Pitocin 5.4/mi in ampoules Syntometrine—a combination of syntocinon 5 units and ergometrine 0.5 mg

Mode of Action: Acts directly on myofibrils producing uterine contraction and stimulates milk ejection by the breasts.

Indications: (i) Pregnancy:
To induce abortion (inevitabie, missed)
To expedite expulsion of hydatidlform molc
For oxytocin challenge test
To stop bleeding following evacuation
To induce labour.
(ii) Labour:
To augment labour
In uterine inertia
To prevent and treat postpartum hemorrhage.
(iii) Postpartum:
To initiate milk let down in breast engorgement.

Contraindications: (i) In late pregnancy:
Grand multipara
Contracted pelvis
History of cesarean section or hysterotomy
Malpresentation.
(ii) During labour:
All contraindications mentioned in pregnancy
Obstructed labour
Incoordinate uterine action.
(iii) Anytime:
Hypovolemic state
Cardiac disease.

Adverse Effects: • Hypertonic uterine activity
- Fetal distress and fetal death
- Uterine rupture
- Hypotension
- Neonatal jaundice.

Dosage and Routes of Administration:
- Controlled intravenous infusion (ten units of oxytocin in one liter of Ringers lactate or 5% dextrose in water)
- Nasal spray for milk letdown.

Nursing Considerations

- Assess the following:
  - Intake and output ratio
  - Uterine contractions and FHR
  - Blood pressure, pulse and respiration.
- Administer the drug by I.V infusion. After having crash cart (emergency trolley) available in the ward.

  Evaluate *the* length and duration of contractions, notify physician of contractions and lasting over one minute or absence of contractions.

  Teach client/family
  - To report increased blood loss, abdominal cramps or increased temperature.

ii. Ergot Derivatives

Ergot alkaloids are either natural or semi synthetic.

Preparations: • Ergometrine (Ergonovine) 0.25 mg or 0.5 mg ampoules and 0.5-1 mg tablets
- Methergine (Methyle ergonovine) 0.2 mg ampoules and 0.5-1 mg tablets
- Syntometrine Ergometrine 0.5 mg + Syntocinon 5.0 unit's ampoules.

Ergometrine and methergine can be used parenterally or orally. As the drug produces titanic uterine contractions, it should only be used after delivery of the anterior shoulder or following delivery of the baby. It should not be used in induction of labour or abortion. Syntometrine should always be administered intramuscularly.

Mode of Action: Ergometrine acts directly on the myometrium. It stimulates uterine contractions and decreases bleeding.

Indications: • Therapeutic—To stop the atonic uterine bleeding following delivery, abortion or expulsion of hydatidiform mole.

- Prophylactic—As a prophylaxis against excessive hemorrhage; it may be administered after the delivery of the anterior shoulder (active management of third stage), with crowning or following delivery of the baby.

Contraindications: • Suspected plural pregnancy—If given accidentally with the delivery of the first baby, the second twin is likely to be compromised by the titanic contractions of the uterus.

- Organic cardiac disease—It may cause sudden squeezing of blood out of the uterine circulation into the general circulation causing overloading of the right heart and precipitating failure.
- Severe pre-eclampsia and eclampsia—There maybe sudden rise of blood pressure.
- Rh-negative mother—There is more chance of fetomaternal micro-transfusion.

Note: For women with heart diseases or hypertension oxytocin is a better substitute.

Adverse Effects/Side Effects: • Because of its vasoconstrictive action, it may precipitate rise of blood pressure.

- Prolonged use in puerperium may interfere with lactation by decreasing the concentration of prolactin.
- Prolonged use may lead to gangrene of the toes due to its vasoconstrictive effect.

Nursing Considerations

- Assess the following:
  - Blood pressure, pulse and respiration
  - Watch for signs of hemorrhage
- Administer the drug orally or IM in deep muscle mass and have emergency cart readily available.
- Evaluate the therapeutic effect—decreased blood loss.
- Teach client/family to report increased blood loss, abdominal cramps, headache, sweating, nausea, vomiting or dyspnea.

iii. Prostaglandins (PGs)

Prostaglandins are synthesized from one of the essential fatty acids, arachidonic acid, which is widely distributed throughout the body. In the female, these are identified in the menstrual fluid, endometrium, decidua and amniotic membrane.

Preparations: • PGE2—Prostin E2 (dinoprostone)

- PGF2alpha—Prostin F2a (dinoprost tromethamine)
- PGE1—Misoprostol

Mode of Actions: Both PGE2 and PGF2a have an oxytocic effect on the pregnant uterus. They also sensitize the myometrium to oxytocin. PGFcL acts predominantly on the myometrium, while PGE2 acts mainly on the cervix.

Indications: • For induction of abortion during second trimester and expulsion of hydatidiform mole.

- For induction of labour in intrauterine death of fetus.
- In augmentation or acceleration of labour.
- To stop bleeding from the open uterine sinuses as in refractory cases of atonic PPH.
- Cervical priming.

Contraindications: Hypersensitivity, uterine fibrosis, cervical stenosis, pelvic surgery, pelvic inflammatory disease, respiratory disease.

Side effects/adverse reactions: Headache, dizziness, hypotension, leg cramps, joint swelling, blurred vision.

Dosage and Routes of Administration:

- Tablets—containing 0.5 mg Prostin E2
- Vaginal suppository—containing 20 mg PGE2 or 50 mg PGF2a
- Vaginal pessary—containing 3 mg PGE2
- Injectable ampoules or vials of Prostin E2, 1 mg/ml Prostin F2a, 5 mg/ml,
- Misoprostol (POE1) 50 mg, given four hourly by oral, vaginal or rectal route for induction of labour.

Nursing Considerations

- Assess the following:
  - Respiratory rate, rhythm and depth.
  - Vaginal discharge, itching or irritation indicative of infection
- Administer antiemetic or antidiarrheal preparations prior to give this drug and put suppository at high in vagina, if vaginal preparations are used after warming the suppository by running warm water over package
- Evaluate for length and duration of contractions, notify physician of contractions lasting over one minute or absence of contractions and fever and chills
- Teach client/family
- To remain supine for 10 to 15 minutes after vaginal insertion.

ANTIHYPERTENSIVE DRUGS

Antihypertensive drugs are used in hypertensive disorders of pregnancy. The commonly used drugs are:

- Adrenergic inhibitors—Methyldopa
- Adrenergic blocking agents—Labetalol, propranolol
- Vasodilators—Hydralazine, Diazoxide, sodium nitroprusside
- Calcium channel blockers—Nifedipine.

i. Methyldopa

Preparations: Aldomet, Dopamet

Mode of action: Stimulates central a-adrenergic receptors or acts as false transmitter, resulting in reduction of arterial pressure.

Indications: Hypertension

Contra indications: Active hepatic disease, congestive cardiac failure, blood dyscrasias, psychiatric disorders.

Side Effects/Adeverse Reactions: • Nausea, vomiting, diarrhea, constipation

- Bradycardia, orthostatic hypotension, angina, weight gain
- Drowsiness, dizziness, headache, depression
- Leukopenia, thrombocytopenia coomb's test may be positive.

Dosage and Route of Administration:

- Orally—250 mg BID to 1 gm TID
- IV infusion—250 to 500 mg.

Nursing Considerations

- Assess the following:
  - Blood values—Neutrophils, platelets,
  - Renal studies—Protein, BUN, creatinine
  - Liver function tests
  - Blood pressure before beginning treatment and periodically thereafter.

  Perform/Provide storage of tablets in tight containers.
- Evaluate the following:
  - Decrease in blood pressure (therapeutic response).
  - Allergic reaction—Rash, fever, pruritis, urticaria.
  - Symptoms of congestive heart failure (edema, dyspnea, wet rales).
  - Renal symptoms—Polyuria, oliguria, frequency.
- Teach client/family:
  - To avoid hazardous activities.
  - Administer one hour before meals.
  - Not to discontinue drug abruptly or withdrawal symptoms may occur.
  - Not to use over the counter (OTC) medications (non-precription) for cough, cold or allergy, unless directed by physician.
  - Compliance with dosage schedule even if feeling better.
  - To rise slowly to sitting or standing position to minimize orthostatic hypotension.
  - Not to skip or stop drug unless directed by physician.
  - Notify physician of untoward signs and symptoms.

ii. Labetalol

Preparations: Trandate, Normodyne

Mode of action: Nonselective 3 blocker

Indication: Hypertension

Contraindications: Hepatic disorders, sinus bradycardia, bronchial asthma.

Side effects/adverse reactions: Orthostatic hypotension, bradycardia, chest pain, ventricular dysrhythmias, drowsiness, headache, nightmares, lethargy, agranulocytosis, thrombocytopenia, sore throat, dry burning eyes.

Dosage and routes of administration: Orally—100 mg TID up to 800 mg daily.

- IV infusion (Hypertensive crisis)—1-2 mg / mm until desired effect.

Nursing Considerations

- Assess the following:
  - Intake output and weight daily.
  - Blood pressure and pulse check q4h.
  - Apical or radial pulse before administration.
- Administer the drug:
  - P0, before food and HS. or SF. IV, keep client recumbent for 3 hours.
- Perform/Provide storage in dry area at room temperature.
- Evaluate the following:
  - Therapeutic response—Decreased BP after 1 to 2 weeks.
  - Edema in feet, legs daily.
  - Skin turgor and dryness of mucous membranes for hydration status.
- **Teach client/family:**
  - Not to discontinue drug abruptly, taper over 2 weeks.
  - Not to use over the counter medications containing α-adrenergic stimulants, such as nasal decongestants and cold medications, unless directed by physician.
  - To report bradycardia, dizziness, confusion or depression.
  - To avoid alcohol, smoking and excess sodium intake.
  - Take medication at bedtime to prevent the effect of orthostatic hypotension.
  - Wear support hose to minimize effects of orthostatic hypotension.

iii. Propranolol (Inderal)

Action: 3-adrenergic blocker—Decreases preload, after load, which is responsible for decreasing left ventricular end diastolic pressure and systemic vascular resistance.

Indications: Hypertension, prophylaxis of angina pain.

Contraindications: Bronchial asthma, renal insufficiency, diabetes mellitus, cardiac failure.

Side Effects/Adverse Reactions

- Maternal:
  - Severe hypotension, sodium retention, bradycardia, bronchospasm, cardiac failure.
  - Bradycardia and impaired fetal responses to hypoxia, IUGR with prolonged therapy, neonatal hypoglycemia.

Dosage and Routes of Administration: Orally 80 to 240 mg in divided doses.

Nursing Considerations

- Assess the following:
  - BP, pulse and respirations during therapy.
  - Weight daily and report excess weight gain.
  - Intake output ratio.
- Administer the drug administer with 240 ml of water on empty stomach.
- Evaluate the following:
  - Tolerance if taken for long period.
  - Headache, light-headedness, decreased BP.
- **Teach client/family:**
  - That there may be stinging sensation when the drug comes in contact with mucous membranes.
  - The drug may be taken before stressful activity exercise.
  - Client compliance with treatment regimen.
  - To make position changes slowly to prevent fainting.

iv. Hydralazine

Preparations: Apresoline, Hydralyn, Rolazine

Mode of action: Vasodilates arteriolar smooth muscles by direct relaxation, reduction in blood pressure with reflex increase in cardiac function.

Indications: Essential hypertension.
Contra indications: Coronary artery disease, mitral valvular rheumatic heart disease.

Adverse effects

- Maternal:
  Hypotension, tachycardia, arrhythmia, palpitation, acute rheumatoid state, and muscle cramps, headache, dizziness, depression, anorexia, diarrhea, pruritis.

Dosage and Routes of Administration:

- Orally—100 mg/day in 4 divided doses
- IV/IM bolus 20-40 mg q4-6h

Nursing Considerations

- Assess the following:
  - BP every 15 minutes initially for 2 hours then every hour for 2 hours, and then q4h, pulse q4h.
  - Blood studies—Electrolytes, CBC and serum glucose.
  - Intake—Output and weight daily.
- Administer the drug to patient in recumbent position, keep in that position for one hour after administration.

- Evaluate the following:
  - Edema in feet and legs daily.
  - Skin and mucous membrane for hydration.
  - Rales, dyspnea, orthopnea.
  - Joint pain, tachycardia, palpitation, headache and nausea.
- Teach client/family:
  - To take with food to increase bioavailability.
  - To notify physician if chest pain, severe fatigue, muscle or joint pain occurs.

v. Nifedipine

Preparation: Adalat, procardia

- Calcium channel blocker

Mode of action: Produces direct arteriolar vasodilatation by inhibition of inward calcium channels in vascular smooth muscles.

Indications

- Hypertension, angina pectoris.

Contraindications: Simultaneous use of magnesium sulphate could be hazardous due to synergistic effect.

- Second or third degree heart block.

Side Effects/Adverse Reactions:

- Flushing, hypotension, palpitations, bradycardia, inhibition of labour, headache, fatigue, drowsiness, nausea, vomiting.

Dosage and Routes of Administration

Orally—5-10 mg, tid

Nursing Considerations

- Assess the blood levels of the drug, therapeutic levels 0.025-0.1 g/ml.
- Administer the drugs before meals, and HS
- Evaluate the therapeutic response, cardiac status, BP, pulse, respiration and ECG.
- Teach client/family:
  - To limit caffeine consumption.
  - To avoid OTC drugs unless directed by the physician.
  - Stress patient compliance to all aspects of drug use.

vi. Diazoxide

Preparation: Hyperstat

Action: Vasodilator

Indication: Hypertensive crisis, when urgent decrease of diastolic pressure is required.

Contraindications:

- Diabetes, heart disease
- Diuretics should be used simultaneously.

Side Effects:

- Maternal:
  - Fluid and sodium retention
  - Inhibition of uterine contraction
  - Hyperglycemia
  - Severe hypotension
  - Palpitations.
- Fetal
  - Hypoxia.

Dosage and Routes of Administration

IV—30 to 50 mg, may be repeated every 10 to 15 minutes or continuous infusion.

Nursing Considerations

- Assess the following
  - BP q5min for 2 hours, then q/hr for 2 hours and then q4h.
  - Pulse, jugular venous distention q4h.
  - Serum electrolytes, CBC, serum glucose.
  - Weight daily and intake output.
- Administer the drug to patient in recumbent position, keep in that position for one hour after administration.
- Perform/Provide protection from light
- Evaluate the following:
  - Therapeutic response—primarily decreased diastolic pressure.
  - Edema in feet and legs.
  - Hydration status.
  - Dyspnea and orthopnea.
  - Postural hypotension—Take BP sitting and standing.
- Teach patient/family:
  - To limit caffeine consumption.
  - To report side effects if present.
  - To comply with the regimen.

vii. Sodium Nitroprusside

Preparations: Nipride, Nitropress

Action: Peripheral vasodilator, directly relaxes arteriolar, venous smooth muscle, resulting in reduction of cardiac preload and after load.

Indications: Hypertensive crisis.

- To decrease bleeding by creating hypoertension during pregnancy.

Contraindications
- Should be used in critical care unit for short time.
- Compensatory hypertension is possible.

Side Effects/Adverse Reactions
- Maternal
  - Nausea, vomiting, severe hypotension.
  - Restlessness, decreased reflexes, loss of consciousness.
- Fetal
  - Toxicity due to metabolites—Cyanide and thiocyanate.

Dosage and Route of Administration
- IV infusion 0.5 to 10 mg/kg/minute.

Nursing Considerations
- Assess the following:
  - Serum electrolytes, BUN and creatinine.
  - Hepatic function (AST, ALT and alkaline phosphatase).
  - BP and ECG.
  - Weight and intake output.
- Administer the drug using an infusion pump only and wrap bottle with aluminum foil to protect from light.
- Evaluate the following:
  - Therapeutic response—Decreased BP, absence of bleeding.
  - Edema—Feet and legs.
  - Hydration status

DIURETICS

Diuretics are used in the following conditions during pregnancy.
- Pregnancy induced hypertension with massive edema
- Eclampsia with pulmonary edema
- Severe anemia in pregnancy with heart failure
- Prior to blood transfusion in severe anemia
- As an adjunct to certain antihypertensive drugs, such as hydralazine or diazoxide.

Common Preparations

i. Furosemide (Lasix)

Action: A loop diuretic; Acts on loop of Henle by increasing excretion of sodium and chloride.

Dosage: 40 mg tab, daily following breakfast for 5 days a week. In acute conditions, the drug is administered parenterally in doses of 40 to 120 mg daily.

Side Effects
- Maternal
  - Side effects include weakness, fatigue, muscle cramps, hypokalaemia, hyponatraemia, hypocalcaemia, hypochloraemic alkalosis and postural hypotension.
- Fetal
  - May occur due to decreased placental perfusion leading to fetal compromise. Thrombocytopenia and hyponatraemia are other hazards.

Contraindications
- Hypersensitivity to suphonamides, hypovolemia.

Interactions/Incompatibilities
- Increased toxicity—Lithium, skeletal muscle relaxants, and digitalis
- Decreased effects of antidiabetics
- Increased anticoagulant activity
- Increased action anticoagulants.

Nursing Considerations
- Assess the following:
  - Weight, intake and output daily to determine fluid loss.
  - Respiration—Rate, depth and rhythm.
  - BP—Lying and standing.
  - Electrolytes—Sodium, chloride, potassium, BUN, blood sugar, CBC, serum creatinine, blood pH and ABGs.
  - Glucose in urine, if patient is diabetic.
- Administer and drug in AM to avoid interference with sleep and do potassium replacement, if serum potassium is less than 3.0. and with food, if nausea occurs, absorption may be decreased slightly.
- Evaluate the following:
  - Improvement in edema of feet, legs and sacral area.
  - Signs of metabolic acidosis—Drowsiness, restlessness.
  - Signs of hypocalcaemia, postural hypotension, malaise, fatigue, tachycardia and leg cramps.
  - Rashes and temperature elevation.
- *Teach patient/family:*
  - To increase fluid intake 2-3 L/day unless contraindicated.
  - To rise slowly from lying or sitting position.
  - To report adverse reactions, such as muscle cramps, nausea, weakness or dizziness.

- To take with food or milk.
- To take early in day to prevent nocturia.

ii. Hydrochlorothiazide

Preparations: Esidrex, hydrodiuril, hydrozide.

Action: Sulphonamide derivative. Acts on distal tubule by increasing excretion of water, sodium, chloride and potassium.

Indications: Edema, hypertension

Dosage and Route
- P.0, 25-100 mg/day.

Side Effects/Adverse Reactions
- Polyuria, glycosuria, frequency
- Nausea, vomiting, anorexia
- Rash, urticaria, fever
- Increased creatinine, decreased electrolytes.

Contraindications
- Hypersensitivity to thiazides or sulphonamides.

Nursing Considerations
- Assess the following:
  - Weight, intake and output to determine fluid loss.
  - Rate, depth and rhythm of respiration.
  - BP—lying and standing.
  - Electrolytes—Potassium, sodium and chloride. BUN, blood sugar, CBC, serum creatinine, blood pH and ABGs.
  - Glucose in urine, if patient is diabetic.
- Administer the drug in AM to avoid interference with sleep and make potassium replacement, if serum potassium is less than 3.0 with food if nausea occurs.
- Evaluate the following:
  - Improvement in edema.
  - Improvement in CVP.
  - Signs of metabolic acidosis, drowsiness and restlessness.
  - Signs of hypokalemia, postural hypotension, malaise, fatigue, tachycardia, leg cramps and weakness.
  - Rashes and temperature elevation.
- Teach patient/family
  - To increase fluid intake to 2-3 L/day unless contraindicated.
  - To notify physician of muscle weakness, cramps, nausea and dizziness.
  - Drug may be taken with food or milk.
  - To take early in day to avoid nocturia.

iii. Spironolactone (Aldactone)

Mode of action: The drug antagonizes aldosterone by competitive inhibition in the distal tubules, thereby preventing the potassium excretion and decreasing the sodium reabsorption.

Dosage: Initially 25 mg P0 may be increased to 100 mg in divided doses.

Advantages: There is no potassium loss. It has some hypotensive action.

Nursing Considerations
- Assess the following:
  - Weight, intake and output daily to determine fluid loss.
  - Blood pressure—Lying and standing as postural hypotension may occur.
  - Serum electrolytes (sodium, potassium, chloride), BUN, blood glucose, serum creatinine and CBC.
- Administer the drug in AM to avoid interference with sleep and do potassium replacement, if serum potassium is less than 3.0 with food—if nausea occurs.
- Evaluate the following:
  - Improvement in edema—Feet, legs and scral area daily.
  - Signs of metabolic acidosis—Drowsiness, restlessness.
  - Signs of hypokalaemia—Postural hypotension, fatigue, tachycardia, leg cramps and weakness.
- *Teach client/family:*
  - To increase fluid intake.
  - To rise slowly from lying or sitting position.
  - To take with food or milk for GI symptoms.
  - To take early in day to prevent nocturia.

TOCOLYTIC AGENTS

These drugs can inhibit uterine contractions and used to prolong the pregnancy. In women who develop premature uterine contractions, in addition to putting them to absolute bed rest and sedating, tocolytic drugs are administered in an attempt to inhibit uterine contractions.

The commonly used drugs are—Isoxsuprine (duadilan), ritodrine hydrochloride (yutopar) and magnesium sulphate.

i. Isoxsuprine (Duadilan)

Action: Acts directly on vascular smooth muscle causes cardiac stimulation and uterine relaxation.

Dosage and routes: Initial IV drip 100 mg in 5 percent dextrose. Rate 0.2 ug per minute. To continue for at least two hours after the contractions cease.

Maintenance

- IM 10 mg six hourly for 24 hours, Tab 10 mg 6-8 hourly.

Side Effects

- Hypotension, tachycardia, nausea, vomiting, pulmonary edema, cardiac arrhythmias, adult respiratory distress syndrome, hyperglycemia, hypokalaemia, lactic acidosis.

Contraindications

- Hypersensitivity, postpartum.

Nursing Considerations

- Assess the following:
  - BP and pulse during treatment.
  - Take BP—Lying and standing—orthostatic hypotension is common.
  - Intensity and length of uterine contractions.
  - Fetal heart tones.
- Administer the drug:
  - With meals to reduce GI upset.
- Perform/Provide storage at room temperature.
- Evaluate the therapeutic response, i.e.
  - Reduced uterine contractions
  - Absence of pre-term labour
  - Increased pulse volume
- *Teach patient/family*
  - To avoid hazardous activities until stabilized on medication. Dizziness may occur.
  - To make position changes slowly, or fainting may occur.
  - To notify physician if rash, palpitations or severe flushing develops.

ii. Ritodrine Hydrochloride (Yutopar)

Action

- Uterine relaxant—Acts directly on vascular smooth muscle. Causes cardiac stimulation and uterine relaxation.

Dosage and Routes

- Initial:
  - IV drip 100 mg in 5 percent dextrose. Rate, 0.1 mg per minute gradually increased by 0.05 mg per minute q10 min until desired response. To continue for at least 2 hours after the contractions cease.
- Maintenance:
  - Tab 10 mg 6 to 8 hourly.
  - P.O 10 mg given half hour before termination of IV, then 10 mg q2h x 24 hrs, then 10- 20 mg q4h, not to exceed 120 mg/day.

Side Effects/Adverse Reactions

- Hyperglycemia, headache, restlessness, sweating, chills, and drowsiness.
- Nausea, vomiting, anorexia and malaise.
- Altered maternal and fetal heart tone and palpitations.

Contraindications

- Hypersensitivity, eclampsia, hypertension and dysrhythmias.

Nursing Considerations

- Assess the following:
  - Maternal and fetal heart tones during infusion.
  - Intensity and length of uterine contractions.
  - Fluid intake to prevent fluid overload, discontinue if this occurs.
- Administer the drug in only clear solutions after dilution 150 mg in 500 ml D5W or NS, give at 0.3 mg/ml and using infusion pumps or monitor carefully.
- Perform/Provide that the positioning of patient in left lateral recumbent position to decrease hypotension and increase renal blood flow.
- Evaluate the therapeutic response, i.e.
  - Decreased intensity
  - Length of contraction
  - Absence of pre-term labor
  - Decreased BP.
- *Teach patient/family*
  - To remain in bed during infusion.

ANTICONVULSANTS

The commonly used anticonvulsant is magnesium sulphate. Diazepam, phenytoin and phenobarbitone are also used.

i. Magnesium Sulphate

Action: Decreases acetylcholine in motor nerve terminals, which is responsible for anti- convulsant properties, thereby reduces neuromuscular irritability. It also decreases intracranial edema and helps in diuresis. Its peripheral vasodilatation effect improves the uterine blood supply. Has depressant action on the uterine muscle and CNS.

Use: It is a valuable drug lowering seizure threshold in women with pregnancy-induced hypertension. The drug is used in pre-term labour to decrease uterine activity.

Dosage and route: For control of seizures, 20 ml of 20 percent solution IV slowly in 3-4 minutes; to be followed immediately by 10 ml of 50 percent solution IM, and continued 4 hourly till 24 hours postpartum. Repeat injections are given only if the knee jerks are present, urine output exceeds 100 ml in previous 4 hours and the respirations are more than 10/minute. The therapeutic level of serum magnesium is 4-7 mEq/L. 4 gm IV slowly over 10 mm., followed by 2 gm/hr, and then 1 gm/hr in drip of 5 percent dextrose for tocolytic effect.

Side effects

Maternal: Severe CNS depression (respiratory depression and circulatory collapse), evidence of muscular paresis (diminished knee jerks).

- Fetal: Tachycardia, hypoglycaemia.

Antidote

- Injection calcium gluconate 10 percent 10 ml IV.

Nursing Considerations

- Assess the following:
  - Vital signs q 15 mm. after IV dose. Do not exceed 150 mg/mm.
  - Monitor magnesium levels.
  - If using during labor, time contractions, determine intensity.
  - Urine output should remain 30 ml/hr or more, if less notify physician.
  - Uterine contractions when used as tocolytic agent.
  - Reflexes—knee jerk, patellar reflex.
- Administer the drug only after calcium gluconate is available for treating magnesium toxicity. When using infusion pumps or monitors carefully; IV at less then 150 mg/mm; circulatory collapse may occur. Use only dilutions.
- Perform/Provide the following:
  - Seizure precautions—Place client in single room with decreased stimuli, padded side rails.
  - Positioning of client in left lateral recumbent position to decrease hypotension and increase renal blood flow.
- Evaluate the following:
  - Mental status, sensorium, memory.
  - Respiratory status—Respiratory depression, rate and rhythm: Hold drug if respirations are less than 12/mm.
  - Hypermagnesaemia—depressed patellar reflex, flushing, confusion, weakness, flaccid paralysis, dyspnea.
  - Respiratory rate, rhythm and reflexes of newborn if drug was given within 24 hours prior to delivery.
  - Reflexes—Knee jerk and patellar reflex decrease with magnesium toxicity. Discontinue infusion if respirations are below 12/minute, reflexes severely hypotonic, urine output below 30 ml/hour or in the event of mental confusion or lethargy or fetal distress.
- *Teach client/family:*
  - On all aspects of the drug—Action, side effects and symptoms of hypomagnesaemia.
  - To remain in bed during infusion.

ii. Diazepam (Valium)

Action: Depresses subcortical levels of CNS, anticonvulsant, and antianxiety.

Dosage and Route of Administration

- P0, 2 to 10 mg tid—qid
- IV, 5 to 20 mg (bolus), 2 mg/mm, may repeat q5—l0min, not to exceed 60 mg, may repeat in 30 mm if seizures reappear.

Side Effects

- Mother: Hypotension, dizziness, drowsiness, headache.
- Fetus: Respiratory depressant effect, which may last for even three weeks after birth. Hypotonea and thermoregulatory problems in newborn.

Nursing Considerations

- Assess the following:
  - BP in lying and standing positions; if systolic pressure falls 20 mmHg, hold drug and inform physician.
  - Blood studies—CBC.
  - Hepatic studies.
- Administer the drug through: IV into large vein to decrease chances of extravasation. P0 with milk or food to avoid G.I symptoms.

- Provide an assistance with ambulation during beginning therapy since drowsiness and dizziness may occur and use safety measures include side rails.
- Evaluate the therapeutic response:
  - Mental status, sensorium, sleeping pattern.
  - Physical dependence, headache, nausea, vomiting.
- *Teach patient/family*
  - That drug may be taken with food.
  - To avoid alcohol ingestion.
  - Not to discontinue medication abruptly.
  - To rise slowly as fainting may occur.

iii. Phenytoin (Dilantin)

Action: Inhibits spread of seizure activity in motor cortex.

Dosage and Route of Administration:
- Eclampsia—10 mg/kg IV at the rate not more than 50 mg/minute, followed 2 hours later by 5 mg/kg.
- Epilepsy—300-400 mg daily orally in divided doses.

Side Effects
- Maternal
  - Hypotension, cardiac arrhythmias and phlebitis at injection site.
- Fetal
  - Prolonged use by epileptic patients may cause craniofocal abnormalities, mental retardation, microcephaly and growth deficiency.

Nursing Considerations

Assess the following:
- Blood studies—CBC, platelets every 2 weeks until stabilized.
- Discontinue drug if neutrophils < 1600/mm^2.
- Administer the drug after diluting with normal saline, never in water.

- Evaluate the following:
  - Mental status, sensorium, affect, memory.
  - Respiratory depression.
  - Blood dyscrasias—Sore throat, bruising.
- *Teach patient/family*
  - All apects of drug administration, when to notify physician.

iv. Phenobarbitone (Luminal)

Action: Decreases impulse transmission and increases seizure thresholds at cerebral cortex level.

Dose and Route of Administration
- 120-240 mg/day in divided doses.

Side Effects
- Maternal
  - Sedation, drowsiness, hangover headache, hallucinations.
- Fetal

  Withdrawal syndrome.

Nursing Considerations
- Assess the following:
  - Blood studies, liver function tests during long-term treatment.
  - Therapeutic level 15-40 mg/ml.
- Evaluate the following:
  - Mental status, mood, senorium, affect and memory.
  - Respiratory depression.
  - Blood dyscrasias—Fever, sore throat bruising, rash.
- *Teach patient/family*
  - All aspects of drug administration and when to notify physician.

ANTICOAGULANTS

i. Heparin Sodium

Action: Prevents conversion of fibrinogen to fibrin.

Indications: Deep vein thrombosis, thromboembolism, disseminated intravascular coagulation, patients with prosthetic valves in the heart.

Dosage and Routes
- Administered parenterally; only 5,000-7,000 JU to be administered initially as IV push, followed by 2,500 units subcutaneously every 24 hours.

Side Effects

Leukopenia, thrombocytopenia, osteoporosis, hemorrhage, alopecia.

Nursing Considerations
- Assess the following:
  - Blood studies—Hematocrit, platelets, occult blood in stools.
  - Partial prothrombin time.
  - Blood pressure—Signs of hypertension.
- Administer the drug at same time each day to maintain steady blood levels and avoid all IM injections that may cause bleeding.
- Evaluate the following:
  - Therapeutic response—Decrease of deep vein thrombosis.

- Bleeding gums, petechiae, ecchymosis, black tarry stools, hematuria.
- Fever, skin rash, urticaria.
- *Teach patient/family*
  - To avoid use of drugs unless prescribed by physician.
  - To use soft bristle toothbrush to avoid bleeding gums.
  - To comply with instructions.
  - To report and sign of bleeding—gums, under skin, urine, stool.

ii. Warfarin Sodium (Cumadin)

Action: Interferes with blood clotting by indirect means—depresses hepatic synthesis of vitamin K—dependent coagulation factors (II, VII, IX, X).

Indications
- Deep vein thrombosis, pulmonary embolism.

Dosage and Route
- 10-15 mg orally daily for 2 days, followed by 2-10 mg at the same time each day depending upon the prothrombin time.

Side Effects
- Maternal
  - Hemorrhage
- Fetal
  - Skeletal and facial deformities, optic atrophy, microcephaly.

Nursing Considerations
- Assess the following:
  - Blood studies—Hematocrit, platelets, occult blood in stools.
  - Prothrombin time.
  - BP—Watch for signs of hypertension.
- Administer the drug at same time each day to maintain steady blood levels alone—do not give with food and avoid all IM injections that may cause bleeding.
- Perform/Provide i.e. storage in tight container.
- Evaluate the following:
  - Therapeutic response—decrease of deep vein thrombosis.
  - Bleeding gums, petechiae, echymosis, black tarry stools, hematuria.
  - Fever, skin rash, urticaria.
- *Teach patient/family:*
  - To avoid over the counter (OTC) preparations unless prescribed by physician.
  - Drug may be held during menstruation.
  - To use soft—bristle tooth brush.
  - Stress client compliance.
  - To report any sign of bleeding.

ANALGESIA AND ANAESTHESIA IN OBSTETRICS

Anatomical and Physiological Considerations: Nerve supply of the genital tract—uterus is under both nervous and hormonal control. Hypothalamus controls the uterine activity which balances the effects of two autonomic divisions. Hormonal control is generally agreed that intact nerves supply is not essential for the initiation and progress of labour. Total spinal block does not inhibit uterine activity provided blood pressure is not allowed to fall and normal delivery can occur in the paraplegic patient. It is believed that some hormones are essential for the control of uterine activity. Oxytocin, a hormone derived from posterior pituitary maintains the uterine activity during labour. Progesterone is the pregnancy stabilizing hormone. Labour commences when it is withdrawn. Adrenaline with its beta activity inhibits the contraction of the uterus while its alpha activity excites it.

Labour may be easy and trouble free with good psychological approach. Unprepared and untreated patient feel more pain during uterine contractions. Drugs are useful for the relief of pain but they are not much important than the proper preparation and training for child birth. The intensity of labour pain depends on the intensity and duration of uterine contractions, the degree of dilatation of cervix, the distension of perineal tissue, the parity and pain threshold of the woman. The most distressing time during the whole labour is just prior to full dilatation of the cervix.

The ideal procedure should produce efficient relief from pain without depressing the respiration of the fetus and should not depress the uterine activity causing prolonged labour. The drug must be nontoxic and safe to the mother and fetus. But there is no such drugs are available fulfilling all these conditions. Every cases of labour does not require analgesia and only sympathetic explanation may be all that is required.

Methods to Relief of Pain

1. Hypnosis This method is not reliable. So not proved popular for general use.
2. Sedatives and analgesics

3. Inhalation agents
4. Regional analgesics
5. Psycho prophylaxis

Sedatives and Analgesics

There are certain factors to control the dose of sedative and analgesics.

1. The threshold of pain Varies in individuals. Some patients may feel pain though the uterine contractions are weak. In such patients pain must be controlled even if this involves a temporary depression in uterine action.
2. Primigravida or Multigravida, Multiparous woman need less analgesics due to added relaxation of the birth canal and rapid delivery.
3. Maturity of the fetus; Minimal dose is indicated while the fetus is thought to be premature to avoid asphyxia.

Sedatives Chloral hydrate, barbiturates berizodiazepines etc may be employed in the early part of the first phase. That is up to 8 cm dilatation of cervix to primigravida and up to 6 cm dilatation of cervix to multigravida.

Cliloral hydrate 2 gm orally along with equal amount of potassium bromide will provide mild sedation in early labour. Barbiturates Pheno-barbitofle butobarbitofle quinal barbitone and 5cdium amytal are commonly used. These are less depressing to fetal respiration than morphine. The first phase controlled by sedatives and analgesics and second phase is controlled by inhalation agents. The ideal is to avoid the risk of delivery of a depressed baby.

Sedatives Like chloral hydrates, barbiturates benzodiazepine, pethidine, pethidine with antagonists, pentazocine (Fortwin), combination of narcotics and tranquilhisers. Narcotics produce less respiratory depression and prevent vomiting. But these are disadvantages like hypotension and delay in second stage.

Inhalation Method

Nitrous oxide and air has no effect on fetus and does not interfere with uterine contractions. Nowadays nitrous oxide and air is not wet because this mixture produces hypoxia. Premixed nitrous oxide and oxygen 50 and 50 percent oxygen mixture used by Entonox apparatus has been approved for used by midwife. Trichioroethylene (Trilene) is a useful drug in labour. This agent is intermittently in 0.35 percent to 0.5 percent through the apparatus the Tecota mark 6 trichioroethylene inhaler.

Methoxyflurane (penthrane) is a good analgesic agent and more effective than trichloroethylene. It is given by means of a "cardiff" inhaler in concentration of 0.35 percent in air.

Regional Anesthesia

When complete relief of pain is needed throughout labour, epidural analgesia is safest and simplest method of producing it. Being a time consuming method it is not practiced for labour.

Continuous Lumbar Epidural Block

A lumbar puncture needle is introduced (Tuohy needle) between 2nd and 3rd vertebrae after preparing the area like lumbar puncture with the patient in left lateral position. When the epidural space is ensured, a plastic catheter is passed through the epidural needle for continuous epidural anesthesia. Repeated doses of 4 to 5 ml of 0.5 percent bupivacaine or 1 percent lignocaine are used to maintain the analgesia. This method is used only when labour is well established. BP pulse and fetal heart sound should be checked and recorded every 15 minutes following the induction of analgesia and hypotension if occurred should be treated immediately.

Contraindications to Epidural Anesthesia

1. Sepsis at the site of injection
2. Hemorrhagic disease or anticoagulant therapy.
3. Supine hypotension
4. Neurological diseases.

Caudal epidural analgesia: Patient is in left lateral position and sacral region is prepared with full aseptic precaution. Sacral hiatus is identified and a mulleable needle is pushed through it, first piercing the skin and sacrococcygeal ligament at right angle and depressing the needle towards the natal deft (pertaining to the birth) at an angle of 40° to the skin. The needle is gently advanced to the sacral canal. Stylet is withdrawn and aspiration test is carried out to ensure that dura or vein is not punctured. A fine nylon epidural catheter is passed through the needle and needle is then withdrawn 16 to 20 ml of 1 per cent lignocaine is passed through the catheter and relief of pain is established within 10 to 20 minutes. Bupivacaine 0.5% can be used for prolonged analgesia. This method is rarely used because the approach to the epidural space through sacral hiatus dirtier, harder and fails more often.

Paracervical nerve block: A long needle is passed in the lateral fornix and 4 to 5 ml of lignocaine with adrenaline are injected at the site of the cervix and the procedure is repeated on the other side. This dose is sufficient to relieve pain for about an hour or two and injections can be repeated if necessary. Bupivacaine 0.25 percent is effective for 3 hours in order to avoid complications a specially constructed guard tube is used and the needle is inserted through that tube. Although the paracervical block may be useful from 5cm dilatation of the cervix, it is most useful towards the end of the first stage of labour to remove the desire to beardown earlier. Paracervical nerve block can only relieve the uterine contraction and the perineal discomfort is removed by the pudental nerve block.

Perineal infiltration: Perineal infiltration anesthesia is given extensively prior to episiotomy. A 10 ml syringe with a fine needle and about 8 to 10 ml of 1 percent lignocaine hydrochloride (Xylocaine) are required. The proposed area of perineum site is infiltrated in a fan wise manner, starting from the middle of the fourchette. Each time prior to infiltration aspiration test is done to exclude blood is mandatory. Episiotomy is to be done within 2 to 5 minutes following the infiltration. For outlet forceps or ventose traction perineal and labal infiltration is required.

Pudendal nerve block: It does not relieve the pain of labour but affords perineal analgesia and relaxation. Pudendal nerve block is mostly used for forceps and vaginal breech delivery. Simultaneous perineal and vulval infiltration is needed to block the perineal branch of the posterior cutaneous nerve of the thigh and the labial branches of the ilioinguinal and genitofemoral nerves. This method is less dangerous to the mother and fetus than general anesthesia.

The pudendal nerve is blocked by either by the transvaginal or transperineal route and transvaginal route is commonly preferred.

Spinal anesthesia: Spinal anesthesia can be used to alleviate the pain of delivery and during the third stage of labour. Brief of minimal spinal anesthesia is far safer than prolonged spinal anesthesia. The advantages of spinal anesthesia are less fetal hypoxia unless there is less hypotension and minimal blood loss. Technique is not difficult and no inhalation anesthesia is required, but post spinal headache occurs in 5 to 10 percent of patients.

Spinal anesthesia canbe obtained by injecting 1 ml of hyperbaric lignocaine (5%) into the subarachnoid space of the third or fourth lumbar interspace with the patient lying or her side with a slight head uplift. BP and respiratory rate should be checked every three minutes for the first ten minutes and every 5 minutes there after. Oxygen should be supplied in respiratory depression and hypotension. If marked BP fall occurs vasopressor drugs may be needed.

Undesirable Side Effects of Spinal or Epidural Anaesthesia

- Hypotension due to blocking of sympathetic fibers leading to vasodilatation and low cardiac out put
- Respiratory depression may occur
- Post spinal headache due to low or high CSF pressure and leaking of CSF
- Meningitis due to faulty asepsis
- Transient of permanent paralysis
- Toxic reaction of local anaesthetic drugs
- Nausea and vomiting are seen in some patients
- There will be marked hypotension, apnoea and dilated pupils which should be immediately intubated and 100 percent oxygen should be given IV fluids and vasopressin may also have to be given.

Psychophrophylaxis

For natural child birth. It is a psychological method of antenatal preparation of patient to prevent or minimize the pain and difficulty during labour. For most women labour is a time of apprehension, fear and agony. As a result of suitable antenatal preparation majority of women have easy and painless labour.

The goal of this technique is not to use any drug during the first and second stages of labour or to minimize the dose of narcotics or to avoid regional anesthesia.

Pethidine (Meperidine)

It is synthetic narcotic analgesic agent, well absorbed by all routes of administration.

Action: Inhibits ascending pain pathways in central nervous system, increases pain threshold and alters pain perception.

Indications

- Moderate to severe pain in labor, postoperative pain, abruptio placentae, pulmonary edema.

Dosage and Route of Administration

- Injectable preparation contains 50 mg/ml, can be administered SC, IM, IV. Its dose is 50 to 100 mg TM combined with promethazine 25 mg.

Contraindication

Pethidine should not be used intravenously within 2 hours and intramuscularly within 3 hours of the expected time of delivery of the baby, for fear of birth asphyxia. It should not be used in cases of preterm labor and when the respiratory reserve of the mother is reduced.

Side Effects/Adverse Reactions

- Mother
  - Drowsiness, dizziness, confusion, head–ache, sedation, euphoria, nausea and vomiting.
- Fetus
  - Respiratory depression, asphyxia.

Nursing Considerations

- Assess the following:
  - Urinary Output—may cause urinary retention
- Administer the drug with antiemetic (promethacin) to prevent nausea and vomiting. When pain is beginning to return— determine dosage interval by patient response.
- Perform/Provide
  - Storage in light—resistant container at room temperature.
  - Assistance with ambulation.
  - Safety measures—Side rails, night light, call bell within easy reach.
- Evaluate the following:
  - Therapeutic response—Decrease in pain.
  - CNS changes—Dizziness, drowsiness, euphoria.
  - Allergic reactions—Rash, urticaria.
  - Respiratory depression, notify physician if respirations are <12/minute.
- *Teach patient/family*
  - To report symptoms of CNS changes, allergic reactions.

Fentanyl

Fentanyl is a synthetic narcotic analgesic agent.

Action: Inhibits ascending pain pathways in CNS, increases pain threshold and alters pain perception.

Indications

- Moderate to severe pain in labor, postoperative pain and as adjunct to general anesthetic

Dosage and Routes

- 0.05-0.1 mg IM q 1 to 2 hours pm. Available in injectable form, 0.05 mg/mi.

Contraindications

- Hypersensitivity to opiates.

Side Effects/Adverse Reactions

- Dizziness, delirium, euphoria, nausea, vomiting, muscle rigidity, blurred vision.

Nursing Considerations

- Assess the vital signs and note muscle rigidity
- Administer the drug by injection (IM or IV), give slowly to prevent rigidity and having ready only with resuscitative equipment available.
- Perform/Provide the following:
  - Storage in light resistant container at room temperature.
  - Coughing, turning and deep breathing for postoperative patients.
  - Safety measures—Side rails, night light, call bell within reach.
- Evaluate the following:
  - CNS changes—Dizziness, drowsiness, hallucination, euphoria, LOC, pupil reaction.
  - Allergic reaction—Rash, urticaria.
  - Respiratory dysfunction—Respiratory depression: Notify physician if respirations are >12/minute.
- *Teach patient/family*
  - To report any symptoms of CNS changes, allergic reactions.

Promethazine (Phenergan)

Promethazine is an antihistamine, H1—receptor antagonist belonging to the phenothiazine group.

Action: Decreases allergic response by blocking histamine, sedative and antiemetic.

Indications

- Treatment of vomiting in pregnancy.
- Sedation during labor.
- Pregnancy induced hypertension.
- Combined with pethidine to prevent vomiting.
- In Rh isoimmunization to decrease the production of antibodies.
- Allergic reactions.

Dosage and Route of Administration

- Available for oral use as 12.5, 24 and 50 mg tablets and for parenteral use as 25 and 50 mg/ml solutions. The dose is 25 mg, 8 hourly orally and 25 mg intramuscularly, to be repeated as necessary.

Contraindications

- Acute asthma attack.
- Lower respiratory tract disease.

Side Effects/Adverse Reactions

- Drowsiness, dizziness, poor coordination, fatigue, anxiety, confusion, neuritis, parasthesia.

Nursing Considerations

- Assess the following:
  - Urinary output—Be alert for urinary retention, frequency, dysuria; drug should be discontinued if these occur.
- Administer the drug with coffee, tea and cola (caffeine) to decrease drowsiness or with meals if GI symptoms occur when given orally and should be given deep IM in large muscle; rotate site.
- Perform/Provide the following:
  - Hard candy or gum, frequent rinsing of mouth for dryness.
  - Storage in light resistant container.
- Evaluate the following:
  - Therapeutic response.
  - Respiratory status—wheezing, chest tightness.
  - Cardiac status—Palpitation, hypotension, increased pulse.
- *Teach patient/family*
  - That drug may cause photosensitivity, to avoid prolonged sunlight
  - To notify physician if confusion, or hypotension occurs
  - To avoid concurrent use of alcohol or other CNS depressants
  - To avoid drinking or other hazardous activity, if drowsiness occurs.

Anesthesia for Caesarean Section

Problems of Anesthesia for Caesarean Section

- Caesarean section maybe done either as elective or emergency procedure2
- The mother may have a full stomach raising the probability of aspiration
- Many drugs pass through the placental barrier and may depress the baby
- Uterine contractibility may be diminished by volatile anaesthetic agents like ether, halothane etc
- Hypoxia and hypercapnia may occur.

General anesthesia Preoperative medication with sedatives or narcotics is not required as they may cause respiratory depression to fetus. Patient is given 30 ml of antacid (magnesium trisilicate) by mouth to reduce the gastric acidity to lesion the aspiration pneumonitis (Mendelsons syndrome). Patient is given 0.65 mg of atropine intravenously, and 100 percent oxygen for at least 3 minutes prior to the induction of anesthesia.

Induction of anesthesia is done with intravenous injection of thiopentone sodium 200 to 250 mg a 2.5 percent solution intravenously and maintained with 50 percent nitrous oxide. Fifty percent oxygen and a trace of halothane. After delivery of the baby, the nitrous oxide concentration should be increased to 70 percent and narcotics are injected intravenously to supplement anesthesia.

EFFECTS OF MATERNAL MEDICATIONS ON FETUS AND BREASTFEEDING INFANTS

During early embryogenesis, the drugs taken by the mother reach the conceptus through the tubal or uterine secretions by diffusion. The harmful effect on the blastocyst is usually death. In case of survival, there is chance of congenital anomalies.

From 2nd to 12th week (period of organogenesis), drugs taken by the mother can cause serious damages. Gross congenital malformations and even death of the fetus may result, depending on the route, length of time and dose of exposure.

From the second trimester onwards, transfer of drugs takes place through the uteroplacental circulation. The drug transfer across the placenta is increased due to the lowered serum albumin concentration, which results from hemodilution. As the albumin-binding capacity of the drugs is decreased, more free drug is available for placental transfer. In addition, the metabolism of the drugs may be hampered by the increase in plasma steroids. Increased utero-placental blood flow, increased placental surface area and decreased thickness of the placental membrane are the additional causes for increased drug transfer.

Fetotoxic or teratogenic drugs are prescribed only when the benefits outweigh the potential risks. Prior counseling is mandatory and minimum therapeutic dosage is used for shortest possible duration.

Maternal Medications with Established Teratogenic Properties and their Effects

- Cytotoxic drugs—Multiple fetal malformations and abortion.
- Androgenic steroids, Hydroxy progesterone—Masculinization of the female off-spring.
- Lithium—Increased congenital malformations when used in the first trimester, neonatal goiter, hypotonia and cyanosis.
- Diethyl stillbestrol—Vaginal stenosis, cervical hoods and uterine hypoplasia in female fetuses.

Possible Teratogens

- Antithyroid drugs—Goiter, mental retardation.
- Oral antidiabetic drugs—Abnormalities in the eyes, central nervous system, skeletal system and neonatal hypoglycemia.
- Vitamin D—Cardiopathies, hypercalcaemia and mental retardation.
- LSD (lysergic acid diethylamide)—Chromosomal abnormality and stunted growth.
- Anticonvulsants (Phenytoin, valproate) — Mental retardation, cardiac abnormalities, limb defects, neonatal bleeding, epilepsy.

Fetotoxic Drugs

- Aspirin—High doses in the last few weeks can cause premature closure of ductus arterious, persistent pulmonary hypertension and kernicterus in the newborn.
- Corticosteroids (prednisolone)—Doses above 10 mg daily may produce fetal and neonatal adrenal suppression.
- Aminoglycosides (antibiotics, e.g. amikacin, streptomycin)—Auditory or vestibular damage.
- Chloramphenicol—Peripheral vascular collapse (gray baby syndrome).
- Tetracycline—Dental discoloration (yellowish) and deformity, inhibition of bony growth.
- Long acting sulphonamides—Neonatal hemolysis, jaundice and kernicterus.
- Nitrofurantoin (furadantin)—Hemolysis in newborn with 06 PD deficiency, if used at term.
- Vitamin K (large doses)—Hyperbilirubinemia and kernicterus.
- Alcohol and smoking—Intrauterine growth retardation, pre-term labor, mental retardation.
- Narcotics—Depression of CNS—Apnea, bradycardia and hypothermia.
- Anesthetic agents—Convulsion, bradycardia, acidosis, hypoxia, hypertonia.
- Antihistamines—Tachycardia, vomiting, diarrhea.
- Anticoagulants—Optic atrophy, microcephaly, chondrodysplacia punctate.
- Diuretics—Fetal compromise due to diminished placental perfusion.
- Beta-blockers (antihypertensive drugs) — IUGR, fetal bradycardia and impaired fetal responses to hypoxia.

Maternal Drug Intake and Breastfeeding

Maternal drug intake of nursing mothers has adverse effects on lactation and also on the baby as it may be present in the breast milk.

Milk concentration of some drugs such as iodides may even exceed those in the maternal plasma so that therapeutic doses in the mother may cause toxicity to the infant. Certain drugs in breast-milk may cause hypersensitivity in the infant when used in therapeutic doses.

Transfer of drugs through breast milk depends on the following factors:

- Chemical properties
- Molecular weight
- Degree of protein binding
- Ionic dissociation
- Lipid solubility
- Tissue pH
- Drug concentration
- Exposure time.

Drugs that are nonionized, of low molecular weight and lipid soluble compounds are usually excreted through breastmilk. Drugs identified as having effects on lactation and the neonates are listed below:

- Bromides—Rash, drowsiness and poor feeding
- Iodides—Neonatal hypothyroidism
- Chloramphenicol—Bone marrow toxicity
- Oral pill (combined preparations)— Suppression of lactation
- Bromocriptine (parlodel)—Suppression of lactation
- Ergot—Suppression of lactation
- Metronidazole (Flagyl)—Anorexia, blood dyscrasias, irritability, weakness, neurotoxic disorders

- Anticoagulants—Hemorrhagic tendency (warfarin appears safe in therapeutic doses)
- Isoniazid—Anti-DNA activity and hepatotoxicity
- Antithyroid drugs and radioactive iodine—Hypothyroidism and goiter, agranulocytosis
- Antimetabolites (methotraxate)—Anti-DNA activity, immunosuppression
- Diazepam, opiates, phenobarbitone— Sedation effect with poor sucking reflex

Breast feeding is discouraged for mothers on medications that are harmful for the infant.

Lactation Suppressants

Commonly used drug to suppress lactation is bromocriptine mesylate, which suppress postpartum lactation by inhibiting prolactin secretion. The drug should be administered 1 to 5 days after delivery.

DRUGS ACTING ON THE UTERUS

Uterine Depressants

Uterine depressants inhibit uterine contractions by relaxing smooth muscles of uterus. Most of the uterine depressants act on the beta- 2 adrenergic receptors.

Commonly used drugs: Are magnesium sulfate, ritodrine hydrochloride, terbutaline and isoxsuprine.

Clinical uses: Prevention of threatened miscarriage and uncomplicated premature labor.

Untoward effects: Can cause maternal tachycardia, hypertension, hyperglycemia, and pulmonary edema.

Nursing implications

- Place the patient on her left side
- Monitor fluid intake and output
- Monitor lung sounds for pulmonary edema
- Monitor heart rate, and blood pressure
- Monitor fetal heart sounds
- If complications occur, stop intravenous infusion of the drug immediately.

Uterine Stimulants

Uterine stimulants cause contraction of uterine smooth muscles. The three different groups of drugs that cause uterine contractions are oxytocin, ergot alkaloids and prostaglandins.

Commonly used drugs: Oxytocin, methylergonovine maleate, ergonovine maleate, and dinoprostone (used as vaginal suppository or gel).

Clinical uses: To induce rapid labor, control hemorrhage, prevent uterine bleeding after cesarean section or parturition, and induce abortion.

Untoward effects: These drugs can cause GI irritation, and hypertension.

Nursing implications

- Record the patient's blood pressure before administration of the drug
- Monitor, patient's uterine contractions, heart rate, and blood pressure (BP should not exceed 140/90 mm Hg or an increase of 20 mm Hg in systolic from the patient's baseline)
- Monitor fetal heart sounds
- The pain and cramping caused by administration of uterine stimulants may not be completely relieved by analgesics
- Magnesium sulfate (intravenous) is the effective antidote for severe contractions caused by uterine stimulants
- Live birth from an abortion is possible.

13 Family Welfare Programme

INTRODUCTION

Family planning is a way of thinking and living that is adopted voluntary upon the basis of knowledge, attitude, and responsible decisions by individuals and couple, in order to promote the health and welfare of the family group and thus contribute effectively to the social development of the country (WHO 1971).

Family planning refers to practices that help individuals or couples to attain certain objective which include:

- To avoid unwanted births;
- To bring about wanted births;
- To regulate the interval between pregnancies;
- To control the time at which births occur in relation to the ages of the parent; and
- To determine the number of children in the family.

Some people feel that "Fertility Regulations" is perhaps more acceptable than the word "Family Planning". As a rule, family planning conjures up in the minds of the people of developing countries the idea of population control. Fertility regulation implies a situation where fertile couples space out their children and have the number of children they want. Infertile couples can be assisted to become fertile. Since the word 'family planning' is widely accepted for a long time it has been continued to use.

Family planning is very necessary in communities where the birth rate is high and medical services and financial resources are poor. Infant mortality rate is high because the parents cannot give proper care to the children on their limited resources. Moreover, involuntary parenthood creates emotional and social problems. Other indications for family planning are medical conditions such as cardiac disease, hypertension and chronic renal disease. Patients with these conditions cannot afford large families because of their impaired health. They also need to space out these pregnancies. Family planning is still a novelty to some people. As such the people need to be educated about it. They should be made to understand that family planning does not mean limiting one's family. It means judicious spacing children, so that their essential needs in life can be provided for by their parents. The children's health, their nutrition, their education, to mention a few needs, can only be taken care of if a decision on the spacing and total number of the children desired is taken in relation to the financial and health status of the parents. Family planning is becoming widely accepted in some developing countries including India.

Evolution of Fertility Regulations Methods (Contraceptions)

Fertility control is not a new concept. The ancient religious leaders exorcized in favour of having few children. In Rigveda, it is mentioned "A man with many children succumbs to miseries". This is probably the oldest statement suggesting against a large family. In virtually every culture which is of historical importance, as also in 'Hindu Dharma', of India, there existed a desire for birth control by natural as well as artificial means. The written history of contraception and antifertility measures goes as far back as to the "Atharva Veda", Brihadaranyopanishat and Kausikasutra, there is reference to prayers, surgical measures like crushing of testicle, vasectomy, and hysterectomy and medicaments for producing sterility and infertility, both in the male and the female. Some of the main preventive or birth limiting measures in ancient Indian Society (Bhagwan Dash, 1975) are:

- Delay in marriages
- Prohibition of cohabitation, on certain days
- Sex taboos limiting the frequency of cohabitation.

There is evidence of using local contraceptive, oral contraceptives for male and female (Read. Author's text on "Community Health Nursing")

- In fact many methods have been used throughout history to prevent pregnancy. In ancient Egypt, for example, women used domes formed of hollowed lemon halves to cover the cervix. Other cultural groups have used tampons or followed elaborate rituals to prevent conceptions. In many countries a parturient woman is not allowed to go out until forty days after delivery. Sexual intercourse is prohibited during the period of lactation, which in many developing countries lasts two to three years. In addition, after the mandatory forty days period of rest, the woman usually goes to live with her parents in-law until the infant is weaned. This segregation of the wife from the husband is a method of birth control by total abstinence. In addition to the above, men and women wore rings amulets etc. to protect themselves against an unwanted pregnancy.

Today contraception means choosing and using a method to delay, prevent or space pregnancy. It affords many alternatives and choises during the reproductive years. Contraception is an important factor in many women's lives, with needs varying according to the particular stage of life continuum, and should also be viewed in wider context of sexual and reproductive health. It has been argued that control of their own fertility is the largest single factor affecting the independence of women. The capacity to enjoy and control sexual and reproductive behaviour is key element of sexual health. Unintended pregnancies can have long lasting effects on the quality of life of parents and children.

Methods of Fertility Regulation (Contraceptions)

The methods of fertility regulation can be divided into appliances and nonappliance methods. The nonappliance methods include:

1. Total abstinence
2. Periodic abstinence
3. Temperature method
4. Coitus interruptus, coitus reservatus, coitus interfemoris.

Examples of the appliance methods are the use of the condom by the male and diaphragms, cervical caps and vimules, jellies, serosol foams etc., by the female. Jellies and aerosol foams are spermicidal. They can be used alone or in combination with the cervical cap, vimule or diaphragm by the female and the condom by the male and the female (Table 13.1).

Nonappliance Methods

Total abstinence: This method has the advantage of cheapness. It costs nothing except self denial on the part of the couple. It is absolutely reliable in that the failure rate is nil if it can be used successfully. It is, however, difficult to use it and it is doubtful whether the modern Indian couple will subscribe to it except on health grounds.

Periodic abstinence: This method depends on the avoidance of sexual intercourse during the period surrounding ovulation, i.e. two or three days before and after ovulation is deemed to have taken place. It is only practicable in women who have regular menstrual periods. Even in such women it is not easy to predict when fertilization of the ovum will take place. In addition it is known that ovulation is, in some women, stimulated by sexual intercourse, as in the rabbit. For the above reasons the failure rate of this method of birth control is high.

The temperature method: This form of periodic abstinence based on the prediction of the time of ovulation by taking the basal body temperature daily and avoiding sexual intercourse around the time of ovulation, i.e. when there is a rise of about 0.5°C in the basal body temperature. It is not a practicable method in a place where there is a high level of illiteracy. The illiterates will not be able to read the thermometer or chart the temperature even if they know which end of the thermometer to put in tho mouth. For the educated it is a good method but even the educated woman finds it a little bothersome.

Coitus interruptus: This is a method that has been in vogue for about two centuries. Intercourse takes place but the penis is withdrawn just before ejaculation of the semen. It is a method that can lead to a great deal of psychological upset in both sexual partners. Sometimes it is difficult for the

Table 13.1: Methods of contraception

Method	*Failure rate: Accidental pregnancy rate (Typical use: First year) (%)*	*Postpartum use*	*Risks and disadvantages*	*Benefits*
Abstinence	0	Is the method of choice for first 4-6 wk, especially for operative deliveries, complications, and lacerations	May be unacceptable to woman or partner; may cause relationship problems when there is disagreement	Promotes healing and involution
Oral contraceptives (two types) 1. Regular pill: combined oestrogen plus progestin 2. Minipill: progestin only	3	May interfere with lactation by decreasing milk supply; if lactating, use minipill or wait until lactation is well established	Minor side effects are breast tenderness, nausea, irregular bleeding (especially with minipill); major risks are rare in women age 36 and younger who do not smoke; blood clots, Liver tumour, cerebrovascular accident, myocardial infarction, gallbladder disease; requires regular monitoring by health-care provider	May be acceptable for healthy women aged 36-50 yr who do not smoke; menses are lighter and shorter, and there are fewer cramps; may protect against breast, ovarian, and uterine disease
Norplant	0.04	No studies are available of use during first 6 wk; lactating concerns same as those for the birth control pill	Requires insertion and removal of implants in arm by trained health-care provider; change in bleeding pattern common; risks similar to minipill; expensive	Contains progestin only; circulating hormone level less than that with minipill; lasts 5 yr; little monitoring required after insertion
Depo-Provera	0.04	Not recommended first 6 wk; does not prevent lactation; can be passed to infant via breast milk; no known harmful effects on newborn	Must be given by health-care provider; irregular menses common; risks similar to those of minipill	Injected intramuscularly every 12 wk; lasts for 3 mo
Intrauterine device (IUD)	3	Is not recommended during postpartum period	Must be inserted by a health-care provider during menses; has an increased risk of pelvic infection; may increase menstrual flow and cramps	One in place, requires little monitoring by woman; for suitable candidate, may be inserted during first menses after childbirth
Diaphragm with spermicide	18	Is not recommended; decreased levels of oestrogen make the vagina thinner and drier than normal and insertion difficult; must be refitted after a pregnancy; proper fitting is not possible until involution is complete	Causes irritation, allergic reactions, bladder irritation, must be inserted before intercourse and left in place for 6 hr; some positions may dislodge	Not appropriate during the early postpartum period

Contd...

Contd...

Method	*Failure rate: Accidental pregnancy rate (Typical use: First year) (%)*	*Postpartum use*	*Risks and disadvantages*	*Benefits*
Cervical cap with spermicide	18	Same as diaphragm	Are same as for diaphragm, except may leave in place longer; may increase risk of cervical neoplasia; few health-care providers fit caps	Not recommended during the postpartum period
Sponge	28	May cause irritation related to decreased levels of oestrogen; may increase risk of pelvic infection	Is difficult to remove; causes irritation and allergic reactions; linked to toxic shock syndrome	Is available over the counter; may be left in place longer than diaphragm; is disposable
Spermicide alone	21	May cause irritation because of decreased levels of oestrogen	May cause allergic reactions; is messy; insert just before intercourse	Available over the counter, affords some protection against sexually transmitted diseases
Foams with condoms, used together	3	Has no contraindications	Irritation and allergic reactions are rare; must be inserted/put on just before intercourse; is messy; may decrease sensation sexually transmitted diseases	As effective as the pill when used together; foam is lubricant; available over the counter; protect against
Condoms alone	12	Have no contraindications	Irritation and allergic reactions are rare; must be inserted/put on just before intercourse; is messy; may decrease sensation use correctly	Available over the counter; used together; foam is lubricant; available over the counter; protect against sexually transmitted diseases
Natural family planning, fertility awareness, periodic abstinence	20	Are not recommended; requires signs and symptoms of hormone fluctuation during normal cycling; this cycling does not occur during the postpartum period, especially during lactation	No risks; require practice and education from trained professional; require self-monitoring and record keeping as well as varying periods of abstinence	Require no devices or chemicals; may be acceptable for couples who do not wish to use other methods because of religious or other reasons
Withdrawal	18	Has no contraindications	Requires interruption of sexual response cycle; fluid with sperm is often released before ejaculation	Requires no devices or chemicals;
Vasectomy or male sterilization	0.15	Has no contraindications	Is permanent; requires minor surgery	No further monitoring required after verification that all sperm in system have been ejaculated
Bilateral tubal ligation or female sterilization	0.4	May be performed during cesarean delivery; may be performed soon after vaginal delivery	Is permanent; may present surgical complications	Requires no further monitoring

partners to separate when orgasm is imminent. The method calls for a great deal of self control on the part of the two partners and requires a great deal of motivation for continued use.

Coitus reservatus: In this method, penetration of the vagina takes place, but there is little or no motion and the man does not ejaculate into the vagina. It is not a good method.

Coitus interfemoris: The erect penis is placed between the thighs of the female, so ejaculation, if it occurs, does so outside the vagina.

Appliance Methods

Barrier methods Barrier methods prevent spermatozoa coming into contact with the ovum. They comprise male and female condoms, caps and diaphragms which are used with spermicides (Figs 13.1 to 13.5).

Physical Methods

Male condoms In India it is known as 'NIRODH'. The condom is rolled on to the erect penis and must applied before any genital contact occurs as some semen may escape prior to ejaculation. The condom is fitted on the erect penis before intercourse. The air must be expelled from the teat end to make room for the ejaculate. The condom must be held carefully when withdrawing it from the vagina to avoid spilling seminal fluid into the vagina after intercourse. A new condom should be used for each sexual act.

Condom prevents the semen from being deposited in vagina. The effectiveness of condom may be increased by using it in conjunction with a spermicidal jelly inserted into vagina before intercourse. It serves as additional protection in the unlikely event that the condom should slip off or tear.

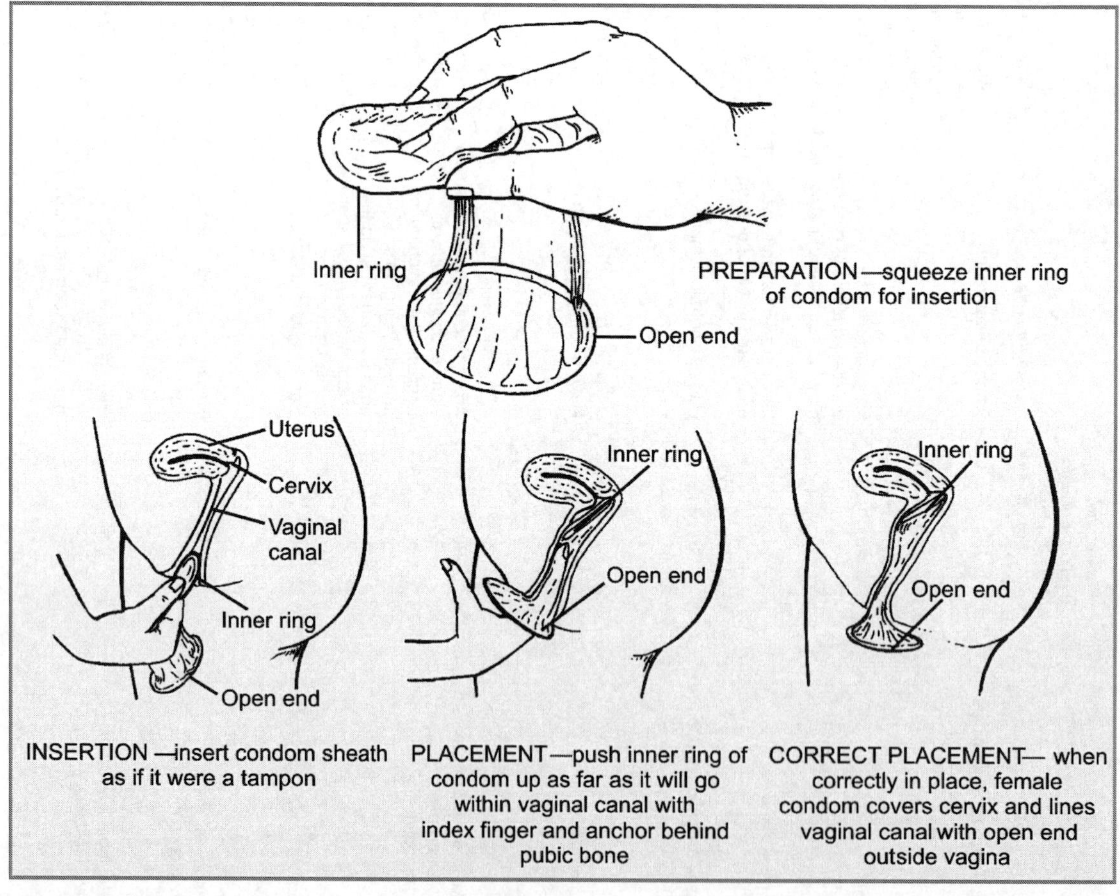

Fig. 13.1: The female condom is a prelubricated transparent sheath that forms a second skin inside the vagina when inserted properly shields the vaginal and urethral areas from contact with the penis while capturing semen during intercourse

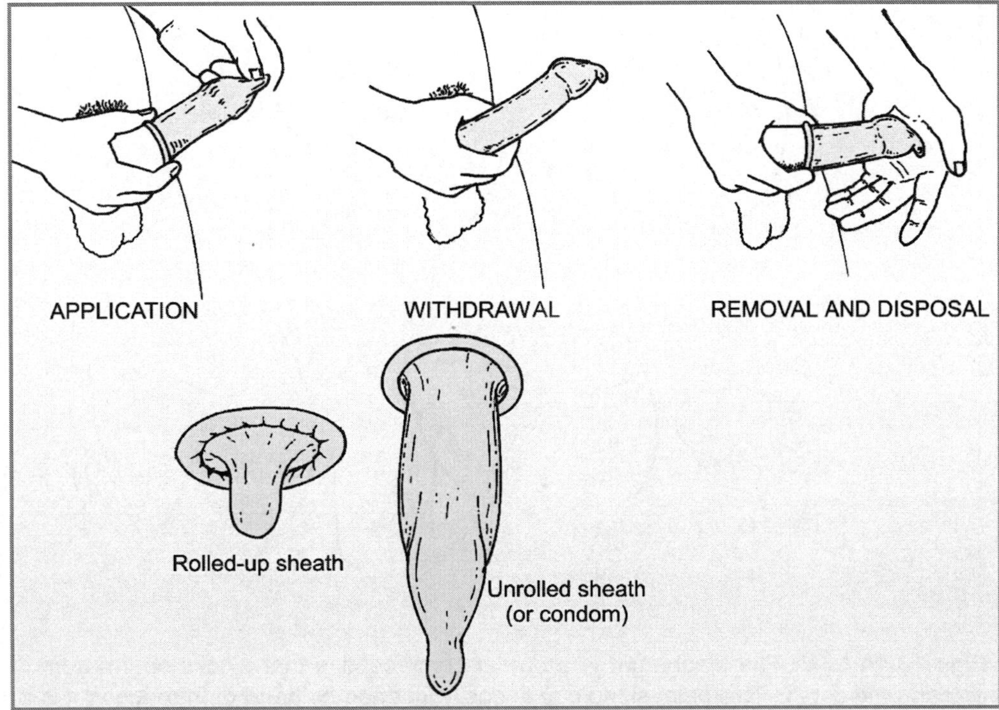

Fig. 13.2: Male condoms prevent the deposit of sperm in the vagina: There are many types of condoms, and packaging becomes an important part of marketing. The male condom is a sheer rubber sheath before use

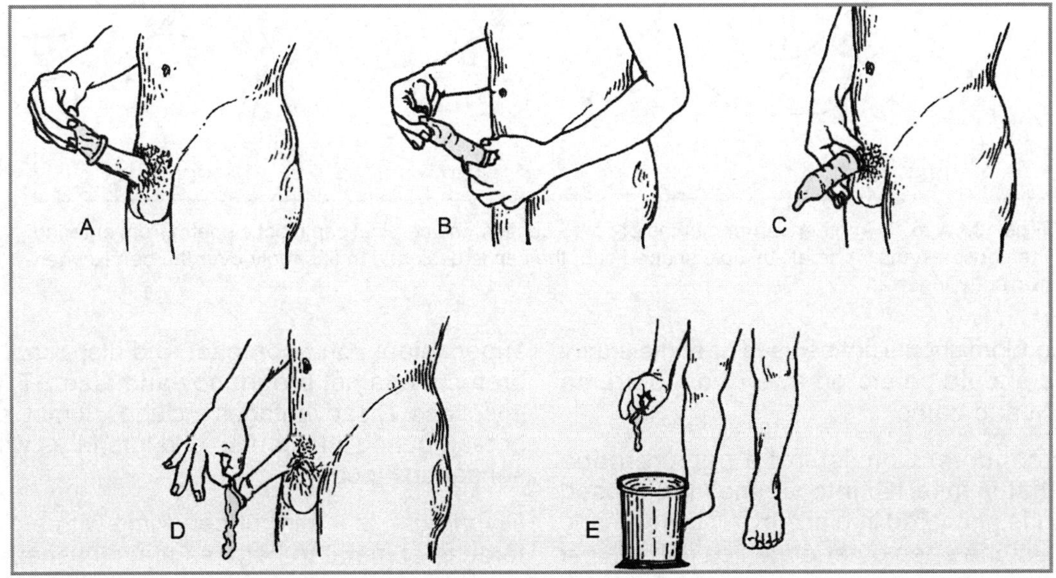

Figs 13.3A to E: How to use a condom safely

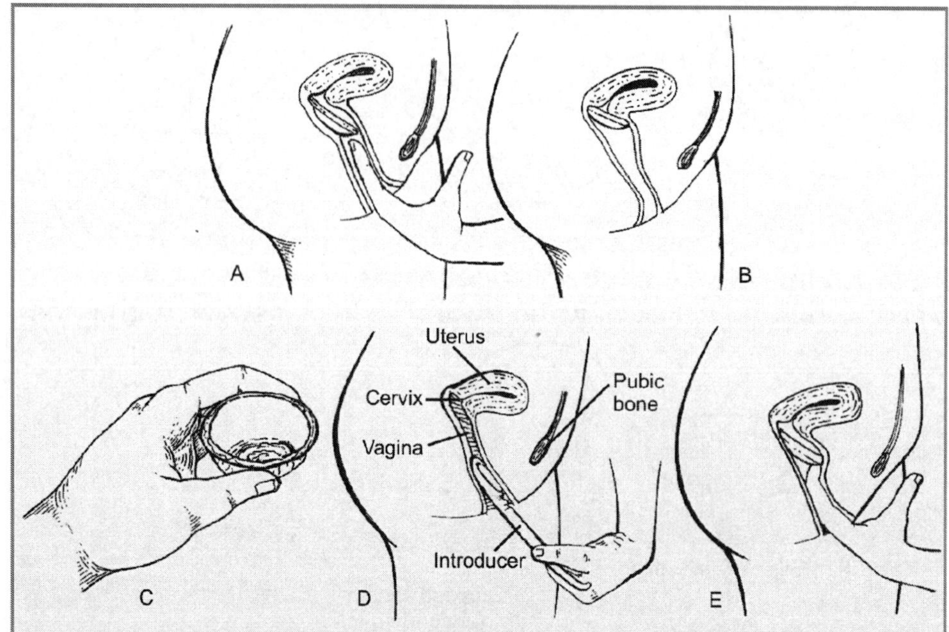

Figs 13.4A to E: The diaphragm is a barrier contraceptive that blocks sperm from entering the cervix: This palm-sized cup is easily inserted by hand or introducer, it is designed to be used with spermicidal cream or gel

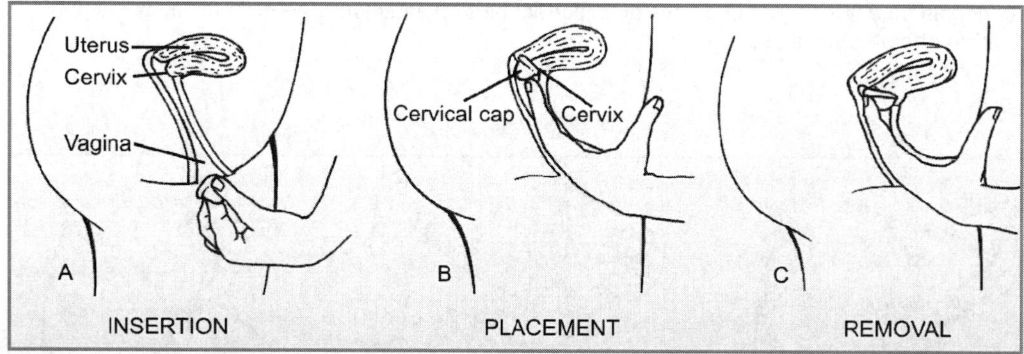

Figs 13.5A to C: Another barrier method of contraception, the cervical cap blocks sperm from entering the cervical canal: A small, thimble shaped cup, the cap is designed to fit snugly over the cervix when correctly inserted

The condom should not be used after the expiry date and should be stored away from extreme heat, light and damp.

Female condom: Consists of a polyurethane sheath that is inserted into vagina. The closed inner and is anchored in place by a polyurethane ring. Whilst the open outer edge lies flat against the vulva.

General advantages of condoms include the easy availability of condoms safe and inexpensive, easy to use, do not require medical supervision; light, compact and disposable and protects against pregnancy and also STD, HIV infections. Disadvantages includes, it may slip off or tear, during intercourse and interferes with sex sensations locally.

Diaphragm: is a thin rubber dome with a circumference of metal to help maintain its shape. It is available in a range of types and sizes and the woman is individually fitted.

The diaphragm is a shallow cup made of synthetic rubber or plastic material. It ranges diameter from 5-10 cm (2-4 inches). It has a flexible rim made of spring or metal. When in place, the rim of the diaphragm should lie closely against the vaginal walls and rest between the posterior fornix and the symphysis pubis. Before insertion, spermicide should be applied. After insertion the woman must check that her cervix is covered. In order to preserve spontaneity during intercourse. The diaphragm can be inserted every evening as a matter of routine. This should be done after bathing, if applicable rather before.

If intercourse occurs more than 3 hours after insertion, then additional spermicide is required. The diaphragm must be left in place for at least 6 hours after the last intercourse. On removal, the diaphragm should be washed with a mild soap, dried and inspected for any damage. A new diaphragm should be fitted annually and following any alteration in weight by more than 3 kilograms. In case of postpartum, period, preferably new diaphragm should be used after assessing size of the same.

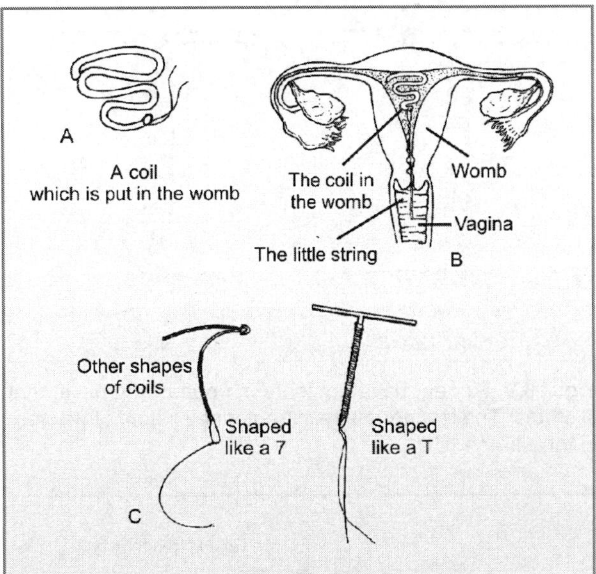

Fig. 13.6: The intrauterine contraceptive device

Chemical Methods

There are spermicides which include:

- Foams, foam tablets, foam aerosoles
- Creams, jellies and pastes squeezed from a tube
- Suppositories-inserted manually
- Soluble films-Cfilm-inserted manually.

These preparations kill spermatozoa, but as they are not able to penetrate the cervical mucus and thus probably only active in the vagina, they are not recommended for use on their own. They must be applied immediately before or in the case of pessaries 10 minutes before intercourse.

The main drawbacks of spermicides are they have a high failure rate; they must be used almost immediately before intercourse and repeated before each sex act; they must be introduced into those regions of the vagina where sperms are likely to be deposited and they may cause mild burning or irritation, besides messiness. And spermicides are not as effective when used alone.

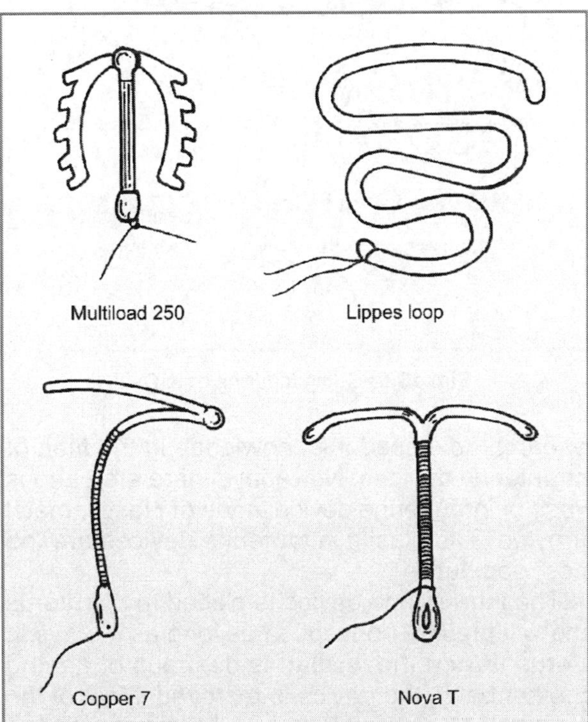

Fig. 13.7: Some intrauterine contraceptive devices

The Intrauterine Contraceptive Device (IUCD or IUD) (Figs 13.6 to 13.11)

Intrauterine contraceptive devices have been known for many years. Arabian camel owners used to insert a stone into the uterus of the camel to prevent conception 2000 years ago. Intrauterine contraceptive devices in the human were at first widely used but later were condemned because of the many complications which resulted from their use. Around 1940 they became popular again because intensive scientific

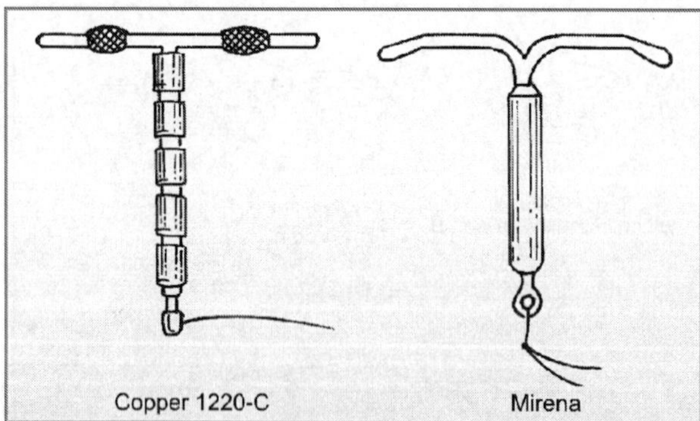

Fig. 13.8: Recent developments in copper and hormonal systems: The levonorgestrel intrauterine system of delivery in the Mirena IUD

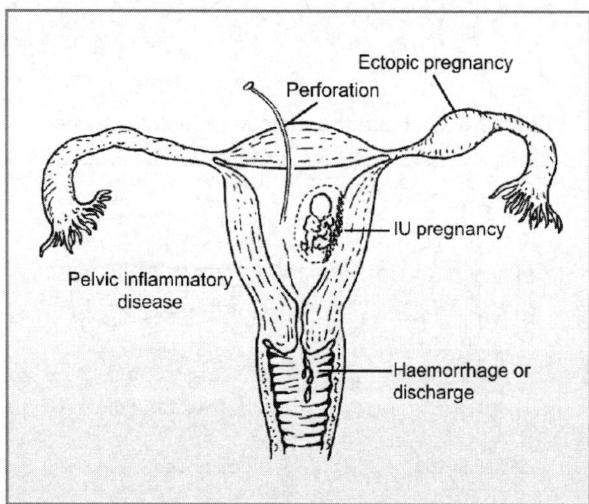

Fig. 13.9: Complications of IUDs

research advanced the knowledge in the filed of intrauterine devices. Nowadays there are various types of intrauterine device made of plastic, metal or nylon. The plastic intrauterine devices are the most popular.

The intrauterine device is placed in the uterus and will prevent conception as long as it stays in uterus. When the woman is desirous of having another baby, the device is removed. Most of the devices are easy to insert and remove and the insertion can usually be done in the out-patients department without anaesthesia. A device can stay for as long as the patient desires but it may be desirable to remove it at the end of five years and insert another. The patient is closely followed up in the family planning clinic. Certain intrauterine devices, such as the Copper-T and Copper 7 (gravigard) which rely on elemental copper for

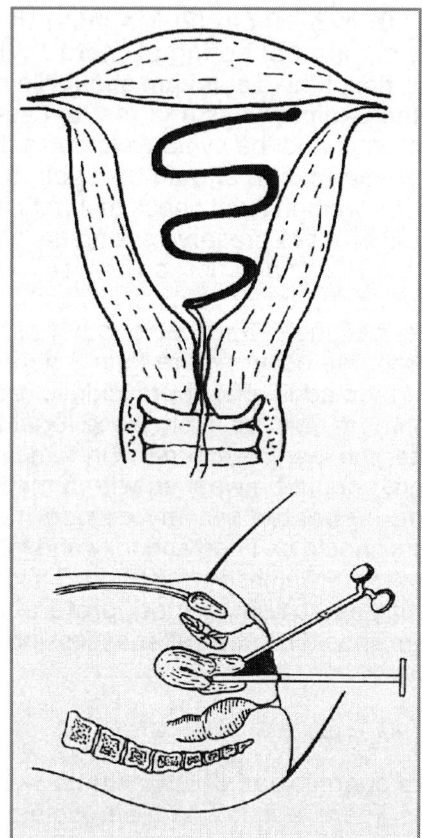

Fig. 13.10: Insertion of the IUD

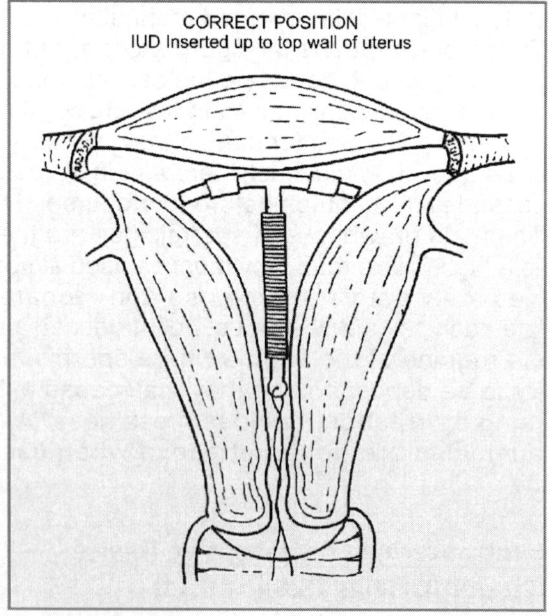

Fig. 13.11: The intrauterine device (IUD) causes an inflammatory reaction to the uterus, preventing implantation of the fertilized ovum

their high efficacy, may need to be removed and replaced by new ones as frequently as once in 2,3 or 4 years, depending on the amount of elemental copper. The advantages of the intrauterine device far outweighs the disadvantages. The disadvantages are:

- It is expensive in terms of the organization of clinics and personnel.
- The patient has to see a physician or nurse to be able to use it.
- It may fail and conception may take place even with the device in situ this is, however, rare and occurs in only about 3 per cent of all women wearing the device.

The advantages are:

- The device itself is cheap.
- Once it is inserted, the patient does not have to spend money monthly as in the case of the pill.
- It does not interfere with the act of coitus; the patient does not have to remember to carry it around with her; the need for continued motivation on the part of the user is removed.
- It is reasonably effective being so in about 97 to 98 per cent of cases.

The IUCD creates an inflammatory response, with the increased number of leucocytes destroying spermatozoa and ova. Gamete viability is further impaired by alterations of uterine and tubal fluids. Copper affects endometrial enzymes, glycogen metabolism and oestrogen uptake, thus rendering the endometrium hostile to implantation.

A copper T can be inserted upto 5 days following the earliest estimated date of ovulation that is day 19 in a 28 day cycle. Some prefer to insert a routine IUCD from day 4 to day 14. The woman may experience some discomfort during the procedures, which should be performed using aseptic technique. Depending upon the type of IUCD used, it may be left in place from 3 to 10 years and longer in some instances.

Side Effects or Complications of Intrauterine Devices

1. Abnormal uterine bleeding: This may take the form of menorrhagia or it may be in the form of prolonged bleeding immediately after insertion of the device. The abnormal uterine bleeding usually stops after the first or second menstrual period.
2. Vaginal discharge may be troublesome in the first few weeks following insertion of the device. It is easily treated and does not constitute a serious problem.
3. Lower abdominal pain and backache. This may be complained of by the patient. Usually both symptoms disappear even without treatment, after two or three menstrual cycles.
4. Pelvic inflammatory disease: This may occur after insertion of the device but this is not common and it is easily treated.
5. Expulsion of the device: The device is usually expelled during a menstrual flow but it can also be expelled without any association with menstrual flow but it can also be expelled without any association with the menses. Sometimes, the device may be expelled into the vagina and the patient may not be aware of this. Pregnancy may result from such unnoticed expulsions. The patient must be asked to feel the nylon thread at the end of the device once in a while. This will enable her to know whether the device has been displaced or not.
6. Pregnancy: The device may fail even when it is in utero and pregnancy may occur. This is very uncommon and only occurs in about 2 to 3 percent of women wearing the device. Pregnancy rates vary with different types of device. The figures quoted apply to the Lippes loop.

The majority of patients wearing the device may not have any of the complications listed above. When complications are reported to the nurse midwife, she should at once refer the patient to the physician. Intrauterine contraceptive devices are contraindicated in the presence of pregnancy, uterine fibroids, chronic cervicitis with or without cervical erosion, pelvic inflammatory disease or in patients suspected of having carcinoma of the cervix.

All patients attending family planning clinics should have routine cytological screening before any method of contraception is used.

Hormonal Methods

Hormonal contraceptives used are the most effective spacing methods of contraception. Oral contraceptives of combined types are almost hundred per cent effective in preventing pregnancy. Hormonal contraceptive currently in use and/or under study may be classified as follows:

- Oral pills
  - Combined pill, e.g. Mala-N, and Mala-D
  - Progestogene only pill (POP)
  - Post coital pill – IUD, Hormonal
  - Once a month (long acting pill)
  - Long acting estrogen with short acting progesterone
  - Male pill
- Depot (slow release) formulation
  - Injectables—DMPA (Deport-medroxy progesterone acetate NET-EN (norethisterone-enanthate)
  - Subcutaneous implants—Norplant, Norplan (R) –2
  - Vaginal rings.

Steroid hormonal contraceptives: Steroid hormones are used to prevent conception. They can be administered orally (oral contraceptives the pill) or parenterally, by intramuscular injection, or subfascially, by implantation. The intramuscular administration may be monthly, three-monthly or six monthly.

Oral contraceptives: There are many preparations of oral contraceptives. They usually contain an oestrogen or a progestrogen or both. The oestrogen preparations often used are ethinyl oestradiol and mestranol. The progestogen preparations are numerous. Many of them are derived from the 19-nortestorone series and others are derived from 17-hydroxy-progesterone. Three main types of oral contraceptive therapy are used in family planning clinic.

These are:

1. The combined therapy;
2. The sequential therapy;
3. The continuous low-dose therapy.

Combined therapy: A tablet containing oestrogen and progestogen is given daily from the 5th day of the menstrual cycle until the 22nd day, when an iron containing nonsteroidal, noncontraceptive tablet is given from the 23rd day to the 4th day of the next menstrual cycle, after which the combined tablet is repeated as in the previous cycle. There is usually a withdrawal bleeding coinciding with the menstrual period around the 28th day of a preceding cycle or on the first day of a subsequent cycle.

Sequential therapy: In this method, an attempt is made to stimulate the pattern of the menstrual cycle. From the 5th day of a cycle a tablet containing oestrogen is given daily until the 14th day. Thereafter, a tablet containing oestrogen and progestogen is given daily until the 22nd or 23rd day, after which a nonsteroidal, noncontraceptive tablet is given from that day until the 4th day of the next cycle.

Low-dose therapy: Small daily doses of oestrogens or progestogens are given starting from the 5th day of a cycle and continuing until the woman no longer desires to prevent pregnancy or when complications if any, arise.

Mode of Action of Oral Contraceptives

The combined and sequential therapies act by inhibiting ovulation through their effect on the hypothalamus and the anterior pituitary. They also act directly on the endometrium, bringing about a disharmony between glandular and stromal development. They make the intrauterine environment unsuitable for implantation of the fertilized ovum. They affect sperm capacitation making it difficult for the spermatozoon to fertilize the ovum. They also have an effect on the cervical mucus but not to the same extent at the low dose progestogens.

The low-dose progestogens act not necessarily by inhibiting ovulation but by their direct effect on the cervix. They alter the physical and chemical properties of the cervical mucus and make it impenetrable to the spermatozoa. They cause diminished spinbarkeit and cause the cervical mucus to be thick and viscous.

The Effects of Oral Contraceptives on Health

The effects may be beneficial or harmful. The beneficial effects are as follows:

1. Relief of dysmenorrhoea. This is because primary or essential dysmenorrhoea occurs only in ovulatory cycles. Abolition of ovulation by oral contraceptive therapy prevents dysmenorrhea.
2. Diminution of menstrual blood flow. Women who are known to have heavy menstrual bleeding have normal menstrual loss when they take oral contraceptives regularly. In addition, women who have irregular menses prior to taking oral contraceptives have the menstrual periods restored to a normal rhythm.

3. Improvement in acne. Progestogen only contraceptives improve acne by decreasing the production of sebum due to suppression of sebaceous gland activity.
4. Postponement of menstruation. Contraceptives, if taken continuously, may be used to postpone a menstrual period which is likely to interfere with an important social engagement, e.g. a wedding.
5. Inhibition of the midcycle (Mittelshmerz) pain. Because oral contraceptives inhibit ovulation they also abolish the midcycle ovulation pain.
6. Increase in libido. Oral contraceptives may or may not increase libido. Increase in libido may be psychological due to removal of the fear of pregnancy resulting from a sexual act.
7. Doubtful relief of premenstrual tension. It is believed that oral contraceptives relief premenstrual tension. There is some doubt about this, oral contraceptives have been used to advantage for other conditions.

The harmful effects: The harmful effects of oral contraceptives are sometimes exaggerated. There are many possible harmful effects but only the important ones, about which there is no doubt will be mentioned.

Effects on the reproductive system

1. Prolonged amenorrhoea after cessation of therapy or during therapy. This is uncommon but it is known to occur.
2. Infection with candida (monilia) albicans. Moniliasis or candidiasis is not an uncommon finding in women taking oral contraceptives.
3. Abnormal menstrual bleeding patterns may be caused by oral contraceptives. These may take the form of intermenstrual bleeding or spotting.
4. Abolition or suppression of lactation. Oral contraceptives tend to suppress lactation in a woman who is breastfeeding her infant.
5. Enlargement of pre-existing uterine fibroids. Oestrogen causes enlargement of pre-existing fibroids.
6. Carcinoma: The carcinogenic effect of oral contraceptives has not been proven beyond doubt. In the case of carcinoma of the cervix, the nurse midwife should remember that the patients who may want oral contraceptives are those at risk of developing carcinoma of the cervix by virtue of their high parity and possibility of postpartum chronic cervicitis, etc.
7. Tenderness and lumps in the breast. Oral contraceptives are known to cause tenderness and enlargement of the breasts.

Effects on the cardiovascular system

1. Elevation of arterial blood pressure this is usually blamed on the oestrogen component of oral contraceptives.
2. Interference with blood clotting mechanism resulting in:
   a. Thromboembolism;
   b. Pulmonary embolism;
   c. Ischaemic cerebrovascular disorder;
   d. Retino-vascular disease.

Oral contraceptives are said to be associated with an eight fold increase of venous thrombosis of pulmonary embolism. The risk is further increased by smoking and advancing age (above the age of 40 years), whether there is a cause-and-effect relationship between oral contraceptive therapy and the development of thromboembolic phenomena is still highly debatable. It is generally believed that the oestrogen component of oral contraceptives is responsible for the blood clotting defects. This is why tablets containing a low dose of oestrogen, e.g. 35 to 50 micrograms per tablet, are given. Oral contraceptives should not be prescribed for women who are prone to thrombophlebitis or women who have very bad varicose veins.

Metabolic effects: These are seen in three major endocrine glands and the liver. The three endocrine glands are:

1. The adrenals
2. The thyroid
3. The pancreas.

The effects of oral contraceptives on the adrenal and thyroid glands are not very serious. The effects on the pancreas are serious, especially is known diabetics. Diminished glucose tolerance is found in women taking oral contraceptives. Impairment of glucose tolerance is more severe in women who have latent or overt diabetes and who are taking oral contraceptives. Oral contraceptives should not be given to diabetic women. It is therefore necessary to exclude glycosuria in all the women attending the family planning clinics. If there is glycosuria, a fasting blood sugar estimation followed by a glucose tolerance test should be done.

Effects on the liver: Oral contraceptives cause some alteration in liver function. The degree of alteration depends on the dose of oral contraceptives. Jaundice occurs in about 1 in 10,000 women on oral contraceptives. Oral contraceptives should not be given to women who have recurrent cholestatic jaundice (or pruritus) of pregnancy. They should not be given to women who have gallbladder problems.

In addition to the above, oral contraceptives affect the metabolism of lipids (fats), vitamins such as B6 (pyridoxine), folic acid/pteroylglutamic acid), vitamin B12 (cyanocobalamine), thiamine, riboflavine (vitamin B1), ascorbic acid (vitamin C) and vitamin A (retinol).

Effects on salt and water metabolism: Steroid hormonal contraceptives bring about a decrease in the excretion of sodium and chloride and cause water retention.

Effects on the kidneys: The progestogen component of oral contraceptives may lead to ureteral dilatation and therefore cause a symptomatic pyelonephritis. The ureteral dilatation disappears when oral contraceptives are stopped.

Effects on the respiratory system: These effects are not very clear.

Effects on their central nervous system

1. Nausea and vomiting: Nausea and vomiting and other gastrointestinal symptoms may occur during the first few days of the initial two or three months of the treatment cycles. Thereafter, the symptoms tend to disappear. It is believed the gastrointestinal upset is due to the oestrogen component of the oral contraceptive.
2. Depression sometimes occurs in women taking oral contraceptives, especially those containing a high dose of progestogen.
3. Headaches associated with migraine. Oral contraceptives are said to cause migraine headaches in women who previously did not have migraine. Paradoxically, oral contraceptives are said to relieve headaches in women previously known to have migraine.
4. Decreased libido: Some women on oral contraceptives complain of loss of libido. It is tought that the loss of libido is due to the progestogen component.

Effects on the skin: Oral contraceptives are known to cause chloasma or melasma, a condition of hyperpigmentation over the forehead, the molar eminences and the lower parts of the cheeks. It is thought that the oestrogen components of the oral contraceptive is responsible for the skin changes. In some cases oral contraceptives have been associated with the male type of alopecia.

When examined in isolation the adverse effects of oral contraceptives are frightening. They are, however, not as bad as they sound. Quite apart from the fact that the adverse effects are not always encountered in every woman taking oral contraceptives, these adverse effects should be weighed against the risks of an unwanted pregnancy. An unwanted pregnancy can lead to a great deal of emotional upset. In addition, an attempt to procure an abortion, especially by unqualified personnel, may have serious consequences. Such an attempt may lead to a great deal of morbidity and physical disability. If the patient survives the complications of uterine perforation, haemorrhage and infection, she may be sentenced to permanent sterility because of blockage of the Fallopian tubes. She may also end up with chronic inflammatory disease with acute exacerbations.

In view of some of the complications of oral and other contraceptives, it is important that a good history be obtained from a woman before enrolling her in the fertility regulation clinics. A thorough clinical examination should be carried out after history taking. The clinical examination should include recording of the weight and blood pressure and breast examination. In addition, the urine should be tested for sugar, albumin and acetone. A pelvic (vaginal) examination must be made and, if possible, vaginal and cervical smears taken for cytological examination. The packed cell volume or haemoglobin should be estimated.

Evaluation of Oral Contraceptives

When taken correctly, oral contraceptives are very effective in preventing pregnancy. The theoretical effectiveness of the combined therapy is about 100 per cent but the use effectiveness is much less. The combined therapy is the most efficacious of the three methods of therapy. The low-dose progestogens are the least efficacious. They, however, cause fewer symptoms than the other types of therapy. The combined and sequential therapies are not suitable for lactating women.

The injectable steroid hormonal contraceptives: As previously stated, there are long acting and short acting injectable hormonal contraceptives.

Long-acting injectable contraceptives: Two preparations are used.

Depot medroxy progesterone acetate (DMPA) of Depot Provera is an Upjohn product. It is usually given in doses of 150 mg at intervals of twelve weeks. The first injection is given at intervals of 12 weeks.

Norethisterone oenanthate (Net Oen) (The trade names are Noristerate, Norigest) is a product of Schering Berling AG. It is given in doses of 200 mg. The first injection is given on the 5th day of the menstrual cycle. Subsequent injections are given at intervals of 8 weeks for the first 3 injections. Thereafter, injections are given at intervals of 8 weeks for the first 3 injections. Thereafter, injections are given at intervals of twelve weeks.

DMPA and Net Oen are given by deep, intramuscular injection into the glutal muscle. When both preparations are given as described above they are very effective in preventing pregnancy. They can safely be administered to lactating mothers. They do not inhibit lactation. If anything, they increase the milk flow. They can be given to some women who may not tolerate oral contraceptives.

One major drawback of long acting injectable contraceptives is that they cause prolonged amenorrhoea after cessation of therapy, DMPA is more guilty in this respect than Net Oen. The long-acting injectable contraceptives sometimes also cause abnormalities in the bleeding pattern of the women taken them. These abnormalities may take the form of spotting, or menorrhagia. Other side effects include non-menstrual symptoms such as headache and depression. Hypertension has been observed in a small proportion of women who were normotensive before the commencement of therapy. It must be realized that the side effects of the long acting injectables are not always serious. The advantages of IMPA and Net Oen far outweigh their disadvantages. In view of the possiblility of prolonged amenorrhoea after cessation of therapy, it is preferable to give DMPA and Net Oen to women who, though young (under 35 years), have had the desired member of children and do not wish to be sterilized.

Clinical Injectable Contraceptives

Cycloprovera is the preparation given at monthly intervals. One-millilitre ampoule of cycloprovera contains 50 mg of depot medroxy progesterone acetate and 10 mg of oestradiol cypionate. The monthly dose is 25 mg of DMPA and 5 mg of oestradiol cypionate, i.e. half a milliliter of the preparation. It is given by deep injection into the gluteal muscle.

Although cycloprovera causes less amenorrhoea than DMPA it is not entirely free from the side effects caused by DMPA and Net Oen.

Subfascial Implants: Implantation of pellets of a progestogen preparation can be done using the fascia lata (fascia covering the thigh muscles). Subfascial implantation, depending on the dose, may last as long as two years before the contraceptive effects wear off. As a rule this method of steroid hormonal therapy is not used in family planning clinics. It is not easy to carry out and it can hardly be delegated to nurses or auxillaries, both of whom could give an intramuscular injection.

Other Methods

Pregnancy termination In some countries, pregnancy termination is used as a method of fertility regulation or birth control. In many countries pregnancy termination is not permitted by law. Attitudes are however, changing in some of these countries. Because the laws on induced abortions are changing in some developing countries it may be profitable for the nurse midwife to be conversant with some of the methods of pregnancy termination.

It must be emphasized that induced abortion carried out, even in a well equipped hospital, is not without risks. However, it carries much less risk than induced abortions done clandestinely in squalid surroundings.

The earlier in pregnancy abortion is induced the fewer the risks involved. Thus, induced abortion in the first trimester carries much less risk than that done in the second trimester. (Please see MTP Act 1971 of India).

Methods of Pregnancy Termination in the First Trimester

Menstrual regulation or menstrual extraction This is a method of terminating early pregnancies, e.g. at 6 to 8 weeks. It is achieved by the use of the Karman plastic syringe and plastic cannulae of varying sizes.

The detailed description of the method of menstrual regulation is beyond the scope of this book. Sufficient it to say that menstrual regulation is simple and straight forward. It can be done as an outpatient procedure.

Dilatation and curettage: First trimester pregnancy termination can be achieved by dilatation of the cervix and curettage of the uterus. It is not always easy to achieve dilatation of the cervix in early pregnancy. Cervical laceration and uterine perforation are risks which must be avoided. Menstrual extraction or suction evacuation is to be preferred to dilatation and curettage.

Suction evacuation: In cases unsuitable for menstrual regulation on account of the large uterine size more than 6 to 8 weeks but 12 weeks or less suction evacuation can be carried out. Like menstrual regulation, suction evacuation is a simple and straightforward procedure which can be done in out patients.

Mid-trimester pregnancy termination: Mid-trimester pregnancy termination should be avoided if possible. In the event of a woman reporting an unwanted pregnancy after the 12th week of gestation it is preferable to advice her to carry the pregnancy to term unless it is established that continuation of the pregnancy is injurious to her mental and physical health.

Apart from surgical intervention in the form of abdominal hysterotomy intra-amniotic abortifecients such as prostaglandins, hypertonic saline and urea can be used to effect mid-trimester pregnancy termination. To facilitate the intra-amniotic instillation of the abortifacients it is advisable to wait until about the 16th week of gestation when the uterus is surely palpable abdominally and there is sufficient liquor amnii.

Surgical methods of contraception: These methods are only used in cases where both partner agree not to have any more children or where the health of one or both of them makes further pregnancies undesirable.

Two methods are commonly employed. They are:

1. *Female sterilization* (Figs 13.12A to C) This implies bilateral tubal ligation or salpingectomy. This can be done during the operation of caesarean section, or on the second or third post partum day if the patient had a vaginal delivery, or as an elective procedure in a non-pregnant woman. Before female sterilization is done, the position regarding future pregnancies must be adequately explained to the husband and his wife because the operation is, as a rule, irreversible, great thought must be given to the problem before the operation is performed. The consent of the husband and wife must be obtained. It must also be remembered that

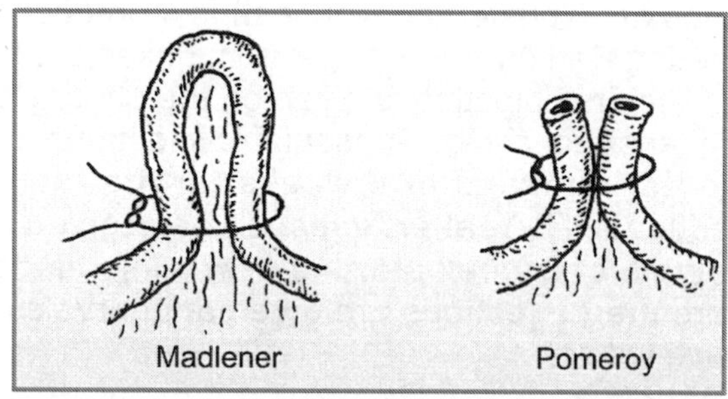

Fig. 13.12A: Sterilization by tubal ligation and excision

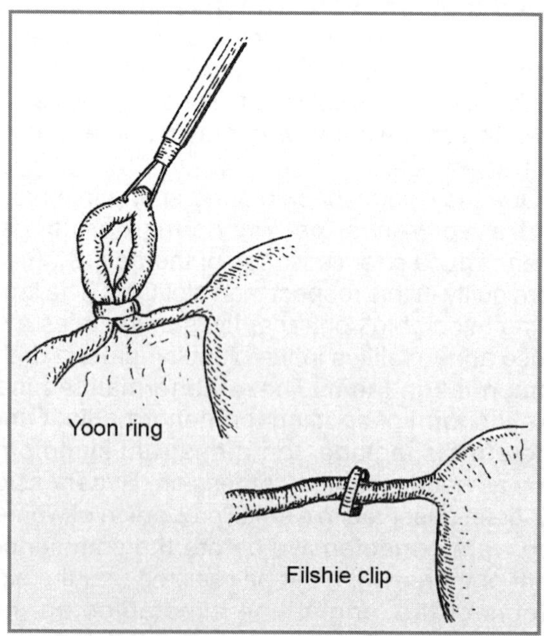

Fig. 13.12B: Sterilization by clip occlusion

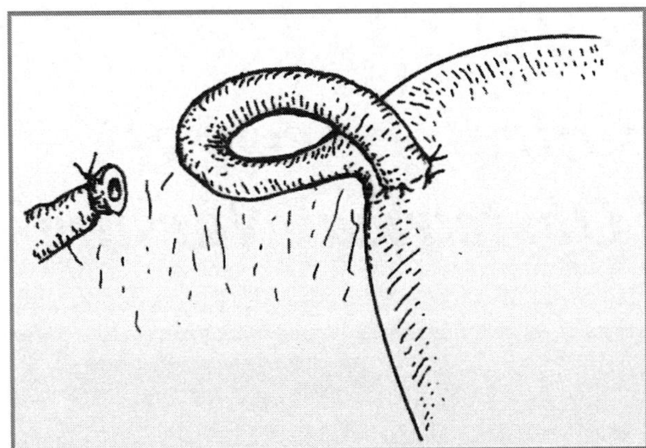

Fig. 13.12C: Burial of tubal stumps

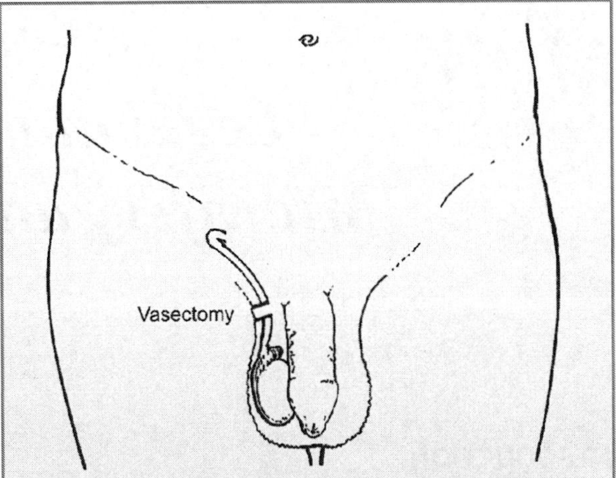

Fig. 13.13: Vasectomy involves excision of a segment of the vas deferens

very occasionally female sterilization in the form of tubal ligation alone may fail. Only removal of the uterus can guarantee 100 per cent contraception.

Tubal ligation can be achieved at laparatomy, laparoscopy, culdoscopy and posterior colpotomy. The laparoscopic, culdoscopic and colpotomy methods can be done in an outpatient theatre. The patients are usually discharged home on the same day after a few hours observation in the hospital.

The conventional technique of laparotomy may be used, i.e. one in which a large abdominal incision is made and the patient is hospitalized for at least 1 week. On the other hand the mini-laparatomy technique involving a very small incision about 2.5 cm long may be employed. The advantage of the mini-laparotomy technique is that it leaves a very small scar and obviates the need to hospitalize the patient for more than a few hours for observation.

2. *The male sterilization* (Fig. 13.13): This implies what is known as vasectomy. In this operation, the vas deferens on each side is divided and ligated. This prevents the passage of spermatozoa into the seminal vesicles and so conception does not take place after intercourse. The operation is very popular in India and other parts of Asia. After vasectomy the husband and wife are enjoined to abstain from intercourse for six to eight weeks or to use some form of contraceptive protection during that period.

To ensure normal healing of the wound and to ensure the success of vasectomy, the patient should be given the following advice:

- The patient should be told that he is not sterile immediately after the operation; at least 30 ejaculations may be necessary before the seminal examination is negative.
- To use contraceptives until aspermia has been established.
- To avoid taking baths for at least 24 hours after the operation.
- To wear a T-bandage or scrotal support for 15 days and keep the site clean and dry.
- To avoid cycling or lifting heavy weights for 15 days, there is, however no need for complete bed rest.
- To have the stitches removed on the 5th day after the operation.

Recently “No-scalpel Vasectomy” is a new technique that is safe, convenient and acceptable to males.

14 CHAPTER

Legal and Ethical Aspects of Midwifery and Obstetrical Nursing

INTRODUCTION

Law is a societal institution that governs relationship among members of this society. In our society, competent adults are responsible and accountable for their behaviour when other may be at risk of harm; adults are expected to meet certain standards of behaviour that ordinary reasonable prudent persons would use under similar circumstances.

Legal matters can cause considerable professional anxiety. There are many laws operate, are poorly understood and constraints of the law are often blamed by health care professionals for their being forced to adapt defensive practice to protect them from accusations of misconduct, complaints or negligence. Each nurse who is practicing nursing and midwifery is accountable for their own practice in whatever environment they practice. Each nurse-midwife shall act, at all times in such a manner as to justify public trust and confidence to uphold and enhance the good standing and reputation of the profession, to serve the interest of the society and above all to safeguard the interest of the society and above all to safeguard the interest of individual patients and clients.

Accountability: The term 'accountability' variously use words such as responsibility, answerable and obligations. The nature of nurse's responsibility is that expects accountability to be much wider than to the clients. There is a clear objective to the profession itself and to society in general.

A profession "of good standing" comprises members who are skilled, knowledgeable and act consistently in the interests of their clients. Keeping upto date, increasing the knowledge base of nursing/midwifery through research and audit, ensuring a high standard of education and training at preregistration and postregistration level, operating firm but fair self regulation through a robust and open professional conduct process are all ways in which a profession retains the confidence of the public.

In midwifery practice, the nurse hears the words "high risk" they usually think of client with complications of pregnancy. But this term take on a new meaning when it refers to legal issues in perinatal nursing. Nurses working in the field face the highest risk of law suit compared with nurses in other speciality areas. To avoid becoming a victim of the malpractice crisis, it is imperative to understand the mindset of those individuals filing the lawsuits, which include:

- Reasons for lawsuits—social attitudes, and well educated public
- Reason for increasing lawsuits—nursing as a profession
- High-risk practice area—perinatal nursing.

Reason for Lawsuits

The way society thinks affects the propensity to use. Certain attitudes increase the likelihood of lawsuits, which includes the following:

- *Need to blame*: When a person refuses to accept responsibility for his or her own actions, the result is fixation of blame on another person. For, e.g. giving wrong advices to clients leads to problems.
- *Expectation of perfection*: People think that everything can be cured by modern medical technology. The medical profession must take partial responsibility. For conveying that attitude to the public. The truth is that there generally be a treatment than a proposed treatment regimen, will produce the desired

outcome. Clients who feel medical system has wrongfully failed, there are likely to pursue legal recourse.

- *Lack of personalism:* The sophisticated equipments in use today likely to advanced monitoring techniques that have substantially improved the quality of client care. Yet the client's perceptions of the quality of care is often quite the opposite. Automatically there is lack of personal touch with the client, may lead to move on lawsuit.
- Well educated public clients are better educated now regarding their health care. They want and get more information about diagnosis, medication and prognosis. By being more involved in their own health care, they also are very away when an adverse outcome occurs. Client faced with a poor result will probably ask what went wrong, and should be told by the proper person. Clients today are likely to be aware when they have been treated negligently. In fact, one of the worst thing a health care provider can do when faced with a bad result is attempt to cover up the truth, because a client who later learns he or she has been the victim of a deception is very likely to take legal action. Angry clients are potential plaintiffs. (A plaintiff is the party who claims he or she was injured and initiates a lawsuit).

Reason for Increase in Lawsuit against Nurses

Some years back, if a nurse was involved in a lawsuit, it was most likely as a witness, who has knowledge of the events resulting in the lawsuit. Now, nurses are more likely to be involved. There is an increase in the number of nurses named as defendants in lawsuits (A defendant is party in the lawsuit who is sued and accused of wrong doing). There are several reasons why nurses involvement in lawsuits has evolved in this manner.

Nurses used to be merely medical men "handmaidens" whose function was to follow orders. There was no independence or autonomy. Nurses did not make decisions or perform independent assessments. Nursing has changed, though. Now nurses are recognized as professionals. Nursing is now well recognized as a practice that is independent of the practice of medicine.

With this recognition of nurses as professionals claim accountability. By presenting ourselves to the public as independent professionals, we also declare that we are responsible for our own actions. Today's nurse operates with autonomy and makes independent judgements regarding client care. It has increased the risk of being named as defendant in a lawsuit.

The plaintiff attorney's responsibility is to find sufficient financial resources to compensate the plaintiff in whatever amount the jury determines failure. The nurse becomes another 'pocket' to dip into in order to satisfy the judgement. The nurse might also be named as a defendant in an attempt to hold the hospital liable by the doctrine of "respondent superior" (let the master respond). For, e.g. employer as deep pocket.

The Reasons for High-Risk Practice area—Perinatal Nursing

There are many reasons for perinatal nursing a high risk practice area are as follows:

- *Nurses held to higher standard of care,* wherever nurses practice in a speciality area than required, increased skill, training, and experience beyond that which is taught in nursing school or college, those nurses will be held to higher standard of care. Perinatal nursing is highly specialized area.
- *High expectations of outcomes*
  Usually, obstetric clients do not perceive themselves as sick, and therefore, completely unprepared for any bad results of their pregnancy. When a bad result occurs, it is absolutely devastating to the expectant parent. In such a situation, it is often impossible for the parent to accept that sometimes things like this just happen. When this fact is added to our society's general tendency to fix blame, often the physician and/or nurses bear the brung of the accusation of wrong doing in the form of a lawsuit.
- *Defective infant survival rate*: Although there is reduction in the defective infant survival rate due to advanced perinatal technology many of the babies suffer severe medical consequences (For, e.g. MR, cerebral palsy, seizures, etc.). Which leads to costly monitoring and treatment. For which also parents blame the health care providers.

In addition, long statute of limitations for minors, sever potential plaintiffs, long involvement in treatment in and nursing autonomy issues also leads to increased lawsuits.

Theories of Liability

Lawsuits can arise based on several different theories. While the most common is the allegation of negligence in the form of medical malpractice, causes of action can also be based on wrongful death, wrongful birth, and wrongful life.

Torts are civil wrongs against a person and may be either intentional there must be harm resulting from the action either physical emotional are concerned.

Negligence is the failure to act as a reasonably prudent person would have in specific circumstances.

Negligence

Negligence is an unintentional action or in action that breaches a duty of care owed to another person forcibly causes harm to that person. It is the failure to act as a reasonable person. Four legal elements constituting negligence must be present for a court towards compensation.

They are:

- A duty of care because of the forcibility of harm
- Breach of that duty of care
- Casual relations of breach to harm, and
- Actual harm.

Once the nurse client relationship established, the nurse has a duty to treat the client in accordance with acceptable standard of care. A breach of a nurse's duty is the failure to abide by or live up to the acceptable standard of care. The breach of duty consists of either an act or an omission. The duty to a client can be breached by doing something that should not have been done, or by not doing something that should have been done. The term injury, and damages (harm) are often used inter-changeably in lawsuits. More exactly, the damage usually refer to the monitory value of the injury. Forcibility means that the type of injury that was sustained must be the type of consequences which one would reasonably expect from a particular negligent act. Proving the proximate causation element in probably the most difficult part of malpractice action. The plaintiff must prove that the breach of duty was the direct and proximate cause of the injury and that injury was forcible consequence of the breach of duty.

Malpractice and Nursing Profession

Malpractice is the greatest legal concern of health care practitioners. It is negligence applied to the acts of a professional. In other words, malpractice occurs when a professional failed to act reasonably prudent professional under specific circumstances. Malpractice is classified as an unintentional tort. This means that it is not necessary to prove that the professional intended to be negligent. In malpractice, both doing things that should not be done (commissions) and not doing things that should be done (omissions) may be the basis for legal actions.

When a patient brings a malpractice claim against a nurse defendant, evidence is presented to the jury to determine if the element of liability are present. At questions in whether the nurse met the prefailing standard of care in what the reasonably prudent nurse, under similar circumstances would have done. It is a peer standard of care is decided by the jury on a case by case basis and is developed through use by expert witness testimony; documents, including national standards of practice, the patient record; and other pertinent evidence such as the direct testimony of the patient, the nurse and others.

The prerequisition for a malpractice action is that the defendant (nurse has specialized knowledge and skills and through the practice of that specialized knowledge caused the plaintiffs (patients) injury. In order for a plaintiff patient to prove that the nurse defendant is liable for the injury all elements cause of action for negligence must be proved. The elements are the same for any professional accused of malpractice. The elements necessary for a malpractice actions are as follows:

The professional nurse has assumed the "duty of care" i.e. responsibility patient's care.

The professional nurses breaches the duty of care by failing to meet the standard of care.

- The failure of professional nurse to meet the standard of care proximity causes the injury
- The injury is proved.

A review of malpractice cases where the liability of the nurse has been successfully litigated showed the categories of cases as follows:

- The nurse failed to carry out the medical order
- The nurse carried out an order incorrectly
- The nurse implemented a faulty medical order
- The nurse failed to make an accurate assessment
- The nurse failed to act on an assessment
- The nurse failed to report an inadequate patient care.

- The nurse failed to secure adequate care for a patient
- The nurse abandoned a patient needing care.

The lesson to be learned from such malpractice cases is that professional nurses must carefully consider the legal implications of practice and by willing and capable of conforming that care to legal expectations.

Malpractice can be defined as negligence by a professional that causes an injury. It is a specialized form of negligence based on breach of a standard care known to a person because of education in a professional field. It is an extension of the ordinary reasonable prudent person standard to behaviour for professionals.

Professionals including physicians, nurses, lawyers, teachers, through specialized education and experience gained knowledge and skills that are unique. For this witness expert in the profession must provide testimony in malpractice cases as to whether the standard of care was met. The public recognizes these specialized skills and trusts the professionals to apply them reasonably and prudently for the benefit of clients.

Malpractice is a breach of professional duty to a client brought about by an unintentional but unreasonable action or inaction that forcibly results in harm to the client. Eg, failure to monitor SFGA infant for signs of hypoglycaemia with resultant brain damage.

Common Causes of Malpractice

Lawsuits brought against doctors (physician surgeon obstetrician, paediatrician etc.) and nurses differ reflecting the well recognized differences between these professions and their responsibilities. A possible cause for an allegations against doctor might be one of the following:

- Failure to diagnose a high-risk pregnancy.
- Delay in performing a caesarean section.
- Improper vaginal delivery or failure to perform caesarean section.
- Improper use of forceps
- Incidents surroundings induction of labour and the use of oxytocin.
- Delay in arriving at hospital
- Non attendance at the delivery.

Many lawsuits against nurses are the results of problems arising out of medication functions. Considering the amount of time, nurses spend in various aspects of medication administration, this should come as no suspense. Allegations against nurses include but are not limited to, improper client identifications, wrong medication, dosage, route or time; and failure to monitor for side effects.

Nurses are expected to monitor that clients at appropriate time intervals that depend upon the client's condition. Failure to adequately monitor a client can lead to a change of client abandonment. Nurses monitoring the client according to directives of doctors, institutional policies and procedure and also without specific directives it is often upto nursing judgement.

Labour and delivery poses a unique monitoring challenge, in that there are two clients to monitor the mother and the baby. The delivering mother must be adequately monitored to prevent any maternal complications during antenatal period. Any substantial increases or decreases in the mother's blood pressure could affect the baby's welfare. The same is true for any other alterations of vital signs, such as elevated temperature or pulse. Any variations from the norm must be reported and corrected to prevent possible harm to the baby. The foetus is the other client to be monitored, especially during labour. Many lawsuits have arisen as a result of problems related to foetal monitoring.

Other causes of malpractice is perinatal nursing and the kidnapping infants from nurseries in hospital (most of these appeared in media). Nurses sometimes wonder what their responsibility is to prevent newborn kidnapping. One obligation that can be imposed on nursing is to be alert in one's unit for suspicious persons or behaviour and to question any unrecognized person claiming to be employee or significant to family should be reported to authorities. Another important one is that exchanging of the newborn, to be seriously viewed.

Consent

Treating a client without obtaining the proper consent can lead to a charge of assault and/or battery. These terms are of on used together, but do have different meanings. Assault is the threat of an unauthorized touching. Battery is the unauthorized touching of a client.

Informed Consent

Informed consent is a well-recognized doctrine based on the client's right to autonomy. Clients have a right to decide what medical treatment they will have performed. To make an intelligent decision regarding medical treatment, clients have a right to sufficient information so that they can make an educated choice. Clients have a right to know what treatment is proposed, the expected outcome, the risks and what alternative treatment is available.

Informed consent occurs most frequently when the client and the physician are discussing the proposed course of treatment. The physician should document informed consent in the medical record. The nurse is usually the one who obtains the client's signature on the consent form.

Sometimes nurses are confused as to their proper role in this informed consent process, and understandably so, nurses should realize that informed consent is not the same as the consent form. The consent form serves as written proof that informed consent took place.

The courts have generally held that it is the physician's duty to obtain informed consent. But the responsibility for obtaining the client signature on the consent form can safely be delegated to the nurse, as the nurse follows the correct procedure for doing so.

The nurse should approach the client with the consent form and ask the client if the physician has explained the procedure and answered all of the client's questions. If the client answers affirmatively, the nurse should then ask the client to read and sign the consent form for the hospital record. The nurse can then witness the client's signature. By doing so, the nurse is attesting to the fact that the client voluntarily signed the form.

If the client states that the physician has neither explained the procedure nor answered the client's questions, the nurse must realized that the client has not given informed consent. The nurse should not have the client sign the consent form, but should notify the physician that the client still has questions. Having a client sign a consent form when the nurse knows that informed consent has not been given is substandard nursing practice and result in the nurse being included with the physician in a lawsuit for assault or battery. Major elements of informed consent will include:

- Consent must be given voluntarily.
- Consent must be given by an individual with capacity and competence to understand.
- The patient must give enough information to be the ultimate decision maker.

Implied Consent

Sometimes a client is incapable of giving consent for treatments, such as in an emergency situation. No one would want to withhold life saving treatment from a client just because he or she was unconscious and could not give consent. The law presumes that if a person were capable of giving consent to life saving treatment, he or she would do so. This promise resulted in the doctrine of implied consent. In an emergency situation in which the client cannot consent to treatment, consent will be "implied by law," thereby protecting health care professionals from lawsuits for assault and battery.

Implied consent also applies to situations where the client has not objected to a current course of treatment. This is often referred to as "implied-in-fact" consent. If you ask a labour and delivery client to hold out her arm so you can start in intravenous line, and she does so, consent is implied.

Consent to Treat Minors

A minor is defined in most states as a person who has not reached his or her eighteenth birthday. Once a person reaches the age of 18, he or she has legal capacity to consent for medical treatment. Nurses must check their own state's laws regarding minors, since they vary from state to state.

Treating a minor without the consent of the parent or guardian constitutes assault and battery. Some exceptions to this exist. First, in an emergency situation, the doctrine of implied consent covers any treatment given to save the minor's life. Parental consent is not necessary in an emergency situation. In fact, parents sometimes lack legal capacity to refuse lifesaving treatment on behalf of their minor children, even if for religious reasons.

Second, an emancipated minor can consent to treatment. The definition of emancipation varies from state to state, but usually includes minors who are married, have a child, are in the military or are self supporting. In most states, minors can also consent for pregnancy related treatment.

When treating an emancipated minor, not only is parental notification and consent not necessary, it might lead to a charge of breach of confidentiality of privileged information.

Right to Refuse Treatment

Generally speaking, competent adults have a right to refuse any medical treatment they do not want, even if it means they will die without it. Sometimes pregnant women wish to refuse treatment, even though the baby might suffer as a result of the mother's decision. This problem has led to an ethical dilemma. When is it appropriate to force unwanted treatment on the mother to benefit the baby.

This has not been an easy issue to resolve because someone's rights are violated regardless of which decision is made. The problem for the courts and for society is to make the determination of whose rights take precedence in a particular case.

Courts have been known to order a mother to undergo a caesarean section in spite of religious opposition, when there was a high likelihood that the baby would suffer damage or die during a vaginal delivery. Yet other forms of treatment, particularly those which pose a greater risk to the mother, have not been imposed.

Another issue closely related to this one is whether or not a woman should be penalized for behaviour that poses a risk to the foetus. The most prevalent example is that of substance abuse during pregnancy. How far can society go to protect the foetus? Some have advocated incarceration of pregnant drug abusers, while as many others have spoken to the inappropriateness and ineffectiveness of such a directive. Again, the dilemma arises as we try to determine whose rights are superior, and to what extent the other's rights can be violated (see Ethical Dilemmas).

There are no good answers to this conflict at this time, only more questions. Nurses should keep abreast of developments in this area.

Abortion

Nursing's Role in Abortion

Abortion is probably the most controversial issue any of us has faced in our lifetime. Those who favour abortion right believe as passionately in their position as those who oppose abortion.

In the nursing profession there are those who mirror the societal conflict. Many nurses consider themselves pre-choice, and many consider to themselves pro-life. Nurses on both sides of the issue are confronted with client care situations in which a woman is either having an abortion performed, or is being treated for complications of an abortion. How can the nurse who morally opposes abortion deal with the above scenarios?

Nurses cannot be forced to participate in procedures they find morally offensive. Nurses have a right to refuse to assist with abortion. However, a nurse cannot attempt to stop an abortion from being performed.

The nurse also has a legal obligation to take care of a client who has undergone an abortion, or who is being treated for complications of an abortion. To refuse care to a client in this situation is to make a character judgement upon which the provision of nursing care is based. Nurses are not allowed to do that. If a nurse refused to treat a client after an abortion, and the client suffered because of the lack of nursing care, the nurse could be sued for abandonment of the client.

Minor Requesting Abortion

Several recent cases have addressed the issue of minor's rights to consent to abortion. Many states have attempted to pass laws limiting minor's access to abortion without parental approval. The states differ tremendously on this issue, and the laws are in a constant state of change. Even when a law is passed, often an injunction is filed to block it before the law goes into effect. Then the higher court either upholds the law or decides that it is unconstitutional.

This will be a difficult area for nurses to remain current, but if a nurse is working in a setting where abortions are performed on minors, it is imperative that the nurse find a way to keep abreast of this constantly changing issue.

Malpractice Prevention

The best defense to a malpractice action is prevention. But malpractice prevention is no accident. It requires conscious attention to the two "Ds" of malpractice defense—demeanor and documentation.

Demeanor

The manner in which a nurse treats a client sets that stage for the likelihood of a lawsuit in the event of an adverse outcome. Nurses must never underestimate the power of rapport with the client in malpractice prevention.

Nursing care is delivered by human beings and consequently is subjected to human error. When a negligent error results in an injury, the lawsuit climate is created. Whether or not the client takes the next stand to the lawyer is likely to depend on the nurse's demeanor while treating the client. Simply put, given two identical poor client outcomes, the risk of a lawsuit might not be equal.

What determines whether or not an adverse outcome proceeds to a lawsuit? The nurse's rapport with the client. Remember the formula:

Adverse Outcome + Uncaring Demeanor = Lawsuit

Developing good rapport with your clients is an important part of malpractice prevention. A lawsuit is often circumvented when the staff treats the client with warmth and caring.

Communication Skills

The ability to develop good rapport with clients is dependent on the nurse having good interpersonal communication skills. Listening is by far the most important communication skill. It is imperative that the nurse learn to listen to what the client says.

In one case, the jury found the nurse negligent when the client's husband's repeated requests to call the physician were ignored. The nurse told the husband that the client was only dilated 7 cm., therefore there was no need to notify the physician. The husband told the nurse that his wife had previously delivered a baby while only dilated 8 cm, but the nurse still ignored the request that the physician be called. The woman delivered only a few minutes later, with no physician in attendance.

Besides listening to the client, the nurse must also be carefully attend to the client's nonverbal communications.

Communication is a two way street. Information communicated from the nurse to the client must be done in an understandable and appropriate manner. Discharge instructions should be communicated orally and is writing.

The manner in which communication occurred between a nurse and a client has been at issue in court cases. In another case, the court indicated that a reasonably prudent nurse would not make disparaging remarks to a client.

Documentation

Documentation is by far the best defense once a lawsuit is file. The medical record is a legal document and is admissible in court as evidence. It enjoys a privileged status in that it is presumed to be an accurate account of what transpired. This is because it was written at the time of the occurrence, by someone with knowledge of the events, and before litigation was initiated.

The documentation in the medical record must able to stand on its own in proving that the standard of care was met. Omission of information from the medical record leads to the charge that the standard of care was violated. Unfortunately for the nurse, filling in the gaps in the medical record later in court will not suffice to prove that the standard of care was met. Spoken words have at best questionable credibility in a courtroom.

A case is only as good as the proof that is presented in court. Spoken words are often felt to be self serving and therefore cannot prove the case. Why should a jury believe that you provide continuous nursing care when your documentation indicates otherwise? Given the opportunity, the jury will choose to believe what is documented in the medical record instead of the spoken words they hear in court.

From a litigation stand point, the jury often assumes that if something was not charted, it was not done. Nurses should give themselves credit for care they provided by thoroughly documenting it in the medical record.

Documentation Format

In recent years, there has been a trend away from straight narrative charting to flow sheets. Sometimes nurses question whether or not these flow sheets are sufficient to defend them if they are sued. It is not the format, but the completeness of the documentation that determines how good it is. A complete and thorough flow sheet is better than an incomplete, vague narrative note, and a complete narrative not defends better than an incomplete flow sheet. The key is to provide all of the pertinent information about the client. The format is secondary.

When using flow sheets, the nurses should be careful to not let the small spaces on the flow sheet discourage thorough reporting of information. If the flow sheet is not adequately telling the whole story, it must be supplemented with a narrative note. Nurses do not get into legal trouble by documenting too much it is usually too little documentation that causes problems. A general documentation rule by which to live is, when in doubt as to how much to document, document more not less.

Documentation Tips to Stayout of Court

Write legibly: An illegible entry cannot serve its intended purpose, which is to communicate information. And it will not be relied on to provide a defense in court if the party cannot read it.

Use ink: The medical record is a legal document. When written it is intended to be permanent. To ensure its permanency, you should always use ink. Using pencil is dangerous because anyone could erase your entry and replace it with something else.

Never obliterate an entry: If you make an error in the chart, follow your institution's policy for error correction, which usually entails drawing one line through the incorrect entry, so it can still be read and inserting the correct information. An obliterated entry can be used by your opponent to imply that pertinent information has been removed from the record, and you might not be able to prove otherwise because no one can read what you obliterated.

Fill in all blanks and lines: A flow sheet should be completely filled otherwise some one else could come in later and fill in accurate information that makes him or her look good and you look bad. In a narrative note, no lines should be left blank, in spite of a request by a co-worker to do so in order that he or she can fill it in later.

Date and time all entries: Sometimes it is very important what time something happened. If a nurse notifies a physician of a problem with a client, the nurse should document when the problems began and when the physician arrived. Documenting this sequence can prove that the nurse acted properly, and refute a charge by the physician that it was the physician and not the nurse who first noticed the problem.

Document thought processes: When faced with a situation where nursing judgment comes into play and decision have to be made, document the process by which the decision is reached. Doing so can assure that the jury knows that the judgment that was made was the correct one in that situation.

Be objective: Document what you see and hear, not just conclusions. Do not document "client tell," unless you saw the client fall, document your observation, e.g. "client found on floor".

Describe behaviours, do not make personal judgments: Do not document "client is hostile", or "client is drunk". Instead, describe the behaviour and leave the conclusion to the imagination of the reader. A record that describes a client who has "reddened eyes, staggering gait, slurred speech, and admits to consuming a case of beer, "informs the reader, but makes no personal judgment about the client's character.

Never air grievance in the chart: The chart is not a battleground for wars among the staff. Documenting conflicts gives the plaintiff's attorney the opportunity to prove to the jury that someone was guilty of wrong doing because one staff member pointed the finger at another.

Document the client's noncompliance with treatment: In the event a client chooses to refuse to comply with medical advice, the client should not be able to sue the health care team for injuries, brought on by his or her own noncompliance. Documenting the noncompliance in the medical record is imperative to defeat a lawsuit brought by the noncompliant client. If a client with threatened premature labour is sent home with strict instructions to stay in bed, and the client admits to playing tennis, this admission should be documented. In the event of this client's baby has problem the defence will put the blame back on the woman in proving that the medical staff did not violate any standard of care.

Document your assessment: This proves that you attended to your client appropriately. If the client is attached to a foetal monitor, include the information in the medical record. If your do not document the results your assessments, the jury might assume, they were not done.

Document your interventions: When your assessment shows something abnormal about your client's condition, your duty is to address the problem. The chart must include what you did for the client at that point. For example, if a client complains of pain, and you administer pain medication, that fact must be documented. If your client's blood pressure drops and you notify the physician, document that you did so. The record must reflect not only that problems were assessed, but that the appropriate interventions were instituted.

Document physician contacts: When a physician is notified, document the physician's name, the time the conversation took place, what was told to the physician, and the physician's response. Many disputes erupt between nurses who claim they called the physician and the physicians who allege they were never notified.

If you are sued, your documentation can be your best friend, or your worst enemy. Time spent documenting is time well spent in the prevention of a lawsuit.

Ethical Decision-Making

As a nurse, you must know the "right" thing to do. Rightness or wrongness can be applied to any nursing decision made or action taken. Many people, including your clients, your instructors, and yourself, will evaluate your nursing care. Doing the right or best things for each client is the objective of all nursing care.

The definition of the correct thing varies from person-to-person; it is not what an individual feels like doing. Rightness involves ethics and morality. Everyone uses personal standards to judge whether attitudes, behaviour, actions, and decisions are good or bad. The profession of nursing also has standards of moral behaviour that describe how a nurse should behave and act when practicing nursing.

Ethics, Morals and Values

When you ask yourself what you should do in a situation and why, you are asking moral questions. An understanding of morals, ethics and values can help you to provide nursing care that is right for the client and done the right way.

Morals are what a person should and ought to do. However, these responsibilities and obligations raise the question of right, best, or correct choices. More questions suggest that there are at least two answers available. Sometimes, several options, some good and some bad are possible. Even when refusing to decide, a person has made a choice (to do nothing). You must keep a professional attitude, even when your client makes a decision with which you disagree. Professional caring behaviour is exhibited by attitude, as well as by actions.

Ethics are the reasons we should or ought to do something. Thus a woman may decide to breastfeed her infant because she values the close interactions with her baby, believes that mother's milk is best (not only because the health professionals say so but because she has read and understands the difference between breast and formula milk), or perhaps because her family or culture says it is the thing to do. Each reason involves the ethical principle of autonomy (self determination or choice by the woman). Her reasons include values held by her and members of her family.

Values are the attitudes or beliefs that describe how you feel about something or towards someone else. Values are also attitudes or beliefs that are practice as you interact with other people or that guide the decisions you make in life. You have many values; you grew up with them.

Ethical Mandate for Nursing

There is an ethical dimension to every nursing situation. People interacting with other people need to act responsibly, they need to act responsibly; they need to respect one another, and they need to care about each other. Self respect and caring for oneself play a large role in this interaction. All of these behaviours, are based on ethical principles; respect for human dignity, caring, and competence in professional practice. Because you will deal with people, you will need to know and understand ethics and to practice in ethical manner. You will need to understand how your and your client's morals and values influence the decisions or choices you make.

Determination of "Right" (See Pregnant Client Rights, Responsibilities)

Personal Values

As you were growing up, many people gave you advice and direction on the right or wrong thing to do or say. Parents and families are important sources for learning values. Other then religious groups, schoolmates, books and television. Even your neighbourhood and the money among your family had, were important influences on the values you now have.

Personal values that could influence the practice of maternal-infant nursing include ideas about life in general, procreation, sex within marriage, parenting, love, telling the truth, the golden rule, suffering and pain. You will be asked to care for many women who share your personal values. You will also take care of women who do not share your values. For example, what should you do when a 14 year old preparing for the birth of her first child asks you to "put her to sleep" so she won't feel any more pain, but you know that "sleep" might injure the infant? The first step in analyzing, a conflict is to remember that respect for another person and their values does not mean you have to agree with them. Your professional judgement is also worthy of respect, though you must remember that it may be a value with which the client disagree.

Professional Values

The nursing profession has its own standards of proper conduct (moral behaviour) for nurses. These values or moral standards are stated in the code for nurses with interpretive statements. The code says nurses should practice with respect for human dignity and support client choice. Nurses should also practice in a competent and responsible manner (accountability) and protect clients from the "unethical, illegal or immoral actions" of anyone else. Again, respecting client choice does not always mean that she has made the right decision for herself or her infant. A need for objective, professional judgment remains.

The nursing profession expects nurses to understand and practice safe care. Nurses should always balance safety with client preferences. In the example of the 14 year old in labour, the nurse should explain the danger of general anesthesia for the baby and then try to find another, safer method of relieving the girl's pain. This approach provides safe care for both baby and girl without harming either.

The code states that nurses are morally obligated to provide care without discrimination. You may disagree with a choice a client or family has made, but you cannot abandon them. If a choice is appropriate, or correct for a woman you must care for her, at least until another nurse is available to provide care.

Personal and professional values sometimes conflict. Nurses are expected to overcome personal bias and provide respectful care to all clients. It is also wrong for you to impose your values on clients, especially without knowledge or admitting it. When you most deeply held values are called into question, however, you may be supported in refusing to care for a patient. The church amendment was passed by the federal government in the wake of the early abortion controversy. This amendment allows health professionals who are morally opposed to abortion and other legal health care options to refuse to care for women selecting them. However, your employer needs to know about your beliefs ahead of time so another health professional can be found to provide care.

The Pregnant Client's Bill of Rights

The pregnant client has the right to participate in decisions involving her well-being and that of her unborn child, unless there is a clear cut medical emergency that prevents her participation.

1. The pregnant client has the right, prior to the administration of any drug or procedure, to be informed by the health professional caring for her of any potential direct or indirect effects, risks, or hazards to herself or her unborn or newborn infant that may result from the use of a drug or procedure prescribed for or administered to her during pregnancy, labour, birth, or lactation.
2. The pregnant client has the right, prior to the proposed therapy, to be informed not only of the benefits, risks, and hazards of the proposed therapy but also of known alternative therapy, such as available childbirth education classes, that could help to prepare the pregnant patient physically and mentally to cope with the discomfort or stress of pregnancy and the experience of childbirth, thereby reducing or eliminating her need for drugs and obstetric intervention. She should be offered such information early in her pregnancy in order that she may make a reasoned decision.
3. The pregnant client has the right, prior to the administration of any drug, to be informed by

the health professional who is prescribing or administration of any drug, to be informed by the health professional who is prescribing or administering the drug to her that any drug she receives during pregnancy, labour, and birth, no matter how or when the drug is taken or administered, may adversely affect her unborn baby, directly or indirectly, and that no drug or chemical has been proved safe for the unborn child.

4. The pregnant client has the right, if caesarean birth is anticipated, to be informed prior to the administration of any drug, and preferably prior to her hospitalization, that minimizing her and, in turn, her baby's intake of non-essential preoperative medicine will benefit her baby.
5. The pregnant client has the right, prior to the administration of a drug or procedure, to be informed of the areas of uncertainty if there is no properly controlled follow-up research that has established the safety of the drug or procedure with regard to its direct or indirect effects on the physiologic, mental, and neurologic development of the child exposed, via the mother, to the drug or procedure during pregnancy, labour, birth, or lactation (this would apply to virtually all drugs and the vast majority of obstetric procedures).
6. The pregnant client has the right, prior to the administration of any drug, to be informed of the brand name and generic name of the drug in order that she may advise the health professional of any past adverse reaction to the drug.
7. The pregnant client has the right to determine for herself, without pressure from her attendant, whether she will accept the risks inherent in the proposed therapy or refuse a drug or procedure.
8. The pregnant client has the right to know the name and qualifications of the individual administering a medication or procedure to her during labour or birth.
9. The pregnant client has the right to be informed, prior to be administration of any procedure, whether that procedure is being administered to her for her or her baby's benefit (medically indicated) or as an elective procedure (for convenience, teaching purposes, or research).
10. The pregnant client has the right to be accompanied during the stress of labour and birth by someone she cares for and to whom she looks for emotional comfort and encouragement.
11. The pregnant client has the right after appropriate medical consultation to choose a position for labor and for birth that is least stressful to her baby and to herself.
12. The obstetric client has the right to have her baby cared for at her bedside if her baby is normal and to feed her baby according to her baby's needs rather than according to the hospital regimen.
13. The obstetric client has the right to be informed in writing of the name of the person who actually delivered her baby and the professional qualifications of that person. This information should also be on the birth certificate.
14. The obstetric client has the right to have her and her baby's hospital medical records complete, accurate, and legible and to have their records, including nurses' notes, retained by the hospital until that child reaches at least the age of majority or, alternatively, to have the records offered to her before they are destroyed.
15. The obstetric client has the right to have her and her baby's hospital medical records complete, accurate, and legible and to have their records, including nurses' notes, retained by the hospital until the child reaches at least the age of majority or, alternatively, to have the records offered to her before they are destroyed.
16. The obstetric client, both during and after her hospital stay, has the right to have access to her complete hospital medical records, including nurses' notes, and to receive a copy on payment of a reasonable fee and without incurring the expense of retaining an attorney.

It is the obstetric client and her baby, not the health professional, who must sustain any trauma or injury resulting from the use of a drug or obstetric procedure. The observation of the rights listed above will not only permit the obstetric patient to participate in the decisions involving her and her baby's health care but will help to protect the health professional and the hospital against litigation arising from resentment or misunderstanding on the part of the mother.

The Pregnant Client's Responsibilities

In addition to understanding her rights, the pregnant client should also understand that she too has certain responsibilities include the following:

1. The pregnant client is responsible for learning about the physical and psychological process or labour, birth, and postpartum recovery. The better informed expectant parents are, the better they will be able to participate in decisions concerning the planning of their care.
2. The pregnant client is responsible for learning what comprises good prenatal and intranatal care and for making an effort to obtain the best care possible.
3. Expectant parents are responsible for knowing about those hospital policies and regulations that will affect their birth and postpartum experience.
4. The pregnant client is responsible for arranging for a companion or support person (husband, mother, sister, friend) who will share in her plans for birth and who will accompany her during her labour and birth experience.
5. The pregnant client is responsible for making her preferences known clearly to the health professionals involved in her case in a courteous and cooperative manner and for making mutually agreed on arrangements regarding maternity care alternatives with her physician and hospital in advance of labour.
6. Expectant parents are responsible for listening to their chosen physician or midwife with an open mind, just as they expect him or her to listen openly to them.
7. Once they have agreed to a course of health care, expectant parents are responsible, to the best of their ability, for seeing that the program is carried out in consultation with others with whom they have made the agreement.
8. The pregnant client is responsible for obtaining information in advance regarding the approximate cost of her obstetric and hospital care.
9. The pregnant client who intends to change her physician or hospital is responsible for notifying all concerned, well in advance of the birth if possible, and for informing both of her reasons for changing.
10. In all their interactions with medical and nursing personnel, the expectant parents should behave towards those caring for them with the same respect and consideration they themselves would like.
11. During the mother's hospital stay, the mother is responsible for learning about her and her baby's continuing care after discharge from the hospital.
12. After birth, the parents should put into writing constructive comments and feelings of satisfaction or dissatisfaction with the care (nursing, medical, and personal) they received. Good service to families in the future will be facilitated by those parents who take the time and responsibility to write letters expressing their feelings about the maternity care they received.

All the previous statements assume a normal birth and postpartum experience. Expectant parents should realize that if complications develop in their cases, there will be an increased need to trust the expertise of the physician and hospital staff they have chosen. However, if problems occur, the childbearing woman still retains her responsibility for making informed decisions about her care or treatment and that of her baby. If she is incapable of assuming that responsibility for making informed decisions about her care or treatment and that of her baby. If she is incapable of assuming that responsibility because of her physical condition, her previously authorized companion or support person should assume responsibility for making informed decisions on her behalf.

Moral Development as Moral Authority

Piaget and Kohlberg spent many years in studying how human beings develop intellectually and morally. Kohlberg's cross cultural theory of moral development offers some insight into how individuals make moral choices (choices of right or wrong).

Kohlberg's first level of moral development, preconventional, has two stages. In the first stage persons determine what the right thing is based on whether they will receive a reward or punishment. People functioning at this stage of moral development may decide that driving the speed limit is wrong because they will get a ticket (punishment) if they are caught speeding. At the second stage, people do good things for others so they can get something in return, even though they are not really interested in helping others.

Most adults in our society function at the second level of moral development, the conventional level. At this level of Kohlberg's model, "right" defined by individuals in positions of authority. For example, a staff nurse may decide to follow a physician's advice for a patient because the nurse believes the physician is always right. The law becomes the moral authority for right or wrong; for example, a man might drive 55 miles per hour on highway, not because he might get a ticket, but because it is the law and the law is right.

Nurses who place their moral authority in others (e.g., head nurse, doctor, client, law or hospital rules) often practice in an ethical manner. They also have fewer options for action because they believe that authority figures are always right. Even when thinking another choice is better, this nurse will still follow the authority figure. Many suggest that nurses functioning at the conventional level of morality are better prepared to care for others than nurses at the preconventional level. The latter often practice in fear of punishment, especially a lawsuit, and may not be able to make decisions in the best interests of their clients. Fear rather than concern for the client drives their decision making.

At both of these levels of moral development, nurses may face conflict when others hold values and moral positions different from their own. They will favour the action that will avoid punishment or that agrees with the authority figure, however, even if the client disagrees.

The preconventional level of morality allows individuals to choose from ethical principles, rather than other persons or fear, as guides for right and wrong. The major guide at this level is utilitarianism, the action or choice that will result in the greatest good for the greatest number of people. Few individuals function consistently at this level, however.

Systems of Ethical Thought

There are many different values, moral standards and ethical principles in the world. Ethical principles are familiar ideas such as to tell the truth, to practice the golden rule, do good and not harm and for nursing, client autonomy, quality and sanctity of life, and justice and mercy.

The ethical principle of respect for persons is based on the idea that persons should never be treated as objects or used for gain. Kant proposed this idea more than 200 years ago, but we forget it occasionally in health care. You must remember that every human being, despite age, physical or mental condition, work status, or educational level, is worthy or respect.

Clients too young or too weak to speak for themselves need special protection in health care. When caring for newborns and children, you will need to use special caution in deciding their best interests. Nurses often ask parents to make decisions for their infant on the assumption that they will do what is best for their own child. There may be occasions when this assumption is not true, and you may need to seek another person to represent the in far such as a court appointed guardian.

A person may justify, based on ethical principles, why a particular action or response is chosen. For example, when a premature infant is born with little hope of survival, health professionals often ask whether they should treat the infant or allow him to die. Often, this decision, although very emotional and heart-wrenching, is reached on the basis of the quality of life the infant will have if life sustaining treatment is begun. Other persons use the ethical principle of vitalism, or life at all costs, to justify any and all treatment, even though this treatment sometimes causes great harm to the ill neonate. Thus, a nurse must weigh the risks and benefits of treatment versus non-treatment, as well as ethical and moral principles. Most decision making in health and illness requires some balancing of principles and some balancing of risks or harms and benefits.

Utilitarianism

Nurses sometimes cause immediate harm or pain for clients when caring for them. It hurts a newborn baby when he is given an injection of vitamin K. A caesarean section to save an infant in distress is major surgery for the mother. How are these hurts justified? One system of ethical thought holds that persons should do no harm. Some deny harm by saying that procedures do not really hurt.

This system of ethical thought suggests that immediate or short term pain or harm can be tolerated when greater harm is avoided. Immunization, medication to cure disease, or surgery can hurt but can also save lives. This system of thought views these interventions as good ends and therefore they are justified.

Utilitarianism is also defined as actions or decisions that promote the greatest happiness or usefulness for the treatest number of people. Concepts of justice may be viewed as part of utilitarianism. For example, several years ago visiting hours for maternity wards reflected the same rules used in the rest of the hospital, meaning that any child under 15 could not visit the mother or new sibling and that fathers could only come 2 to 3 hours a day. The general hospital rules were established to avoid infections from children to already ill clients and to control traffic patterns and congestion in busy hospital corridors. Recently, hospital maternity awards have recognized the value in sibling visitation, unrestricted visiting hours for fathers and grandparents, and rooming in for family development, and the utilitarian based hospital rules were changed.

Natural Law

Some describe and use a third system of ethical thought to justify health care actions and decisions. Natural law evaluates the correctness of actions on the basis of what is natural or the natural purpose of human beings and body organs. For example, contraception is viewed as morally wrong by some conservative religious traditions. They claim the purpose of sexual intercourse is to reproduce. Therefore, any action or device used to interfere with procreation is viewed as wrong by these groups and individuals. Natural law may also be the basis for opposition to artificial insemination, in vitro fertilization, surrogate motherhood, and medicated childbirth.

Natural law for some would justify refusal of the use of any biomedical technology or care. However, this refusal is rarely interpreted as total opposition because nurses have the capacity to help these individuals recover from illness and maintain their health. In addition, groups that refuse technologic interventions are as healthy or healthier during the childbearing than those who demand them. When a person is dying, however, these persons are willing to let nature take its course rather than prolong the dying. They could argue that care and comfort should be the goals of medical and nursing care, rather than invasive treatments, surgery, and medications intended to cure when a cure is no longer possible.

The naturalistic fallacy is a false view of nature. In nature, animals get stick and die without health care. Some see nature as good, so whatever happens naturally is good. Others claim this is false. Animals starve to death, That does not mean it is right for them or for humans. For people with these beliefs, all health care can be seen as a violation of nature.

Some health care providers turn the naturalistic fallacy into a technologic fallacy. For example, a baby is dying, but technology is available to keep him alive in a handicapped condition. Some way the technology must be used at all costs. Others say that the technologic imperative is false; it may allow interns to be trained, but it uses persons for the needs of others rather than focuses on the client's well being. The technologic imperative may do more harm than good. It may cause suffering iatrogenic illness rather than relieve it. Therefore merely having the machinery does mean we should use it. Sometimes there are other reasons for using technology, including making money for the hospital, giving in terms practice giving doctors medical triumphs, or making nurses feel good, but these do not offset the suffering of the client and the violation of the ethical norms of health care.

Ethical Pluralism

We live in a society that supports ethical pluralism (e.g. several systems of ethical justification for making the right decision or choice). We have just reviewed principles of vitalism, utilitarianism, and natural law. We have also discussed the value systems we hold and differing levels of moral development that explain some of our choices in life and in health care. Because of these different systems, it is easy to understand how, at times, Intelligent, sensitive, and caring individuals may make decisions that seem contradictory.

Ethical Decision Making

It implies that you have taken the time to understand the choices available. You have gathered information to make sure you understand all the ethical principles and values involved. You have tried to understand the consequences of your choices and then have selected the option that best fulfils what you and others define as good or right. Ethical decision making does not automatically imply that every one agrees with you choice. At the very least, however, all individuals involved should understand why the choice was made. It is not easy to make the good or right decisions as a nurse, but it is required notheless.

Process for Ethical Decision Making

Ethical decision making is a complex process because it is based on moral reasoning, analyzing, weighing, justifying, choosing, and evaluating attitudes, behaviours and actions. This process of critically examining the moral and ethical dimensions of nursing care takes into account personal and professional values, levels of most development, and ethical theories used to justify choices of action. All individual affected by the decision are included in this process because of the shift away from the health professional's knowing what is best for clients (paternalism) and the shift toward clients' defining their own goals of health care and sharing the decision making with professionals. To make good decisions as a nurse, you need to know and understand yourself what you value, what you believe, and to what you are committed in nursing care.

Good decisions require time. It is hard to think critically in an emergency, especially when quick action is needed to save a life. Even when a lot of time is available, however, you must use it to think critically about the options available for nursing care. You must be willing to ask questions and to gather information that will help you to understand as much about the client and her situation as possible. You must also be willing to listen to the client's preferences and reasons for making a decision. You must help her sortout the risks, benefits, costs, good, and harms of each choice.

Good decision making also requires that you know whether you personal values influence the information you share with a client about her condition and therapy bias her for or against an option. You must understand how you decide what is right or wrong. If fear of lawsuit or loss of your job is primary force in what you decide to do as a nurse, for example, your clients may lose some autonomy in decision making. Understanding the client's sources of moral authority can also help in sorting through conflicts. If the client lacks the capacity to make a decision, whether by age (infant) severe pain (difficult labour) or unconsciousness (anesthesia) others (for example, parents, spouses and physicians) will need to be involved so good decisions can be made.

The decision model available can be used to analyze the ethical dimensions of midwifery care and nursing practice. It includes elements of decision theory, moral reasoning, applied ethics, and factors that might hinder decision making in clinical practice. Use this model to analyze the ethical dimensions of your practice as a nurse. It works best when a group of individuals analyze the same case, but it can also be issued by an individual.

Ethical Concerns in Maternal-Infant Nursing/Perinatal Nursing

We have focused on ethical decision making because many of the major concerns or issues in bioethics today can be found in midwifery and nursing. Issues related to contraception or family planning, abortion, and genetics precede childbearing. Issues related to how, with whom, and when to conceive are evident when considering conception. People with traditional moral standards insist that conception should occur only within marriage but in and outside of marriage, millions of people do not consider conception; they just get pregnant. The issues of unwanted pregnancy are ethical and moral ones. Because of the rise in world population and strain on resources, the area of preventive care in childbearing assumes greater importance. Issues of appropriate use of biomedical technology during pregnancy, labour and birth, and in the care of seriously ill neonates highlight the technologic imperative.

Biomedical technology has progressed rapidly in maternal-infant care in recent decades. The availability of caesarean births in this century saved many babies and women from death. However, it is now said that this procedure is used too often and may cause more harm than good for some women. Electronic foetal monitoring promised hope of saving babies in distress during labour; yet when used inappropriately, it can cause psychologic harm, as well as financial harm, to the woman and her infant. Nurses are caught by the technologic imperative. Health care providers and families believe they must save infants because they can do it. Many ethicists, professionals, and clients suggest otherwise, however.

Technology is useful as an adjunct to clinical decision making. It never was intended to replace it. The technologic imperative is a naturalistic fallacy. You must remember that technology is useful in monitoring the foetal heart rate but must never forget to care for the woman and child attached to the machine.

In all aspects of family care during child bearing, you will be faced with the daily concerns of respect for human dignity, allocation of scarce resources, and ethical practice. These are the "ordinary ethics" for ordinary nursing practice. Many have suggested that the true measure of our morality as human beings is what we do when no one else is looking. Your ethics determine what you do from minute to minute in caring for childbearing families rather than what you do when a special situation occurs (e.g., whether to treat an immature infant).

Much of what you will learn in midwifery and nursing is based on the idea that pregnancy and childbearing are natural, normal events. They are happy events for many families but not for all. Because childbearing is a healthy process, the nurse needs to orient care giving to the health of the clients and the prevention of disease. Because health during pregnancy is the responsibility of the pregnant woman or couple, the nurse's primary role is to offer information, support the healthy behaviours of the woman or couple, and encourage self-care. Self-care requires that women be motivated to be healthy and that they receive information that they can understand and use. This sharing of information involves the ethical principles of truth-telling, informed consent with minimal bias, and respect for the humanness of each client and family. Sharing knowledge requires you to have an adequate and up-to-date knowledge base, as well as competence in nursing practice and especially competence in ethics and health care.

Selected Ethical Dilemmas

Birth of a disabled child Naturally, the birth of a healthy child is the ideal, but this ideal is not always achieved. For some parents a child of the "wrong" sex or "wrong" colouring is a disappointment. Others must face a baby partially or overwhelmingly deformed. When the child is healthy, the system clearly acts as an advocate and does everything in its power to help the infant thrive. Children with many handicaps raise questions about whether life should be maintained regardless of the subsequent quality of that life. Currently, it is recognized that 2.5% of premature infants will have permanent moderate-to-severe neurologic impairment. An even larger number will have learning disabilities and subtle functional behavioural disorders not apparent until the child reaches school age.

If you are unsure about whether to treat an infant, the best overall rule is to act. Erring on the side of action is always better than forever regretting inaction caused by the pressures of the situation.

However, action can create problems. Although the courts see no difference between withholding and withdrawing treatment, the consensus within the health care field is that once a treatment is started, it is difficult to stop it. Court input is often necessary before stopping a treatment. The important point to demonstrate is that continuation of the treatment is medically futile. When the infant is terminally ill, action may not be indicated because intervention will only prolong dying. The legal standard against which you are judged is always that behaviour expected of a reasonable and prudent person acting in a similar situation. Because many hospitals have Infant Care Review Committees and "do not resuscitate" policies, potential conflict cases can be carefully reviewed and decisions made thoughtfully.

If the parents of an infant refuse to consent to medically indicated treatment, they can be charged with child abuse. The hospital must go to court to get authorization for the treatment of the ill infant. The court will apply either the "best interests" or the "substituted judgment" standard to determine which action should be taken on behalf of the infant. The court will either name a guardian or authorize the treatment or non-treatment itself. The parents will be responsible for payment for the treatment of their infant, even if they do not consent to it.

With holding treatment: Three situation in which the condition of the newborn is so grave that treatment would not be indicated are specified in the child abuse amendments legislation. The three conditions that are exceptions to treatment are the following:

1. The infant is chronically and irreversibly comatose.
2. The provision of such treatment would merely prolong dying, not to be effective in ameliorating or correcting all of the infant's life threatening condition, or otherwise be futile in terms of the survival of the infant.
3. The provision of such treatment would be virtually futile in terms of the survival of the infant and the treatment itself under such circumstances would be inhumane.

Withdrawal of food and water from adults who are in a chronic vegetative state is increasingly recognized as a valid choice the courts. Removal of food and fluid in neonates has yet to be addressed. The child abuse law requires "appropriate nutrition, hydration, and medication for all infants, including those comatose and born dying". In the legal cases involving adults the court has made a distinction between removing food and discontinuing artificial feeding techniques such as gastrostomy and nasogastric tubes. The argument is that the feeding tube is a medical treatment and can be removed it its continuation is futile and the patient would refuse if competent. Competence means being able to make informed decisions. Infants have never been competent, and premature infants may not be able to take food naturally because of an inability to such. Conceivably, the courts would again argue that food rather than medical treatment is being discontinued.

Index

D

K

L

M

Q

R

S

T

U